PRACTICAL
GENERAL
PRACTICE

For Churchill Livingstone:
Commissioning Editor: Timothy Horne
Development Editor: Carole McMurray
Project Manager: Mahalakshmi Nithyanand
Designer: Charles Gray

PRACTICAL GENERAL PRACTICE

GUIDELINES FOR EFFECTIVE CLINICAL MANAGEMENT

SIXTH EDITION

Edited by

Alex Khot MA MB BChir DCH
General Practitioner, East Sussex, UK

Andrew Polmear MA MSc FRCP FRCGP
Former Senior Research Fellow, Academic Unit of Primary Care, The Trafford Centre for Graduate Medical Education and Research, University of Sussex, Brighton, UK

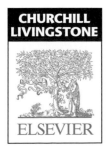

CHURCHILL
LIVINGSTONE

ELSEVIER

Edinburgh   London   New York   Oxford   Philadelphia   St Louis   Sydney   Toronto   2010

CHURCHILL
LIVINGSTONE
ELSEVIER

First Edition 1988
Second Edition 1992
Third edition 1999
Fourth edition 2003
Fifth edition 2006
Sixth edition 2011 © Elsevier Limited. All rights reserved.

ISBN 978 0 7020 3053 6
Reprinted 2011, 2012, 2013

British Library Cataloguing in Publication Data
A catalogue record for this book is available from the British Library

Library of Congress Cataloging in Publication Data
A catalog record for this book is available from the Library of Congress

Notice
Knowledge and best practice in this field are constantly changing. As new research and experience broaden our knowledge, changes in practice, treatment and drug therapy may become necessary or appropriate. Readers are advised to check the most current information provided (i) on procedures featured or (ii) by the manufacturer of each product to be administered, to verify the recommended dose or formula, the method and duration of administration, and contraindications. It is the responsibility of the practitioner, relying on their own experience and knowledge of the patient, to make diagnoses, to determine dosages and the best treatment for each individual patient, and to take all appropriate safety precautions. To the fullest extent of the law, neither the Publisher nor the Editor assumes any liability for any injury and/or damage to persons or property arising out of or related to any use of the material contained in this book.

The Publisher

Contents

Disclaimer

The clinical advice and the organisational details contained in this book refer to the United Kingdom, unless otherwise stated. The book is intended for the use of medical practitioners and not for patients.

While strenuous efforts have been made to ensure the accuracy of the information in this book, it is the responsibility of the doctor who is caring for the patient to make his or her own judgment on the best treatment for that patient at that time. Some of the information contained in this book will become out of date. Some of it may even be wrong, written as it is by mere human beings. In particular, we recommend that prescribing details are checked with the British National Formulary or equivalent, or with the manufacturers' data sheets. We do not even attempt to list contraindications or adverse effects, nor do we always point out when a product is unlicensed for the use we are suggesting.

The authors, editors and publishers cannot accept liability for information that is subsequently shown to be wrong.

Alex Khot and Andrew Polmear work as members of Khot & Polmear LLP, a limited liability partnership, registered in England. The registered address is 27 Links Road, Portslade, Brighton BN41 1XH and the registered number OC320449.

Preface

In the preface to the first edition of this book, we wrote about our belief that it was possible 'to draw up guidelines of management which are logical and justifiable on the evidence'. The subsequent development of evidence-based medicine and of clinical guidelines shows that we were not alone in our belief, and the evidence on which guidelines can now be based is far more extensive than it was then. For this reason, we have continued to use other authors to write some of the chapters, and they have indeed brought a new breadth to the book.

We want to stress that this is a manual of clinical practice, not a collection of national guidelines. The purpose of the book is to help the doctor decide what to do with a patient during the consultation. Each section is structured to try to mirror the thought processes of the doctor (see *The structure of the book*) in a way that few national guidelines are. It is not a textbook designed to give the reader an all-round knowledge of the subject. Furthermore, we are deeply suspicious of textbooks as instruments of stagnation. We urge our readers to realize that this book will have started to go out of date by the time it goes on sale. Our hope is that the reader will use it as a template on which to write new information and new management strategies.

In addition, the book acts as an avenue into the general practice literature. The extensive references are there not only to justify the statements in the text but also to enable the reader to access the article, via PubMed or via the website we quote, and read the full details of the study or guideline.

This new edition maintains the ways of functioning established in editions:

1. The search for evidence has been conducted systematically. Each author has searched for national guidelines, in the UK and abroad. If a reliable guideline was not found, a search for evidence was conducted by working through *The Cochrane Library, Clinical Evidence, Evidence-Based Medicine, Bandolier, Drug and Therapeutics Bulletin, Effective Health Care*, Medline and other sources of evidence, until reliable information was found.

2. Where no evidence is found to guide the authors in their recommendations we have relied on experience, drawn from as many different sources as possible: formal consensus panels, individual doctors and from patients. We do not think that a book that is evidence-based is weakened by the use of the evidence from individuals' experience when more formal research evidence is lacking.

3. Contributors to two chapters come from Australia and New Zealand. The chapters that they have contributed, therefore, contain practical information, about patient organisations for instance, local to those authors, as well as the equivalent information for the UK. Using overseas authors has showed us that the core of the book is applicable to any country where a system of primary care exists that resembles that in the UK. We have also learnt that the local details differ so much that a single book cannot contain them. We have not found a

way round the present compromise and ask that you excuse our inconsistency. Our move to an international version is not due to unbounded ambition, but to our realisation that previous editions have sold well abroad, and that we need to respond to what is clearly a need in countries other than the UK. Indeed, the book has already been translated into Spanish.

Alex Khot
Andrew Polmear

The structure of the book

ASTERISKS AND BULLETS

Central to the structure are instructions preceded by an asterisk:

* Ask the patient x, y and z;
* Examine for a, b and c;
* Take blood for d, e and f, etc.

At the same time the reasons for these steps are explained, either in the same sentence or above, signalled by a round bullet:

● Patients with x are...
● Treatment can be expected to ...
● Nurses are better than GPs at ...

LISTS

Where we present a list in no particular order we use

(a) chest pain; or
(b) hypotension; or
(c) heart failure.

Where there are subdivisions of another heading we use square bullets:

■ Multiple sclerosis
■ Giant cell arteritis
■ Stroke

Where the order is important we number the list:

1. Sit the patient up.
2. Give oxygen.
3. Give diamorphine ...

BOXES

These are used to highlight information that might otherwise get lost in the text: guidelines, a list of tests as a 'work-up' for a patient with a particular condition, or patient organisations.

REFERENCES

Our aim is to reference every statement of fact. Where such a statement is not accompanied by a reference, the reader can assume it is taken from the reference in a box at the start of that section.

Acknowledgements

We would like to thank the staff at Butterworth-Heinemann for their help and support, especially Carole McMurray, Mahalakshmi Nithyanand and Timothy Horne in the production of this edition; Alison Taylor, Catherine Jackson, Caroline Makepeace, Melanie Tait, Mary Seager, Geoff Smaldon and Heidi Allen for previous editions; and Sue Deeley, our original editor, whose faith in our book from the start made the whole project possible.

As editors we would like to thank the contributors for their work and for their willingness to shrink their masterpieces into the required format. In turn the contributors would like to thank Anne Livesey (child protection), Sue O'Connell (Lyme disease) Karen Edmond, Sian Bennett and Paul Seddon (paediatrics) Peter Larsen-Disney (gynaecology), Des Holden (obstetrics), Luis Nacul (chronic fatigue syndrome) Professor R West (smoking cessation), Bruce Macleod (ophthalmology), Martin Kenny (haematology) and Rose Turner (palliative care).

The editors also wish to thank Mike Cohen, Ross Lawrenson, Stephen Cox, William Rhoton and Fernando Petersen-Aranguren, Lisa Argent, Jane Gunn, David Lewis, Ben Essex, Brian McAvoy, Steven Laitner, Ngaire Kerse, Matthew Parsons, and Catherine and John Neden for their contributions to chapters 7, 8, 10, 11, 13, 15 16, 17, 24, and 27, respectively, in previous editions.

Andrew would like to thank his wife Margaret for her support over the 22 years that he has been writing and editing this book. Alex would like to thank Betty for her support and his daughters, Laura and Anna, for their tolerance in having an intermittently 'mentally absent' father since 1987.

List of Contributors

EDITORS

Alex Khot MA, MB, BChir, DCH
General Practitioner, Portslade on Sea, East Sussex, UK

Andrew Polmear MA, MSc, FRCP, FRCGP
Former Senior Research Fellow, Academic Unit of Primary Care, The Trafford Centre for Graduate Medical Education and Research, The University of Sussex, Brighton, UK

CONTRIBUTORS

CHAPTER 3

Jackie Cassell FRCP, FFPH, MSc, Dip GUM, DFFP
Professor in Primary Care Epidemiology
Brighton and Sussex Medical School,
University of Sussex, UK

Gary Brook MD, FRCP, BSc, DTM&H, DCH, DRCOG, Dip GUM
Clinical Lead in GUM/HIV Services, North West Hospitals Trust
Patrick Clements Clinic
Central Middlesex Hospital
London, UK

CHAPTER 6

Hilary Pinnock MB, ChB, MD MRCGP
General Practitioner, Whitstable Medical Practice, Kent and Senior Clinical Research Fellow,

Allergy and Respiratory Research Group, Centre for Population Health Sciences: GP Section, University of Edinburgh, UK

CHAPTER 9

Kevork Hopayian MD, BSc, FRCGP, DCH, DRCOG
General Practitioner, Leiston, Suffolk, UK

CHAPTER 12

Sam Rowlands LLM MD FRCGP FFSRH DRCOG DCH
Department of Sexual Health, Worcestershire Primary Care Trust, UK; Honorary Associate Professor, Institute of Clinical Education, University of Warwick, UK

CHAPTER 14

Steve MBJM Kane-ToddHall BM, BCh, MA (Oxon), FRACGP, DFSRH, DRCOG, Dip. Ther.
General Practitioner, Narangba, Australia

CHAPTER 17

Euan Lawson MRCGP
General Practitioner, Centre for Medical Education Lancaster University

CHAPTER 20

Philip Cotton MD, FRCGP
Senior Lecturer, Medical School, Glasgow, UK

CHAPTER 22

Geoffrey Mitchell MB BS, PhD, FRACGP, FAChPM
Professor of General Practice and Palliative Care,
University of Queensland Medical School,
Australia

CB Del Mar MA, MD, MB BChir, FRACGP, FAFPHM
Professor of Primary Care Research, Faculty of
Health Science and Medicine, and Pro Vice
Chancellor (Research), Bond University,
Queensland, Australia.

CHAPTER 23

Aziz Sheikh MD, BSc, MSc, MB BS, FRCGP, FRCP, DCH,
DRCOG
Professor of Primary Care Research and
Development, Allergy & Respiratory Research Group
Centre for Population Health Sciences
The University of Edinburgh, UK

Alison Worth PhD, BSc, RGN, HV
Senior Research Fellow, Allergy and Respiratory
Research Group
Centre for Population Health Sciences: GP Section
University of Edinburgh Medical School

Michael Gallagher BSc, MSc, PhD
Research Fellow
Centre for Research on Families and Relationships
(CRFR), University of Edinburgh

CHAPTER 25

Rehabilitation
Jane Crawford-White DipCOT, BSc (Hons), SROT
County Manager Community Rehabilitation
Cambridge Community Services
Cambridge, UK

Disability
Nick Lennox MB BS, B Med SC, Dip Obst, FRACGP
Professor & Director, Queensland Centre for
Intellectual and Developmental Disability,
School of Population Health, University of
Queensland, Australia

List of abbreviations

5-FU	5-fluorouracil	**BMI**	body–mass index
5-HT	5-hydroxytryptamine	**BMJ**	*British Medical Journal*
A/C	albumin/creatinine ratio	**BNF**	*British National Formulary*
AA	attendance allowance	**BP**	blood pressure
AAA	abdominal aortic aneurysm	**BSER**	brainstem evoked response
ABI	ankle–brachial index	**BTB**	breakthrough bleeding
ABPM	ambulatory pressure monitoring	**CABG**	coronary artery bypass graft
ACBS	Advisory Committee on Borderline Substances	**CCF**	congestive cardiac failure
		CDH	congenital dislocation of the hip
ACE	angiotensin converting enzyme	**CDSC**	Communicable Disease Surveillance Centre
AD	Alzheimer's disease		
ADHD	attention deficit (hyperactivity) disorder	**CEG**	clinical effectiveness guidelines
		CF	cystic fibrosis
AF	atrial fibrillation	**CHD**	coronary heart disease
AFP	alpha-fetoprotein	**CI**	confidence interval
AI	aortoiliac	**CIN**	cervical intraepithelial neoplasia
AIDS	acquired immune deficiency syndrome	**CJD**	Creutzfeld–Jakob disease
ALP	actinomyces-like organism	**CMO**	Chief Medical Officer
ALT	alanine transferase	**CMV**	cytomegalovirus
AOM	acute otitis media	**CNS**	central nervous system
APTT	activated partial thromboplastin time	**COAD**	chronic obstructive airways disease
APV	acellular pertussis vaccine	**COC**	combined oral contraceptive
AS	ankylosing spondylitis	**COMA**	Committee on Medical Aspects of Food and Nutrition Policy
ASO	antistreptolysin O (titre)		
ASW	approved social worker	**COPD**	chronic obstructive pulmonary disease
a-v	arteriovenous	**CPAP**	continuous positive airways pressure
AV	atrio-ventricular	**CPHM**	Consultant in Public Health Medicine
b.d.	twice daily (*bis die*)	**CPK**	creatine phosphokinase
BA	Benefits Agency	**CPN**	community psychiatric nurse
BBT	basal body temperature	**CPR**	cardiopulmonary resuscitation
BCC	basal cell carcinoma	**CRP**	c-reactive protein
BCG	bacillus Calmette–Guérin	**CSA**	child sexual abuse
BMA	British Medical Association	**CSF**	cerebrospinal fluid
BMD	bone mineral density	**CSM**	Committee on Safety of Medicines

CSOM	chronic suppurative otitis media	**FSH**	follicle stimulating hormone
CT	computerized tomography	**FT$_3$**	free tri-iodothyronine
CTD	connective tissue disease	**FT$_4$**	free thyroxine
CVA	cerebrovascular accident	**FTU**	fingertip unit
CVB	chorionic villus biopsy	**FVC**	forced vital capacity
CVD	cardiovascular disease	**GA**	general anaesthetic
CXR	chest X-ray	**GCA**	giant cell arteritis
D&C	dilatation and curettage	**GCS**	Glasgow Coma Scale
DC	direct current	**GGT**	gamma-glutamyl transferase
DEET	diethyltoluamide	**GI**	gastrointestinal
DEXA	dual energy X-ray absorptiometry	**GMC**	General Medical Council
DLA	disability living allowance	**GORD**	gastro-oesophageal reflux disease
DMARD	disease-modifying antirheumatic drug	**GP**	general practitioner
DMPA	depot medroxyprogesterone	**GPC**	General Practitioners' Committee
DNA	deoxyribonucleic acid		(of the BMA)
DoH	Department of Health	**GTN**	glyceryl trinitrate
DRO	disablement resettlement officer	**GTT**	glucose tolerance test
DSM	Diagnostic and Statistical Manual	**GUM**	genitourinary medicine
DSS	Department of Social Security (now the Department of Work and Pensions)	**H$_2$**	histamine receptor type 2
		HAART	highly active antiretroviral therapy
DTB	*Drug and Therapeutics Bulletin*	**Hb**	haemoglobin
DTP	diphtheria, tetanus and pertussis	**HbA$_{1c}$**	glycated haemoglobin
DU	duodenal ulcer	**HBeAg**	hepatitis B virus e antigen
DVLA	Driver and Vehicle Licensing Agency	**HBIG**	hepatitis B immunoglobulin
DVT	deep vein thrombosis	**HBsAg**	hepatitis B virus surface antigen
DXR	deep radiotherapy	**HCG**	human chorionic gonadotrophin
DXT	deep radiotherapy	**HDL**	high density lipoprotein
ECG	electrocardiogram	**HGV**	heavy goods vehicle
ED	extended delivery	**Hib**	*Haemophilus influenzae* b
EDD	expected date of delivery	**HIV**	human immunodeficiency virus
EEG	electroencephalogram	**HMSO**	Her Majesty's Stationery Office
EIA	enzyme immunoassay	**HNIG**	normal human immunoglobulin
ELISA	enzyme-linked immunosorbent assay	**HNPCC**	hereditary non-polyposis colorectal cancer
EMA	endomysial antibody		
ENT	ear, nose and throat	**HR**	heart rate
EPA	enduring power of attorney	**HRT**	hormone replacement therapy
ERPC	evacuation of the retained products of conception	**HSE**	Health and Safety Executive
		HSV	herpes simplex virus
ESR	erythrocyte sedimentation rate	**HTN**	hypertension
FAP	familial adenomatous polyposis	**HV**	health visitor
FBC	full blood count	**HVS**	high vaginal swab
FBS	fetal blood sample	**IBS**	irritable bowel syndrome
FDA	Food and Drugs Administration (USA)	**IDD**	insulin dependent diabetes
FEV$_1$	forced expiratory flow volume in 1 second	**IFG**	impaired fasting glycaemia
		IgG	immunoglobulin G
FHSA	Family Health Services Authority	**IgM**	immunoglobulin M
FM3	Form Med 3	**IGT**	impaired glucose tolerance
FM5	Form Med 5	**IHD**	ischaemic heart disease
FM6	Form Med 6	**im**	intramuscular
FOB	faecal occult blood	**IMB**	intermenstrual bleeding
FP	femoropopliteal	**INR**	international normalized ratio
FPA	Family Planning Association	**IOP**	intraocular pressure

IQ	intelligence quotient	**NIDD**	non-insulin dependent diabetes
ISA	intrinsic sympathomimetic activity	**NNH**	number needed to harm
ISDN	isosorbide dinitrate	**NNT**	number needed to treat
ISMN	isosorbide mononitrate	**NRT**	nicotine replacement therapy
ITP	idiopathic thrombocytopenic purpura	**NSAID**	non-steroidal anti-inflammatory drug
iu	International Units	**NSF**	National Service Framework
IUCD	intrauterine contraception device	**NSPCC**	National Society for the Prevention of Cruelty to Children
IUD	intrauterine device		
IUGR	intrauterine growth retardation	**NSU**	non-specific urethritis
IUS	intrauterine system	**o.d.**	every day
iv	intravenous	**o.m.**	every night (*omni nocte*)
IVU	intravenous urogram	**OA**	osteoarthritis
JVP	jugular venous pressure	**OME**	otitis media with effusion
KUB	kidneys, ureter and bladder	**OR**	odds ratio
LBC	liquid-based cytology	**ORS**	oral rehydration salts
LDL	low-density lipoprotein	**OT**	occupational therapy/therapist
LFT	liver function test	**OTC**	over the counter
LH	luteinizing hormone	**p.r.n.**	as necessary
LHRH	luteinizing hormone releasing hormone	**PA**	posteroanterior
		PAM	postauricular myogenic response
LMP	last menstrual period	**PCO**	primary care organization
LNG-IUS	levonorgestrel releasing intrauterine system	**PCOS**	polycystic ovary syndrome
		PCP	*Pneumocystis carinii* pneumonia
LOC	loss of consciousness	**PE**	pulmonary embolus
LR	likelihood ratio	**PEFR**	peak expiratory flow rate
LSCS	lower segment caesarean section	**PEG**	percutaneous endoscopic gastrostomy
LTOT	long-term oxygen therapy	**PET**	positron emission tomography
LVF	left ventricular failure	**PF**	peak flow
MA	Maternity Allowance	**PFI**	pill-free interval
MAOI	monoamine oxidase inhibitor	**PHLS**	Public Health Laboratory Service
MASTA	Medical Advisory Service for Travellers Abroad	**PHN**	post-herpetic neuralgia
		PID	pelvic inflammatory disease
MCP	metacarpophalangeal	**PIH**	pregnancy-induced hypertension
MCV	mean cell volume	**PIP**	proximal interphalangeal
MDA	Misuse of Drugs Act	**PKU**	phenylketonuria
MDI	metered dose inhaler	**PMR**	polymyalgia rheumatica
MI	myocardial infarction	**PMS**	premenstrual syndrome
miu	millions of international units	**POP**	progestogen-only pill
MMR	measles, mumps and rubella	**PPH**	post-partum haemorrhage
MMSE	Mini-mental State Examination	**PPI**	proton pump inhibitor
MR	modified release	**ppm**	parts per million
MRI	magnetic resonance imaging	**PSA**	prostate-specific antigen
MS	multiple sclerosis	**PSV**	public service vehicle
MSBP	Munchausen's syndrome by proxy	**PTA**	post-traumatic amnesia
MSU	mid-stream urine	**PUVA**	psoralens with UVA
MTP	metatarsophalangeal	**PV**	plasma viscosity
NE	norethisterone enantate	**PVD**	peripheral vascular disease
NETOEN	1,9-nortestosterone	**q.d.s**	to be taken four times a day (*quarter die sumendum*)
NHS	National Health Service		
NI	National Insurance	**RA**	rheumatoid arthritis
NICE	National Institute for Clinical Excellence	**RAST**	radioallergosorbent testing
		RCGP	Royal College of General Practitioners

RCP	Royal College of Physicians	T_4	thyroxine
RCT	randomized controlled trial	**TB**	tuberculosis
RDC	research diagnostic criteria	**TCA**	tricyclic antidepressant
REM	rapid eye movement	**TENS**	transcutaneous electrical nervous stimulation
RIDDOR	Reporting of Injuries, Disease and Dangerous Occurrences Regulations	**TFT**	thyroid function test
RMO	Regional Medical Officer	**TIA**	transient ischaemic attack
RMS	Regional Medical Service	**TIBC**	total iron-binding capacity
RNA	ribonucleic acid	**TM**	temporomandibular
RR	relative risk (according to context)	**TOP**	termination of pregnancy
RR	respiratory rate (according to context)	**TPHA**	*Treponema pallidum* haemagglutination (test)
RRR	relative risk reduction	**TSH**	thyroid stimulating hormone
RUQ	right upper quadrant	**TURP**	transurethral resection of the prostate
SBE	subacute bacterial endocarditis	**TV**	*Trichomonas vaginalis*
sc	subcutaneous	**U&Es**	urea and electrolytes
SCC	squamous cell carcinoma	**UPSI**	unprotected sexual intercourse
SD	standard deviation	**URTI**	upper respiratory tract infection
SHBG	sex hormone binding globulin	**USS**	ultrasound scan
SIDS	sudden infant death syndrome	**UTI**	urinary tract infection
SK	solar keratosis	**UV**	ultraviolet
SLE	systemic lupus erythematosus	**UVA**	ultraviolet wavelength A
SLR	straight leg raising	**UVB**	ultraviolet wavelength B
SMP	statutory maternity pay	**UVC**	ultraviolet wavelength C
SpA	spondylarthropathies	**VA**	visual acuity
SPECT	single photon emission computerized tomography	**VAT**	value added tax
SPF	sun protection factor	**VDRL**	Venereal Disease Reference Laboratory
SSD	Social Services department	**VF**	ventricular fibrillation
SSM	superficial spreading melanoma	**VTE**	venous thromboembolism
SSP	statutory sick pay	**VZIG**	varicella-zoster immunoglobulin
SSRI	selective serotonin reuptake inhibitor	**WB**	withdrawal bleed
stat	immediately	**WBC**	white blood cell (count)
STD	sexually transmitted disease	**WHO**	World Health Organization
STI	sexually transmitted infection		
t.d.s.	to be taken three times a day (*ter die sumendum*)		

Chapter 1

General

CHAPTER CONTENTS

© 2011 Elsevier Ltd.
DOI: 10.1016/B978-0-7020-3053-6.00001-5

MEDICAL CERTIFICATES (SOCIAL SECURITY, STATUTORY SICK PAY AND MATERNITY BENEFITS)

ADVICE

Dept for Work and Pensions (DWP) booklet *Medical Evidence for SSP, SMP and Social Security Incapacity Benefit Purposes: A Guide for Registered Medical Practitioners* leaflet IB 204. Available: www.dwp.gov.uk/medical/guides_new.asp

Patients are deemed unfit for work because of:

(a) illness; or

(b) the danger of their passing on infection; or

(c) the fact that they are receiving treatment on a regular basis (e.g. dialysis, chemotherapy or radiotherapy).

In practice, GPs issue certificates for a number of reasons (Ford 1998):

(a) They agree with the patient's self-assessment.

(b) They want to avoid conflict.

(c) It is quicker than debating the issue with the patient.

(d) They feel unable to disprove the patient's claims.

(e) There is external pressure (e.g. from the Job Centre or the employer).

However, certifying a patient as unfit to work carries potential adverse consequences.

● *Poor mental health.* Once unemployed for 12 weeks or more there is a greater risk of depression, anxiety and physical illness. The risk of suicide is higher (Lewis and Sloggett 1998), especially so for men aged under 35.

● *Poor long term prospects of work.* An individual who has been off work for 12 months is unlikely to return to work for 7 years; and, if off for more than 2 years, the person is more likely to retire than ever return to work. Possible reasons for this are that they acquire a poor employment record and so are less employable, and also they interpret the stress of being unemployed as 'sickness' and request further certificates (Ford, Ford and Dowrick 2000).

STATUTORY SICK PAY

To qualify for *Statutory Sick Pay* (SSP), a patient must be employed, be under age 65 and have been sick for 4 consecutive days. This includes days when the patient would not normally have worked. Periods of sickness that are less than 8 weeks apart count as one. An employee not eligible for SSP may claim *Incapacity Benefit* (IB) or, from October 2008, *Employment and Support Allowance* (ESA), instead. More information for patients is available from local Jobcentre Plus offices.

Self-certification: if patients are sick for 4–7 days they should, on the last day of illness, certify themselves on *form SC1* if claiming IB or ESA, or *form SC2* if claiming SSP. The GP is not required to fill in a certificate for the first 7 days of illness.

If issuing a certificate:

❉ Use the *Statement of Fitness for Work (Form Med 3)*.

❉ Use *form Med 3* (FM3) if the patient has been seen and examined not more than 1 day before. Otherwise use *form Med 5* (FM5).

❉ Assess whether the patient is fit to work at his or her normal occupation, or whether he or she could be fit to work if certain adjustments were made. If unemployed, consider the patient's fitness for his or her last job, or the job for which they were registered with the Employment Service.

THE STATEMENT OF FITNESS FOR WORK

When can the statement be issued?

The statement may be issued by a doctor:

(a) on the day the doctor assesses the patient, either in person or on the telephone; or

(b) on a later date if the doctor considers that it would have been reasonable to have issued the statement on the day of assessment; or

(c) as a result of a written report from another doctor or registered health professional.

How does the doctor indicate whether the patient is fit to work within certain conditions?

The doctor must state either that the patient is not fit for work, or that the patient may be fit for work if one or more measures are taken.

If choosing to state the latter, the doctor must give details of those measures and must, in the comments box, give the employer sufficient information about the patient's ability to function, so that the employer can judge the feasibility of the patient's returning to work.

For how long may the statement be issued?

The doctor states the duration of the period in which the patient is unfit for work either:

(a) by stating a period of time, which may be for no more than 3 months at a time in the first 6 months of illness, but which may be for a period of any length after the first 6 months, including for 'an indefinite period'; or

(b) by specifying a start and end date. This may be done if:

- the statement covers a previous period when no statement was issued; or
- the statement is for < 14 days and the doctor does not wish to see the patient again; or
- the doctor judges that specifying a date for the return to work will help to motivate the patient.

Does the doctor need to sign the patient off as 'fit for work'?

No. The doctor must specify whether he or she needs to see the patient again. If the doctor has stated that another assessment is required, and the patient is found fit for work, the doctor does not need to certify the patient as 'fit for work'. A final statement is only needed if the patient will return to work on a date other than that on the original statement.

THE MEDICAL SERVICES OF THE DEPARTMENT FOR WORK AND PENSIONS (DWP)

The Medical Services may be involved:

(a) at the request of an employee because the employer has refused to pay SSP. This happens when an employer does not accept that the employee is unfit to work;

(b) where an employer asks for a second opinion, as in the case of prolonged or frequent illness, e.g. more than four periods of illness of 4–7 days each in any one year;

(c) where an adjudication officer at the local office cannot find sufficient reason to grant IB or ESA to a patient who is claiming it.

WHEN THE GP DISAGREES WITH THE DECISION

When an adjudication officer declares that a patient is fit for work, a GP may only continue to issue form Med 3 if the patient's condition has deteriorated or the diagnosis has changed. It is important to detail the change in the 'comments section.' If neither of these circumstances applies, *and the patient disagrees that he or she is fit for work of any kind*, the patient should appeal against the decision of the adjudication officer to the Independent Tribunal Service.

The GP can assist the appeal by:

(a) writing in support of the patient;

(b) asking a consultant for an opinion;

(c) referring the patient to the Disability Employment Adviser for an opinion;

(d) advising the patient to obtain support from a trade union or local rights organization.

EMPLOYMENT REHABILITATION

As soon as it becomes clear that a patient will never be fit to return to previous work, consider whether rehabilitation or a change of job would be advisable. It is worth raising this topic before the BA applies the Work Capability Assessment.

OPTIONS WHEN THE PATIENT MAY BE FIT FOR ALTERNATIVE WORK

(a) Issue form Med 3 stating what changes need to be made in order to enable the patient to work; or

(b) Continue to issue form Med 3 and refer, with the patient's consent, to the Disability Employment Adviser at the Job Centre. Write a letter or complete *form DP99* (available from the Job Centre) or just write a note in the 'comments' section of form Med 3. The Adviser can arrange for the patient to be registered as disabled, which can lead to a number of facilities including retraining and placement in sheltered work-shops or in vacancies reserved for the disabled. The Adviser also has access to schemes that provide special equipment and assistance with fares, and to the Job Introduction Scheme (which finances a disabled person in a job for a 6-week trial); or

(c) Continue to issue form Med 3 and recommend that the patient takes on 'permitted work', which is part-time or light work as therapy. This can be done without loss of benefits provided the patient earns less than £20 a week, or less than £92 a week (2009) while working for fewer than 16 hours a week. Prior approval by a doctor is not required. Prior approval from the local Job Centre is necessary before starting work to avoid accusations of 'moonlighting'. While work earning up to £20 a week may continue indefinitely, work up to £92 a week may only continue without loss of benefit for up to 26 weeks, or longer if supervised by a professional caseworker.

FOOD HANDLERS (DEPARTMENT OF HEALTH 1995)

- Food handlers with diarrhoea or vomiting that is likely to be infectious should refrain from work and not return until 48 hours after the diarrhoea or vomiting has ceased. Indicators of infection are the presence of fever, or more than one episode of diarrhoea or vomiting. They should be notified as suspected food poisoning. Negative stool samples will only be needed from those with *Salmonella typhi* or *paratyphi* (six samples) or toxin-producing *Escherichia coli* (two samples 48 hours apart).
- Food handlers with hepatitis A may return to work 7 days from the *onset* of symptoms.
- Food handlers with a skin lesion:
  - (a) patients with a clean wound may work provided the wound is covered with a waterproof plaster;
  - (b) patients with a discharging lesion in a non-exposed site may work provided they pay meticulous attention to hand washing;
  - (c) patients with a discharging lesion in an exposed site (hands, face, neck or scalp) should remain off work until it is healed. The same advice applies to patients with boils and whitlows.
- Food handlers with discharging eyes, ears, mouth or gums should remain off work until the affected area is healed.
- Food handlers with respiratory diseases do not pose a risk of food-borne infection. However, the patient who is coughing or sneezing over food should not be working.

Before certifying such a patient as unfit to work, ask whether alternative work with the same employer is possible. If so use form Med 3, certifying that the patient is fit to work but in the 'comments' section add that the patient is not to handle food.

These recommendations also apply to healthcare professionals and to those working with very young children.

MATERNITY AND PATERNITY BENEFITS

GUIDANCE

DWP. *A Guide to Maternity Benefits.* Leaflet NI 17A from local Jobcentre Plus offices

Most working women will be entitled to *Statutory Maternity Pay* (SMP) or *Maternity Allowance* (MA). The regulations are complex, and it is up to the woman's employer to tell her the details. A woman not entitled to SMP or MA should claim incapacity benefit from 6 weeks before the expected date of delivery (EDD) until 2 weeks after the birth.

The woman should:

(a) inform her employer at least 4 weeks before she intends to stop work (she must not stop work earlier than 14 weeks before the expected delivery, i.e. when 26 weeks pregnant);

(b) hand in medical evidence of the expected date of confinement (form Mat B1, see below).

Both SMP and MA are paid for a maximum of 26 weeks from, at the earliest, 11 weeks before the expected week of confinement (i.e. 29 weeks pregnant). A woman may delay starting the time during which she draws her allowance until, at the latest, 1 day after the baby's birth.

SMP or MA may be paid for a shorter period if a woman:

(a) continues to work into the last 6 weeks of pregnancy (i.e. after 34 weeks of pregnancy); or

(b) claims late.

A potential father who wishes to claim *Statutory Paternity Pay* should notify his employer by the 15th week before the baby is due.

A *Sure Start Maternity Grant* is available to women if they or their partner are on income support or certain other benefits.

FORM MAT B1

∗ A *form Mat B1(A)* should be issued either by the GP or by the midwife not earlier than 20 weeks before the expected week of delivery (i.e. after 20 weeks of pregnancy). Examination may have been before this time.

∗ If maternity allowance is claimed after confinement, use *form Mat B1(B)*.

PREGNANCY AND EMPLOYMENT

GUIDANCE

Health and Safety Executive. *New and Expectant Mothers at Work; a Guide for Health Professionals.* Published 2003. Available: www.hse.gov.uk (choose 'New and Expectant Mothers')

● Employers are required by UK law to identify factors at work that pose potential hazards for pregnant, breastfeeding or postpartum employees. They must make these hazards known to all female employees of childbearing age.

● Once a hazard is identified, the employer is obliged to remove it, or adjust the woman's hours or conditions of work, or find her alternative work or give her paid leave.

If you consider that work poses a hazard:

∗ Issue a Med 3, stating 'you may be fit for work' and, in the comments section, detail the adjustments needed or the problem identified.

This is often better for the patient, for both financial and psychological reasons, than certifying that she is unfit for work.

EXAMPLES OF HAZARDS

■ *Absolute:* deep sea diving, working with lead or radiation, lambing.

■ *Relative:* (where adjustments could allow the patient to continue to work):

(a) heavy lifting
(b) excessive hours
(c) working alone
(d) working at heights
(e) travelling long distances
(f) risk of violence
(g) lack of privacy for breastfeeding or expressing milk.

INFORMATION FOR PATIENTS

HSE Infoline 08701 545500
    HSE website www.hse.gov.uk (choose 'New and Expectant Mothers')
    The Public Services website www.direct.gov.uk (search on 'Pregnancy and Employment')

FINANCIAL BENEFITS FOR PATIENTS

The GP may be the first professional with whom a person, eligible for benefits, comes into contact. A basic understanding of the UK system will help the GP guide the patient in the right direction. For more detailed assistance, direct the patient to:

■ the local Jobcentre Plus (for those of working age);

■ the website of the Department of Work and Pensions (www.dwp.gov.uk) or www.direct. gov.uk;

■ the free Benefit Enquiry Line 0800 88 22 00;

■ the telephone numbers for individual benefits listed in the UK phone book under Jobcentre Plus.

PATIENTS WITH A LOW INCOME AND/OR LITTLE SAVINGS (REGARDLESS OF HEALTH)

In 2009 the threshold for savings was £16,000. These patients are entitled to:

(a) *Income Support* if aged < 60 and working < 16 hours a week, or living with a partner who is working < 24 hours a week.

(b) *Pension Credit* if aged 60 or over.

(c) *Jobseeker's Allowance* if below state pension age and working for < 16 hours a week while seeking work.

(d) *Housing* and *Council Tax Benefit.*

(e) *Child Tax Credit* for those with at least one child < 16 or in full-time education.

(f) *Working Tax Credit* for those:

■ aged ≥ 25 and working ≥ 30 hours per week; or

■ aged ≥ 16 and either disabled or looking after a child, and working > 16 hours a week. Contact the Tax Credit Helpline on 0845 300 3900 or www.taxcredits.inlandrevenue.gov.uk

(g) Certain NHS benefits: free prescriptions, dental treatment and sight tests, vouchers for glasses. Help with hospital travel costs can be claimed directly from the hospital if the patient has proof of eligibility, or via the Jobcentre Plus.

(h) Payments from *The Social Fund*: funeral payments, cold weather payments, maternity payments, budgeting loans, crisis loans and community care grants, which are designed to help people who would otherwise not manage to stay in the community to do so. These grants are discretionary, and may help with the purchase of beds, bedding, cooker, refrigerator, vacuum cleaner, clothes, shoes, furniture, heaters, washing machine, house repairs, removal costs, etc. They may be loans, and applicants considered too poor to repay them may be turned down.

PATIENTS WHO ARE ILL OR DISABLED (REGARDLESS OF INCOME)

These patients may be eligible for:

(a) *Incapacity Benefit* (IB), which is paid to those of working age when SSP ends or from the 4th day of illness if the patient is ineligible for SSP. Receipt of Incapacity Benefit in the first 28 weeks is dependent on a doctor issuing a medical certificate; thereafter, it depends on the Medical Services of the DWP performing the Personal Capability Assessment. A new applicant after October 2008 will receive an Employment and Support Allowance instead.

(b) *Disability Living Allowance* (DLA), which is for those aged under 65 who need help with personal care or who are aged 3 or over and have severe difficulty walking or aged 5 or over and need help getting around. People who did not qualify for the old Attendance and Mobility Allowances may qualify for the DLA, e.g. those over 16 who are unable to prepare a main cooked meal or who have difficulty taking medication reliably. To qualify, a patient must have needed help for 3 months (except in the case of the terminally ill) and be likely to need help for at least a further 6 months.

(c) *Attendance Allowance* (AA), which is for people aged 65 or over who need help with their bodily

functions or to stop them being a danger to themselves or to others. Bodily functions include hearing, seeing, eating, dressing, washing and going to the toilet. The need must have existed for 6 months before applying (except in terminally ill patients, see below). It is not necessary actually to have someone provide that care.

(d) *DLA and AA in terminal illness.* Patients likely to die within 6 months can claim DLA or AA immediately, whether or not they need looking after. They need not know that they are terminally ill. Patients should submit the ordinary DLA or AA claim form, ticking the box to apply under the *Special Rules*, accompanied by the doctor's report on form DS 1500.

(e) *Carer's Allowance*, which is for those, aged at least 16, who care for at least 35 hours a week for someone who is getting or waiting to hear about: AA, DLA, or a Constant Attendance Allowance associated with Industrial Injuries Disablement Benefit, or with a War Disablement Pension. It is not paid to someone who is receiving more than a minimal earning from another job. Married women and women who are separated from their husbands can now claim.

(f) *Council Tax – The Reduction for Disabilities Scheme.* Residents are entitled to a council tax discount if certain features of the home are essential, or of major importance, for the well-being of a disabled person. Examples are an additional bathroom or space dedicated to a wheelchair. Details are set out in *Council Tax: A Guide to Your Bill* available at www.local. odpm.gov.uk (choose 'Council Tax').

(g) *Industrial Injuries Disablement Benefit*, which is for those disabled by an accident at work or by disease related to their work. Benefit can be paid from 15 weeks after the onset of disablement. Patients who suffer even a minor injury should seek a declaration from the Jobcentre Plus on form BI 100A, in case they need to claim benefits later. Only 1% disablement is required for some respiratory conditions. Conditions include: asthma, chronic bronchitis, deafness, pneumoconiosis (including silicosis and asbestosis), tenosynovitis and vibration white finger.

(h) *Reduced Earnings Allowance*, which is available for those whose earnings have been reduced because of an accident or illness caused by work, but only if it occurred before 1.10.1990.

(i) *War Disablement Pension*, which is for those injured or disabled through serving in the

Armed Forces and for certain other categories injured or disabled because of war. In addition to the pension, the disabled person is entitled to priority treatment for the disability from the NHS and payment of funeral expenses if death is due to the disablement. There is provision for a widow or widower's pension, and allowances for children, parents and other relatives in certain circumstances.

(j) *Criminal Injuries Compensation*. The injury must be severe enough to need sutures or to have caused a fracture, or hospital admission, and can include compensation for mental injury. Minor injuries, such as scratching or bruising are unlikely to qualify but a combination of minor injuries may if they last for at least 6 weeks and necessitate at least two visits to a doctor. Patients should apply to the Criminal Injuries Compensation Authority, Tay House, 300 Bath Street, Glasgow G2 4LN, tel. 0845 602 3890. www.cica.gov.uk. Note that Northern Ireland has a separate scheme. Claims should normally be made within 2 years of the injury. They should be accompanied by the relevant police crime reference number.

(k) *Vaccine damage payments*, which are for people severely disabled as a result of immunization, performed in the UK, against diphtheria, tetanus, pertussis, polio, measles, mumps, rubella, TB, *meningococcus* group C, *Haemophilus influenzae* type b, pneumococcus, or smallpox prior to 1971. Claims should be made on a form available from the Vaccine Damage Payments Unit, Palatine House, Lancaster Road, Preston PR1 1HB or downloaded from www. direct.gov.uk (search on 'Vaccine Damage').

FREE PRESCRIPTIONS

(a) aged < 16 or ≥ 60; or
(b) aged 16–18 and in full-time education; or
(c) pregnant or delivered of a baby in the last 12 months; or
(d) on a low income with little savings; or
(e) family in receipt of certain benefits, e.g. Income Support; or
(f) patients with certain conditions:
- permanent fistula requiring continuous surgical dressing or requiring an appliance;
- epilepsy requiring continuous anticonvulsant drugs;

- diabetes mellitus, except where treated by diet alone;
- hypothyroidism;
- hypoparathyroidism;
- diabetes insipidus or other forms of hypopituitarism;
- hypoadrenalism for which specific substitutional therapy is indicated;
- myasthenia gravis;
- continuing physical disability which makes it impossible to go out without the help of another person.

FREE NHS SIGHT TESTS

(a) age < 16 or 16–18 and in full-time education;
(b) age ≥ 60;
(c) registered blind or partially sighted;
(d) diabetes;
(e) glaucoma or aged > 40 with a first-degree relative with glaucoma;
(f) receiving, or their partner gets, Income Support or certain other benefits;
(g) people on low income; they need to apply in advance (using form HC1) for an HC2 or HC3 certificate; or to apply on form HC5 for reimbursement within 2 weeks of the test;
(h) under the care of a hospital ophthalmologist;
(i) requiring complex lenses.

FREE NHS DENTAL TREATMENT

(a) aged < 16 or 16–18 and in full-time education. Being aged < 18 entitles patients to free treatment but not free appliances;
(b) pregnant or delivered of a baby in the last 12 months;
(c) receiving, or their partner gets, Income Support or certain other benefits;
(d) on low income; they need to apply in advance (using form HC1) for an HC2 or HC3 certificate; or to apply on form HC5 for reimbursement within 2 weeks of the test;
(e) resident in a residential care or nursing home and receiving help from the local authority with the fees.

PATIENTS WHO ARE CHRONICALLY ILL OR DISABLED AND ON LOW INCOME WITH LITTLE SAVINGS

These patients are, in addition, eligible for:

(a) *Independent Living Fund*. This is intended to assist severely disabled people, aged 16–65, to remain at home, if they wish, rather than enter residential care. It is for those receiving DLA at the higher rate or a Constant AA who are not able to pay for the care they need to live at home. Savings of the patient (and partner) must be < £23,000 (2009). Application forms are available from the Independent Living Fund, PO Box 7525, Nottingham NG2 4ZT, tel. 0845 601 8815, www.ilf.org.uk.

(b) *Community Care Grants*. These are to help people live independently or to assist them in a time of exceptional stress. They are more likely to be awarded to patients on low income, especially if they are supported by a letter from their GP detailing the medical need.

IF YOU DISAGREE WITH THE DWP DECISION

∗ Advise your patient to get booklet GL24, *If you think our decision is wrong*. It is available from the local Job Centre and on www.direct.gov.uk. It includes an appeal form. The appeal must be made within 3 months of the original decision.

∗ Advise your patient to seek guidance from an advice centre or solicitor.

∗ Support the patient's appeal by supplying a medical report.

Further advice is available from:

(a) local Job Centre offices or Citizens' Advice Bureaux; www.adviceguide.org.uk

(b) *Disability Rights Handbook*, published by the Disability Alliance, Universal House, 88–94 Wentworth Street, London E1 7SA, tel. 020 7247 8776, www.disabilityalliance.org

(c) *Welfare Benefits and Tax Credits Handbook*, published by the Child Poverty Action Group (CPAG), 94 White Lion Street, London N1 9PF, tel. 020 7837 7979, www.cpag.org.uk Benefit claimants are eligible for a reduction in price.

FITNESS TO DRIVE

ADVICE

At-a-Glance Guide to the Current Medical Standards of Fitness to Drive. DVLA, 2007. Available: www.dvla. gov.uk (choose 'Medical Rules')

● It is the duty of licence holders to inform the DVLA if they suffer from:
  (a) a prescribed, relevant or prospective disability; or
  (b) a previously notified disability that has become worse.

● The patient should notify the Drivers Medical Group, DVLA, Swansea, SA99 1TU, tel. 0845 850 0095, or, in Northern Ireland, Driver Licensing Medical Section, County Hall, Castlerock Road, Coleraine BT51 3TB, tel. 028 7034 1340, www. dvlni.gov.uk. Using the questionnaire that can be downloaded from the website will speed up the process.

● The inclusion of prospective disability means that the patient is obliged to notify the DVLA as soon as an illness is diagnosed if that illness could lead to the patient being unfit to drive in the future. Insulin-dependent diabetes is an example. The DVLA is likely to issue a licence for 1, 2 or 3 years, which permits them to review the case. Temporary disabilities (e.g. fractured bones) that are not expected to last more than 3 months are exempt.

● It is the duty of the doctor to inform patients with a disability of their obligation to notify the DVLA and the vehicle insurance company. Record that such advice has been given in the patients' notes.

● Epilepsy is the commonest cause of collapse at the wheel, followed by blackouts, diabetes and cardiac conditions. In almost all these cases the majority of patients are aware of their condition, and, if they have not notified the DVLA, their insurance is liable to be invalid. Doctors unable to demonstrate that they warned patients of the need to notify the DVLA could be liable to legal action.

● If there is doubt about a case, contact:
  (a) England, Wales and Scotland: the Medical Adviser, Drivers Medical Group, DVLA,

Longview Road, Swansea SA99 1TU, tel. 01792 761119, email medadviser@dvla.gsi.gov.uk.

(b) Northern Ireland: Driver and Vehicle Licensing, Castlerock Road, Coleraine BT51 3TB, tel. 028 7034 1369.

CONFIDENTIALITY

Patients' names should not normally be disclosed to the DVLA without their consent. If, however, there is any doubt about whether the patient will inform the DVLA, the UK General Medical Council recommends the following steps (reproduced with permission) (General Medical Council 2000):

1. The DVLA is legally responsible for deciding if a person is medically unfit to drive. The Agency needs to know when driving licence holders have a condition which may now, or in the future, affect their safety as a driver.

2. Therefore, where patients have such conditions you should:
   (a) make sure that patients understand that the condition may impair their ability to drive. If a patient is incapable of understanding this advice, for example because of dementia, you should inform the DVLA immediately;
   (b) explain to patients that they have a legal duty to inform the DVLA about the condition.

3. If patients refuse to accept the diagnosis or the effect of the condition on their ability to drive, you can suggest that the patients seek a second opinion, and make appropriate arrangements for the patients to do so. You should advise patients not to drive until the second opinion has been obtained.

4. If patients continue to drive when they are not fit to do so, you should make every reasonable effort to persuade them to stop. This may include telling their next of kin.

5. If you do not manage to persuade patients to stop driving, or you are given or find evidence that a patient is continuing to drive contrary to advice, you should disclose relevant medical information immediately, in confidence, to the medical adviser at the DVLA.

6. Before giving information to the DVLA you should try to inform the patient of your decision to do so. Once the DVLA has been informed, you should also write to the patient, to confirm that a disclosure has been made.

The doctor has a similar responsibility to breach confidentiality in the case of a patient whose licence has been revoked on medical grounds and who continues to drive. In this case, with the provisos above, the doctor should notify the police.

WHAT TO DO IF THE DOCTOR OR PATIENT DISAGREES WITH THE DVLA's DECISION

The patient has the right of appeal, within 6 months in England and Wales and within 21 days in Scotland. This may be costly. An informal letter to the Medical Adviser from the doctor may be more appropriate (Rouse 1995).

COMMON MEDICAL PROBLEMS THAT AFFECT DRIVING

If a patient's medical condition poses a danger to the public, he or she must stop driving and notify the DVLA whether or not the condition is listed in Tables 1.1–1.6.

The details of the more common conditions listed are taken from the DVLA publication *At-a-Glance Guide to the Current Medical Standards of Fitness to Drive*, September 2007. A more recent and detailed version is available at www.dvla.gov.uk (choose 'Medical Rules'), which includes the regulations that apply to holders of a Group 2 licence for driving lorries, buses and taxis.

* Advise patients to notify their insurance company of any relevant medical condition, even if it is not necessary to notify the DVLA. Failure to do so could lead to a refusal by the company to support the patient if an accident occurs that is related to the condition.

DRIVING AND THE ELDERLY

- Drivers over the age of 70 have to renew their licence every 3 years, making a declaration of health.
- Elderly patients are more likely to have impaired concentration, memory loss and slower reaction

Table 1.1	Neurological problems	
CONDITION	NOTIFICATION OF DVLA	LIKELY ADVICE ON DRIVING TO BE GIVEN BY THE DVLA MEDICAL ADVISER OR THE GP AS APPROPRIATE
Epilepsy	Notify	Stop driving. The licence is likely to be restored when free from seizures for 1 year. No need to stop driving if an attack occurred while asleep and there was a previous attack while asleep > 3 years ago and no subsequent attacks have occurred while awake. The patient must comply with treatment
A 'provoked' seizure	Notify	Stop driving. Restoration of the licence is likely once the provoking factor has been removed
Withdrawal of anticonvulsants	No need to notify	Recommend stopping driving once starting to withdraw treatment and for 6 months after stopping. The risk of a seizure is 40% greater in the first year than if treatment is continued
A solitary fit	Notify	Stop driving. The licence is likely to be restored after 1 year if there are no more fits and medical exam is satisfactory
Chronic neurological disorders	Notify	Continue driving if performance is not impaired
Disabling giddiness	Notify	Stop driving. Restart if symptoms are controlled
Stroke	Notify only if there is residual neurological deficit after 1 month (other than mild limb weakness)	Stop driving for 1 month. Restart if recovery is satisfactory
Multiple frequent TIAs	Notify	Stop driving until free from attacks for 3 months
Simple faint(s) with clear provoking factors and unlikely to occur while sitting or lying	Do not notify	No restrictions
LOC: probable syncope; no provoking factors but risk of recurrence low	Notify	Stop driving for 4 weeks
LOC: probable syncope but no provoking factors and risk of recurrence high (e.g. heart disease)	Notify	Stop driving for 6 months (or 4 weeks if the cause has been treated)
LOC with no clinical pointers	Notify	Stop driving for 6 months
Unwitnessed LOC or altered awareness with seizure markers (e.g. incontinence, bitten tongue or amnesia for > 5 minutes)	Notify	Stop driving for 1 year

Other conditions dealt with in the *At-a-Glance Guide:* narcolepsy, encephalitis, meningitis, transient global amnesia, supratentorial and infratentorial tumours, serious head injury, intracranial haemorrhage, intracranial abscess, subdural empyema, hydrocephalus, shunts, neuroendoscopic procedures and cerebral implants.

times, as well as being more likely to have other conditions that make them unfit to drive.

- The GP may need to assess elderly patients at the latter's request when they are applying for renewal of a driving licence, or at the request of the insurance company.
- Modifications to the car may enable the patient with locomotor problems to drive. It may be

easier to ask a partner to perform the medical examination.

- If there is doubt, a single trial driving lesson from a professional instructor will give the patient an impartial opinion. Patients who have lost confidence or have not driven for some time may benefit from a course of lessons.

Table 1.2 Cardiovascular problems

CONDITION	NOTIFICATION OF DVLA	ADVICE ON DRIVING
Angina at rest, due to emotion or while driving	No need to notify	Stop driving until symptoms are controlled
Myocardial infarction and acute coronary syndrome	No need to notify	Stop driving for 4 weeks (1 week in non ST elevation MI treated with successful angioplasty)
Elective angioplasty	No need to notify	Stop driving for 1 week
CABG	No need to notify	Stop driving for 4 weeks
Arrhythmias	No need to notify unless symptoms are distracting or disabling	Stop driving if arrhythmia is causing incapacity until symptoms have been controlled for at least 4 weeks
Pacemaker insertion or box change	Notify	Stop driving for at least 1 week
Aortic aneurysm ≥ 6 cm	Notify	Recommence driving only after successful treatment and no evidence of further enlargement

Other conditions dealt with in the *At-a-Glance Guide* that require action: left ventricular assist devices, catheter ablation, implanted ventricular defibrillator, chronic aortic dissection, congenital heart disease.

Table 1.3 Diabetes mellitus

CONDITION	NOTIFICATION OF DVLA	ADVICE ON DRIVING
On insulin	Notify	Will be allowed to drive but licence will require renewal every 1, 2 or 3 years. Should stop driving if frequent hypoglycaemic episodes occur or if awareness of hypoglycaemia is lost
On oral drugs or diet alone	No need to notify	Need not stop driving unless other disabilities develop, e.g. visual or lower limb problems

Table 1.4 Psychiatric problems

CONDITION	NOTIFICATION OF DVLA	ADVICE ON DRIVING
Severe anxiety or depression	Notify	Stop driving. Licence may be restored once a period of stability has been reached
Acute or chronic psychosis	Notify	Stop driving. Licence may be restored after at least 3 months of stability and the patient is compliant with treatment
Dementia	Notify	Stop driving. Licence may be restored if symptoms are mild and progression is slow
Learning disability	Notify	Do not start driving. Licence may be granted if the disability is mild
Behaviour disorder if seriously disturbed	Notify	Stop driving. Licence may be restored if behaviour is satisfactorily controlled
Developmental disorders e.g. autism or ADHD	Notify	A licence will be granted unless specific symptoms render the patient a hazard
Personality disorders	Notify	A licence will be granted unless specific symptoms render the patient a hazard

Table 1.5 Drug and alcohol misuse

CONDITION	NOTIFICATION OF DVLA	ADVICE ON DRIVING
Alcohol misuse (sufficient to cause disturbed behaviour or physical harm)	Notify	Stop driving. Licence may be restored after at least 6 months abstinence or controlled drinking
Alcohol dependency	Notify	Stop driving. Licence may be restored after abstinence for 1 year
Cannabis, ecstasy, LSD, etc.	Notify if dependent or using them persistently	Stop driving. Licence may be restored after abstinence for 6 months
Heroin, cocaine, etc.	Notify if dependent or using them persistently	Stop driving. Licence may be restored after abstinence for 1 year or stabilization on a maintenance programme
Benzodiazepine misuse (either illicit use or very high prescribed doses)	Notify	Stop driving. Licence may be restored after abstinence for 1 year
A drug- or alcohol-related seizure	Notify	Stop driving. Licence may be restored after 1 year

Multiple drug use, including alcohol, renders a patient unfit to drive.

Table 1.6   Visual problems

CONDITION	NOTIFICATION OF DVLA	ADVICE ON DRIVING
Reduced acuity	Notify if unable to meet the requirements (see next column)	Stop driving if unable to read an 'old' number plate at 20.5 metres or a post 1.9.2001 plate at 20 metres
Severe bilateral cataract or post cataract surgery with continuing disability	Notify	Stop driving if unable to read a number plate as above. This lies between 6/9 and 6/12 on the Snellen chart
Monocular vision	Notify	May drive once the patient has adapted to the disability
Visual field defects	Notify	Stop driving until DVLA confirms that the national requirements are met: a field of at least 120^0 horizontally plus binocular vision $20°$ above and below the horizontal meridian
Diplopia	Notify	Stop driving. Restart only on confirmation to the DVLA that it is controlled by glasses or a patch

Other conditions dealt with in the *At-a Glance Guide* that require action: night blindness and blepharospasm. The *At-a-Glance Guide* also deals with renal, respiratory and sleep disorders and discusses the question of age, which is not a bar per se but may be associated with other factors which would be.

DRIVING AND THE DISABLED

A DISABLED PATIENT WHO WISHES TO DRIVE

> **INFORMATION**
>
> The Department for Transport on www.dft.gov.uk (choose 'Access for Disabled People')
>   The Forum of Mobility Centres, tel. 0800 559 3636, www.mobility-centres.org.uk
>   RADAR (Royal Association for Disability and Rehabilitation), 12 City Forum, 250 City Road, London EC1V 8AF, tel. 020 7250 3222, www.radar.org.uk
>   Mobilise (previously the Disabled Drivers' Motor Club and the Disabled Drivers' Association), tel. 0150 848 9449, www.mobilise.info

Most patients who are disabled can drive cars with suitable modifications, including paraplegics, hemiplegics and those who are wheelchair-bound. They should be aware of the following:

- *DVLA*. Whether already holding a driving licence or applying for one for the first time, the first step is for the patient to notify the DVLA (see page 9) of the disability.
- *Driving Assessment Centres*. There are 16 Disabled Drivers' Assessment Centres in the UK that will assess the patient's disability and

advise on modifications to vehicles. They are private firms, and are listed in Annex 2 of the DVLA *At-a-Glance Guide* on www.dvla.gov.uk/at_a_glance/content.htm Their umbrella organization is the Forum of Disabled Drivers' Assessment Centres, tel. 0080 559 3636, www.mobility-centres.org.uk

- *Car modification firms*. Once advice has been obtained, the assessment centre will provide a list of firms able to carry out modifications. The Disabled Living Foundation (www.dlf.org.uk) also has a list.
- *Finance*. The Disability Living Allowance (see page 6) entitles the driver to other advantages: exemption from vehicle excise duty, a Blue Badge, and access to the Motability Scheme, which helps applicants to buy or hire cars or outdoor electric wheelchairs or scooters. Contact, for the car schemes: Motability Operations, City Gate House, 22 Southwark Bridge Road, London SE1 9HB, tel. 0845 456 4566; and for the wheelchair and scooter schemes: route2 mobility, Montgomery House, Newbury Rd, Enham Alamein, Andover, Hants SP11 6JS, tel. 0845 607 6260, www.motability.co.uk
- *Electrically propelled invalid carriages* fall into two classes: class 2 (maximum speed 4 mph) and class 3 (maximum speed 8 mph). A driving licence is not required, and so the Medical Rules do not apply, but patients are advised to consult

their GP for advice about their suitability. The DVLA suggests that a driver of such a vehicle should have to be able to read a number plate at 12.3 metres.

THE BLUE BADGE

- Patients over the age of 2 are eligible for a Blue Badge if they have:
  - (a) a permanent and substantial disability that causes very considerable difficulty in walking. As a guideline, patients normally able to walk more than 50 metres unaided are unlikely to be considered suitable; or
  - (b) have a severe disability in both upper limbs, regularly drive a motor vehicle but cannot turn the steering wheel even if that wheel is fitted with a turning knob; or
  - (c) are registered blind; or
  - (d) receive the higher rate mobility component of the DLA; or
  - (e) receive a war pension mobility supplement; or
  - (f) use a motor vehicle supplied for disabled people by a Government Health Department.
- The patient may use the badge either as a driver or as a passenger.
- The patient should apply to the local Social Services department for the Badge.
- More information is to be found on www.dft.gov.uk (search on 'Blue Badge').

Refusal to support the patient's application for the badge may cause friction between doctor and patient. Minimize this by:

(a) walking with the patient to establish his or her limits;

(b) pointing out that the final decision lies not with the GP but with the issuing office, to whom complaints should be made.

EXEMPTION FROM THE WEARING OF A CAR SEAT BELT

Advise patients who ask for an exemption certificate as follows:

* Recommend the booklet *Medical Exemption from Compulsory Seat Belt Wearing* obtainable from the Department of Health, PO Box 777, London SE1

6XH; or to go to www.thinkroadsafety.gov.uk and choose 'Site Map' then 'Seat Belts' then 'Medical Exemption From Compulsory Seat Belt Wearing'.

* Explain that (except in specific cases) a fee is payable for the examination, but that a free examination may be arranged by the Department of Transport (see the above leaflet).
* Explain that it is very unlikely that a certificate will be issued. There are few conditions, if any, which permit patients to drive and yet render them unfit to wear a seat belt.
* Accompany the patient to the car and explain how the repositioning of attachments or the 'Clever Clip' to reduce pressure across the chest or abdomen may solve the problem.

Certificates. If you do intend to issue a certificate, use the official *Certificate of Exemption from Compulsory Seat Belt Wearing* obtainable from the Department of Health, PO Box 777, London SE1 6XH; tel. 08701 555455 or email doh@prologistics.co.uk.

FITNESS TO FLY

GUIDANCE

British Airways Health Services. *Health and Medical Information* on www.britishairways.com/health (choose 'Health and Medical Information')

Medical Guidelines for Airline Travel, 2nd edition 2003. Aerospace Medical Association, www.asma.org

Assessing fitness to fly: guidelines for medical professionals from the Aviation Health Unit, Civil Aviation Authority. Available: www.caa.co.uk/fitnesstofly

- An ill or disabled passenger who is contemplating flying should notify the airline in advance on a form obtainable from the travel agent or the airline. Urgent cases should be discussed by telephone with the airline medical service.
- Such a passenger should inform his or her insurer in writing of all pre-existing medical conditions.
- Patients who might need medication during the flight must carry it in their hand luggage together with a medication list. They should

warn airport security staff if carrying needles, syringes or lancets.

- Patients who fly frequently can obtain a frequent traveller's medical card (FREMEC), which will be recognized by many airlines. This saves completing new forms for every flight and means that the airline will know what assistance will be needed at the airport and on board.

- Patients with a pacemaker or an implantable cardiac defibrillator (ICD) should warn security staff and those with an ICD should ask to be hand searched. There is a theoretical risk that even a hand-held electronic wand might trigger a shock (Possick and le Barry 2004).

Airlines stress that each case is considered on its merits but that the following rules are likely to apply to passengers on British Airways (the US Aerospace Medical Association guidance tends to be more strict).

- *Locomotor disability*. Patients with arthritis or other lower limb problems may need the extra legroom of First Class unless the airline can provide economy seating with extra space. Electric buggies and hoists can get patients on to the plane. Airlines will normally accommodate a stretcher, at a price, but any patient on a stretcher must be accompanied by a trained person. Special wheelchairs can be used to transfer patients from seat to toilet, but cabin staff cannot assist a patient in the toilet because they are food handlers.

- *Hypoxia*. Patients who cannot tolerate mild hypoxia are either unfit to fly or will need oxygen during the flight. These patients include those with a stroke in the last 3 days, even if recovering, a grand mal fit in the last 24 hours or anaemia below 7.5 g/dl. Patients with chronic respiratory disease who cannot walk 50 metres on the flat, or climb one flight of stairs, without severe dyspnoea, are unfit to fly. For those with cardiovascular disease, see below. Patients with arteriosclerotic dementia may become confused. A patient may not fly within 10 days of a sickle-cell crisis and anyone with the disease, although not the trait, must alert the airline that they may need in-flight oxygen. See box below for advice about which patients should alert the airline about the possible need for oxygen during the flight. Patients may not carry their own oxygen on board.

> **PATIENTS WHO SHOULD ALERT THE AIRLINE IN ADVANCE OF THEIR POSSIBLE NEED FOR IN-FLIGHT OXYGEN**
>
> *Assessing fitness to fly:* guidelines for medical professionals from the Aviation Health Unit, Civil Aviation Authority. Available: www.caa.co.uk/docs/923/FitnesstoFlyPDF)
>
> - Those using oxygen at home or with a baseline P_aO_2 < 70 mm Hg.
> - Congestive heart failure NYHA class III–IV.
> - Angina CCS class III–IV.
> - Cyanotic congenital heart failure.
> - Primary pulmonary hypertension.
> - Other cardiovascular diseases associated with hypoxaemia.
> - Severe chronic respiratory disease.
> - Sickle-cell disease.
> - Severe anaemia (in which the decision has been taken to allow the patient to fly).
> - NYHA = New York Heart Association.
> - CCS = Canadian Cardiovascular Society.

- *Difficulties due to gas expansion*. Gas in the body is likely to expand by about 30% during the flight. Patients who cannot tolerate this include those:
  - (a) with blocked Eustachian tubes and sinuses;
  - (b) with a tonsillectomy or middle ear surgery in the last 2 weeks;
  - (c) within 10 days of bowel or chest surgery;
  - (d) within 3 weeks of a gastrointestinal bleed; and those with an active peptic ulcer;
  - (e) within 7 days of air encephalography or intracranial or intraocular surgery; and not within 6 weeks if gas has been used in the treatment of retinal detachment;
  - (f) within 24 hours of laparoscopy;
  - (g) with a pneumothorax. A patient with a spontaneous pneumothorax should wait 1 week after an X-ray shows resolution. A patient with a traumatic pneumothorax should wait 2 weeks after X-ray resolution;
  - (h) who have been scuba diving in the 12 hours before the flight;
  - (i) with a recently applied plaster cast (patients should wait for 24 hours before a flight of less than 2 hours and 48 hours before a longer flight, unless the cast is capable of expansion).

- *Time zones.* Epilepsy may be precipitated by fatigue when flying, and patients should increase rather than decrease their medication as they change to the new time zone. Insulin-dependent diabetics should carry everything they need in their hand luggage in case of delays, including all their insulin since it would be inactivated if the hold temperature fell below freezing. They should take enough food with them for them to be able to keep to their own time zone during the flight.

Melatonin is remarkably effective in reducing jet-lag (Herxheimer and Petrie 2001), although it is not licensed in the UK. Between 0.5 and 5 mg should be taken at bedtime on arrival at the destination. Patients with epilepsy and those on warfarin should avoid it. Otherwise it is recommended, especially for those crossing at least five time zones, particularly if travelling east.

- *Cardiovascular disorders:*
  - (a) uncomplicated myocardial infarction within 7 days;
  - (b) complicated myocardial infarction within 4–6 weeks;
  - (c) unstable angina;
  - (d) decompensated congestive heart failure;
  - (e) uncontrolled hypertension;
  - (f) coronary artery bypass graft within 10 days;
  - (g) uncontrolled cardiac arrhythmia;
  - (h) severe symptomatic valvular disease.
- *Respiratory disorders.* Asthma should not present a problem if well controlled. Medication should be carried in hand luggage. COPD is not a problem if the patient can pass the walking test (see above). In cases of doubt, where the patient is keen to fly, refer to a respiratory physician for assessment by hypoxic challenge.
- *Diabetes.* (For further information visit www.diabetes.org.uk)
  - (a) pre-planning and discussion with the diabetic team is important;
  - (b) equipment medication (including insulin) should be kept in hand luggage;
  - (c) insulin should not be packed in hold luggage as it may be exposed to temperatures that may degrade it and there is a potential for loss of baggage;
  - (d) travelling east the day will be shortened. If the day is shortened by more than 2 hours it may be necessary to take fewer units of medium or long acting insulin;
  - (e) travelling west the travel day will be lengthened. If this is more than 2 hours it may be necessary to take more short acting or intermediate acting insulin.
- *Pregnancy.* A pregnant woman may fly up to and including the 36th week of pregnancy. A woman with a multiple pregnancy may not fly after the 31st week. If a woman is > 28 weeks pregnant she should carry with her a medical certificate confirming her EDD and that a doctor considers she is fit to fly. Newborn babies should not fly in the first 2 days of life while their alveoli are still expanding.
- *Deep vein thrombosis (DVT).* A patient with an acute DVT may not fly. All travellers should keep well hydrated, avoid excess alcohol and sedatives, exercise their legs half-hourly and walk about the cabin as much as possible. Older patients on long-haul flights, women on HRT, combined oral contraceptives or who are pregnant or post-partum, and others at high risk should consider the use of graduated compression stockings. In one study, below-knee UK class II stockings (ankle pressure 18–24 mmHg) reduced the incidence of asymptomatic DVTs in travellers on long-haul flights, with an average age of 62 but no other risk factors, from 10% to nil (Scurr, Machin, Bailey-King, *et al.* 2001; Anderson 2001). In addition, they should ask for an aisle seat so they can walk about more easily. High-risk cases are sometimes advised to consider taking aspirin or low molecular weight heparin, although the NNT for a high risk patient to prevent one symptomatic DVT is 8600. For a low risk patient it is 34,000 (Bandolier 2003). The Department of Health in March 2007 (www.dh.gov.uk and search on 'Deep Vein Thrombosis') defines high risk as:
  - (a) those who have ever had a DVT or pulmonary embolus (PE);
  - (b) anyone with a family history of clotting conditions;
  - (c) those with an inherited tendency to clot (thrombophilia);
  - (d) people with cancer or who have had treatment for cancer in the past;
  - (e) those who have undergone major surgery in the last 3 months;

(f) those who have had a hip or knee replacement within the last 3 months;

(g) anyone who has suffered a stroke.

Note that the risk of DVT applies to all forms of transport in which the passenger sits relatively immobile for 4 hours or more, not just to flying.

- *Other conditions:*

  (a) Contagious patients may not fly.

  (b) Psychiatric patients should be accompanied by someone competent to handle them if they are unsettled by the stress of flying.

  (c) Airlines will not accept the terminally ill if they are liable to die on the flight.

  (d) Patients with offensive conditions are not welcomed by airlines.

  (e) Patients with wired jaws must be able to release the mechanism in the event of vomiting.

For further information contact the UK Civil Aviation Health Unit, tel. 01293 573674, email aviationhealthunit@caa.co.uk.

FITNESS TO SCUBA DIVE

REVIEW/STUDY

Review: Sykes JJW. Medical aspects of scuba diving. BMJ 1994; 308: 1483–8.

Study: Glen S, White S, Douglas J. Medical supervision of sport diving in Scotland: reassessing the need for routine medical examinations. Br J Sports Med 2000; 34: 375–8.

- In the UK a routine medical certificate of fitness to dive is unnecessary. Divers complete an annual Medical Declaration Form and only those answering 'yes' to one or more questions need to contact their local medical referee. The form, and details of local medical referees, can be found on www.uksdmc.co.uk. General practitioners are, however, still likely to be asked for advice on this subject.

- The combination of cold water, high pressure and strenuous exercise makes great demands on the diver. The 'buddy' system of diving means that any diver must be capable of rescuing another.

- An Australian study found that many scuba divers were diving despite medical contraindications (Taylor, O'Toole and Ryan 2002).

The following conditions are likely to exclude an applicant from diving:

(a) asthma, unless it is well controlled, not triggered by cold, emotion or exercise, and where a 'rescue' inhaler has not been needed in the previous 48 hours;

(b) spontaneous pneumothorax in the last 5 years, pulmonary cysts or other respiratory disease;

(c) cardiac disease (this is the cause of almost half the deaths in divers over 40 years old). Hypertensives may usually dive if their BP on first application is 160/90 or below (whether on treatment or not) and there is no end organ damage;

(d) orthopaedic problems including acute and chronic back pain;

(e) problems with balance;

(f) diabetes, unless there have been no 'hypos' in the last year; *and* no hospitalization due to the diabetes in the last year; *and* control is good with no renal, neuropathic, vascular or ocular complications, other than background retinopathy;

(g) neurological disorders including epilepsy and other causes of loss of consciousness. However, a person with epilepsy may be considered fit if there have been no fits for 5 years and no medication is taken;

(h) a recent history of head injury as follows: with post traumatic amnesia (PTA) < 1 hour: no diving for 3 weeks; PTA 1–24 hours: no diving for 2 months; PTA > 24 hours: no diving for at least 3 months;

(i) poor vision and, especially, a history of eye surgery. Contact lens wearers should use soft lenses to avoid corneal oedema;

(j) problems with Eustachian tubes, drums, middle or inner ear disease, other than presbyacusis;

(k) upper airways disorders, including laryngectomy;

(l) certain upper GI problems including severe reflux;

(m) certain haematological disorders: sickle-cell disease, polycythaemia, acute anaemia;

(n) neuromuscular disorders;

(o) psychiatric difficulties;

(p) obesity (BMI > 30) although an individual who can demonstrate adequate agility in the pool may be considered fit;

(q) pregnancy.

More information from the UK Sport Diving Medical Committee is available on www.uksdmc.co.uk.

MENTAL CAPACITY

GUIDANCE

The Law Society and the BMA. *Assessment of Mental Capacity; Guidance for Doctors and Lawyers.* London: British Medical Association, 2nd edition, 2004.

Mental Capacity Act 2005: Code of Practice. Available: www.justice.gov.uk (choose 'Guidance' then 'Mental Capacity').

British Medical Association. Adults with Incapacity (Scotland) Act. See www.bma.org.uk (search on 'Incapacity').

- The underlying principle, at least in England and Wales, is that people should be enabled and encouraged to take for themselves those decisions that they are able to make. Capacity is judged by whether a person is able to make that particular decision at that particular time. A patient may be capable of making one sort of decision but not another, and of making a decision one day, during a 'lucid interval', and not the next.
- The Mental Capacity Act, which came into force in England and Wales in 2007, has formalized previous best practice and common law principles. It relates to adults (aged 16 and over) who are unable to make decisions for themselves. Those decisions may be about healthcare and personal care, or about property, financial affairs or where to live. The main reasons for such incapacity are dementia, learning disability, mental illness, drug or alcohol intoxication, head injury or stroke. However, the presence of such a condition does not necessarily mean that the person is incapable.
- The situations in which the Act becomes relevant for a healthcare professional are:

(a) when providing care or treatment for a patient who might be incapable of giving consent;

(b) when asked to give an opinion on the capability of a patient by a third party.

The Code of Practice (see box above) contains detailed advice about the implications of the Act. For a GP the key points are as follows.

The two-stage test of capacity. A person is incapable of making a decision if:

(a) he or she has an impairment in or disturbed functioning of the way the brain or mind works; and

(b) he or she cannot make the required decision. This may be because he or she fails to:

　(a) understand information relevant to that decision; or

　(b) retain that information; or

　(c) use or weigh up that information; or

　(d) communicate that decision.

'Relevant information' includes what the decision is, why it is needed and what the consequences will be.

The 'best interests' principle. If making a decision on behalf of someone who is incapable, it must be in his or her best interests. This may be different from 'what the person would have wanted' and from what the person making the decision would like to happen. Certain principles are laid down in deciding what is in the person's best interests. Consider:

(a) all possibilities, without discrimination;

(b) all relevant circumstances;

(c) the possibility of deferring the decision to another time if the patient's condition may improve;

(d) the possibility of improving communication so that the patient can understand and communicate back; their wishes, feelings, beliefs and values;

(e) the views of relevant others, including family and carers, not necessarily solely the next of kin.

Who makes the decision?

- For most day-to-day actions or decisions, the decision-maker will be the carer most directly involved with the person at the time.
- Where the decision involves the provision of medical treatment, the doctor or other member of healthcare staff responsible for carrying out the particular treatment or procedure is the decision-maker.

- Where nursing or paid care is provided, the nurse or paid carer will be the decision-maker.
- If a Lasting Power of Attorney (or Enduring Power of Attorney) has been made and registered, or a deputy has been appointed under a court order, the attorney or deputy will be the decision-maker, for decisions within the scope of their authority.
- If the decision involves the drawing up of a care plan, a team may make the decision.

Who should be consulted when a major decision is made on behalf of a person without capacity?

- Anyone the person has previously named as someone they want to be consulted;
- anyone involved in caring for the person;
- anyone interested in their welfare (for example, family carers, other close relatives, or an advocate already working with the person);
- an attorney appointed by the person under a Lasting Power of Attorney; and
- a deputy appointed for that person by the Court of Protection.

PROCEDURE AND CAUTIONS

* Record the steps taken to come to your decision. If a doctor takes reasonable steps to come to a judgment that a person is incapable and makes a decision in his or her best interests, the Act protects that doctor from legal liability (but see below).
* Beware of assuming that the person is capable just because he or she agrees with the management you are proposing. It is convenient to do so but it is against the meaning of the Act. However, if, after assessment, you judge that the person is incapable, and that the management is in the person's best interests, then it may go ahead.
* Do not assume the person is incapable just because you disagree with their decision.
* Information about a patient remains confidential even when they are incapable; but confidentiality may be broken if it is necessary to do so to protect the person, or others, from harm. For this reason it is ethical to tell relevant people of your decision and the reasons for it; but try first to obtain the patient's permission. They may be able to give meaningful permission even though incapable of making other decisions. Failing that permission, give relevant

people the information they need to act in the best interests of the person who is incapable.
* If there is more than one reasonable decision that is in the patient's best interests, choose the least restrictive solution.
* Modify the thoroughness of your assessment according to the urgency of the situation. The decision to treat an unconscious patient in an emergency can usually be made instantaneously. Conversely, the assessment of capacity to make a will, to marry or to enter into any other formal contract should be made and recorded formally.
* Do not witness a patient's signature without being clear that he or she is capable of making the decision to sign.
* If a patient refuses to co-operate with your assessment you can attempt to explain the reasons for co-operating but you cannot force an assessment on the patient. If force is needed it can only be done under the provisions of the Mental Health Act (see page 472).
* Once an assessment has been made, and the patient has been judged to be incapable, only use restraint (e.g. while giving an injection) where this is necessary to protect the person from harm and is a proportionate response to the risk of harm.
* Do not overrule an Advance Decision to refuse treatment made by a patient who, at that time, was capable of making the decision.
* If there are no relevant persons to consult (other than professional carers) and a decision is needed about major medical treatment, or where the person should live, consult an Independent Mental Capacity Advocate (IMCA). This is compulsory if the person without capacity will stay in hospital longer than 28 days, or in a care home for more than eight weeks.

SUMMARY

- Does the patient have a mental or physical condition that might impair capacity to make a decision?
- Is the patient incapable of making that decision at this particular time?
- Is there anything that can be done to improve the patient's ability to make that decision? This may include postponing the decision to another time.
- What decision would be in the patient's best interests? If several decisions are possible, which would be the least restrictive?

WITHHOLDING LIFE–SUSTAINING TREATMENT

An advance directive that the person wishes life-sustaining treatment to be withheld must be respected if the situation described in the directive has occurred. Otherwise a decision should be made on the patient's best interests. The assessment may legitimately lead to the conclusion that it would be in the best interests of the patient to withdraw or withhold life-sustaining treatment, even if this may result in the person's death. The person or team making the decision must not be influenced by the fact that they, or others, would prefer the patient to die.

A Lasting Power of Attorney does not give the attorney the right to decide whether life-sustaining treatment should be withheld unless the document explicitly states this.

If your decision that it is in the patient's best interest to withhold, or not to withhold treatment is disputed, apply to the Court of Protection for a decision.

THE LIMITS TO PROTECTION FROM LIABILITY

There are two main exceptions to this protection:

(a) if a patient, judged to be incapable, is confined (for instance in a nursing home) against his or her wishes. In such a situation an order from the Court of Protection is needed, unless detention under the Mental Health Act is more appropriate. Even attorneys and deputies appointed by the Court of Protection cannot give permission for an action that takes away a person's liberty.

(b) if restraint is used which is not justified to protect the patient or others from harm; or which is disproportionate to the risk.

TESTAMENTARY CAPACITY (THE CAPACITY TO MAKE A WILL)

Patients who are mentally disordered can make a valid will provided they understand:

(a) the nature and effect of making a will; and

(b) the extent of the property being disposed of; and

(c) the claims others may have on that property; and

(d) provided their decision is not the result of the mental disorder, for instance, the result of a delusion.

These are known as the Banks v. Goodfellow points, from a landmark judgement in 1870 (Jacoby and Steer 2007). The decision need not appear sensible to others, especially if it is consistent with the patient's previous personality.

If asked to assess a patient's testamentary capacity, proceed as follows:

* Ask the solicitor making the request to provide details of the patient's property and who might be considered to have a claim to it. Ask for details of any previous wills as well as of the new will.

* Ask the solicitor or patient for the patient's written permission for the assessment and for the subsequent disclosure of the result.

* Check that the patient is not suffering from a mental disorder, or if a mental disorder is found, that it is not influencing the patient's judgment as regards the will.

* Check that the patient understands the Banks v. Goodfellow points (above).

* Record the answers verbatim.

* Make a judgment about the patient's capacity.

* If in doubt ask for a second opinion, e.g. from an old age psychiatrist.

Note: A GP may be asked to witness a will without the solicitor or patient or family making it clear that they hope the doctor's signature will be taken to mean that the doctor thought the patient had the capacity to sign. Do not witness a will without having formally assessed that capacity.

POWERS OF ATTORNEY

Under a power of attorney, the chosen person (the attorney or donee) can make decisions that are as valid as one made by the person (the donor). This may be:

■ an *Ordinary Power Of Attorney*, which ceases to have effect if the patient (the donor) becomes mentally incapable; or

■ an *Enduring Power Of Attorney* (EPA), introduced in 1985, which continues if the donor is mentally incapable, provided it is registered with the Public Guardian. (In Scotland, an ordinary power of attorney signed after January 1991 remains valid even if the donor becomes mentally incapable.) These powers of attorney only cover financial matters, not, for instance, consent to treatment; or

■ a *Lasting Power of Attorney* (LPA) introduced in 2007. As well as property and affairs (including financial matters), LPAs can cover personal welfare (including healthcare and consent to medical treatment) for people who lack capacity to make such decisions for themselves. Attorneys must still make decisions in the person's best interests, as above.

For an EPA or LPA the donor must understand:

(a) that the attorney will be able to assume complete authority over the person's affairs;

(b) that the attorney will be able to do anything with the donor's property that the donor could have done;

(c) that the authority will continue if the donor becomes mentally incapable; and

(d) that the authority will be irrevocable while the donor remains incapable.

When consulting an attorney appointed under a LPA about a medical or care decision, check that the LPA covers personal care, that there are no restrictions on the decisions that the attorneys can take, and that it has been registered with the Public Guardian.

THE CAPACITY TO HANDLE FINANCIAL AFFAIRS: COURT OF PROTECTION

If a person, by reason of mental disorder, becomes incapable of managing his or her affairs, and has not previously signed an EPA or LPA, it may be necessary for someone, usually the nearest relative, to apply to the Court of Protection for the appointment of a deputy (usually a family member or friend but occasionally a professional) to do so. The medical practitioner should apply the two-stage test of capacity (see above) before completing the appropriate form.

The deputy will have power to manage the person's property and affairs and, if the Court so decrees, to make decisions regarding personal welfare. (If the patient's affairs are confined to the drawing of social security benefits, arrangements can be made with the Social Security authorities without involving the Court.)

If a patient becomes mentally disordered and has not made a will, the family may apply to the Court of Protection for a statutory will to be drawn up. The Court will attempt to draw up the will as the patient would have drawn it up had he or she been capable.

THE CAPACITY TO MAKE A GIFT

If the gift is substantial, the same degree of capacity is required as for making a will. However, if the gift is small relative to the patient's estate, case law has established that a lower degree of understanding is adequate.

THE CAPACITY TO CONSENT TO MARRY AND ENGAGE IN SEXUAL INTERCOURSE

Those with a mental disorder. In order to be able to consent to marry, a person with a mental disorder must be able to understand broadly what marriage entails. Similarly, those who are mentally disordered can consent to sexual intercourse if they understand what is proposed and its implications, e.g. pregnancy, and are able to exercise choice. This later condition requires that they are not under the undue influence of the other person and that they would be capable of saying no if they were not enjoying the experience.

Children. A special case exists when a doctor becomes aware that a young person under 16 is sexually active. If the patient is under the age of 13 there would need to be very special reasons why a doctor would not inform the parents, the child protection service and the police. When the child is aged 13–15 the doctor would similarly need to inform the relevant people if the activity was abusive or seriously harmful. In other circumstances the doctor would have to judge the case on its merits and would hope to be able to act with the young person's consent (General Medical Council 2007). Note that this advice may be in conflict with that of some local Child Protection Committees (Coombes 2005).

THE CAPACITY TO CONSENT TO MEDICAL TREATMENT

GUIDANCE

The BMA's views on the capacity to consent to and refuse medical treatment can be found on www.bma.org.uk (search on 'Consent Tool Kit').

This is required when a doctor examines, investigates or treats a patient. Often that consent is implicit. A patient who attends for a blood test may be understood to be giving implicit consent. Explicit consent may be verbal or written. In verbal consent the doctor should record that it has been given.

In more serious interventions the patient must be able to:

(a) understand what the treatment is and why it is proposed;

(b) understand the benefits, risks and alternatives;

(c) understand the consequences of not having the treatment;

(d) retain the information long enough to make a decision; and

(e) make a free choice; and

(f) understand that the patient may change his or her mind at any time.

The amount of information will vary according to the patient's ability to deal with it and the seriousness of the situation.

If competent, an adult can refuse a procedure whether the decision appears rational or irrational. However, if the decision appears to contradict the patient's own previously expressed attitudes it calls into question the patient's competence.

If an adult is unable to consent, because, for instance, of coma or mental incompetence, no-one else can do so, but treatment can be carried out if it is in the patient's best interests (see above). The opinions of the relatives are important in deciding on that best interest, but a consent form signed by a relative carries no legal force.

Age

Patients aged 16 and above can consent to treatment. Those under 16 can either consent to treatment themselves if they have 'sufficient discretion to be able to make a wise choice in their best interests', or their parents can consent for them. In England and Wales a child's consent to treatment cannot be overridden by the parents if the doctor judges that the child has the above discretion. The BMA advises that, to be judged capable, a child should have:

(a) the ability to understand that there is a choice and that choices have consequences;

(b) the willingness and ability to make a choice (including the option of choosing that someone else make treatment decisions);

(c) understanding of the nature and purpose of the proposed procedure;

(d) understanding of its risks and side-effects;

(e) understanding of the alternatives to the proposed procedure and the risks attached to them and the consequences of no treatment;

(f) freedom from pressure.

The level of capacity will need to be higher if the child or young person is making a decision about complex treatment than if the issue is a simple one.

If a child, or young person under 18 (England and Wales) or 16 (Scotland), refuses treatment, however, his or her decision can be overruled by the parents or by a court even if the patient is judged by the doctor to be competent. It is then for the doctor to weigh up the harm caused by violating the young person's wishes against the harm of not providing the treatment.

Do not hesitate to ask for a second opinion, e.g. from a doctor working in child protection, or for advice from your defence body, if there is conflict between a competent child and the child's parents.

Children and young people have the same right to confidentiality as adults. Obtain their permission to share information with their parents if the patient is seen alone. If the patient refuses permission to divulge information, only override that wish if:

(a) there is an overriding public interest in the disclosure; or

(b) you judge the child not to have the capacity to decide and you think it is in the child's best interests to disclose; or

(c) disclosure is required by law (General Medical Council, *0-18 years: Guidance for All Doctors*, September 2007).

If you judge that the child has capacity, the parents may not see the child's medical records without the child's consent.

The rights of a 'parent'

In England and Wales, for a child born after 1.12.2003, either biological parent can give consent provided both are registered on the birth certificate. Before that date both parents have that right only if married at the time of conception or after. Otherwise, only the mother has the right unless the father has formally acquired the right through a Parental Responsibility Agreement with the mother or a Parental Responsibility Order through the courts. Step-parents and registered civil partners can acquire parental responsibilities in the same way. Divorce makes no difference to a parent's rights.

Only one parent need give permission but in controversial circumstances (e.g. male circumcision for non-medical reasons) the consent of both would be wise.

If no parent is available and treatment is urgent, the doctor may proceed in the child's best interests.

Guardians or the Local Authority or a court may have parental rights.

ADVANCE DECISIONS (ADVANCE DIRECTIVES, STATEMENTS OR LIVING WILLS)

ADVANCE STATEMENTS

The BMA's views can be found on www.bma.org.uk (choose 'Ethics' then 'Publications' then 'Guidance').

Dyer C. Living wills will have to specify treatments that patient is refusing. BMJ 2004; 328: 1035.

Mental Capacity Act 2005: Code of Practice. Available: www.justice.gov.uk (choose 'Guidance' then 'Mental Capacity').

These are statements where a person makes a decision about medical treatment in case he or she becomes incapable of making that decision later. A patient may decline specific treatments. A patient cannot insist on specific treatment but can authorize one, should it be offered. It is legally binding if:

(a) it is in writing, is signed and witnessed and is clear what the patient means; and

(b) the patient was aged 18 or older when it was made; and

(c) it is applicable to the current situation; and

(d) the patient was competent when the directive was made; and

(e) it specifies the treatment which the patient is refusing (including artificial nutrition and hydration); and

(f) it states that the decision holds even at the risk of death; and

(g) the patient was informed about the treatment in question; and

(h) it was made without undue pressure from others.

It is good practice for the decision to have been witnessed by someone independent; for the issue to have been discussed with a health professional; and for the decision to be reviewed regularly. An incomplete advance decision is not useless; it can be accepted as an indication of the patient's wishes when considering his or her best interests. A verbal advance decision, recorded by someone else, also carries weight, but is not sufficient to allow the withholding of life-sustaining treatment.

A more flexible approach is for the patient to sign a LPA, specifying that the attorney has power to make a decision to withhold life-sustaining treatment. This allows the attorney to make a decision that takes into account modern treatments that were not available when the patient signed the advance decision.

The Act states that doctors should not withhold 'basic care' (e.g. symptom control) even in the face of a decision which specifies that the patient should receive no treatment.

Despite an advance decision, a doctor in the UK cannot do anything whose *prime* purpose is to hasten death.

If there is doubt about the validity of an advance decision, err on the side of preserving life. If there is doubt and time permits, obtain an order from the Court of Protection.

INFORMATION AND THE RELEVANT FORMS ARE AVAILABLE FROM

Dignity in Dying. 181 Oxford Street London W1D 2JT. Tel. 0870 777 7868, www.dignityindying.org.uk (choose 'Living Wills').

The Patients Association, www.patients-association. com (choose 'Help and Advice' then 'Advice Publications').

VICTIMS OF CRIME OR ACCIDENTS

IMMEDIATE MANAGEMENT

The doctor's role is to support, treat and ensure the safety of the patient, as well as to gather information for legal purposes.

* Ensure privacy.
* Offer a woman a female doctor or chaperone if she has been assaulted by a man.
* Check whether the patient intends to report the assault to the police. Respect the patient's decision, except in the case of child abuse, which must be reported. Explain that reporting is necessary if the victim wishes to claim Criminal Injury Compensation.
* Discuss whether the patient is safe to return home. If not, recommend a woman's refuge (via the duty Social Worker) or urgent homeless accommodation from the Council Housing Department.
* For legal purposes:
  (a) document the date, time and place of the event;
  (b) document any injuries in detail, both physical and psychological;
  (c) arrange for a photograph to be taken, unless the police have already done so.
* Tell the patient about Victim Support.
* At subsequent meetings look for evidence of post-traumatic stress disorder (see page 461).
* Sexual assaults: see below.

VICTIM SUPPORT

Local schemes and the witness service in the crown court may be found in the local directory. The UK Victim Support line is 0845 30 30 900. The website is www.victimsupport.com
   Support after Murder and Manslaughter (SAMM). Cranmer House, 39 Brixton Road, London SW9 6DZ, tel. 020 7735 3838, www.samm.org.uk

RAPE AND INDECENT ASSAULT

● The implications of the examination of an alleged victim of a sexual offence are so great that it is best for this to be done by a doctor trained and experienced in such work (Clinical Effectiveness Group (Association for Genitourinary Medicine and the Medical Society for the Study of Venereal Diseases) 2001). The police or the patient may, however, request a GP to perform the examination if there is no other option. The police will provide a kit for taking samples.

● The forensic examination may be useful up to 7 days after the assault. If it is performed it should be done *before* the medical examination.
● Even when the patient presents for medical advice and says that she does not wish to report the event to the police, record as many of the findings below as possible. She may change her mind.
● Laboratory evidence will only be accepted in court if there is a 'chain of evidence', i.e. at every hand-over each specimen is signed for, with the date and time.
● Strict attention to procedure is essential:
  (a) Obtain written consent from the woman concerned, or from the parents or guardian if under 16 years of age. Include the wording that this is 'a declaration of consent to medical examination for non-treatment purposes'.
  (b) Examine the patient where lighting and facilities are adequate.
  (c) Obtain:
    ■ a detailed history: this may determine how you look for forensic evidence;
    ■ the date of her last menstrual period;
    ■ how long ago she last had intercourse other than the alleged assault;
    ■ any drugs or alcohol taken.
  (d) Record everything.
  (e) Note the appearance and mental state of the patient.
  (f) The patient should undress on a large sheet of new brown paper, which can be folded and sent to the laboratory. The state of the underclothing should be noted, and whether any stains are visible. All clothing worn at the time of the alleged incident should be sent in a clean polythene or paper bag for analysis.
  (g) The whole body should be examined for injuries or stains. Scrape off stains if possible, or remove with a moistened swab if unable to remove dry. Label each one with details of which part of the body it came from.
  (h) Examine genitalia and:
    ■ remove stains as above;
    ■ comb the pubic hair and send any loose hairs;

- pluck a pubic hair from the patient and send that separately.

(i) Aspirate vaginal fluid before digital examination; also fluid from the anus if anal intercourse is alleged. Smear on to a microscope slide only if there will be a delay of more than 24 hours before it is examined. Spermatazoa survive in the vagina for up to 6 days and in the rectum for up to 3 days.

(j) Note specifically the state of the vulva, hymen, vagina, anus and mouth.

(k) Take swabs for sexually transmitted diseases (see below).

(l) Take fingernail scrapings.

(m) Take 10 ml clotted blood.

(n) Take saliva.

FULL STI SCREEN

- Culture for gonococcus and tests for *Chlamydia trachomatis* from any site of penetration.
- Vaginal slides for microscopy for yeasts, bacterial vaginosis, and *Trichomonas vaginalis*. Also culture for trichomonas.
- Blood for syphilis serology and save serum. Offer testing for hepatitis B, C and HIV.

Examination of an alleged assailant follows the same pattern. Informed consent is essential.

Once the examination is complete, discuss with the patient the need for:

(a) emergency contraception (see page 365);

(b) prophylactic antibiotics against chlamydia and the gonococcus, e.g. ciprofloxacin 500 mg stat and doxycycline 100 mg bd for 7 days; or ciprofloxacin 500 mg and azithromycin 1 g orally stat. Women who are pregnant or breast feeding should be offered amoxicillin 3 g stat plus probenecid 1 g stat and erythromycin 500 mg bd for 14 days (Clinical Effectiveness Group (Association for Genitourinary Medicine and the Medical Society for the Study of Venereal Diseases) 2001);

(c) follow-up for counselling – inform the patient of the service offered by the nearest Rape Crisis Centre, or the victim support scheme;

(d) a blood test 3 months later for syphilitic serology and, at 3 and 6 months, for HIV and hepatitis B and C antibodies;

(e) prophylaxis against hepatitis B and HIV (see pages 40 and 78). The risk of HIV transmission depends on the risk that the assailant is HIV positive and the nature of the assault. The risk of HIV transmission following rape of a woman in a high prevalence area has been estimated at 1 in 14000; the risk to a man raped by three homosexual men in London at 1 in 77 (Welch and Mason 2007). If the assailant is known to be HIV positive then the risk from vaginal intercourse is 1 in 1000 (but higher if there is trauma) and from receptive anal intercourse 1 in 33.

(f) a follow-up appointment 2 weeks later to repeat the examination for STIs, for any woman who declines antibiotic prophylaxis.

MALE VICTIMS OF SEXUAL ASSAULT

The procedure to be followed is as described for women, with obvious anatomical differences.

PATIENT ORGANIZATIONS

Look in the telephone directory for details of the local rape crisis centre or on www.rapecrisis.co.uk

Abused Empowered Survive Thrive, supporting adult survivors of childhood or adult sexual abuse; www.aest.org.uk

Independent Care after Incestuous Relationships and Rape, Helpline 01255 675351. PO Box 10215, Birmingham B42 2WZ

Survivors, 12A Evelyn Court, Grinstead Road, London SE8 5AD, Helpline 0845 1221201 for male rape victims, www.survivorsuk.org

HAVOCA (Help for Victims of Child Abuse); Ross Cottage, Northwick Road, Pilning, Bristol, BS35 4HB; www.havoca.org

Advice for professionals on how to collect evidence: www.careandevidence.org

DOMESTIC VIOLENCE

GUIDANCE

Heath I. *Domestic Violence: The General Practitioner's Role*. Royal College of General Practitioners. London, 1998. Available: www.rcgp.org.uk (search for 'Domestic Violence').

Shakespeare J, Davidson L. *Domestic Violence in Families and Children; Guidance for Health Care Professionals.* Royal College of General Practitioners. London, 2002. Available: www.rcgp.org.uk (search for 'domestic violence').

Domestic Violence: A Resource Manual for Health Care Professionals. Department of Health, 2000. Available: www.dh.gov.uk/assetRoot/04/06/53/79/04065379.pdf

- Domestic violence accounts for 25% of all violent crime in the UK. 45% of female homicide victims are killed by present or former male partners, though only 8% of male victims are killed by current or former female partners.
- One in four women and one in seven men have experienced domestic violence.
- 50% of those reporting violence live with children under the age of 16. In families where there is repeated assault on the woman, 45% of the children are aware of the violence.
- The association between domestic violence and child physical abuse is high (studies range from 30 to 66%). Children are frequently abused by the same perpetrator as the mother.
- Violence often starts or intensifies during pregnancy and is associated with death, severe morbidity, fetal death, miscarriage, depression, suicide, parasuicide and alcohol and drug abuse.
- On average a woman is assaulted by her partner 35 times before reporting it to the police.
- Domestic violence involves not only physical assault but also psychological and emotional abuse. Such abusive behaviour can include, for example:
  - (a) constant criticism and belittling comments;
  - (b) verbal abuse and threats (including threats to harm the children);
  - (c) isolation and control of contact with family and friends;
  - (d) restrictions on entry/exit from home;
  - (e) intimidation;
  - (f) controlling and coercive behaviour;
  - (g) denial of privacy;
  - (h) oppressive control of finances;
  - (i) destruction of personal property and valued possessions.

- Being the target for someone's violence is demeaning and demoralising and in attempting to survive it, women tend to lose their self-esteem and begin to accept the counter accusation that they are somehow to blame.
- Battered Women Syndrome (BWS) is a psychological condition that is characterized by psychological, emotional and behavioural deficits arising from chronic and persistent violence. The central features of BWS include 'learned helplessness', passivity and paralysis.
- Common features of post-traumatic stress disorder (PTSD) in domestic violence include: anxiety, fear, experiencing flashbacks or persistently re-experiencing the event, nightmares, sleeplessness, exaggerated startle responses, difficulty in concentrating, feelings of shame, despair and hopelessness.
- For a woman to extract herself from an abusive relationship there is a high price to pay, including: loss of the only intimate relationship she has, loneliness, disruption of the children's relationship with their father, and an economic price including possible homelessness.
- Fewer than 20% of cases are identified by the GP (Ramsay, Richardson, Carter *et al.* 2002). There is insufficient evidence to show whether screening or case-finding leads to better outcomes; but it can lead to high rates of detection (Wong, Wester, Mol *et al.* 2006).
- Doctors trained to enquire about domestic abuse detect most cases when patients present with multiple somatic symptoms or mental complaints; while doctors not so trained detect fewer cases, mainly as a result of disclosure by the patient or as a result of injury (Wong, Wester, Mol, *et al.* 2006).
- In England most women do not object to being asked about domestic violence. In a study in Cambridge general practice, a maternity unit and an accident and emergency unit, only 8% found such questioning unacceptable (Boyle and Jones 2006).
  - ∗ Consider domestic violence when the woman:
    - (a) admits past or present abuse;
    - (b) presents with unexplained bruises, whiplash injuries consistent with shaking, possible slap injuries, burns or multiple injuries;

(c) presents with injuries in areas hidden by clothing and not easily revealed because of apparent shyness, especially in Asian women;

(d) presents with injuries to the face, chest, breast and abdomen;

(e) has evidence of sexual abuse;

(f) has an injury that is not consistent with the explanation;

(g) presents some time after the injury;

(h) alleges an accident in a hesitant, embarrassed or evasive manner;

(i) has a history of repeated accidental injuries;

(j) presents with physical symptoms for which no explanation can be found (especially in women whose first language is not English);

(k) is accompanied by her partner who insists on staying close and answers for her;

(l) has injuries during pregnancy;

(m) has a history of miscarriage (miscarriage is 15 times more likely in women experiencing domestic violence);

(n) has a history of psychiatric illness, especially attempted suicide, alcohol or drug dependence;

* *Confidentiality.* Reassure the patient that anything she talks about is confidential (unless you are directed to disclose information by a court or if the public interest demands it). The concept of confidentiality may be unfamiliar to immigrant women.

* Ask directly but gently about violence. Possible questions are:

(a) I notice you have a number of bruises. Could you tell me how they happened? Did someone hit you?

(b) You seem frightened of your partner. Has he ever hurt you?

(c) Many patients tell me they have been hurt by someone close to them. Could this be happening to you?

(d) You mention your partner loses his temper with the children. Does he ever lose his temper with you? What happens when he loses his temper?

(e) Have you ever been in a relationship where you have been hit, punched, kicked or hurt in any way? Are you in such a relationship now?

(f) You mentioned your partner uses drugs/alcohol. How does he act when drinking or on drugs?

(g) Does your partner sometimes try to put you down or control your actions?

(h) Sometimes, when others are over-protective and as jealous as you describe, they react strongly and use physical force. Is this happening in your situation?

(i) Your partner seems very concerned and anxious. That can mean he feels guilty. Was he responsible for your injuries?

* Record clearly:

(a) Data from previous medical record which is suggestive of prior abuse.

(b) Time, date and place and witnesses to assault or accident.

(c) If patient states that abuse is the cause of injury, preface patient's explanation by writing: 'Patient states … '.

(d) Avoid subjective data that might be used against the patient (for example, 'It was my fault he hit me because I didn't have the kids in bed on time').

(e) If patient denies being assaulted, write: 'The patient's explanation of the injuries is inconsistent with physical findings' and/or 'The injuries are suggestive of battering'.

(f) Record size, pattern, age, description and location of all injuries. A record of 'Multiple contusions and lacerations' will not convey a clear picture to a judge or jury, but 'Contusions and lacerations of the throat' will back up allegations of attempted strangling. If possible, make a body map of injuries. Include signs of sexual abuse.

(g) Record non-bodily evidence of abuse, such as torn clothing.

* *Photographs.* Consider taking photographs or advising the patient to have photos taken of the visible injuries.

* *Let the patient tell you her story.* Gather as much information as possible. Try to include the following:

(a) The history of the abuse (include past and present physical, emotional and/or sexual abuse).

(b) Attempts by the patient to remedy her situation (for example, through police, courts, separation, refuges, and so on).

(c) Sources of emotional support.

(d) The current living situation. Is there some place, other than home, where she can go to recuperate if it is dangerous for her to return home?

(e) Present danger:
- Is the abuser verbally threatening her?
- Is the abuser frightening friends and relatives?
- Is the abuser threatening to use weapons?
- Is the abuser intoxicated?
- Does the abuser have a criminal record?
- Are the children in danger?

PROVIDE INFORMATION

(a) Explain to the patient that violence in the home is as illegal as violence on the street and that she is the victim of a crime and has legal rights.

(b) Explain the physical and emotional consequences of chronic battering.

(c) Provide written information about legal options and help offered by:
- Police domestic violence units;
- The National Helpline (see below);
- Local authority social services departments;
- Local authority housing departments;
- Department of Social Security.

(d) Offer help in making contact with other agencies.

DEVISE A SAFETY PLAN

A patient should not be pressurized into following any particular course of action. Only the patient can decide what is right for her in her particular situation. Her individual autonomy, self-esteem and self-determination should be encouraged and respected. Even if the patient decides to return to the violent situation, she is not likely to forget the information and care given and, in time, this may help her to break out of the cycle of abuse. However, beware of the danger of the needs of some

ethnic minority patients being ignored under the guise of 'respect' for different cultures.

(a) If she does not wish to return to the abuser, advise her on the services available from local agencies and offer help with contacting them.

(b) If she chooses to return to the abuser:
- give her the phone number of the local women's refuge or the local Women's Aid;
- advise her to keep some money and important financial and legal documents hidden in a safe place, in case of emergency;
- help her to plan an escape route in case of emergency.

(c) If children are likely to be at risk, seriously consider referral to social services, if possible with the patient's consent.

PATIENT INFORMATION AND SUPPORT

National helpline (tel. 0808 2000 247). This offers women and children access to emergency refuge accommodation, an information service, safety planning and translation facilities. www.womensaid.org.uk, www.refuge.org.uk

Male advice and enquiry line tel. 0808 801 0327, www.mensadviceline.org.uk

Samaritans tel. 08457 909090

OCCUPATIONAL DISEASE REPORTING

ADVICE

RIDDOR: Information for Doctors. London: Health and Safety Executive, 1995. Available from HSE Books, PO Box 1999, Sudbury, Suffolk CO10 2WA, tel. 01787 881165, www.hsebooks.com or download free from www.hse.gov.uk/pubns/hse32.pdf

Since 1.4.1996, doctors have not been obliged to notify occupational diseases. They are, however, required to inform the employers, in writing and with the patient's consent, if patients develop a reportable disease known to be linked with their occupation. The doctor need not decide whether the disease is, in each particular case, caused by the occupation. Employers are, in turn, obliged to notify the local office of the Health and Safety Executive (HSE). The self-employed are obliged to report the disease themselves. Reports should be made to the Incident Contact Centre, Caerphilly Business Park, Caerphilly CF83 3GG, tel. 0845 3009923, www.hse.gov.uk/riddor.

If the patients do not consent to the notification of employers, they might agree to the notification of their employer's occupational health service or to direct notification to the Employment Medical Advisory Service of the HSE. Addresses are contained in the RIDDOR booklet above.

Some examples of reportable diseases that are commonly not reported are:

(a) occupational asthma;

(b) irritant dermatitis;

(c) folliculitis, acne or skin cancer in workers exposed to mineral oil, tar, pitch or arsenic;

(d) vibration white finger in workers using vibrating or percussive machinery;

(e) tenosynovitis in workers doing movements of the hand or wrist;

(f) bursitis (e.g. 'housemaid's knee') in workers involved in kneeling;

(g) writer's cramp and all repetitive strain injuries;

(h) occupational deafness;

(i) hepatitis B in health workers.

References

Anderson, R., 2001. Deep-vein thrombosis in long-haul flights (letter). Lancet 358, 837.

Bandolier, 2003. DVTs and all that. Bandolier, 2003 (April), pp. 110–112.

Boyle, A., Jones, P.B., 2006. The acceptability of routine inquiry about domestic violence towards women: a survey in three healthcare settings. Br. J. Gen. Pract. 56, 258–261.

Clinical Effectiveness Group (Association for Genitourinary Medicine and the Medical Society for the Study of Venereal Diseases), 2001. National Guidelines on the Management of Adult Victims of Sexual Assault. http://www.bashh.org/guidelines.

Coombes, R., 2005. Guidance on reporting under age sex is confusing. BMJ 331, 918.

Department of Health, 1995. Food Handlers' Fitness to Work. HMSO, London.

Ford, F., 1998. Sickness Certification: Time to scrap Med 3? Br. J. Gen. Pract. 48, 1353.

Ford, F., Ford, J., Dowrick, C., 2000. Welfare to work: the role of general practice. Discussion Paper. Br. J. Gen. Pract. 50, 497–500.

General Medical Council, 2000. Confidentiality: Protecting and Providing Information. September 2000; Appendix 2. GMC, London. http://www.gmc-uk.org.

General Medical Council, 2007. 0-18 years: Guidance for All Doctors. September.

General Practitioners' Committee, 2004. Medical certificates and reports: the new GMS and PMS contracts: guidance for GPs. BMA, July.

Herxheimer, A., Petrie, K.J., 2001. Melatonin for the prevention and treatment of jet-lag (Cochrane Review). In: The Cochrane Library, Issue 4. Update Software, Oxford.

Jacoby, R., Steer, P., 2007. How to assess capacity to make a will. BMJ 335, 155–157.

Lewis, G., Sloggett, A., 1998. Suicide, deprivation and unemployment: record linkage study. BMJ 317, 1283–1286.

Possick, S.E., le Barry, M., 2004. Evaluation and management of the cardiovascular patient embarking on air travel. Ann. Intern. Med. 141, 148–154.

Ramsay, J., Richardson, J., Carter, Y.H., et al., 2002. Should health professionals screen women for domestic violence? Systematic review. BMJ 325, 314.

Rouse, E., 1995. DVLA Senior medical adviser's reply. BMJ 311, 1163.

Scurr, J.H., Machin, S.L., Bailey-King, S., et al., 2001. Frequency and prevention of symptomless deep-vein thrombosis in long-haul flights: a randomised trial. Lancet 357, 1485–1489.

Taylor, D.M., O'Toole, K.S., Ryan, C.M., 2002. Experienced, recreational scuba divers in Australia continue to dive despite medical contraindications. Wilderness Environ. Med. 13, 187–193.

Welch, J., Mason, F., 2007. Rape and sexual assault. BMJ 334, 1154–1158.

Wong, S.L.F., Wester, F., Mol, S.S.L., et al., 2006. Increased awareness of intimate partner abuse after training: a randomised controlled trial. Br. J. Gen. Pract. 56, 249–257.

Chapter 2

Infectious diseases: immunization, travel and related issues

CHAPTER CONTENTS

© 2011 Elsevier Ltd.
DOI: 10.1016/B978-0-7020-3053-6.00002-7

GUIDANCE

Immunisation Against Infectious Disease 2006 (known as the 'Green Book'), published by the DoH, the Scottish Home and Health Department and the Welsh Office. Available from The Stationery Office, PO Box 29, Norwich NR3 1GN and authorized bookshops and from www.tsoshop.co.uk. The full text plus updates is also available on www.dh.gov.uk/greenbook

More information, designed for patients rather than doctors, is available on www.immunisation.nhs.uk

Department of Health. *Health Information for Overseas Travel*, 2nd edition. London: The Stationery Office, 2001; known as the 'UK Yellow Book'. The full text is available on www.dh.gov.uk (search on 'Overseas Travel'). The Department warns that some of the Yellow Book is out of date and is being revised. It should not to be confused with the US Yellow Book, *CDC Health Information for International Travel 2008*, which is available on wwwn.cdc.gov/travel/contentYellowBook.aspx

A ROUTINE SCHEDULE OF IMMUNIZATION

See Appendix 1.

INCUBATION AND INFECTIVITY PERIODS OF COMMON DISEASES

See Appendix 2.

NOTIFICATION OF INFECTIOUS DISEASES

See Appendix 4.

THE ORGANIZATION OF AN IMMUNIZATION PROGRAMME IN PRIMARY CARE

Ensure that:

(a) an effective call and recall system is in place;

(b) there is an effective system for the ordering and proper care of vaccines;

(c) there are dedicated immunization clinics at times that are feasible for the patients; and

(d) written material about the vaccines is available; and that parents and patients have time to study them and discuss any concerns, before giving consent.

PROCEDURE WHEN GIVING AN IMMUNIZATION

* Establish that the immunization is needed.
* Check that the patient is fit and that there are no contraindications. Minor illness does not mean that the immunization need be postponed. More severe illness may, but only because of the difficulty of distinguishing subsequent symptoms of the illness from an adverse effect of the immunization.
* Check that consent has been obtained. In childhood immunizations this usually consists of:

(a) written consent to the programme in general; and

(b) verbal consent to the specific immunization at the time. Bringing a child to an immunization clinic has been viewed as giving consent, but parents may not realize which vaccines are going to be given. In order to be considered 'informed', parents must have been given information about the benefits and possible adverse effects of the vaccine and had a chance to discuss them.

* Explain how to treat the more likely adverse effects: e.g. paracetamol or ibuprofen for pain or fever.
* Explain that information about those who have been immunized will be kept and used to monitor the safety and efficacy of the vaccination programme. This is a requirement of current Data Protection guidance.
* Check that the vaccines are not out of date and that the cold chain has not been interrupted. This means that you are satisfied that the vaccines have not, at any stage, frozen or warmed to $> 8°C$.
* Check that facilities for resuscitation are available. This includes a resuscitation pack containing adrenaline that is in-date.
* Record the date, vaccine and batch number in each patient's medical record.
* Do not clean the limb unless it is obviously dirty.
* Use a long (25 mm, blue hub) needle (either 23 gauge or 25 gauge). This reduces the incidence of adverse reactions, presumably because it is more likely to reach muscle than the short (16 mm, orange hub) needle (Diggle, Deeks and Pollard 2006).
* If more than one injection is to be given, give them into different limbs. If the same limb must be used, give injections at least 2.5 cm apart. Record the site of each vaccine given.
* Give vaccines intramuscularly unless the patient has a bleeding disorder, when deep s.c. injection should be used. Exceptions to this are BCG, Japanese encephalitis, varicella, yellow fever and cholera.
* Use the deltoid or the antero-lateral thigh. Using the buttock risks inadvertent injection into fat which may reduce the effect of the immunization.
* Consider how to reduce the trauma of the event for the child. Infants who were given 25% sucrose solution to drink 2 minutes before the injection and who continue to suck on the bottle, or on a pacifier, while being held by their parents, while the injection was given, cried significantly less (Reis, Roth, Syphan, et al. 2003).
* Do not insist that the patient wait in the clinic for 20 minutes after the immunization. There is no evidence in favour of this time-honoured custom. An exception to this might be the patient with a history of syncope after injections.

WHO IS ENTITLED TO GIVE CONSENT? (DEPARTMENT OF HEALTH 2006)

The following applies in England and Wales. Minor differences exist in the other three countries of the UK.

(a) Anyone who is mentally capable and aged 16 and over.
(b) Any child under 16 who is judged by the person administering the immunization to be competent to make such a decision. Such a child who gives consent cannot be over-ruled by the parents; and the parents would have difficulty in over-ruling such a child who refuses consent: only a court has the power to do so.
(c) Those with parental responsibility for a child who is not competent to give consent. This means:

  ■ the mother, or
  ■ the father if married to the mother at the time of conception or birth of the child or subsequently, or if, after 1.12.2003, his name appears on the child's birth certificate as the father, or if he has signed a Parental Responsibility Agreement (PRA) with the mother. A step-parent only has capacity if there is a PRA or a court has granted a Parental Responsibility Order.

The responsible parent need not be present at the time of the immunization. That role, and the consent that goes with it, can be deputized, e.g. to a grandparent or childminder. Similarly, in older children, if the parents have been notified that an immunization will be given at school on a certain day and the child attends without the parents having notified an objection, the school may assume that consent is being given.

If two responsible parents disagree, a court decision is needed before immunization can take place.

Consent need not be in writing, but the clinician should record that it has been given.

HOW TO CHECK THAT THE COLD CHAIN HAS BEEN MAINTAINED AND THAT VACCINES ARE LIKELY TO BE VIABLE

* Check that the vaccine is in its original packaging, so that batch number and expiry date can be checked.
* Check that the vaccine is not out of date.

* Check that the vaccines have been kept in a dedicated refrigerator with a max/min thermometer whose readings have been recorded and have not gone below 2°C or above 8°C.
* If transported in a cool box to the clinic, check that the box also has a max/min thermometer which shows that the correct range has been adhered to. Check that vaccine has not frozen because it was packed too close to the ice.
* Dispose of multidose vials at the end of the clinic.

CONTRAINDICATIONS

It is important to be clear about the genuine contraindications to immunization (see under individual vaccines) and not to be deflected from immunizing children, for instance, because of:

(a) eczema;

(b) a family history of allergy;

(c) a personal history of allergy unrelated to the vaccine in question;

(d) a personal history of epilepsy or febrile convulsions;

(e) a minor infection, without fever or systemic upset; or

(f) a non-allergic reaction to a previous immunization.

Serious concomitant infection may be grounds for postponing immunization but only because of the difficulty of distinguishing adverse effects of the vaccination from symptoms due to the infection.

ADVERSE REACTIONS

Previous editions of the Green Book listed severe local or systemic reactions as relative contraindications to further immunization with that vaccine. The 2006 edition reverses this advice, pointing out that these reactions are not allergic and may not recur with subsequent doses.

Anaphylaxis is usually the only absolute contraindication. Two situations in which immunization should be deferred until the child is stable are:

1. where encephalopathy or encephalitis occurred within 7 days of the previous immunization, no cause was found, and the child had not recovered after 7 days; or

2. where seizures and fever occurred within 72 hours of the previous immunization, no cause was found, and the child had not recovered after 24 hours.

This tightening of the grounds on which immunization might be refused or deferred comes from the realization that the danger of infection in an unimmunized child puts him or her at greater risk than repeating the immunization. Except in the case of anaphylaxis, repetition of most other apparent adverse effects seems to occur no more than would be expected by chance.

VACCINE DAMAGE PAYMENTS

Vaccine damage payments are for those suffering 60% or more disablement as a result of immunization with one of the recommended childhood vaccines administered in the UK under the age of 18. Payment can also be made for damage due to polio, rubella and meningococcal C vaccines given after the age of 18, and for damage due to vaccines given as part of the management of an outbreak of infectious disease in the UK.

Claim forms are available from the Vaccine Damage Payments Unit, Palatine House, Lancaster Road, Preston PR1 1HB, tel. 01772 899944, or downloaded from the government website, www. direct.gov.uk (search on 'Vaccine Damage Payments').

LIVE VACCINES

These are:

(a) BCG;

(b) measles;

(c) mumps;

(d) oral typhoid;

(e) oral polio;

(f) rubella;

(g) varicella;

(h) yellow fever.

They should not normally be given:

(a) *to pregnant women* (this is a theoretical risk only, and may be outweighed by the risk of infection);

(b) *to the immunocompromised*. This includes the following:

■ patients who have received high dose systemic steroids in the last 3 months. This means children who have received 2 mg/kg/ day for at least 1 week or 1 mg/kg/day for at least 1 month, or adults who have received the equivalent of 40 mg prednisolone per day for > 1 week or 20 mg/day for at least 1 month. Lower doses may suppress immunity, especially if combined with cytotoxic drugs. Discuss each case with the specialist concerned;

- patients on biological therapies e.g. infliximab;
- patients with malignancy of the reticuloendothelial system;
- patients who are immunosuppressed due to radiotherapy or chemotherapy in the last 6 months, or are in some other way immunodeficient.

(c) *within 3 weeks of each other*. If they must be given within 3 weeks, they should be given on the same day. This is, however, only based on the observation that smallpox immunization may be less effective if given within 3 weeks of another live vaccine. If it is unavoidable, immunizations should be given within three weeks of each other rather than omitted;

(d) *as MMR with immunoglobulin. Normal human immunoglobulin (HNIG)* should be given at least 3 weeks before MMR or at least 3 months after. Contrary to previous advice this does not apply to other live vaccines (Department of Health 2001) because HNIG in the UK is unlikely to contain immunoglobulin to these organisms.

SPECIAL CASES

(A) THE PATIENT WHOSE IMMUNIZATION STATUS IS UNCERTAIN OR INCOMPLETE (HEALTH PROTECTION AGENCY 2004)

* If the patient is uncertain, treat as though unimmunized.
* If the patient is certain but any immunization is incomplete, restart where the course left off.
* If a course was begun with a vaccine that is not now available, continue the course with the new vaccine. For instance: partially vaccinated with OPV, complete the course with IPV; partially vaccinated with wP, complete the course with aP.
* There are a few situations where a patient is too old to need the full course. If the patient has not been immunized with Hib and is aged 1–10, give a single dose. Omit if over 10 years old.

If the patient has not been immunized with MenC and is aged 4 months to 1 year, give only two doses. If aged 1–25 years old give a single dose. Omit if aged 25 or over. However, two doses of MMR, at least 3 months apart, should be given to the unimmunized, regardless of age, as should full courses (five doses) of Td/IPV.

(B) HIV-POSITIVE PATIENTS

Patients carrying HIV may receive live vaccines, except BCG, oral typhoid and yellow fever. Furthermore, they should receive immunization against varicella, unless already immune, and against influenza and pneumococcus.

However, if severely immunosuppressed (CD4 count < 200/µl in an adult or older child, < 500/µl in a child under 6 years old), avoid MMR and varicella.

The Immunisation Guidelines for HIV-infected Adults (2006) published by the British HIV Association are available on www.bhiva.org (choose 'Guidelines').

(C) OTHER IMMUNOSUPPRESSED PATIENTS

* Ensure that the full course of routine immunization has been given. If further immunization is needed, discuss timing with the physician in charge. Time their administration when immunosuppression is least, in order to:
  (a) maximize the chance that immunity will develop;
  (b) in the case of live vaccines, reduce the risk of fulminating infection.
* In addition, give influenza and pneumococcal vaccination and warn the patient to avoid contact with chickenpox and exposed shingles. If exposure does occur, consider urgent immunoglobulin (see page 38).

(D) CLOSE CONTACTS OF IMMUNOSUPPRESSED PATIENTS

* Check that the full course of routine immunizations has been given. Make good any deficiencies.
* Immunize against varicella (unless already immune) and influenza, to reduce the risk of catching the disease and passing it to the patient.

(E) PATIENTS WITHOUT AN ACTIVE SPLEEN

* Give Hib, influenza, MenC and pneumococcal vaccine.
* Give oral phenoxymethylpenicillin prophylaxis against streptococcal and neisserial infection.

The lifetime risk of overwhelming infection post-splenectomy seems to be 5%. Most of these are preventable (Newland, Provan and Myint 2005).

(F) PATIENTS WITH A COCHLEAR IMPLANT

* Give pneumococcal vaccine.

(G) PATIENTS ON HAEMODIALYSIS

* Give hepatitis B vaccine at double the normal dose for four doses.

(H) PATIENTS WITH HAEMOPHILIA

* Give hepatitis A and B vaccines.

(I) PATIENTS WITH CHRONIC MEDICAL CONDITIONS: DIABETES, OR HEART, LUNG, LIVER OR RENAL DISEASE

* Give influenza and pneumococcal vaccines.

(J) CLINICAL STAFF

* Check that they have documented evidence of two MMR doses or of antibodies to measles and rubella.
* Give BCG if Mantoux-negative and in close contact with patients with tuberculosis.
* Give hepatitis B vaccine if working with blood or body fluids contaminated with blood, or at risk of sharps injuries, or of being bitten by a patient.

(K) NON-CLINICAL STAFF WHO ARE IN CONTACT WITH PATIENTS

* Check that they are immunized with MMR, as for clinical staff.
* If no clear history of chickenpox or shingles, check for varicella antibodies and immunize if negative.
* Give hepatitis B vaccine if they may come into contact with contaminated sharps.

SPECIFIC INFECTIOUS DISEASES AND IMMUNIZATIONS

DIPHTHERIA IMMUNIZATION

INDICATIONS

(a) Infants, preschool children and school leavers (see Table 2.1).
(b) Travellers to areas where diphtheria is endemic or epidemic. Ordinary travellers need to be fully immunized according to the schedule in Table 2.1. Those who will be in close contact with local people need an additional booster.
(c) Healthcare and laboratory workers exposed to diphtheria.
(d) Contacts of a diphtheria case. Previously immunized contacts need a booster dose. Non-immune contacts need full immunization. Both groups need prophylactic penicillin or erythromycin.

Note: In patients likely to be exposed to the risk of diphtheria over a length of time, e.g. healthcare workers, check antibody levels at least 3 months after their most recent immunization and give 10-yearly boosters of low-dose vaccine. It will have to be given combined with tetanus and polio even if these are not needed, since diphtheria vaccine does not come alone.

Table 2.1	Routine schedule of immunizations
AGE	**IMMUNIZATION**
2 months	DTaP/ IPV/ Hib and PCV
3 months	DTaP/ IPV/ Hib and Men C
4 months	DTaP/ IPV/ Hib and Men C and PCV
12 months	Hib/MenC
13–15 months	MMR and PCV
3 years 4 months–5 years (preschool)	DTaP/ IPV, or dTaP/ IPV, and MMR
13–18 years	Td/ IPV plus MMR (two doses) and Men C (one dose) if not already given
18–24 years	Men C (one dose) if not already given
65 onwards	Flu annually and PCV once
Girls aged 12–13	Cervarix

aP = acellular pertussis; D = diphtheria; d = low dose diphtheria; flu = influenza; Hib = *H. influenzae* b; IPV = inactivated polio vaccine; Men C = meningococcal C; MMR = mumps, measles and rubella; PCV = pneumococcal vaccine; T = tetanus.

CONTRAINDICATIONS

(a) Confirmed anaphylactic reaction to a previous dose or to neomycin, streptomycin or polymyxin B.

(b) Fever and a seizure within 72 hours of the immunization with incomplete recovery at 24 hours and no cause found: defer until stable.

(c) Encephalitis or encephalopathy within 7 days of the previous immunization with incomplete recovery at 7 days and no cause found: defer until stable.

(d) Any other unstable neurological condition.

Note that a severe local reaction or a severe systemic reaction to a previous dose without anaphylaxis (e.g. fever, convulsions, screaming, or a hypotonic–hyporesponsive episode) is not a contraindication.

PRACTICALITIES

∗ Use low-dose vaccine in adults and children over 10 years old. Full strength vaccine in those over 10 years old is more likely to lead to severe reactions.

∗ Isolated diphtheria vaccine is not available. Give in combination with other vaccines even if these other vaccines are not indicated; they may be redundant but they will not be harmful.

(a) *Infants:* give as part of routine childhood immunization.

(b) *Infants, children and adults in whom the primary course has been interrupted:* resume the course, giving the remaining doses at monthly intervals. Children over 10 and adults should receive Td/IPV.

(c) *Children and adults who have not received their booster doses:* give the first dose 3 years after the completion of the primary course, but reduce this interval to one year if necessary to get a child back on schedule. Give the second dose 10 years after the first dose but reduce this to 5 years if necessary to get the patient back on schedule.

(d) *Children who have been given their first booster dose at the age of 18 months:* ignore this dose and give two more boosters as per Table 2.1.

HAEMOPHILUS INFLUENZAE TYPE B (Hib)

INDICATIONS

(a) As per national schedule (at 2, 3, 4 and 12 months), see Table 2.1. A child who misses these doses should be immunized up to the age of 10. If diphtheria, tetanus and polio have been given, give a single dose of Hib/MenC vaccine.

(b) *Household contacts* of invasive Hib disease if aged under 10 and not already immunized.

(c) *Non-household contacts* aged under 10 at a creche, nursery or playgroup if not already immunized.

(d) *A patient with invasive Hib disease*, regardless of age, unless subsequent serology shows that immunity has been acquired.

(e) *High-risk patients:* children and adults with a non-functioning spleen, or otherwise immunocompromised, should receive a single booster of Hib/MenC provided they have been fully immunized against Hib. If not, the primary course should be completed if under 10 or, if aged 10 or over, two doses of Hib/MenC should be given 2 months apart.

CONTRAINDICATIONS

(a) Acute illness.

(b) Confirmed anaphylactic reaction to a previous dose or to neomycin, streptomycin or polymyxin B.

A deteriorating neurological condition is grounds for deferring immunization but a severe reaction to a previous dose without anaphylaxis (e.g. fever, convulsions, screaming, or a hypotonic–hyporesponsive episode) is not a contraindication.

CHEMOPROPHYLAXIS

Rifampicin is indicated:

(a) in households where there is a case of invasive Hib infection and another member of the household is at risk. At-risk groups are: children under 4, the immunocompromised and those without a functioning spleen. In such cases all members of the household need chemoprophylaxis to protect those at risk;

(b) in schools, nurseries etc, where two or more cases have occurred in 120 days. Although the risks are small and the evidence of benefit slight, rifampicin should be offered to teachers and children in contact with the case.

Note: Rifampicin is contraindicated in children under 3 months of age, pregnant or breast feeding women and people with severely impaired hepatic function. Dose: 20 mg/kg/day (maximum 600 mg daily) once daily for 4 days.

PRACTICALITIES

(a) *Infants:* give as part of routine childhood immunization.

(b) *Infants and children under 10 in whom the primary course has been interrupted:* resume the course, giving the remaining doses at monthly intervals. Children over 10 and adults do not need Hib. Over the age of 1 a single primary dose of Hib gives satisfactory immunity but children who have missed Hib have probably missed DTaP/IPV as well and so will need to have sufficient doses to complete the primary course of those vaccines. However, single Hib vaccine exists for those under the age of 10 who have completed the other immunizations.

(c) *Children and adults with asplenia:* if aged < 10, give the primary immunization schedule. If already immunized, give a single booster of Hib after the age of 1. Give unimmunized older children and adults a single dose of Hib.

HEPATITIS A: ACTIVE IMMUNIZATION

INDICATIONS

Immunization is recommended for:

(a) laboratory staff working with the virus;

(b) haemophiliacs and any others treated with coagulation factors (give the injection s.c.);

(c) those with chronic liver disease, including hepatitis B or C, because of the severity of hepatitis A infection in an already compromised liver;

(d) travellers to areas of poor sanitation, especially if travelling to areas of high or medium risk repeatedly or for more than 3 months;

(e) individuals who are at risk because of their sexual behaviour including men who have sex with men;

(f) injecting drug users.

Immunization should be considered for:

(a) close contacts of those with hepatitis A. Take advice from the Consultant in Communicable Disease Control or, in Scotland, from the Consultant in Public Health Medicine (CPHM);

(b) outbreaks in schools, nurseries and closed communities. Take advice as in (a);

(c) residents of institutions for those with learning difficulties;

(d) workers at risk, e.g. sewage workers, laboratory workers exposed to hepatitis A, and those working in institutions for those with severe learning disabilities.

CONTRAINDICATIONS

(a) Severe febrile illness.

(b) Anaphylactic reaction to the vaccine or, in the case of Epaxal only, to egg.

PRACTICALITIES

Give one dose of vaccine intramuscularly into the deltoid. This gives immunity for 3 years. A second dose 6–12 months later gives immunity for 10–20 years. A further dose may be given at 20 years if the risk continues.

HEPATITIS A: PASSIVE IMMUNIZATION

INDICATIONS

Human normal immunoglobulin (HNIG) may be given to patients in any of the categories for whom active immunization is recommended, but in the UK supplies are now scarce. Its main use is in the protection of contacts when jaundice in the index case appeared more than 1 week before, and so the slower onset of immunity following active immunization may mean it fails to offer protection. Even this indication is not strong. A randomized controlled trial from Kazakhstan found that, when immunization of contacts was given at an average of 10 days post exposure, the benefit from immunoglobulin over active vaccination was slight (3.3% vs 4.4% developed hepatitis) and not statistically significant (Victor, Monto, Surdina, *et al.* 2007). The benefit from passive immunization lasts for about 4 months.

CONTRAINDICATIONS

If possible, live viruses should be given at least 3 weeks before or at least 3 months after. This does not apply to yellow fever vaccine.

HEPATITIS B

* By global standards the prevalence of hepatitis B in the UK is very low, at 0.05% for some rural areas rising to 1% in some inner city areas with high immigrant populations.
* Because of the low prevalence the emphasis in the UK is to test and immunize those at risk rather than the whole population.
* Hepatitis B may present as acute hepatitis or the initial episode may be asymptomatic. The diagnosis may, therefore, be first made in the patient who presents with jaundice or abnormal LFTs, similar to the diagnosis of hepatitis C (see page 41).

THE TESTS ARE COMPLICATED BY THE DIFFERENT IMPLICATIONS OF THE DIFFERENT ANTIGENS AND ANTIBODIES

Briefly:

(a) *The presence of viral antigen* (HBsAg, HBeAg) suggests active viral replication. HBsAg appears as early as 14 days after the onset of infection and is the most reliable marker of hepatitis B infection. HBeAg appears later and disappears earlier. If present it suggests that the patient is highly infectious.

(b) *The presence of antibody* (anti-HBsAg, anti-HBe, anti-HBc) suggests recovery from infection or represents successful immunization. The finding of antibody in the absence of antigen means that the patient is not a carrier and is not infectious. The finding of antibody in the presence of antigen suggests that the patient has acute or continuing infection.

ACTIVE IMMUNIZATION

Indications

(a) Occupational exposure
 ■ All health personnel in contact with blood products or with possibly HBsAg-positive patients. Most at risk are those working in mental institutions, renal units, liver units, and those working in high-risk areas abroad.
 ■ Others at risk by virtue of occupation: staff of prisons and of institutions for those with learning difficulties, dental workers, morticians and embalmers, and prostitutes. The risk for police and ambulance crews is not increased, but individuals within those services may be considered to be at increased risk. Foster parents who accept children in an emergency should be offered immunization especially where those children may be immigrants from areas of high prevalence (see below).

(b) Lifestyle exposure
 ■ Those with multiple partners, especially male homosexuals (in 1990, 50% of male homosexuals attending a London STD clinic were positive).
 ■ Injecting drug users (in the UK, 50% are positive), or those likely to progress to injecting.
 ■ Sexual partners and other close family contacts, themselves negative, of patients who are HBsAg positive or whose risk of contracting hepatitis B is high (e.g. injecting drug users).
 ■ Prisoners.

(c) *Babies* born to mothers who are chronic carriers of hepatitis B virus or who acquire it during pregnancy. The UK National Screening Programme recommends that all pregnant women be offered antenatal screening for hepatitis B (NHS Executive 1998). If screening is omitted during pregnancy it should be offered at the time of delivery and a result obtained within 24 hours.

(d) *Travellers* to areas of high prevalence for long periods who might therefore require medical or dental treatment there or expose themselves to the risk of sexual transmission.

(e) *Immigrants*. Members of families who have immigrated from high-risk areas. These are South and Central America, sub-Saharan Africa and Asia, with South East Asia (especially Vietnam) having the highest incidence (50%). Families adopting or fostering a child from a high-risk area.

(f) Patients at risk. Patients undergoing high-risk treatment, e.g. repeated transfusions, haemodialysis; patients entering institutions for those with learning difficulties (50% of Down's syndrome inpatients, for instance, may be positive). Home carers of dialysis patients are also at risk. Patients with severe liver disease should be immunized, because the consequences of infection would be greater in an already damaged liver. So too should those positive for hepatitis C. The fact that they have acquired hepatitis C suggests that they have risk factors for the acquisition of hepatitis B as well.

Note: Those not yet exposed to the risk of hepatitis B should be immunized without prior screening for hepatitis B antibodies. As immunity takes 6 months to develop, immunization should be started well before exposure.

Those with a substantial chance of already being positive should be screened before immunization to avoid an unnecessary course of injections.

CONTRAINDICATION

Previous anaphylactic reaction to the vaccine.

PRACTICALITIES

* Give three injections at 0, 1 and 6 months. In cases of urgency, give the third injection at 2 months with a booster at 12 months. In even more urgent cases give it at 0, 7 and 21 days with a booster at 1 year.
* Give a booster with the preschool immunizations to children born to hepatitis B-infected mothers.
* Give 1 ml (0.5 ml in children) into the deltoid or antero-lateral thigh (injection into the buttock is less effective).
* Test for antibodies 1–4 months later. For those whose risk is occupational this is a requirement of the COSHH regulations. 10% will still be negative, mainly those over 40 years old.
* Give further courses as follows:
  (a) Non-responders (< 10 mIU)/ml) need a repeat course of vaccine. Test also for markers of current or past infection.
  (b) Poor responders (10–100 mIU/ml) need a single booster. Test also for markers of current or past infection.
  (c) The 'Green Book' recommends a single booster 5 years later in those who remain at risk or if exposure to the virus occurs.

* Warn those with levels of less than 100 mIU/ml and no markers of current or past infection that they would need hepatitis B immunoglobulin if exposed to risk.

HEPATITIS B: PASSIVE IMMUNIZATION

INDICATIONS

(a) Those who are accidentally inoculated or who contaminate eye, mouth or fresh wounds with infected blood (see page 78). All these patients will require active immunization as well. The episode should be managed in consultation with the local Public Health Laboratory or Health Protection Unit (see 'Needlestick injuries' page 77).
(b) Babies born to mothers who are HBeAg-positive, or HBsAg-positive without e markers (or where e marker status is unknown), or who had acute hepatitis B during pregnancy (as well as active immunization, see above).
(c) Sexual contacts of patients with acute hepatitis B and of carriers who are highly infectious (i.e. HBsAg and HBeAg-positive but anti-HBe-negative).

CONTRAINDICATIONS

Immunization with live virus should be avoided in the 3 weeks before and the 3 months after administration of immunoglobulin. This does not apply to yellow fever, and possibly not to a booster of oral polio vaccine.

PRACTICALITIES

* Give hepatitis B immunoglobulin (HBIG) as soon as possible after exposure as well as active immunization. If a patient declines active immunization, give a second dose of immunoglobulin 4 weeks later. In someone previously immunized, give a booster dose of vaccine unless they are known to have antibody levels above 100 mIU/ml.
* *Newborn babies* (see (b) above). Give 200 IU of hepatitis B immunoglobulin within 1 hour of birth, or at the latest within 48 hours. Start active immunization at the same time (in a contralateral site).

* *Sexual contacts.* Test the partner for hepatitis B antibodies at the time of giving HBIG. If negative, give a rapid course of active immunization.
* *A person who is accidentally inoculated.* Give 500 IU of HBIG within 48 hours of the injury, although passive immunization up to 7 days later may still be worthwhile. Consider the need for prophylaxis against HIV (see page 75).

HEPATITIS C

GUIDELINES

Royal College of General Practitioners. *Guidance for the Prevention, Testing, Treatment and Management of Hepatitis C in Primary Care.* 2007. Available: www.smmgp.org.uk/html/guidance.php
    Department of Health. *Hepatitis C – Essential Information for Professionals and Guidance on Testing* 2004. Available: www.dh.gov.uk (search on 'Hepatitis C')

* The prevalence of hepatitis C infection in the UK is between 0.4% and 1%. A full-time GP will have between 8 and 18 infected patients of whom nearly 90% will be current or ex-drug injectors.
* 80% of infected patients are undiagnosed and only 1–2% are likely to be receiving the appropriate treatment recommended by NICE. Untreated, one in five progress to advanced fibrosis and cirrhosis over 20–30 years.
* The Department of Health National Action Plan and the RCGP guidelines (above) call for a major improvement in the management of this condition in primary care. Antiviral treatment offers hope of cure for 50–80%, approaching 100% if given in the acute phase.

SCREENING

* Offer screening for hepatitis C virus (HCV) to the following patients (CMO 2004a):
  (a) injecting drug users (whether currently injecting or not);
  (b) non-injecting users of drugs such as cocaine, especially if they have shared pipes or straws;
  (c) those who are HIV- or hepatitis B-positive;
  (d) immigrants from countries with high prevalence of HCV;
  (e) needlestick victims (the risk of HCV transmission when the index case is positive seems to be 2%);
  (f) sexual partners of positive patients;
  (g) children of positive mothers;
  (h) patients transfused in the UK before September 1991 or given blood products before 1986;
  (i) recipients of organ or tissue transplants in the UK before 1992;
  (j) those on haemodialysis for renal failure;
  (k) those who have been pierced or tattooed in places without proper infection control procedures;
  (l) those who have received medical or dental treatment in countries where hepatitis C infection is common and infection control poor;
  (m) any patient with unexplained abnormal liver function tests, especially elevated ALT.

HEPATITIS C PRETEST COUNSELLING (DEPARTMENT OF HEALTH 2004A)

Explain:
(a) the nature of hepatitis C infection and its implications: that it is common, serious and usually curable, especially in the early stages.
(b) the implications:
   ■ of a positive test: that 25% of people clear the virus spontaneously but that 75% have continuing infection. That a further test will distinguish these two states;
   ■ of a negative test: that it rules out hepatitis C infection unless the exposure was in the last 3 months (rarely 6 months). A second test 6 months later will be needed to make sure.
(c) the need for risk reduction, whatever the test shows;
(d) details of the test and how the result will be given (i.e. in person);
(e) the fact that a positive test will make life insurance more expensive.

* Obtain consent to the test only after these issues have been explained and understood.

* Check throughout the discussion the effect it is having on the patient in order to judge whether extra support will be needed.

THE TESTS

* Take blood for HCV antibodies. With the patient's agreement, test for antibodies to hepatitis A and B and HIV as well. Most patients at risk of hepatitis C will be at risk of those infections as well and their presence will influence management.

* If the patient is HCV antibody-positive, test for HCV RNA. It saves time and a further venepuncture if a second sample is sent with the first, requesting 'HCV RNA if the patient is antibody-positive'.

* If the patient is HCV antibody-negative and exposure was within the last 3 months, repeat the test 3 months after exposure.

* If the patient fails to attend to hear the result, seek him or her out. One in five patients tested in the UK do not hear their result.

INTERPRETATION OF THE RESULTS AND FURTHER ACTION

● *Antibody-positive, but HCV RNA-negative:* the patient has probably cleared the virus spontaneously. Check the tests after a further 6 months to be sure. Reinforce advice about reducing future risk. If still HCV RNA-negative after 6 months, no further action needed. However, if the risk continues plan a repeat test every 6–12 months.

● *Antibody-negative and exposure was within the last 3 months:* repeat the test 3 months after exposure. If still negative, explain that the patient has not contracted hepatitis C. Reinforce advice about reducing future risk. However, if the risk continues plan a repeat test every 6–12 months.

● *Antibody-positive, and HCV RNA-positive*

* Refer to the local specialist. Drug treatment (pegylated interferon and ribavirin) is now recommended by NICE for all, regardless of the stage of the infection.

* Explain that the patient has contracted HCV, that further tests will be needed but that

treatment is available which is successful in the majority of patients.

* Encourage the patient to do the following to reduce the chance of progression to liver damage:
  (a) reduce alcohol intake or stop completely;
  (b) stop smoking;
  (c) diet if overweight.

* Offer immunization against hepatitis A and B unless the patient is already immune. Either of those infections would further compromise a liver already infected with HCV.

* Explain the importance of the following, for the sake of the patient's health and to protect others:
  (a) moving to safer injecting;
  (b) using condoms;
  (c) explaining to sexual partners or those who have shared injecting equipment that they might wish to be screened;
  (d) informing any doctor or dentist involved of the HCV result, and not donating blood or carrying a donor card;
  (e) informing an employer if the patient's occupation (e.g. surgery) and HCV status poses a risk to others. This action is for the patient rather than the GP.

Note: A doctor is obliged to reveal a positive test, or a test whose result is awaited, but not a negative test, to an insurance company which has the consent of the patient to request a medical report.

* Reassure the patient that the risk of passing the infection to close family members, other than sexual partners, is virtually nil, but that it is wise not to share toothbrushes or razors, and to mop up any spilt blood with care. Even the risk to a regular sexual partner in a stable relationship is small.

SURVEILLANCE

A patient with continuing HCV infection who is not receiving antiviral treatment needs follow-up annually with LFTs. This can be managed in primary care with the opportunity it offers for further advice about risk reduction. After 20 years, 20% of patients will have developed cirrhosis but the rate of progression is unpredictable. It seems possible that all patients with continuing infection will develop cirrhosis if they live long enough.

INFORMATION FOR PATIENTS AND PROFESSIONALS

UK Hepatitis C Resource Centre, 195 New Kent Road, London SE1 4AG, or 276 Bath Street, Glasgow G2 4JR; helpline 0870 242 2467 10 am to 4 pm; www. hepccentre.org.uk

The NHS Hepatitis C website: FACE IT www.hepc. nhs.uk. Info line 0800 451451 7 am to 11 pm.

Hepatitis C – Your Questions Answered 2004. Available: www.dh.gov.uk (search on 'Hepatitis C')

INFLUENZA

As this book goes to press the development of the global H1N1 pandemic means that any comments on the pandemic will be out of date by the time it is published. This section therefore confines itself to seasonal influenza.

- UK studies show that immunization can prevent, or reduce the severity of, influenza with a reduction of hospital admissions by 60% and of mortality by 40% compared to controls (CMO 2001a).
- The UK target for 2007/8 was that at least 70% of people age 65 and over should be immunized.

INDICATIONS (CMO 2004B)

(a) Those aged 6 months and over with:
  - chronic respiratory disease, including asthma requiring continuous or repeated use of inhaled or systemic steroids or with previous exacerbations requiring hospital admission;
  - cardiovascular disease requiring regular medication or follow-up;
  - chronic renal or liver disease;
  - diabetes mellitus;
  - immunosuppression whether due to disease or to treatment, including systemic steroids equivalent to 20 mg prednisolone daily for more than a month.
(b) All aged 65 years and over.
(c) Those living in long-stay residential and nursing homes and other long-stay facilities where the residents are at high risk.
(d) Health and social care workers involved in direct patient care.

(e) Carers, where the welfare of the person cared for would be at risk if the carer falls ill.
(f) Poultry workers.

Those outside these groups may request immunization, and GPs may give it, but the Chief Medical Officer (CMO) warns that excessive immunization of people outside the target groups could lead to vaccine shortages. Furthermore, the evidence does not support the immunization of healthy adults since it only reduces the number of cases of clinical influenza by 25%, the number of working days lost by half a day, with no effect on complications or hospitalizations (Demicheli, Rivetti, Deeks and Jefferson 2004). In contrast, the immunization of those aged > 75 is associated with a significant reduction in mortality (Armstrong, Mangtani, Fletcher, *et al.* 2004).

CONTRAINDICATIONS

Previous anaphylactic reaction to egg or to influenza vaccine or to neomycin, kanamycin or gentamicin.

Pregnancy is not a contraindication in a woman in an at-risk category, but a thiomersal-free vaccine should be used, if available. If not, a vaccine containing thiomersal may be used rather than omit the vaccination.

PRACTICALITIES

Give one injection yearly to adults between September and early November. Children (under 13 years old) need two injections 4–6 weeks apart as a primary course, followed by yearly boosters.

PROPHYLAXIS AND TREATMENT (NICE 2003)

Prophylaxis: if influenza is circulating in the community give oseltamivir, within 48 hours of exposure, to the following close contacts of a person with a flu-like illness:

(a) at-risk adults and children over 1 year old (see above);
(b) residents of care institutions.

Oseltamivir is not needed if the patient has already been immunized in that season with a vaccine that corresponds to the virus circulating in the community. If that immunization was given less than 14 days before, treat as though unimmunized.

Treatment: give oseltamivir or zanamivir, within 48 hours of the onset of symptoms, to at-risk individuals (see above) who develop a flu-like illness at a time when influenza is circulating in the community. Do not use zanamivir in children under 13 years old. Note the BNF caution about the use of zanamivir in those at risk of bronchospasm. *Amantadine* is no longer recommended.

Influenza is deemed to be circulating in the community when virological studies confirm its presence and new GP consultations for flu-like illness reach 30 per 100,000 population per week. A weekly National Influenza Report is published on www.hpa.org.uk (choose 'Topics A–Z' then 'I').

LYME DISEASE

● Over 300 laboratory confirmed cases are reported annually of which about 20% are reported to have been acquired abroad. It is thought that up to six times that number occur and are diagnosed clinically or the diagnosis is not made (HPA 2005).

● It is most likely in people exposed to tick bites in the UK or travellers returning from walking or camping holidays in the north-eastern US, France, Germany, Austria, Scandinavia and Eastern Europe. In the UK, areas known to harbour the infection are Exmoor, the New Forest, the South Downs, parts of Wiltshire and Berkshire, Thetford Forest, the Lake District, the Yorkshire moors and the Scottish Highlands. However, no area can be assumed to be immune: infected ticks have even been found in London parks.

● The diagnosis of early disease is clinical but it is easily missed. Half of cases have the typical erythema migrans, the other half have less specific rashes. Only half of patients recall a tick bite. Fewer than half of those presenting with established Lyme disease, beyond the acute stage, recall a rash.

● Serology for acute Lyme disease is insensitive. It is useful to confirm a case but cannot rule it out if negative (Stanek and Strle 2003). Even if eventually positive it is likely to be negative in the first 2 weeks after the bite.

● Late disease may present with atypical rheumatological, neurological and possibly neuropsychiatric symptoms. The knee is the joint most often affected. Unilateral facial palsy may be the first neurological sign. The diagnosis at this stage is serological.

PREVENTION

∗ Warn those exposing themselves to risk how to avoid tick bites (see page 59). The essentials are:

(a) to cover exposed parts of the body;

(b) to use an insect repellent containing DEET on exposed areas, including the head;

(c) to search the skin daily for ticks. The nymphs are no bigger than a pinhead. Check especially sites that are warm, moist and thin-skinned (axillae, groin, navel, neck). Do not confine the search to areas of the body that have been touched by vegetation: ticks can attach themselves to clothing and climb up until they find a congenial area of skin before biting.

TREATMENT OF A TICK BITE

∗ *If still attached*, remove the tick with a pair of fine forceps. Grasp it underneath its body, i.e. between its body and the patient's skin, and pull steadily upwards. Grasping the body itself will squash the tick and mean that the mouth parts have to be removed by hand under a magnifying glass. If no forceps are available, loop a cotton thread around the mouthparts of the tick (i.e. between the body of the tick and the skin) and pull firmly upwards.

∗ *If a patient presents in the 72 hours after a tick bite* in an endemic area, a single dose of doxycycline 200 mg can prevent 87% of cases. However, even in a hyperendemic area of New York, this amounts to a NNT of 36, which might not be considered worth the 19% increase in the incidence of adverse effects (Stanek and Strle 2003). The other extreme is to treat only those who develop disease. A compromise is to treat those, seen within 72 hours of the bite, who know that the tick has been attached for at least 24 hours or in whom the tick, when removed, was engorged with blood (Wormser 2006).

TREATMENT OF ESTABLISHED DISEASE

* *Antibiotic treatment.* Give doxycycline 100 mg b.d. or amoxicillin 500 mg t.d.s. or cefuroxime 500 mg b.d. for 2 weeks after discussion with the local infectious disease specialist. Early treatment is important to avoid the systemic complications. Late use of antibiotics may be unsuccessful.

* *In patients with high fever,* or fever that does not respond to 48 hours of antibiotics, suspect another type of tick-borne infection, possibly coexisting with Lyme disease, e.g. Ehrlichiosis or Babesiosis (Wormser 2006).

* *Watch for a Jarisch-Herxheimer reaction;* it occurs in 15% within 24 hours of the start of treatment.

* *Warn the patient not to expect immediate cure.* The rash takes 1–2 weeks to disappear after the start of treatment. Systemic symptoms, e.g. malaise, fatigue, muscle and joint pains, are present in 25% of treated patients 3 months later.

* *Reassure the patient that,* if treated in the acute phase, the later complications of arthritis, palsies and cardiac lesions are very unlikely to occur (Wormser 2006).

* If a specialist with expertise in Lyme disease is not available locally in the UK, contact Southampton Laboratory Level B, South Laboratory Block, Southampton General Hospital, Southampton SO16 6YD, tel. 02380 796 408, email: reglab-se@hpa.org.uk

INFORMATION FOR PATIENTS

Borreliosis and Associated Diseases Awareness – UK (BADA-UK), PO Box 70, North Walsham NR28 0WX, www.bada-uk.org
   Lyme Disease Action. PO Box 235, Penryn, Cornwall TR10 8WZ, www.lymediseaseaction.org.uk

MEASLES, MUMPS AND RUBELLA (MMR)

INDICATIONS

(a) All children between 13 and 15 months of age, plus a preschool booster.

(b) Older children who have not previously been given MMR.

(c) Women of child-bearing age who are seronegative for rubella.

(d) Seronegative health workers likely to be in contact with pregnant women.

(e) Unimmunized children in contact with a case of measles. Give MMR within 3 days of contact. However, immunocompromised children and adults who are not immune to measles should be given human normal immunoglobulin (HNIG), not MMR, as should children debilitated by severe illness. Give HNIG within 6 days of contact. Prophylactic active immunization is ineffective in contacts of mumps and rubella because antibodies develop too slowly.

(f) Pregnant women in contact with measles who believe they are not immune. Measles in pregnancy carries a risk of intra-uterine death. Give HNIG within 6 days of contact, only delaying to check for measles antibody first if the HNIG can still be given within 6 days.

(g) Adults who have not been immunized nor had the diseases, as follows:

■ Those born 1980–1990 and immunized in the UK. They will have received measles and rubella vaccines without the mumps component. Offer two doses of MMR 1 month apart.

■ Those born 1970–1979 and immunized in the UK. They will have received measles vaccine without the rubella and mumps components. Offer two doses of MMR 1 month apart.

Those born before 1970 are likely to have natural immunity to all three diseases.

ADVERSE EFFECTS

(a) *Malaise, fever and a rash* 1 week after the injection. Febrile convulsions occur at this stage in 1:1000 immunizations. Parents of a child with an increased tendency to convulsions should be warned of this and of the need to reduce the child's temperature. They can be reassured that in the UK the child is ten times more likely to convulse after catching measles than after immunization.

(b) *Parotid swelling* occurs in 1%, usually in the third week.

(c) *Arthralgia or arthritis* occurs rarely 2–3 weeks after immunization.

(d) *Meningoencephalitis* due to the mumps component occurred in 1:400,000 cases until 1992, when the mumps virus strain was changed. No cases have been reported since.

(e) *Thrombocytopenia*, usually transient, occurs in 1:32,000 after the first dose but less frequently after the second. The rate of thrombocytopenia after natural infection is higher, being 1:3000 for rubella and 1:6000 for measles. Thrombocytopenia after natural infection tends to be more severe. Children who develop thrombocytopenia within 6 weeks of a first dose of MMR should be tested for antibodies to measles, mumps and rubella. If non-immune, the booster dose of MMR should be given.

(f) *Autism.* The evidence available is overwhelmingly against a connection between MMR and autism (CMO 2001b). The evidence is listed on www.mmrthefacts.nhs.uk. The CMO warns that children should not be given separate doses of measles, mumps and rubella vaccines as there is no evidence of benefit and a clear risk of harm.

Children with any of the above reactions following their first dose are less likely to develop the same reaction after the second. This is because the reactions are the direct effect of the live viruses. By the second dose the child will have partial immunity.

(g) *Anaphylaxis* is a rare complication (3–14 per million doses) and is a contraindication to a second dose.

CONTRAINDICATIONS

(a) As for all live vaccines (see page 34). If given to a woman, pregnancy should be avoided for 1 month. However, the risk to the fetus if a woman is inadvertently immunized is slight.

(b) A previous anaphylactic reaction to MMR.

(c) A previous anaphylactic reaction to gelatin or neomycin. Contact dermatitis is not a contraindication.

(d) Anaphylactic reaction to egg is *not* now a contraindication because anaphylaxis after the vaccine is rare even in children who are hypersensitive to eggs. If there is concern, the vaccine can be given in hospital.

MENINGOCOCCAL INFECTION

INDICATIONS FOR MENINGOCOCCAL VACCINES

(a) *Children in the first year of life* (Group C) (two doses and one reinforcing dose at 12 months, see Table 2.1).

(b) *Children over the age of 1, or young adults aged < 25, if not previously immunized* (Group C) (one dose, see Table 2.1).

(c) *Close contacts* of a patient with meningococcal infection (other than B) if not already immunized. Give MenC vaccine if the case has meningococcal C, or (ACW135Y) for infection with groups A, W135 or Y. They should also receive antibiotic prophylaxis (see below). There is no vaccine against group B.

(d) *To control outbreaks*, especially of group C organisms, in institutions such as schools.

(e) *Travellers* going to sub-Saharan Africa during the dry season, and likely to be in contact with local people, and those travelling to Mecca, who will need written proof of vaccination in the last 3 years (Groups ACWY). The Foreign and Commonwealth Office has produced a leaflet for Hajjis available on www.fco.gov.uk/hajj

(f) *Laboratory staff* working with *N. meningitidis* (usually Group C).

(g) *Patients with an absent or dysfunctional spleen* (Group C) (CMO 2002). If fully immunized as a child, give a booster dose when splenic dysfunction is first diagnosed. If the patient is a child over the age of 1 or an adult who has not been immunized, give two doses of Hib/MenC 2 months apart.

CONTRAINDICATIONS

Previous anaphylactic reaction to the following vaccines: meningococcal C, diphtheria toxoid, or tetanus toxoid or to the CRM_{197} carrier protein.

PRACTICALITIES

(a) *Infants aged 2–4 months:* give three doses as part of routine childhood immunization.

(b) *Infants aged 5 months to 1 year* only need two doses.

(c) *Patients aged 1–25* only need a single dose.

ANTIBIOTIC PROPHYLAXIS

On the advice of the local health protection unit, give close contacts rifampicin or ciprofloxacin (according to local policy). Rifampicin is given for 2 days at: adults, 600 mg b.d.; children 1–12 years, 10 mg/kg b.d.; 3 months to 1 year, 5 mg/kg b.d. Ciprofloxacin is given to adults only as a single dose of 500 mg.

IMMEDIATE TREATMENT OF A SUSPECTED CASE

* Give parenteral benzyl penicillin: 300 mg (children under 1); 600 mg (children 1–9 years) or 1.2 g (adults). This reduces mortality without making subsequent diagnosis more difficult (CMO 2004a).

METHICILLIN RESISTANT *STAPHYLOCOCCUS AUREUS* (MRSA)

RECOMMENDATIONS

Royal College of Nursing. 2007. *Methicillin Resistant Staphylococcus Aureus (MRSA): Guidance for Nursing Staff.* Available: www.rcn.org.uk (search on 'MRSA')
Nathwani D, Morgan M, Masterton RG, *et al.* on behalf of the British Society for Antimicrobial Chemotherapy Working Party on Community-onset MRSA Infections. 2008. Guidelines for UK practice for the diagnosis and management of methicillin-resistant *Staphylococcus aureus* (MRSA) infections presenting in the community. J Antimicrob Chemo doi:10.1093/jac/dkn096

- 30% of the population is colonized by *Staphylococcus aureus*. In the UK about 1% carry MRSA (Loeb, Main, Walker-Dilks, *et al.* 2003).
- MRSA rarely causes infection in healthy people; and when it does the infection is almost always a skin infection.
- People at risk of developing more severe infections from MRSA are those with chronic illness, those who have had recent surgery or instrumentation, those recently hospitalized or who have received an antibiotic in the last year, residents of nursing homes, shelters or prisons, vets, pet owners and pig farmers, those who are

HIV-positive or otherwise immunodeficient, and injecting drug users.
- MRSA spreads in the community as a result of close skin-to-skin contact, open cuts or abrasions, poor hygiene and crowded conditions.

ADVICE TO A PATIENT WHO IS A CARRIER OF MRSA IN THE COMMUNITY

- Do not restrict your social life.
- Cover any wound or sore with a plaster.
- Wash your hands carefully after handling the part of you that is infected or colonized. Use soap and water and wash for as long as it takes to sing the whole 'Happy Birthday' song twice (30 seconds). If your hands are becoming sore, use an alcohol wash or wipe.
- Avoid sharing personal items, e.g. towels or razors, with anyone else.
- If you know you are going to come into contact with anyone at risk of severe infection, warn them. They should not stop seeing you but it would be wise for them to wash their hands if they have touched you or surfaces close to you.
- Antibiotics are not required unless you become ill from the MRSA (Loeb, Main, Walker-Dilks, *et al.* 2003). Your body's natural immunity will clear the organism in time.

* Consider taking a swab if a member of an at-risk group (above) develops a superficial infection that could be staphylococcal.
* If the swab shows MRSA and the patient is well enough to remain at home, give an antibiotic combination according to the sensitivities: first-line treatment is usually rifampicin 300 mg b.d. PLUS doxycycline 100 mg b.d. or fucidic acid 500 mg t.d.s. or trimethoprim 200 mg b.d.
* Explain the situation and the above advice and recommend the leaflet on www.hpa.org.uk (search on 'MRSA').
* Liaise with the community nurses, who will have received advice from the hospital ward staff if the MRSA was acquired in hospital, and are likely to have their own local guidelines.
* In addition, consider trying to eradicate it in a carrier if the patient is vulnerable or may require admission to a hospital or nursing home for other reasons. The patient should use antiseptic

washes for the body and hair with shampoo (e.g. chlorhexidine or triclosan) daily for 5 days, chlorhexidine or mupirocin nasal cream t.d.s. for 5 days, and hexachlorophene powder to axillae and groins if they carry the organism (Smyth 2008). Repeat swabs at intervals to monitor clearance.

* Wash your hands on leaving the house after touching the patient or objects in the patient's vicinity. Explain that other visitors need not do so but a doctor is frequently in contact with vulnerable patients. Carry a bottle of alcoholic gel to wash with if soap and water is unlikely to be available.

THE GP's RESPONSIBILITY TO ALL PATIENTS

The Royal College of Nursing recommends that a nurse should wash her or his hands after every patient contact. The finding from the West of Ireland that GPs have a MRSA carriage rate of 8% suggests that GPs should follow the same advice (Mulqueen, Cafferty, Cormican, et al. 2007). As with all infection control measures, attention to detail is important:

* Wash the hands thoroughly.
* Do not wear rings.
* Dry on a paper towel rather than re-using a wet hand towel.
* Ensure that sleeve cuffs do not touch the patient.

PERTUSSIS (WHOOPING COUGH)

INDICATIONS

All children up to the age of ten as per the schedule (see Table 2.1). A child under ten who has not received all four doses of pertussis vaccine should be given them, as DTaP/IPV or DTaP/IPV/Hib, even if some or all of those other vaccines are not needed.

SIDE-EFFECTS

Suspicion has, in the past, been raised of an association between whole-cell pertussis vaccine and encephalopathy, sudden infant death syndrome, and the development of asthma and allergy. Reviews have found no evidence to suggest that any association is other than one of chance. No such suspicions have been raised about the acellular vaccine.

CONTRAINDICATIONS

A confirmed anaphylactic reaction to a previous dose or to neomycin, streptomycin or polymyxin B.

A deteriorating neurological condition, including poorly controlled epilepsy, is grounds for deferring immunization but a severe reaction to a previous dose from which the child has recovered (e.g. fever, convulsions, screaming or a hypotonic–hyporesponsive episode) is not a contraindication, nor is a previous severe local reaction or a personal or family history of epilepsy.

PRACTICALITIES

(a) *Infants:* give as part of routine childhood immunization (see Table 2.1).

(b) *Infants and children under age 10 in whom the primary course has been interrupted:* resume the course, giving the remaining doses at monthly intervals. Children over 10 and adults do not need immunization.

(c) *Children under 10 who have not received their booster dose:* give it 3 years after completion of the primary course.

(d) *Children who have been given their booster dose at the age of 18 months:* ignore this dose and give a booster age 3–5 as per Table 2.1.

(e) *Contacts, aged < 10,* who have received their primary immunization but not their booster dose: give their booster dose immediately. Give prophylactic antibiotics (azithromycin for 3 days or clarithromycin for 4 days) to contacts aged < 10 if not fully immunized (Altunaiji, Kukuruzovic, Curtis, et al. 2007).

(f) *Antibiotics* (as above) given to the index case will reduce his or her infectivity (Altunaiji, Kukuruzovic, Curtis, et al. 2007).

PNEUMOCOCCAL INFECTION (CMO 2004b)

INDICATIONS FOR VACCINATION

(a) Infants see Table 2.1.

(b) Everyone aged 65 and over.

(c) Those (aged at least 2 months) at high risk (see below).

High-risk groups are those with:

(a) asplenia or severe splenic dysfunction;

(b) HIV infection or other cause of immunodeficiency, including adults on, or likely to be on, systemic steroids equivalent to prednisolone 20 mg daily for > 1 month;

(c) diabetes mellitus requiring oral drugs or insulin;

(d) chronic heart, lung, renal or liver disease;

(e) a cochlear implant or a CSF shunt;

(f) previous invasive pneumococcal infection at age < 5 years old.

Patients with hypo- or asplenism should also receive immunization against *H. influenzae* b, influenza and meningococcal C infection. They also need penicillin (phenoxymethylpenicillin 250 mg b.d.) until at least age 16, and should take special care to avoid malaria and tick bites (McMullin and Johnston 1993).

CONTRAINDICATIONS

Anaphylactic reaction to a previous dose.

PRACTICALITIES

- At-risk children at least 2 months old but under the age of 5:

  (a) starting < 6 months old: give three doses 1 month apart plus a booster age 13 months;

  (b) starting 7–11 months old: give two doses 1 month apart plus a booster age 13 months;

  (c) starting age 1–5 years old: give one dose (but two doses, 2 months apart for those with asplenia, splenic dysfunction or immunosuppression).

For all the above use the 13-valent conjugate vaccine (PCV). Then after the child reaches the age of 2 give a single dose of 23-valent polysaccharide vaccine (PPV) at least 2 months after the last dose of conjugate vaccine.

- At-risk children age 5 or over and adults: give a single dose of 23-valent polysaccharide vaccine.

- Give the immunization at least 2 (and preferably 4–6) weeks before splenectomy. Revaccination 5 yearly should be considered in those at greatest risk, e.g. asplenia splenic dysfunction or nephrotic syndrome. In other patients it is associated with severe reactions and is not otherwise recommended.

POLIO (HPA 2004)

INDICATIONS FOR VACCINATION

(a) The whole population should receive the basic course of five injections of inactivated poliomyelitis vaccine (IPV) (see Table 2.1).

(b) Travellers to endemic or epidemic areas should have had a booster in the previous 10 years. At the time of writing (2008) polio is endemic in only four countries: Nigeria, India, Pakistan and Afghanistan.

(c) Healthcare workers at high risk need a single booster dose every 10 years.

CONTRAINDICATIONS

Anaphylactic reaction to a previous dose or to neomycin, streptomycin or polymyxin B.

A deteriorating neurological condition is grounds for deferring immunization but a severe reaction to a previous dose without anaphylaxis (e.g. fever, convulsions, screaming or a hypotonic–hyporesponsive episode) is not a contraindication.

PRACTICALITIES

(a) *Infants:* give as part of routine childhood immunization.

(b) *Infant and children under age 10 in whom the course has been interrupted:* resume the course, giving the remaining doses of the primary course at monthly intervals, followed by boosters after 3 years after the primary course with a second booster 10 years later. DTaP/IPV/Hib should be used while under age 10; Td/IPV when aged 10 or over. These boosters can be brought forward to 1 year after the primary course and 5 years after the first booster if that will bring the child back on schedule. A course which was begun with oral polio vaccine can be completed with IPV.

(c) *Adults and children > 10 in whom the course has been interrupted:* resume the course, as above, but using Td/IPV.

(d) *Children who have been given their booster dose at the age of 18 months:* ignore this dose and give a booster age 3–5 as per Table 2.1.

(e) *Household contacts*, and possibly other close contacts, should receive oral polio vaccine, on the advice of the local health protection unit.

It is preferred to IPV in this situation because it reduces the symptomless excretion of wild virus by promoting immunity in the gut. Immunocompromised individuals should, however, receive IPV.

TETANUS

- Everybody should be immunized against tetanus. Older people are more likely not to have been immunized. In the UK from 1984 to 2002, 74% of cases of tetanus occurred in patients aged 45 and over.
- Immunity is likely to be lifelong, so further routine boosters (after the basic five) are unnecessary.

INDICATIONS

(a) The whole population requires the basic course of five injections.
(b) Travellers to remote areas, where passive immunization would not be available if they sustained a tetanus-prone wound, should be given a booster if their last booster was more than 10 years ago, even if they have received all five injections.

CONTRAINDICATIONS

(a) Anaphylactic reaction to a previous dose or to neomycin, streptomycin or polymyxin B.
(b) A deteriorating neurological condition is grounds for deferring immunization but a severe reaction to a previous dose without anaphylaxis (e.g. fever, convulsions, screaming or a hypotonic–hyporesponsive episode) is not a contraindication.

PRACTICALITIES

(a) *Infants:* give as part of routine childhood immunization (see Table 2.1).
(b) *Infants, children and adults in whom the primary course has been interrupted:* resume the course, giving the remaining doses at monthly intervals. Children over 10 and adults should receive Td/IPV.

(c) *Children under the age of 10 who have not received their booster doses:* give the first dose 3 years after the completion of the primary course, but reduce this interval to 1 year if necessary to get a child back on schedule. Give the second dose 10 years after the first dose but reduce this to 5 years if necessary to get the child back on schedule.
(d) *Older children and adults who have not received their booster doses:* give the first dose 5 years after the completion of the primary course, and the second dose 10 years after the first dose.
(e) *Children who have been given their first booster dose at the age of 18 months:* ignore this dose and give two more boosters as per Table 2.1.

TETANUS–PRONE INJURY

This is defined as a wound or burn that:

(a) was sustained more than 6 hours before surgical treatment (and that needs treatment); or
(b) is showing one or more of the following:
- a significant degree of devitalized tissue;
- a puncture-type wound; particularly one in contact with soil or manure;
- a wound containing a foreign body;
- evidence of systemic sepsis.

MANAGEMENT

* Clean the wound thoroughly.
* If the wound meets the above criteria for a tetanus-prone injury, immunize as follows:
* Non-immunized or incompletely immunized patients. Give:
  (a) a tetanus toxoid booster (combined with low-dose diphtheria) or a primary course as appropriate; and
  (b) tetanus immunoglobulin. This is available from Bio Products Laboratory (020 8258 2342), or from the Scottish National Blood Transfusion Services (0131 536 5300). Give one vial (250 IU) i.m. or two vials if more than 24 hours have elapsed, the wound is heavily contaminated or is a burn, or the patient weighs over 90 kg.
* *Patients of unknown immune status.* If patients are uncertain whether a primary course has been given, assume that they will have received

primary immunization only if they were born in the UK after 1960, or were in the Armed Forces in or after 1938.

* *Fully immunized patients:* only give immunoglobulin if the risk is especially high, e.g. heavily contaminated or extensively devitalized tissue.

TUBERCULOSIS (TB)

- TB has increased by 40% in England and Wales from 1987 to 2004, with an annual rate of 13/100,000 population (Department of Health 2004b). In black Africans living in the UK the rate is 210/100,000 and in those of an ethnic origin from the Indian subcontinent it is 121/100,000 (see page 188). HIV-positive patients who have latent TB develop active TB at a rate of 5–10% per year, while HIV-negative people progress from latent to active TB at a rate of 5–10% per lifetime (Goodman and Lipman 2008).

- Once the diagnosis of TB is suspected the patient is referred to the appropriate specialist unit. The role of the GP is in the detection of those who need BCG (see below) and in the early diagnosis of TB in those with respiratory symptoms and signs and who are at increased risk of having TB: immigrants from Africa or Asia or their contacts; those with HIV; the homeless or malnourished. Diagnosis in a patient with sputum begins with the sending of three sputum samples, of which one should be early morning, specifying TB.

INDICATIONS FOR BCG

It is only indicated in those at higher risk who have not already been immunized.

* *Neonates* living in the UK in an area where the incidence is at least 40 per 100,000 per year; or with a parent or grandparent born in a country of high incidence; or with a family history of TB in the last 5 years.

* *Infants, or children aged up to 16 years old*, with a parent or grandparent who was born in a country where the incidence is at least 40 per 100,000 per year. If the child is under 6 years old BCG may be given without prior tuberculin

testing. From the age of 6 tuberculin testing is recommended followed by interferon-gamma testing (NICE 2006).

* *Contacts of patients* with open respiratory tuberculosis:

  ▪ *workers in contact with potential cases*, e.g. health workers and staff in prisons, old people's homes and hostels for the homeless or for refugees. However, immunization of those aged 35 and over is not recommended because of the absence of evidence of benefit;

  ▪ *veterinary and abattoir staff* in contact with potential cases;

  ▪ *immigrants aged under 16* from areas of high prevalence, i.e. where the incidence is at least 40 per 100,000 per year and who have not already received BCG. Immigrants aged 16–35 should be offered BCG if from sub-Saharan Africa or from another country with an incidence of > 500 per 100,000;

  ▪ *travellers* to high prevalence areas (Asia, Africa, Central and South America) who intend to stay for more than a month, and to healthcare workers travelling to work in those areas regardless of duration. Again, immunization of those aged 35 and over is not recommended because of the absence of evidence of benefit.

SIDE-EFFECTS

Local ulceration or abscess formation, especially if the dose has been given subcutaneously instead of intradermally. Axillary adenitis is common, and usually subsides within weeks.

CONTRAINDICATIONS

(a) As for all live vaccines including those who are HIV-positive (see page 34).

(b) When the patient has already received BCG vaccination, or has a past history of TB, or has a positive Mantoux skin test.

(c) When there has been a previous anaphylactic reaction to BCG.

(d) A neonate in a household where there is a case of active TB.

(e) A generalized septic skin condition. Patients with eczema may be vaccinated, but avoid eczematous patches.

PRACTICALITIES

* Refer to a chest clinic, where a tuberculin test will be performed before administering BCG except in infants and young children.
* Once BCG has been given, do not use that arm for any other immunization in the next 3 months because of the risk of axillary lymphadenitis.

VARICELLA (CHICKENPOX) AND HERPES ZOSTER: ACTIVE IMMUNIZATION

INDICATIONS

(a) Healthcare workers who are in contact with patients or with varicella virus in a laboratory setting. This is to protect both the workers themselves and other patients to whom they might pass on the infection (CMO 2003). This includes receptionists in general practice.
(b) Others who are not immune and who will be in contact with an immunocompromised patient, e.g. the family of a patient undergoing chemotherapy. Separation of the non-immune person from the patient is an alternative but this is not practical within the nuclear family.

CONTRAINDICATIONS

As for all live viruses.

PRACTICALITIES

Healthcare workers who are in contact with patients, and who do not have a clear history of chickenpox or shingles should be tested for varicella antibodies. Those who are negative (likely to be 10%) should receive two doses of vaccine 4–8 weeks apart. Children < 12 years old need a single dose only.

* Use the same procedure for the close contacts of immunodeficient patients.
* Warn all who receive the vaccine to:
  (a) avoid salicylates for 6 weeks;
  (b) look for a post-vaccine rash from 4 weeks after the first vaccination to 6 weeks after the second.

ADVERSE EFFECTS

A localized or generalized vaccine rash, which is papular or vesicular, may occur in 5–10% in the month following vaccination. Staff with a generalized rash should avoid patient contact until it has crusted (although only three cases of spread have been reported in 16 million doses) (Breuer 2005). Staff with a localized rash can continue to work (except with high-risk patients) provided it can be covered.

VARICELLA (CHICKENPOX) AND HERPES ZOSTER: PASSIVE IMMUNIZATION (VZIG)

Check that:

(a) the person in contact with a case of varicella or zoster is in one of the at-risk categories below; and
(b) that contact was significant both in terms of proximity and timing; and
(c) there is time to give VZIG, if ordered, within 10 days of contact.

Persons at risk:

(a) The immunosuppressed. This includes HIV-positive patients if they have HIV-related symptoms or a low CD4 count. It also includes those on systemic corticosteroids, or those who have taken them in the last 3 months, at the equivalent of prednisolone 40 mg daily for at least a week (children 2 mg/kg/day for at least a week).
(b) Non-immune pregnant women, to protect them from severe illness. It may not protect the fetus from congenital varicella syndromes. These syndromes are most common at below 20 weeks gestation. Pregnant women beyond 20 weeks gestation have the lowest risk, among the at-risk groups, and supplies of VZIG may not be available for them.
(c) Neonates, if:
  ■ the mother develops chickenpox between 7 days before and 7 days after delivery; or
  ■ there has been contact with chickenpox or zoster in the first 7 days of life and the mother

is not known to be immune. Check maternal serology before giving immunoglobulin. (There is no risk to the baby if the mother develops zoster, since she clearly has had chickenpox in the past and the infant will be protected by maternal antibodies.)

Contact is significant if the person has been face to face with, or spent at least 15 minutes in the same room as, someone with:

(a) chickenpox; or

(b) disseminated zoster; or

(c) exposed zoster; or

(d) localized zoster that is not exposed, but where the patient with the zoster is immunosuppressed (and so may be shedding more virus).

Timing. The index cases should be considered to be contagious from 2 days before the rash until the lesions have crusted. The exception to this is localized zoster, when the index case is only contagious from the onset of the rash.

PRACTICALITIES

* Arrange an urgent test for VZ antibodies on potential candidates (other than infants) while discussing the case with the local microbiologist who can advise about the availability of VZIG. The immunoglobulin is in short supply and can be returned if antibodies are present. It must be given within 10 days of contact, and preferably within 7 days. If the result is not available at 7 days after contact, and there is no history of chickenpox, give VZIG without further delay, except in pregnant women, when a delay up to 10 days after contact is acceptable.

* Rely on a history of a previous episode of chickenpox in pregnant women, but ignore it in the immunosuppressed, who may have been immune but lost it.

* Explain to the patient receiving VZIG that it is only a partial protection. About 50% of non-immune contacts will still develop chickenpox.

For the treatment of acute herpes zoster see page 574.

ADVICE FOR TRAVELLERS AND IMMUNIZATION FOR TRAVEL ABROAD

ADVICE

DoH. *Health Information for Overseas Travel*, 2nd edition, 2001. London: The Stationery Office. Known as the Yellow Book, it is available from The Stationery Office, PO Box 29, Norwich NR3 1GN and authorized bookshops and from www.tsoshop.co.uk. The full text is available on www.nathnac.org (choose 'Health Professionals' then search on 'Yellow Book')

National Travel Health Network and Centre Health Information Sheets are regularly updated and are available on www.nathnac.org

General advice for doctors and travellers can be found on www.dh.gov.uk. It includes information about entitlement to medical treatment abroad.

Country by country advice is available from the National Travel Health Network and Centre on www.nathnac.org and from www.fitfortravel.nhs.uk

Information about issues other than health (e.g. terrorism, crime, typhoons) can be obtained from the Foreign and Commonwealth Office on www.fco.gov.uk/travel

* Check that the potential traveller is fit. Most serious illness occurring abroad is due to pre-existing cardiovascular or pulmonary disease, not to tropical diseases. Some elderly travellers do not realize the stress that travel imposes.

* Explain that most countries outside the European Economic Area (EEA) do not have reciprocal health agreements with the UK. Travel insurance is needed. Within the EEA and Switzerland treatment needed while abroad is covered by the use of the European Health Insurance Card (EHIC), which should be obtained before travelling from www.dh.gov.uk or by phoning 0845 606 2030. Applicants will need to have their NHS or National Insurance number to hand. Application may also be made by post on a form obtainable from a Post Office but the applicant should allow 21 days for the EHIC to arrive.

* The EHIC gives the card holder the same right to state-provided treatment as though a resident

of that country. Note that this will not necessarily cover all the cost nor extra items, such as repatriation back to the UK for which insurance is still needed. It will not cover the traveller at all if the main purpose of the trip is to obtain treatment.

* Check that the traveller has received all the routine immunizations recommended for the UK. Consider giving the following boosters if the last immunization was over 10 years ago and the planned travel poses more risk than is present in the UK: polio, tetanus and diphtheria. The combined Td/IPV vaccine should be used even if only one or two of the immunizations is needed.

* *DoH leaflets*. Recommend that the patient reads the latest edition of the NHS leaflet *Health Advice for Travellers* available on www.dh.gov.uk/travellers. Patients can obtain copies free of charge by phoning 08701 555455. It is not published sufficiently frequently for the immunization recommendations to be up to date, and updates are available on page 460 of CEEFAX (BBC2).

* *Prevention*. Stress the importance of preventive measures against gastroenteritis, insect bites, sunburn, accidents and sexually transmitted diseases. Excellent advice is contained in the above leaflet. Travellers should know that accidents are the greatest cause of morbidity and mortality in travellers, and that more become HIV-positive than contract typhoid or malaria.

* Recommend the appropriate immunizations from an up-to-date source, see the beginning of this section. For a suggested table of how the necessary immunizations can be scheduled see Appendix 3.

* *Unusual itineraries*. Advise patients with unusual itineraries or with other health problems to contact MASTA (Medical Advisory Service for Travellers Abroad) on www.masta.org for a personal health travel brief, given online for a very small charge.

* *Medical equipment*. Advise patients travelling to remote areas to purchase a sterile medical equipment pack, also obtainable from MASTA.

* *Altitude illness*. Warn climbers and walkers who are planning to go above 2500 metres about the danger. Nine per cent suffer from altitude sickness in the high Alps (Maggiorini, Buhler,

Walter, *et al.* 1990), and over 50% can expect to get it on the trek to Everest base camp if they fly in (Norboo and Ball 1988). Acclimatization is the best prevention but if there is insufficient time prescribe acetazolamide 125 mg twice daily from 2 days before the ascent to 2 days after starting the descent, or until acclimatization has occurred. Recommend a 2-day trial of the drug at this dosage before leaving the UK to assess adverse effects. Higher doses (750 mg daily) may be more effective but with greater risk of adverse effects. Warn of the risk of paraesthesiae in the hands and feet in the first 2 days of treatment. It is not a reason to stop the drug. Dexamethasone 4 mg 6 hourly can be given to those intolerant of acetazolamide or who want to ascend too soon to start it. Dexamethasone may be started only hours before the ascent (Barry and Pollard 2003).

* *Advise skiers and snowboarders* that the evidence is now in favour of the wearing of helmets in the prevention of head injuries, with a 60% reduction in risk (Sulheim, Holme, Ekeland, *et al.* 2006).

* *Deep vein thrombosis (DVT)*. Warn those at increased risk of DVT about the hazard posed by longhaul travel (say, over 8 hours) whether by plane, bus, train or car. Explain the need for exercises and avoidance of constricting clothing. For those at greatest risk recommend class 2 below knee graduated compression stockings. Consider, in conjunction with a haematologist, the need for injections of low molecular weight heparin in those with a previous DVT or pulmonary embolus.

TAKING MEDICINES OUT OF THE UK

* Recommend that a patient who plans to take prescription drugs abroad should take them in their original, labelled bottles, as well as a copy of the prescription (or the slip for ordering repeat prescriptions). In some countries it is an offence to enter with drugs which the patient will consider harmless, e.g. codeine or a hypnotic, without such documentation.

Controlled drugs are a special case:

* Advise the patient that there are limits on the quantity of controlled drugs that can be taken out of the UK. To find out what these limits are

and for further information see the leaflet published by HM Revenue and Customs, *Taking Medicines With You When You Go Abroad*, HMRC reference notice 4, available on www.hmrc.gov.uk (search on 'Drugs Abroad').

* Provide a letter detailing the patient's condition and drugs taken.

* Explain that if they are within the limit then there is no need to declare these drugs to customs in the UK.

* Advise the patient who has to carry more than the accepted limit of controlled drugs, to apply for a licence from the Home Office at least 14 days before travelling. Details of how to apply can be found at the web address above.

* Advise the patient to contact the relevant Embassy, High Commission or the Home Office Drugs Branch, for information about individual countries' restrictions: Home Office Drugs Branch, Room 239, 50 Queen Anne's Gate, London SW1 9AH, tel. 020 7217 8457/8446.

TRAVELLERS' DIARRHOEA

* Explain that:
  (a) oral rehydration is the most important aspect of treatment. A study of healthy adults has shown that ordinary liquids are as good as sugar and salt replacement drinks (Hill and Ryan 2008). However, those with more severe fluid loss, or children, might benefit from specific oral rehydration products. If commercial sachets of replacement sugar and salt are not available, travellers can add eight level teaspoonfuls of sugar and a half a level teaspoonful of salt (but no more) to one litre of boiled or bottled water;
  (b) the patient should continue to eat if food can be tolerated. It can shorten the duration and amount of diarrhoea;
  (c) loperamide, bought over the counter, can reduce abdominal cramps and diarrhoea but it should not be used if there is high fever, blood in the stool, nor in young children;
  (d) medical help should be sought if there is significant fever, confusion, blood in the stools or if the diarrhoea does not settle in 72 hours (adults) or 24 hours (small children and the elderly).

* *Treatment.* Offer travellers to areas of poor hygiene:
  (a) ciprofloxacin to be taken if diarrhoea occurs (see page 63 for doses). For areas of high campylobacter prevalence, e.g. South Asia and South East Asia, azithromycin may be a better choice. The number of days of diarrhoea and the severity of the illness are significantly reduced but with an increase in minor adverse effects (De Bruyn, Hahn, Borwick 2000); and
  (b) tinidazole or metronidazole to those going to areas where giardiasis is likely, e.g. the Indian subcontinent.

* *Prophylaxis.* Offer prophylaxis only to those travellers for whom gastroenteritis would have serious implications, e.g. travelling politicians or athletes or those already ill with another condition. This is because of the problems of antibiotic resistance if this were widely used. A fluroquinolone, e.g. ciprofloxacin 750 mg once, is the first choice for most areas (Hill and Ryan 2008). Prevention of gastroenteritis through handwashing, cautious eating, and drinking bottled drinks or drinks treated with water purifying tablets is more ecologically friendly.

Note: Drugs prescribed in the UK for use abroad should be on a private prescription.

A SUGGESTED SCHEDULE OF IMMUNIZATIONS (Table 2.2)

Note: Advice on immunizations which are routinely recommended for those not travelling (e.g. hepatitis A and B, polio, BCG) is included in the previous section.

CHOLERA

● An oral cholera vaccine has replaced the old, ineffective, parenteral vaccine.

● The WHO does not recommend routine cholera immunization for travellers. Overall, the risk of cholera in a UK traveller to the developing world is 2 per million. Only give it as a result of official advice in the event of an epidemic or to those travelling rough or working in endemic areas where they will be exposed to risk, e.g. refugee camps.

Table 2.2	A suggested table of immunizations for travel
Day 0	Rabies, Japanese encephalitis, tick-borne encephalitis, hepatitis B
Day 7	Rabies, Japanese encephalitis
Day 14	Tick-borne encephalitis
Day 28	Rabies, Japanese encephalitis, hepatitis B
At some point in the above schedule (either together or spread out over the month). Immunization early in the month (at least 1 week before departure) will allow time for immunity to develop.	Cholera, hepatitis A, meningococcal ACWY, polio, tetanus and diphtheria (as Td/IPV), typhoid, yellow fever

This schedule is for an adult who has been fully immunized as a child according to the UK recommendations. Few travellers will need all the immunizations; they should only be given if appropriate to the travel planned.

If exposure to risk continues, further immunizations against hepatitis B will be needed at 2 months and at 1 year from the first dose, and against tick-borne encephalitis at 9–12 months after the last dose.

- Cholera vaccination is not an official requirement for entry into any country. Reports continue of officials requiring it at remote borders. If a traveller suspects that this may happen, issue a signed statement on headed notepaper that cholera vaccination is not needed. Appendix 1 of Health Information for Overseas Travel has a sample document.

JAPANESE ENCEPHALITIS (JE)

JE is a potential hazard for those travelling during the monsoon season (May to October) to rural areas of the Indian subcontinent, South East Asia and the Far East. The risk is all year in southern regions of the Far East (Malaysia, the Philippines and Indonesia). Normal tourist and business trips pose little hazard. Only two cases have been documented among UK travellers, and none since 1994. Vaccine should therefore only be offered to those planning to stay in a rural setting, in an endemic area, for over 4 weeks, at the time when transmission is most likely. An area that contains rice fields or pig farms is the most hazardous.

* Warn travellers to take precautions against mosquito bites (see under malaria).

* Warn the patient that use of the vaccine is unlicensed and that allergic reactions occur, both immediate and delayed. The patient should remain under observation for 30 minutes after each dose and should complete the course at least 10 days before travelling. Overall, the risk of a systemic reaction (headache, fever, nausea, aching muscles etc) is 10–30%.

* The injection schedule varies according to the product used and the duration of protection required. The National Travel Health Network and Centre recommends three doses for the non-immune traveller, which means starting the course at least 40 days before travelling, to allow 10 days observation for adverse effects (www.nathnac.org/healthprofessionals/japanese-encephalitis.html).

* Obtain vaccine from Aventis Pasteur or from MASTA, on a named patient basis.

MALARIA

GUIDELINES

Chiodini P, Hill D, Lalloo D, et al. Guidelines for Malaria Prevention in Travellers from the United Kingdom 2007. London. Health Protection Agency, January 2007.

Hughes C, Tucker R, Bannister B, et al. Malaria prophylaxis for long-term travellers. Commun Dis Pub Health 2003, 6, 200–208.

Both are available on www.hpa.org.uk

The HPA guidelines recommend that advice to travellers be given under four headings (ABCD): Awareness of risk; Bite prevention; Chemoprophylaxis and prompt Diagnosis and treatment.

* Assess the degree of risk for a traveller by asking about the destination, duration, likely activities and style of travel. Those travelling for longer periods are the most at risk, partly because they are less likely to take preventative measures, as well as antimalarials, for the whole trip (Chen, Wilson and Schlagenhauf 2006).

* Explain to patients that they cannot rely on prophylactic drugs as their sole protection against malaria. In high-risk parts of Africa in the 1990s > 3% of travellers taking chloroquine developed malaria each month (Huzly, Schonfeld, Beuerle and Bienzle 1996). Recommend that patients:

(a) cover arms and legs from dusk till dawn when out of doors;

(b) use an effective mosquito repellent on exposed skin and under thin clothes, e.g. DEET (diethyltoluamide) and, if using the 20% concentration, re-apply it every 2 hours;

(c) sleep with closed windows, having sprayed the room with a 'knock-down' spray. If this is not possible, sleep under permethrin-impregnated mosquito netting; the permethrin should be renewed every 6 months. If that is not available, burn a mosquito coil overnight or vaporize a synthetic pyrethroid on an electric mat. Do not use electronic buzzers, which do not work (Croft 2004).

∗ Explain that fever occurring within 1 year, and especially within 3 months, of possible exposure could be malaria, whatever precautions were taken, and medical help should be sought.

∗ *High-risk patients.* Warn certain patients that they are especially at risk: those without a functioning spleen and pregnant women, in whom the disease is usually more severe and in whom it may lead to abortion or stillbirth.

DRUG PROPHYLAXIS

∗ Explain that patients must start all tablets 1 week before departure (except mefloquine, where a start 2½ weeks before departure is recommended, and proguanil plus atovaquone (Malarone), or doxycycline, where 1 or 2 days before is enough). However, it is better to start the drugs late than not to take them at all. They should be continued for 4 weeks after leaving the area, except in the case of Malarone, where 7 days is enough.

∗ Warn the patient that fever occurring while taking the tablets, or for up to 1 year after stopping the tablets, may still be due to malaria.

∗ Advise the traveller to obtain in the UK all necessary prophylactic tablets before setting out. Medication obtained abroad or over the internet may be substandard or even fake.

∗ Follow the current recommendations of the Malaria Reference Laboratory and Ross Institute, available from a number of sources, including the British National Formulary.

● A decision about whether to take drug prophylaxis will depend not only on the area to be visited but also on the type of travel. Backpacking, or visiting remote areas, will increase the risk; staying exclusively in air-conditioned hotels will reduce it. Business travellers, however, should realize that they may be taken on an unexpected visit into the country by their hosts. The longer the stay the greater the malarial risk, whereas the adverse effects of prophylactic drugs usually occur in the first few weeks.

● The recommendation for areas without drug resistance or where resistance is low is likely to be chloroquine or chloroquine plus proguanil or proguanil alone.

● For travellers to highly chloroquine-resistant areas, the choice is between:

(a) mefloquine;

(b) Malarone (proguanil plus atovaquone);

(c) doxycycline.

  ■ The choice between the three drugs above may be dictated by the traveller's medical history or personal preferences. All regimens have a relatively high incidence of adverse effects, as does placebo, though their nature differs (Schlagenhauf, Tschopp, Johnson, *et al.* 2003). Severe events tended to be more common with mefloquine (11%; 95%CI 6 to 15) and chloroquine and proguanil (12%; 95%CI 7 to 18), than with Malarone (7%; 95%CI 2 to 11) and doxycycline (6%; 95%CI 2 to 10).

  ■ Mefloquine is contraindicated by a history of epilepsy or psychiatric illness, especially depression. The serious nature of the neuropsychiatric adverse effects that occur rarely with mefloquine may influence travellers in choosing an alternative. The hazard of vaginal candidiasis can be mitigated by prescribing a single dose of treatment to be used if necessary.

  ■ Chloroquine is contraindicated in those with a history of epilepsy or psoriasis.

  ■ Doxycycline is contraindicated in those unwilling to take the 3% risk of photosensitivity.

  ■ Malarone is especially suitable for those making a short visit to a high-risk area because it only needs to be taken for 1–2 days before entering the malarious area and only continued for 1 week after leaving.

TRAVELLERS WHO PLAN TO STAY LONGER THAN THE PERIOD FOR WHICH THEIR CHOICE OF PROPHYLACTIC DRUG IS LICENSED

All available prophylactic drugs, except proguanil, are licensed for use for a limited period only. This, except in the rare case of retinal toxicity with chloroquine, is because of lack of data about safety rather than evidence about danger. The current recommended periods are:

(a) chloroquine: ophthalmological assessment recommended at least annually after 6 years;

(b) mefloquine: 1 year;

(c) Malarone: 28 days;

(d) doxycycline: 2 years (for acne).

The Health Protection Agency Advisory Committee on Malaria Prevention for UK Travellers (Hughes, Tucker, Bannister, *et al.* 2003) considers that the possible hazards of continuing a well-tolerated drug outside those limits are less than the hazards of stopping prophylaxis or changing to another drug.

IMMIGRANTS AND THEIR CHILDREN

Immunity to malaria is lost after 2 years. A failure to understand this explains why 80% of malaria in the UK is in those travelling to visit relatives and friends, rather than for holiday (Bannister 2007). If immigrants from a malarious area are returning to that area on holiday, they should use prophylactic drugs. If they are returning long-term, they should not take prophylaxis but should be aware that they are at risk from malaria. Children of such immigrants born in the UK should be protected for the first 12 months in a malarious area with an antimalarial.

STANDBY DRUGS FOR TRAVELLERS TO REMOTE AREAS

Travellers who will be more than 24 hours away from medical care, in an area of high risk, may be given antimalarials as standby treatment to take at the onset of fever. Instructions should be given in writing (downloadable from the guidelines on the HPA website – see above) and should include the fact that fever within 7 days of entering the malarious area is not due to malaria. Current recommendations are:

(a) *area of no chloroquine resistance:* chloroquine (150 mg chloroquine base) four tablets on days 1 and 2, and two tablets on day 3;

(b) *area of multidrug-resistant falciparum malaria:* Malarone four tablets as a single dose daily for 3 days; or co-artemether four tablets initially, then at 8 hours then at 24, 36, 48 and 60 hours to make a total of 24 tablets; or quinine (400 mg t.d.s. for 3 days) plus doxycycline (100 mg b.d. for 7 days);

(c) *a pregnant woman:* quinine 600 mg t.d.s. for 5–7 days PLUS clindamycin 150 mg three tablets t.d.s. for 5 days. Chloroquine alone may be used if there is no chloroquine resistance.

Anyone using standby treatment should still contact a health professional as soon as possible thereafter.

TREATING MALARIA

* Admit any patient who is sufficiently ill; otherwise telephone one of the above numbers for advice.

* Notify malaria to the local authority. The PHLS Malaria Reference Laboratory (MRL) requests that doctors also notify the MRL on a blue form available from them. This requests more information than the statutory notification.

MENINGOCOCCAL IMMUNIZATION

● Epidemics of meningitis in the meningitis belt of sub-Saharan Africa, and in Saudi Arabia associated with the Hajj, are usually due to meningococcus groups A or W135.

● The UK Department of Health recommends use of the quadrivalent ACWY meningococcal polysaccharide vaccine for travellers to any high-risk area, especially those in contact with local people, e.g. aid workers or backpackers. Childhood immunization against meningococcus group C offers little protection. The risk among conventional tourists, even in high-risk areas, is very low.

● Travellers entering Saudi Arabia for the pilgrimage to Mecca must provide proof of vaccination with meningococcal ACWY vaccine. Even those with a current certificate of vaccination against meningococcal A and C need to be vaccinated against W and Y strains if going on the pilgrimage.

RABIES

Only 24 cases of classical rabies have occurred in the UK since 1902, all acquired abroad. However, in 2002 a licensed bat handler died from rabies following a bite from a bat in the UK (Smith, Morris and Crowcroft 2005).

PRE-EXPOSURE

* Immunize anyone at risk from rabies by nature of their occupation in the UK or abroad.
* Immunize travellers to an endemic area for at least a month or who are likely to be exposed to local animals, e.g. trekkers, campers, etc.

IMMUNIZATION SCHEDULE

* Give a total of three doses, on days 0, 7, and 28. Boosters after 1 year and then every 3–5 years are necessary for those at continuing risk, especially if remote from medical care. Testing for seroconversion is only recommended in those working with live rabies virus.

POST-EXPOSURE

* If a patient is bitten, licked or scratched by a potentially rabid animal, the wound should be thoroughly scrubbed with soap and water for 5 minutes then treated with disinfectant. Primary suturing should be avoided in case it facilitates the passage of virus to the nerves.
* Ascertain the risk of rabies in the country concerned from www.who-rabies-bulletin.org; or telephone the Health Protection Agency

Virus Reference Department, Colindale on 020 8200 4400, or the Communicable Disease Surveillance Centre, 020 8200 6868; or Health Protection Scotland, 0141 300 1100; or the Public Health Laboratory, Belfast City Hospital 028 9032 9241.

* If recommended, give the vaccine on days 0, 3, 7, 14 and 30. Stop if the animal is under observation and still well after 15 days. Fully immunized patients need only receive the boosters at days 0 and 3.
* If the risk is high, give human rabies immunoglobulin 20 IU/kg, into and around the wound. If the wound is healed, or it cannot take the whole volume, give the rest intramuscularly into the antero-lateral thigh, away from the site of primary immunization. It may be given up to 7 days after the start of active immunization. Fully immunized patients do not need immunoglobulin.

TICK–BORNE ENCEPHALITIS (TBE)

Patients at risk are those walking or camping in certain forested areas of Europe from April to October. Countries most affected are Alsace, Austria, Croatia, Czech Republic, Germany, Hungary, Poland, Slovakia, Slovenia, Switzerland, the western parts of the former USSR and Siberia and north and east China.

* Advise walkers to tuck long trousers into socks and to spray exposed skin with an insect repellent containing DEET and clothes with one containing permethrin.
* Warn travellers to avoid unpasteurized milk; it can be caught from the milk of an infected animal.
* Instruct those at risk to inspect the skin for ticks daily. If found, ticks should be pulled off (intact) by applying steady traction (see page 59). Do not rupture the tick; mouth parts will be left in the skin. Only 1–2% are likely to be infected and 90% of patients who contract the virus remain asymptomatic. Specific immunoglobulin is no longer available in Europe and it would probably be inadvisable to accept it if offered it in Asia, merely because of a tick bite.
* Offer vaccine to those planning to walk, camp or work in forested regions in the infected areas in spring or summer. The vaccine is effective and

safe. It has been used in Austria as part of the national routine vaccination programme for over 25 years. However, there has never been a case of TBE *reported* in a traveller returning to the UK and travellers may reasonably decide to rely on tick-avoidance measures instead of the vaccine.

TYPHOID

200 cases a year are diagnosed in England and Wales, the main source being the Indian subcontinent. If at first sight that seems high, it only equates to an attack rate of 10 per 100,000 travellers to all at-risk areas.

INDICATIONS FOR IMMUNIZATION

(a) All travellers outside Europe, North America and Australasia, if they are likely to be in close contact with the local population or staying where sanitation standards are poor. It is recommended for travellers to some Eastern European countries if planning to eat in local restaurants.
(b) Laboratory workers handling specimens from suspected cases.

A single injection of Typhim Vi or Typherix gives 70% protection for 3 years. Thereafter, a 3-yearly booster is necessary. It may be given in combination with immunization against hepatitis A. If the oral vaccine (Ty21a) is used, three doses are needed on alternate days, with annual boosters, in those still exposed, for a further 3 years. This makes the oral vaccine less attractive to patients and doctors alike. Furthermore, it is a live vaccine and the contraindications common to all live vaccines apply.

PREVENTING SPREAD OF TYPHOID IN THE UK

* Notify the local Health Protection Unit (HPU) by telephone as soon as a case of typhoid is suspected.
* Work with the HPU to identify any contacts who would pose a risk to others if they developed the infection:
  ■ food handlers;
  ■ healthcare workers;
  ■ children under 5 years old attending a nursery; or older contacts who have difficulty with personal hygiene.

Immunization is not recommended for contacts in the UK.

YELLOW FEVER

INDICATIONS

(a) Laboratory workers at risk.
(b) Travellers to endemic areas of Africa and South America.

A single injection gives excellent immunity for at least 10 years.

SIDE-EFFECTS

● Mild local and systemic reactions occur in 10–30%, 5–10 days after the injection.
● Two rare severe syndromes have been reported: yellow fever vaccine-associated neurological disease (YEL-AND) and yellow fever vaccine-associated viscerotropic disease (YEL-AVD). The former is usually not fatal but the mortality rate of the latter is over 60%. The risk of one or other syndrome is only about 7 per million (always in those with no previous immunity) but this risk increases to 37 per million in those over 60 years old (Marfin, Eidex, Kozarsky *et al.* 2005).

CONTRAINDICATIONS

(a) As for all live vaccines (see page 34). A specific contraindication is the presence of a disorder of the thymus or a history of thymectomy.
(b) Children aged 5 months and under. The contraindication for children aged 6–9 months is relative and should depend on the degree of risk posed.
(c) Pregnancy; however, if a pregnant woman is travelling to a high-risk area and is over 6 months pregnant, the safer course would be to have the vaccination.
(d) Previous anaphylactic reaction to the vaccine, or to any of its components, or to egg.

PRACTICALITIES

Vaccination can only be given at yellow fever vaccination centres, where the certificate will be issued. Details of centres are available on www.nathnac.org. Enter the site and click on the link to 'Yellow Fever Centres'. Travellers in whom the immunization is contraindicated need an exemption certificate in order to enter those countries where immunization is a requirement.

SYMPTOMS IN TRAVELLERS RETURNING FROM ABROAD

ADVICE

DoH. *Health Information for Overseas Travel*, 2nd edition, 2001. London: The Stationery Office. Available from PO Box 29, St Crispins, Duke Street, Norwich NR3 1GN and authorized bookshops and from www.tsoshop.co.uk. The full text is available on the professionals' home page at www.nathnac.org

Background information: Freedman DO, Weld LH, Kozarsky PE *et al.* 2006. Spectrum of disease and relation to place of exposure among ill returned travelers. N Eng J Med 354, 119–133.

The history must include:

(a) the dates and places visited;
(b) visits to rural areas;
(c) contact with animals;
(d) swimming in inland waters;
(e) sexual contact with local people;
(f) what immunizations were given, what prophylaxis was taken and for how long.

Note: Remember that the patients may be contacts of travellers, and not the travellers themselves.

Note: One study of returned travellers found that a history of exposure was of little value in the prediction of parasitic disease (Whitty, Carroll, Armstrong, *et al.* 2000).

FEVER

REVIEWS

Humar A, Keystone J. 1996. Evaluating fever in travellers returning from tropical countries. BMJ 312, 953–956.

Looke DFM, Robson JMB. 2002. Infections in the returned traveller. MJA 177, 212–219.

INITIAL PROBABILITIES IN A PATIENT RETURNING FROM THE DEVELOPING WORLD WITH FEVER

- Malaria 35% (but only 6% in those returning from the Caribbean).
- Dengue 10% (but < 1% in those returning from sub-Saharan Africa).
- Infectious mononucleosis 3%.
- Rickettsial infections 3%.
- Typhoid or paratyphoid fever 3%.

These figures are taken from a study of 17,353 ill returned travellers who presented to 30 clinics of tropical disease or travel medicine in six continents (Freedman, Weld, Kozarsky, *et al.* 2006). Almost half of those travellers were Europeans. The probabilities in primary care are likely to be different, with more minor and undiagnosed cases, but no figures for primary care exist. This same caveat applies to the boxes describing probabilities for the aetiology of other symptoms in this section.

WORK-UP

(a) FBC with request for thick and thin films for malaria (to reach the laboratory within 1 hour of being taken).
(b) LFTs.
(c) Culture blood and stool.
(d) Serology for dengue and blood for virus isolation, in consultation with the microbiologist.

* Consider a cause unrelated to travel, e.g. respiratory or urinary infection.
* In children the commonest cause is travel-associated diarrhoea (West and Riordan 2003). If diarrhoea is present, proceed as for diarrhoea (below).
* Consider the diseases below.

MALARIA

* There are about 2000 cases of malaria imported into the UK each year, and failure to diagnose malaria is regularly referred to in the Medical Defence Associations' reports. *Falciparum* accounts for over half of UK cases, and can kill within 24 hours. Conversely, the first presentation of *falciparum* may be up to

12 months after exposure. *Vivax* may cause illness as late as 18 months after return.

* Assume that fever in a traveller from sub-Saharan Africa is due to malaria until proven otherwise. Malaria can be contracted by patients in an aircraft on the runway in an endemic area. Malaria does exist even in countries for which prophylaxis is not recommended, e.g. the North African coast.
* If the first blood film is negative, continue to send blood films at least daily for 3 days unless the fever abates or another diagnosis is reached.
* Do not rule out malaria because the patient is afebrile when seen. Fever may be intermittent.

VIRAL HEPATITIS

● The patient may present with fever, without jaundice. There are only about 20 cases of hepatitis A a year in travellers returning to England and Wales, and even fewer with hepatitis B.

TYPHOID AND PARATYPHOID FEVER

● These account for over 400 cases a year in the UK, about half of whom have acquired the disease abroad. They should be suspected in anyone with fever within 3 weeks of returning from an area where typhoid is endemic (e.g. the Indian subcontinent), once malaria has been excluded.
● Blood cultures are most likely to be positive in the first week of illness but they are negative in 40–60% of cases. Urine and stool cultures become positive after the first week of illness but are even less sensitive than blood cultures (Bhutta 2006).
● The Widal test is no more sensitive than blood or stool culture and much less specific: a positive test is associated with active infection in as few as one half of cases. More modern serological tests are more promising.

LEGIONNAIRES' DISEASE

The fever may be associated with headache, myalgia and cough. 25% of cases have watery diarrhoea as a prodrome. About half of cases in the UK are contracted abroad, usually from air conditioning systems, showers, hot tubs or spas. Men over 50 years of age are especially at risk. There will probably be no chest signs, but the CXR will be abnormal.

The diagnosis can be confirmed by sputum culture, urine antigen tests or three serum samples for antibodies, 3–6 weeks apart.

AMOEBIC LIVER ABSCESS

* Suspect it in anyone who has visited the tropics or subtropics within the last year. The majority of cases have pain in the right hypochondrium but some have no focal signs.

LASSA FEVER AND OTHER VIRAL HAEMORRHAGIC FEVERS

* Suspect it in anyone with persistent fever who has been in an endemic area within the last 3 weeks. Endemic areas:
  ■ Lassa fever: West Africa from Senegal to Nigeria;
  ■ Ebola fever: Democratic Republic of the Congo and Sudan;
  ■ Marburg fever: Uganda;
  ■ Crimean/Congo haemorrhagic fever: East and West Africa, Central Asia and the former USSR.
* Arrange for an immediate domiciliary visit by the Consultant in Communicable Disease Control or the Consultant in Infectious Diseases. **Do not admit the patient directly into a general hospital**. If the patient is admitted to a High Security Infectious Disease Unit, the ambulance service will do so as a category III removal.

ACUTE SCHISTOSOMIASIS

The fever may be associated with abdominal pain, cough, urticaria and eosinophilia. Assume that all rivers, lakes and fresh water in sub-Saharan or southern Africa are colonized with snails infected with schistosomiasis.

TUBERCULOSIS

Tuberculosis may be acquired abroad. Suspect it readily in immigrants from areas of high risk; 70% of TB in the UK is in those born abroad.

(National Travel Health Network and Centre Health Information Sheet – Tuberculosis 2008, available on www.nathnac.org)

OTHER INFECTIONS

(a) *Dengue* is common in the Caribbean, Central and South America, the eastern Mediterranean and tropical Asia. Unlike malaria, it is transmitted by mosquitoes that bite during the day. Classic dengue can be recognized by the abrupt onset of fever, headache, vomiting, muscle and joint pains and rash. It does not occur more than 3 weeks after return and usually occurs within 1 week of contact. It usually resolves within 7 days, often after a biphasic course.

(b) *Leptospirosis* is worldwide and caught from inland water.

(c) *Brucellosis* is caught from drinking unpasteurized dairy products.

(d) *Rickettsial* infections are tick-borne. They are common in the Mediterranean. Serology is usually negative in the acute phase and antibiotic treatment (e.g. doxycycline) is justified if the typical rash is present especially if there is an eschar.

(e) *Visceral leishmaniasis* is also found in the Mediterranean; ten cases a year occur in the UK.

(f) *Relapsing fever* accounts for ten cases a year in the UK.

(g) *Meningococcal* infection may be imported from Africa, the Arabian peninsula, North India or Nepal.

DIARRHOEA

INITIAL PROBABILITIES IN A PATIENT RETURNING TO THE UK WITH ACUTE DIARRHOEA RELATED TO TRAVEL ABROAD (BASED ON REPORTS TO THE HEALTH PROTECTION AGENCY IN 2004)

- Salmonella 52%.
- Campylobacter 29%.
- Giardia 7%.
- Shigella 6%.
- Cryptosporidium 2%.
- Others 6%.

* Send fresh stool for microscopy for ova, cysts and parasites, and for culture, specifying the places visited. If the stool contains blood and mucus it is especially important that it should reach the laboratory *fresh*, for microscopy for amoebae.

* Warn the patient that if a pathogen is isolated they will be contacted by the local environmental health department.

* *Mild symptoms:* treat with codeine phosphate, loperamide or diphenoxylate as needed.

* *Moderate to severe symptoms:* treat with ciprofloxacin 750 mg once or 500 mg b.d. for 3 days without waiting for the stool result. This has been shown to speed recovery and reduce severity in travellers' diarrhoea but at the possible price of antibiotic related side-effects (De Bruyn, Hahn and Borwick 2000). A better choice in travellers who have returned from areas where campylobacter is especially common, such as South Asia and South East Asia, is azithromycin 1000 mg once or 500 mg daily for 3 days. Children and pregnant women may be given trimethoprim 200 mg b.d. for 5 days.

* *Diarrhoea suggestive of giardiasis:* treat with metronidazole 2 g daily for 3 days or tinidazole 2 g as a single dose, even if stool microscopy is negative. Giardiasis is suggested by a long incubation period (2 weeks or longer), by watery stool with a lot of flatus, an absence of fever, and a prolonged course (usually over 10 days). Symptoms respond promptly to the above antibiotics, providing a more reliable test than stool examination.

* *Diarrhoea continuing for > 2 weeks:* send two further stool samples for microscopy and culture, as well as blood for FBC and films for eosinophilia and parasites, U&Es, and LFTs. Discuss with the laboratory the need for serology for parasites and testing for *Clostridium difficile* toxin. Refer to a gastroenterologist or specialist in infectious diseases if the cause is still not clear.

Note: Falciparum malaria commonly presents with diarrhoea as well as fever. In a traveller with these symptoms from an endemic area, exclude this before treating the patient for gastroenteritis.

Note: Gastroenteritis may trigger an exacerbation of inflammatory bowel disease or lead to lactose intolerance, which may then continue as prolonged diarrhoea.

JAUNDICE

* Send blood for LFTs and hepatitis serology; viral hepatitis is the most common cause.
* Send blood for thick and thin films for malaria if the patient has returned from sub-Saharan Africa and is febrile.
* Remember that leptospirosis, typhoid, dengue, relapsing fever and yellow fever can present as jaundice.

PHARYNGITIS

* Send a throat swab for diphtheria.
* Remember that Lassa fever may present with pharyngitis and fever.

SEXUALLY TRANSMITTED DISEASES

* Screen all returning travellers who admit to casual, unprotected sexual contact abroad for STD (including HIV).
* Consider chancroid, lymphogranuloma venereum and granuloma inguinale in returning travellers with genital ulcers or inguinal lymphadenopathy. Genital herpes and syphilis are, however, much more common.

SKIN LESIONS

INITIAL PROBABILITIES IN A PATIENT RETURNING FROM THE DEVELOPING WORLD WITH A SKIN LESION

- Insect bite (with or without superinfection) 19%.
- Cutaneous larva migrans 13% (30% in travellers returning from the Caribbean).
- Allergy 11%.
- Skin abscess 10%.
- Superficial mycosis 6%.
- Animal bite requiring post-exposure prophylaxis 5%.
- Leishmaniasis 4%.
- Myiasis 3%.
- Swimmer's itch (schistosomiasis) 3%.
- Impetigo or erysipelas 3%.
- Mites 2%.

EOSINOPHILIA

In a large study, eosinophilia was found in 5% of travellers returning from the tropics; a definite diagnosis was made in a third of them (Schulte, Krebs, Jelinek, *et al.* 2002). However, when the eosinophilia exceeded 15% of the total white count, a positive diagnosis was found in two thirds. Conversely, over half of those with helminthic infestation did not have eosinophilia. Only a third of all those with eosinophilia were asymptomatic; the others suffered mainly from fatigue, diarrhoea and skin lesions. Helminth infestations were most common (e.g. strongyloidiasis, filariasis, hookworm, schistosomiasis, cutaneous larva migrans and ascariasis) followed by protozoal infection (amoebiasis, malaria, blastocystis and giardiasis).

- Send three stools for ova, cysts and parasites.
- Discuss with the laboratory the feasibility of serological tests for schistosomiasis, filariasis, strongyloidiasis, toxocariasis and angiostrongyliasis.
- Once the stools have been sent discuss with the patient the use of a broad-spectrum anthelminthic, e.g. mebendazole.

SCREENING OF IMMIGRANTS AND THOSE WHO HAVE SPENT A LONG TIME ABROAD

SCREENING RETURNING TRAVELLERS

ADVICE

DoH. *Health Information for Overseas Travel*, 2nd edition, 2001. London: The Stationery Office. Available: PO Box 29, St Crispins, Duke Street, Norwich NR3 1GN and authorized bookshops, and from www.tsoshop.co.uk. The full text is available on the professionals' home page at www.nathnac.org

- The Department of Health encourages the screening of returning travellers by GPs, both for their reassurance and for the number of positive results that it yields. One study found positive results in one in four asymptomatic people returning from at least 3 months in the tropics. However, routine screening of returned travellers has not been shown to be cost-effective.

- The results of screening must be interpreted with care (Ellis 1990). A negative blood film does not exclude malaria between episodes of fever. Conversely, the finding of worms in the stool is of no great significance since, with the exception of *Strongyloides*, they will die out without treatment in temperate climates.
- Traditional advice to conduct a full history and examination has not been shown to be useful, at least in the detection of parasitic disease. Exposure correlates poorly with positive findings and relevant findings on examination are rare in asymptomatic patients (Whitty, Carroll, Armstrong, *et al.* 2000).

WORK-UP

(a) Fresh stool microscopy for cysts, ova and parasites.
(b) FBC and differential for eosinophilia.
(c) MSU.
(d) Schistosomal serology.
(e) Specific tests for those at special risk (see below).

SCHISTOSOMIASIS

* Check serology, eosinophil count and microscopy of stool and urine of those who have stayed in endemic areas (Middle East, China, Japan, South East Asia, sub-Saharan Africa and South America). Allow at least 3 months after exposure for seroconversion to take place. A study of Australian travellers to Botswana, Malawi and Zimbabwe found that half considered that they had exposed themselves to a risk of schistomal infection and, of these, 8.5% (95%CI 4.2 to 15.2) were infected (Hipgrave, Leydon, Walker and Biggs 1997).

SEXUALLY TRANSMITTED DISEASES

* Test for STD, including hepatitis B, and offer HIV testing for those at risk.

STRONGYLOIDES

Any patient who has ever been in conditions of extremely poor hygiene, e.g. Far East prisoners of war, should have fresh stool sent to test for *Strongyloides* as well as serological testing. Without treatment, subsequent suppression of the patient's immunity can lead to symptomatic disease.

In all screening cases, take the opportunity to check BP, weight, cervical cytology and mammography where appropriate. These are more likely to reveal a (non-tropical) condition that needs treatment (Carroll, Dow, Snashall, *et al.* 1993).

SCREENING OF IMMIGRANTS

Immigrants unable to provide proof of BCG and normal CXR at the port of entry will be notified to the Consultant in Communicable Disease Control for the area in which they intend to stay. Studies show that screening for TB at the point of entry (in immigrants from endemic areas and all refugees and asylum seekers), is often not performed (DTB 2002). GPs should offer screening as above, and also any immunizations not given in the country of origin.

References

Altunaiji, S., Kukuruzovic, R., Curtis, N., et al., 2007. Antibiotics for whooping cough (pertussis). Cochrane Database Syst. Rev. 3, CD004404.

Armstrong, B., Mangtani, P., Fletcher, A., et al., 2004. Effect of influenza vaccination on excess deaths occurring during periods of high circulation of influenza: cohort study in elderly people. BMJ 329, 660–663.

Bannister, B., 2007. Malaria in the UK: new prevention guidelines for UK travellers. Br. J. Gen. Pract. 57, 4–6.

Barry, P., Pollard, A., 2003. Altitude illness. BMJ 326, 915–919.

Bhutta, Z.A., 2006. Current concepts in the diagnosis and treatment of typhoid fever. BMJ 333, 78–82.

Breuer, J., 2005. Varicella vaccination for healthcare workers. BMJ 330, 433–434.

Carroll, B., Dow, C., Snashall, D., et al., 1993. Post-tropical screening: how useful is it? BMJ 307, 541.

Chen, L.H., Wilson, M.E., Schlagenhauf, P., 2006. Prevention of malaria in long-term travellers. JAMA 296, 2234–2244.

CMO, 2001a. CMO's letter 16 July 2001 (PL/CMO/2001/4). http://www.doh.gov.uk/cmo/cmoh.htm.

CMO, 2001b. CMO's letter 9 March 2001 (PL/CMO/2001/1). http://www.doh.gov.uk/cmo/cmoh.htm.

CMO, 2002. CMO's letter 4 January 2002 (PL/CMO/2002/1). http://www.doh.gov.uk/cmo/cmoh.htm.

CMO, 2003. Chickenpox (varicella) immunisation for health care workers. CMO's letter. Department of Health.

CMO, 2004a. CMO Update. Department of Health, London. http://www.dh.gov.uk/cmo.

CMO, 2004b. Update on the influenza and pneumococcal immunisation programmes. PL/CMO/2004/4. Department of Health, London.

Croft, A., 2004. Malaria: Prevention in travellers. Clinical Evidence. BMJ Publishing Group, London.http://www.clinicalevidence.com.

De Bruyn, G., Hahn, S., Borwick, A., 2000. Antibiotic treatment for travellers' diarrhoea. Cochrane Database Syst. Rev. 3, CD002242.

Demicheli, V., Rivetti, D., Deeks, J., Jefferson, T., 2004. Vaccines for preventing influenza in healthy adults (Cochrane Review). In: The Cochrane Library, Issue 3. John Wiley & Sons, Ltd, Chichester, UK.

Department of Health, 2001. Health Information for Overseas Travel, 2nd ed. Stationery Office, London.

Department of Health, 2004a. Hepatitis C: Essential Information for Professionals and Guidance on Testing. Department of Health, London. http://www.dh.gov.uk/publications.

Department of Health, 2004b. Stopping Tuberculosis in England: An Action Plan from the Chief Medical Officer. Department of Health, London. http://www.dh.gov.uk/publications.

Department of Health, 2006. Immunisation against Infectious Disease (the Green Book). Department of Health, London. http://www.dh.gov.uk.

Diggle, L., Deeks, J.J., Pollard, A.J., 2006. Effect of needle size on immunogenicity and reactogenicity of vaccines in infants: randomised controlled trial. BMJ 333, 571–574.

DTB, 2002. BCG, TB and the UK. Drug Ther. Bull. 40, 78–80.

Ellis, C., 1990. The returning traveller. Practitioner 234, 831.

Freedman, D.O., Weld, L.H., Kozarsky, P.E., et al., 2006. Spectrum of disease and relation to place of exposure among ill returned travellers. N. Engl. J. Med. 354, 119–130.

Goodman, A., Lipman, M., 2008. Tuberculosis. Clin. Med. 8, 531–534.

HPA, 2004. Vaccination of Individuals with Uncertain or Incomplete Immunisation Status. CDSC, Immunisation Department, HPA, London. http://www.hpa.org.uk.

Hill, D., Ryan, E., 2008. Management of travellers' diarrhoea. BMJ 337, 863–867.

Hipgrave, D., Leydon, J., Walker, J., Biggs, B., 1997. Schistosomiasis in Australian travellers to Africa. Med. J. Aust. 166, 294–297.

HPA, 2005. Lyme Disease: The Health Protection Agency. http://www.hpa.org.uk (choose 'topics A-Z' then 'L').

Hughes, C., Tucker, R., Bannister, B., et al., 2003. Malaria prophylaxis for long-term travellers. Commun. Dis. Public Health 6, 200–208.

Huzly, D., Schonfeld, C., Beuerle, W., Bienzle, U., Malaria chemoprophylaxis in German tourists: a prospective study on compliance and adverse reactions. J. Travel Med. 3, 148–155.

Loeb, M., Main, C., Walker-Dilks, C., et al., 2003. Antimicrobial drugs for treating methicillin-resistant *Staphylococcus aureus* colonization. Cochrane Database Syst. Rev. 4, CD003340 10.1002.DOI:14651858.CD003340.

McMullin, M., Johnston, G., 1993. Long term management after splenectomy. BMJ 307, 1372–1373.

Maggiorini, M., Buhler, B., Walter, M., Oelz, O., 1990. Prevalence of acute mountain sickness in the Swiss Alps. BMJ 301, 853–855.

Marfin, A.A., Eidex, R.S., Kozarsky, P.E., et al., 2005. Yellow fever and Japanese encephalitis vaccines: indications and complications. Infect. Dis. Clin. North Am. 19, 151–168.

Mulqueen, J., Cafferty, F., Cormican, M., et al., 2007. Nasal carriage of methicillin-resistant Staphylococcus aureus in GPs in the West of Ireland. Br. J. Gen. Pract. 57, 811–813.

Newland, A., Provan, D., Myint, S., 2005. Preventing severe infection after splenectomy. BMJ 331, 417–418.

NHS Executive, 1998. Screening of pregnant women for hepatitis B and immunisation of babies at risk: Health Service Circular HSC 1998/127.

NICE, 2003. Guidance on the use of oseltamivir and amantadine for the prophylaxis of influenza. http://www.nice.org.uk.

NICE, 2006. Tuberculosis: clinical diagnosis and management of tuberculosis and measures for its prevention and control. Clinical Guideline 33. http://www.nice.org.uk.

Norboo, T., Ball, K., 1988. High altitude pulmonary oedema in the Himalayas: a preventable condition. Practitioner 232, 557–560.

Phillips-Howard, P., Blaze, M., Hurn, M., Bradley, D., 1986. Malaria prophylaxis: survey of the response of British travellers to prophylactic advice. BMJ 293, 932–934.

Reis, E., Roth, E., Syphan, J., et al., 2003. Effective pain reduction for multiple immunization injections in young infants. Arch. Pediatr. Adolesc. Med. 157, 1115–1120.

Schlagenhauf, P., Tschopp, A., Johnson, R., et al., 2003. Tolerability of malaria chemoprophylaxis in non-immune travellers to sub-Saharan Africa: multicentre, randomised, double blind, four arm study. BMJ 327, 1078–1083.

Schulte, C., Krebs, B., Jelinek, T., et al., 2002. Diagnostic significance of blood eosinophilia in returning travellers. Clin. Infect. Dis. 34, 407–411.

Smith, A., Morris, J., Crowcroft, N., 2005. Bat rabies in the United Kingdom. BMJ 330, 491–492.

Smyth, S., 2008. MRSA carriage. Br. J. Gen. Pract. 58, 125.

Stanek, G., Strle, F., 2003. Lyme borreliosis. Lancet 362, 1639–1647.

Sulheim, S., Holme, I., Ekeland, A., et al., 2006. Helmet use and risk of head injuries in alpine skiers and snowboarders. JAMA 295, 919–924.

Victor, J.C., Monto, A.S., Surdina, T.Y., et al., 2007. Hepatitis A vaccine versus immune globulin for postexposure prophylaxis. N. Engl. J. Med. 357, 1685–1694.

West, N., Riordan, F., 2003. Fever in returned travellers: a prospective review of hospital admissions for a 2 1/2 year period. Arch. Dis. Child. 88, 432–434.

Whitty, C., Carroll, B., Armstrong, M., et al., 2000. Utility of history, examination and laboratory tests in screening those returning to Europe from the tropics for parasitic infection. Trop. Med. Int. Health 5, 818–823.

Wormser, G.P., 2006. Early Lyme disease. N. Engl. J. Med. 354, 2794–2804.

Chapter 3

Sexually transmitted infections and HIV

CHAPTER CONTENTS

GENERAL APPROACH

- Sexually transmitted infections (STIs) frequently coexist, so patients diagnosed with one STI generally need further investigation to exclude other infections.
- Genitourinary (GUM) or sexual health clinics provide full screening, immediate microscopy and assistance for patients in the treating and informing of partners (partner notification or contact tracing). This is important in limiting the spread of disease, and patients diagnosed with an STI should be routinely referred to GUM for further management.
- Late diagnosis of HIV is a major cause of avoidable mortality in infected individuals, and GPs have an important role in making earlier diagnoses, which improves prognosis and can limit ongoing transmission.

PATIENTS REQUIRING INVESTIGATION BY THE GP

(a) Those who are eligible for a local or national screening programme (e.g. for chlamydia).
(b) Those who require treatment urgently and cannot attend GUM immediately (e.g. symptomatic pelvic inflammatory disease out of hours).
(c) Those who are unwilling or unable to attend a GUM clinic after discussion and recommendation, and require testing for STIs or HIV.

© 2011 Elsevier Ltd.
DOI: 10.1016/B978-0-7020-3053-6.00003-9

(d) Those presenting with a possible STI-related problem in a primary care setting which has training and experience in managing STIs including partner notification (e.g. through Locally Enhanced Service schemes, or GPs with a special interest).

PATIENTS REQUIRING MANAGEMENT BY THE GP

(a) Those who have tested positive for an STI at the surgery and wish to be managed in primary care or cannot attend GUM immediately.

(b) Those who present as contacts of an STI and decline to attend GUM for testing, treatment and partner notification advice, after discussion and recommendation of this course of action.

CONTACT TRACING (PARTNER NOTIFICATION)

- This is usually best done by GUM, or at least with their support and advice.
- As a minimum, screening of all contacts of acute STIs over the last 3 months should be attempted. For syphilis and HIV there is no arbitrary limit, and partner notification will depend on who is contactable, and the earliest likely time of infection.
- If the patient is diagnosed with non-specific urethritis (NSU), chlamydia, syphilis, *Trichomonas vaginalis* or gonorrhoea, the partner should be treated even if tests are negative.

PRINCIPLES OF TREATMENT

- Give appropriate antibiotics, bearing in mind any recent travel history.
- Advise complete abstinence from all sexual contact until both patient and partner are treated.
- Follow-up after completion of antibiotics for compliance and possibly retesting (which is indicated only in pregnancy or where symptoms persist).

WORK-UP FOR CASES TO BE MANAGED IN PRIMARY CARE

- * Take a full sexual history, focusing on the last two partners (irrespective of time interval), or all partners in the last 3 months (if more than two).
- * Current practice is moving towards testing asymptomatic individuals without examination, and reserving examination for those who are symptomatic.
- * Where examination is indicated, examine the genitalia for discharge, ulcers or warts (including the vagina and cervix in females), the mouth for ulcers, and perform proctoscopy if there are anal symptoms or a history of anal intercourse.

Diagnostic tests in women

- ▪ *Gonorrhoea*: cervical, urethral swabs; also oropharyngeal and rectal swabs if symptomatic at those sites, if a partner has gonorrhoea, or if suggested by the sexual history.
- ▪ *Chlamydia*: endocervical chlamydia swab (rotate well) (unless first-catch urine or self-taken vulvovaginal swab is being used for screening).
- ▪ *Trichomonas vaginalis, bacterial vaginosis and candida*: high vaginal swabs may detect candidal infection, but are only useful in the diagnosis of *Trichomonas vaginalis* if inoculated into a trichomonal culture medium. Swabs without immediate microscopy are of limited use for diagnosing bacterial vaginosis.
- ▪ Check that cervical smears are up to date.

Diagnostic tests in men

- ▪ *Gonorrhoea and chlamydia:* urethral swabs (insert 1–4 cm and rotate), and a slide for the laboratory if there will be a delay in swab transport. Oral and rectal swabs may be indicated by the sexual history.

Tests to be done in all patients suspected of having an STI

- * Check syphilis serology and repeat it 3 months after exposure if there has been a significant risk.
- * Check hepatitis B serology in patients who have been exposed in countries with high incidence, if a sexual partner comes from an endemic area, in homosexual men, and where the patient and his/her partner has a history of injecting drug use. Consider the need for immediate hepatitis B immunization.
- * Discuss and offer HIV testing to all patients. Where a patient does not wish to attend a GUM clinic, consideration should be given to testing in primary care.

SPECIFIC MANAGEMENT OF STIs

See also entries on pelvic inflammatory disease (page 331), bacterial vaginosis (page 331), candidiasis (page 330) and sexual assault (page 23).

GONORRHOEA

GENITAL GONORRHOEA (UNCOMPLICATED)

GUIDELINE

British Association for Sexual Health and HIV. *National Guideline on the Management of Gonorrhoea in Adults.* Available: www.bashh.org (choose 'Guidelines')

Gonorrhoea is strongly concentrated among individuals with high risk sexual behaviours and their partners. Referral to or, at the least, advice from GUM is therefore strongly recommended, and screening for other STIs should be routinely undertaken. Antibiotic resistance patterns are changing rapidly, and it is advisable to check with the GUM clinic for current recommendations.

* Cefixime 400 mg oral as a single dose or: ceftriaxone 250 mg i.m. as a single dose; or spectinomycin 2 g i.m. as a single dose. (At the time of writing, resistance patterns are changing rapidly.)
* Treat all patients for chlamydia infection. The co-infection rate is 40%.
* Seek advice for all pregnant women.
* Trace and treat contacts over the previous 3 months.
* Follow-up at least once to confirm compliance, resolution of symptoms and partner notification.

CHLAMYDIA INFECTION (UNCOMPLICATED)

GUIDELINE AND REVIEW

British Association for Sexual Health and HIV. *National Guideline on the Management of Chlamydia trachomatis Genital Tract Infections.* Available: www. bashh.org (choose 'Guidelines')

Nucleic acid amplification tests (NAAT) are now standard for swab or urine samples. Their sensitivity is over 95%. Treatment and partner notification should be undertaken on strong suspicion (e.g. mucopurulent cervicitis or pelvic inflammatory disease) before the result is back. Endocervical swabs should be rotated firmly, and male urethral swabs should be rotated 1–4 cm inside the urethra.

* Give:
  (a) azithromycin 1 g as a single oral dose; or
  (b) doxycycline 100 mg b.d. for 7 days; or
  (c) erythromycin 500 mg b.d. for 14 days.
* In pregnancy, give:
  (a) erythromycin 500 mg b.d. for 14 days or 500 mg q.d.s. for 7 days; or
  (b) amoxicillin 500 mg t.d.s. for 7 days; and
  (c) a test of cure performed 3 weeks after completing therapy.
* Patients should be referred to GUM to discuss partner notification with a trained health adviser – the UK chlamydia pilots suggest that this is acceptable to patients diagnosed in primary care. A cut-off for 4 weeks is used for symptomatic men – for all others, the lookback should be for 6 months or to the last partner (whichever is the longer).

SCREENING FOR CHLAMYDIA

A screening programme for genital chlamydia has been implemented in England aimed at covering 17% of people under 25 years old every year (NHS 2009).

Screening is particularly important for:

- women seeking termination of pregnancy and their partners;
- sexually active women and men under the age of 25, especially teenagers;
- men and women aged 25 and over with a new sexual partner or two or more partners in a year.
* Offer screening with an endocervical swab because it is slightly more sensitive and stable, but agree to urine testing (where available) by a NAAT test if the woman prefers it.
* Repeat the screen if the woman changes her partner.

NON-SPECIFIC URETHRITIS (NSU)

GUIDELINE AND REVIEW

British Association for Sexual Health and HIV. *National Guideline on the Management of Non-gonococcal Urethritis.* Available: www.bashh.org (choose 'Guidelines')

* Test all patients who have urethritis for gonorrhoea and chlamydia.
* First line treatment, if tests for chlamydia and gonorrhoea are negative, is doxycycline 100 mg twice a day for 7 days, or azithromycin 1 g orally stat. Follow-up at 2 weeks. For symptomatic patients, all partners during the past 4 weeks should be treated, and treatment of the regular partner is recommended in all cases.
* Patients should abstain from sexual intercourse until they and their sexual partner have completed treatment.
* Refer unresolving cases to GUM, and all cases where you are unable to complete partner notification. Some men have recurring urethritis due to non-infectious causes – in these cases specialist advice and diagnostics, followed by reassurance, are important.

TRICHOMONAS VAGINALIS

GUIDELINE AND REVIEW

British Association for Sexual Health and HIV. *National Guideline on the Management of Trichomonas vaginalis.* Available: www.bashh.org (choose 'Guidelines')

* *Trichomonas vaginalis* (TV) infection is almost exclusively sexually transmitted, through urethral or vaginal inoculation. It is sometimes diagnosed on cervical cytology, where there is a false positive rate of about 30%, so tests should be repeated.
* *Trichomonas* infection is strongly associated with other STIs, and full screening should be undertaken.

* Metronidazole 2 g orally stat, or metronidazole 400 mg b.d. for 5–7 days, will clear 95% of infections. The stat dose is as effective as the 7-day course but is more likely to be associated with adverse effects (Forna and Gulmezoglu 2000). Test of cure is required only if symptoms persist, in which case the patient should attend GUM. Alcohol should be avoided during and for 48 hours after treatment.
* Symptomatic disease in early pregnancy can be controlled with clotrimazole pessaries 100 mg daily for 7 days, or Aci-gel, before systemic treatment in the second trimester.
* Current partners should be screened for STIs.

ANOGENITAL WARTS

GUIDELINE AND REVIEW

British Association for Sexual Health and HIV. *National Guideline on the Management of Anogenital Warts.* Available: www.bashh.org (choose 'Guidelines' then 'HPV Guideline')

* Most anogenital warts cause minor irritation, or are simply cosmetic. However, they cause a good deal of psychological distress. Patients should be given an explanation of their condition, emphasizing that the majority of anogenital warts are caused by human papilloma virus (HPV) types 6 and 11, which are not associated with cervical neoplasia.
* Many carriers of HPV have no visible lesions.
* Condom use may prevent transmission of warts to uninfected partners. Their use with regular partners, however, has not been shown to affect the outcome of treatment in patients with visible warts.
* Perianal warts are associated with anal sex (although they can occur without) and should suggest the need for anorectal samples for other STIs, and GUM referral.
* None of the existing treatments is satisfactory, and all have high recurrence rates. Patients should be made aware of this. The evidence base for distinguishing first and second line treatments is weak.

- Pregnancy: pregnant women can be treated using cryotherapy, trichloroacetic acid or other ablative therapies in a specialist setting. However, warts often worsen during pregnancy and improve afterwards. The risk of transmitting warts or laryngeal papillomata to the neonate is small, and Caesarean section is indicated only in rare cases of giant vulval warts or gross cervical warts.

SOFT, NON-KERATINIZED WARTS

* Prescribe podophyllotoxin 0.5% (twice daily for 3 days, repeated weekly for up to 4 weeks). Patients using podophyllotoxin at home must take great care to follow the instructions, in order to avoid chemical burns. It should not be used in pregnancy, and is not licensed for extragenital lesions, such as anal warts.

* Imiquimod 5% cream is an immune response modifier which can be used three times weekly for up to 16 weeks. It should not be used in pregnancy.

KERATINIZED WARTS

- Use ablative therapy such as cryotherapy which is available at GUM clinics.

HERPES GENITALIS

GUIDELINE AND REVIEW

British Association of Sexual Health and HIV. *National Guideline on the Management of Genital Herpes.* Available: www.bashh.org (choose 'Guidelines')

- New diagnoses of primary herpes may be due to HSV type 1 or type 2. After childhood, HSV1 is equally likely to be acquired in the genital or oral areas (Langenberg, Corey, Ashley, *et al.* 1999). Much genital herpes is due to orogenital contact and can therefore occur in patients who may not consider themselves as 'sexually active'. Primary herpes is often asymptomatic, and patients often present many years later with symptoms which are due to recurrence.

- Autoinoculation (e.g. from labial herpes) can only occur during primary episodes. Patients who have developed herpes for the first time but had no recent sexual contact should be referred to a consultant in GUM who will be familiar with such cases, and able to advise patients at a time of considerable distress and uncertainty.

- Genital herpes can be acquired from asymptomatic partners, sometimes in a long-term relationship. Some patients never develop symptoms, although those with HSV2 will usually develop symptoms at some point (Langenberg, Corey, Ashley, *et al.* 1999).

- Initial episodes are typically far more severe, and of longer duration, than recurrences. Recurrences tend to decrease over time, but are more frequent with HSV type 2 (Benedetti, Zeh and Corey 1999).

- Diagnosis is by culture or PCR testing and typing of the virus using a swab from the base of an ulcer, sent rapidly to the laboratory in special transport media.

- In primary episodes, patients can benefit from practical counselling in relation to the natural history, and issues in relationships (including risk to the partner). This can be provided at the GUM clinic. Psychological stress does not increase recurrences (Green and Kocsis 1997).

- Partner notification is guided by the individual case and history of symptoms in the partner. Health advisers in the GUM clinic are experienced in this issue and can help with this.

MANAGEMENT OF A FIRST SYMPTOMATIC EPISODE

* *Oral antiviral therapy*, commenced within 5 days of the episode or while new lesions are forming, reduces the severity and duration of that first episode. Options are aciclovir 200 mg five times daily, valaciclovir 500 mg b.d., or famciclovir 125 mg b.d. with a duration of 5 days.

* *Offer analgesia*, and recommend saline bathing. Topical anaesthetics can be used although they occasionally cause sensitization. It may be easier to pass urine in a tepid bath.

* *Admit* patients with urinary retention, meningism or severe systemic symptoms.

* *Offer counselling*, including a discussion of the risk of asymptomatic shedding and its implications for relationships, and the need to inform healthcare workers in the case of later pregnancy. Health advisers at the GUM clinic are experienced in this area.

MANAGEMENT OF RECURRENCES

● Most recurrences cause minor symptoms, of a few days duration.

● Severe recurrences may be shortened by oral antiviral agents as above. There is no evidence that topical antiviral creams are effective. Saline bathing, vaseline or lidocaine gel may aid symptoms.

● *Suppressive therapy*. Depending on patient preference, relationship status, and severity of symptoms, it may be appropriate to offer systemic antiviral treatment to reduce the duration and severity of attacks and frequency. This can reduce anxiety, help in adjustment and improve quality of life, usually in patients with six or more recurrences a year. Suppressive therapy should be undertaken for a defined period of time before review, and is best undertaken by or in collaboration with the GUM clinic.

PATIENT SUPPORT GROUP

The Herpes Viruses Association, 41 North Road, London N7 9DP, tel. 0845 123 2305, info@herpes.org.uk, www.herpes.org.uk

SYPHILIS

Like gonorrhoea, syphilis is concentrated among individuals at high behavioural risk and their partners, and untreated syphilis also has major long-term sequelae. Suspected or diagnosed syphilis must be referred to the GUM clinic, where further investigation, treatment and partner notification will be undertaken. Long-term partner notification is required, and these patients may be at very high risk for other STIs and bloodborne viruses.

HIV AND AIDS

PREVENTION AND EARLY DIAGNOSIS

● Prevention of HIV is an essential part of contraceptive care, travel care, and well person clinics. Testing for HIV should now be universally offered as part of antenatal care, so that women avoid vertical transmission, and access services.

ADVISING ON SAFER SEX AND AVOIDING HIGH-RISK ACTIVITIES

■ Hugging, kissing and mutual masturbation are safe.

■ HIV has been transmitted through oral sex, but this is rare. A condom can be used for receptive oral sex, to improve protection. Condoms can be lubricated with KY Jelly or similar lubricants but *not* oils or vaseline, which reduce their strength by 95%.

■ High-risk sexual activities include penetrative vaginal or anal sex without a condom.

■ Other high-risk activities include sharing needles or syringes for i.v. drug use.

■ Sex with local residents in high prevalence areas of the world (e.g. Africa, South America, Thailand, parts of South America), or with people otherwise at high risk (e.g. men who have sex with men) increases the risks in the event of condom breakage or unprotected sex.

By the end of 2007, an estimated 77,400 adults over 15 were living with HIV in the UK, of whom 28% remained unaware of their infection. HIV incidence is increasing among men who have sex with men (MSM). In 2007, 3160 MSM were diagnosed with HIV in the UK, of whom 82% probably became infected in the UK. Of the 4260 cases of new heterosexually acquired HIV, the estimated number of people infected within the UK has increased from 540 new diagnoses in 2003 to 960 in 2007, and has doubled, from 11% to 23%, as a proportion of all heterosexual diagnoses during this period. The majority were probably acquired in sub-Saharan Africa.

MSM, migrants from countries with high HIV incidence, and injecting drug users, remain the populations at greatest risk of HIV infection.

A high proportion of deaths are now avoidable and attributable to late diagnosis, and early diagnosis is now recognized as a mainstay both of transmission prevention and of clinical care.

HIV testing is now recommended on GP registration in high prevalence areas (mainly London, see hpa.org.uk for details), and for a range of 'indicator diseases' in which HIV is much more likely than in the general population. These indicator diseases include all sexually transmitted infections, as well as many other conditions likely to present to the GP, such as severe psoriasis or seborrhoeic dermatitis, chronic diarrhoea, unexplained weight loss or lymphadenopathy, bacterial pneumonia, recurrent herpes zoster, unexplained blood dyscrasia, peripheral neuropathy, pyrexia of unknown origin, aseptic meningitis, mononucleosis-like syndrome and dementia (British Association for HIV, British Association for Sexual Health and HIV, British Infection Society 2008).

Note re. insurance reports: The BMA and RCGP advise doctors *not* to answer the lifestyle questions on insurance reports, even with consent. These questions allocate a person to an at-risk group, which is discriminatory, while only high-risk behaviour is relevant.

THE HIV ANTIBODY TEST

- The HIV test is 99.9% sensitive and specific 3 months after exposure to the virus (Sloand, Pitt, Chiarello and Nemo 1991), although the 'window period' before becoming positive can occasionally be longer (e.g. after post-exposure antiretroviral prophylaxis).
- If HIV primary infection is suspected, P24 antigen and plasma pro-viral DNA or HIV RNA testing may be appropriate, as prognosis may be improved by antiretroviral therapy at this time. GUM specialist advice should be sought.
- A positive antibody test should be repeated to exclude identification errors.

HIV TESTING

- HIV testing is now more accepted as part of good clinical care, and in the UK is offered to all pregnant women and patients with TB. Primary care practitioners are now encouraged to undertake HIV testing, particularly where this is unlikely to occur in another setting.

- Patients who do not wish to have the result recorded in their notes in primary care should be referred to the GUM clinic.
- The patient should understand that having the test is entirely voluntary.
- Written information about the test and its pros and cons is available on www.tht.org.uk (choose 'HIV Testing').

PRETEST DISCUSSION

- Patients should have an HIV test only with their informed consent, and normally need to come back in person for the result.
- Issues to be covered in pretest discussion for HIV:
  (a) the difference between HIV infection and AIDS, how the virus is transmitted, whether the patient has any misapprehensions;
  (b) the latency between transmission and seroconversion. Ensure that the patient is not in the 3-month 'window period' (occasionally longer). If so, discuss the need to postpone or repeat the test;
  (c) the importance of screening for other STIs and of making plans for safer sex whatever the test result.

PRETEST DISCUSSION

Advantages of the test
1. Effective therapies are available which extend life expectancy to near-normal.
2. Knowing the result means that partners can be protected if it is positive or make decision to move to safer sex if negative.
3. Decisions about pregnancy can be made.
4. Anxiety due to uncertainty about HIV status is ended.
5. Informed decisions about medical issues, such as live vaccines, can be made.

Other considerations
1. If positive, the patient will need to cope with a difficult diagnosis. He or she will need to consider whom to tell.
2. A positive (but not a negative) result may affect insurance, and possibly employment prospects.

POST-TEST DISCUSSION

Negative results

* Discuss any concerns that have given rise to the test, and how the patient plans to protect him- or herself in future. Discuss the window period and whether further testing will be needed for full reassurance.

Positive results

* Ensure that you have time and there will be no interruptions to the interview. Tell the patient early in the interview, to allow time for reflection and questions.
* Establish what the patient knows and expects to happen, and ensure that he or she understands the difference between HIV infection and AIDS. Ensure the patient understands that there are now many very effective therapies that dramatically improve prognosis.
* Explain that the virus is not passed on by normal domestic or work contact, and obtain the leaflet *Keep Safe*, available free from the Department of Health (Department of Health 2003).
* Refer to a specialist clinic, which may be the GUM service or the Infectious Diseases Unit, for specialist follow-up and support. Clinics will fit in a newly diagnosed patient urgently.
* Discuss and advise on concerns about transmission to others (see box 'Advising on safer sex and avoiding high-risk activities'), and the need for protected sex.
* Find out what the patient's plans are for the rest of the day, and ensure that he or she arranges to meet someone for support.
* Arrange to see the patient again in a few days – do not overload with information and issues at this initial interview.
* Give information on patient helplines.

PATIENT INFORMATION

Keep Safe – the Department of Health leaflet. Available: www.dh.gov.uk (search on 'Keep Safe'). Further copies can be obtained by faxing 01623 724524.

Patient support

The National AIDS Helpline (NAH) on 0800 867 123 for free and confidential advice and information about

---

HIV/AIDS, other sexually transmitted infections or sexual health matters. A 24-hour 7-days a week telephone service, NAH can also give details about local services, including sexual health clinics and support agencies for people with HIV/AIDS, their partners, family and friends. A Minicom Service is available for people with hearing difficulties 0800 521 361 from 10 am to 10 pm, 7 days a week. For details of minority ethnic language service call the NAH number.

Terence Higgins Trust, tel. 0845 12 21 200 (Helpline) Monday – Friday 10 am–10 pm Sat and Sun 12 noon–6 pm. www.tht.org.uk, email; info@tht.org.uk

Positively Women: Women living with HIV answer the helpline from Monday to Friday, 10 am–1 pm and 2 pm– 4 pm. PW will ring you back free of charge. www.positivelywomen.org.uk

African AIDS: Helpline 0800 0967 500. Monday–Friday (except bank holidays), 10 am until 6 pm. There is an answer phone service outside these hours). Also www.blackhealthagency.org.uk and www.africaninengland.org

MANAGING THE HIV–POSITIVE PATIENT IN THE COMMUNITY

In the last few years, communication between specialist HIV clinicians and primary care has improved, and patients are often managed in collaboration. This allows GPs to gain experience in the condition, while encouraging patients to access care for unrelated conditions, and to use out of hours care and community nursing appropriately. Following publication of the Standards for HIV Clinical Care (BHIVA, RCP, BASHH, BIS 2009) there has been an emphasis on provision of HIV care within a managed service network, which will be expected to support primary care and others in providing non-specialist HIV services.

ROUTINE CARE

* Regular estimates of viral load and CD4 measurements are important in advising patients to start highly active antiretroviral therapy (HAART) at the optimal time (usually when the CD4 count is less than $350 \times 10^6/l$). These are best done through the specialist HIV services (usually GUM). Syphilis serology, baseline hepatitis B and C serology, FBC, LFT, should be repeated yearly, while

cytomegalovirus (CMV) antibodies and toxoplasma antibodies should be assessed at baseline. Lipids, blood sugar, calcium/phosphate and possibly other monitoring tests are needed if on therapy. Women should have yearly cervical smears because of the increased incidence of carcinoma.

* Advise patients which symptoms should be treated seriously, including fever, weight loss, diarrhoea, lymphadenopathy, shortness of breath or cough, paraesthesiae, headache, mouth ulceration, and visual disturbances.

* Avoid BCG and yellow fever vaccines – seek specialist advice for other live vaccines but otherwise vaccinate as usual. Hepatitis B vaccination should be offered if seronegative.

* Advise the patient to avoid exposure to toxoplasmosis (uncooked meat and unwashed salads), and to cryptosporidium if severely immunosuppressed (unboiled tap water).

* Encourage patients with a CD4 count less than 200 to take prophylaxis against *Pneumocystis carinii* pneumonia (PCP) in the form of co-trimoxazole 960 mg daily or thrice weekly, or dapsone 100 mg daily, or nebulized pentamidine 300 mg every 4 weeks.

* Ensure the patient has adequate psychological support in adjusting to his or her diagnosis.

* The issue of pregnancy and contraception, together with safe sex, needs to be discussed with women on an ongoing basis. Effective interventions are now available which can reduce the risk of transmission to the baby to under 1%. Specialist advice should be sought at an early stage.

* Risk reduction in relation to sexual partners needs to be regularly reviewed. Transmission of HIV to uninfected partners, or transmission of resistant strains, is possible and safe sex must be practised.

SYMPTOMS NEEDING SPECIAL CONSIDERATION

● *Cough*, especially dry cough with breathlessness in a patient with minimal chest signs, and (initially) a normal CXR can indicate PCP. This requires urgent specialist care. Patients are also at increased risk of community acquired pneumonia, tuberculosis (TB), and bacterial chest infection.

● *Headaches* can suggest cerebral toxoplasmosis, non-Hodgkin's lymphoma, tuberculoma or, importantly, cryptococcal meningitis, which may *not* be accompanied by neck stiffness or headache.

● *Diarrhoea* can indicate opportunistic bowel infection, including cryptosporidium or microsporidium, although often no cause is found and symptomatic treatment is required.

● *Dysphagia* can indicate oesophageal candidiasis, treatable with fluconazole 100 mg o.d. for 14–21 days, or (in the severely immunocompromised) CMV ulceration.

● *Visual disturbances* including flashes and floaters, can suggest CMV retinitis. This should be referred urgently.

VENEPUNCTURE

● The same universal precautions should be taken as with patients of unknown serostatus (gloves, avoid resheathing needles, place in appropriately sealed packaging and transport in safe containers). Avoidance of resheathing needles should be standard practice.

● Some laboratories require 'high risk' stickers – this will depend on local policy. 'High risk' does not require stating the diagnosis of HIV for transport purposes, which is unnecessary for routine tests and can generally be avoided in other cases. This practice is an unnecessary risk to patient confidentiality.

● Spills should be mopped up with hypochlorite (10 parts water to 1 part household bleach), or undiluted Milton.

POST–EXPOSURE PROPHYLAXIS FOR HEALTHCARE WORKERS (INCLUDING NEEDLESTICK INJURIES)

GUIDELINE

DoH. *HIV Post-exposure Prophylaxis: Guidance from the UK Chief Medical Officer's Expert Advisory Group on AIDS.* London: Department of Health, revised 2008. http://www.dh.gov.uk/en/Publicationsandstatistics/Publications/PublicationsPolicyAndGuidance/DH_088185. Also available from Department of Health Publications, PO Box 777, London SE1 6XH.

Systematic review: Bandolier Extra. *Needlestick Injuries.* Available: www.medicine.ox.ac.uk/bandolier/extra.html (search on 'Needlestick').

The risk of acquiring HIV infection following percutaneous exposure to HIV-infected blood is on average around 3 per 1000, and less than 1 in 1000 after mucocutaneous exposure. The risk is increased in cases of deep injury, visible blood on the device causing the injury, a needle which had entered an artery or vein, or terminal illness in the source patient. An 80% reduction in the transmission rate can be achieved by appropriate prophylaxis, and all districts should have an arrangement for 24-hour access to such supplies for exposed healthcare workers.

The risk of acquiring hepatitis is, in most parts of the world, greater than that of HIV.

MANAGEMENT

* After *any* exposure to blood (whether or not the source patient is known to be HIV- or hepatitis B- or C-positive), wash the wound liberally with soap and water, but do not scrub. Antiseptics should not be used.

* Telephone for advice on local arrangements for 24-hour access to HIV prophylaxis, and specialist advice on risk assessment, based on the nature of the exposure, the risk posed by the source and the immune status of the contact. The local consultant in Communicable Disease Control (via the Public Health Department), consultant microbiologist/virologist or consultant in GU medicine will be able to advise if you do not have information to hand. Drug starter packs are usually held at the local Accident and Emergency department.

* Take blood for baseline HIV and hepatitis B and C serology.

* If the risk is assessed as potentially significant, antiretroviral drugs should be commenced as soon as possible, preferably within 1 hour. Medication should be continued for a total of 4 weeks if subsequent risk assessment confirms this is appropriate. The contents of starter packs are under constant review.

* Unless the source is already known to be negative for hepatitis B, or the contact known to be fully immunized, give active immunization against hepatitis B (see page 38). Passive immunization with hepatitis B immunoglobulin (HBIG) can be given within 48 hours, but may still be worthwhile up to 7 days after exposure.

However HBIG is expensive, in short supply and only available for immunocompromised/pregnant patients exposed to known hepatitis B. Patients already immunized against hepatitis B need a booster of active immunization.

* If the source patient is of unknown status, he or she should routinely be approached (by someone other than the exposed patient) to ask for consent for testing.

* Arrange follow-up, by Occupational Health, the GUM department or another appropriate department, for the exposed worker, in order to consider testing for HIV and hepatitis B and C in confidence at a later stage.

SUMMARY OF POST-EXPOSURE PROPHYLAXIS

1. Clean the wound.
2. Get advice. If significant risk exists, offer:
   (a) antiretroviral drugs within 1 hour;
   (b) active immunization with hepatitis B vaccine;
   (c) passive immunization with hepatitis B immunoglobulin if donor is HBV+ve and recipient immunocompromised or pregnant.
3. Take blood for baseline serology of contact and source (with consent).
4. Arrange follow-up.

POST-EXPOSURE PROPHYLAXIS FOLLOWING SEXUAL OR OTHER NON-OCCUPATIONAL EXPOSURE

Post-exposure prophylaxis for HIV may be required following sexual exposure. Examples may include some cases of sexual assault, and condom failure between HIV discordant couples or unprotected anal sex in men who have sex with men. In these circumstances, prophylaxis against hepatitis B should also be considered.

Policies and regimens for HIV post-exposure prophylaxis, including indications for use after sexual exposure, are to be found on the BASHH website (http://www.bashh.org/documents/58/58.pdf). The consultant at the local GUM clinic should be able to give immediate advice and assist in risk assessment. Prophylaxis, if required, should be started as soon as possible and certainly within 72 hours.

NOTIFICATION AND SURVEILLANCE

Microbiology laboratories voluntarily notify positive HIV results (confidentially and anonymously) to the Communicable Disease Surveillance Centre (CDSC), Centre for Infections, 61 Colindale Avenue, London NW9 5EQ, or Health Protection Scotland (http://www.hps.scot.nhs.uk/). These establishments then write to the clinician concerned asking for further clinical details. Doctors may also notify cases directly. If the patient has not been referred on for further specialist management, the GP who receives a positive test result may be invited to provide information for the voluntary, confidential, anonymized database. Details of HIV and AIDS surveillance, together with recent data, can be seen at http://www.hpa.org.uk.

References

Benedetti, J.K., Zeh, J., Corey, L., 1999. Clinical reactivation of genital herpes simplex infection decreases in frequency over time. Ann. Intern. Med. 131, 14–20.

BHIVA, RCP, BASHH, BIS, 2009. Standards for HIV clinical care. http://www.bhiva.org/cms1191535.asp.

British Association for HIV, British Association for Sexual Health and HIV, British Infection Society, 2008. UK National Guidelines for HIV Testing.

Department of Health, 2003. Online. http://www.doh.gov.uk (search on 'Keep Safe').

Forna, F., Gulmezoglu, A.M., 2000. Interventions for treating trichomonas in women (Cochrane Review). In: The Cochrane Library, Issue 3. Update Software, Oxford.

Green, J., Kocsis, A., 1997. Psychological factors in recurrent genital herpes. Genitourin. Med. 73, 253–259.

Langenberg, A.G., Corey, L., Ashley, R.L., et al., 1999. A prospective study of new infections with herpes simplex virus type 1 and type 2. N. Engl. J. Med. 341, 1432–1438.

NHS, 2009. National Chlamydia screening programme. http://www.chlamydiascreening.nhs.uk/ps/commissioners/summary.html.

Sloand, E.M., Pitt, E., Chiarello, R.J., Nemo, G.J., 1991. HIV testing. State of the art. J. Am. Med. Assoc. 266 (20), 2861–2866.

Chapter 4

Childhood problems

CHAPTER CONTENTS

© 2011 Elsevier Ltd.
DOI: 10.1016/B978-0-7020-3053-6.00004-0

CHILD HEALTH PROMOTION

OVERVIEW

Hall DM, Elliman D. 2003. *Health for All Children: Report of the Third Joint Working Party on Child Health Surveillance*, 4th edition. Oxford University Press, Oxford

See Appendix 5 for an account of the screening procedures that may be carried out at different ages. Current thinking, however, is moving away from a rigid screening protocol towards a more holistic approach, with an emphasis on child health promotion.

REDUCING THE RISK OF COT DEATH

* Instruct all parents about the following:
  (a) *Sleeping position.* Lie the infant on the back, not on the side, nor prone. The prone position is associated with an eight-fold increased risk of cot death, the side position a two-fold increase. There is no evidence that placing babies on their back results in an increased risk of death by choking or vomiting (Chief Medical Officer's Expert Group 1993).
  (b) *Overheating.* Make sure that the infant does not overheat; clothing and bedding should be no more than for an older child. Avoid duvets. Make the bed up, with the feet touching the bottom of the cot, so that the infant cannot slip down under the bedclothes. Keep the head uncovered. The bedroom should be maintained at 16–20°C. Do not let the baby sleep near a radiator or in direct sunlight.
  (c) *Smoking.* Smoking in pregnancy is associated with an increased risk of cot death. Parental smoking combined with falling asleep with the baby whilst sharing a bed, in a chair or makeshift bed increases the risk of cot death considerably. Smokers should smoke outside the house.
  (d) *Sharing a bed.* Parents are advised not to sleep with the baby in the bed, although there is some controversy about this. Having a cuddle or feed is acceptable but babies are safest sleeping in their own cot in the parents' room for their first 6 months. The risk of overlaying when sharing a bed is markedly increased when a parent has taken sedative medication or alcohol, or is extremely tired, or is a smoker.
  (e) *Illness.* When they feel their baby is unwell to use Baby Check (see below).

PARENTS WHO HAVE ALREADY LOST A CHILD FROM SUDDEN INFANT DEATH SYNDROME (SIDS)

* Recommend The Foundation for the Study of Infant Deaths; 24 hour helpline 020 7233 2090, www.fsid.org.uk. The CONI system (Care Of the Next Infant) is run locally in the UK by the health visiting service.

* Suggest they obtain a copy of Baby Check, available to download from www.fsid.org.uk. then search for 'Baby Check'. It is a simple guide for parents to use to assess their baby if they suspect that the child is unwell.

ADVICE FOR PROFESSIONALS

Foundation for Sudden Infant Death, www.fsid.org.uk

UNEXPECTED DEATH IN A BABY OR CHILD

New procedures have been in place since April 2009 in England and Wales. Following an unexpected child death GPs should expect to be invited to participate in multiagency meetings to review the causes of the death and the family's needs.

PREVENTION OF UNINTENTIONAL INJURY

A 'Health of the Nation' target was to reduce accidents in children by one third by the year 2005.

* Be aware of sources of potential injury at every contact with a family (Health Development Agency 2001). Alert the health visitor to any causes for concern.

NUTRITION

BREASTFEEDING (see also page 401)

● Although 65% of women are breastfeeding on discharge from hospital, only 30% are still feeding after 4 months. Inadequate milk supply is the most common reason put forward for stopping breastfeeding (Department of Health and Social Security 1988).

● Human milk is the recommended nutritional source for infants, exclusively for the first 6 months of postnatal life and in combination with complementary foods until the age of 2. Extensive research, especially in recent years, documents the many advantages to infants, mothers, families and society from breastfeeding and the use of human milk for feeding.

● Encourage the mother to have confidence in herself and her abilities. All possible measures should be taken to ensure adequate lactation.

* *Too frequent weighing of the baby* in the first few months may undermine confidence; opinion is divided as to when it should be done. A minimum is to weigh at birth and at 10 days, and thereafter only if there is concern about the adequacy of the supply of breast milk or suspicion that the baby is not thriving. At 3–4 days weight loss should be no more than 10%; at 7 days the baby should have started to gain weight; and by 10–12 days birthweight have been regained.

* Advise against:
  (a) *complementary feeding* – unless essential;
  (b) *additional water*, which is rarely necessary (even in hot weather), and may increase the risk of gastrointestinal infection.

SUPPORT GROUPS

National Childbirth Trust, www.nctpregnancyandbabycare.com
  La Leche League, www.laleche.org.uk

VITAMIN K

ADVICE

Department of Health. *Vitamin K for Newborn Babies.* PL CMO (1998)3: availabl: www.dh.gov.uk (search on 'Vitamin K')

See also page 400.

● Supplemental vitamin K (i.m. or oral) at birth helps reduce mortality from haemorrhagic disease of the newbornim; i.m. vitamin K is more effective than oral vitamin K in preventing early mortality.

● One study has suggested a link between i.m. vitamin K, but not oral, and cancer in childhood. This has not been confirmed in a number of better designed studies.

● All babies should receive one dose of vitamin K (oral or i.m.) at birth. Formula fed babies will receive enough vitamin K. Breastfed or predominantly breastfed babies require long-term prophylaxis.

Oral preparation. Doses of phytomenadione 10 mg/ 1 ml (mixed micelles), 0.2 ml should be given in the first week and breastfed babies should receive another dose at 4 weeks of age.

WEANING

The Committee on Medical Aspects of Food and Nutrition Policy 2000 (COMA) recommends that:

(a) breastfeeding should be encouraged for 6 months, preferably longer;

(b) early weaning should be discouraged;

(c) foods regarded as potentially allergenic should be avoided until 6 months of age, e.g. cows' milk, gluten, eggs, soya proteins, wheat and citrus fruits.

General/behavioural principles

(a) Foods should be offered by spoon, in small quantities. An infant who refuses the food should not be pressed to take it.

(b) Time should be put aside for feeding and infants allowed to feed at their own pace.

(c) New foods should be introduced slowly and in small quantities initially.

(d) Snacks should not be offered between meals.

Warn the parents to avoid nuts and other foods that could be inhaled.

Encourage parents to reduce the fat intake from 1 year onwards.

INFANT FORMULA FEEDING

● Formula milks should only be used if human milk feeding is not possible (e.g. through maternal choice, or a mother with HIV infection or hepatitis C). There are many different commercial formulations and the nutrient composition of each breast milk substitute is slightly different, reflecting the uncertainty about the infant's need for nutrients, specifically protein–energy ratio, fat blend and amount of calcium and phosphorous. Infant formulas do not contain any of the biologically active immune substances, nor the hormones or growth factors found in human milk.

● Formula milk, rather than cows' milk, should be given until the infant is at least 12 months old.

● Follow-on milks may be recommended in certain situations, e.g. persistently poor weight gain, or where cows' milk is introduced as the main milk at 6 months. Follow-on milks are lower in protein than whole milk and are fortified with iron and vitamins A, C and D.

✳ Advise the parents to use whey dominant milks, where the whey:casein ratio is similar to human milk (e.g. SMA Gold, Cow and Gate Premium, Ostermilk, Aptamil). There is no justification for changing older or 'hungrier' babies onto casein-dominant milks (e.g. SMA White, Cow and Gate Plus, Ostermilk Number 2, Milumil), where the whey:casein ratio is similar to cows' milk.

✳ Cows' milk is low in iron and vitamins A, C, D and E. 'Doorstep' milk can be used to mix feeds, etc. but should not be used as the main milk until 1 year. After 1 year, whole milk is recommended until the age of 5. Infants fed on cows' milk during the first year of life have a high risk of serious iron deficiency.

✳ Feed volume. The infant requires about 150 ml/kg per day. Traditionally this is given as 5–6 feeds a day, but 'on demand' feeding does not result in fatter babies. When a baby regularly finishes the feed offered, this can be increased by 30 ml per feed. Parents should beware of misinterpreting hand sucking or crying as a request for a feed.

✳ Changing milks because the baby is 'not satisfied' or has 'colic' is of no value, and may increase anxiety. If the baby is genuinely not satisfied, the feed volume should be increased. If the baby is still not satisfied solids could be considered if the baby is over 4 months old.

✳ Additional supplements (e.g. vitamins and fruit juices) are not necessary.

✳ Soya milks do not protect the infant against atopy and should not be given for colic or unconfirmed cows' milk intolerance.

OTHER ASPECTS OF INFANT/PRESCHOOL NUTRITION

Vitamins

● Premature infants should take multivitamin supplements from the time they are tolerating full feeds until they reach approximately 2 kg. Premature infants should take oral iron supplements from the time they are tolerating full feeds (after 2 weeks of age) until 6–12 months of age.

● It is recommended that all children over the age of 1 year should take a multivitamin supplement. Traditionally this has been given as vitamin A, C and D (Healthy Start children's vitamin drops) from health clinics.

- All breastfed babies and babies in high-risk groups (Asian children and Caribbean children on exclusion diets) should start multivitamins before the age of 6 months.
- All pregnant and lactating women should take vitamin D supplements.

Iron

- Studies estimate the prevalence of iron deficiency in preschool children to be between 5 and 40%, and in school-age children between 5 and 10%. Iron deficiency anaemia is defined as a haemoglobin < 11 g/dl, together with other evidence of iron deficiency or a ferritin of < 10 mcg/l. Iron deficiency is not necessarily accompanied by anaemia. Iron deficiency is more common in children:
  - (a) born prematurely; or
  - (b) of low birth weight; or
  - (c) who started drinking 'doorstep' milk early; or
  - (d) who drink tea; or
  - (e) who have poor nutrition.
- Iron deficiency not only causes anaemia, but also can affect behaviour, development and susceptibility to infection.
- * Consider ordering an FBC and serum ferritin in children with those problems.
- * If iron deficiency is found, treat with a 3-month course of ferrous sulphate oral paediatric solution 5 mg/kg per day.

Sugar

See nutritional advice below.

Salt

- * Advise against adding salt to food cooked for a baby under 6 months. After 6 months the salt added should be kept to a minimum, with no added salt at the table.

Fibre

- * Advise against rigorously high-fibre diets, as they do not supply adequate nutrition to a growing child and can cause diarrhoea.

Drinks

- * Advise the parents (after weaning) to:
  - (a) give drinks only with or after meals, and to restrict the milk intake to below 1.5 pints a day to avoid reducing appetite. Encourage water;
  - (b) offer drinks by feeder cup or beaker from 6 months;
  - (c) remove the cup from in front of the child after he or she has had enough;
  - (d) discourage tea, which impairs iron absorption. Fruit juices should be diluted with water.

DENTAL AND ORAL DISEASE

- 40% of 5-year-olds in the UK have active tooth decay.
- Young children who attend the dentist 'only when they have trouble with their teeth' have more diseased teeth than children who attend for regular check-ups.
- * Encourage the parents to:
  - (a) avoid the use of sugared dummies and juices in a 'dinky feeder' or night comforter;
  - (b) wean their children on to food and drinks which are free from non-milk extrinsic sugars;
  - (c) discourage bottle feeding after 12 months;
  - (d) restrict the intake of any sugary food and drinks to mealtimes;
  - (e) beware of 'hidden sugars' in food and drink, even in commercially prepared baby foods;
  - (f) restrict the intake of acidic drinks (fruit juices or carbonated drinks) to meal times, and dilute any fruit juices with water;
  - (g) brush children's teeth once they appear using a small toothbrush with a children's fluoride toothpaste (500 parts per million (ppm) concentration). No more than a pea-sized blob is required;
  - (h) commence early and regular dental visits; 6 months of age is the ideal time to seek advice from a dentist on a child's need for fluoride supplements;

(i) encourage dental attendance at least once a year.

* Prescribe and promote the use of sugar-free medicines, especially when they are needed long-term.

* Refer children with suspected or overt dental disease to a dentist.

FLUORIDE

Topical fluoride is of more value in toothpaste than as oral supplementation. Fluoride supplements should be given only where the water supply contains less than 0.7 ppm.

ASPECTS OF SCREENING

For an account of the UK child screening programme see Department of Health (The Child Health Promotion Programme) www.dh.gov.uk. For the neonatal and 8-week examinations see check-list chart, Appendix 5.

Below are discussed aspects of screening which may involve the GP.

EXAMINATION OF THE HIP FOR CONGENITAL DISLOCATION OF THE HIP (CDH)/DEVELOPMENTAL DISPLACEMENT OF THE HIP (DDH)

● *Screening for CDH/DDH does not detect all cases at birth.* Regular examination and awareness is necessary until the child is walking normally.

● *High-risk groups:* first-born children, girls, those with a family history of CDH/DDH, breech delivery, congenital positional deformities of the feet or other joints, oligohydramnios, fetal growth retardation, cerebral palsy or other disorders of the motor system.

  * Check that all babies in the above high-risk groups are being followed up. This may include ultrasound examination, which has been shown to significantly reduce the need for abduction splinting (Elbourne, Dezateux, Arthur *et al.* 2002).

Note: Overexamination may be harmful, and only one professional should screen on each occasion.

Examination under 3 months

* Use the modified Ortolani/Barlow manoeuvres. The infant should lie supine on a flat surface in a warm room. The hips should be partially abducted and fully flexed. The pelvis should be stabilized with one hand by holding a thumb over the symphysis pubis and fingers under the sacrum. The leg on the side being checked is held with the other hand. With the upper part of the tibia resting between the examiner's forefinger and thumb, the femur is gripped so that the middle finger is held over the greater trochanter and the thumb over the lesser trochanter. Assess one hip at a time.

  (a) Abduct the hip by pressing medially on the greater trochanter with the middle finger. If the hip is posteriorly dislocated it will relocate into the acetabulum with a clunk (Ortolani positive).

  (b) Place the thumb on the inside of the thigh and press laterally, trying to push the head of the femur backwards out of the acetabulum. The dislocatable or subluxable hip 'clunks' over the posterior edge of the acetabulum (Barlow positive).

* *Ligamentous clicks* without movement are of no importance in themselves, but are associated with an increased incidence of CDH/DDH at later testing. Review at 6 weeks; if still present refer to an orthopaedic surgeon.

Signs and examination over 3 months of age

* Look for the following:

  (a) shortening of the leg; compare the level of the knees;

  (b) the thigh lying in partial lateral rotation, flexion and abduction;

  (c) flattening of the thigh on the affected side when prone;

  (d) asymmetrical skin creases;

  (e) a large gap between the thighs, in patients with bilateral dislocation;

  (f) reduced abduction.

* *6–9 months.* Abduct the hip when flexed to 90°. If CDH/DDH is present, resistance will be felt before 45° is reached. If CDH/DDH is unilateral, abduction will be asymmetrical. In some children, a clunk may be felt as the head

relocates. In either situation, refer to an orthopaedic surgeon.

* *18–24 months.* Refer any child with a waddling gait suggestive of CDH/DDH.

UNDESCENDED TESTIS

Tekgul S, Riedmuller H, Gerharz E, *et al.* 2008. *Guidelines on Paediatric Urology.* European Society for Paediatric Urology and the European Association of Urology. http://www.uroweb.org/fileadmin/ user_upload/Guidelines/Paediatric%20Urology.pdf

* About 6% of boys have one or both testes undescended at birth. 0.8% are still undescended at one year and spontaneous descent after that is rare (Prem 2006).
* One boy in 120 with an untreated undescended testis will develop malignancy.
* Examine all boys at the neonatal examination, and at 6–8 weeks. Refer to a surgeon at this point if one or both testes are not clearly descended. The surgeon may well choose not to see the child until shortly before his first birthday and not to operate until his second year.
* The older child. Examine with the child squatting and lying down. Examination of the standing child is very likely to give rise to error.

CONGENITAL HEART DISEASE

* The birth prevalence of congenital heart disease (CHD) is 8 per 1000.
* Examine the baby shortly after birth and at 6–8 weeks for symptoms and signs of CHD. Any murmur heard in the first 48 hours of life is likely to be significant, and warrants early referral. Any murmur heard at 6 weeks also warrants referral, but not urgently if the child is well. Consider CHD in any child who fails to thrive or has tachypnoea (particularly if it interferes with feeding), or, persistent sternal recession; recurrent 'chest infection', sweating or cyanosis. Subsequent routine examination is not necessary, but the opportunity can be taken to examine the heart when examining the child for other reasons.

* Always check the femoral or foot pulses.
* *High risk of congenital heart disease.* Ensure that all children at risk have an ECG and echocardiogram in the first few weeks of life. These are children:
  (a) with conditions that put them at higher risk, e.g. Down's syndrome;
  (b) with a sibling with congenital heart disease.

'INNOCENT' MURMURS

* Innocent murmurs occur in 50% or more of children. They are more often present in the febrile child. Characteristically:
  (a) they are of low intensity, and are even quieter sitting up;
  (b) they have a musical quality;
  (c) they are localized to a small precordial area;
  (d) there are no other symptoms or signs of heart disease.
* Arrange an echocardiogram or refer if there is any suspicion of underlying disease.

GROWTH

* The infant usually regains his or her birth weight by the end of the second week, and then gains 150–200 g per week. A doubling of birth weight is achieved by the age of 4–5 months. Growth then slows, and the birth weight is tripled by 12–13 months. Only 2–3 kg is gained in the second year.
* There is no reason to assume that every baby should continue on the same centile from birth onward.
* Most babies who cross centile lines in the first few months are adopting their own genetically determined growth pattern.
* It is rare for significant changes in weight to be the only clue to serious abnormality.
* All measurements should be plotted on:
  (a) the 1990 nine-centile charts, available from the Child Growth Foundation and now in most parent-held child health records in UK; or
  (b) the new WHO 0–5 years growth charts which were launched nationally in April 2009. They are based on the growth patterns of exclusively breastfed babies and show that these babies gain weight more slowly than formula fed babies.

Charts and measuring equipment are available from:

(a) the Child Growth Foundation, 2 Mayfield Avenue, London W4 1PW, tel. 020 8995 0257 or 020 8994 7625, www.childgrowthfoundation.org

(b) www.health-for-all-children.co.uk

Recommendations for routine growth monitoring

* *Check weight:* at birth, then regularly at routine well baby checks. Too frequent weighing may pick up small fluctuations and increase anxiety. The latest Hall report (Hall 4) recommends weighing and plotting at immunizations, at 8, 12 and 24 months and between 3 and 4 years.
* *Check height/length* if there are concerns about wellbeing or growth. Only check routinely at age 5. Only check length at the neonatal or 6-week check if there was a low birth weight or if there is some other concern about health.
* *Check head circumference:*
  (a) *before discharge from hospital* (excessive moulding, etc. should be noted, and the head circumference repeated a few days later);
  (b) *at 6–8 weeks of age.* If the plotted results follow the centile lines, no further routine measurements are necessary.

Recheck only if there is concern about the child's growth, health or development.

Where there is concern about growth

* Measure and plot the child's length, weight and head circumference. Include birth weight and head circumference, and any other clinic weights, on the chart. Use the charts in the Personal Child Health Record or obtain them from www.health-for-all-children.co.uk
* Enquire about the child's diet, general behaviour and the character of the stool (irritability and steatorrhoea are indicators of malabsorption).
* Examine the infant fully both to reassure the parents and to exclude cardiac, renal or other system disorders. Check the urine for protein, and send a specimen for culture. Refer if the child appears unwell.
* Assess the environment in which the child is being raised, and the parents' relationship with the child.

* Ask the advice of the health visitor in all cases, but particularly if there is reason to suspect 'non-organic failure to thrive'.

Abnormal patterns of growth

* *Slow weight gain.* Consider referral if the weight gain is slow and crosses two channels (a channel is the space between two centile lines). Refer more urgently if there are unexplained symptoms or, in addition, a fall-off in head circumference.
* *Single measurement of length/height.* Refer any child who has a single length or height measurement above the 99.6 centile or below the 0.4 centile.
* *Slow gain in height.* Refer if the child's height crosses two channel widths. Review a preschool child after a year if the child's height crosses one channel width. Review a school age child after a year if the height crosses half a channel width or more.
* *Single measurement of head circumference.* Refer if a single measurement is above the 99.6 centile or below the 0.4 centile. The exception may be when development is normal and the baby's head circumference is commensurate with the parents' head circumference centiles.
* *Head circumference crossing centiles upwards.* Refer urgently if the child shows symptoms or signs of hydrocephalus or other abnormality. If there are no accompanying symptoms or signs, take two measurements over a 4-week period, and then decide whether to refer.
* *Head circumference crossing centiles downwards.* If the child is thriving there is no cause for concern. Refer if the growth line is below the second centile and falling from it.

HEARING DEFECTS

● If nothing is done, children with sensorineural hearing loss suffer impairment of language acquisition. Educational difficulties follow and lead to social isolation, an increased risk of mental health problems and reduced prospects for independence in later life.

● The estimated birth prevalence of congenital severe (≥ 40 dB) hearing impairment is 1.16 per 1000. (A number acquire this severe loss of hearing bringing this figure to 1.3 per 1000. These children need a hearing aid.)

- At least a further 0.3 per 1000 have a hearing loss which is less than 40 dB but is sufficient for the child to need a hearing aid.
- If all high-risk factors are considered, between 40% and 70% of all cases could be identified by testing 5–10% of all babies.
- The following are at a high risk of congenital deafness:
  (a) survivors of intensive care, gestation < 33 weeks or birth weight < 1500 g, severe asphyxia at birth, meningitis, marked jaundice requiring exchange transfusion, or treatment with aminoglycosides;
  (b) survivors of severe intrauterine growth retardation;
  (c) those with a family history of deafness which may be genetic;
  (d) children of mothers who suffered from rubella, CMV or other relevant infections during pregnancy;
  (e) children with dysmorphic syndromes, particularly those affecting the head and neck.

Paediatric departments should follow-up all high-risk infants and assess their hearing. All babies now have an automated otoacoustic emissions test, and those with an unsatisfactory response have a second screening. Those who fail this should have two automated auditory brainstem response tests.

- * Refer any high-risk infant not followed up, or where there is concern. Parents' recognition of deafness is often accurate.
- * Refer any child not performing as below. Older children are best seen first by the health visitor.
  (a) *3 months:* infants smile at the sound of parents' voices, even when they cannot see them, and turn the head in response.
  (b) *6 months:* infants turn immediately and accurately across the room to a parent's voice.
  (c) *9 months:* infants listen attentively to sounds and try to localize very quiet sounds. They enjoy making a loud tuneful babble.
  (d) *12 months:* infants respond to their own names.

VISION DEFECTS

- * Examine the eyes of all babies after birth and at 6–8 weeks. Check the pupils, the alignment of the eyes and the red reflex. Use the ophthalmoscope set on +3, held 30 cm from the baby's eye.
- * *Neonates.* Check that the following infants have been examined by an ophthalmologist:
  (a) *those born prematurely* under 1250 g and/or under 32 weeks gestation;
  (b) *those with a family history of inherited eye disease;*
  (c) *those with a permanent squint* urgently, to exclude retinoblastoma and cataracts.
- * *Infants.* Refer if any of the following are present:
  (a) a lack of fixation or following movements;
  (b) nystagmus;
  (c) photophobia;
  (d) opacities (best seen with an ophthalmoscope as above);
  (e) delayed development possibly due to visual problems. Children aged 6–9 months should: look at, recognize and follow their parents with their eyes; examine their hands and feet; look at and reach towards small objects.
- * *School age.* Any child picked up during routine screening or by an optician should be referred for full assessment by an ophthalmologist. Early treatment may reduce the development of amblyopia (Dutton and Cleary 2004).

Squint

- Premature babies and those who had a stormy perinatal course are more prone to squint. If one parent has a history of squint the risk factor for the child increases by 25%. If both parents have a history of squint the risk factor increases by 70%.
- A true squint involves deviation from the object of regard by one or both eyes.
- A squint that is present within the first year of life is regarded as an infantile squint, either in-turning (esotropia) or out-turning (exotropia). It may be intermittent and may only appear at times or on cover testing (eso- or exophoria).
- The end result of a missed squint may be severe amblyopia (poor visual development because of competitive inhibition) or, worse still, missed pathology.

- Amblyopia is best corrected in the first 4 years of life. After that it can be difficult to guarantee a good visual result. Remember the old adage 'A true squint never goes away'.
- ✳ Take parents' concerns about a squint seriously and refer if there is any doubt. Establish what exactly they mean by a squint. They may mean that the child tends to screw up the eyes not squint.
- ✳ Refer for orthoptic assessment if there is any suspicion of a squint within the first year of life. Refer urgently if there is a persistent squint in the first 6 months of life. It may be the sign of an abnormality of the globe such as retinoblastoma, cataract, etc.

Older children presenting with squint (e.g. at 2–3 years of age) are often found to have a significant refractive error.

- The commonest squint is an esotropia or esophoria (i.e. a constant or latent in-turning) which can be controlled with glasses.
- Some have no refractive error but a muscle imbalance that can only be corrected by surgery.
- Initially management is directed at correcting any refractive error and amblyopia. Only when there is a non-responsive squint or residual squint is surgery needed.
- Divergent squints are sometimes associated with short sight (myopia) and the child is often photophobic and screws up the affected eye in bright light.

A squint may be indicated by the following:

(a) *appearance*. The squint may be apparent on examination. However, broad epicanthic folds can give the appearance of a convergent squint (pseudosquint). When a true squint is present the child may hold the head at a tilt to maintain binocular fixation;

(b) *corneal reflections*. These should be identical in position in both eyes. With the child focusing on a small toy, check the reflection of a diffuse focal light, e.g. a small torch held 40 cm away from the eye or the reflection of a window behind the observer;

(c) *cover test*. This is used to exclude a latent squint. Encourage the child to look at a toy while one eye, then the other, is occluded. If a squint is present in the occluded eye it will move to take up fixation when uncovered. Ideally, fixation

should be tested with both a near object (about 30 cm) and one at 6 m;

(d) *eye movements*. These should be assessed in the horizontal and vertical planes.

- ✳ If a squint is found, look for an intact red reflex with an ophthalmoscope.

DISORDERS OF DEVELOPMENT AND BEHAVIOUR

- The more common disorders are: cerebral palsy, 1.5–3 per 1000; Duchenne muscular dystrophy, 3 per 10,000; severe learning disability (previously called mental handicap), 3.7 per 1000; Down's syndrome, 1 per 600; persisting speech and language impairments, 2 per 1000; autistic spectrum disorder, 1–2 per 1000.
- The GP who remains vigilant despite normal routine screening results is more likely to detect the milder manifestations of the above. False reassurance is a common cause for a delay in diagnosis.

For developmental charts, see Appendix 6.

LEARNING DIFFICULTIES

See page 627.

SPEECH AND LANGUAGE

- Early detection and intervention where speech and language are delayed may avoid irreversible impairment of language acquisition and limit the negative experiences which seriously affect subsequent health and progress (Garrett and Nye 2003).
- ✳ Discuss with the health visitor whether emotional deprivation may be contributing to the poor language development.
- ✳ Refer any child where there is parental concern about speech to a speech therapist.
- ✳ Refer children as follows:
  (a) *18 months*: not using any words; unable to identify common objects;
  (b) *2 years*: words are not joined together; simple instructions are not understood;
  (c) *3 years*: not using sentences; speech is not understood outside the family; simple concepts are not understood;

(d) *4 years:* difficulty in following a story; sentences are immature; poor understanding of simple concepts, e.g. colour; or difficulty in holding a conversation.

∗ Refer preschool children with a stammer. 5% of children stammer at some stage; 74% recover without professional help. However, because early treatment is more effective than treatment later, the British Stammering Association (BSA) recommends that all children who stammer should have an early assessment by a speech and language therapist. Referral can be made by Nursery staff, by a health visitor or direct by the parents themselves, who can find details of the local Speech and Language Therapy Service from the Primary Care Trust. Certainly, a child with a stammer that affects at least 2% of syllables and that has been present for, say, 6 months, should be referred. The Lidcombe programme has been shown to reduce the frequency of stammering after 9 months by 77% in such children compared to 43% in controls (Jones, Onslow, Packman, *et al.* 2005). The BSA website www.stammering.org has guidance for parents on how to manage their child with a stammer.

AUTISM AND ASPERGER'S SYNDROME

Baird G, Cass H, Slonims V. 2003. Diagnosis of autism. BMJ 327, 488–493.
    Parr J. 2008. Autism. *Clinical Evidence.* http:// clinicalevidence.bmj.com

● Autism is characterized by a triad of symptoms: impairment in social interaction, impairments in communication, and restricted interests and repetitive behaviour. 50% of autistic people have severe learning disability (IQ< 50), 25% have moderate learning difficulties (IQ 50–75).

● Asperger's syndrome is usually diagnosed later in life, and is characterized by abnormalities of gaze, poverty of expression, a lack of feeling for others, lack of humour, extreme egocentrism and an idiosyncratic attachment to objects. Intelligence and language are normal.

● Children in whom the condition is suspected should be referred early to a community paediatrician or child development team. In confirmed cases, early diagnosis allows behavioural management which can limit inappropriate behaviour.

∗ Refer all children under the age of 2 for assessment, who:

(a) lack a social smile, lack appropriate facial expression, have poor attention, poor social interaction;

(b) ignore people, sit or play alone, lack eye contact, lack appropriate gestures or emotional expression, who are not pointing things out or looking at others.

Children aged 2–3 years

∗ Refer those who:

(a) have no babble, pointing or other gesture by 12 months;

(b) no single words by 18 months;

(c) no two word spontaneous (not echoed) phrases by 24 months;

(d) any loss of any language or social skills at any age.

∗ Consider autism if they show:

(a) *Impaired social communication:* language not used as a tool for exchange; poor comprehension, talking incessantly about one topic; inappropriate laughing and giggling; echolalia – copying words like a parrot; no eye contact.

(b) *Impaired social interaction:* aloofness/ indifference to others, not playing with others; only joining in if an adult assists or insists; one-sided interaction with no response to another child; 'odd interactions', e.g. inappropriate questions.

(c) *Impairment in other interests:* over-sensitivity to sound or touch; hitting, biting, or aggression; lack of creative or pretend play; play becomes stereotyped or obsessional and ritualized; inability to cope with change; repetitive playing with toys, e.g. lining up dolls; playing with switches.

Later childhood

- Communication impairments:
  - (a) abnormal language development especially muteness and inappropriate rhyming;
  - (b) echolalia;
  - (c) use of the third person to refer to oneself;
  - (d) limited vocabulary for age or social group;
  - (e) limited language in communication.
- Social impairments:
  - (a) inability to join in with or play with other children, inappropriate attempt at joining in (disruptive or aggressive behaviour);
  - (b) lack of awareness of social and classroom 'norms', e.g. dress, or how to participate;
  - (c) abnormal relationship to adults (too intense or no relationship);
  - (d) extreme reactions to invasion of personal space or to being hurried.

Management

- Once the diagnosis has been made the role of the GP is to support the family, to ensure that they are in touch with the appropriate specialists, and that they have all the information they need.
- Each child will need a programme tailored to his or her particular needs. Different educational programmes have been developed to help children develop basic skills before they attend school. While evidence for their effectiveness is sparse they do appear to give parents more confidence that they can help their child.
- There is no evidence that dietary interventions are useful.
- Most children with autism do not need medication but a minority have symptoms which can be helped. Methylphenidate may reduce hyperactivity, risperidone may reduce aggression and SSRIs may help depression, anxiety and repetitive behaviour.

Patient contact: National Autistic Society, 393 City Road, London EC1V 1NG, tel. 020 7903 3599; fax 020 7833 9666; e-mail: nas@nas.org.uk; www.nas.org.uk
   Patient leaflet: Parr J. 2008. Autism. *Clinical Evidence.* http://clinicalevidence.bmj.com

DYSLEXIA

REVIEW

Snowling MJ. 1996. Dyslexia: a hundred years on. BMJ 313, 1096

- Dyslexia is a specific learning difficulty which results in a significant and persistent difficulty with reading, spelling, written prose and sometimes arithmetic. The individual may also have difficulties with orientation in time, short-term memory, sequencing, auditory or visual perception and motor skills.
- It is estimated that around 350,000 UK schoolchildren suffer from dyslexia, of whom 75% are boys.
- Early recognition and management may allow greater attainment of educational potential and limit the stress and frustration that occurs when the problem is not recognized and the child falls behind at school.

The preschool child

(a) *Speech or language delay* (see page 90):
   * Refer the child to a speech therapist if there is any delay in speech, especially where there is difficulty in naming objects correctly, remembering two instructions or recognizing similarities in rhyming words or parts of words.
   * Encourage the parents to inform the school of any *past* difficulties when the child begins schooling. Many children with early language delay who speak normally by the time they go to school subsequently have difficulty learning to read or write.

(b) *Poor hand/eye coordination and visual perceptual problems*: The child may appear to be developing normally, but has marked difficulty copying shapes and patterns, catching a ball, dressing in the right order, tying shoelaces, clapping in rhythm, etc.
   * Refer the child to a community paediatrician.

The school–age child

Refer children with:

(a) a lack of educational achievement, particularly in learning to read, write and spell; difficulty in answering questions on paper;

(b) a lack of understanding of time and tense;

(c) poor concentration in reading and writing;

(d) secondary emotional symptoms (e.g. disruptive behaviour, psychosomatic symptoms).

The older child failing at school

* Refer to the appropriate specialist if specific disabilities are apparent, e.g. problems with:

  (a) visual function;

  (b) auditory ability;

  (c) speech or language difficulties;

  (d) motor coordination.

* *If no specific disabilities are apparent*, refer for assessment either by a chartered psychologist or community paediatrician. Include a report from the school with the referral.

* Advise the parent to get further advice from one of the support organizations.

* Encourage the parents to support the child, for example by:

  (a) helping him or her to maintain self-image;

  (b) encouraging involvement in hobbies where the child can succeed;

  (c) supporting the child in schoolwork, with an awareness that the child is more likely to be tired than others.

* Where the child is suffering significantly at school, encourage the parent to apply to the school to have the child assessed with a view to making a 'Statement of Special Educational Needs'.

PATIENT CONTACT

The British Dyslexia Association, www.bdadyslexia. org.uk

ATTENTION DEFICIT (HYPERACTIVITY) DISORDER (ADHD)

GUIDELINES

Scottish Intercollegiate Guidelines Network (SIGN). June 2001. *Attention Deficit and Hyperkinetic Disorders in Children and Young People.* www.sign.ac.uk

NICE. 2008. *Attention Deficit/Hyperactivity Disorder (ADHD).* National Institute for Clinical Excellence. www.nice.org.uk

Keen D, Hadjikoumi I. *ADHD in Children and Adolescents.* http://clinicalevidence.bmj.com

● ADHD is characterized by the presence of inattention, hyperactivity and impulsivity for at least 6 months. For the detailed Diagnostic and Statistical Manual (DSM) diagnostic criteria, see the ADDnet website in the box below. Other conditions frequently co-exist with ADHD, including developmental disorders and psychiatric disorders.

● In the UK, the estimated prevalence of ADHD is 1.7% of boys of primary school age (Taylor, Sandberg, Thorley and Giles 1991). Only about one third grow out of their condition completely (Bellak and Black 1992). Only about 10% of children in the UK with ADHD are diagnosed.

● Not all are characterized by hyperactivity. A subgroup occurs who are inattentive and do particularly badly at school.

● Hyperactivity in preschool years is associated with conduct disorders in school-age children.

● Dietary alteration may have value in a very small number of children, especially where ingestion and effect are obvious. Exclusion diets are demanding and tedious, and should only be attempted with a dietician's support.

GP management

The child with ADHD may already have seen a number of different agencies (psychologists, social workers, etc.) and may have been recognized as having special educational needs. Where there is concern that a more specific diagnosis and treatment may help:

* Refer to a local specialist who has an interest in the problem. This may be a child or adolescent psychiatrist or paediatrician. Include a report by

the parents of their child's symptoms, copies of all psychologists' and psychiatrists' reports as well as an up-to-date report from the school.

* Do not start drug treatment. A GP may, however, continue treatment once started.

   (a) Methylphenidate (ritalin) and dexamphetamine have been shown to be markedly effective in improving behaviour, but do have side-effects. They may affect appetite and growth, and sleep if given too late in the day.

   (b) Clonidine is less commonly used; there is some evidence to support its use (Hazell and Stuart 2003; Tourette's Syndrome Study Group 2002).

   (c) Atomoxetine may be effective when first line drugs fail.

   (d) A number of other drugs are used, e.g. risperidone, venlafaxine, or buproprion, but there is little research evidence to support their use.

* Check FBC and ferritin if there is clinical suspicion of anaemia. There is evidence of reduced serum ferritin in this condition, that lower levels correlate with more severe symptoms (Konofal, Lecendreux, Arnulf, *et al.* 2004) and limited evidence that behaviour may be improved with iron supplementation (Sever, Ashkenazi, Tyano, *et al.* 1997).

* Conduct disorders/delinquency should be referred. There may be benefit from drug therapy and family and parent interventions (Woolfenden, Williams and Peat 2001).

* Assess the mental health of the parents. They may benefit from drug therapy or training programmes (Barlow and Coren 2001).

* Recommend that the parents contact national or local organizations (see box below).

* Explain to the parents that treatment may or may not involve drugs, but includes:

   (a) an understanding of the condition, particularly that it is innate and not their child being naughty;

   (b) behavioural modification, e.g. where the child is positively rewarded for good behaviour;

   (c) alteration of the environment, e.g. to reduce distractions.

* Reassure the parents that the drugs used are not addictive and that there is some evidence that alcohol and drug misuse is less common in treated subjects (Wilens, Faraone, Biederman, *et al.* 2003).

PARENT SUPPORT GROUPS

ADDISS, The National Attention Deficit Disorder Information and Support Service, www.addiss.co.uk

   Hyperactive Children's Support Group, 71 Whyke Lane, Chichester, West Sussex PO19 7PD, tel. 01243 551313, fax 01243 552019, www.hacsg.org.uk

Parent leaflets

Keen D, Hadjikoumi I. ADHD in children and adolescents. Patient leaflets: ADHD: what is it? and ADHD: what treatments work? Available http://clinicalevidence.bmj.com

   Royal College of Psychiatrists. ADHD hyperkinetic disorder; leaflet 5. Available www.rcpsych.ac.uk/mentalhealthinfoforall/mentalhealthandgrowingup.aspx

---

DYSPRAXIA (DEVELOPMENTAL COORDINATION DISORDER)

Between 6 and 10% of children in the UK are affected. Children have extreme difficulty in learning motor skills and there may be other difficulties with language, perception and thought. It is commoner in infants who were pre-term. In preschool children there may be:

(a) a history of lateness in reaching milestones, e.g. sitting, walking, etc.;

(b) a difficulty in running, hopping or jumping;

(c) a need to be taught how to do things which other children learn instinctively;

(d) difficulty in dressing;

(e) slowness and hesitancy in actions;

(f) difficulty in gripping a pencil;

(g) difficulty in sorting shapes, jigsaws, etc.;

(h) difficulty in catching or kicking a ball.

The school-age child may:

(a) have all the problems above;

(b) avoid activities that involve coordination;

(c) be unable to remember or follow instructions;

(d) have other difficulties, e.g. in reading and writing or a reduced attention span.

* Refer for assessment by a local specialist.

* Advise the parents to contact the Dyspraxia Foundation for further advice on management and assessment. They publish a number of information sheets and books for parents and professionals.

PATIENT SUPPORT

Dyspraxia Foundation, 8 West Alley, Hitchin, Herts SG5 1EG; http://www.dyspraxiafoundation.org.uk

CHILD PROTECTION

RESOURCES

Department of Health. *The Children Act Report 2004.* www.opsi.gov.uk, search on 'Children Act 2004'

HM Government. *Every Child Matters.* www.dcsf. gov.uk/everychildmatters

HM Government. 2006. *Working Together to Safeguard Children.*

Hobbs CJ, Hanks HGI, Wynne JM. 2000. *Child Abuse and Neglect: A Clinician's Handbook.* Churchill Livingstone, Edinburgh.

Eminson M, Postlethwaite RJ (Eds). 2000. *Munchausen Syndrome by Proxy Abuse: A Practical Approach.* Arnold, London.

National Institute for Health and Clinical Excellence. July 2009. *When to Suspect Child Maltreatment.* NICE CG 89, www.nice.org.uk

HM Government. 2008. *Safeguarding Children in Whom Illness is Fabricated or Induced.* www.dcsf. gov.uk

Every area in England has a Local Safeguarding Childrens' Board (LSCB) which produces and oversees local child protection procedures. It includes a PCT representative and a named GP.

Consider discussing queries with the local named GP for child protection or the local designated doctor.

PHYSICAL ABUSE (NON–ACCIDENTAL INJURY)

Physical abuse should be considered when:

(a) the explanation is inconsistent with the injuries;

(b) parents /carers delay seeking help for an injury;

(c) an injury is combined with hostile or inappropriate parental / carer interactions with their child;

(d) the child appears wary ('frozen watchfulness').

The following injuries should arouse suspicion and further intervention:

(a) bruises in the shape of fingers, grip marks or an implement (e.g. belt or stick);

(b) burns or scalds that may have arisen from being held against a hot object or in scalding water;

(c) any injury in a child who is not independently mobile unless clearly an unavoidable accident;

(d) probable cigarette burn or strap injuries;

(e) a torn frenulum in an infant (from ramming a bottle into the baby's mouth);

(e) long bone or rib fracture in an infant;

(f) injuries on non-bony prominences of head, neck or buttocks;

(g) multiple unexplained lacerations, abrasions or scars.

Note that this list is not exhaustive.

CHILD SEXUAL ABUSE (CSA)

This includes exposure to indecent acts, pornography, masturbation of an adult, being used for intracrural intercourse, or being penetrated orally, vaginally or anally. Children may present with:

(a) symptoms of anal or genital trauma or infection, such as soreness, pain, bleeding or discharge;

(b) emotional disturbance – e.g. loss of concentration, recurrent abdominal pain, enuresis, soiling, anorexia or self-harm;

(c) sexualized behaviour or inappropriate sexual knowledge for their age.

NEGLECT AND EMOTIONAL MALTREATMENT

Neglect is a common form of maltreatment in the UK. It is insidious and adversely affects children in many ways, including retardation of growth and development. Poor general health may be a feature.

All forms of abuse involve emotional maltreatment. Emotional abuse is complex and its long-term effects on children can result in impaired social, emotional and intellectual functioning, disturbed attachments and long-term mental health difficulties.

The symptoms of neglect and emotional abuse vary with the age of the child and may include:

(a) *infants:* failure to thrive, recurrent and persistent minor infections, severe nappy rash, generally delayed development, anxiety and a lack of social responsiveness;

(b) *preschool children:* unkempt or dirty, excessive or under weight, short stature, delayed language development, a poor attention span, overactivity, aggressive and impulsive behaviour, indiscriminate friendliness and desire for physical contact from strangers;

(c) *school children:* poor hygiene and unkempt appearance, poor school progress, lack of self-esteem, poor coping skills, social and emotional immaturity, few friendships, challenging behaviour, self-stimulating or injurious behaviour, soiling, secondary bed wetting.

Neglect may include parental failure to bring the child to medical appointments or to seek medical advice when needed.

FACTITIOUS AND INDUCED ILLNESS (FORMERLY MUNCHAUSEN'S SYNDROME BY PROXY)

There is a spectrum of parental behaviour in seeking advice about their children's health ranging from neglect of symptoms through a normal response to over-anxiety, exaggeration or even invention or induction of symptoms. The latter are known as factitious or induced illness. Children may be abused by unnecessary lengthy or invasive investigations as well as by the actions of the carer.
  Alerting features include:

(a) claims of illness and seeking multiple opinions or 'doctor shopping' when the child is well;

(b) repeated episodes of unexplained illness, e.g. seizures, or haematuria, only witnessed by the carer;

(c) exaggerated invalidism in which a child with a medical condition or disability is brought up with a greater degree of mental or physical incapacity than is actually present;

(d) parental gain, such as parents claiming disability living allowance for a child inappropriately.

MANAGEMENT OF SUSPECTED CHILD ABUSE

(a) A full history should be taken from the informant and recorded.

(b) The parent's explanation for any injuries should be noted.

(c) The child should be fully examined, except in suspected CSA, and the examination fully documented. In suspected CSA, detailed examination should be done by a doctor with experience in child protection and carried out only after a multiagency discussion. Repeated ano-genital examinations are not in a child's best interest but sometimes medical symptoms mean that a GP will need to look briefly at the genital or anal area.

IF ABUSE IS LIKELY

The urgency of action will be determined by:

(a) the severity of injuries and need for immediate medical attention; and the type of abuse. Physical abuse needs more urgent action than sexual or emotional abuse, which need a planned response;

(b) the child's safety, e.g. if the abuser is still living in the house the risk to the child is greater. Also important is the age of the child; a younger child is at greater risk.

ACTIONS

* Contact the Social Services Office (now usually referred to as Social Care) when there is suspicion of abuse, after treatment of any acute injuries.

* Discuss immediate plans with the parents. Detailed discussion is usually unwise, and it may be best to say no more than that there is a need to seek further advice.

* Arrange for a second examination by another doctor:

  (a) if possible physical abuse, by the consultant or registrar on call;

  (b) if possible CSA, the social worker will arrange this;

  (c) for failure to thrive, refer to the health visitor and arrange for outpatient assessment by a consultant paediatrician; for developmental delay refer to the health visitor/community paediatrician;

(d) if emotional abuse and fabricated illness are suspected refer to a child psychiatrist after discussion with the social worker.

WHAT MAY HAPPEN NEXT

Social care and the police child protection team (CPT) will consider doing the following;

(a) draw together information about the child and family;

(b) have a strategy discussion involving health professionals but not parents;

(c) do a home visit;

(d) decide whether to make a more detailed assessment (Section 47 enquiry);

(e) consider the need to remove the child to a safe place. If the child is not admitted to hospital this is arranged by a social worker or the NSPCC or the police.

There is now provision for the child to be examined in the home, without removal from it (see below).

Case conference

(a) Must be held within statutory time limits.

(b) GP will be expected to provide a report or to attend the case conference.

(c) If the case conference decides that the child and siblings need to be the subject of child protection plans (formerly this step was called putting their names on the Child Protection Register), a key worker will be appointed and a core group of professionals will be set up to take things forward.

(d) Primary care professionals should keep the key worker informed about any further worries.

WHERE ACCESS TO THE CHILD IS REFUSED

* Contact the Social Services Department (SSD) or the NSPCC, who can apply to the court for a Child Assessment Order. The order will only be granted if the circumstances meet the same criteria as are needed for an Emergency Protection Order (see below). The order lasts for a maximum of 7 days, and the court will direct the nature and type of assessment to be carried out and whether the child should be kept away from home for the purposes of the assessment.

* *Police protection.* If the situation is more urgent, the police have the right of entry, and can remove a child for a maximum of 72 hours.

POSSIBLE OUTCOMES

'PLACE OF SAFETY'

The court may issue an Emergency Protection Order where there is reasonable cause to believe that the child is likely to suffer significant harm if:

(a) the child is not removed to another place; or

(b) the child's removal from where he or she is accommodated is not prevented.

Application is usually from the SSD or NSPCC, but may be made by anyone. The Order is limited to 8 days, and a single extension of 7 days may be granted. The parents can appeal if they were not present initially, but not within the first 72 hours. The court will direct the nature and type of assessment.

CHILD PROTECTION PLAN (FORMERLY THE CHILD PROTECTION REGISTER)

This is decided at the case conference. It has statutory legal standing under the Children Acts, but does not confer legal rights to the local authority; it signifies the level of concern and the need for monitoring and has an expectation of co-operation from parents. The child protection plan is the responsibility of social care (social services department), and involves the child being seen by one of a specified group of professionals every 10 days to check on their welfare plus regular meetings. A child protection plan can last up to 6 months before it has to be reviewed in another case conference. If parents fail to co-operate with this the local authority will decide whether to apply to the family courts for a legal order.

SUPERVISION ORDER

This will only be granted if the requirements for Care Orders are met (see below). The court can make a Supervision Order rather than a Care

Order. A Supervision Order can apply for a maximum of 3 years, but is usually reviewed regularly. It does not give the local authority parental responsibility, which is given to a person appointed by the court and supervised by the person taking out the order. Certain conditions may be applied, e.g. regular weighing, regular attendance by the social worker, etc.

CARE ORDER

The court may issue a Care Order if:

(a) the child is suffering or is likely to suffer significant harm; and

(b) the harm or likelihood of harm is attributable either to the care given or likely to be given to the child if the Order were not made or to the child being beyond parental control.

A Care Order commits a child to the care of the local SSD, usually until the age of 17. Being 'in care' is now legally termed being 'accommodated' by the local authority.

Parental responsibility is shared with the SSD, who have the power to decide how much the parents may exercise their parental responsibility. The SSD must allow reasonable contact and try to promote such contact. The parents or the local authority can return to the court and apply for a revocation of the Care Order. In some cases, the child may be allowed home on trial by the local authority.

While a court is considering its decision, it may make an Interim Supervision or Care Order.

MEDICAL REPORTS AND CONFIDENTIALITY

Under the Children Acts 1989–2006, a GP may be asked to submit a written report. The DoH gives the following guidelines for reports:

(a) confine the report to the facts;

(b) present objective and measurable evidence of the child's health and development;

(c) where subjective views are given, they should reflect balanced professional judgment;

(d) comment and advice should be in the context of the local authority and the court's considerations about whether to apply for, or make, an order;

(e) the more comprehensive and comprehensible the report, the less likely it is that the GP will be called to give verbal evidence in person;

(f) the child's needs are paramount.

PRIVATE FOSTERING ARRANGEMENTS

● It is estimated that 8–10,000 children under the age of 16, are fostered by an adult, who is not a relative, as a private arrangement between parent and carer. Anecdotal evidence suggests that children in private foster care are at a high risk of abuse. This includes:

(a) children whose immigrant parents are working;

(b) adolescents estranged from their families;

(c) children from overseas attending language schools, independent schools, etc., and refugee children;

(d) children brought to the UK with an intent to adopt.

● Local authorities have duties under the Children Acts to satisfy themselves that the welfare of the child is not at risk by checking the suitability of the placement, making regular visits to the child, and offering advice where required.

∗ Notify social services of any child in private foster care, especially if they are felt to be at risk of abuse or neglect.

DIVORCE/MARITAL STRIFE: THE EFFECTS ON THE CHILDREN

REVIEW

Hartnup T. 1996. Divorce and marital strife and their effects on children. Arch Dis Child 75, 1–3

● One in three marriages in the UK ends in divorce, with the result that one in five to six children is affected.

● One third of the children of divorced parents suffer long-term psychological effects similar to those resulting from traumatic experiences. Children are likely to be worse 1 year after the divorce than at the time.

● There is some evidence that support and cognitive therapy significantly reduces mental health problems (Woclik, Sandler, Millsap, et al. 2002).

∗ Advise parents, if the opportunity arises, that children need:

(a) clear information in language that is appropriate to their age;

(b) to maintain the best possible relationships with both their parents;

(c) to express their feelings and talk about what troubles them;

(d) to be kept clear of conflict between the parents;

(e) consistency and continuity.

* Consider recommending that the parents contact *Resolution*. They are a group of family lawyers (5000) committed to a non-confrontational approach. Tel. 08457 585671, www.resolution. org.uk

* Refer a child who is exhibiting abnormal behaviour or mental health problems to the Child and Adolescent Mental Health Unit.

INFORMATION FOR PARENTS AND CHILDREN

P Hall. 2007. *Help Your Children Cope with Your Divorce: A 'Relate' Guide.* Vermilion

R Stones. 2002. *Children Don't Divorce.* Happy Cat Books

D Sanders. *Kids in the Middle.* http://publications. dcsf.gov.uk, search for 'Kids In The Middle'

McGhee C. *Separation and Divorce: Helping Parents Help Children.* Can be downloaded from www. resolution.org.uk

Royal College of Psychiatrists. *Separation and Divorce.* Leaflet 14, available on www.rcpsych.ac.uk/ mentalhealthinfoforall/mentalhealthandgrowingup. aspx

---

INFANCY

PRETERM INFANTS

There is an increasing tendency for these infants to be discharged early, often on reaching 1.8 kg. They may still be tube fed and/or on oxygen.

FEEDING

* Check that the baby is being given vitamins and iron (see page 84).

* Continue vitamins until 2 years old depending on the adequacy of the diet (continue later in the fussy eater).

* Continue iron until mixed feeding is achieved, usually around 6 months – again longer if the diet is inadequate.

* Preterm infants with chronic lung disease may need calorie-supplemented milk (e.g. by adding Duocal or using ready-made high-energy infant formula).

WEIGHT AND DEVELOPMENT

Preterm infants will, by the age of 2 years, reach a stage of development and a weight that is appropriate for their date of birth, regardless of their gestational age. Infants who have undergone prolonged ventilation are usually significantly behind in gross motor development, but should eventually catch up.

* Plot weight/length and OFC and expect the developmental stage appropriate for corrected age until the age of 2. For instance, if the infant is 6 months old and 3 months premature, plot as 3 months.

IMMUNIZATION

Give routine immunizations at the usual times (8, 12 and 16 weeks from *birth*). Neonatal convulsions without progressive neurological disorder are not a contraindication to pertussis immunization (but see page 48). The support of the neonatologist may reassure the parents.

RESPIRATORY INFECTION

Preterm infants with chronic lung disease are at high risk of infection, both viral and bacterial, especially with *Moxarella*. Antibiotics should be given more freely, e.g. co-amoxiclav.

FEEDING PROBLEMS

Advice when the child is being weaned can avoid subsequent feeding problems. The following 'rules' may help.

(a) Mealtimes should be organized and unhurried. If necessary, the child should be fed before the family eats, but any advantage gained should be balanced against the benefit of the whole family eating together.

(b) A variety of foods should be offered, of an interest to the child and in small portions.

Finger foods of fun sizes and shapes may help encourage children to take an interest in feeding themselves. However, there is little value in striving too hard to change a child who is resistant and growing well on a bland but nutritious diet.

(c) The child should not be forced to eat, or hovered over while eating. However, a parent should remain by or within the sight of the child.

(d) Food rejected should be put aside and brought back if requested. A new meal should not be prepared, nor milk offered as a calorie substitute. Snacks between meals should be avoided or minimized if mealtimes are problematic and high calorie snacks should not be used as substitutes. Some parents resort to these because they think a child may 'fade away'!

(e) Anger at rejection or bad behaviour should be avoided. It is likely to lead to a battle, which the child will always win.

THE CHILD WHO IS UNWILLING TO TAKE SOLID FOOD

The child is usually well nourished, but taking large quantities of milk.

* Advise parents to reduce the milk intake by about a half and to introduce a variety of foods. The above rules apply, and it is important that the parents do not weaken because they feel the child will starve. A further reduction of milk may be necessary if the initial reduction is unsuccessful.

THE CHILD WHO WON'T TAKE LUMPY FOODS

* Advise the parents, using the rules above, and encourage a combination of homogenized and finger foods with the steady introduction of more solid foods.
* Refer if the problem persists. Other factors may be a problem, e.g. large tonsils, or oesophageal or neurodevelopmental problems.

VOMITING IN INFANCY

Vomiting is common in infancy, and does not usually indicate severe illness.

* Refer any child with:
  (a) bile-stained vomitus;
  (b) forceful vomiting;
  (c) persistent vomiting, especially when it continues through to the next feed;
  (d) weight loss/weight crossing centiles;
  (e) abdominal distension;
  (f) localized tenderness;
  (g) any child who is unwell.

Note: Congenital pyloric stenosis is most common at the age of 4–6 weeks, and is unlikely to develop after that.

Possible causes of vomiting are:

(a) *overfeeding*;
(b) *possetting*; the infant brings up small amounts on winding;
(c) *gastro-oesophageal reflux* (Dalby-Payne and Elliot 2005); the infant brings up large amounts on winding and after lying down, sometimes with a small amount of altered blood. Consider thickening the feeds and giving a raft antacid. Both have been shown to be effective within 1–2 weeks. There is limited evidence that lying the baby in the prone or left lateral positions improves reflux but both positions may be associated with a higher risk of sudden infant death syndrome. If there is no improvement, especially if there is poor weight gain, refer to a paediatrician. Troublesome severe reflux may require a prokinetic agent (e.g. domperidone), H_2 antagonist or proton pump inhibitor or fundoplication;
(d) *upper respiratory infection*; the vomitus contains small amounts of mucus;
(e) *viral enteritis*;
(f) *cows' milk protein intolerance*, occasionally (see 'Changing milks' below).

EXCESSIVE CRYING ('COLIC')

'Colic' is correlated more closely with socioeconomic factors than with physical ones (Crowcroft and Strachan 1997).

The classic picture starts when the infant is about 2 weeks of age, and lasts until about 4 months. The infant cries for long periods, is apparently in distress, and may draw the legs up, go pale and pass flatus. In some, there is a marked diurnal variation, 'evening colic', in which the infant is usually well in the morning but as the day progresses the crying becomes worse until, by the evening, the infant appears inconsolable.

* Establish the parents' perceptions of the problem, and assess whether there are other factors affecting them (e.g. overcrowding, marital strife, etc.).

* Exclude important causes, e.g. infantile spasms, recurrent volvulus, intussusception or acute infection (especially otitis media and urinary tract infection). Look also for less severe causes, e.g. excoriated skin, oral thrush, anal fissures.

* Reassure the parents that the problem will only last a short time, and that it is not caused by poor feeding, allergy, or poor handling. While there is no easy cure, behaviour modification may help (see below).

* Encourage the continuation of breastfeeding and discourage a change or supplementation with formula milk.

* Encourage the parents to get as much time off and rest as is possible. This will mean taking turns in looking after the infant and enlisting the help of friends and relatives.

* Contact the health visitor, who is very important in supporting and monitoring the situation and for advising on day-care facilities for other siblings.

* Follow-up is essential both by the GP and health visitor.

* Consider prescribing *dicycloverine* but there is limited evidence that it may be of benefit (Kilgour and Wade 2004).

* *Sedation* should be used only as a last resort. It is essential that the dose is adequate, and that the sedative is only used in conjunction with a change in management and for short periods.

* Admit to hospital if the situation has progressed so far that the parents are distraught and desperately need reassurance and/or the child is felt to be at risk.

BEHAVIOURAL MODIFICATION

Explain that sometimes the cycle of crying sets up a vicious circle of unintentional overstimulation, leading to a tired, distraught infant. A more structured sleeping and feeding routine has been shown to help (Sleep, Gillham, St James-Roberts, *et al.* 2002). This involves:

(a) feeding the infant between 22.00 and 24.00;

(b) trying not to rock, hold or feed babies to sleep, with the intention of minimizing night-time interaction and emphasize the difference between day and night lighting;

(c) after 3 weeks, if the baby is well and gaining weight, to lengthen the interval between night feeds and resettling the baby without feeding. The intention is to reduce the reflex of 'waking' and 'feeding'. However, parents are not advised to let their children cry for long periods.

Conversely, some infants respond to an increase in care or increased carrying (St James-Roberts 1992).

CHANGING MILKS

● There is some evidence that changing to a whey hydrolyzate formula reduces crying (Crowcroft and Strachan 1997). However, changing milks should be avoided on the whole, as only a very small number of children are truly intolerant of cows' milk. Problems with tolerating cows' milk comprise:

(a) *lactose intolerance:* this is usually temporary, causing persistent diarrhoea following gastroenteritis. The watery stools are positive for lactose on chromatography. Change to a soya formula and reintroduce cows' milk formula after 6 weeks.

(b) *cows' milk protein intolerance:* this is manifest by excessive crying, usually with vomiting and diarrhoea, sometimes containing blood; occasionally by constipation. A short trial of soya formula or hydrolyzed formula (e.g. Nutramigen) results in dramatic improvement: there is no other convenient diagnostic test. It may be possible to reintroduce cows' milk formula after 3–6 months.

(c) *true milk allergy:* usually manifests as an urticarial rash or anaphylaxis in an atopic child and family. Refer for assessment (skin testing or radioallergosorbent testing (RAST) may be needed if there is doubt) and for dietetic advice. Hydrolyzed formula is recommended as soya allergy often coexists. Wean onto a milk-free diet then review at 1 year. The condition gradually improves over preschool years but other food allergies may coexist.

WATERING/DISCHARGE FROM THE INFANT EYE

OVERVIEW

Young DH, MacEwan CJ. 1997. Managing congenital lacrimal obstruction in general practice. BMJ 315, 293–296

* Reassure the parents that 20% of infants develop the symptoms of lacrimal obstruction, and that 99% of these resolve by 1 year.
* Examine to exclude other causes, especially infection. Consider taking a swab for pathogens including chlamydia if under 1 month old.
* Advise parents that:
  (a) topical antibiotics should be used only if there is clear evidence of infection;
  (b) lid cleaning of debris may decrease the risk of secondary infection; and
  (c) massage of the lacrimal sac is often recommended, but its value has not been assessed.
* Refer at the age of 1 year if symptoms are still present, but explain that surgical intervention may not be necessary and the surgeon may delay operating until 2 years of age.

NAPPY RASH

The following are important in preventing napkin dermatitis:

(a) frequent nappy changes (5–6 times per day, i.e. when urine is voided);
(b) periods without nappies;
(c) general skin care.

GENERAL SKIN CARE

(a) *Hygiene*: at each change, the nappy area should be washed with water and gently dried.
(b) *Local emollients*, e.g. aqueous cream, should be applied at the earliest sign of irritation.
(c) *Bath oil* should be used if the skin is dry or easily irritated.

MANAGEMENT

* Decide whether this is ammoniacal dermatitis or is due to *Candida*. In both conditions, encourage the parents to allow the infant to be exposed for as long as possible each day.
* *Ammoniacal dermatitis*. Distinctive sign: redness does not extend into the creases. Advise the parents to:
  (a) change the nappy even more frequently, e.g. every 2 hours if wet;
  (b) boil towelling nappies vigorously to kill ammonia-producing bacteria; and
  (c) use a barrier cream, e.g. white soft paraffin or zinc ointment, at each nappy change.
* *Candida dermatitis*. Distinctive sign: redness extends deep into the creases, with spotty satellite lesions. Prescribe a topical antifungal agent at each nappy change. Resistant cases: check for oral *Candida* and treat; consider an antifungal combined with steroid.

CONSTIPATION

Infants are very different from older children in the number and volume of stools that they pass, and vary enormously from one infant to another. Only consider that the child has constipation if the stool is especially hard or is associated with pain or bleeding.

* Exclude an anal fissure.
* Consider adding juice from strained fruit to feeds. If necessary, give 2.5 ml of lactulose daily to a newborn and up to 10 ml daily to a 1-year-old.

Delay in passing the first meconium stool and subsequent constipation raises the possibility of Hirschsprung's disease.

AT THE TIME OF WEANING

Short-term but distressing constipation can occur on the introduction of a varied diet. Strained fruit should be added to the diet. High-fibre diets should not be encouraged, as they can lead to iron and calorie deficiencies.

DIARRHOEA WITH OR WITHOUT VOMITING

REVIEW

Dalby-Payne J, Elliot E. 2007. Gastroenteritis in children. *Clinical Evidence.* http://clinicalevidence.bmj.com/

Guideline
National Institute for Health and Clinical Excellence. 2009. *Diarrhoea and Vomiting Caused by Gastroenteritis: Diagnosis, Assessment and Management in Children Younger than 5 Years.* CG 84. NICE, London. www.nice.org.uk/CG084

Telephone assessment may be appropriate if the parents report that:

- the child is well and taking fluids orally;
- the child is passing a normal amount of urine, and has warm hands and feet;
- the skin is not pale or mottled;
- there are no symptoms suggesting a diagnosis other than gastroenteritis;
- the social circumstances are appropriate for home care; and
- the child is not in a high-risk group (see box).

CHILDREN AT INCREASED RISK OF DEHYDRATION, AS DESCRIBED BY NICE

- Infants, especially those < 6 months and those of low birth weight.
- Children who have passed > 5 stools in the last 24 hours.
- Children who have vomited more than twice in the last 24 hours.
- Children not taking extra fluid orally.
- Infants who have stopped breastfeeding during this illness.
- Children with signs of malnutrition.

Face to face assessment is needed if these criteria are not met.

* Exclude:
  (a) surgical emergencies;
  (b) pneumonia;
  (c) meningitis;
  (d) otitis media in children under the age of 5;
  (e) urinary tract infection (UTI);
  (f) chronic constipation with overflow.
* Refer:
  (a) if the child is dehydrated; or
  (b) the child is ill out of proportion to the diarrhoea and vomiting.
* If satisfied that the illness is consistent with a diagnosis of viral gastroenteritis and that the child is well enough to stay at home:
  (a) treat with hydration;
  (b) do not use antiemetics, antidiarrhoeal agents or antibiotics (except as below);
  (c) explain the need for family hygiene to avoid spread of the infection, e.g. hand washing and safe nappy disposal. The child should stay away from school or childcare facility until free from diarrhoea and vomiting for 48 hours and should not swim in a public pool for 2 weeks;
  (d) warn the parents what are the 'red flag' symptoms and signs (see box) that would require them to seek urgent help. Make sure they understand how to access that help.

'RED FLAG' SYMPTOMS AND SIGNS AS DEFINED BY NICE

Red flag symptoms:
- unwell or deteriorating;
- altered responsiveness (e.g. irritable or lethargic).

Red flag signs:
- sunken eyes;
- tachycardia;
- tachypnoea;
- reduced skin turgor.

ANTIBIOTICS

* *Giardia:* give metronidazole for 3 days.
* *Campylobacter:* erythromycin may help in *Campylobacter* infection if there is systemic upset or blood is still present in the stools.
* *Salmonella* or *Shigella infection:* children with these organisms who are systemically ill need admission for what is a septicaemia.

MAINTENANCE OF HYDRATION

- Oral rehydration salts (ORS) are used because sodium and water are actively absorbed from the bowel. This absorption is increased considerably if an energy source is presented to the bowel wall. They are probably more effective than intravenous rehydration.
- Preparations marketed in the UK are for mild to moderate diarrhoea, and have a lower sodium concentration (35–60 mmol/l) and higher glucose concentration (up to 200 mmol/l) than WHO-recommended ORS. They can be flavoured with dilute fruit squashes.

* *Bottle-fed children*. Tell the parents to:
  1. Use the solution as the only oral fluid, with no solids. If the child is dehydrated or in danger of becoming so give 50 ml/kg over 4 hours before returning to the child's normal amounts. If not dehydrated plan to give at least as much as the child would normally drink in a day.
  2. Give small amounts often (even 5 ml every 10 minutes if the parents say that the child vomits everything consumed).
  3. Continue the ORS until the diarrhoea is settling.
  4. Then feed the child as follows: for an infant under 6 months, either reintroduce full strength milk, or 'regrade' (see below). Opinion is divided on the need for regrading in order to avoid lactose intolerance in this age group; for an infant over 6 months, reintroduce full strength milk. There is evidence that lactose free feeds reduce the duration of diarrhoea in children with mild to moderate dehydration.

* *Breastfed children*. Breast feeding should continue, with ORS used as supplementary fluid replacement.

* *Weaned children* may continue to eat if they have an appetite. Small, frequent meals of bland foods (e.g. boiled rice) are appropriate. There is some evidence that lactobacillus (yoghurt) reduces the duration and intensity of infectious diarrhoea (Van Niel, Feudtner, Garrison, *et al.* 2002).

> **REGRADING**
>
> Give 1/4 then 1/2 then 3/4 then full strength milk. Complete the sequence over 24–36 hours.

RECURRENCE OF DIARRHOEA

If diarrhoea recurs after reintroducing milk, regrade as above.

NOTIFICATION

* Send a stool sample for culture for bacteria and viruses and for ova, cysts and parasites if:
  (a) the stool contains blood;
  (b) the diarrhoea is prolonged;
  (c) the child has an underlying illness or is especially ill;
  (d) the child has recently been abroad to a country where gastroenteritis is endemic;
  (e) more than one member of the family is affected at the same time.

* Notify the environmental health officer as 'food poisoning' if one of the following organisms is isolated: *Shigella, Salmonella, Giardia, Campylobacter, Cryptosporidium* and *E. coli* 157.

* Notify the environmental health officer as 'suspected food poisoning', without waiting for the culture result, if two or more members of a family are affected at the same time.

PROLONGED DIARRHOEA (MORE THAN 2 WEEKS)

* Refer any child with prolonged diarrhoea who is failing to thrive.

* Otherwise:
  (a) Repeat a stool culture (send a fresh specimen and request culture and microscopy).
  (b) Check fresh stool for reducing sugars. Use Clinitest tablets (add 10 drops of water and 5 drops of liquid stool to the Clinitest tablet.) If the stool contains more than 0.5% reducing sugars, prescribe a lactose-free formula feed (e.g. Pregestimil) for 3–6 weeks. Explain to the parents that this intolerance of lactose is

likely to be temporary. No other food containing milk should be given. The advice of a dietician is recommended. Refer to hospital outpatients if symptoms have not resolved after 6 weeks.

(c) Check urine for organisms (especially in young children).

(d) If stool cultures are negative and the above tests are normal, try to reintroduce food and only return to a liquid diet if the diarrhoea worsens.

CRYPTOSPORIDIUM

This is contracted from animals by milk or water, but can be transferred within families by the faeco-oral route. It can last up to 90 days and does not respond to antibacterial therapy.

TODDLER'S DIARRHOEA

Many young children (commonly boys) suffer from prolonged watery diarrhoea with undigested food in the stool that starts, or is first noticed, after an attack of apparently infectious diarrhoea. Peas, carrots, sweetcorn and baked beans are especially likely to appear. The child remains well. Once cultures and tests for acid and sugars are negative, the likely diagnosis is 'toddler's diarrhoea'. This is due to a rapid transit time.

* Reassure the parents that:
  (a) the condition is benign and that the child will continue to flourish, despite diarrhoea;
  (b) the condition usually improves by the age of 5 years.
* Advise the parents to review the child's diet. An increase in dietary fibre and dietary intake of fat (to 35–40% of total energy intake) with a reduction in fruit juices (especially apple juice), may be effective (Hoekstra 1998).
* Review the child regularly and monitor the growth. Refer if there is any parental anxiety or if the child is failing to thrive.
* Loperamide 2.5–5 ml t.d.s. should be considered if the diarrhoea is difficult to manage, e.g. on starting nursery school. The drug is only effective for the time it is taken.

FEVER IN CHILDREN UNDER FIVE

The non-specific nature of many infections in infants and young children, and their potential for serious illness, has led the National Institute for Health and Clinical Excellence to issue guidance on the management of fever in this age group (NICE 2007).

ASSESSMENT

(a) *Is the illness clearly life-threatening?* If so, admit immediately, usually by dialling 999.
(b) *How ill is the child?* The guideline describes the 'traffic light' system of assessment in which children who are basically well are in the green category; children who are mildly to moderately ill are in the amber; and children with one or more markers of serious illness are in the red. The guideline lists symptoms and signs which should be elicited in this assessment.
(c) *Are there any specific pointers to a cause for the fever?* This is mainly a question of history and examination, with urine examination the one worthwhile investigation that can be performed outside hospital (see page 118).

MANAGEMENT ACCORDING TO THE ASSESSMENT ABOVE

* *Green category*. Treat symptomatically at home. Explain to the parents when they should seek further help.
* *Amber category*. Decide whether to treat at home or refer to a paediatric specialist. If not referring give the parents in writing details of the 'safety net': what to look out for, who to contact, when to come for a follow-up assessment. Liaise with any other healthcare professionals who might be contacted, e.g. the out-of-hours service.
* *Red category*. Refer to a paediatric specialist urgently.

SYMPTOMATIC TREATMENT

* Advise against tepid sponging.
* Make sure the child is neither over- nor underdressed.

∗ Recommend paracetamol or ibuprofen, but not both, if the child is uncomfortable. Do not recommend them to reduce the fever for its own sake, nor to prevent a febrile convulsion.

CONVULSIONS

CONVULSIONS ASSOCIATED WITH A FEVER

> **REVIEWS**
>
> Offringa M, Moyer VA. 2001. Evidence based management of seizures associated with fever. BMJ 323, 1111–1114.
> Mewasingh LD. 2008. Febrile seizures. *Clinical Evidence* http://clinicalevidence.bmj.com

∗ Look for signs of meningitis and encephalitis. The probability of bacterial meningitis is low (range 0–4%) and a normal physical examination and history make bacterial meningitis highly improbable.
∗ Admit:
   (a) any child thought to have suffered a febrile convulsion under the age of 18 months, even if he or she appears fully recovered;
   (b) any child who is unwell or who has suffered a 'complicated' febrile convulsion, e.g. one lasting 15 minutes, focal or with postictal paralysis;
   (c) any child who suffers from more than one fit in the same febrile illness.
∗ If the child is over 18 months of age and appears to have recovered fully, instruct the parents to telephone you should the child become unwell again later (DTB 1987).
∗ *Information for parents* (Valman 1993):
   (a) Febrile convulsions are common between the ages of 6 months and 5 years, affecting 4% of the childhood population (Verity and Golding 1991).
   (b) About 30% of sufferers will have another convulsion, but only 1% go on to develop epilepsy.
   (c) The majority of convulsions, although frightening, last less than 5 minutes.
   (d) *Further febrile illness:* start paracetamol immediately. The child should be kept cool or

sponged down with tepid water if the fever is high (Kinmouth, Fulton and Campbell 1992). If a fit occurs, advise the parents to:
   ■ turn the child into the prone position – do nothing more;
   ■ call for a doctor or an ambulance if it lasts more than 5 minutes;
   ■ call for a doctor if recovery is not complete, or if there is any other cause for anxiety;
   ■ inform their doctor even when recovery appears complete so that he or she can make a decision about the need for a visit.
   (e) Simple febrile convulsions have no effects on behaviour, school performance or intellect.

RECURRENT FEBRILE CONVULSIONS

∗ Prescribe rectal diazepam if a child has had recurrent or a single prolonged febrile convulsion. Show the parents how to use it at the start of a seizure.
∗ Discuss with the parents the question of referral for consideration of prophylaxis with continuous oral anticonvulsants. The risk of recurrence is 20–30%; but four children would have to be treated with valproate, or eight with phenobarbital, to prevent one seizure. Adverse effects from both drugs make the benefit doubtful (Rantala, Tarkka and Uhari 1997). Adverse effects include cognitive impairment, hyperactivity, irritability and aggressiveness. Furthermore, anticonvulsants do not appear to reduce the risk of later epilepsy.

CONVULSIONS NOT ASSOCIATED WITH A FEVER

∗ Admit any child under the age of 6 months with obvious fits, absences or abnormal behaviour possibly caused by a seizure.
∗ Admit a child of any age with a history of a seizure and evidence of raised intracranial pressure or other worrying signs.
∗ Refer to outpatients:
   (a) any child with suspected absence seizures (which can be confirmed in the surgery by encouraging the child to hyperventilate, thereby inducing absences);

(b) a child over the age of 6 months with a history of a non-febrile convulsion who, when seen, is well (check the blood pressure and examine the fundi).

Note: If a child has had three or more convulsions within a few weeks, consider treating with carbamazepine while awaiting the urgent appointment.

STATUS EPILEPTICUS

If the child is still fitting when the doctor arrives:

● Rapid and decisive management is important: prolonged seizures (more than 30 minutes) in a child predispose to long-term epilepsy.

* Lie the patient prone and ensure that the airway is clear.

* Give diazepam rectally, 0.2–0.3 mg/kg, i.e. 1 mg per year of age. Use rectal tubes 5 mg and 10 mg, or use an i.v. preparation in a syringe (without the needle). In a child over the age of 1 year in whom you can get intravenous access, lorazepam is now the preferred intravenous drug.

* Arrange for immediate admission.

BLADDER AND BOWEL PROBLEMS

TOILET TRAINING

● 10% of 5-year-olds still wet the bed (boys more than girls); by the age of 10, about 4% of children still regularly wet the bed (boys much more than girls). If one parent was not dry at night until 6 years old, then children have a 40% chance of not being so either.

* Advise parents that:
  (a) 2 years is the most sensible age to start training for both bladder and bowels;
  (b) before starting, the child should learn to sit on the toilet or potty and know the difference between being wet and dry.

* *Bladder training* should follow automatically if the child can recognize the difference between wet and dry. In those who appear not to do so, trainer pants will help. Imitating parents is an effective way of encouraging children. It is important not to force the child, who may then use toileting as a powerful weapon. Children who void

appropriately should be rewarded with praise or cuddles.

* *Bowel training.* Advise the parents to sit the child on the potty during the day after meals. This should be fun for the child, who is the focus of attention. If stool is passed in the potty, the child should be rewarded, but if passed in a nappy after the child has given up, this should be ignored or turned into an encouragement to do a 'poo for mummy or daddy next time'.

PATIENT INFORMATION

Green C. 2006. *New Toddler Taming: A Parents' Guide to the First Four Years.* Vermillion, London

BEDWETTING

REVIEW

Kidoo D. Nocturnal enuresis. *Clinical Evidence.* http://clinicalevidence.bmj.com/

● Nocturnal enuresis affects 15–20% of 5-year-old children, 5% of 10-year-old children, and 1–2% of people aged 15 years and over. 15% of affected children become dry each year, without treatment.

● Nocturnal enuresis is not diagnosed in children younger than 5 years, and treatment may be inappropriate for children younger than 7 years.

* Enquire:
  (a) at what age the parents were dry;
  (b) whether the child is now wetting having been previously dry;
  (c) whether the child wets during the day;
  (d) about upsets in the family and stresses at school;
  (e) whether there are any 'payoffs' when wetting occurs, e.g. cuddles, etc.

* Exclude infection, especially in cases of secondary enuresis.

* Discuss the problem with the health visitor.

* **Refer to outpatients any child over the age of 4 years with daytime symptoms.**

Younger children (aged 5–7)

At this age, the problem is likely to be delayed maturation. It seems reasonable for the parents not to struggle to get the child out of nappies at night if a behavioural approach fails. Fluid restriction and lifting may help to reduce the problem without curing it.

* Advise the parent to praise the child for any dry beds. Star charts are helpful at this age, although not under the age of 5 years.
* Prescribe desmopressin acetate tablets 200 mcg for nights away from home, holidays, etc., but not as continuous treatment.

Older children (aged 7–15)

Desmopressin, tricyclic antidepressants and alarms seem to be effective. Alarms are more trouble to set up but may be associated with longer lasting improvement (Glazener and Evans 2002; 2003a).

* Advise the parents:
  (a) to establish a means of positive encouragement or reinforcement whenever a child has a dry bed, with an increased reward if the child has three consecutive dry beds (usually this is done using a star chart or an equivalent sticker chart);
  (b) to ignore wet beds and praise dry ones;
  (c) that 'lifting' the child when the parents go to bed may save a wet bed.
* If not successful, refer to the local authority enuresis clinic for a bedwetting alarm.

Note: Some older children may be able to wake themselves and go to the toilet using an alarm clock set to a time just before they usually wet.

* If the use of a buzzer alarm fails, prescribe desmopressin acetate melt 120 mcg or tablets 200–400 mcg at night for 3 months. Then assess

after a week without treatment. If the response is not maintained, consider a further 3-month course. It probably does not affect the ultimate outcome. If not responding, refer to an enuresis clinic.

Note: The CSM warns that, in order to avoid hyponatraemia, patients on desmopressin should:

(a) avoid excessive drinking, especially at night;
(b) omit desmopressin if there is vomiting or diarrhoea;
(c) keep to the recommended starting doses;
(d) avoid other drugs which increase vasopressin secretion, e.g. tricyclic antidepressants.

It is rare to use a tricyclic antidepressant, e.g. imipramine 25–50 mg at night. It may work by lightening sleep. Improvement usually takes 3–4 weeks, and treatment should be continued for at least 4 months. This is only likely to reduce the bedwetting by one day a week (Glazener and Evans 2003b). The controversy relates to the danger of the drug in overdose.

An alternative rationale and increasingly common approach to treatment (the three systems approach) is recommended by the Enuresis Resource and Information Centre (Butler 2002).

(a) *Presumed lack of vasopressin:* if the child has severe wetting within the first few hours of sleep try desmopressin for 3 months and then gradually withdraw.
(b) *Bladder irritability:* if the child also has symptoms of urgency and frequency during the day try oxybutynin.
(c) *Lack of arousal from sleep:* if the child sleeps very deeply and is unaware of a full bladder, try an alarm.

Adolescents 16 years and over

* Refer for urological assessment.

CONSTIPATION AND SOILING

REVIEWS

Constipation. Clinical Knowledge Summaries. http://www.cks.nhs.uk
  Rubin G, Dale A. 2006. Chronic constipation in children. BMJ 333, 1051–1055

Soiling is abnormal after the age of 4 years. The majority of soilers are constipated, with a loaded rectum.

* Distinguish, from the history, between *encopresis* (normal stool passed in the wrong place) and *soiling* (leaking liquid stool into pants).
* Enquire as to:
  (a) whether the child has ever been continent;
  (b) the frequency, size and nature of the stool;
  (c) the attitude of the parents and child.
* Examine:
  (a) the abdomen for faecal masses;
  (b) the anus for fissure; and
  (c) the rectum for faecal masses.

Empty rectum

* Intentional defecation to offend the parent (encopresis) – refer to a child psychiatrist.
* Poor training – should respond to a star or 'poo' chart, provided the emotional rewards are sufficient.
* Stress – this may be factor in regression, and should respond to a star chart.

Full rectum

The most common cause is a full, distended rectum with loss of the urge to defecate. Liquid faeces seep around the obstruction, which also comes away piecemeal.

* Explain the problem to the parents and child. Normal rectal sensation will only return once the rectum has been empty for a time.
* Empty the rectum using:
  (a) increased fluids;
  (b) soften the retained stool with lactulose 1 ml/kg/day in two divided doses and or docusate 5 mg/kg/day in two divided doses;
  (c) a stimulant laxative, e.g. senna as a syrup 0.5 ml/kg/day at night (2–6 years, 2.5–5 ml; 7–12 years, 5–10 ml), increasing the dose by 5 ml each week until a significant result is achieved;
  (d) Macrogol (Movicol) sachets 1 daily increasing to a maximum of 4 daily. This is only licensed for children aged over 5.

If severely constipated and still loaded after a month on the above routine, refer to hospital.

* *Maintenance.* Once the rectum has been cleared, a maintenance dose of both stimulant (e.g. senna 5–10 ml at night) and softener laxative (e.g. lactulose 0.5 ml/kg/day in two divided doses) should be given and the diet of child and parents discussed.
* *Retraining* is necessary: the child should be encouraged to use the toilet after every meal, and rewarded with heavy praise when he or she defecates in the appropriate place. Rewards for clean pants may encourage retention to continue; a star or 'poo' chart should be started, which also acts as a reward.
* Review the child and charts regularly. Reduce the dose of laxative when continence has been maintained for 3 months. Reassure both child and parents that accidents are inevitable because it takes a long time for the bowel to regain activity.
* If the above routine fails, refer to a paediatrician.

PARENT ADVICE

Royal College of Psychiatrists. *Soiling or Wetting.* Leaflet 8, www.rcpsych.ac.uk/mentalhealthinfoforall/mentalhealthandgrowingup.aspx

SLEEP PROBLEMS

REVIEWS

Ramchandani P, Wiggs L, Webb V, *et al.* 2000. A systematic review of treatments for settling problems and night waking in young children. BMJ 320, 209–213.
  Montgomery P, Dunne D. 2007. Sleep disorders in children. *Clinical Evidence.* http://clinicalevidence.bmj.com/

Parent information
Green C. 2005. New toddler taming: a parents' guide to the first four years. Vermillion, London

* Check that the development of a sleeping difficulty in a child with a previously good sleep pattern is not due to an underlying emotional problem. If it is, assessment and referral should focus on the emotional problem rather than on the behavioural approach outlined below.

ASSESSMENT OF THE PROBLEM

Difficulty in getting a child to sleep, or recurrent waking, are common problems. They require a lot of time and understanding from the GP, and an alteration in the way the parents manage the situation.

* Try to see both parents together. Ask whether there are other factors that are making the situation worse, e.g. living in a bedsit or with grandparents.
* Explain to the parents that for a plan to succeed:
  (a) both parents must agree on the approach;
  (b) that approach must be followed consistently;
  (c) for the parents' sake, the workload should be shared as far as possible;
  (d) neighbours should be told.
* *Sleep diary*. Ask the parents to fill in a diary for a few days, noting the following:
  (a) the time the child wakes in the morning;
  (b) the time and lengths of naps during the day;
  (c) the time the child went to bed in the evening;
  (d) the time the child settled in bed;
  (e) the times and duration of waking during the evening, the mood of the child, and the action taken by the parents;
  (f) the times and lengths of waking at night, the mood of the child, and the action taken by the parents on each occasion.

DIFFICULTY IN GETTING A CHILD TO SETTLE

Children who won't go to sleep at an appropriate time may be:

(a) alert because of naps during the day;
(b) tired, but overstimulated just before bedtime. Use of the computer or watching TV may stimulate melatonin secretion;
(c) finding the room is too hot or cold;
(d) frightened or anxious about being left alone;
(e) confused because of shifting ground rules, e.g. one parent puts the child to bed but the other parent gets him or her up again on coming home later;
(f) attention-seeking. Dry-eyed crying suggests that the child is attention-seeking rather than distressed.

* Advise the parents as follows:
  1. Establish a bedtime routine (e.g. warning the child that bedtime is coming, then a ritual undressing, bath, story, then tucked up in bed).
  2. Be consistent and firm in the routine and refuse to play 'after hours' or to read more stories.
  3. Leave the room once the child is tucked up, saying that they will be back in 5 minutes. Keep coming back until the child is asleep. Once this works, make the intervals longer.
  4. Parents should not run in if crying starts, as the child will usually settle within a short time; they should also avoid picking the child up and so providing further stimulation. They should behave normally; a normal background noise encourages the child to feel secure that the parents are still there.
  5. Avoid chastisement, but introduce appropriate rewards for good behaviour.
* *Very distressed parents*. Ask them if they feel at the end of their tether or if they have felt tempted to hit the child. They may benefit from extended family or social care or use of hypnotics in addition to an alteration in management. Hypnotics need to be in adequate doses to avoid a paradoxical response, e.g. alimemazine tartrate 2 mg/kg. This is the dose recommended for preoperative premedication, and some children may be heavily sedated. Explanation of this to the parents may avoid subsequent difficulties when they present the prescription to the chemist. The hypnotic should not be continued for more than 7 days.

If the above fails

* Advise the parents on the controlled crying technique (see below).

WAKING AT NIGHT

Children and adults normally cycle into a lighter phase of sleep every 60–90 minutes through the night. Children may make a noise and rapidly condition their parents to respond. The child may receive feeds or other attention, and this perpetuates the cycle.

There is some evidence that 'controlled crying' (see below) reduces infant sleep problems and maternal depression at 2 months after starting but not at 4 months (Hiscock and Wake 2002).

* Encourage the parents to keep a sleep diary (as above).
* Advise the parents on the controlled crying technique, and tell them to warn neighbours before starting it.

Controlled crying

No child should be allowed to cry him- or herself to sleep without comfort. Instead, recommend the following.

1. Leave the child to cry for 5–10 minutes, depending on the degree of distress.
2. Go into the room, cuddle and comfort, and when the cries give way to sobs put the child to bed and say goodnight.
3. The child will probably immediately start crying again. Leave him or her for 2–5 minutes longer than last time before going in again.
4. Once the child is comforted, withdraw again.
5. Subsequent episodes of crying should be left for additional 2–5 minute periods before responding.
6. **The parent must try to rest.**
7. If the crying time is about 30 minutes, sedation should be considered (see above).
8. Heap praise on the child when he or she starts to sleep for longer periods.

The child who comes into the parents' bed at night

The principles are the same as above. Advise the parents to explain to the child that he or she is going to stay in his or her own bed.

1. Put the child back the moment he or she appears.
2. On reappearance, the child is given a warning and returned.
3. At the third reappearance, the child should be returned, the door wedged partially open (but not enough for the child to get through) and the controlled crying technique started.

OTHER SLEEP PROBLEMS

Nightmares

Nightmares are common in children over the age of 5, and occur during rapid eye movement (REM) sleep.

* Reassure the parents that comforting the child is usually all that is required, and that the phase will pass.
* Refer to a child psychiatrist if nightmares:
  (a) have a recurring theme;
  (b) are frequent;
  (c) follow a frightening experience.

Meanwhile, consider encouraging the child to express his or her feelings, e.g. through art.

Night terrors

Night terrors occur during deep non-REM sleep, often about 2 hours after falling asleep. They are common in children under the age of 5, but can occur at any age. Classically the child screams in terror, sits up or tries to walk around, appearing to hallucinate. After a short while he or she falls asleep and wakes the next day with no memory of the event.

* Reassure the parents that the child will grow out of this and that it does not indicate any severe psychological disorder.
* *Anticipation.* Many children have terrors at 'set times'. If this is so, the sleep pattern can be altered if the child is fully woken 15–30 minutes before the likely event for 1 week.
* *Sedation* may be valuable if terrors are frequent and do not respond to the anticipatory technique. Prescribe a short-acting benzodiazepine nightly for 4 weeks, then tail it off. Benzodiazepines reduce non-REM sleep.

Sleep walking

* Advise the parents to:
  (a) ensure that the bedroom is safe and secure; and
  (b) attempt to wake the child fully 15–30 minutes before the most likely time of attack, for 1 week.
* *Sedation* should only be considered if severe problems occur during the episodes. Prescribe diazepam 5 mg at night, for 1–3 months.

POOR SLEEP ROUTINES IN ADOLESCENTS (KOTAGAL AND PIANOSI 2006)

Adolescents suffer from problems specific to their age.

- Their rise in melatonin output, necessary for sleep, will not occur until about 10.30 pm.
- They often go to sleep much later, for a number of reasons: TV or computer in the bedroom, caffeine in commercial drinks, nicotine and illegal stimulants, and the emotional turmoil of adolescence.
- They need on average at least 9 hours sleep at night.
- During term-time they often have to get up at 7.00 am, having not had enough sleep.
- At weekends, being chronically sleep deprived, they sleep till mid-day, thus disturbing their sleep pattern for a further week.

* Explain the principles of sleep hygiene, see page 463.
* In those with daytime sleepiness, check for:
  - the characteristic cataplectic episodes of narcolepsy. One third of cases begin before the age of 15;
  - delayed sleep phase syndrome, in which the patient is unable to fall asleep until 2 or 3 am;
  - obstructive sleep apnoea.

TEMPER TANTRUMS

PARENT INFORMATION

Green C. 2005. *New Toddler Taming: A Parents' Guide to the First Four Years.* Vermillion, London

Children soon learn what behaviour will irritate their parents. Usually such contrary behaviour is wilfulness (the children testing out their developing strength against the will of the parents), but it can be repayment for not getting their own way in other matters.

* Ask the parents:
  (a) what *the child* does during a tantrum;
  (b) what *they* do during and after the tantrum;
  (c) what causes the tantrums.
* Assess whether inconsistent handling of the child by the parents is contributing to the problem.

PRINCIPLES OF MANAGEMENT

(a) *Avoiding provocation.* Parents need to realize that telling the child what is wanted is more likely to be successful than subsequent chastisement. Parents need to be consistent in their behaviour and emotions towards the child.

(b) *Withdrawal of attention.* Ignoring a tantrum may not be easy, but walking out of the room achieves the same result. It is important that the child is not left in a potentially dangerous situation. The child should be left for 3–4 minutes only.

(c) *Time out.* The child should be removed from the room to a safe but boring part of the house, or told to sit on a chair in the middle of the room and not get off it until allowed. Again the process should only last for 3–4 minutes or until the child has calmed down. If a room is used, it must never be locked, the lights must stay on and a parent should remain outside.

(d) *'Punishment'* by withholding an expected reward, for example: deny the child a favourite television programme; refuse the child permission to play with friends.

(e) *Not giving in* is essential for any plan to work.

(f) *Rewarding good behaviour.* This is best done with praise and cuddles or permission to watch previously banned programmes, etc. Warn parents about relatives who may confuse a child with undeserved rewards and threaten the management plan.

* If defiance is continued, assess whether:
  (a) the parents are consistent;
  (b) the rewards and 'punishments' are appropriate;
  (c) withdrawal of privilege is threatened but not carried out.
* If still failing to deal with the problem, refer to a child psychiatrist, a clinical psychologist or a family consultation centre.

'BREATH-HOLDING' ATTACKS

BLUE ATTACKS

These occur in children who become angry, cry, and then hold the glottis closed. The child quickly becomes cyanosed and then loses consciousness. Recovery is very quick.

* Reassure the parents that it is not epilepsy, nor is it serious.
* Explain that flicking cold water in the child's face can sometimes abort attacks.
* Advise the parents to avoid being 'held to ransom' or becoming overprotective.

WHITE ATTACKS (REFLEX ANOXIC SEIZURES)

A child who is surprised or hurt may suddenly fall unconscious, and become pale, limp and apnoeic. If this continues long enough the child may have an anoxic seizure.

* Advise the parents to leave the child prone when this happens.
* Reassure them that their child will not suffer damage, but may be more likely to faints when older.
* Stress that this is not epilepsy.
* Refer if episodes are frequent or the parents need reassurance.

RESPIRATORY PROBLEMS

* Children may have as many as 20 colds in the first 18 months, and still get six a year at age 7. There is no place for antibiotics.
* The best guide to whether a small child has pneumonia is the child's general condition, not chest signs. If the child is ill enough to suggest pneumonia, then admission is better than blind antibiotics.
* Discourage the parents from smoking anywhere near the child.

THE CATARRHAL CHILD

It takes about 6 weeks for the cilia to recover after each cold. It is not surprising that for much of the year the child has nasal catarrh.

* Reassure the parent that if the child is well, catarrh is not a sign of illness and does not necessarily need treatment.
* Treat any allergic component (see page 535).
* Encourage nose blowing and discourage sniffing.
* *Decongestants*. Prescribe topical nose drops (e.g. xylometazoline 0.05%), but only for 10 days at a time. Oral decongestants (e.g. pseudoephedrine) are less effective and cause hyperactivity. Advise parents not to give a dose before bedtime.
* Check the ear drums and the hearing.
* Refer any child with:
  (a) nasal discharge from soon after birth. Primary ciliary dyskinesia occurs in 1 in 20,000 in the UK;
  (b) unilateral discharge – to exclude a foreign body;
  (c) purulent discharge – again there may be a foreign body or sinus infection;
  (d) adenoidal obstruction. This is likely in a child with persistent mouth breathing and an apparently clear nose. Even then, natural improvement will occur by the age of 6–7. Refer only if there is sleep apnoea, otitis media with effusion (OME), or obstruction severe enough to interfere with speech or eating.

COUGH

* Advise the parents, if the child is well and there are no chest signs, that the cause is probably viral and that the cough may last 2 weeks or more. At 2 weeks 25% of children still have a cough (Hay and Wilson 2002). If a child has had a cough for 1 month or more, arrange a CXR to exclude foreign body inhalation and low-grade pneumonia.

CHILDREN UNDER 18 MONTHS
Wheeze following viral infection

Upper respiratory tract infection (URTI) followed by wheezing, coughing and breathlessness with signs of hyperexpansion and prolonged expiration – about 50% of infants who suffer repeated episodes of this go on to develop asthma.

* Admit all ill children, especially if they are too breathless to feed.
* Beta-agonist or ipratropium. In a well child (with no significant difficulty in feeding), it is worth assessing the response to a beta-agonist e.g. salbutamol 2.5 mg t.d.s orally or 200–400 mcg via face mask and spacer. Note that beta-agonists are not licensed in this age group and are only effective in a small number of children. If a beta-agonist is not effective, ipratropium 40–80 mcg by mask and spacer may be.

Bronchiolitis

> Lozano JM. 2007. Bronchiolitis. *Clinical Evidence*. BMJ Publishing Group, London

A diagnosis of 'probable bronchiolitis' can be made if an URTI occurs with:

(a) progressive dry cough in an ill infant;

(b) raised respiratory rate (≥ 40);

(c) subcostal recession and hyperexpansion with prolonged expiration;

(d) bilateral crackles;

(e) difficulty in feeding.

* Manage at home (Isaacs 1995) if the infant:
    (a) is able to feed;
    (b) is aged over 3 months;
    (c) has a respiratory rate $< 50/\text{min}$;
    (d) has no other complicating factors.
* Management consists of support and monitoring. Antibiotics are of no, and steroids of little, value, and bronchodilators usually ineffective.
* Otherwise, admit. The child is likely to need oxygen and nasogastric or i.v. fluids. The infant who presents with apnoea should always be admitted.

Whooping cough

* Admit if apnoea occurs, or if there is major distress from coughing. Do so even if the infant seems well when you arrive at the house. (Believe the parents' history of an apnoeic attack – the next one could be fatal.) Admit all infants with suspected whooping cough, if under 1 month old.
* If there is no evidence of respiratory distress, the child can be managed at home. Consider giving the child, and any other susceptible children (especially infants) who have been in contact, a course of clarithromycin (see page 48).
* *Cough* does not respond to conventional cough suppressants.

Recurrent 'chest infections'

* Arrange a CXR.
* Check whether the child is thriving.
* Consider referring to exclude cystic fibrosis.

CHILDREN OVER 18 MONTHS OF AGE

Dry cough, worse at night, with or without wheezing

Always consider that the child might have asthma.

* Enquire about wheezing, recurrent chest infections and exercise-induced wheezing and coughing.
* Consider a trial of:
    (a) a beta-agonist although there is no clear evidence of benefit (Chavasse, Seddon, Bara, *et al.* 2002);
    (b) inhaled steroids (see below).

Sudden onset of coughing with no previous URTI

* Exclude an inhaled foreign body. Arrange a CXR (ensure that the film is taken on expiration).
* Note that a normal CXR does not exclude a foreign body: if the history is suggestive (e.g. choking then cough in a young child) refer for bronchoscopy.

Chronic cough, mouth breathing, sniffing and snoring

The symptoms may be due to a postnasal drip in a child with catarrh (see page 535).

ASTHMA IN CHILDREN UNDER 5 YEARS

For the management of asthma in children over 5, see page 179 and Appendix 11B and 11E.

Asthma in young children does not always follow the picture of older children and adults. There are two clinical patterns:

(a) acute wheezy episodes (usually with viral infections);

(b) recurrent day-to-day symptoms (presumed atopic asthma).

The treatment of these two patterns is different. Children with pattern (a) do not require inhaled steroids unless the episodes are very frequent (e.g. one per month). Even then they are of limited effectiveness (McKean and Ducharme 2001).

PRESUMED ATOPIC ASTHMA

Aims of treatment

(a) Child to be as symptom-free as possible day and night.

(b) For beta-agonists to be needed no more than once a day.

(c) To avoid adverse effects of treatment, particularly with regard to growth and development.

Diagnosis

The diagnosis is a clinical one. If in doubt, consider a trial of oral prednisolone for 3 days (at the same dose as the rescue course, see Appendix 11E) or inhaled steroid (for 6 weeks minimum), in children over the age of 12 months. The diagnosis is hard to make in children under 12 months. A personal or family history of atopy makes the diagnosis of asthma more likely (Chavasse, Bastian-Lee, Richter, *et al.* 2001). In time a clearer pattern will emerge. Meanwhile refer if symptoms are sufficiently troublesome.

✴ Consider a CXR or referral if:

(a) the response to simple treatment is poor; or

(b) the child has a productive cough or recurrent chest infections or focal lung signs; or

(c) symptoms date back to the neonatal period; or

(d) there is failure to thrive.

Patient/parent management

Involve both the parents and child closely in the management of the condition. Management includes:

(a) understanding the condition;

(b) monitoring symptoms, peak flow and drug usage;

(c) having a prearranged plan of action should symptoms deteriorate;

(d) avoidance of precipitants (see page 179).

Stress that parents who smoke risk worsening their child's symptoms.

Drug treatment

- In the child with definite asthma, introducing inhaled steroids early, probably protects against decline in lung function (Agertoft and Pedersen 1994).
- However, the younger the child, the more difficult it is to diagnose asthma and the greater the potential concerns about inhaled steroids.
- The efficacy of treatment depends on the age of the child and whether the child can inhale adequate amounts of drug. The delivery system must be tailored to the child. More than 50% of children receiving treatment with conventional metered dose inhalers (MDI) derive little or no benefit because of poor inhalation technique. The following broad guidelines apply:

  (a) *0–2 years* need an MDI via a spacer, preferably with a face mask;

  (b) *2–5 years* need an MDI via spacer;

  (c) *5–8 years* can use a dry powder inhaler or an MDI with a spacer;

  (d) *over 8 years* can use a dry powder inhaler or an MDI.

See Appendix 11C for a stepwise guide to the management of asthma in children under 5, and Appendix 11B for the management of asthma in older children.

ACUTE ASTHMA IN YOUNG CHILDREN

✴ Admit anyone who:

(a) is too breathless to talk;

(b) is too breathless to feed;

(c) has a respiratory rate of > 50 breaths per minute;

(d) has a pulse > 140 beats per minute;

(e) is using accessory muscles to breathe.

Life-threatening features are:

(a) cyanosis;

(b) a silent chest;

(c) exhaustion;

(d) agitation or drowsiness.

Those not requiring immediate admission to hospital

1. Give an inhaled beta-agonist 10–20 puffs by MDI using a spacer, with each puff being breathed in before the next puff is given; or by nebulizer 3–4 hourly (dose: < 1 year (unlicensed), salbutamol 1.25 to 2.5 mg, 1–5 years, 5 mg).

2. Give 20 mg of prednisolone orally (in the soluble form).

3. *If there is a poor response or a relapse within 3–4 hours*, arrange admission.

4. *If the response is good*, continue the beta-agonist every 3–4 hours. If still requiring 3–4 hourly inhalations after 12 hours, continue oral prednisolone (dose: < 1 year, 1–2 mg/kg/day; 1–5 years, 20 mg/day) and consider referral to hospital.

On recovery

Consider the following:

(a) Was there an avoidable cause?

(b) Was the attack sudden, or did the patient deteriorate slowly?

(c) Did the patient/relatives respond appropriately?

(d) Was the patient complying with treatment?

(e) Was the medical management appropriate?

(f) Should the child have a course of steroids at home for acute use?

(g) Does the child need regular inhaled steroids if not already on them?

FOLLOW–UP

* Assess symptoms regularly. Particular questions to ask are:

    (a) Does the child cough or wheeze at night?

    (b) Does the child cough or wheeze with exercise?

    (c) Is exercise limited?

* Assess inhalation technique occasionally, and if symptoms deteriorate.

* Monitor the frequency of repeat prescriptions.

* Continue the education of child and parent.

CYSTIC FIBROSIS

All patients suffering from cystic fibrosis (CF) should be managed by a regional cystic fibrosis clinic in conjunction with a district paediatrician and their GP.

The principles of management are that:

(a) patients have regular physiotherapy to reduce retention of secretions;

(b) aggressive antibiotic therapy is prescribed at the first sign of infection;

(c) improved nutrition improves the prognosis. Patients with CF have higher than normal energy requirements and require 120–150% of the normal daily calorie intake to maintain body weight and to grow.

INFECTION

Unlike normal children, respiratory viral infections are frequently associated with bacterial infection, from infancy onwards.

* Treat any respiratory infection associated with a cough with a broad spectrum oral antibiotic covering *Staphylococcus* and *Haemophilus* (e.g. co-amoxiclav or cefadroxil) for 14 days. Doses of penicillins/cephalosporins need to be double the normal because of increased excretion, e.g. cefadroxil 125 mg b.d. under 1 year, 250 mg b.d. 1–5 years, 500 mg b.d. 6–12 years, 1 g b.d. 13+ years.

* If cough persists, refer or arrange sputum/cough swab culture and discuss with specialist.

Note: Look for non-specific evidence of respiratory infection, e.g. weight loss or fever.

* *Pseudomonas aeruginosa.* Start an antibiotic, and discuss/refer immediately if *Pseudomonas* is isolated for the first time. Treat aggressively:

    (a) if the child is well, treat with ciprofloxacin orally for 2 weeks and start nebulized Colomycin/tobramycin;

    (b) if the child has symptoms as above, admit for intravenous antibiotics.

This strategy will clear new *Pseudomonas* infection in more than 50% of children. Chronic *Pseudomonas* infection requires long-term nebulized antibiotics.

NUTRITION

* Consider oral supplements to provide the necessary calorie intake.
* Prescribe pancreatic enzyme supplements to improve fat and protein absorption. If the stools are frequent, foul-smelling or floating, the supplements should be increased.

DIABETES

* Ensure that the patient maintains a high calorie intake. Control the blood sugar with adjustment of the insulin dosage, not with dietary restriction.

FERTILITY

Almost all men with CF are sterile, but many women remain fertile. The issue should be discussed with patients in early adolescence (Sawyer 1996).

DORNASE ALFA

Dornase alfa helps reduce sputum viscosity by breaking down the DNA from dead neutrophils. It is given once a day (2.5 mg) by jet nebulizer. It should be initiated and initially monitored by a specialist, and prescribing should only be devolved to the GP with an agreed protocol.

PATIENT ORGANIZATION

Cystic Fibrosis Trust, 11 London Road, Bromley, Kent, BR1 1BY, tel. 020 8464 7211; www.cftrust.org.uk

UPPER AIRWAYS OBSTRUCTION

Do not examine the throat of a child with stridor.
* Admit if:
    (a) *the child is toxic or drooling.* Assume that this is haemophilus epiglottitis or bacterial tracheitis; death can occur within hours; or

(b) *the obstruction is severe and/or the child is becoming exhausted.* The child will be distressed, with a very rapid pulse and intercostal recession; or

(c) *inhalation of a foreign body is suspected.* This is characterized by the sudden onset of stridor in an afebrile child, with no preceding illness; or

(d) the child has just returned from an area where diphtheria is common.

Note: If you suspect croup and the child's stridor is worsening rapidly, consider giving nebulized adrenaline 4 ml of 1:1000 while waiting for the ambulance: relief is short-lived. Give steroids (see below). Make all actions taken clear in the admission note.

MILD/MODERATE CROUP

Johnson D. 2005. Croup. *Clinical Evidence.* BMJ Publishing Group, London

* Children with mild stridor and a barking cough who are basically well can be managed at home.
* Glucocorticoids improve the child's condition within 6 hours. Fewer return visits or readmissions are required.

FOR ALL CHILDREN WITH CROUP

* Give a single dose of oral or intramuscular dexamethasone 0.15–0.6 mg/kg (Geelhoed, Turner and Macdonald 1996), or oral prednisolone 1 mg/kg (Ausejo, Saenz and Pham 1999). Dexamethasone at 0.15 mg/kg is probably as effective as 0.6 mg/kg. Giving oral dexamethasone to children with mild croup has an NNT of 10; that is, giving the drug to 10 children with mild croup will save one child from re-consulting with significant croup. Nebulized budesonide has also been used but seems less effective than oral steroids (Luria, Gonzalez-del-Rey, DiGiulio *et al.* 2001). There is no evidence that giving nebulized budesonide as well as dexamethasone is of any benefit.
* Reassure the parents and encourage them to comfort and settle the child (anxiety makes the stridor considerably worse).

* Tell the parents not to bother with steam inhalations: they are of no benefit (Scolnik, Coates, Stephens *et al.* 2006).
* Do not give antibiotics. The aetiology is viral.
* Advise the parents to contact you if there is any deterioration. Explain that the barking cough is likely to be worse at night for about 3 nights.

RECURRENT OR CONTINUING CROUP

* *Recurrent croup* without preceding infection has been linked to allergy and upper airway hyperreactivity. Consider a trial of beta-agonist + inhaled corticosteroid.
* *Continuing croup:* refer. Children with stridor or an odd cry without upper respiratory infection may have laryngomalacia, subglottic stenosis or a laryngeal web.

URINARY TRACT INFECTIONS (UTI)

GUIDELINE

NICE. 2007. *Urinary Tract Infection in Children: Diagnosis, Treatment and Long-term Management.* National Institute for Health and Clinical Excellence, CG54, www.nice.org.uk

* 11% of girls and 3.6% of boys have a UTI in childhood. Without adequate investigation, 75% of them will suffer from recurrent UTIs.
* 25–55% of children with UTI have associated urinary tract abnormalities (7–10% have obstruction, 12–20% have renal scarring, 30% have vesico-ureteric reflux).
* Renal scarring. Of those with renal scarring, up to 23% will develop hypertension by early adulthood and 10% will develop end-stage renal disease.
* Children under 2 are at the greatest risk of renal damage if they develop infection, yet this group is least likely to be investigated with a urine culture. These children are likely to present with non-specific symptoms such as fever, vomiting and diarrhoea, or failure to thrive without urinary symptoms.

* If renal damage is present in a child aged < 5, then both subsequent UTIs and vesico-ureteric reflux may further damage the kidneys. An onset of scarring after the age of 5 is rare.

URINE TESTS

When screening the urine of a child without urinary symptoms, a dipstick for leucocyte esterase (LE) and nitrites (N) is sufficient. If both are positive, their sensitivity is 88% and their false positive rate is 4% (Gorelick and Shaw 1999). If there is a stronger reason to suspect infection, or the child is clearly unwell, laboratory microscopy and culture (M+C) are needed (see below).

* Obtain a urine sample as follows:
  (a) in the very young child, use a urine collection pad (Vernon 1996), a urine bag, or obtain a clean catch;
  (b) in potty-trained children, loosely stretch cling film over the potty and take urine from the pool;
  (c) in the older child, obtain a mid-stream specimen. Cleaning the genital area, in girls and boys, before catching the specimen can improve the positive predictive value of the test from 13% to 41% (Vaillancourt, McGillivray, Zhang, *et al.* 2007).
* Decide whether to send the specimen for microscopy and culture or whether to test with a dipstick.

CHILDREN UNDER 3 YEARS OLD BUT OLDER THAN 3 MONTHS

■ NICE suggests that the urine should be sent for microscopy and culture, but that a dipstick may be appropriate in those at intermediate, rather than high, risk of serious illness if the child is being kept at home and there will be a delay in receiving the microscopy result.

CHILDREN AGED 3 YEARS AND OVER

■ If the child is at high risk of having serious illness (see box), send for urgent M+C and refer to a paediatrician urgently.

■ If the child is at intermediate risk of having serious illness, send for M+C. If there will be a delay in obtaining the microscopy result, perform a dipstick test and interpret as below.

■ If the child is at low risk of having serious illness, perform a dipstick test in the first instance.

(a) If leucocyte esterase (LE) positive, and nitrite (N) positive: start antibiotics. Only send for M+C if there is a history of recurrent infections.

(b) If LE negative and N positive: send for M+C and start antibiotics.

(c) If LE positive and N negative: send for M+C and only start antibiotics if there is other good evidence of a UTI.

(d) If LE negative and N negative: look for other causes of the illness. This is unlikely to be a UTI.

REFERRAL AND TREATMENT

∗ *Infants under 3 months old* with a suspected urinary tract infection should be referred immediately.

∗ *Infants and children aged 3 months or older with suspected lower urinary tract infection*: treat at home with antibiotics for 3 days. Trimethoprim or a cephalosporin are likely to be appropriate; amoxicillin is not. Ask the parents to re-attend if the child is still unwell 24 hours after starting treatment.

∗ *Infants and children aged 3 months or older with suspected upper urinary tract infection:* admit if seriously ill especially if unable to take oral antibiotics. Consider giving antibiotics at home for 10 days if less unwell.

The NICE guideline suggests the following rule:
■ Bacteriuria and either fever $\geq 38°C$ or loin pain or tenderness: upper UTI.
■ Bacteriuria but temperature $< 38°C$ and no loin symptoms or signs: lower UTI.
The weakness of this guidance for primary care is that the GP usually has to make a decision before the result of the urine M+C is known.

DECIDING WHETHER THE CHILD IS AT RISK OF HAVING SERIOUS ILLNESS

NICE Guideline No. 47 *Feverish Illness in Children* promotes the 'traffic light system' for identifying children likely to have serious illness. In the red category, at high risk of having serious illness, are those who appear ill to a healthcare professional, among many other features. In the amber category are those at intermediate risk of having serious illness, who appear less ill but are still not normal.

CONFIRMED UTI

The growth of a single pathogen at $10^5/ml$ is significant, but a pure growth at 10^4 or fewer may also be. Pyuria strengthens the diagnosis, but is not necessary for it.

∗ Treat as above.

∗ Encourage complete emptying of the bladder and avoidance of constipation.

∗ Refer for imaging unless previously investigated. Refer infants urgently. Include the details of the urine culture.

∗ Refer to a paediatrician for further investigation children:

(a) with an atypical infection (seriously ill, poor urine flow, abdominal mass, raised serum creatinine, failure to respond to antibiotics within 48 hours, or infection with an organism other than *E. coli*); or

(b) with recurrent infection that meets the following criteria:
■ three episodes of lower UTI; or
■ two episodes of UTI in at least one of which the infection was in the upper urinary tract.

∗ Organize a follow-up urine specimen 1 month after the infection. There is no agreement on the value of this or of further routine urine cultures.

∗ Exclude urinary infection in future episodes of unexplained fever, abdominal pain, etc., without stopping prophylactic antibiotics if the child is taking them.

ANTIBIOTIC PROPHYLAXIS

NICE recommends against the use of prophylactic antibiotics for the prevention of recurrence. A large study from primary care in the US supports this view, showing that antibiotic prophylaxis was not associated with a decreased risk of UTI but was associated with increased risk of antibiotic resistance (Conway, Cnaan, Zaoutis, *et al.* 2007).

VULVOVAGINITIS

REVIEW

Joishy MJ, Ashtekar CS, Jain A, Gonslaves R. 2005. Do we need to treat vulvovaginitis in prepubertal girls? BMJ 330, 186–188

- Studies indicate that the vaginal microflora of asymptomatic prepubertal girls commonly contains anaerobic and aerobic bacteria. Symptomatic prepubertal girls have a similar spectrum of bacteria but are more likely to grow *Staphylococcus aureus*, β haemolytic *Streptococcus* Group A and possibly *Haemophilus influenzae*.
- The clinical features of vulvovaginitis include: vaginal discharge, redness (especially of the introitus) and soreness.
- Vulvovaginitis in prepubescent girls is usually due to non-specific bacterial infection associated with poor hygiene or with threadworms (probably secondary to the night-time itching).
- Foreign body is uncommon and likely to cause a particularly offensive smell and sometimes altered blood in the discharge.
- Sexual abuse should be considered if:
  - (a) the genital or anal examination looks abnormal; or
  - (b) there are reports of sexualized behaviours; or
  - (c) the child's demeanour is unusual; or
  - (d) there are other family concerns; or
  - (e) a swab grows *Chlamydia* or a sexually transmitted organism; or
  - (f) there are other unexplained symptoms.

Discuss with a community paediatrician.

- * Advise daily baths, wiping from front to back after using the toilet, and not wearing tight-fitting clothing.
- * Take a swab from the introitus and await the result. Ideally only treat if there is a pure or predominant growth of a pathogen.
- * Treat with oral antibiotics if the culture is positive or while awaiting the results, if symptoms are severe.
- * *Persistence or recurrence.* Treat with mebendazole if itchy. Threadworm is likely.
- * Refer to a gynaecologist, if symptoms persist, to look for a foreign body.

PATIENT INFORMATION

Suggest the parent downloads the information sheet on vulvovaginitis from www.rch.org.au/kidsinfo/factsheets.cfm

THE CHILD WHO APPEARS SMALL OR TALL

When there is anxiety about a child's growth, establish:

(a) the height and weight of the child, and plot them on the new nine-centile chart; and

(b) the expected final adult height of the child (see below).

EXPECTED ADULT HEIGHT BASED ON THE HEIGHT OF THE PARENTS

The expected adult height is calculated as follows:

- *for a boy* – the mean of the parents' heights plus 7 cm;
- *for a girl* – the mean of the parents' heights minus 7 cm.

Plot the value on the relevant growth chart as age 19 (i.e. adult).

MEASUREMENT OF HEIGHT

Correct measurement of height is essential.

(a) The child should not wear shoes and the heels should be against the wall with an assistant or parent holding the feet down gently.

(b) With the child standing straight, the thighs and pelvis should be held gently to the wall.

(c) The jaw and external auditory meatus should be in a horizontal line.

(d) The child should be gently stretched upwards with traction under the angle of the jaw, and the height measured.

MANAGEMENT

- A quarter of children with a height at least 2.5 standard deviations (SD) below the mean (which is close to the 0.4 centile) had organic disease in the Wessex growth study (Voss, Mulligan, Betts *et al.* 1992).
- * Refer if the child:
  - (a) is above the 99.6 or below the 0.4 centile;
  - (b) is crossing centile channels;
  - (c) differs significantly from the centile corresponding to the expected adult height.

PUBERTY

For the stages of puberty, see Appendix 7.

EARLY PUBERTY

Most will be girls who will be found to have idiopathic precocious puberty. Once other pathology is excluded, the only treatment is explanation and support and occasionally consideration of gonadotrophin analogues (± antiandrogenic drugs) in an attempt to achieve a higher final height.

- * Refer any child who develops secondary sexual characteristics before the age of 8.
- * Refer any child where one secondary sexual characteristic develops out of proportion to the others and out of proportion to the growth rate. This suggests an abnormal source of hormone secretion. Examples would be isolated breast development without the development of pubic hair and apocrine sweat in girls, and penile enlargement without increase in testicular volume in boys.
- * Refer any child who is passing through the stages of puberty abnormally fast if this is causing concern either for social reasons or because of worries about final height.
- * *Precocious unilateral or bilateral breast development.* This usually occurs before the age of 2 and rarely reaches stage 3. It is very unlikely to be due to organic disease but referral is probably wise.
- * *Pubic hair development under age 8 in girls or age 9 in boys.* This is almost always due to an adrenal androgen surge, but again referral is probably wise.

DELAYED PUBERTY

Most will be boys with constitutional delay of growth and puberty.

Refer any child without secondary sexual characteristics by the age of 14. Even if the delay is shown to be constitutional, these children suffer from psychological problems, increased liability to osteoporosis and a short spine in comparison to leg length. These problems can be avoided by the use of low-dose sex hormones or anabolic steroids (Stanhope, Albanese and Shalet 1992).

RECURRENT PHYSICAL SYMPTOMS

Children commonly develop somatic symptoms where no organic cause can be found. This may reflect psychological distress. It is important to:

- (a) exclude likely physical causes;
- (b) help the family change the focus from physical to underlying psychological issues;
- (c) encourage the child to express his or her feelings;
- (d) encourage continuing school attendance. Avoiding school makes eventual attendance harder.

RECURRENT ABDOMINAL PAIN

In the majority of children with recurrent abdominal pain, the pain is not due to organic pathology. There seems to be a spectrum, with children at one end who seem to have nothing more than an awareness of peristaltic movements, and children at the other end with 'periodic syndrome'. Children at this extreme may vomit, go unusually pale and may be febrile. There is a close connection with migraine.

FEATURES OF BENIGN RECURRENT ABDOMINAL PAIN

- (a) The pain is central, episodic and variable in character.
- (b) The pain is not usually associated with fever, vomiting or with any disturbance in bowel habit.
- (c) The child continues to thrive.

(d) The timing of the pain varies, but tends to be less frequent at weekends and during school holidays.

* Examine the child fully, plot the height and weight and check the urine for protein and infection.

* Refer any child who has symptoms of general illness or bowel disturbance, or where the picture differs significantly from that described above.

* Assess whether there are problems at home or school; whether the child is using the pain as a way of avoiding stress or to gain attention; whether there is evidence of emotional disorder.

* Reassure the parents that the symptoms are not due to a grumbling appendix. Explain that the pain is real but not due to any abdominal pathology and does not require any further investigations. Use the analogy that to have a headache does not mean that there is something wrong with the brain and that, similarly, to have abdominal pain does not necessarily indicate that there is something wrong in the abdomen.

* Follow-up regularly, and repeatedly reassure the child and parents. Indeed parental factors predict the persistence of abdominal pain better than factors related to the child, especially whether the parents accept that psychological factors play a large part.

* Consider a trial of peppermint oil for 2 weeks. A RCT in 42 children found an improvement in 71% compared to 43% on placebo (Berger, Gieteling and Benninga 2007). However, prescribe it in a way that reduces, rather than strengthens, the parents' conviction that organic illness is present.

* Consider using prophylactic pizotifen for children with 'periodic syndrome' (as in Migraine, page 292) (Abu-Arafeh and Russell 1995; Dignan, Symon, AbuArafeh, et al. 2001).

* Refer if the parents are dissatisfied or if the pain does not settle.

RECURRENT HEADACHE

Headache is common in children, and the incidence increases with age; 80–90% of secondary school-age children suffer from recurrent headaches!

The incidence of migraine in this age group is about 5%, but many children suffer severe non-migrainous headaches. About 25% of severe adult migraine sufferers can remember having severe headaches by the age of 10 years.

* Check the blood pressure and examine the fundi.

* Refer if there is any anxiety about organic pathology. This is more likely in children under 5, where the headache is not relieved by simple analgesics, the frequency and severity is increasing, the child is not thriving or has signs of intellectual slowing, or where there are neurological signs.

* If there is no evidence of organic pathology, reassure the parents that the child does not have a tumour or blood clot causing the headaches.

* *Migrainous headaches.* If associated with recurrent abdominal pain, pallor, paraesthesiae, visual disturbances or vomiting, the diagnosis is likely to be migraine. Advise the parents to treat the attack at an early stage with soluble paracetamol and to encourage the child to lie down. Mild hypoglycaemia is a common trigger; try snacks, especially before vigorous exercise, and avoid long gaps between food. Children with frequent migraines may benefit from prophylaxis, e.g. pizotifen or propranolol, for 6 months in the first instance (see also Migraine page 292).

* *Non-migrainous headaches* are commonly tension-related. Reassure the child of their benign nature and encourage them to take paracetamol early in the headache.

Examination of lifestyle and an alteration in behaviour may help. A number of children suffer headaches at the end of a busy day when many factors may have contributed, including hunger. One RCT in adolescents has shown significant improvement in migraine frequency with self-administered stress management therapy (McGrath, Humphreys, Keene, *et al.* 1992).

Note: Eye strain is only rarely a cause of headaches, and many children are prescribed glasses unnecessarily for minor refractive errors.

NIGHT CRAMPS/JOINT PAINS

Night cramps are felt more in the legs than in the arms, and are felt *between* (not *in*) the joints. They are not growing pains, but may reflect stresses in the child's life akin to headaches. They are generally more common during term-time than during school holidays. The pains commonly wake the child up from sleep.

* Investigations are neither necessary nor helpful.
* Emotional support, e.g. cuddles and massage, are all that is needed. Analgesics are not required but may provide a necessary placebo.
* Refer if there is any suspicion of juvenile idiopathic arthritis, particularly if the child:
  (a) is reluctant to join in with physical activities;
  (b) has a change in mood, e.g. tired and withdrawn;
  (c) is unwilling to use one limb in particular;
  (d) has pain, stiffness (especially in the morning) or joint swelling;
  (e) has a number of joints affected especially in the lower limb.
* Arrange for FBC, ESR, rheumatoid factor and antinuclear antibodies.

TIC DISORDERS

Chowdhury U, Heyman I. 2004. Tourette's syndrome in children. BMJ 329, 1356–1357

Tics are abrupt and recurrent motor or vocal actions. They may be preceded by a sensory urge and suppressed for some time. They are sudden and purposeless.

Tics can be divided into:

(a) simple tics, e.g. blinking, grunting, clearing one's throat, shrugging;
(b) complex tics, e.g. licking, jumping or touching objects.

Tourette's syndrome is the most severe form with multiple motor and vocal tics lasting a year or more. The complex vocal tic involving involuntary swearing occurs in less than 15% of those with Tourette's syndrome.

Tics affect 4–18% of children at some stage.

* *Mild tics.* Reassure and explain to the parents and teachers that this is an organic disorder of the brain and that it will resolve in time. Assess whether the child is bullied or reprimanded at school. Refer if there are emotional difficulties arising from the tic.
* *Complex tics.* Refer for assessment by a child psychiatrist. Medication may help: dopamine agonists (e.g. pergolide) antagonists (e.g. haloperidol) or the α2 agonist, clonidine. It is important to exclude obsessive compulsive disorder and ADHD as well as psychopathology.

PATIENT ORGANIZATION

Tourette Syndrome (UK) Association. PO Box 26149, Dunfermline KY12 7YU, tel. 0845 458 1252, email: enquiries@tsa.org.uk, www.tsa.org.uk

SCHOOL REFUSAL

● About one in of all school pupils are absent from school at any one time, and one fifth of these have no legitimate reason for being away. The latter fall into three main groups: truants, children voluntarily withheld by parents and school refusers.
● School refusal may be based on a fear of separation from one or both parents or fear of school attendance. School-refusing children generally work well at school, and are expressing an underlying neurotic disorder. School refusal tends to occur in three main age groups: 5–7, 11 (after changing to secondary school) and in adolescence.
* Exclude an underlying cause if the presentation is of physical illness.
* Ask specifically about bullying (see below).
* Refer to a specialist unit according to what is locally available.
* Encourage the child to go back to school. This involves convincing the parents of the importance of doing so. Even severe emotional problems can improve rapidly on re-establishing attendance.

BULLYING

● Bullying is more common in boys and in the youngest pupils in a school.
● The commonest type of bullying is name-calling, followed by being physically hit, being

threatened and having rumours spread about the bullied individual.

- Research suggests an incidence of about one in five for being bullied (with higher figures for children who attend remedial classes or who are of Asian origin) and up to one in ten for bullying others.
- Being bullied is one of the factors most strongly associated with suicidal behaviour in adolescents. Both bullies and victims are at increased risk of suicide (Kaltiala-Heino, Rimpela, Marttunen, *et al.* 1999).
- Bullying by fellow pupils is a primary responsibility of the school; every school should have an anti-bullying policy.
- 'Passive victims' of bullying tend to be: cautious, sensitive, quiet, more anxious and insecure, have fewer friends, feel unhappy and lonely, have low self-esteem, have a negative view of themselves and their situation, look upon themselves as failures, feel stupid, ashamed and unattractive.
- 'Proactive victims' (a smaller group) have a combination of anxious and aggressive reactions that provoke other children who then retaliate in a negative fashion. These children may have concentration difficulties, be overactive and often behave in ways that cause irritation and tension around them.
* Suspect bullying in children who present with:
  (a) sleeping difficulties;
  (b) bed wetting;
  (c) feeling sad;
  (d) headaches;
  (e) stomach aches;
  (f) irritability, poor concentration;
  (g) depression, suicidal ideation, deliberate self-harm;
  (h) somatic symptoms;
  (i) anxiety;
  (j) social dysfunction.
* Encourage the child to tell their parents and teacher. Reassure them they were right to tell and that the adults will try to work together to keep them safe.
* Encourage the parents to approach the school directly. Consider involving a school counsellor/nurse or practice counsellor (Dawkins 1995).

* Refer to a specialist child and adolescent mental health service children who:
  (a) are severely depressed;
  (b) have suicidal thoughts;
  (c) are self-harming;
  (d) show social withdrawal;
  (e) refuse to eat;
  (f) are severely anxious or have insomnia;
  (g) are developing school refusal.

They may benefit from a number of interventions especially cognitive behavioural therapy (Stein, Jaycox, Kataoka, *et al.* 2003).

INFORMATION FOR PATIENTS

The Royal College of Psychiatrists. *The Emotional Cost of Bullying*, leaflet 18, available on http://www.rcpsych.ac.uk (search for 'Bullying').

Bullying UK, http://www.bullying.co.uk

The Bullying Project provides online mentoring support programmes, as well as educational resources http://www.bullying.org

---

SURGICAL PROBLEMS

STRAWBERRY NAEVUS

Strawberry naevi usually appear shortly after birth and grow very rapidly for the first 4–5 months of life. They then involute and become pale. Full resolution may take many years.

* Reassure parents that surgery is not warranted and that the lesion naturally regresses.
* Advise them how to stop any bleeding, should it occur, by applying pressure.
* *Exceptions:*
  (a) large haemangiomas on the nose, lip, eyelid or cheek may grow very large and need steroid treatment or surgery;
  (b) haemangiomas on the eyelid: refer early to prevent amblyopia;
  (c) haemangioma on the face with stridor: refer urgently (suggests laryngeal haemangioma).

INGUINAL HERNIA

These usually present in the first 3–4 months of life and are less common with increasing age.

* Refer for urgent outpatient appointment; early operation is recommended to avoid incarceration or strangulation.

HYDROCELE

These are the most common cause of scrotal swelling. There are two types:

(a) slack, often bilateral, which disappear within the first year;

(b) tense, often unilateral, which exist after the first year and need surgery lest spermatogenesis is impaired.

UNDESCENDED TESTIS

See page 87.

THE FORESKIN

● The foreskin has a protective role and is not usually retractile until 1 year. 'Adhesions' are present in 60% of boys aged 6. They are physiological and regress spontaneously.

● Retraction of the foreskin should be encouraged from the age of 6 in order to clean out smegma, but not to break down the 'adhesions'. These will continue to separate naturally throughout childhood and adolescence. Tearing them forcibly risks causing scarring (Anon 1993). Surgical separation or circumcision should only be considered if they are causing symptoms.

CIRCUMCISION

● The General Medical Council (GMC) and British Medical Association have developed guidelines relating to the circumcision of boys (Beecham 1997; BMA 2003). They stress that, among other issues:

(a) the doctor should have the necessary skills and experience both to operate and to treat the patient's postoperative pain;

(b) the doctor should explain the risks and benefits of the operation and obtain consent, preferably from both parents.

(c) *non-therapeutic circumcision.* It is legal in the UK for boys but not girls, but responsibility for demonstrating that circumcision lies in the child's best interest lies with the parents, both of whom must give consent.

● Adverse effects of circumcision occur in 0.03–7.4% according to circumstances. Bleeding is the most common immediate adverse effect, with scar formation, reduced penile sensation, and a poor cosmetic appearance the commonest late complications. Circumcision while still in nappies can give rise to meatal ulceration and subsequent stricture.

● The following issues may be raised by parents (Malone and Steinbrecher 2007):

(a) *prevention of HIV infection.* While this may be worthwhile in communities in which men do not use condoms it is not grounds for circumcision in the UK. Transmission of sexually transmitted diseases other than HIV is probably not reduced (Dickson, van Rhoode, Herbison, *et al.* 2008);

(b) *prevention of urinary tract infection.* The risk of UTI is greater in uncircumcized boys with an increase in risk of between three and seven times. Most of the infections occur in infancy. However, these infections only occur in those with recurrent infections and/or those with an abnormal urinary tract, e.g. high grade vesico-ureteric reflux. Treatment should be directed at the urinary tract abnormality not at the foreskin, and not in those without those extra risk factors;

(c) *prevention of penile cancer.* Penile cancer is more common in uncircumcized men but only in those with a pathological phimosis. Surgery for the phimosis is justified anyway in its own right.

Common indications for circumcision which may be justified are:

(a) *balanitis:* prescribe antibiotic ointment (e.g. fusidic acid) to be massaged into the preputial orifice. After three attacks, consider circumcision;

(b) *phimosis:* true phimosis is uncommon. It is usually due to balanitis xerotica obliterans, which manifests as a scarred appearance at the prepuce. Circumcision should be considered only if there is difficulty passing urine or if a full erection is impeded. Almost all cases of physiological tightness of the preputial orifice will resolve naturally. It is still present in 8% of 7-year-olds. Even ballooning of the foreskin does not necessarily mean that circumcision is necessary. Sometimes aligning the preputial orifice with the meatus before starting to pass urine, by pulling back on the foreskin, will avoid the problem;

(c) *paraphimosis:* this should be reduced as soon as possible. Shrink the glans with an ice pack, and use a lubricant to reduce the paraphimosis. Admit if irreducible;

(d) *redundant prepuce:* a long prepuce may occasionally lead to recurrent irritation and discomfort.

HYPOSPADIAS

Refer immediately if the child is not producing a good stream of urine. Non-urgent cases should be seen by the age of 6 months so that subsequent surgery can be planned.

UMBILICAL HERNIA

* Tell the parents that:
  (a) umbilical hernias increase in size in the first 6 months of life but they do not strangulate;
  (b) bandaging with an old penny is of no value.
* At 1 year, if the hernial orifice:
  (a) is less than 1 cm in diameter then spontaneous resolution is likely;
  (b) is greater than 1 cm in diameter then surgical intervention may be necessary.
* Consider hypothyroidism: check that the child is growing and gaining weight normally.

BAT EARS

If operation is desired, do not refer until the child is aged 3 years; the cartilage is not firm enough for surgery until then.

ORTHOPAEDIC PROBLEMS

EXAMINATION OF THE HIP FOR CONGENITAL DISLOCATION

See page 86.

CLUB FEET

Marked congenital talipes equinovarus is easily recognized at birth. Much more common is positional talipes due to the position of the foot *in utero.*

* Refer if the foot cannot be moved into the normal position.
* *Positional talipes.* The foot is easily moved into the normal anatomical position. Reassure the parents that it will correct itself. Exercises may help – teach the parents to stretch the medial border of the foot and to push the foot into eversion and dorsiflexion on a regular basis, e.g. when bathing the baby each day.

IN-TOEING

This may be due to:

(a) *metatarsus adductus (varus)* or hooking of the forefoot which usually straightens by the age of 3 years. Referral is only needed if the deformity cannot be corrected by passive straightening;

(b) *femoral neck anteversion.* These children walk with their kneecaps facing each other because of anteversion of the femoral neck. Examine the child prone with the knees flexed and the feet in the air. Internal rotation (turning the leg outwards) is increased from 70° to as much as 90°. Conversely, external rotation (turning the leg inwards) is considerably reduced. Refer extreme cases for orthopaedic opinion. Reassure the parents of less extreme cases that the femoral anteversion resolves by the age of 8–9 years;

(c) *tibial torsion* occurs when the normal growth and rotation of the tibia is out of step with the femur. Inward rotation leads to in-toeing.

  * Reassure the parents that it resolves by the age of 3–4 years, but consider rickets in at-risk children.

BOW LEGS AND KNOCK KNEES

Bow legs and knock knees rarely need treatment. Many infants have outward curving of the tibia, and spontaneous resolution usually occurs by the age of 2 years. Children may then become knock kneed, which reaches a maximum by the age of 4 years. They then improve spontaneously, achieving normal alignment by about 6 years of age.

* Refer:
  (a) if the child is unwell, especially if the bones are tender or joints swollen as in rickets;

(b) the legs are asymmetrical;

(c) there is anterior curvature of the tibiae;

(d) if in bow legs the knee to knee distance is greater than 3 cm; or

(e) if in knock knees the medial malleoli are more than 7 cm apart when the child lies down with the knees together and the patellae facing forwards. Referral might be made at lesser measurements if the distance is increasing.

FLAT FEET

* Refer if there is neurological abnormality, muscle weakness or a lack of movement at the tarsal joints.

* Reassure if the child is asymptomatic, there is a full range of active and passive movements at all joints, and the arch is seen normally when the child stands on tiptoe. The arch is likely to be normal by the age of 10.

CURLY TOES

* Reassure the parents that the toes can be straightened if necessary.

* Refer the child to have the toes straightened only if the deformity is fixed and sufficiently severe for one toe to impinge on another in a way that is likely to cause symptoms.

THE LIMPING CHILD

The child who presents with a painful limp and complains of pain in the knee should be assumed to have a problem in the hip until proved otherwise. Depending on the age of the child, the problem may be due to:

(a) *congenital dislocation of the hip*. This is painless and usually obvious once the child begins to walk;

(b) *Perthes'* avascular necrosis of the femoral head, which usually occurs between age 5 and 10;

(c) *slipping of the upper femoral epiphysis*, which usually occurs between age 10 and 15;

(d) *acute septic arthritis and acute osteomyelitis*, which can occur at any age and are surgical emergencies;

(e) *transient synovitis of the hip* (irritable hip) – this is the most common cause of limp due to hip pain

and is commonest between age 4 and 10. 90% resolve in 7 days, but it cannot reliably be distinguished in general practice from more serious causes of hip pain, and all patients should be referred.

* Refer all these to hospital urgently.

OSGOOD SCHLATTER'S DISEASE

* Explain the benign nature of the condition. It will resolve spontaneously, leaving only a prominent tibial tubercle.

* Explain that exercise may make the pain worse but will not cause progressive damage. Patients may do any sport that they can manage without excessive pain.

* Do not X-ray or refer.

SCOLIOSIS

This occurs more commonly in girls than in boys.

* Examine all children over the age of 10 years, when the opportunity arises. Examine from behind, as follows:

(a) stand the child up with the feet together;

(b) assess whether the hips are level (i.e. there is no compensation);

(c) ask the child to touch his or her toes with the knees straight;

(d) look for a 'rib hump'. This will be most marked when the spine is flexed.

* Refer to an orthopaedic surgeon if there is any suggestion of 'rib hump' or curvature.

PREVENTIVE HEALTHCARE IN ADOLESCENTS

OVERVIEWS

Viner R. 2005. ABC of adolescence. BMJ 330: several sections across different issues

National Adolescent & Student Health Unit and the Royal College of General Practitioners. 1996. The Health of Adolescents in Primary Care. Royal College of General Practitioners, London. Available from RCGP, 14 Princes Gate, Hyde Park, London SW7 1PU, tel. 020 7581 3232

- Teenagers prefer to reduce their risk of being excluded from their peer group, or of looking immature, than take notice of any perceived health risk.
- Health behaviours in adolescence are continued into adulthood. These include: smoking, drinking alcohol, drug abuse, violence, sexual intimacy, exercise and obesity. Over 90% of adult smokers started smoking as teenagers.
- Health in adolescence can have a considerable impact on the development of adult conditions.
- Health risk behaviours cluster. Those who smoke are more likely to take drugs, drink alcohol, engage in risky sexual behaviour and be involved in violence.
- * Ensure that adolescents are aware of the confidentiality policies and practices of the practice. Teenagers rate confidentiality and access as the most important aspects of medical care.
- * Ensure that the practice is giving the message to adolescents that they are seen as an important group for whom specific services exist.
- * Target the younger adolescent as the key risk periods for smoking, taking drugs and taking sexual risks are before the age of 14. At this age teenagers are still 'concrete' thinkers and health promotion messages should concentrate on the 'here and now' not what might happen in adulthood.
- * Be aware that rational health promotion messages are often ineffective in adolescents. Helping a teenager to develop self-esteem is more likely to lead to healthy behaviour than negative messages about the dangers of sex or smoking.
- * Recommend teenage-friendly health promotion sites e.g.:
  - (a) www.teenagehealthfreak.org; and
  - (b) www.lifebytes.gov.uk

PATIENT INFORMATION

Royal College of Psychiatrists. *Help is at Hand: Surviving Adolescence*, and *Surviving Adolescence – A Toolkit for Parents.* www.rcpsych.ac.uk

SUBSTANCE MISUSE (see Chapter 17)

- *Alcohol.* About 20% of 12–13-year-olds report drinking alcohol. This increases to 40–50% by age 14–15 and to over 70% by the age of 17. About 40% of adolescents report binge drinking.
- *Smoking.* The proportion who smoke regularly rises from about 1% at age 11 to 24% by the age of 15.
- *Drugs.* 30–50% of 16–17-year-olds report trying cannabis. Regular use is less common: 10% report weekly use, and 3% daily use. Inhalants (paint, glue or petrol) may be misused by around 5% of adolescents.
- * Recognize that change takes time and that the patient may spend a considerable time with no serious thought about behaviour change before giving it serious thought, and then eventually starting to modify behaviour.
- * Arrange to see the adolescent regularly.
- * Discuss moderation as a harm reduction strategy.
- * Recommend the web sites above and www. talktofrank.com

MENTAL HEALTH PROBLEMS (see Chapter 16)

The prevalence of mental health problems among 11–15 year olds is estimated to be around 11%. These include:

(a) depression, which affects 8–10% of adolescents. The presentation may be that of depressed mood but is more likely to be masked, e.g. behavioural problems, substance misuse, school phobia or failure at school, tiredness or other somatic symptoms;

(b) school phobia (see page 123);

(c) learning difficulties. Dyslexia and other specific learning problems are often an undiagnosed cause of adolescents leaving school early;

(d) conduct disorders where the adolescent persistently disrupts and violates the rights of others or social norms;

(e) ADHD. About 80% of children with ADHD continue to have the disorder during adolescence and up to 50% of adolescents continue with it into adulthood;

(f) anxiety and panic are common during adolescence. Generalized anxiety may present as excessive worrying accompanied with difficulty in concentrating, irritability, sleep problems and tiredness.

* Suspect mental health problems in adolescents presenting with:

  (a) signs of depression (low mood, tearfulness, lack of interest in usual activities);

  (b) somatic symptoms, e.g. headache, stomach ache, backache, and sleep problems;

  (c) self-harming behaviour;

  (d) aggression;

  (e) isolation and loneliness;

  (f) deviant behaviour such as theft and robbery;

  (g) change in school performance or behaviour;

  (h) use of psychoactive substances, including over-the-counter medications;

  (i) weight loss or failure to gain weight with growth;

  (j) self-neglect.

SELF-HARM AND SUICIDE (see Chapter 16)

● Self-harm. 7–14% of adolescents self-harm at some time and 20–45% of adolescents report having suicidal thoughts. Suicide rates are far higher in boys than girls and are rising.

● Depression is common in most who go on to die by suicide. So also is a history of behavioural disturbance, substance misuse, family problems (divorce, separation or death of a parent), a family history of psychiatric disorder and a history of self-harm. 25–50% of those who go on to commit suicide have self-harmed in the past.

● Self-harm is often an impulsive act (with only a few minutes prior thought) and may be associated with alcohol and drug consumption.

* Ask an adolescent who has self-harmed what's going on. It is often an attempt to relieve unbearable tension, or to 'get back at' other people. It may have been triggered by events at home, at school or with friends of the same or opposite sex.

* Refer all adolescents who have self-harmed to the Child and Adolescent Mental Health Unit.

* Refer urgently those who are at high risk of suicide. These are especially those whose act was parasuicide rather than repetitive self-harm and who:

  (a) carried the act out in isolation;

  (b) timed it so that intervention was unlikely and took precautions to avoid discovery;

  (c) made preparations in anticipation of death (e.g. leaving indication of how belongings to be distributed, suicide note or message);

  (d) told others beforehand about thoughts of suicide;

  (e) had considered the act for hours or days beforehand;

  (f) did not alert others during or after the act.

PATIENT INFORMATION

Royal College of Psychiatrists. *Self-harm in Young People.* Leaflet 26, available: www.rcpsych.ac.uk/mentalhealthinfoforall/mentalhealthandgrowingup.aspx

CONTRACEPTION

● The median age for sexual intercourse is around 16 for boys and girls.

● Half those under the age of 16 and a third aged 16–19 used no contraception the first time they had sex.

● Teenagers are relatively poor users of contraception but condoms remain the contraceptive of choice. The combined use of oral contraceptives and condoms (to protect against pregnancy and STIs) is thought to be the most effective approach.

● *Emergency contraception.* Less than 50% of adolescents know about the 72 hour limit on oral emergency contraception.

● 4000 girls under 16 have terminations in the UK each year.

* Consider:

  (a) making condoms easily available without the need for counselling or appointments;

(b) having easily accessible health promotion material that covers emergency contraception and young people's legal rights to contraception;

(c) offering contraceptive methods that are attractive to young people (e.g. flavoured condoms), useable just at the time of intercourse, and cheap and easily obtainable;

(d) advise use of combined oral contraception and condoms ('double dutch').

SEXUALLY TRANSMITTED INFECTIONS

● Chlamydia rates in 16–19-year-olds increased two- to three-fold in the period 1995–2001. 30–40% of sexually active teenagers in high-risk groups are infected. Gonorrhoea has shown similar increases.

● Teenage girls are more susceptible to chlamydia infection than adults possibly because of a more immature cervix.

● Note that:

(a) vaginal discharge is the commonest presentation for chlamydia and gonorrhoea in girls under the age of 13;

(b) chlamydia and gonorrhoea are asymptomatic in 70–80% of adolescent girls who are infected. Pelvic inflammatory disease can also be asymptomatic;

(c) gonorrhoea may present as pharyngeal and rectal infections.

∗ Consider adolescent girls to be at higher risk of STIs if they:

(a) practise unsafe sex;

(b) have multiple, sequential sexual partners or concurrent partners;

(c) have mental health problems;

(d) are taking drugs.

References

Abu-Arafeh, I., Russell, G., 1995. Prevalence and clinical features of abdominal migraine compared with those of migraine headache. Arch. Dis. Child. 72 (5), 413–417.

Agertoft, L., Pedersen, S., 1994. Effects of long-term treatment with inhaled corticosteroids on growth and pulmonary function in asthmatic children. Respir. Med. 88, 373–381.

Anon, 1993. Medical indications for childhood circumcision. Drug Ther. Bull. 31, 99–100.

Ausejo, M., Saenz, A., Pham, B., et al., 1999. The effectiveness of glucocorticoids in treating croup: meta-analysis. BMJ 319, 595–600.

Barlow, J., Coren, E., 2001. Parent-training programmes for improving maternal psychosocial health (Cochrane Review). In: The Cochrane Library, Issue 4. Update Software, Oxford.

Beecham, L., 1997. GMC issues guidelines on circumcision. BMJ 314, 1573.

Bellak, L., Black, R.B., 1992. Attention deficit disorder in adults. Clin. Ther. 14 (2), 138–147.

Berger, M.Y., Gieteling, M.J., Benninga, M.A., 2007. Chronic abdominal pain in children. BMJ 334, 997–1002.

BMA, 2003. Law and ethics of male circumcision – guidance for doctors 2003. http://www.bma. org.uk/ap.nsf/Content/ malecircumcision2003.

Butler, R.J., 2002. Nocturnal enuresis resource pack. Bristol ERIC.

Chavasse, R.J., Bastian-Lee, Y., Richter, H., et al., 2001. Persistent wheezing in infants with an atopic tendency responds to inhaled fluticasone. Arch. Dis. Child. 85, 143–148.

Chavasse, R., Seddon, P., Bara, A., et al., 2002. Short acting beta agonists for recurrent wheeze in children under 2 years of age. (Cochrane Review). In: The Cochrane Library, Issue 3.

Chief Medical Officer's Expert Group, 1993. Report of the CMO's Expert Group on the Sleeping Position of Infants and Cot Death. HMSO, London.

Conway, P., Cnaan, A., Zaoutis, T., et al., 2007. Recurrent urinary tract infections in children. JAMA 298, 179–186.

Crowcroft, N.S., Strachan, D.P., 1997. The social origins of infantile colic: questionnaire study covering 76,747 infants. BMJ 314, 1325–1328.

Dalby-Payne, J., Elliot, E., 2005. Gastro-oesophageal Reflux in Children. Clinical Evidence. BMJ Publishing Group, London.

Dawkins, J., 1995. Bullying in schools: doctors' responsibilities. BMJ 310, 274–275.

Department of Health and Social Security, 1988. Present Day Practice in Infant Feeding. Report on Health and Social Subjects 32. HMSO, London.

Dickson, N.P., van Rhoode, T., Herbison, P., et al., 2008. Circumcision and risk of sexually transmitted infections in a birth cohort. J. Pediatr. 152, 383–387.

Dignan, F., Symon, D.N., AbuArafeh, I., et al., 2001. The prognosis of cyclical vomiting syndrome. Arch. Dis. Child. 84, 55–57.

DTB, 1987. The management of febrile convulsions. Drug Ther. Bull. 25 (3), 9–11.

Dutton, G.N., Cleary, M., 2004. Should we be screening for and treating amblyopia? BMJ 327, 1242–1243.

Elbourne, D., Dezateux, C., Arthur, R., et al., 2002. Ultrasonography in the diagnosis and management of developmental hip dysplasia (UK Hip Trial): clinical and economic results from a multicentre randomized control trial. Lancet 360, 2000–2017.

Garrett, L.J., Nye, C., 2003. Speech and language therapy interventions for children with primary speech and language delay or disorder. In: Cochrane Library, Issue 3. Update software, Oxford.

Geelhoed, G.C., Turner, J., Macdonald, W.B., 1996. Efficacy of a small single dose of oral dexamethasone for outpatient croup: a double blind placebo-controlled clinical trial. BMJ 313, 140–142.

Glazener, C.M.A., Evans, J.H.C., 2002. Desmopressin for nocturnal enuresis in children (Cochrane Review). In: The Cochrane Library, Issue 4. Update Software, Oxford.

Glazener, C.M.A., Evans, J.H.C., 2003a. Alarm interventions for nocturnal enuresis in children (Cochrane Review). In: The Cochrane Library, Issue 4. Update Software, Oxford.

Glazener, C.M.A., Evans, J.H.C., 2003b. Tricyclic and related drugs for nocturnal enuresis in children (Cochrane Review). In: The Cochrane Library, Issue 3. Update Software, Oxford.

Gorelick, M.H., Shaw, K.N., 1999. Screening tests for urinary tract infection in children: a meta-analysis. Pediatrics 104 (5), e54.

Hazell, P.L., Stuart, J.E., 2003. A randomized controlled trial of clonidine added to psychostimulant medication for hyperactive and aggressive children. J. Am. Acad. Child Adolosc. Psychiatry 42, 886–894.

Hay, A.D., Wilson, A.D., 2002. The natural history of acute cough in children aged 0–4 years in primary care; a systematic review. Br. J. Gen. Pract. 52, 401–409.

Health Development Agency, 2001. What works in preventing unintentional injuries in children and young adolescents. http://www.hda-online.org.uk/evidence (choose 'Search For Evidence' then search on 'Injuries In Children').

Hiscock, H., Wake, M., 2002. Randomised controlled trial of behavioural infant sleep intervention to improve infant sleep and maternal mood. BMJ 324, 1062–1065.

Hoekstra, J.H., 1998. Toddler diarrhoea: more a nutritional disorder than a disease. Arch. Dis. Child. 79, 2–5.

Isaacs, D., 1995. Bronchiolitis. BMJ 310, 4–5.

Jones, M., Onslow, M., Packman, A., et al., 2005. Randomised controlled trial of the Lidcombe programme of early stuttering intervention. BMJ 331, 659–661.

Kaltiala-Heino, R., Rimpela, M., Marttunen, M., et al., 1999. Bullying, depression and suicidal ideation in Finnish adolescents. BMJ 319, 348–351.

Kilgour, T., Wade, S., 2004. Infantile colic. Clinical Evidence. BMJ Publishing Group, London.

Kinmouth, A.L., Fulton, Y., Campbell, M.J., 1992. Management of feverish children at home. BMJ 305, 1134–1136.

Konofal, E., Lecendreux, M., Arnulf, I., et al., 2004. Iron deficiency in children with attention deficit disorder. Arch. Pediatr. Adolesc. Med. 158, 1113–1115.

Kotagal, S., Pianosi, P., 2006. Sleep disorders in children and adolescents. BMJ 332, 828–832.

Luria, J.W., Gonzalez-del-Rey, J.A., DiGiulio, G.A., et al., 2001. Effectiveness of oral or nebulized dexamethasone for children with mild croup. Arch. Pediatr. Adolesc. Med. 155, 1340–1345.

McGrath, P.J., Humphreys, P., Keene, D., et al., 1992. The efficacy and efficiency of self-administered treatment for adolescent migraine. Pain 49, 321–324.

McKean, M., Ducharme, F., 2001. Inhaled steroids for episodic viral wheeze of childhood (Cochrane Review). In: The Cochrane Library, Issue 4. Update Software, Oxford.

Malone, P., Steinbrecher, H., 2007. Medical aspects of male circumcision. BMJ 335, 1206–1209.

NICE, 2007. Feverish Illness in Children. Clinical Guideline 47. Available http://www.nice.org.uk

Prem, A.R., 2006. Common paediatric problems. BMJ 333, 486–489.

Rantala, H., Tarkka, R., Uhari, M., 1997. A meta-analytic review of the preventative treatment of recurrences of febrile seizures. J. Pediatr. 131, 922–925.

St James-Roberts, I., 1992. Managing infants who cry persistently. BMJ 304, 997–998.

Sawyer, S.M., 1996. Reproductive and sexual health in adolescents with cystic fibrosis. BMJ 313, 1095–1096.

Scolnik, D., Coates, A.L., Stephens, D., et al., 2006. Controlled delivery of high vs low humidity vs mist therapy for croup in emergency departments: a randomized controlled trial. JAMA 295, 1274–1280.

Sever, Y., Ashkenazi, A., Tyano, S., et al., 1997. Iron treatment in children with attention deficit hyperactivity disorder. Neuropsychobiology 35, 178–180.

Sleep, J., Gillham, P., St James Roberts, I., et al., 2002. A randomized controlled trial to compare alternative strategies for preventing infant crying and sleep problems in the first 12 weeks: the COSI study. Primary Health Care Research and Development 3, 176–183.

Stanhope, R., Albanese, A., Shalet, S., 1992. Delayed puberty. BMJ 305, 790.

Stein, B.D., Jaycox, L.H., Kataoka, S.H., et al., 2003. A mental health intervention for schoolchildren exposed to violence- a randomized controlled trial. JAMA 290, 603–670.

Taylor, E., Sandberg, S., Thorley, G., Giles, S., 1991. The Epidemiology of Childhood Hyperactivity. Maudsley Monographs, No. 33. Oxford University Press, Oxford.

Tourette's Syndrome Study Group, 2002. Treatment of ADHD in children with tics: a Randomised controlled trial. Neurology 58, 527–536.

Vaillancourt, S., McGillivray, D., Zhang, D., et al., 2007. To clean or not to clean: effect on contamination rates in midstream urine collections in toilet-trained children. Pediatrics 119, 1288–1293.

Valman, H.B., 1993. Febrile convulsions. BMJ 306, 1743–1745.

Van Niel, C.W., Feudtner, C., Garrison, M.M., et al., 2002. *Lactobacillus* therapy for acute infectious diarrhea in children: a meta-analysis. Pediatrics 109, 678–684.

Verity, C.M., Golding, J., 1991. Risk of epilepsy after febrile convulsions: a national cohort study. BMJ 303, 1373–1376.

Vernon, S.J., 1996. Comments on managing urinary tract infection in children were inadequate. BMJ 313, 491–492.

Voss, L.D., Mulligan, J., Betts, P.R., et al., 1992. Poor growth in school entrants as an index of organic disease: the Wessex growth study. BMJ 305, 1400–1402.

Wilens, T.E., Faraone, S.V., Biederman, J., et al., 2003. Does stimulant therapy of attention deficit/hyperactivity disorder beget later substance abuse? A meta-analytic review of the literature. Pediatrics 111, 179–185.

Woclik, S.A., Sandler, I.N., Millsap, R. E., et al., 2002. Six-year follow-up of preventative interventions for children of divorce. JAMA 288, 1874–1881.

Woolfenden, S.R., Williams, K., Peat, J., 2001. Family and parenting interventions in children and adolescents with conduct disorder and delinquency aged 10–17 (Cochrane Review). In: The Cochrane Library, Issue 4. Update Software, Oxford.

Chapter 5

Cardiovascular problems

CHAPTER CONTENTS

© 2011 Elsevier Ltd.
DOI: 10.1016/B978-0-7020-3053-6.00005-2

HYPERTENSION

GUIDELINES

Williams B, Poulter N, Brown M, *et al.* 2004. British Hypertension Society guidelines for hypertension management 2004 (BHS-IV): summary. BMJ 328, 634–40. Available: www.bhsoc.org
    National Institute for Health and Clinical Excellence. 2006. *Hypertension: Management of Hypertension in Adults in Primary Care.* NICE clinical guideline 34, June 2006. Available: www.nice.org.uk

- 37% of adults in the UK have hypertension, using the new UK definitions (see below) (Primatesta, Brookes and Poulter 2001). For details of the diagnosis of hypertension see *Evidence-based Diagnosis in Primary Care* by A. F. Polmear (editor), published by Butterworth-Heinemann, 2008.
- The rule of halves was described in the US in 1972 (Wilber and Barrow 1972). It states that half of hypertensives are not known to have a raised BP; of those with known hypertension, half are not on treatment and half of those on treatment are poorly controlled. Figures for the UK in 1998 (Primatesta, Brookes and Poulter 2001) show that, using the new definitions (see below), half of those with hypertension knew they were hypertensive; of these, two thirds were on treatment and a third of those were controlled. Even using a threshold and target of 160/95, 71% knew they had hypertension; of these, 59% were on treatment; and 65% of these were controlled.

- If hypertension is found it should trigger a search for other risk factors for cardiovascular disease. These factors tend to cluster and their risks are multiplicative.
- *The benefits of treatment*: treating mild hypertension reduces the risk of a cardiovascular event by 25%. For patients with mild-moderate hypertension and a 10-year CHD risk of at least 15% the number needed to treat for 5 years is 40 (i.e. treating 40 such patients for 5 years will prevent one cardiovascular event).

DETECTION

All adults should have their blood pressure measured at least every 5 years. Those not qualifying for treatment but whose blood pressure is at least 130/85 need review annually. Patients with a BP of at least 140/90 but below 160/100 are deemed to have mild hypertension by WHO standards (Guidelines Committee 2003) (Table 5.1).

Note: Where a threshold or target level of blood pressure is given, e.g. 160/100 (Table 5.2), it means that action should be taken if the systolic is 100 or over OR the diastolic is 100 or over.

Two points about these targets:

(a) *any* reduction in blood pressure carries benefit, even if the target is not reached;
(b) the lower the blood pressure the greater the benefit, at least down to 115/75 (Nash 2007). Below this there is no evidence either way.

PRACTICALITIES

(a) The patient should be seated, but in older patients and in diabetics check the blood pressure both standing and sitting.

Table 5.1	Classification used by the British Hypertension Society, the European Society of Hypertension and the WHO, based on clinic readings (Williams B, Poulter N, Brown M, *et al.* 2004)	
CATEGORIES	**SYSTOLIC BP**	**DIASTOLIC BP**
Optimal	< 120	< 80
Normal	120–129	80–84
High normal	130–139	85–89
Mild hypertension (grade 1)	140–159	90–99
Moderate hypertension (grade 2)	160–179	100–109
Severe hypertension (grade 3)	≥ 180	≥ 110
Isolated systolic hypertension grade 1	140–159	< 90
Isolated systolic hypertension grade 2	≥ 160	< 90

Table 5.2	Whom to treat with drugs? – The UK NICE/BHS guidelines thresholds (National Institute for Health and Clinical Excellence 2006)		
CONDITIONS		**THRESHOLDS**	**TARGETS**
Threshold for drug treatment if at low risk of cardiovascular disease (CVD)		160/100 or above	Minimum: < 150/90 Optimal: ≤ 140/90
Threshold if at high risk i.e. (a) target organ damage; or (b) with CVD; or (c) with a 10-year risk of CVD of 20% or more; or (d) with diabetes		140/90 or above	≤ 140/90 but the lower the better Target in diabetes, CVD or renal impairment: ≤ 130/80

(b) On the first occasion measure the BP in both arms. A significant difference is found in 20% of hypertensives. If there is a difference of > 5 mmHg use the arm with the higher reading for future measurements.

(c) Measure the systolic and diastolic pressures (phase V) to the nearest 2 mm. If > 140/90, repeat the measurement towards the end of the consultation. If markedly different from each other, take at least one more. Take the average. Repeated readings by a nurse give the most reliable clinic results, occasional readings by a doctor the least (Little, Barnett, Barnsley, *et al.* 2002).

(d) *Timing.* In mild uncomplicated hypertension, do not start treatment until three readings have been taken over a 3-month period. 25% of blood pressures will settle in that time. Those that settle to below treatment levels need lifelong annual follow-up. If the initial diastolic is > 200/110 mmHg or there is evidence of end-organ damage, cardiovascular disease or diabetes, three readings over 2 weeks would be more appropriate. Consider immediate treatment if the pressure is > 220/120.

(e) Follow-up 6 monthly, once the patient is established on treatment. It is as good as – monthly (Birtwhistle, Marshall, Godwin, *et al.* 2004).

AGE LIMITS

Continue treatment beyond the age of 80 and consider starting it beyond 80 in a patient who is sufficiently fit, especially if there is target organ damage (NICE 2004). The HYVET study of patients with a mean age of 84 at enrolment showed that treatment reduced the risk of stroke, heart failure and all cause mortality with fewer serious adverse effects than placebo (Beckett, OPeters, Fletcher, *et al.* 2008).

HOME BLOOD PRESSURE MEASUREMENT

- Hypertensives regularly record lower pressures at home or with ambulatory monitoring (ABPM) than in the clinic. Home readings are, on average, 5 mmHg lower than clinic readings and ambulatory monitoring readings are 15 mmHg lower (Guidelines Committee 2003).
- 13% of patients show an exaggerated rise in BP when it is measured in the clinic ('white coat hypertension') (Bobrie, Chatellier, Genes, *et al.* 2003).
- A similar number (9%) show the opposite phenomenon; that is, lower readings in the clinic than at home ('masked hypertension') (Bobrie, Chatellier, Genes, *et al.* 2003).
- Cohort studies show that home readings predict prognosis better than clinic readings when there is a mismatch (Bobrie, Chatellier, Genes, *et al.* 2003; Ohkubo, Imai, Tsuji, *et al.* 1998).
- All randomized controlled trials of the benefits of antihypertensive treatment have been conducted using clinic readings. A recent RCT has shown that, while home monitoring can be useful in identifying those with white coat hypertension, its use in judging whether medication should be adjusted, in those in whom a decision to treat has been made, leads to undertreatment (Staessen, Den Hond, Celis, *et al.* 2004). Until an RCT using home readings establishes the superiority of home readings in monitoring treatment, clinic levels should be used routinely.

∗ Consider asking a patient to record home levels if:
(a) levels are borderline and the decision about whether to treat is difficult;
(b) white coat hypertension is suspected because of fluctuating readings, or obvious anxiety, in the clinic;

(c) the patient has evidence of target organ damage which is greater than would be expected from the clinic baseline BP.

* If using home readings, adjust threshold and target levels down by 5 mmHg since the BHS thresholds and targets refer to readings taken in clinic settings.

* Supply the patient with an automated machine that uses the upper arm and that prints or stores the results. Instruct the patient to become familiar with the machine and then to take two readings twice a day for 7 days, each time after sitting for 5 minutes. Take the average. Only ask for more readings if there are wide fluctuations or the readings continue to show a tendency to decline towards the normal range over the 7 days (Pickering, Miller, Ogedegbe, *et al.* 2008). This gives a result akin to the reliability of ABPM (Brueren, Schouten, De Leeuw, *et al.* 1998). Wrist and finger devices are inaccurate.

WORK-UP

(a) A history of family and personal risk factors for stroke or coronary heart disease. Check whether relevant drugs (e.g. NSAIDs) or excess alcohol are taken.

(b) Examination, including:
- fundi (essential only in severe hypertension) (van den Born, Hulsman, Hoekstra, *et al.* 2005);
- femoral pulses;
- palpation of kidneys and auscultation for presence of bruit;
- signs of left ventricular hypertrophy.

(c) Urinalysis for protein and blood.

(d) Blood:
- creatinine and electrolytes;
- fasting blood sugar
- serum lipids.

(e) Look for left ventricular hypertrophy using ECG and CXR, with echocardiography in borderline cases or where the finding of hypertrophy would affect management (Collins, Peto, MacMahon, *et al.* 1990).

(f) Calculate the patient's 10-year CVD risk using a recognized calculator, e.g. the revised Joint British Societies calculator on www.bhsoc.org (choose 'Guidelines'). Note the change from the older version which calculated CHD risk. A 20% 10-year CVD risk means that the lower threshold for treatment applies and that primary prevention of CVD is needed.

NON-DRUG TREATMENT

Non-drug treatment can lower the systolic pressure by 4–10 mmHg (Stevens, Obarzanek, Cook 2001; Writing Group of the PREMIER Collaborative Research Group 2003). More important, it lowers the risk of CVD. It should be offered to all with hypertension, whether or not drugs are being prescribed.

Encourage all patients to:

(a) *lose weight* if overweight. A loss of 8.8 kg is associated with a fall in blood pressure of 5/7 mmHg (Stevens, Obarzanek, Cook 2001);

(b) *alcohol:* reduce excessive consumption;

(c) *diet: salt.* Reduce intake of salt to < 5 g per day Giving advice on salt reduction leads to a fall of between 1 and 10 mmHg in systolic pressure, with larger falls in older patients (Hooper, Bartlett, Davey Smith and Ebrahim 2003). Common sources of salt are nuts, crisps, canned foods and bread. Low salt versions are available;

(d) *diet: the DASH diet.* This is a diet rich in fruit, vegetables and oily fish and low in total and saturated fat. It can reduce BP by 11/5. Details of the DASH diet are available on www.nhlbi.nih.gov (search on 'Healthy Eating');

(e) *diet: coffee.* Discourage *excessive* coffee drinking. A meta-analysis found that BP was 2/1 higher in coffee drinkers with a mean intake of five cups a day (Jee, He, Whelton, *et al.* 1999);

(f) *the contraceptive pill:* consider stopping but not until other adequate contraceptive measures are in place;

(g) *exercise.* Brisk walking for 30 minutes every day is as beneficial as more vigorous exercise three times a week. Brisk walking for an hour, three or four times a week may be even better (Cleroux, Feldman and Petrella 1999). After only 2 weeks of aerobic exercise the mean fall is 5/4 (Whelton, Chin, Xin and He 2002);

(h) *stress.* Patients often blame a stressful life for their hypertension. In fact a Bandolier review shows that stress management does not lead to lower pressures and it is worth being clear about this with patients so that they focus their energies on more worthwhile strategies (at least for lowering blood pressure) (Bandolier 2002);

(i) *smoking:* ask about smoking. If appropriate offer advice and refer to the smoking cessation services. This is a New Contract requirement. Stopping will not reduce the BP but it will lower the cardiovascular risk;

(j) *aspirin:* give 75 mg daily if CVD is present or the patient is aged 50 or over with a CVD risk of at least 20% or with target organ damage, or with diabetes, provided the BP is controlled to 150/90 (Hansson, Zanchetti, Carruthers, *et al.* 1998);

(k) *statins:* give them if the patient has CVD or diabetes or has a risk of CVD that is sufficiently high. The NSF for CHD recommends a threshold of 10-year risk of CHD of > 30%. The BHS recommends a threshold of CVD risk of ≥ 20% in a patient up to at least 80 years old with a baseline cholesterol ≥ 3.5 mmol/l.

DRUG MANAGEMENT

PRINCIPLES (BROWN, CRUICKSHANK, DOMINICZAK, *ET AL.* 2003)

- About half of patients fail to take their antihypertensives as prescribed. Patients have many reservations about drug treatment (Benson and Britten 2002). Getting them to voice those reservations gives the clinician a chance to alter any erroneous ideas they may have. A study of London black Caribbean patients found that common misconceptions were:
  - once the BP was controlled, they were cured and didn't need the medication; and
  - that they could sense when their BP was raised and so could judge when they needed to take the medication (Connell, McKevitt and Wolfe 2005).
- Most of the benefit comes from lowering the blood pressure rather than choosing one class of drugs over another (Turnbull 2003). Used in an appropriate patient, each class of drugs lowers the blood pressure by roughly the same amount, with the exceptions that atenolol appears to be slightly less effective (ASCOT; Dahlof, Sever, Poulter, *et al.* 2005) and a thiazide-type diuretic slightly more effective (ALLHAT; ALLHAT

officers and coordinators for the ALLHAT Collaborative Research Group 2003).

- Commonly used drugs produce a similar average fall of 9.1/5.5 mmHg at standard doses (Law, Wald, Morris and Jordan 2003). Most patients with hypertension therefore need more than one antihypertensive drug.
- Combining two drugs from different classes reduces the blood pressure five times more than doubling the dose of one drug (Wald, Law, Morris, *et al.* 2009).
- Even in trial settings two out of three patients fail to reach BP targets.
- The choice of drugs should be influenced by age, by comorbidity, by adverse effects, by possible synergistic effects between classes of drugs and by the individual's response to each drug. Ethnic origin also influences the choice of medication; younger white patients tend to have high levels of renin and angiotensin II; older patients and those of African origin tend to have low renin levels and so respond less well to drugs that block the renin–angiotensin system. However, the influence of ethnic origin on response to medication is slight. At least 80% of blacks and whites have similar responses to ACE inhibitors and beta-blockers (Anon. 2004).
- Follow the scheme outlined below, but do not persevere with a drug that has produced no benefit (i.e. a drop in BP of < 5 mmHg.). Instead switch to a drug with a different mode of action, e.g. from A to C or D. Persevere with a drug that shows some, but inadequate benefit: it may be synergistic with a drug from a different group.
- * Divide drugs into those that suppress the renin system ['A' (ACE inhibitors and angiotensin receptor blockers)] and those that work independently of it ['C' (calcium channel blockers) and 'D' (diuretics)] (Brown, Cruickshank, Dominiczak, *et al.* 2003). The steps given in Table 5.3 are recommended, but tailor it to the needs of the individual patient.

Beta-blockers have been relegated to step 4 because trials show atenolol to be slightly less effective than other drugs in reducing CVD risk, and less effective than other drugs in reducing the risk of developing diabetes, especially if combined with a diuretic. However, they may be used earlier than described in the table in certain patients:

Table 5.3	Drug management in hypertension	
	AGE < 55 AND NON–BLACK	**AGE ≥ 55 OR BLACK**
Step 1	A	C or D
Step 2	A and C or D	
Step 3	A and C and D	
Step 4	Add an alpha-blocker, or a beta-blocker, or spironolactone or another diuretic or refer	

(a) women of childbearing potential;

(b) patients with high sympathetic drive;

(c) patients with another reason to need a beta-blocker (e.g. angina, post myocardial infarction, heart failure, migraine).

Furthermore, they may be continued in a patient already well controlled on a beta-blocker who is not at high risk of developing diabetes. Patients at high risk are those with a close family history of type 2 diabetes, the obese, those with IGT or IFG, South Asians and Afro-Caribbeans).

* If withdrawing a beta-blocker, step the dose down slowly.

* If in doubt about using a beta-blocker, consider using one other than atenolol. There is some evidence that they do not suffer the same disadvantages (Ong 2007).

PRACTICALITIES (Table 5.4)

■ *Drug doses.* Traditional advice is to increase drug dosage, at monthly intervals, to the maximum recommended dose before abandoning it as ineffective or adding another drug. However, a recent meta-analysis (Law, Wald, Morris and Jordan 2003) has shown that higher doses give diminishing extra benefit while increasing adverse effects. Reducing the drug dose to half the standard dose produces on average only a 20% loss of benefit. Conversely, the adverse effects of two drugs at low dosage seem to be less than would be predicted from the adverse effects of each drug alone.

■ *Drug combinations* which include appropriate drugs at the right dose may aid adherence and now have the approval of the BHS (Brown, Cruickshank, Dominiczak, *et al.* 2003).

Either:

* use low doses of up to three drugs, only increasing to higher doses if necessary, before moving to step 4; or

* start each drug low and increase it to the higher dose before moving to the next step.

DRUG TREATMENT OF PATIENTS WITH OTHER MEDICAL PROBLEMS

(a) *Hyperlipidaemia:* the effect of beta-blockers and low-dose thiazides is so small that the presence of hyperlipidaemia does not alter the general drug recommendations (Lakshman, Reda, Materson, *et al.* 1999).

Table 5.4	Typical drug from each class with doses, main cautions and possible additional benefits			
DRUG	LOW DAILY DOSE	STANDARD DAILY DOSE	MAIN CAUTIONS	ESPECIALLY INDICATED IN
Ramipril	2.5 mg	5–10 mg	Renovascular disease, aortic stenosis, high doses of diuretics, low serum sodium	Previous MI, cerebrovascular disease, diabetic renal disease, heart failure
Bendroflumethiazide	1.25 mg	2.5 mg	Hypokalaemia, renal and hepatic impairment, gout	Heart failure
Amlodipine	5 mg	10 mg	Unstable angina, aortic stenosis	Stable angina, Raynaud's disease, migraine
Doxazosin	4 mg	16 mg	Heart failure, orthostatic hypotension	Prostatic hypertrophy
Spironolactone	25 mg	50 mg	Hyperkalaemia, renal failure	Oedema, heart failure, post MI
Long-acting propranolol	80 mg	160 mg	Asthma, COPD, uncontrolled heart failure, heart block, sportsmen and women	Angina, post MI, heart failure, tachyarrhythmias, migraine

(b) *Angina:* use a beta-blocker or a calcium-channel blocker.

(c) *The elderly:* use a thiazide; then a calcium-channel blocker or ACE inhibitor.

(d) *Heart failure:* use a diuretic, an ACE inhibitor, a beta-blocker then an alpha-blocker.

(e) *Diabetics:* use an ACE inhibitor, a low-dose thiazide, an alpha-blocker or calcium-channel blocker (Curb, Pressel, Cutler, *et al.* 1996).

(f) *Smokers:* do not use a beta-blocker.

(g) *Peripheral vascular disease:* use a thiazide, calcium-channel blocker, or alpha-blocker.

(h) *Migraine:* use a beta-blocker and/or calcium-channel blocker; then all other alternatives.

(i) *Those active in sports:* avoid beta-blockers.

(j) *Raynaud's syndrome:* use a calcium-channel blocker.

(k) *Supraventricular arrhythmias:* use a beta-blocker and/or calcium-channel blocker.

(l) *Renal failure:* get specialist advice. ACE inhibitors may improve renal function, but will need to be given in lower dosage.

(m) *Gout:* avoid thiazides.

(n) *Asthma:* avoid beta-blockers.

OTHER POINTS ABOUT THE DRUGS

Thiazides

* Recheck creatinine and electrolytes 1 month after starting a thiazide then repeat annually. Repeat more frequently if the patient is unwell, is taking digoxin or another drug which might affect renal function. A rise of creatinine of up to 30% is acceptable provided it remains < 200 μmol/l (Martin and Coleman 2006).

* Diabetes is not a contraindication. In the SHEP study a thiazide was associated with the development of diabetes in an extra 4.3% of patients over 4 years but it protected those who developed diabetes against an increase in cardiovascular mortality (Kostis, Wilson, Freudenberger, *et al.* 2005).

* Ask specifically about erectile difficulties in men. The incidence in patients on thiazides is double that in those on placebo (17% vs 8%), but patients rarely volunteer this information. The difficulties appear early, and may not be sufficiently troublesome to warrant stopping treatment (Grimm, Grandits, Prineas, *et al.* 1997).

Calcium–channel blockers (CCBs)

● The possibility has been raised but not proven that CCBs may increase the risk of death from cardiovascular and non-cardiovascular causes (Psaty, Smith, Siscovick, *et al.* 1997). A more recent meta-analysis has found no evidence for this but, compared with CCBs, low-dose diuretics were associated with reduced risks of cardiovascular disease events (RR, 0.94; 95%CI, 0.89 to 1.00) and CHF (RR, 0.74; 95%CI, 0.67 to 0.81) (Psaty, Lumley and Furberg 2003). Short-acting nifedipine is not recommended in hypertension because of the possibility of an increased risk of myocardial infarction in patients who have CHD (Beevers and Sleight 1996).

* Use a long-acting preparation, e.g. diltiazem 120–180 mg slow release b.d. or verapamil 120–240 mg b.d. or 240–480 mg slow release daily. Their hypotensive effect is the same as nifedipine, with fewer side-effects. Use brand names. Different generic products have different bioavailabilities.

* Use a dihydropyridine calcium-channel blocker, e.g. nifedipine slow release or amlodipine, if:

(a) beta-blockers are also being given;

(b) there is peripheral vascular disease with skin ischaemia. It will not, however, help intermittent claudication;

(c) there is a risk of heart failure, which might be worsened by a non-dihydropyridine.

Note: Beta-blockers are not necessary to counteract the tachycardia caused by nifedipine; this settles in 48 hours anyway (McLeay, Stallard, Watson, *et al.* 1983).

ACE inhibitors and related drugs

● Starting them:

(a) the first dose should be taken at night. Even then, first-dose hypotension due to once-daily agents may not occur until 6–8 hours after the first dose, and may last for 24 hours;

(b) recheck serum creatinine and electrolytes 1 week after starting the drug, and after any dose increase, then annually.

   ■ A rise of serum creatinine of < 30% is acceptable provided it remains < 200 μmol/l (Martin and Coleman 2006). A greater rise suggests renal artery stenosis or chronic kidney disease. Above that, reduce or stop the drug and recheck weekly till the creatinine has returned to its previous level. Look for underlying renal disease.

- A rise of serum K^+ to 5.5–5.9 mmol/l is acceptable but recheck more frequently. Stop the drug if the level reaches 6 mmol/l and refer (Martin and Coleman 2006).

* Use them in insulin-dependent diabetics; they improve insulin resistance (whereas thiazides and beta-blockers may worsen it).

* Avoid them in patients with peripheral vascular disease. As a group they have a 33% incidence of renal artery stenosis (Choudhri, Cleland, Rowlands, *et al.* 1990).

* Use an angiotensin II receptor antagonist in patients who need an ACE inhibitor but cannot tolerate it because of cough (DTB 1995).

Beta-blockers

* Use:
  (a) a once-daily selective agent, e.g. atenolol 50 mg (but see below) or metoprolol SR 200 mg;
  (b) a drug with intrinsic sympathomimetic activity (ISA) in patients with sinus bradycardia, e.g. acebutolol 400 mg o.d.

* Keep in touch with guidance on whether atenolol poses a risk. A meta-analysis comparing atenolol with other antihypertensives (none of them beta-blockers) found that it was associated with an increase in mortality [1.13 (95%CI 1.02 to 1.25)] and, in this respect, was no better than placebo (Carlberg, Samuelsson and Lindholm 2004).

* Perform a peak flow before and after starting treatment if the history suggests the possibility of COPD. If there is a significant fall, stop the drug. However, cardioselective beta-blockers may be tolerated in mild to moderate reversible airways obstruction (Salpeter, Ormiston, Salpeter and Wood-Baker 2004).

* Warn the patient not to stop a beta-blocker suddenly, especially one without ISA. Even those without known coronary heart disease (CHD) have a four-fold increased risk of myocardial infarction or angina in the subsequent 4 weeks.

Alpha-blockers

Total cholesterol falls by an average of 4%, with a beneficial rise in HDL cholesterol.

* Start with a low dose, e.g. terazosin 1 mg, or doxazosin 1 mg, taken at night in case of first-dose hypotension.

* Use with caution in the elderly, who may experience continued postural hypotension.

PATIENT ORGANIZATION

The Blood Pressure Association, 60 Cranmer Terrace, London SW17 0QS, tel. 020 8772 4994, www.bpassoc.org.uk

Poor control

* Gently ask about adherence. A question like 'how difficult do you find it to take all of your tablets?' is more likely to elicit a truthful answer than 'do you ever forget to take them?'.

* Consider the white-coat effect. If the BP seems to fluctuate or the patient seems tense, arrange for home readings (see page 135).

* If neither of these applies, this is resistant hypertension (see below).

RESISTANT HYPERTENSION

Calhoun DA, Jones D, Textor S, *et al.* 2008. Resistant hypertension: diagnosis, evaluation and treatment. A scientific statement from the American Heart Association Professional Education Committee of the Council for High Blood Pressure Research. Hypertension, published online on April 7 2008 and available on http://hyper.ahajournals.org

It is defined as hypertension not controlled by three drugs, where the patient is taking them and the BP is raised at home as well as at the clinic.

- It is common, being found in 20–30% of patients.
- It is likely to be multifactorial: older age, obesity, alcohol excess, other drugs,

secondary hypertension, and a genetic resistance to the antihypertensives being used.

* Check that this is true resistance, not poor adherence or the white coat effect.
* Look for other drugs that may be contributing: NSAIDs, selective COX-2 inhibitors, steroids, the oral contraceptive, and liquorice ingestion in sweets or chewed tobacco.
* *Look for an underlying medical cause:*
  ■ obesity;
  ■ obstructive sleep apnoea (OSA) – ask about snoring, episodes of apnoea at night and daytime sleepiness. One small study found that 83% of patients with resistant hypertension had OSA;
  ■ chronic kidney disease. One study found that fewer than 15% were controlled on an average of three drugs;
  ■ renal artery stenosis. It is common in older hypertensives, although it is not necessarily the cause of the poor control;
  ■ diabetes;
  ■ primary hyperaldosteronism – look for hypokalaemia, although in most patients with the condition it is normal. The best test is to measure plasma aldosterone and plasma renin activity. In primary hyperaldosteronism the ratio of aldosterone to renin is raised (Hammer and Stewart 2009). One study found primary hyperaldosteronism in 11% of patients with resistant hypertension, of whom fewer than half had hypokalaemia (Douma, Petidis, Doumas, *et al.* 2008);
  ■ Cushing's disease – look for the typical clinical features;
  ■ phaeochromocytoma – suggested by a history of episodes of headache, sweating, palpitations associated with an often dramatic rise of blood pressure. The best test is the plasma free metanephrines, but if this is not available measure 24-hour urinary catecholamines (Hammer and Stewart 2009).

If a cause for resistance is found that can be managed in primary care, continue management, even if it means proceeding to step 4. Otherwise, refer. Hypertension clinics are capable of controlling half of those referred with resistant hypertension.

REFERRAL

* Refer patients in whom there is reason to suspect secondary hypertension: onset age under 30, fluctuating BP levels, evidence of renal disease, resistant hypertension.
* Refer urgently anyone with accelerated hypertension (grade IV retinopathy).

STABLE ANGINA

GUIDELINE

Scottish Intercollegiate Guidelines Network. *Management of Stable Angina: A National Clinical Guideline.* SIGN Guideline No. 96 2007. Available on www.sign.ac.uk

WORK-UP

The diagnosis is clinical, based on the history. For details of the diagnosis of chest pain and stable angina see *Evidence-based Diagnosis in Primary Care* by A. F. Polmear (editor) published by Butterworth-Heinemann, 2008. The work-up (below) is designed to elucidate the cause and severity of the angina but, if negative, cannot refute the diagnosis.

* Check for:
  (a) diabetes and a family history of diabetes;
  (b) hypo/hyperthyroidism;
  (c) anaemia/polycythaemia;
  (d) hypertension; treatment is warranted if the blood pressure is 140/90 or above. It should be reduced below 140/85 (Wood, Durrington, Poulter, *et al.* 1998);
  (e) hyperlipidaemia (see page 168) and a family history of cardiovascular disease;
  (f) arrhythmias;
  (g) valvular disease. Any aortic systolic murmur needs assessment for aortic stenosis unless the patient's general condition is too poor to consider even a valvotomy.

WORK-UP – INVESTIGATIONS

(a) Hb.

(b) Thyroid function tests (TFTs).

(c) Fasting blood sugar.

(d) Fasting lipid profile.

(e) Resting ECG. A normal ECG does not exclude the diagnosis but an abnormal ECG makes it more likely.

(f) Exercise ECG in order to assess the severity of coronary artery obstruction. Symptoms are a poor guide to the severity of the disease.

Reasons for not performing an exercise ECG are:

■ the patient is physically incapable of performing the test;

■ the patient has some other illness or condition which would make him or her unsuitable for coronary artery surgery;

■ the diagnosis is in doubt (an exercise ECG has low specificity for making the diagnosis of angina);

■ where symptoms are uncontrolled by medical treatment (such patients should be referred for angiography).

REFERRAL

The National Service Framework for Coronary Heart Disease (DoH 2000) urges the referral of most patients with a new diagnosis of angina. The only exceptions are patients ill with other conditions in whom further investigations for angina would be inappropriate; and patients whose GP has the expertise, and the access to exercise ECG testing, to make referral unnecessary.

* Refer to a cardiologist those patients:

(a) with a positive exercise test, or all new patients if there is no direct access to exercise ECG testing;

(b) with angina not controlled by medication;

(c) whose diagnosis is in doubt;

(d) with aortic stenosis who develop angina, especially if elderly (British Heart Foundation Factfile 1986);

(e) who are candidates for angiography with a view to CABG or angioplasty (Elder, Shaw, Turnbull, et al. 1991). Any patient with a positive exercise ECG should be considered, especially those with angina following myocardial infarction (MI). The MI makes

patients stronger candidates for coronary artery surgery.

* Refer urgently to a Rapid Access Chest Pain Clinic, or for admission, any patient whose angina is unstable, i.e. there has been an abrupt change in symptoms (see below). The recent onset (in the last 2 months) of severe angina should also be treated as unstable.

* Admit, by dialling 999, any patient with cardiac pain lasting > 15 minutes despite GTN. A normal ECG does not remove the need for such admission.

WHICH PATIENTS WITH STABLE ANGINA BENEFIT MOST FROM ANGIOPLASTY OR CABG? (O'TOOLE AND GRECH 2003)

Those with:

(a) left main stem or three vessel disease; ±

(b) abnormal left ventricular function; ±

(c) an abnormal exercise test; ±

(d) more severe anginal symptoms.

It is those patients most likely to benefit symptomatically who also are most likely to achieve a reduction in subsequent major cardiovascular events. A UK study found that if patients, in whom continued medical treatment was a reasonable option, were randomized to angioplasty or continued medical treatment, there was no difference in the rate of MI or death over the next 7 years, although symptoms were better following angioplasty (Henderson, Pocock, Clayton, et al. 2003).

DRUG TREATMENT

ACUTE ATTACKS

* Use glyceryl trinitrate:

(a) sublingually: 300–500 mcg (300 mcg is less likely to cause headaches). The shelf life is only 2–3 months; or

(b) spray: 400 mcg per puff; or

(c) buccal tablets, which may be more effective than sublingual preparations.

PREVENTIVE TREATMENT

Nicorandil can reduce the risk of future major coronary events (see page 143). The benefit from beta-blockers post-MI suggests that they may exert similar protection in angina. Certainly, any patient with angina that is more than occasional should be offered treatment, starting with a beta-blocker, unless contraindicated. One contraindication specific to angina is the presence of Prinzmetal angina, that is, vasospastic angina occurring at rest. It is worsened by beta-blockade and relieved by dihydropyridine calcium-channel blockers.

In patients for whom beta–blockers are not contraindicated

1. Use a long-acting beta-blocker, e.g. atenolol 50 mg daily. Once taken, assess whether the patient is fully beta-blocked. This is indicated by a heart rate of 60 beats/min or less at rest, and a rate of 90 beats/min or less after walking up two flights of stairs. Further increases in dose above the minimum required to achieve beta-blockade will probably be unhelpful. Warn the patient not to stop or omit even one dose. If it is necessary to stop for medical reasons, tail off over 4 weeks.
2. If control is unsatisfactory, add a long-acting dihydropyridine CCB, e.g. amlodipine. If using a long-acting nifedipine, prescribe by brand name because of differences in bioavailability. Non-dihydropyridine CCBs should not be started in general practice in a patient taking beta-blockers because of their effects on the conducting system. However, note the following problems with all CCBs:
   (a) vasodilation may reduce flow through the coronary artery stenosis and make the angina worse;
   (b) reflex tachycardia can occur for the first few days of use;
   (c) aortic stenosis is a contraindication. The coronary blood flow may be further decreased by nifedipine.

Studies are conflicting on whether a combination of beta-blocker and CCB is more effective than either alone. Only persevere with the combination if symptoms improved after the addition of each drug. There is no evidence on whether the addition of a third drug (a long-acting nitrate or nicorandil) would be beneficial and referral to a cardiologist is probably needed.

In patients for whom beta–blockers are contraindicated or whose angina is vasospastic, i.e. more prominent at rest than on exertion

1. *Begin* with a CCB. Consider using verapamil or diltiazem; they are more powerful than dihydropyridines in angina. Start with verapamil or diltiazem 120 mg slow-release b.d. Again, prescribe by brand name. Increase the dose after 2 weeks only if angina is not controlled, and side-effects are not a problem.
2. If control is still unsatisfactory add:
   (a) a long-acting nitrate, e.g. isosorbide mononitrate (ISMN) 20–40 mg b.d.; or
   (b) a modified release ISMN; or
   (c) a sustained-release preparation of GTN, e.g. a buccal preparation (Suscard 1–2 mg t.d.s.) or a nitrate patch containing at least 10 mg of nitrate, if ISMN is not tolerated or fails to control symptoms; or
   (d) a potassium channel activator, e.g. nicorandil 10 mg b.d. increasing to 20 mg b.d. in combination with any other agents that have proved useful (IONA 2002). The higher dose has been shown to reduce major coronary events compared to placebo by 14% over 1.6 years (NNT = 44) but with 10% unable to tolerate the drug, mainly because of headache.

Problems with nitrates

(a) Postural hypotension, syncope and headache. Start with a low dose, and increase once well tolerated.
(b) Reflex tachycardia, which may decrease coronary blood flow and worsen the angina.
(c) Tolerance, which may develop after several weeks. This can be avoided by allowing a nitrate-free period of 8 hours a day. Patches need to be removed at night. Patients on ISMN and isosorbide dinitrate (ISDN) should take the second dose at 4 pm, and not at bedtime. The alternative is to use a once-daily formulation. One study suggests that the increased cost will be offset by greater adherence, resulting in fewer consultations (Brown, Kendall and Halpern 1997).

SECONDARY PREVENTION OF CVD AND OTHER ISSUES

* Enrol the patient in the cardiovascular disease prevention programme and manage for the secondary prevention of cardiovascular disease as set out on page 168.

* Advise the patient about the symptoms of a myocardial infarction or unstable angina and the importance of calling an ambulance if chest pain persists for > 15 minutes despite use of glyceryl trinitrate (GTN).

* *Driving*. Advise patients to notify their insurance company (though not the DVLA) and not to drive until symptoms are controlled. However, Group 2 licence holders (large lorries and buses) and holders of a pilot's licence must inform the appropriate authority and stop driving/flying meanwhile.

* *Immunizations*: recommend influenza annually and pneumococcal vaccination once.

* *Quality of life*. Ask what effect the angina is having on the patient. Look especially for depression, erectile dysfunction and unnecessary invalidism. Consider referring for cardiac rehabilitation any patient whose quality of life is impaired.

PATIENT GROUPS

British Cardiac Patients Association, 2 Station Road, Swavesey, Cambridge CB4 5QJ, tel. 0800 4792800, www.bcpa.co.uk

British Heart Foundation, 14 Fitzhardinge Street, London W1H 6DH, Heart Information Line 08450 70 80 70, www.bhf.org.uk

Heart Surgery in Great Britain, http://heartsurgery.healthcarecommission.org.uk, a website dedicated to helping heart surgery patients make informed choices about their treatment

UNSTABLE ANGINA (ACUTE CORONARY SYNDROME)

GUIDELINE

British Cardiac Society Guidelines and Medical Practice Committee; Royal College of Physicians Clinical Effectiveness and Evaluation Unit. 2001. Guideline for the management of patients with acute coronary syndromes without persistent ECG ST segment elevation. Heart 85, 133–142

● *Definition*. Unstable angina means that there has been an *abrupt* change in symptoms such that angina is occurring at rest, or at significantly lower levels of activity, or that the frequency, duration or severity of the attacks has substantially worsened. The recent onset (in the last 2 months) of severe angina should also be treated as unstable. For details of the diagnosis of acute coronary syndrome see *Evidence-based Diagnosis in Primary Care* by A. F. Polmear (editor) published by Butterworth-Heinemann, 2008.

● *Outcomes*. Even with treatment, 5–7% will have a serious outcome (death, MI or emergency revascularisation) within 1 week and 15% within 1 month (Dahlof, Sever, Poulter, *et al.* 2005). Opinions on the benefit of early invasive treatment vary. A recent large British trial found that invasive treatment improved symptoms in the short and long term, with a reduction in death and MI at 4 months that was lost at 1 year (Fox, Poole-Wilson, Henderson, *et al.* 2002). To support this later point, a large Dutch study found that patients receiving medical treatment did as well at 1 year as those receiving early invasive treatment *provided* that those managed conservatively were offered invasive treatment if they remained unstable or failed an exercise test before discharge from hospital (de Winter, Windhausen, Cornel, *et al.* 2005).

* Admit by emergency ambulance any patient with cardiac pain lasting > 15 minutes despite GTN. This applies whatever the ECG shows.

* Arrange for specialist assessment that day for any other patient with unstable angina.

* While awaiting admission, give:
  (a) GTN, e.g. three sprays over 15 minutes if pain continues; and
  (b) a tablet of soluble or chewable aspirin, 75–300 mg. Continue this after discharge. It can reduce by one third the rate of MI, stroke and death over the next 6 months with a NNT of 20. If the patient cannot tolerate aspirin give clopidogrel. The combination of aspirin and clopidogrel has been shown to reduce cardiovascular events following ACS but at the risk of more bleeding combinations (Boucher, Armstrong, Pharand and Skidmore 2002). If the combination is started in hospital it should be continued for 12 months before reverting to aspirin alone; and

(c) a beta-blocker without ISA, if there is likely to be a delay in arranging admission. This will slightly reduce the rate of myocardial infarction.

* Intensify treatment at home in patients whose angina has gradually worsened but without the abruptness that defines unstable angina. However, warn them to call urgently if symptoms worsen suddenly. In borderline cases, be more ready to admit those who are at higher risk because of:

(a) age > 65;

(b) diabetes or other concurrent illness;

(c) impaired left ventricular function;

(d) new ECG changes, especially T wave inversion or ST depression.

* If not admitting, check for a cause for the deterioration:

(a) physical or emotional stress;

(b) non-compliance with medication;

(c) intercurrent illness;

(d) a deterioration in cardiac function;

(e) anaemia.

At follow-up, check for depression. In one group of patients following acute coronary syndrome major depressive disorder was present in 15–23% and was associated with a three-fold increase in the subsequent mortality. Treatment with antidepressants improves mood, quality of life and level of functioning (Swenson and Clinch 2000).

INVASIVE MANAGEMENT OF PATIENTS > 75 YEARS OLD WITH ACS

Working on intuition rather than evidence, some clinicians still deny the benefits of invasive treatment to the very old, purely on the grounds of age. However, a study from the US (Bach, Cannon, Weintraub, *et al.* 2004), of coronary angiography within 48 hours versus exercise ECG, which resulted in a rate of revasculization that was almost double in the invasive group, shows that patients over age 75 benefit *most* from early invasive management, at a lower cost per life saved than in younger people. The endpoints of death or MI at 6 months gave the following figures:

■ patients < 65: no significant difference between the groups;

■ patients 65 and over: RRR 39%; NNT 21;

■ patients > 75: RRR 56%; NNT 10. This was despite an increase in major bleeding in the invasive group that was most marked in the very old.

Clearly, such invasive management might not be appropriate for patients already ill with other conditions, who were excluded from this trial.

NON–CARDIAC CHEST PAIN

Less than half of patients referred to cardiac clinics and A&E departments with chest pain are found to have coronary artery disease (Bass and Mayou 2002). Many of these patients continue to suffer pain and long-term functional impairment. Their management is often inadequate once the diagnosis of cardiac disease is excluded.

* Be clear from the history, investigations and specialist assessment, that the pain is non-cardiac. Then resist requests for further cardiac referral.

* Try to make a positive diagnosis of the cause of the pain: musculo-skeletal disorders, panic attacks, reflux, depression.

* If a clear diagnosis is possible, treat accordingly (for instance with NSAIDs for musculo-skeletal pain, a PPI for reflux, antidepressants for depression).

* If no clear diagnosis is possible, attempt an explanation along the following lines: that the symptoms are real; that they do not arise from the heart or from any other specific illness; that the brain normally disregards sensations that it receives from all over the body, but that for some reason, in this patient, it is sensitized to sensations from the chest. This explanation might lead on to discussion of how such sensitization may have occurred. The patient may volunteer the memory of some event which seemed to trigger the chest pain.

* Ask who else in the family is worried about the pain and try to see them as well.

* Refer to a psychologist or counsellor patients who accept the above explanation but who still find themselves bothered by the pain. Cognitive-behavioural therapy has been shown to result in a significant reduction in pain after between 4 and 12 sessions (van Peski-Oosterbaan, Spinhoven, van Rood, *et al.* 1999).

* Consider a trial of a tricyclic antidepressant or SSRI in a patient sufficiently troubled by pain, even in the absence of depression.

MYOCARDIAL INFARCTION (MI)

GUIDELINES

Braunwald E, Antman EM, Beasley JW, *et al.* 1999. ACC/AHA guidelines for the management of patients with acute myocardial infarction, 1999 update. Circulation 100, 1016–1030

Scottish Heart and Arterial Disease Risk Prevention (SHARP). *Brief Guidelines for General Practitioners giving Thrombolytic Therapy 2004*, available from SHARP, Dept of Medicine, Ninewells Hospital & Medical School, Dundee DD1 9SY

NICE Technology Appraisal Guidance No. 52. *Guidance on the Use of Drugs for Early Thrombolysis in the Treatment of Acute Myocardial Infarction*. National Institute for Clinical Excellence; London. October 2002. Available: www.nice.org.uk

NICE Clinical Guideline 48. *Secondary Prevention in Primary and Secondary Care for Patients Following a Myocardial Infarction*. National Institute for Clinical Excellence; London. May 2007. Available: www.nice.org.uk

● Every district needs a policy, worked out between the primary and secondary care and the ambulance service, to ensure the provision of the most effective care. The National Service Framework for Coronary Heart Disease (DoH 2000) sets a maximum time of 60 minutes between the patient's first call and the administration of thrombolysis ('call-to-needle' time), when it is indicated. In practice this means that a call for chest pain which sounds cardiac should be answered by a cardiac resuscitation ambulance, able to administer morphine and, unless close to a hospital A&E department, thrombolysis. Attendance by an ambulance within 1 hour of the onset of pain has been calculated to save 140 deaths over the next 30 days per 1000 patients (DTB 2000).
● The SHARP guidelines (above) (United Kingdom Heart Attack Study (UKHAS) Collaborative Group 1998) recommend that

thrombolysis, if indicated, should be given outside hospital if the travelling time to hospital is 30 minutes or more.
● *Primary angioplasty* can achieve results superior to thrombolysis but only in centres experienced in its use. Meta-analysis shows a short-term death rate for primary angioplasty of 7% against 9% for thrombolysis (Keeley, Boura and Grines 2003). Benefits are still apparent at long-term follow-up. To achieve the benefit seen in trials the patient must be assessed within 12 hours of the onset of symptoms, and the transfer to the centre where the procedure will be performed must be achieved in under 2 hours (Andersen, Nielsen, Rasmussen, *et al.* 2003).

IMMEDIATE MANAGEMENT

* Ensure that the ambulance has been called as an emergency by dialling 999 (in the UK). This may enable the service to respond faster than if the same call is telephoned direct to the ambulance control centre. Delay in reaching hospital is associated with a poorer outcome. Those reaching hospital in less than 1 hour from the onset of symptoms appear to derive the most benefit (United Kingdom Heart Attack Study (UKHAS) Collaborative Group 1998; Pai, Haites and Rawles 1987).

If the GP is present:

* insert an i.v. cannula so that more than one i.v. drug can be given easily.
* *pain relief:* for pain relief give either:
  (a) i.v. diamorphine 1 mg/min (maximum 5 mg); or
  (b) i.v. morphine 2 mg/min (maximum 10 mg).
Have nalorphine available in case of respiratory depression. These maximums can be repeated after 15 minutes if pain is not relieved.
* *Antiemesis:* give an antiemetic in the same syringe, e.g. metoclopramide 10 mg or cyclizine 50 mg i.v. Avoid cyclizine in heart failure or hypotension because it causes arterial constriction. Cyclimorph has the further disadvantage of being unrepeatable if more morphine is needed. Doses of cyclizine over 50 mg cause confusion and drowsiness.
* *GTN:* give as the spray or sublingually to oppose coronary vasoconstriction and to reduce

myocardial work. Do not give if the pulse is over 100, or the systolic BP is under 90.

* *Oxygen:* give 100% oxygen routinely.
* *Bradycardia:* if the pulse is below 40, give atropine 300 mcg i.v. and further doses of 300 mcg if needed, up to 1.2 mg, whether the bradycardia is due to heart block or to sinus bradycardia. If the pulse is between 40 and 60, only give atropine if there is evidence of low cardiac output.
* *Aspirin:* give 150–300 mg, either in a chewable or dispersible form. This gives 38 fewer major vascular events per 1000 patients at 1 month (NNT 27) (Antithrombotic Trialists' Collaboration 2002).
* *Defibrillation:* defibrillate a patient who develops ventricular fibrillation while awaiting transfer to hospital. If no defibrillator is available, perform cardio-pulmonary resuscitation while waiting for one to arrive. Approximately 5% of patients experiencing an acute myocardial infarction develop cardiac arrest in the presence of the GP. Out of hospital defibrillation has been shown to save lives (Pai, Haites and Rawles 1987).
* *Thrombolysis:* make an initial judgment about the patient's suitability. All patients with a typical history of MI and ST segment elevation or left bundle branch block should be considered for thrombolysis, regardless of age, if their quality of life warrants it, and if local policy does not prefer acute percutaneous coronary intervention (PCI).
* Thrombolysis is of benefit in the 24 hours after the onset of symptoms, with more benefit the sooner it is given. The short-term decrease in mortality is 18% (NNT 56 in 1 month) but with a 'number needed to harm' (NNH) of 250 for stroke and 143 for an major extracerebral bleed) (Fibrinolytic Therapy Trialists (FTT) Collaborative Group 1994). The NNT is 25 if given in the first hour, rising to 33 if given in the first 6 hours, 50 if given in the first 9 hours and 100 if given in the first 18 hours. The benefit from aspirin is in addition to this. The benefit of thrombolysis is sustained over time, with an NNT at 12 years of 7 (95%CI 4 to 41) (French, Hyde, Patel, *et al.* 1999). Thrombolysis involves hospital admission, whether or not it is given at home first. GPs need special training

(DTB 1994a). It should be given outside hospital only if:

(a) there is strong clinical suspicion of acute myocardial infarction; and
(b) chest pain, unrelieved by GTN spray, has been present for at least 20 minutes and for no more than 12 hours; and
(c) the ECG shows ST elevation or left bundle branch block; and
(d) a defibrillator is available, because of the small but significant increase in risk of ventricular fibrillation (VF) after thrombolysis; and
(e) no contraindications exist.

CONTRAINDICATIONS TO THROMBOLYSIS (LIP, CHIN AND PRASAD 2002)

Absolute

(a) Aortic dissection.
(b) Previous cerebral haemorrhage.
(c) Known cerebral aneurysm or AV malformation.
(d) Intracranial neoplasm.
(e) Any cerebrovascular accident in the last 6 months.
(f) Active internal bleeding (other than menstruation).

Streptokinase should not be given to a patient who has received it more than 4 days previously. The development of antibodies may reduce its effectiveness.

Relative

(a) Uncontrolled hypertension (BP > 180/110) or chronic severe hypertension.
(b) On anticoagulants or known bleeding diathesis.
(c) Trauma within past 2–4 weeks including head injury and prolonged (> 10 minutes) CPR.
(d) Aortic aneurysm.
(e) Recent (within 3 weeks) major surgery, organ biopsy, or puncture of a non-compressible vessel.
(f) Recent (within 6 months) GI, or GU, or other internal bleeding.
(g) Pregnancy.
(h) Active peptic ulcer.

CONTINUING ACUTE MANAGEMENT

Occasionally a patient with a MI will refuse admission, or the decision will be made to keep the patient at home because of other circumstances. More frequently, a patient will be discharged early from hospital so that the bulk of management becomes the responsibility of the GP.

Because the GP may assume management at any stage, a proposed regimen for the patient who is not admitted is described.

* Revisit about 6 hours after the first visit, and again daily for a few days.
* Explain what is happening and what the future programme is.
* Check for pain, arrhythmias, hypotension and heart failure. Clinical evidence of heart failure is associated with a 55% increase in the relative risk of death in the 30 days following MI (Pitt, White, Nicolau, *et al.* 2005). It is strong grounds for admission but, if not admitting, give an aldosterone antagonist (i.e. eplerenone) in addition to an ACE inhibitor, beta-blocker and, if needed, a diuretic (Pitt, White, Nicolau, *et al.* 2005).
* Continue daily *aspirin* (75 mg) indefinitely.
* *ACE inhibitors.* Give an ACE inhibitor, or, to those intolerant of ACE inhibitors, an angiotensin II receptor antagonist. NICE recommends lisinopril 5 mg daily, perindopril 4 mg daily, or ramipril 2.5 mg b.d., in those without heart failure. If tolerated the dose should be doubled after 1–2 weeks. For those with heart failure see page 150.
* Start a beta-blocker on the second day provided it is not contraindicated. The benefit is apparent as early as 1 week later, with a 16% reduction in major cardiovascular events (Yusuf, Peto, Lewis, *et al.* 1985). The drugs with most evidence of benefit are propranolol, timolol and metoprolol but this probably applies to all beta-blockers (Freemantle, Cleland, Young, *et al.* 1999). Most of the benefit is in high-risk patients who have transient arrhythmias or heart failure and then recover well enough to take the drugs.
* *Pericarditis* should be treated with aspirin at full doses, or, if aspirin is contraindicated, an NSAID, e.g. naproxen 500 mg b.d. Occasionally, NSAIDs are needed for up to a year.

* *Physical rehabilitation* should be started after 12–24 hours if the patient is stable. Give the patient written instructions:
  1. Start to walk about from day 2.
  2. By day 7, climb stairs up to four times a day.
  3. By day 14, stroll in the garden or street.
  4. By week 4, walk 1/2 a mile a day, increasing to 2 miles a day by week 6. Resume sexual activities gently (Chua and Lipkin 1993).
  5. From week 6, increase the speed of walking so that 2 miles is covered in less than 30 minutes. Younger patients can then alternate walking and jogging. If a local rehabilitation group is available, the patient should be encouraged to attend from the fourth week 6.
* *Psychological rehabilitation.* Much postinfarction disability is psychological or family-induced. Group sessions and sessions for spouses may be as important as the exercises (Linden, Stossel and Maurice 1996). Nearly half of all patients are depressed 1 week after an infarct, 18% with major depression (Schleifer, Macari-Hinson, Coyle, *et al.* 1989). A study of Dutch men found that anxiety was a more powerful predictor than depression of subsequent cardiac events, rehospitalization and increased use of the cardiac outpatients clinic (Strik, Denollet, Lousberg and Honig 2003).

THE 6–WEEK ASSESSMENT

* Ask about breathlessness and palpitations.
* Look for signs of heart failure or arrhythmias and check the blood pressure.
* Continue aspirin, at 75 mg daily. It is as effective as 300 mg with fewer adverse effects (Antiplatelet Trialists' Collaboration 1994). If allergic, use clopidogrel. If dyspepsia is a problem continue aspirin and add a proton pump inhibitor. If aspirin and clopidogrel are both given, revert to aspirin alone after 4 weeks in the case of acute ST segment elevation, or after 12 months in non-ST segment elevation acute coronary syndrome.
* *Smoking.* Encourage a smoker to stop with the news that stopping even at this late stage probably reduces mortality by 50%. For techniques see page 498.

* *Exercise.* Encourage the continuation of exercise, which will continue to improve cardiac performance and survival and reduce the risk of another infarction by 20%. Exercise can be tennis, jogging, cycling, swimming or circuit training. NICE recommends 20–30 minutes each day, increasing slowly so that it is sufficiently vigorous to make the patient slightly breathless (NICE 2007).

* *Cardiac rehabilitation.* Refer the patient if not already enrolled. Studies show reductions in cardiovascular deaths of 27% (95%CI 2 to 46%) as well as improvements in the quality of life (Jolliffe, Rees, Taylor, *et al.* 2004). Yet only a minority of patients with an MI in the UK or the US receive it (Dalal, Evans and Campbell 2004).

* *Weight.* Advise the obese to lose weight. Obesity increases the risk of further cardiovascular disease by 45%, independently of other risk factors (Bogers, Bemelmans, Hoogenveen, *et al.* 2007).

* *Diet.* Whether the patient needs to lose weight or not recommend a Mediterranean diet. The elements of the diet that seem to be associated with a lower mortality are: moderate alcohol, low meat intake, and high intake of vegetables, fruit, nuts, olive oil and legumes. Dairy products, cereals and fish seem to have no influence on mortality (Trichopoulou, Bamia and Trichopoulos 2009). Other studies have shown benefit from two to four portions per week of oily fish (mackerel, herring, kipper, pilchard, sardine, salmon or trout).

* *Alcohol.* Check that safe limits are not being exceeded (see page 486).

* *Lipids.* Arrange a test for serum lipids at 3 months postinfarction, unless the lipids were assessed within 24 hours of the onset of the infarct. Once blood has been taken, start a statin regardless of baseline value and continue it long term (see page 168).

* *Diabetes.* Unless known to be diabetic, or to have had an assessment of glucose metabolism in hospital, check the fasting plasma glucose. A US study found that half of all patients presenting with acute coronary syndrome had abnormal glucose metabolism; of them only half knew they had diabetes (Conaway, O'Keefe, Reid, *et al.* 2005).

* *Depression.* Look again for depression. Even at 1 year, 25% are depressed.

* *Other drugs.* Check that the patient continues to take an ACE inhibitor and a beta-blocker unless contraindicated. The use of an ACE inhibitor reduces mortality (odds ratio 0.83) in a meta-analysis of trials lasting from 2 to 42 months, giving an NNT of 42 (Domanski, Exner, Borkowf, *et al.* 1999). The benefit of beta-blockade does not appear to diminish with time, with an NNT of 42 to save one life over 2 years (a relative reduction in risk of 23%) (Freemantle, Cleland, Young, *et al.* 1999).

* Recommend an annual influenza immunization. One study found that it halved the rate of death, reinfarction or readmission over 6 months' follow-up (Gurfinkel, de la Fuente, Mendiz, *et al.* 2002).

* Check that the patient has a cardiology appointment for an assessment of the coronary arteries and suitability for invasive treatment (PCI), as well as for an assessment of left ventricular function. The initial screening to assess coronary blood flow is likely to be an exercise ECG (stress ECG). Patients with a negative stress test are unlikely to require coronary artery surgery, and so an unnecessary angiogram can be avoided.

OTHER FACTUAL ADVICE

* Sedentary workers may return to work at 4–6 weeks, light manual workers at 6–8 weeks and heavy manual workers at 3 months.

* Do not fly for 2 weeks, and then only if able to climb one flight of stairs without difficulty. A more cautious policy is to advise against flying for 6 weeks.

* Drivers should not drive for 1 month, but need not now notify the DVLA. They should inform their insurance company. HGV and PSV licence holders must notify the DVLA, and may only continue vocational driving after individual assessment.

AID TO ORGANIZING A PRACTICE-BASED OR PCT-BASED REHABILITATION PROGRAMME

The Edinburgh Heart Manual published by NHS Lothian (see www.theheartmanual.com). It is not available for direct patient use; indeed, it will only be provided to practices once a team member has attended a Facilitator Training Programme.

HEART FAILURE

GUIDELINES

Scottish Intercollegiate Guidelines Network.
*Management of Chronic Heart Failure: A National
Clinical Guideline.* Feb 2007. Available: www.sign.ac.uk
    *Chronic Heart Failure: National Clinical Guideline
for Diagnosis and Management in Primary and
Secondary Care.* NICE Guideline No. 5, Royal College
of Physicians, London, 2003. Available: www.
nice.ac.uk

- In the management of heart failure two 'rules
  of halves' appear to apply. Only about half of
  patients with left ventricular systolic
  dysfunction (LVSD) receive treatment for
  chronic heart failure and only half of these
  receive appropriate therapy. Conversely, only
  about half of patients receiving treatment for
  heart failure have left ventricular dysfunction
  when investigated and only half of those are
  on appropriate therapy (Sharpe and Doughty
  1998). This is, however, not simply a comment on
  poor practice but also reflects the fact that not all
  patients with heart failure have LVSD (Vasan
  2003). For details of the diagnosis of heart failure
  see *Evidence-based Diagnosis in Primary Care* by
  A. F. Polmear (editor) published by Butterworth-
  Heinemann, 2008.
- Every patient deserves a full cardiac diagnosis.
  Clinically, it is easy to miss significant valvular
  and congenital disease with insignificant
  murmurs, constrictive pericarditis and non-
  cardiac causes for heart failure, especially drugs
  (e.g. steroids, non-dihydropyridine calcium-
  channel blockers and NSAIDs).
- The prognosis is poor, with 5-year survivals of
  25% for men and 38% for women (Sharpe and
  Doughty 1998).
- * Organize the care of patients with heart failure
  in the same way as with other chronic
  conditions: a register, 6-monthly review with a
  call and recall system. Audit the completeness
  of the register and the quality of the care
  regularly. The prevalence of heart failure in the
  UK is 1.4% (Davies, Hobbs, Davis, *et al.* 2001).
  A further 0.6% have left ventricular systolic
  dysfunction without overt heart failure.

Check that the practice figures tally with
these or that there are good reasons for not
doing so.
- * Consider referral to a cardiac failure clinic if
  one is available. Such clinics have been shown
  to achieve improvements in patient functioning
  and satisfaction with reductions in
  hospitalizations (Philbin 1999). Exercise
  training is an important part of any such
  programme, with the potential to reduce
  mortality by 35% (ExTraMATCH
  Collaborative 2004).

GROUNDS FOR ADMISSION

(a) Severe symptoms, e.g. severe dyspnoea or
    hypotension.
(b) Acute myocardial infarction.
(c) Severe complicating medical illness, e.g.
    pneumonia.
(d) Inadequate social support.
(e) Failure to respond to treatment.
(f) Uncontrolled arrhythmia.

REFERRAL TO OUTPATIENTS

Refer patients:
(a) aged less than 60; or
(b) with a murmur or known valvular disease; for
    details of the diagnosis of cardiac murmurs see
    Evidence-based Diagnosis in Primary Care by A. F.
    Polmear (editor) published by Butterworth-
    Heinemann, 2008; or
(c) with angina; or
(d) with arrhythmias; or
(e) with severe heart failure; or
(f) with renal impairment, thyroid disease,
    anaemia or other complicating factors; or
(g) where the heart failure is unexplained; or
(h) with diastolic dysfunction or any cause other
    than LV systolic dysfunction; or
(i) who are pregnant or planning a pregnancy.

GP MANAGEMENT

Investigations

- * Confirm the diagnosis with ECG and N-terminal
  BNP (or equivalent). In one study in New Zealand
  primary care, general practitioners diagnosed

heart failure in 70% of a cohort with dyspnoea or oedema when only 25% were finally judged to have heart failure (Wright, Doughty, Pearl, *et al.* 2003). The accuracy of BNP varies according to assay and cut-off value used. Using N-terminal BNP the following figures have been obtained: sensitivity 100%, specificity 70% (Hobbs, Davis, Roalfe, *et al.* 2002). If both BNP and ECG are normal, heart failure is extremely unlikely.

* If one or both are abnormal, check Hb, creatinine, electrolytes, fasting glucose, urinalysis, thyroid function, CXR, and echocardiogram.
* *The echocardiogram* is needed to confirm the diagnosis of heart failure, to detect an unsuspected cause for the failure, e.g. valvular disease (Dargie and McMurray 1994), as well as to quantify the degree of failure. If facilities for BNP testing are not available, the echocardiogram could reasonably be omitted if both CXR and ECG were normal and there were no predisposing factors for heart failure. The chance of heart failure being present would be very small (Hobbs, Davis and Lip 2000).
* *The check for anaemia* is important. One population based study of Canadian patients with new-onset heart failure found that 17% were anaemic and that it was associated with a raised mortality (adjusted hazard ratio 1.34 (CI 1.24 to 1.46)) (Ezekowitz and McAlister 2003).
* Check spirometry or the peak flow. Pulmonary disease may mimic the symptoms and signs of heart failure or coexist.

GENERAL MEASURES

* Explain what is going on and what to do if things get worse.
* Recommend daily weighing at the same time and in the same clothes. Patients should report if they gain more than 2 kg over 2 days.
* Reduce weight, if obese.
* *Diet:* advise a diet with no salty foods or added salt and, unless on ACE inhibitors or spironolactone, one high in potassium (e.g. milk, bananas, oranges, tomato juice and chocolate).
* Restrict fluid intake to 2 litres a day, unless losing fluids from sweat or diarrhoea or vomiting.
* Keep alcohol intake low. In alcoholic heart disease recommend complete cessation.

* Stop smoking; it causes vasoconstriction. Refer to the smoking cessation services.
* Rest in the acute phase, but exercise once stable. Moderate exertion (e.g. bicycling or brisk walking) can reduce dyspnoea in as little as 8 weeks (Lloyd-Williams, Mair and Leitner 2002). It should be carried out for 30 minutes a day on at least 5 days a week. Vigorous exertion should be avoided. Refer to the heart failure rehabilitation service if this facility exists.
* *Vaccination:* recommend influenza vaccination annually and pneumococcal vaccination once.
* Check for depression. It is present in one third and should be treated as thoroughly as if it was not associated with heart failure. Warn patients not to buy St John's wort over the counter (OTC) because of its interaction with prescribed medication, specifically digoxin and warfarin.
* Stop NSAIDs (including COX 2 inhibitors) if taken, unless they are essential. Warn the patient not to buy them OTC.
* Identify the carer or carers and involve them in the management.

CONGESTIVE CARDIAC FAILURE

The following refers to patients with LVSD. Patients with diastolic dysfunction need specialist assessment.

Drug treatment can be based on the patient's condition as classified by the New York Heart Association classification of heart failure symptoms (Table 5.5).

Table 5.5	New York Heart Association classification of heart failure symptoms
Class I – asymptomatic	No limitations of ordinary activity
Class II – mild	Slight limitation of physical activity but comfortable at rest
Class III – moderate	Marked limitation of physical activity. Comfortable at rest but symptomatic on less than ordinary physical activity
Class IV – severe	Inability to carry on any physical activity without discomfort. Symptoms present at rest

Patients of all classes should be given an ACE inhibitor and a beta-blocker. Only patients with evidence of fluid overload need a diuretic and only patients in classes III and IV should be given spironolactone. Digoxin is indicated in patients in Classes III and IV who have not responded adequately to other medication.

ACE INHIBITORS

● All patients with heart failure should be taking an ACE inhibitor, with or without a diuretic, unless there is a contraindication. They increase the ability to exercise, improve well-being and prolong life in all degrees of heart failure (Dargie and McMurray 1994). Their use can reduce mortality by 20% with greater benefits in the higher risk patients (Flather, Yusuf, Kober, et al. 2000). This gives an NNT of 26 to prevent one death over 3 years (Scottish Intercollegiate Guidelines Network 1999).

● They may be used alone in patients with fatigue or mild dyspnoea on exertion without overt heart failure.

∗ Exclude the absolute contraindications of allergy to ACE inhibitors and pregnancy.

∗ Refer for cardiological assessment, as in- or outpatient according to severity, without initiating ACE inhibitors, patients with:

(a) severe heart failure, requiring > 80 mg of furosemide (or equivalent);

(b) low systolic blood pressure (systolic < 80 mmHg);

(c) low serum sodium (< 130 mmol/l) or high potassium (> 5.0 mmol/l);

(d) possible hypovolaemia (low jugular venous pressure (JVP), recent diuresis or fluid loss, high diuretic dose or combined diuretic treatment);

(e) drugs which increase the risk of hypotension: amlodipine, nicorandil, vasodilators;

(f) renal dysfunction (serum creatinine > 200 μmol/l) or known renal artery stenosis;

(g) severe diabetes mellitus with associated renal disease;

(h) severe generalized atherosclerosis (especially if intermittent claudication and arterial bruits are present);

(i) severe chronic obstructive airways disease and pulmonary heart disease (cor pulmonale).

∗ Start ACE inhibitors at home, provided the above contraindications are not present (Mason, Young, Freemantle, et al. 2000).

1. Check creatinine and electrolytes.

2. Stop potassium supplements or potassium-sparing diuretics.

3. Start with a low dose initially, e.g. enalapril 2.5 mg, lisinopril 2.5 mg or ramipril 1.25 mg or perindopril 2 mg. Advise the patient to take the first dose before going to bed to reduce the effect of first-dose hypotension.

4. Repeat the creatinine level after 1 week. A rise suggests renal artery stenosis. Stop the ACE inhibitor and refer.

5. Increase the dose fortnightly, with a check each time of BP and creatinine and electrolytes, until a dose is reached of enalapril 10 mg b.d., lisinopril 20 mg o.d., ramipril 10 mg o.d. or perindopril 4 mg o.d., or side-effects have prevented further increases. Lower doses have not been shown to prolong life. Note that perindopril use involves far less dose titration than other ACE inhibitors.

6. Once the dose is stable, repeat creatinine and electrolytes at 3 months then 6-monthly or sooner if further dose titration is necessary or there is intercurrent infection.

7. Warn the patient to avoid dehydration, for instance in gastroenteritis or in hot weather, as this can cause a sudden deterioration in renal function. If the weight drops by more than 1 kg because of dehydration, the patient should stop the diuretic and drink more fluid.

Note: Potassium-sparing diuretics may be restarted in the rare case where the serum potassium falls to 3.0 mmol/l or below on an ACE inhibitor.

Note: Angiotensin-II receptor blockers may be used in patients intolerant of ACE inhibitors (Pitt, Poole-Wilson, Segal, et al. 2000). They should be started at a low dose and titrated up, e.g. losartan 25 mg rising to 50 mg daily.

Note: Take over the upward titration of an ACE inhibitor in a patient discharged from hospital, unless satisfied that the hospital is doing so. Many patients fall between two stools and never reach an effective dose.

RISES IN CREATININE AND POTASSIUM ON AN ACE INHIBITOR

(a) A rise of creatinine of up to 50% of baseline or to 200 µmol/l (whichever is the smaller) is acceptable, as is a K$^+$ < 6 mmol/l.

(b) If the rise in creatinine is > 100% or to > 350 µmol/l, or the K$^+$≥ 6 mmol/l: stop the ACE inhibitor and refer.

(c) If the rise is between these levels, try the following in order:
1. stop other drugs which may be contributing (e.g. an NSAID, a calcium antagonist, or a K-sparing diuretic) and halve the dose of any other diuretic;
2. halve the dose of ACE inhibitor;
3. refer to cardiologist.

DIURETICS (OTHER THAN SPIRONOLACTONE)

* Use a thiazide in mild failure, e.g. bendroflumethiazide 2.5–5 mg daily, but not in the very elderly or those with impaired renal function: they respond poorly.

* Beyond that dose, or in more severe failure, use a loop diuretic (bendroflumethiazide 10 mg is equivalent to furosemide 20 mg), which will cause less hypokalaemia and impotence than a high-dose thiazide. Increase the dose gradually until diuresis occurs. Once stable, reduce the dose to as low as possible without oedema or breathlessness occurring.

* Recheck the serum creatinine and electrolytes after 4 weeks and then 6-monthly.

* *Combining a loop diuretic with a thiazide.* If diuresis does not occur with furosemide 80 mg/bumetanide 2 mg, consider *adding* bendroflumethiazide 2.5–10 mg or metolazone 2.5–10 mg daily for 3 days in the first instance (Channer, McLean and Lawson-Matthew 1994). Longer use may be associated with electrolyte disturbance. Even in short-term use the diuresis can be excessive and can cause hypokalaemia. Check the patient after 24 hours and again at 3 days with a check of creatinine and electrolytes. Consider a longer course if the patient responds and then relapses after the extra diuretic is stopped.

* *Potassium-sparing diuretics* (amiloride or triamterene) are only indicated in patients not suitable for ACE inhibitors. Add a potassium-sparing diuretic in such patients:
(a) who are on digoxin or otherwise prone to arrhythmias;
(b) whose initial serum potassium is 3.0 mmol/l or below;
(c) who have a potassium-losing condition, e.g. cirrhosis, nephrotic syndrome or chronic diarrhoea;
(d) whose potassium falls to 3.0 mmol/l or below;
(e) who are elderly or chronically sick, with a poor potassium intake;
(f) who have diabetes;
(g) who are on oral steroids;
(h) who are oedematous, until they are no longer having a dieresis (MeReC 1994); or
(i) who are on high doses of loop diuresis, e.g. furosemide 120 mg daily (or bumetanide 3 mg daily) (DTB 1994b).

Aldosterone antagonists

* Add spironolactone 25 mg daily to a loop diuretic and an ACE inhibitor in moderate to severe failure (i.e. when the patient's physical activity is markedly limited). It can reduce the mortality and morbidity by 30% (Pitt, Zannad, Remme, *et al.* 1999) with an NNT of 9 (6–15) over 2 years (McKelvie 2004). NICE recommends that specialist advice be sought but other guidelines think this unnecessary if the creatinine is ≤ 220 µmol/l and the K$^+$≤ 5.0 mmol/l (McMurray, Cohen-Solal, Dietz, *et al.* 2003). The dose may be increased to 50 mg daily but with greater risk of hyperkalaemia. Stop any other potassium-sparing diuretics. Be even more cautious in the very old, whose renal function is more likely to be impaired.

* Warn the patient to avoid salt substitutes with a high potassium content. Warn males about gynaecomastia.

* Hyperkalaemia is a potentially fatal adverse effect (Juurlink, Mamdani, Lee, *et al.* 2004) and is most likely in those with impaired renal function. Only give spironolactone if the creatinine is < 220 µmol/l.

* Check creatinine and electrolytes at 1 week then at 1, 2, 3, 6, 9, and 12 months then 6 monthly. If K$^+$ reaches 5.5 to 5.9 mmol/l or creatinine rises to 200 µmol/l, reduce the dose and monitor closely. If those levels are exceeded, stop and seek specialist advice.

BETA-BLOCKERS

* Consider all patients for beta-blockade once heart failure is controlled. Mortality is reduced by 32%, a benefit which exists for all degrees of severity (Lechat, Packer and Chalon 1998). Benefit in the elderly is as great as in younger patients (Dulin, Haas, Abraham, et al. 2005). The BNF currently recommends that treatment should usually be initiated by 'those experienced in the management of heart failure'. In stable, mild to moderate failure with a pulse > 60, the requisite experience is likely to be found in primary care.

* Check that there is no absolute contraindication: reversible airways obstruction, high degree AV block, or severe hypotension. Do not be put off by more relative contraindications, e.g. diabetes, fixed airways obstruction, mild hypotension (Krum 2009).

* Use a beta-blocker licensed for heart failure, e.g. bisoprolol, carvedilol or nebivolol, or one for which the evidence exists despite the lack of licence, e.g. extended release metoprolol. A study in British general practice found that switching to bisoprolol or carvedilol, mainly from atenolol, was the single most valuable manoeuvre in patients with left ventricular dysfunction (Mant, Hobbs, Glasziou, et al. 2008).

* Start at a low dose, e.g. bisoprolol 1.25 mg daily or carvedilol 3.125 mg b.d. and double the dose every 2–4 weeks until the target dose is obtained (bisoprolol 10 mg daily, carvedilol 25 mg b.d. or 50 mg b.d. if the heart failure is not severe and the patient weighs > 85 kg.). Experience suggests that symptoms frequently worsen initially then subsequently improve and that improvement may not be apparent for 3–6 months. However, a randomized trial showed that initial worsening of symptoms was no worse on carvedilol than on placebo and that some improvement was apparent at 2–3 weeks (Krum, Roecker, Mohacsi, et al. 2003). Overall, adverse effects are mild (Ko, Hebert, Coffey, et al. 2004).

* Monitor heart rate, BP and clinical status at each dose titration, and serum creatinine at some stage. If the pulse is < 50 and symptoms have worsened, halve the dose. Stop and seek specialist advice if symptoms have become severe.

* Check creatinine and electrolytes 1–2 weeks after initiation and 1–2 weeks after reaching the final dose.

* Continue ACE inhibitors and diuretics.

* If at any stage it is necessary to stop the beta-blocker, tail it off gradually to avoid rebound ischaemia and arrhythmias.

DIGOXIN

Digoxin is indicated in:

(a) atrial fibrillation (although not first-line, see page 157);

(b) heart failure persisting despite optimum therapy with diuretics, ACE inhibitors and beta-blockers. Digoxin should be given in combination with an ACE inhibitor. Its use can reduce the need for admission without improving mortality (Hood, Dans, Guyatt, et al. 2004).

Blood level monitoring. Opinion is divided on its value. The NICE guideline is against the routine monitoring of blood levels, on the grounds that the correlation between levels and therapeutic effect is poor. Levels may be needed if toxicity is feared or suspected but interpretation may be difficult since toxicity may occur when the level is in the therapeutic range. However, a post-hoc analysis of the DIG trial showed that patients with a digoxin level 1 month after initiation of 0.5–0.8 ng/ml had a reduced mortality vs placebo (ARR 6.3% (CI 2.1% to 10.5%) while those with a level of 1.2 and above had an 11.8% absolute increase in mortality (CI 5.7% to 18.0%) (Rathore, Curtis, Wang, et al. 2003). This argues in favour of monitoring in order to achieve these lower levels.

Procedure

1. Check creatinine and electrolytes. Correct any hypokalaemia.
2. Give 250 mcg daily or 62.5–125 mcg in the elderly or those with renal impairment.
3. Check serum creatinine and electrolytes:

(a) 1 month after starting treatment; and

(b) if renal function changes. Regular checks of serum creatinine and electrolytes are then needed; or

4. Monitor closely if a drug is added which decreases digoxin elimination, e.g. diltiazem, quinine or amiodarone; or increases its absorption, e.g. omeprazole or tetracycline; or decreases its absorption, e.g. colestyramine or colestipol.

Note: Use digitoxin in mild to moderate renal impairment without a reduction in dose.

INTRACTABLE HEART FAILURE

* Reconsider the diagnosis. Does the patient have:
  (a) thyroid disease;
  (b) infective endocarditis;
  (c) pulmonary infection;
  (d) ventricular dysrhythmia;
  (e) pulmonary thromboembolism;
  (f) inappropriate bradycardia and a need for pacing.
* Review the treatment. Is there:
  (a) overtreatment with diuretics causing uraemia;
  (b) non-compliance with drugs;
  (c) alcohol overuse.
* Is there a role for surgery, e.g. valvular surgery, CABG or transplant?

END-STAGE HEART FAILURE

There comes a point when the decision has to be made whether treatment of heart failure can be optimized further or whether care should now be palliative. Deciding on prognosis in heart failure is difficult and cardiological advice will be needed. The decision is important if the experiences documented in the 1990s are to be improved on: that roughly half of patients dying of heart failure suffer pain, breathlessness, depression, and anxiety for a period that often lasts over 6 months (Gibbs, McCoy, Gibbs, *et al.* 2002).

Once the decision has been made that care is now palliative, rather than attempting to prolong life, the following are essential:

■ continued attention to conventional heart failure treatment to alleviate symptoms;

■ the introduction of specific palliative measures, using lessons learned from the care of cancer patients;

■ full and frank discussion (unless they make it clear they do not want it) with the patient and carers, so that they understand what is happening and what is likely to happen and can make their own choice of how they want it to happen;

■ the patient and carers must be clear whom they should contact in an emergency; and that contact must have access to the information that palliation of symptoms, rather than the prolongation of life, is the main goal;

■ if available, referral to a specialist team, either of specialist heart failure nurses or the community palliative care team;

■ bereavement care of those close to the patient completes the management.

BREATHLESSNESS

* Morphine is the most effective palliation. Give a low oral dose (2.5–5 mg 4-hourly) as peak plasma levels are higher in heart failure.
* Breathless at rest. Consider oxygen therapy at home (40–80% if there is no COPD) (Stewart and Howard 1992).
* Refer for relaxation, breathing exercises, and anxiety management if these are available.

WEAKNESS AND FATIGUE

This is usually secondary to a low cardiac output.
* *Drug reduction*. Consider reducing ACE inhibitors and beta-blockers, and diuretics if there is dehydration.
* *Depression*. Avoid tricylics; SSRIs may be of value.
* *Social factors*. Increase social care if possible and ensure support for the carer(s).

ANOREXIA/NAUSEA

* *Digoxin*. Check serum level and renal function.
* Consider increasing diuretics if there is hepatic congestion.
* *Diet*. Advise the patient to have small, appetizing meals more frequently. Allow small amounts of alcohol before meals.
* *Antiemetics*. Use levomepromazine 12.5 mg nocte. Avoid cyclizine.

OEDEMA

* *Mobilization* is advisable in theory but rarely practicable at this stage.
* *Diuretics.* Avoid increasing diuretics at this stage unless doing so gives symptomatic relief. They are unlikely to have much effect on the oedema.
* Be cautious about advising the patient to raise the feet. This may increase the venous return to the heart and worsen the dyspnoea.
* *Compression stockings/bandages.* These may increase tissue damage and are uncomfortable.

ACUTE PULMONARY OEDEMA

When called urgently to the patient *in extremis*, get someone else to dial for an ambulance while you:

1. sit the patient up with the legs down;
2. give oxygen if available;
3. give a GTN tablet or spray sublingually (for its immediate vasodilator effect);
4. give i.v. diamorphine 1 mg per minute up to 5 mg, or i.v. morphine 2 mg per minute up to 10 mg, mixed with metoclopramide 10 mg i.v. Do not use cyclizine; it raises systemic arterial pressure;
5. give a loop diuretic (i.v. furosemide 50 mg or i.v. bumetanide 1 mg).

* Look for causes of the heart failure that may need treatment in their own right, especially myocardial infarction.
* Admit once the patient is sufficiently stable, for fuller assessment and for continuing treatment.

Note: Digoxin and aminophylline should not be used in acute failure outside hospital.

RIGHT HEART FAILURE

ACUTE RIGHT HEART FAILURE

* The clinical picture of low output state, no pulmonary oedema and a raised JVP may be due to massive pulmonary embolism or to acute right heart failure as in a right ventricle myocardial infarction, or acute cor pulmonale.
* Admit urgently. Position the patient however is most comfortable. Do not give morphine;

respiratory depression and hypotension are very likely to follow. Do not give diuretics: they may precipitate shock (DTB 1990).

CHRONIC COR PULMONALE

* Treat the lung disease. Consider:
  (a) antibiotics for exacerbations of infection;
  (b) inhaled bronchodilators and steroids via a spacing device (see page 190);
  (c) physiotherapy;
  (d) long-term oxygen therapy (see page 191);
  (e) nasal intermittent positive pressure ventilation for those with thoracic deformities and obstructive sleep apnoea.
* Admit readily anyone with an acute exacerbation. Oxygen will dilate the pulmonary vessels and so reduce the pulmonary artery pressure. The danger of hypercapnoea makes this hazardous in the acute situation at home.
* Use diuretics carefully as they may reduce renal blood flow further. They are only required if oedema becomes troublesome.
* Use digoxin only if the patient is in atrial fibrillation.
* Do not start ACE inhibitors outside hospital.

PATIENT RESOURCES

British Heart Foundation, 14 Fitzhardinge Street, London, W1H 6DH. Helpline: 08450 70 80 70: www. bhf.org.uk

British Cardiac Patients Association, 2 Station Road, Swavesey, Cambridge, CB24 5QJ. Tel (Helpline): 01223 846845: www.bcpa.co.uk

ARRHYTHMIAS

Arrhythmias can be treated only after accurate diagnosis. For details of the diagnosis of arrhythmias see 'Palpitations' in *Evidence-based Diagnosis in Primary Care* by A. F. Polmear (editor) published by Butterworth-Heinemann, 2008.

* Perform an ECG in a patient with an established arrhythmia or with a paroxysmal arrhythmia who is currently having an attack. In patients with paroxysmal arrhythmias who are between attacks, the history often suggests the diagnosis. Occasionally the ECG between attacks may

show evidence of pre-excitation, QT prolongation, ventricular hypertrophy or an old, or even recent, myocardial infarction.

* Ask the patient to tap out the rhythm. This may help to decide whether the arrhythmia is regular or irregular. However, patients are surprisingly poor at reporting details of their arrhythmia.

* If the history suggests an arrhythmia but you do not find it on examination, refer. Continuous ambulatory monitoring will detect it if it is occurring at least once every 24 hours. A cardiomemo, which allows the patient to transmit an ECG by telephone during an attack, is more helpful when arrhythmias are less frequent.

ECTOPIC BEATS IN A NORMAL HEART

* Explain their benign nature to the patient. Advise against caffeine, fatigue, smoking and alcohol.

* *Beta-blockers* should be used only if the patient is unable to tolerate the ectopics.

* *Frequent ventricular ectopics (more than 100 per hour)* may be grounds for referral. Patients may have a prolapsing mitral valve, or the older patient may have unsuspected ischaemic heart disease (British Heart Foundation 1995).

* For those still troubled by their symptoms, arrange a single 1-hour session, along cognitive behavioural lines, to attempt to alter the way that the sensations from the heart are perceived. Such a session from a trained nurse, in an Oxford study, was of significant benefit (NNT 3 (95%CI 2 to 7)) (Mayou, Spricings, Birkhead and Price 2002).

ATRIAL FIBRILLATION (AF)

NICE GUIDELINE

The National Collaborating Centre for Chronic Conditions. National Institute for Health and Clinical Excellence. *Atrial Fibrillation: National Clinical Guideline for Management in Primary and Secondary Care.* Royal College of Physicians, June 2006. Available: www.nice.org.uk

● Atrial fibrillation (AF) is associated with increased mortality from stroke and heart failure. In a 20 year follow-up study 89% of the women had a cardiovascular event (leading to hospitalization or death) and 66% of the men (Stewart, Hart, Hole and McMurray 2002).

● UK studies in the 1990s suggest that a quarter of cases of AF are unknown to their general practitioners and that only a quarter to a half of those known to have AF are on warfarin (Hobbs 1999). However, one study suggests that most of those not on warfarin are either ineligible or would decline (Roderick 1998).

● Palpation of the pulse by a trained nurse is a sensitive method of detecting AF although it has lower specificity. This means that few will be missed but that fewer than a quarter of those found by the nurse to have an irregular pulse will have AF (Sudlow, Rodgers, Kenny and Thomson 1998).

● An underlying cause can be found in at least 70% of patients with AF (ACC/AHA/ESC 2001).

● The risk of developing AF is increased five-fold in those with clinical or subclinical hyperthyroidism (Auer, Scheibner, Mische, *et al.* 2001).

WORK-UP OF AF

(a) History of alcohol intake (either chronic or bingeing).

(b) Blood pressure (half of all cases of AF are hypertensive).

(c) TFTs, creatinine and electrolytes.

(d) Examine for heart failure, valvular heart disease, congenital heart disease or acute pericarditis or myocarditis.

(e) ECG (looking for ischaemic heart disease (IHD), LV strain and delta waves).

(f) CXR (for cardiomegaly if echocardiogram not available).

(g) Echocardiogram (for LV systolic dysfunction).

* Admit if rapid AF is associated with:
  (a) chest pain;
  (b) hypotension; or
  (c) more than mild heart failure.

* Refer urgently if seen within 48 hours of the onset of AF and the patient is a candidate for

cardioversion (see below). A single oral dose of amiodarone (30 mg/kg) can achieve cardioversion within 24 hours in 87% against 35% with placebo (Peuhkurinen, Niemela, Ylitalo, *et al.* 2000).

* Refer all other patients to cardiology outpatients for:

(a) an assessment of underlying pathology;

(b) a decision about cardioversion;

(c) a decision about anticoagulation.

CARDIOVERSION VERSUS RATE CONTROL

● *Rate control* is recommended as the treatment of choice in most patients in the US (Snow, Weiss and LeFevre 2003). It has advantages over rhythm control: fewer hospital admissions, fewer adverse drug reactions, possibly a lower mortality (Atrial Fibrillation Follow-up Investigation of Rhythm Management (AFFIRM) Investigators 2002), and it is more cost-effective (Hagens, Vermeulen and TenVergert 2004). UK guidelines suggest an approach tailored to the individual patient (see below).

● *Cardioversion* is most likely to succeed in those with no, or mild, organic heart disease, the young, and those with a short history. However, half of cardioverted patients revert to AF within 3–6 months, the drugs used to maintain sinus rhythm are more toxic than those used for rate control in AF, and cardioversion may be most worthwhile in those with severe symptoms that are due to the AF (ACC/AHA/ESC 2001), even though this is the group in whom it is least likely to succeed. Anticoagulants will be needed for 3 weeks before the procedure and at least 4 weeks after it, unless the onset of the AF is within the previous 48 hours.

● *If successfully cardioverted*, the patient may be offered an antiarrhythmic to prevent recurrence. First line drugs are a standard beta-blocker then, if that fails, a Class 1c drug (flecainide or propafenone) or sotalol, followed by amiodarone. However, if structural heart disease is present, the Class 1c drugs and sotalol are omitted. How long treatment should be continued in a patient in whom AF does not recur is not clear; 6 months is a minimum but 5 years may be safer (Camm 2001). Continued anticoagulation may be recommended despite apparently successful maintenance of sinus rhythm in case the patient is having asymptomatic episodes of AF.

NICE recommends that both options are discussed with the patient, explaining the advantages and disadvantages of each for that particular patient.

Referral for cardioversion is more appropriate for certain patients, either because it is more likely to succeed than in others (the first three categories) or because sinus rhythm offers greater chance of clinical benefit than rate control (the last two categories):

■ younger patients;

■ those presenting for the first time with lone AF;

■ those with AF secondary to a cause that has now been treated;

■ those who are symptomatic;

■ those with congestive heart failure.

Rate control is more appropriate in those in whom cardioversion is less likely to succeed:

■ those over 65 years old;

■ those with structural heart disease or CHD;

■ those whose AF is longstanding (e.g. > 12 months);

■ those in whom previous attempts at cardioversion have failed or been followed by relapse;

■ those in whom an underlying cause, e.g. thyrotoxicosis, has not yet been corrected;

■ those with a contraindication to antiarrhythmic drugs.

ANTICOAGULATION

● All patients with atrial fibrillation are at increased risk of thromboembolism. Overall, atrial fibrillation increases the risk of stroke five times.

● Warfarin reduces that risk by 60% (NNT 33 for 1 year in primary prevention; 13 in secondary prevention), but at the expense of an increased risk of major bleeding (0.3% per year suffer haemorrhagic strokes on warfarin compared to 0.1% in controls and those on aspirin) (Yip, Hart and Conway 2002).

● Aspirin reduces the risk of embolic stroke by 20% with NNTs of 66 (primary) and 40 (secondary prevention) (Yip, Hart and Conway 2002). In a meta-analysis of oral anticoagulants versus aspirin, the former almost halved the stroke risk compared to the latter (van Walraven, Hart, Singer, *et al.* 2002).

Table 5.6   Stroke risk and likely benefit from treatment in patients with atrial fibrillation (Yip, Hart and Conway 2002)

STROKE RISK	STROKE RISK	RECOMMENDATION	NNT FOR 1 YEAR
High: ■ Previous stroke, TIA or other thromboembolic event ■ Age ≥ 75 with diabetes, hypertension, or vascular disease ■ Valvular disease, heart failure, or left ventricular systolic dysfunction on echocardiography	8–12% per year	Warfarin	14–21
Moderate: ■ Age > 65 (but see below) ■ Age < 65 with diabetes, hypertension, PVD or CHD	4% per year	Warfarin; or aspirin. Warfarin may be preferred if more than one risk factor is present	42 125
Low: ■ Aged < 65 with no risk factors	1% per year	Aspirin	500

A more recent review of the same data found that the risk of stroke was not increased with increasing age, over that in an age matched population, provided no risk factors were present. Risk factors included a systolic BP of 140 or above. Older patients without these risk factors can be treated as low risk. This is likely to comprise 16% of the population with AF > 75 years old (van Walraven, Hart, Wells, *et al.* 2003).

- The decision about whether to take warfarin or aspirin must be made with each patient and based on his or her risk, see Table 5.6. When patients are given information about their risk, roughly half the patients wish to take, or not take, warfarin in a way that is contrary to current guidelines (Protheroe, Fahey, Montgomery and Peters 2000).
- The INR should be controlled to between 2 and 3. An INR below 2 does not reduce the risk of intracranial haemorrhage while an INR of 3.5–3.9 has an odds ratio (OR) for intracranial haemorrhage of 4.6 (compared to an INR of 2–3). The OR for intracranial haemorrhage with an INR of 4 or over is 8.8 (Fang, Chang and Hylek 2004).

A simpler scoring system has been developed, called CHADS, or originally CHADS$_2$ to remind the user to score 2 for a history of stroke (Gage, Waterman, Shannon, *et al.* 2001). Its strength is that it reflects the fact that risk factors *multiply* the risk when they coexist.

Scoring the patient's stroke risk using CHADS (Table 5.7)

Score one for each of the following but score two for stroke or TIA:

- **Congestive heart failure (ever).**
- **Hypertension > 160/90 (ever).**
- **Age ≥ 75.**
- **Diabetes.**
- **Stroke or TIA (ever).**

Table 5.7   CHADS – interpreting the score

SCORE	STROKE RISK PER YEAR
0	1.9%
1	2.8%
2	4.0%
3	5.9%
4	8.5%
5	12.5%
6	18.2%

CONTRA-INDICATIONS TO WARFARIN IN AF (MAN-SON-HING AND LAUPACIS 2003)

Absolute contraindications

- Pregnancy.
- Active peptic ulcer or other active source of GI bleeding.
- Current major trauma or surgery.
- Uncontrolled hypertension.
- A bleeding diathesis.
- Bacterial endocarditis.
- Alcoholism.
- Inability to control the INR.

Factors which increase the risk of bleeding slightly but only enough to alter the decision in cases where the benefit is already borderline

- Current NSAID use (add gastroprotection or change to a COX-2 inhibitor).
- Activities that involve a high risk of injury.

Factors often erroneously thought to contraindicate warfarin

- Old age. The INR is no harder to control in the elderly than in younger patients. There is a slight increase in bleeding risk in older patients but with increasing age the benefit from warfarin rises more than the risk.
- Past history of peptic ulcer or GI bleeding, now resolved.
- Hypertension controlled < 160/90
- Patients at risk of falling.
- Previous stroke.
- Alcohol intake of one to two drinks a day.

RATE CONTROL OF ESTABLISHED AF IN GENERAL PRACTICE

* Control the rate if the resting rate is above 90 beats/minute or the patient complains of symptoms associated with a fast rate on exertion.

Use:

(a) a beta-blocker, e.g. atenolol 50 mg daily. If rate control is inadequate after 1 week, add digoxin; or

(b) a rate-limiting calcium antagonist, e.g. diltiazem. If rate control is inadequate after 1 week, add digoxin. Monitor carefully; the diltiazem can increase digoxin levels and precipitate digoxin toxicity. This combination is preferred if there is a need to control the rate on exertion as well as at rest;

(c) if digoxin is contraindicated, add diltiazem to the beta-blocker. The usual concern about causing bradycardia or AV block is less of a problem in AF since that is the aim of the treatment; or

(d) digoxin alone in predominantly sedentary patients.

* Aim for a resting rate of < 80 beats/minute and < 110 beats/minute on exertion although the British Heart Foundation Factfile (British Heart Foundation 2000) allows rates of up to 90 resting and 180 on exertion. Slower rates benefit those with mitral stenosis; faster rates those with poor left ventricular function.

* Check the creatinine and electrolytes. Correct any hypokalaemia. If there is renal impairment use digitoxin, in the usual doses, provided the impairment is not severe.

If there is no urgency:

* give 5 mcg/kg per day (usual starting dose 250 mcg daily) and review after 1 week.

If the situation is more urgent:

* give a loading dose of digoxin of 500 to 1500 mcg (in divided doses over 24 hours), depending on the patient's weight, giving 15 mcg/kg of estimated lean body weight. If the ventricular rate has not slowed satisfactorily after 24 hours, give a further 5 mcg/kg. If that fails, abandon digoxin.

Maintenance

1. Give enough digoxin to control the ventricular rate. In an average-sized patient, start with 250 mcg daily. Halve this if the serum creatinine is even modestly raised. However, a dose of 62.5 mcg daily will be too low unless there is severe renal impairment.

2. Check the serum level before exceeding 500 mcg daily (or 250 mcg daily in the elderly). Aim for a level of 1–2 nmol/l. However, toxicity can occur in hypokalaemia with a therapeutic digoxin level.

3. If therapeutic levels do not control the ventricular rate, add a low dose of a beta-blocker or diltiazem.

Note: Digoxin will not control the rate on exercise or in other situations when sympathetic outflow is high. Check that the patient is calm and resting before taking further action on the basis of a high rate.

Special cases

(a) *Heart failure.* Digoxin and beta-blockers will both be of benefit but the beta-blocker should be introduced more cautiously (and only once the patient is digitalized and stable).

(b) *Thyrotoxicosis.* All patients with otherwise unexplained AF should have their thyroid function checked. Control the rate with beta-blockers temporarily. They are likely to need cardioversion once the thyrotoxicosis is controlled.

(c) *Wolff–Parkinson–White syndrome.* Digoxin and verapamil are contraindicated.

(d) *Sick sinus syndrome.* Digoxin, beta-blockers and calcium antagonists may worsen the situation. Pacing is required.

ORGANIZING THE PRACTICE FOR THE MANAGEMENT OF AF

- The prevalence is 0.4% of the population and 5% of patients > 65 years old (ACC/AHA/ESC 2001).
- Identify patients already known to have AF by searching for patients taking digoxin or already coded as having AF. This will detect about half of those with AF (Sudlow, Rodgers, Kenny and Thomson 1998) (but has the advantage of capturing them quickly). However, only about half of those on digoxin have AF so an examination of the records is needed.
- Find new cases by incorporating a search for an irregular pulse in every routine measurement of BP at Older Person checks, and opportunistically when those aged 65 and older consult, with an ECG in those whose pulse is irregular. This will detect almost all of those with AF (sensitivity > 90%) (Sudlow, Rodgers, Kenny and Thomson 1998) although less than a quarter of those with an irregular pulse will prove to have AF (Sudlow, Rodgers, Kenny and Thomson 1998); hence the need for ECG confirmation. The SAFE study found that opportunistic feeling of the pulse in older patients led to a new diagnosis of AF in 6 out of every 1000 patients age 65 and over (van Weert 2007).
- Once stable and fully assessed, review each patient yearly. Check symptoms, ventricular rate, adverse effects and compliance.
- At the ages of 65 and 75, or if the patient develops diabetes, hypertension or cardiovascular disease, review the risk of thromboembolism in those not on warfarin.

PAROXYSMAL ATRIAL FIBRILLATION

Tailor the treatment to the severity.

(a) *The patient with infrequent attacks and no serious symptoms, or attacks that can be averted by avoiding a precipitating cause, e.g. alcohol or caffeine:* either give
  - no drug treatment, or
  - a pill-in-the-pocket, to be taken at the onset of an attack, if the patient is suitable (see box below). A UK study recommends flecainide or propafenone but only after the drug has been shown to be safe and effective in terminating a paroxysm in that patient in hospital (Camm and Savelieva 2007).

(b) *The patient with more frequent attacks or more severe symptoms:* give a standard beta-blocker. If that is ineffective or not tolerated, choose a second line drug as follows:
  - *no structural heart disease:* a Class 1c drug (flecainide or propafenone), or sotalol then amiodarone;
  - *coronary heart disease:* sotalol, then amiodarone;
  - *left ventricular dysfunction:* amiodarone.

Specialist assessment is recommended before giving a drug other than a standard beta-blocker (see below).

NICE RECOMMENDATIONS FOR THE SUITABILITY OF A PATIENT FOR A 'PILL-IN-THE-POCKET'

- Infrequent episodes.
- Sufficiently reliable to use the treatment correctly.
- No structural heart disease, coronary heart disease or left ventricular dysfunction.
- Satisfactory baseline state: systolic blood pressure > 100 mmHg, resting heart rate > 70 bpm.

NICE warns of the danger of initiating drugs other than standard beta-blockers for paroxysmal AF in general practice without specialist advice, because of the risk that the drug will itself cause ventricular arrhythmias. This is most likely in those with underlying heart disease. In practice the patient will often have been assessed already by a cardiologist and had previous experience of an antiarrhythmic drug without adverse effects, obviating the need for re-referral.

If a paroxysm becomes persistent (arbitrarily defined as lasting at least 7 days), refer for consideration of cardioversion. Refer immediately if the patient develops heart failure or hypotension.

A patient with paroxysmal AF should be considered for antithrombotic treatment according to the presence of risk factors (see page 159) as though the AF were established, regardless of the number and severity of paroxysms.

ATRIAL FLUTTER

Treat as atrial fibrillation. In a US study the mortality over 4775 person-years of follow-up was increased 1.7-fold for flutter over that of controls and 2.4-fold for atrial fibrillation (Vidaillet, Granada, Chyou, *et al.* 2002).

PAROXYSMAL SUPRAVENTRICULAR TACHYCARDIA

If the patient is seen during the attack:

* Get the patient to perform a Valsalva manoeuvre. A quick move from standing into a squatting position will have the same effect.

* Apply carotid sinus massage except where the patient:

  (a) is elderly; or

  (b) has ischaemic heart disease; or

  (c) is likely to be digoxin toxic; or

  (d) has a carotid bruit; or

  (e) has a history of transient ischaemic attacks.

Note: The BNF recommends ECG monitoring during carotid sinus massage.

* Admit if the attack continues and there is no clear history of previous attacks which have terminated themselves. Even if there is such a history, keep the patient at the surgery until the attack does indeed terminate.

* If diagnosed from the patient's history or if the attack has terminated before admission was needed:

  (a) refer for specialist confirmation and initiation of treatment. Referral should be urgent if attacks are associated with chest pain, dizziness or breathlessness;

  (b) if the patient is distressed by frequent attacks, discuss with the cardiologist the possibility of starting an antiarrhythmic drug, e.g. sotalol 80–320 mg daily, while awaiting the cardiology appointment. Sotalol has an amiodarone-like action as well as being a beta-blocker. A baseline ECG, with a further ECG before each dose increase, is recommended to look for prolongation of the QT interval, an indicator that there is a risk of drug-induced *torsade de pointes*. A final decision on the most appropriate drug will depend on the electropathology in the individual patient;

  (c) if sotalol is contraindicated, use verapamil 40–80 mg t.d.s.;

  (d) instruct the patient in the use of the Valsalva manoeuvre, and check that he or she is not smoking or misusing alcohol or caffeine.

VENTRICULAR TACHYCARDIA

* Admit immediately for cardioversion. If the patient is conscious but *in extremis*, give i.v. lidocaine 100 mg while waiting for the ambulance. If the patient is unconscious from circulatory collapse, give a DC shock as for defibrillation. Accompany the patient to hospital. After discharge, prophylaxis will be needed. If amiodarone is chosen, 6-monthly TFTs and LFTs are necessary.

SICK SINUS SYNDROME

This requires pacing. Drugs are likely to make symptoms worse because of the variability of the rhythms.

BRADYCARDIA

* Refer all patients with a bradycardia, other than sinus bradycardia, even if asymptomatic. A pacemaker is likely to be needed and may be life-saving. Untreated second degree and complete atrio-ventricular (AV) block have a mortality of 25–50% in the first year after diagnosis. For this reason, even asymptomatic patients with a rate of 40 or below should be paced.

* Admit a patient in acute AV block with hypotension due to the bradycardia. Give i.v. atropine while waiting for the ambulance.

PROPHYLAXIS OF INFECTIVE ENDOCARDITIS

GUIDELINES

National Institute For Health And Clinical Excellence. *Prophylaxis Against Infective Endocarditis*. NICE Clinical Guideline 64, March 2008. Available: www.nice.org.uk

Gould F, Elliott T, Foweraker J, *et al.* 2006. Guidelines for the prevention of endocarditis: report of the Working Party of the British Society for Antimicrobial Chemotherapy. J Antimicrob Chemother 57

The two guidelines in the box above disagree about the need for any antibiotic prophylaxis in the prevention of bacterial endocarditis. NICE argues against *any* routine prophylactic antibiotics when patients with susceptible cardiac lesions undergo an invasive procedure. The British Society for Antimicrobial Chemotherapy argues for a more selective approach as outlined below. In the absence of evidence to support one or other view, the GP can explain the difficulty to the patient and together decide what action to take.

THE BRITISH SOCIETY FOR ANTIMICROBIAL CHEMOTHERAPY VIEW

DENTAL PROCEDURES

Antibiotic prophylaxis is no longer recommended for patients at lower risk of endocarditis. This change comes from two considerations:

1. the theoretical consideration that bacteraemia from daily activities such as eating and cleaning the teeth hugely exceeds that from a dental procedure; and
2. from a case control study which found that patients with endocarditis were no more likely to have had a dental procedure just prior to the illness than the general population (Strom, Abrutyn, Berlin, *et al.* 1998).

* Stress the importance of good oral hygiene and regular dental appointments for all those with cardiac lesions susceptible to endocarditis.
* Give antibiotic prophylaxis for dental procedures that cause bacteraemia, in patients with:
  - previous infective endocarditis;
  - cardiac valve replacement (mechanical or biological);
  - surgically constructed systemic or pulmonary shunt or conduit.

These procedures include extraction, scaling, gum surgery and any other dental treatment which causes bleeding.

PRACTICALITIES

* Give amoxicillin 3 g orally 1 hour before the procedure.
* If allergic to amoxicillin, use clindamycin 600 mg orally 1 hour before. Azithromycin

suspension 500 mg is an alternative for those who cannot take clindamycin capsules.
* Recommend a pre-operative mouthwash of chlorhexidine gluconate (0.2%) held in the mouth for 1 minute.
* If amoxicillin has already been given in the last 14 days, alternate clindamycin and amoxicillin.
* *General anaesthetic (GA):* If a general anaesthetic is used, give:
  - (a) amoxicillin 3 g orally 1 hour before; or
  - (b) amoxicillin 1 g i.v. immediately before (Littler, McGowan and Shanson 1997);
  - (c) in patients requiring a GA who are allergic to amoxicillin, or who have already received amoxicillin in the last 14 days, give clindamycin 300 mg i.v. over 10 minutes.

OTHER PROCEDURES IN VULNERABLE PATIENTS

In contrast to their stance on prophylaxis before dental procedures, the British Working Party recommends that non-dental procedures be considered to require antibiotic prophylaxis to a wider group of patients with cardiac lesions, namely:

- history of previous endocarditis;
- prosthetic heart valves;
- surgically constructed shunt or conduit;
- complex congenital heart disease (except secundum ASD);
- complex LV outflow abnormalities including aortic stenosis and bicuspid aortic valves;
- acquired valvulopathy and mitral valve prolapse, if there is echocardiographic evidence of substantial leaflet pathology and regurgitation.

The GP may need to remind the surgeon of the need for prophylaxis before various procedures, e.g. cystoscopy (but not catheterization), transrectal prostatic biopsy, Caesarean section (but not vaginal delivery), tonsillectomy and adenoidectomy, other procedures on the upper respiratory tract including nasal packing or nasal intubation, cosmetic piercing of the tongue or cheek, but not the ear or nipple.

* Give amoxicillin 1 g and gentamicin 1.5 mg/kg, both i.v., immediately before the procedure, except for nasal packing or intubation when give

flucloxacillin 1 g i.v. immediately before the procedure, and except for upper respiratory tract procedures when the same antibiotics as for dental procedures should be used.

THE PREVENTION OF CARDIOVASCULAR DISEASE (CVD)

GUIDELINES

British Cardiac Society, British Hypertension Society, Diabetes UK, *et al.* 2005. JBS2: Joint British Societies' guidelines on prevention of cardiovascular disease in clinical practice. Heart 91 (Suppl V), v1–v52

Scottish Intercollegiate Guidelines Network. *Risk Estimation and the Prevention of Cardiovascular Disease: a National Clinical Guideline.* February 2007. Available on www.sign.ac.uk

National Institute for Health and Clinical Excellence. *Lipid Modification: Cardiovascular Risk Assessment and the Modification of Blood Lipids for the Primary and Secondary Prevention of Cardiovascular Disease.* NICE CG 67, May 2008. Available: www.nice.org.uk

THE SCIENCE

- Risk factors for CVD do not just add to each other, they multiply.
- Risk factors tend to cluster. The presence of one or more of the following increases the chance that other risk factors will also be present: hypertension, raised cholesterol, inactivity, obesity, smoking and glucose intolerance (Perry, Wannamethee and Walker 1995).
- The most cost-effective intervention is in those who already have CVD. However, lifestyle changes across the whole population, plus lipid-lowering for those at high risk, would also achieve a major reduction in CVD because of the large numbers involved.
- Lifestyle changes are additive. A large study of Europeans aged 70–90 found the following hazard ratios: Mediterranean-style diet 0.77; any alcohol intake 0.78; moderate physical activity 0.63 and not smoking 0.65. The hazard ratio for someone with all four factors was 0.35 (Knoops, de Groot, Kromhout, *et al.* 2004). This means that following all four of these lifestyle changes would reduce the risk of CVD by 65%.
- According to the MRC/BHF Heart Protection Study (HPS) (Heart Protection Study Collaborative Group 2002), cholesterol lowering with simvastatin 40 mg daily in patients aged 40–80 at the start of the trial lowered the risk of a major cardiovascular event by at least one third, regardless of age, sex and initial cholesterol level. In a patient whose risk of CVD is high, reducing that risk by one third is worthwhile. In a patient at low risk of CVD, the same reduction would lead to a much smaller health gain.
- More aggressive lowering of the cholesterol, e.g. with atorvastatin 80 mg daily, will reduce cholesterol further but with more adverse effects and no demonstrated difference in primary endpoints (Pedersen, Faergeman, Kastelein, *et al.* 2005).
- A systematic approach has been shown to provide more effective care in the management of chronic conditions than an opportunistic approach in some studies but not in others. A nurse-run secondary prevention clinic can improve management in relation to aspirin use, blood pressure control, lipid management, exercise and diet compared to 'usual care' from a GP (Campbell, Ritchie and Thain 1998). Systematic care entails a register from which patients can be called and recalled, an agreed management protocol, a computer template or data entry form for the uniform recording of results and, usually, a dedicated clinic. Against this, a randomized controlled trial of systematic care in Warwickshire showed that, while it improved follow-up and assessment, it made little impact on clinical care (Moher, Yudkin, Wright, *et al.* 2001).

FAMILIAL HYPERCHOLESTEROLAEMIA (FH) (NATIONAL INSTITUTE FOR HEALTH AND CLINICAL EXCELLENCE 2008)

Familial hypercholesterolaemia is present in 1 in 500 of the population in the UK and for men carries a 50% risk of a major coronary event by the age of 50. In women the risk is 30% by the age of 60. This risk is far higher than would be predicted from the cholesterol level alone and requires intensive therapy (high-dose statins and ezetimibe).

The possibility of FH is raised in two situations Opportunistic case-finding:

∗ Ask about family history in every patient with a raised cholesterol, especially if the total cholesterol is > 7.5 mmol/l or the LDL-cholesterol is ≥ 5 mmol/l. These cut-offs should be lowered in younger patients and in females. For instance, for a woman aged up to 24 an LDL-cholesterol ≥ 3.9 mmol/l suggests FH. See the charts in the NICE guideline (National Institute for Health and Clinical Excellence 2008).

Screening because of an affected relative:

∗ Screen children with an affected parent by the age of 10, or by the age of 5 if both parents are affected or if the child has clinical signs, e.g. skin lipid deposits.
∗ Screen adults with a diagnosis of FH in a relative as remote as third degree or with a family history of premature coronary heart disease.

If suspicion of FH is raised:

∗ Recheck the serum lipids with a fasting specimen.
∗ Check for other causes of raised cholesterol (see page 168).
∗ Ask about the family history across three generations. Accept that the patient may need to return with these details after consultation with the family.
∗ Ask about symptoms of CVD.
∗ Examine for evidence of CVD or skin or tendon manifestations of hyperlipidaemia.

Make a clinical diagnosis of FH according to the Simon Broome criteria.

● *FH exists* if the total cholesterol is > 7.5 mmol/l or the LDL-cholesterol is > 4.9 mmol/l AND tendon xanthoma are present (in the patient or a first or second degree relative).

● *FH is possible* if:

(a) the total cholesterol is > 7.5 mmol/l or the LDL-cholesterol is > 4.9 mmol/l AND there is a first degree relative with a myocardial infarction before the age of 60 or a second degree relative with a myocardial infarction before the age of 50; or

(b) the total cholesterol is > 7.5 mmol/l or the LDL-cholesterol is > 4.9 mmol/l in the patient AND also in a first or second degree relative (or > 6.7 or > 4.0, respectively, in a brother or sister under 16 years old).

Referral is needed:

■ *to a specialist with expertise in familial hypercholesterolaemia* for all with a definite or possible clinical diagnosis. Further investigation will include DNA testing for relevant mutations and family screening;
■ *to a cardiologist* if there are symptoms of CHD. Consider referral if the patient has no symptoms but there is a family history of CHD in early adult life or the patient has two or more other risk factors for CHD.

Cholesterol lowering in a patient with a confirmed diagnosis of FH:

∗ give a high-intensity statin (e.g. simvastatin 80 mg daily);
∗ aim for a LDL-cholesterol > 50% below the pretreated level;
∗ if the target is not met, increase the statin to the maximum licensed dose, provided it is tolerated, and/or add ezetimibe;
∗ re-refer if the target is not met;
∗ review annually once stable. Stress that lifestyle changes (see below) are even more important in someone with FH than in the general population.

PRIMARY PREVENTION

1. *Identify those who need intensive management without recourse to a risk score;* that is those with:
   ■ cardiovascular disease (angina, myocardial infarction, stroke, TIA, or peripheral vascular disease);
   ■ familial hyperlipidaemia or another lipid disorder;
   ■ diabetes and aged at least 40;

- chronic kidney disease (CKD) with a glomerular filtration rate (GFR) < 60 ml/min/1.73m^2, indicating stage 3 CKD;
- aged 75 and over, especially smokers and hypertensives.

2. *Assess other patients, aged 40–74, 5 yearly*, using information already contained in the patient's records, and using a chart or computer programme based on the Framingham data, according to:
   - age;
   - sex;
   - lifetime smoking habit;
   - blood pressure. If treated use pre-treatment level;
   - serum lipids if known. If treated use pre-treatment level.

Calculate the 10-year risk of cardiovascular disease using the new Joint British Societies Cardiovascular Risk Assessor computer programme (available on www.bhsoc.org and choose 'Guidelines') or use the charts published in the back pages of the British National Formulary or on www.bhsoc.org.

3. *Arrange a formal assessment* for those with a 10-year CVD risk of at least 20%.

4. *Modify that score following the more detailed assessment and according to other factors* which are not included in such charts:
   - *family history* of CVD in the absence of familial hyperlipidaemia. If there is a first degree relative with a history of premature CVD multiply the risk by 1.5. If there are two such relatives multiply the risk by 2. Premature CVD is when the first occurrence is < 55 years old in a man, or < 65 in a woman;
   - *ethnic origin:* people of South Asian origin (Pakistani, Bangladeshi and Indian) multiply by 1.4; people of Chinese origin multiply by 0.6. Black Caribbeans and Black Africans have a risk close to the British average (Brindle, May, Gill, *et al.* 2006);
   - *obesity*, or waist circumference > 94 cm in men, > 80 cm in women;
   - *socioeconomic status*. The lowest socioeconomic groups are at greater risk, independent of other measurable risk factors (Brindle, McConnachie, Upton, *et al.* 2005);
   - *triglycerides* > 1.7 mmol/l;
   - *age* 75 or over;
   - *premature menopause;*
   - *impaired fasting glycaemia* or impaired glucose tolerance.

5. *Offer intensive management* (see below) to those whose final assessment of 10-year CVD risk is at least 20%, taking into account the modifying factors above. When making this offer, discuss benefits and harms in terms of absolute risk, not relative risk. Patients may understand this better as number needed to treat (or harm), see box on page 168.

6. *Also offer intensive management* to those with a 'lighthouse risk' i.e. a risk factor where the level is so high that it overrules the composite CVD risk score, e.g. total cholesterol/HDL cholesterol > 6, or BP > 160/100, or any raised blood pressure with target organ damage.

7. *Offer lifestyle advice* to those whose 10-year CVD risk is below 20% with an invitation to return for reassessment in 5 years.

LIFESTYLE CHANGES

* *Stop smoking.* Someone who smokes 20 cigarettes a day or less and stops has a risk of CHD 10 years later almost the same as in one who has never smoked. Recovery is, however, less the longer the person has smoked (Doll, Peto, Boreham and Sutherland 2004). Nicotine replacement therapy increases by 1.6 the chance that the patient is not smoking at least 6 months later. This is true for all forms of nicotine replacement and seems to be independent of whether support, other than brief advice, is offered (Silagy, Lancaster, Stead, *et al.* 2004).

* *Alcohol.* Keep alcohol intake within safe limits. A higher intake raises low-density lipoprotein (LDL) cholesterol, triglyceride, blood pressure and calorie intake. Modest alcohol intake (one to three units a day) appears to protect against CHD (relative risk (RR) 0.76, 95%CI 0.64 to 0.91) (Wannamethee and Shaper 1999), but all-cause mortality in this study was unchanged and promoting alcohol for this purpose could be hazardous.

* *Take exercise.* This must be vigorous (for 20 minutes, three times a week) or moderate, e.g. brisk walking (for 30 minutes every day) (Powell and Pratt 1996). The exercise may be broken into separate bouts as long as they are for at least 10 minutes each. In the short term,

the risk of MI is halved (Wannamethee, Shaper and Walker 1998) with less risk of death if it does occur, but this benefit is lost if exercise is stopped. Exercise continued for over 1 year improves the coronary collateral circulation enough to be demonstrable on a thallium scan. Encourage the patient to incorporate the exercise into his or her daily life, rather than rely on visiting a gym or playing football at the weekend. Simple advice from the GP is unlikely to change behaviour. A more supportive programme is needed. One study, using four visits to the physiotherapist, significantly increased activity even though the patients were women over 80 years old (Campbell, Robertson, Gardner, *et al.* 1997).

* *Manage social isolation.* Depression and lack of social support are associated with an increased risk of cardiovascular disease (Bunker, Colquhoun, Esler, *et al.* 2003), as is the combination of high workload and low autonomy at work (Aboa-Eboule, Brisson, Maunsell, *et al.* 2007).

* *Control weight.* Central obesity, rather than a raised body mass index (BMI), carries the greater cardiovascular risk and can be assessed by measuring the waist circumference, with a single cut-off point for each sex. Men with a waist circumference over 94 cm and women over 80 cm are likely to have other risk factors for cardiovascular disease, and men with a waist circumference over 102 cm (women over 88 cm) are two-and-a-half to four-and-a-half times as likely to have other major cardiovascular risk factors (Han, van Leer, Seidell, *et al.* 1995). Small losses of weight are possible in primary care if advice on diet and exercise is accompanied by a behavioural programme.

* *Diet.* Encourage patients to:
  - reduce their meat and fat intake;
  - eat oily fish at least twice a week;
  - eat bread, pasta and potatoes as sources of carbohydrate;
  - eat at least five portions a day of fruit or vegetables;
  - use olive oil and rape seed margarine instead of butter.

For more detailed advice, see page 690. The benefit for an individual of a low fat diet is small, at best, but the potential benefit to a population is large (Hooper, Summerbell, Higgins, *et al.* 2001). Even in a dietician-run programme, the fall in serum cholesterol is unlikely to be more than 3% (Imperial Cancer Research Fund OXCHECK Study Group 1995) or 0.3 mmol/l. Some studies show that a dietician is more effective than a doctor but not more effective than a nurse (Thompson, Summerbell, Hooper, *et al.* 2004). Simple advice in primary care is unlikely to achieve even a 3% reduction. However, the effect of eating fruit and vegetables may be greater than the benefit from the low fat diet. One cohort study found that each extra serving of fruit or vegetable a day was associated with a 4% reduction in the risk of coronary heart disease with no apparent upper limit (Joshipura, Hu, Manson, *et al.* 2001). Advise the patient to avoid adding salt to the food. The (small) reduction in blood pressure is of benefit to all, whether hypertensive or not.

INTENSIVE MANAGEMENT WHEN A 10 YEAR CVD RISK OF AT LEAST 20% IS DETECTED

Lipid–lowering

* Perform the work-up proposed in the box below.

* Start simvastatin 40 mg daily (advised in May 2008). The reduction in major coronary events is likely to be 30%. How useful this is depends on the patient's baseline risk (see box below).

* NICE recommends the 'fire and forget approach': do not subsequently check lipids nor alter the dose. The achievement of cholesterol targets is only recommended in secondary prevention. In contrast, the JBS2 guidelines recommend that serum cholesterol be driven down to the same targets as in secondary prevention: total cholesterol < 4 mmol/l (or a 25% reduction if greater); LDL cholesterol < 2 mmol/l (or a 30% reduction if greater) (Wood, Wray, Poulter, *et al.* 2005).

* Warn the patient to report muscle pain or weakness; in which case check the creatine kinase.

* Continue indefinitely unless adverse effects occur, in which case consider reducing to simvastatin 20 mg daily, or changing to another statin, or using a fibrate or an anion-exchange resin.

✳ On subsequent visits check that the patient is taking the statin. A study from Liverpool found that a quarter of patients took their statin less than 80% of the time and had a higher mortality (Howell, Trotter, Mottram and Rowe 2004).

Blood pressure control

✳ Check blood pressure annually.
✳ Treat if levels are sustained at 140/90 or above.
✳ Aim for a level of < 140/85 or, in those with diabetes < 130/85.

WORK-UP OF A PATIENT WITH A RAISED CHOLESTEROL

■ Check fasting total cholesterol, LDL-cholesterol, HDL-cholesterol and triglycerides at least once after the initial random test.

■ If blood is taken within 3 months of a major illness, re-check outside the 3-month period. Illness can depress the cholesterol.

■ Refer patients with a very high triglyceride (e.g. > 5.0 mmol/l) to a lipid clinic. They may benefit from a fibrate rather than, or in addition to, a statin (BIP Study Group 2000; Haffner 2000).

■ If the cholesterol is still raised, exclude a primary cause:
  (a) check the history for alcohol excess and drugs, e.g. high-dose thiazides, beta-blockers without ISA, oral contraceptives containing levonorgestrel, retinoids and corticosteroids;
  (b) test the urine for protein;
  (c) take blood for TFTs, creatinine, LFTs and fasting sugar. Note that elevated liver enzymes are not a contraindication to the use of a statin. They are not associated with subsequent statin-induced toxicity (Chalasani, Aljadhey, Kesterson, et al. 2004).
  Doubt has, however, been cast on the cost-effectiveness of biochemical screening for underlying causes, which in British general practice yielded 1.8% of positives only in patients with a cholesterol over 6.5 mmol/l. A compromise would be to check the fasting blood sugar in all patients and TFTs in patients with very high cholesterol levels, e.g. over 8 mmol/l.

TALKING TO THE PATIENT ABOUT ABSOLUTE RISKS WHEN TAKING A STATIN
(Tables 5.8 and 5.9)

Table 5.8	Benefits (based on simvastatin 40 mg daily)
PATIENT CHARACTERISTICS	NNT OVER 5 YEARS (HEART PROTECTION STUDY COLLABORATIVE GROUP 2002; CHOLESTEROL TREATMENT TRIALISTS' (CTT) COLLABORATORS 2005)
MI	10
Angina	13
Stroke or PVD or diabetes	15
No CVD but a 30% 10-year CVD risk	32
No CVD but a 20% 10-year CVD risk	48

Table 5.9	Harms
HARM	NUMBER NEEDED TO HARM OVER 5 YEARS (NNH) (LAW AND RUDNICKA 2006)
Rhabdomyolysis	0.00017 or 1 per 30,000 patient-years
Statin-related myopathy	0.0005 or 1 per 10,000 patient-years
Statin-related peripheral myopathy	0.0006 or 1 per 8000 patient-years

Of these only rhabdomyolysis may be irreversible, with a mortality rate of 10%. The chance of dying of rhabdomyolysis may be expressed as being 15 times less likely than being killed in a car accident. Other adverse effects are documented (depression, sleep disturbance, memory loss, sexual dysfunction, diarrhoea) but their frequency is less clear.

SECONDARY PREVENTION

Consider the following measures in those with cardiovascular disease, diabetes, chronic kidney disease, or primary hyperlipidaemia.

✳ Recommend *lifestyle changes* as for primary prevention.
✳ *Lipid-lowering*
  ■ Order the tests recommended under primary prevention and give the same warnings.

- Offer a statin regardless of baseline cholesterol level.
- Start with simvastatin 40 mg daily, or 80 mg daily in those with acute coronary syndrome.
- Recheck the serum lipids after 3 months. If TC ≥ 4 mmol/l or LDL ≥ 2 mmol/l consider offering to increase simvastatin to 80 mg daily. If targets are still not reached, add ezetimibe. Other options are a fibrate, but with a warning about the increased risk of rhabdomyolysis, nicotinic acid or an omega-3 fatty acid.
- If adverse effects occur consider reducing the simvastatin dose, or changing to another statin, or using ezetimibe, or a fibrate or an anion-exchange resin or nicotinic acid.

∗ *Blood pressure.* Treat if levels are sustained at 140/90 or above. Aim for a level of < 140/85 or, in those with diabetes < 130/85.

∗ Give aspirin 75 mg daily for life; if contraindicated use clopidogrel 75 mg daily. If both have been started in hospital, revert to aspirin alone after 4 weeks if the patient had an ST-segment-elevated MI, or after 12 months following a non-ST-segment-elevated acute coronary syndrome. *Aspirin* reduces cardiovascular events by 15% but at a cost of increasing episodes of bleeding by 69% (Sanmuganathan, Ghahramani, Jackson, *et al.* 2001). Benefit outweighs risk when the patient's risk of a major coronary event is at least 15% over 10 years.

∗ *ACE inhibition.* Prescribe an ACE inhibitor to all patients with coronary heart disease. In the HOPE study ramipril 10 mg daily gave a RRR of 22% for a major cardiovascular event, NNT 27 over 5 years (Yusuf, Sleight, Pogue, *et al.* 2000). EUROPA gave similar results with perindopril 8 mg daily regardless of age, blood pressure or any other variables (EURopean trial On reduction of cardiac events with Perindopril in stable coronary Artery disease investigators 2003). However, the PEACE trial was unable to show any benefit from trandolapril (PEACE Trial Investigators 2004).

∗ Prescribe a beta-blocker to all those who have had an MI (see page 148). Start them in patients whose MI was in the last 5 years and who therefore missed the opportunity to have them started in the acute stage. Patients at the highest risk benefit most from beta-blockade, e.g. those aged > 50 with angina, hypertension or heart failure. The reduction in mortality risk (RRR 20%, NNT 48) appears to be long term.

ANNUAL WORK-UP AT A CHD PREVENTION CLINIC

Check: fasting sugar, total cholesterol, urine protein, BP, weight, height and BMI.

Action to be taken when a new abnormal result is found:

A. Fasting sugar

1. If fasting sugar ≥ 7 mmol/l and the patient has symptoms (thirst, polyuria, lethargy) this is diabetes.
2. If fasting sugar ≥ 7 mmol/l and the patient has no symptoms, repeat after 1 week. If still ≥ 7 mmol/l, diabetes is confirmed.
3. If fasting sugar between 6.1 and 6.9 mmol/l inclusive, check blood sugar 2 hours after a 75 g glucose drink (=394 ml of the new Lucozade formulation which contains 73 kcal/100 ml).
   (a) If > 11 mmol/l, diabetes is confirmed.
   (b) If < 7.8 this is impaired fasting glycaemia (IFG). Warn as for IGT below.
   (c) If between 7.8 and 11 inclusive, this is impaired glucose tolerance (IGT). Warn that it carries an increased risk of diabetes, which can be reduced by exercise and diet. Recheck fasting sugar annually.

B. Proteinuria

If + or more, repeat after 1 week on the first morning specimen. If still + or more, check MSU, serum creatinine and electrolytes, and organise a 24-hour urine, or a protein:creatinine ratio on a single urine sample. If the 24-hour urine is > 300 mg/24 hours or the P:C ratio is > 20 or there is haematuria, or the creatinine is raised, this is significant proteinuria.

References

Aboa-Eboule, C., Brisson, C., Maunsell, E., et al., 2007. Job strain and risk of acute recurrent coronary heart disease events. JAMA 298, 1652–1660.

ACC/AHA/ESC, 2001. ACC/AHA/ESC guidelines for the management of patients with atrial fibrillation. Eur. Heart. J. 22, 1852–1923.

ALLHAT officers and coordinators for the ALLHAT Collaborative Research Group, 2003. Diuretic versus alpha-blocker as first step antihypertensive therapy: final results from the Antihypertensive and Lipid-Lowering Treatment to Prevent Heart Attack (ALLHAT). Hypertension 42, 239–246.

Andersen, H., Nielsen, T., Rasmussen, K., et al., 2003. A comparison of coronary angioplasty with fibrinolytic therapy in acute myocardial infarction. N. Engl. J. Med. 349, 733–742.

Anon., 2004. Seventh report of the Joint National Committee on Prevention, Detection, Evaluation, and Treatment of High Blood Pressure and evidence from new hypertension trials. Hypertension 43, 1–7.

Antiplatelet Trialists' Collaboration, 1994. Collaborative overview of randomised trials of antiplatelet therapy I: prevention of death, myocardial infarction, and stroke by prolonged antiplatelet therapy in various categories of people. BMJ 308, 81–106.

Antithrombotic Trialists' Collaboration, 2002. Collaborative meta-analysis of randomised trials of antiplatelet therapy for prevention of death, myocardial infarction, and stroke in high risk patients. BMJ 324, 71–86.

Atrial Fibrillation Follow-up Investigation of Rhythm Management (AFFIRM) Investigators, 2002. A comparison of rate control and rhythm control in patients with atrial fibrillation. N. Engl. J. Med. 347, 1825–1833.

Auer, J., Scheibner, P., Mische, T., et al., 2001. Subclinical hyperthyroidism as a risk factor for atrial fibrillation. Am. Heart J. 142, 838–842.

Bach, R., Cannon, C., Weintraub, W., et al., 2004. The effect of routine, early invasive management on outcome for elderly patients with non-ST-segment elevation acute coronary syndromes. Ann. Intern. Med. 141, 186–195.

Bandolier, 2002. Stress management interventions and blood pressure. Bandolier, October, 104–107.

Bass, C., Mayou, R., 2002. Chest pain. BMJ 325, 588–591.

Beckett, N.S., OPeters, R., Fletcher, A.E., et al., 2008. Treatment of hypertension in patients 80 years of age and older. N. Engl. J. Med. 358.

Beevers, D., Sleight, P., 1996. Short-acting dihydropyridine (vasodilating) calcium channel blockers for hypertension: is there a risk? BMJ 312, 1143–1145.

Benson, J., Britten, N., 2002. Patients' decisions about whether or not to take antihypertensive drugs: qualitative study. BMJ 325, 873–876.

BIP Study Group, 2000. Secondary prevention by raising HDL cholesterol and reducing triglycerides in patients with coronary artery disease: the bezafibrate infarction prevention (BIP) study. Circulation 102, 21–27.

Birtwhistle, R., Marshall, S., Godwin, M., et al., 2004. Randomised equivalence trial comparing three month and six month follow up of patients with hypertension by family practitioners. BMJ 328, 204–206.

Bobrie, G., Chatellier, G., Genes, N., et al., 2003. Cardiovascular prognosis of 'masked hypertension' detected by blood pressure self-measurement in elderly treated hypertensive patients. JAMA 291, 1342–1349.

Bogers, R., Bemelmans, W., Hoogenveen, R., et al., 2007. Association of overweight with increased risk of coronary heart disease partly independent of blood pressure and cholesterol levels: a meta-analysis of 21 cohort studies including more than 300 000 persons. Arch. Intern. Med. 167, 1720–1728.

Boucher, M., Armstrong, P., Pharand, C., Skidmore, B., 2002. The role of clopidogrel in the secondary prevention of recurrent ischaemic vascular events after acute myocardial ischaemia: a critical appraisal of the CURE trial: Canadian Coordinating Office for Health Technology Assessment. Available: www. ccohta.ca.

Brindle, P., May, M., Gill, P., et al., 2006. Primary prevention of cardiovascular disease: a web-based risk score for seven British black and minority ethnic groups. Heart 92, 1595–1602.

Brindle, P., McConnachie, A., Upton, M., et al., 2005. The accuracy of the Framingham risk-score in different socioeconomic groups. Br. J. Gen. Pract. 55, 838–845.

British Heart Foundation, 1995. Ventricular extrasystoles. British Heart Foundation Factfile, London.

British Heart Foundation, 2000. Management of atrial fibrillation - part 1. Factfile 2000;11, available: www.bhf.org.uk.

British Heart Foundation Factfile, 1986. When to refer patients with angina. British Heart Foundation, London.

Brown, M., Cruickshank, J., Dominiczak, A., et al., 2003. Better blood pressure control: how to combine drugs. J. Hum. Hypertens. 17, 81–86.

Brown, R., Kendall, M., Halpern, M., 1997. Cost analysis of once-daily ISMN versus twice-daily ISMN or transdermal patch for nitrate prophylaxis. J. Clin. Pharm. Ther. 22, 67–76.

Brueren, M., Schouten, H., De Leeuw, P., et al., 1998. A series of self-measurements by the patient is a reliable alternative to ambulatory blood pressure measurement. Br. J. Gen. Pract. 48, 1585–1589.

Bunker, S., Colquhoun, D., Esler, M., et al., 2003. Stress' and coronary heart disease: psychosocial risk factors. MJA 178, 272–276.

Camm, J., 2001. Atrial fibrillation: antiarrythmic drugs. Geriatric Medicine June, 61–64.

Camm, A., Savelieva, I., 2007. Some patients with paroxysmal atrial fibrillation should carry flecainide or propafenone to self treat. BMJ 334, 637.

Campbell, N., Ritchie, L., Thain, J., 1998. Secondary prevention in coronary heart disease: a randomised trial of nurse-led clinics in primary care. Heart 80, 447–452.

Campbell, A., Robertson, M., Gardner, M., et al., 1997. Randomised controlled trial of a general practice programme of home based exercise to prevent falls in elderly women. BMJ 315, 1065–1069.

Carlberg, B., Samuelsson, O., Lindholm, L., 2004. Atenolol in hypertension: is it a wise choice? Lancet 364, 1684–1689.

Chalasani, N., Aljadhey, H., Kesterson, J., et al., 2004. Patients with elevated liver enzymes are not at higher risk for statin hepatotoxicity. Gastroenterology 126, 1287–1292.

Channer, K., McLean, K., Lawson-Matthew, P., Richardson, M., 1994. Combination diuretic treatment in severe heart failure: a randomised controlled trial. Br. Heart J. 71, 146–150.

Cholesterol Treatment Trialists' (CTT) Collaborators, 2005. Efficacy and safety of cholesterol-lowering treatment: prospective meta-analysis of data from 90, 056 participants in 14 randomised trials of statins. Lancet 366, 1267–1278.

Choudhri, A., Cleland, J., Rowlands, P., et al., 1990. Unsuspected renal artery stenosis in peripheral vascular disease. BMJ 301, 1197–1198.

Chua, T., Lipkin, D., 1993. Cardiac rehabilitation. BMJ 306, 731–732.

Cleroux, J., Feldman, R., Petrella, R., 1999. Recommendations on physical exercise training. Can. Med. Assoc. J. 160 (Suppl. 9), S21–S28.

Collins, R., Peto, R., MacMahon, S., et al., 1990. Blood pressure, stroke and coronary artery disease. Part 2: Short-term reductions in blood pressure: overview of randomized drug trials in their epidemiological context. Lancet 335, 827–838.

Conaway, D., O'Keefe, J., Reid, K., et al., 2005. Frequency of undiagnosed diabetes mellitus in patients with acute coronary syndrome. Am. J. Cardiol. 96, 363–365.

Connell, P., McKevitt, C., Wolfe, C., 2005. Strategies to manage hypertension: a qualitative study with black Caribbean patients. Br. J. Gen. Pract. 55, 357–361.

Curb, J., Pressel, S., Cutler, J., et al., 1996. Effect of diuretic-based antihypertensive treatment on cardiovascular disease risk in older diabetic patients with isolated systolic hypertension. JAMA 276, 1886–1892.

Dahlof, B., Sever, P.S., Poulter, N.R., et al., 2005. Prevention of cardiovascular events with an antihypertensive regimen of amlodipine adding perindopril as required versus atenolol adding bendrofluazide as required, in the Anglo-Scandinavian Cardiac Outcomes Trial-Blood Pressure Lowering Arm (ASCOT-BPLA): a multicentre randomised controlled trial. Lancet 366, 895–906.

Dalal, H., Evans, P., Campbell, J., 2004. Recent developments in secondary prevention and cardiac rehabilitation after acute myocardial infarction. BMJ 328, 693–697.

Dargie, H., McMurray, J., 1994. Diagnosis and management of heart failure. BMJ 308, 321–328.

Davies, M., Hobbs, F., Davis, R., et al., 2001. Prevalence of left-ventricular systolic dysfunction and heart failure in the Echocardiographic Heart of England Screening study: a population based study. Lancet 358, 439–444.

de Winter, R., Windhausen, F., Cornel, J., et al., 2005. Early invasive versus selectively invasive management of acute coronary syndromes. N. Engl. J. Med. 353, 1095–1104.

DoH, 2000. The National Service Framework for Coronary Heart Disease. Department of Health, London.

Doll, R., Peto, R., Boreham, J., Sutherland, I., 2004. Mortality in relation to smoking: 50 years' observations on male British doctors. BMJ 328, 1519–1528.

Domanski, M., Exner, D., Borkowf, C., et al., 1999. Effect of angiotensin converting enzyme inhibition on sudden cardiac death in patients following acute myocardial infarction: a meta-analysis of randomized clinical trials. J. Am. Coll. Cardiol. 33, 598–604.

Douma, S., Petidis, K., Doumas, M., et al., 2008. Prevalence of primary hyperaldosteronism in resistant hypertension: a retrospective observational study. Lancet 371, 1921–1926.

DTB, 1990. What to do about pulmonary heart disease. Drug Ther. Bull. 29, 90–92.

DTB, 1994a. Should general practitioners give thrombolytic therapy? Drug Ther. Bull. 32, 65–66.

DTB, 1994b. Drugs for heart failure. Drug Ther. Bull. 32, 83–85.

DTB, 1995. Losartan - a new antihypertensive. Drug Ther. Bull. 33, 73–74.

DTB, 2000. Tackling myocardial infarction. Drug Ther. Bull. 38, 17–22.

Dulin, B., Haas, S., Abraham, W., et al., 2005. Do elderly systolic heart failure patients benefit from beta blockers to the same extent as the non-elderly: meta-analysis of > 12, 000 patients in large-scale clinical trials. Am. J. Cardiol. 95, 896–898.

Elder, A., Shaw, T., Turnbull, C., et al., 1991. Elderly and younger patients selected to undergo coronary angiography. BMJ 303, 950–953.

EURopean trial On reduction of cardiac events with Perindopril in stable coronary Artery disease investigators, 2003. Efficacy of perindopril in reduction of cardiovascular events among patients with stable coronary artery disease: randomised, double-blind, placebo-controlled, multicentre trial (the EUROPA study). Lancet 362, 782–788.

ExTraMATCH Collaborative, 2004. Exercise training meta-analysis of trials in patients with chronic heart failure (ExTraMATCH). BMJ 328, 189–192.

Ezekowitz, J., McAlister, F., Armstrong, P., 2003. Anemia is common in heart failure and is associated with poor outcomes. Circulation 107, 223–225.

Fang, M., Chang, Y., Hylek, E., 2004. Advanced age, anticoagulant intensity, and risk for intracranial hemorrhage among patients taking warfarin for atrial fibrillation. Ann. Intern. Med. 141, 745–752.

Fibrinolytic Therapy Trialists' (FTT) Collaborative Group, 1994. Indications for fibrinolytic therapy in suspected acute myocardial infarction: collaborative overview of early mortality and major morbidity results of all randomized trials of more than 1000 patients. Lancet 343, 311–322.

Flather, M., Yusuf, S., Kober, L., et al., 2000. L. Long-term ACE-inhibitor therapy in patients with heart failure or left-ventricular dysfunction: a systematic overview of data from individual patients. Lancet 355, 1575–1581.

Fox, K., Poole-Wilson, P., Henderson, R., et al., 2002. Interventional versus conservative treatment for patients with unstable angina or non-ST-elevation myocardial infarction: the British Heart Foundation RITA 3 randomised trial. Lancet 360, 743–751.

Freemantle, N., Cleland, J., Young, P., et al., 1999. Beta blockade after myocardial infarction: systematic review and meta regression analysis. BMJ 318, 1730–1737.

French, J., Hyde, T., Patel, H., et al., 1999. Survival 12 years after randomization to streptokinase: the influence of thrombolysis in myocardial infarction flow at three to four weeks. J. Am. Coll. Cardiol. 34, 62–69.

Gage, B., Waterman, A., Shannon, W., et al., 2001. Validation of clinical classification schemes for predicting stroke. JAMA 285, 2864–2870.

Gibbs, J., McCoy, A., Gibbs, L., et al., 2002. Living with and dying from heart failure: the role of palliative care. Heart 88 (Suppl. II), II36–II39.

Grimm, R.J., Grandits, G., Prineas, R., et al., 1997. Long-term effects on sexual function of five antihypertensive drugs and nutritional hygienic treatment in hypertensive men and women. Hypertension 29, 8–14.

Guidelines Committee, 2003. European Society of Hypertension - European Society of Cardiology guidelines for the management of arterial hypertension. J. Hypertens. 21, 1011–1053.

Gurfinkel, E., de la Fuente, R., Mendiz, O., et al., 2002. Influenza vaccine pilot study in acute coronary syndromes and planned percutaneous coronary interventions. Circulation 105, 2143–2147.

Haffner, S., 2000. Secondary prevention of coronary heart disease: the role of fibric acids. Circulation 102, 2–4.

Hagens, V., Vermeulen, K., TenVergert, E., 2004. Rate control is more cost-effective than rhythm control for patients with persistent atrial fibrillation - results from the RAte Control versus Electrical cardioversion (RACE) study. Eur. Heart J. 25, 1542–1549.

Hammer, F., Stewart, P., 2009. Rational testing: investigating hypertension in a young person. BMJ 338, 885–886.

Han, T., van Leer, E., Seidell, J., et al., 1995. Waist circumference action levels in the identification of cardiovascular risk factors: prevalence study in a random sample. BMJ 311, 1401–1405.

Hansson, l., Zanchetti, A., Carruthers, S., et al., 1998. Effects of intensive blood pressure lowering and low-dose aspirin in patients with hypertension: principal results of the Hypertension Optimal Treatment (HOT) randomised trial. Lancet 351, 1755–1762.

Heart Protection Study Collaborative Group, 2002. MRC/BHF Heart Protection Study of cholesterol lowering with simvastatin in 20536 high-risk individuals:

a randomised placebo-controlled trial. Lancet 360, 7–22.

Henderson, R., Pocock, S., Clayton, T., et al., 2003. Seven-year outcome in the RITA-2 trial: coronary angioplasty versus medical therapy. J. Am. Coll. Cardiol. 42, 1161–1170.

Hobbs, F., Davis, R., Lip, G., 2000. ABC of heart failure: heart failure in general practice. BMJ 320, 626–629.

Hobbs, F., Davis, R., Roalfe, A., et al., 2002. Reliability of N-terminal pro-brain natriuretic peptide assay in diagnosis of heart failure: cohort study in representative and high risk community populations. BMJ 324, 1498–1500.

Hobbs, R., 1999. Identification and treatment of patients with atrial fibrillation in primary care. Heart 81, 333–334.

Hood, W.J., Dans, A., Guyatt, G., et al., 2004. Digitalis for treatment of congestive heart failure in patients in sinus rhythm. Cochrane Database Syst. Rev. Issue 2.

Hooper, L., Bartlett, C., Davey Smith, G., Ebrahim, S., 2003. Reduced dietary salt for prevention of cardiovascular disease (Cochrane Review). In: The Cochrane Library, Issue 1. Update Software, Oxford.

Hooper, L., Summerbell, C., Higgins, J., et al., 2001. Reduced or modified dietary fat for preventing cardiovascular disease (Cochrane Review). Cochrane Database Syst. Rev. Issue 3.

Howell, N., Trotter, R., Mottram, D., Rowe, P., 2004. Compliance with statins in primary care. Pharm. J. 272, 23–26.

Imperial Cancer Research Fund OXCHECK Study Group, 1995. Effectiveness of health checks conducted by nurses in primary care: final results of the OXCHECK study. BMJ 310, 1099–1104.

IONA, 2002. Effect of nicorandil on coronary events in patients with stable angina. Lancet 359, 1269–1275.

Jee, S.H., He, J., Whelton, P.K., et al., 1999. The effect of chronic coffee drinking on blood pressure. Hypertension 33, 647–652.

Jolliffe, J., Rees, K., Taylor, R., et al., 2004. Exercise-based rehabilitation for coronary heart disease (Cochrane Review). In: The Cochrane Library, Issue 3. John Wiley & Sons, Ltd, Chichester, UK.

Joshipura, K., Hu, F., Manson, J.E., et al., 2001. The effect of fruit and vegetable intake on risk for coronary heart disease. Ann. Intern. Med. 134, 1106–1114.

Juurlink, D., Mamdani, M., Lee, D., et al., 2004. Rates of hyperkalemia after publication of the Randomized Aldactone Evaluation Study. N. Engl. J. Med. 351, 543–551.

Keeley, E., Boura, J., Grines, C., 2003. Primary angioplasty versus intravenous thrombolytic therapy for acute myocardial infarction: a quantitative review of 23 randomised trials. Lancet 361, 13–20.

Knoops, K., de Groot, L.C., Kromhout, D., et al., 2004. Mediterranean diet, lifestyle factors, and 10 year mortality in elderly European men and women: the HALE project. JAMA 292, 1433–1439.

Ko, D., Hebert, P., Coffey, C., et al., 2004. Adverse effects of beta-blocker therapy for patients with heart failure. Arch. Intern. Med. 164, 1389–1394.

Kostis, J., Wilson, A., Freudenberger, R., et al., 2005. Long-term effect of diuretic-based therapy on fatal outcomes in subjects with isolated systolic hypertension with and without diabetes. Am. J. Cardiol. 95, 29–35.

Krum, H., 2009. Consider beta blockers for patients with heart failure. BMJ 338, 1384–1385.

Krum, H., Roecker, E., Mohacsi, P., et al., 2003. Effects of initiating carvedilol in patients with severe chronic heart failure: results from the COPERNICUS Study. JAMA 289, 712–718.

Lakshman, M., Reda, D., Materson, B., et al., 1999. Diuretics and beta-blockers do not have adverse effects at 1 year on plasma lipid and lipoprotein profiles in men with hypertension. Arch. Intern. Med. 159, 551–558.

Law, M., Rudnicka, A., 2006. Statin safety: a systematic review. Am. J. Cardiol. 97 (Suppl. 8A), 52C–60C.

Law, M., Wald, N., Morris, J., Jordan, R., 2003. Value of low dose combination treatment with blood pressure lowering drugs: analysis of 354 randomised trials. BMJ 326, 1427–1434.

Lechat, P., Packer, M., Chalon, S., 1998. Clinical effects of beta-adrenergic blockade in chronic heart failure: a meta-analysis of double-blind, placebo-controlled, randomized trials. Circulation 98, 1184–1191.

Linden, W., Stossel, C., Maurice, J., 1996. Psychosocial interventions for patients with coronary artery disease: a meta-analysis. Arch. Intern. Med. 156, 745–752.

Lip, G., Chin, B., Prasad, N., 2002. Antithrombotic therapy in myocardial infarction and stable angina. BMJ 325, 1287–1289.

Little, P., Barnett, J., Barnsley, L., et al., 2002. Comparison of agreement between different measures of blood pressure in primary care and daytime ambulatory blood pressure. BMJ 325, 254–257.

Littler, W., McGowan, D., Shanson, D., 1997. Changes in recommendations about amoxycillin prophylaxis for prevention of endocarditis. British Society for Antimicrobial Chemotherapy Endocarditis Working Party. Lancet 350, 1100.

Lloyd-Williams, F., Mair, F., Leitner, M., 2002. Exercise training and heart failure: a systematic review of the evidence. Br. J. Gen. Pract. 52, 47–55.

McKelvie, R., 2004. Heart failure: aldosterone receptor antagonists. Clin. Evid. Dec(12), 115–143.

McLeay, R.A., Stallard, T.J., Watson, R.D., et al., 1983. The effect of nifedipine on arterial pressure and reflex cardiac control. Circulation 67, 1084–1090.

McMurray, J., Cohen-Solal, A., Dietz, R., et al., 2003. Practical recommendations for the use of ACE inhibitors, beta-blockers and spironolactone in heart failure: putting guidelines into practice. Eur. J. Heart Fail. 3, 495–502.

Man-Son-Hing, M., Laupacis, A., 2003. Anticoagulant-related bleeding in older persons with atrial fibrillation. Arch. Intern. Med. 163, 1580–1586.

Mant, D., Hobbs, F., Glasziou, P., et al., 2008. Identification and guided treatment of ventricular dysfunction in general practice using B-type natriuretic peptide. Br. J. Gen. Pract. 58, 393–399.

Martin, U., Coleman, J.J., 2006. Monitoring renal function in hypertension. BMJ 333, 896–899.

Mason, J., Young, P., Freemantle, N., et al., 2000. Safety and costs of initiating angiotensin converting enzyme inhibitors for heart failure in primary care: analysis of individual patient data from studies of left ventricular dysfunction. BMJ 321, 1113–1116.

Mayou, R., Sprigings, D., Birkhead, J., Price, J., 2002. A randomized controlled trial of a brief educational and psychological intervention for patients presenting to a cardiac clinic with palpitation. Psychol. Med. 32, 699–706.

MeReC, 1994. Combination diuretics. MeReC Bulletin 5, 37–39.

Moher, M., Yudkin, P., Wright, L., et al., 2001. Cluster randomised controlled trial to compare three methods of promoting secondary prevention of coronary heart disease in primary care. BMJ 322, 1–7.

Nash, I.S., 2007. Reassessing normal blood pressure. BMJ 335, 408–409.

NICE, 2004. Hypertension - Management of Hypertension in Adults in Primary Care. National Institute for Clinical Excellence, London. Clinical Guideline No.18.

NICE, 2006. Hypertension: management of hypertension in adults in primary care. NICE clinical guideline 34. Available www.nice.org.uk.

NICE, 2007. Secondary Prevention in Primary and Secondary Care for Patients Following a Myocardial Infarction. NICE clinical guideline 48. Available: www.nice.org.uk.

NICE, 2008. Familial Hypercholesterolaemia. NICE clinical guideline 71.

Ohkubo, T., Imai, Y., Tsuji, I., et al., 1998. Home blood pressure measurement has a stronger predictive power for mortality than does screening blood pressure measurement: a population-based observation in Ohasama, Japan. J. Hypertens. 16, 971–975.

Ong, H.T., 2007. Beta-blockers in hypertension and cardiovascular disease. BMJ 334, 946–949.

O'Toole, L., Grech, E., 2003. Chronic stable angina: treatment options. BMJ 326, 1185–1188.

Pai, G., Haites, N., Rawles, J., 1987. One thousand heart attacks in Grampian: the place of CPR in general practice. BMJ 294, 352–354.

PEACE Trial Investigators, 2004. Angiotensin-converting enzyme inhibition in stable coronary artery disease. N. Engl. J. Med. 351, 2058–2068.

Pedersen, T., Faergeman, O., Kastelein, J., et al., 2005. High dose atorvastatin versus usual dose simvastatin for secondary prevention after myocardial infarction. JAMA 294, 2437–2445.

Perry, I., Wannamethee, S., Walker, M., 1995. Prospective study of risk factors for development of non-insulin dependent diabetes in middle-aged British men. BMJ 310, 560–564.

Peuhkurinen, K., Niemela, M., Ylitalo, A., et al., 2000. Effectiveness of amiodarone as a single oral dose for recent-onset atrial fibrillation. Am. J. Cardiol. 85, 462–465.

Philbin, E., 1999. Comprehensive multidisciplinary programs for the management of patients with congestive heart failure. J. Gen. Intern. Med. 14, 130–135.

Pickering, T.G., Miller, N.H., Ogedegbe, G., et al., 2008. Call to action on use and reimbursement for home blood pressure monitoring: executive summary. A joint scientific statement from the American Heart Association, American Society of Hypertension, and Preventive Cardiovascular Nurses Association. Hypertension 52, 1–9.

Pitt, B., Poole-Wilson, P., Segal, R., et al., 2000. Effect of losartan compared with captopril on mortality in patients with symptomatic heart failure: randomised trial - the Losartan Heart Failure Survival Study ELITE 2. Lancet 355, 1582–1587.

Pitt, B., White, H., Nicolau, J., et al., 2005. Eplerenone reduces mortality 30 days after randomisation following acute myocardial infarction in patients with left ventricular systolic dysfunction and heart failure. J. Am. Coll. Cardiol. 46, 425–431.

Pitt, B., Zannad, F., Remme, W., et al., 1999. The effect of spironolactone on morbidity and mortality in patients with severe heart failure. N. Engl. J. Med. 341, 709–717.

Powell, K., Pratt, M., 1996. Physical activity and health. BMJ 313, 126–127.

Primatesta, P., Brookes, M., Poulter, N., 2001. Improved hypertension management and control: results from the Health Survey for England 1998. Hypertension 38, 827–832.

Protheroe, J., Fahey, T., Montgomery, A., Peters, T., 2000. The impact of patients' preferences on the treatment of atrial fibrillation: observational study of patient based decision analysis. BMJ 320, 1380–1384.

Psaty, B., Lumley, T., Furberg, C., 2003. Health outcomes associated with various antihypertensive therapies used as first-line agents: a network meta-analysis. JAMA 289, 2534–2544.

Psaty, B., Smith, N., Siscovick, D., et al., 1997. Health outcomes associated with antihypertensive therapies used as first-line agents. JAMA 277, 739–745.

Rathore, S., Curtis, J., Wang, Y., et al., 2003. Association of serum digoxin concentration and outcomes in patients with heart failure. JAMA 289, 871–878.

Roderick, E., 1998. Opportunistic screening for atrial fibrillation is possible. BMJ 9 September 1998; rapid response, 1998.

Salpeter, S., Ormiston, T., Salpeter, E., Wood-Baker, R., 2004. Cardioselective beta-blockers for reversible airway disease (Cochrane Review). In: The Cochrane Library. John Wiley & Sons, Ltd, Chichester, UK, Issue 1.

Sanmuganathan, P., Ghahramani, P., Jackson, P., et al., 2001. Aspirin for primary prevention of coronary heart disease: safety and absolute benefit related to coronary risk derived from meta-analysis of randomised trials. Heart 85, 265–271.

Schleifer, S., Macari-Hinson, M., Coyle, D., et al., 1989. The nature and course of depression following myocardial infarction. Arch. Intern. Med. 149, 1785–1789.

Scottish Intercollegiate Guidelines Network, 1999. Diagnosis and Treatment of Heart Failure due to Left Ventricular Systolic Dysfunction. SIGN, A National Clinical Guideline.

Sharpe, N., Doughty, R., 1998. Epidemiology of heart failure and ventricular dysfunction. Lancet 352 (Suppl. 1), 3–7.

Silagy, C., Lancaster, T., Stead, L., et al., 2004. Nicotine replacement therapy for smoking cessation. Cochrane Database Syst. Rev. (3).

Snow, V., Weiss, K., LeFevre, M., 2003. Management of newly detected atrial fibrillation: a clinical practice guideline from the American Academy of Family Physicians and the American College of Physicians. Ann. Intern. Med. 139, 1009–1017.

Staessen, J., Den Hond, E., Celis, H., et al., 2004. Antihypertensive treatment based on blood pressure measurement at home or in the physician's office: a randomized controlled trial. JAMA 291, 955–964.

Stevens, V., Obarzanek, E., Cook, N., 2001. Long-term weight loss and changes in blood pressure: results of the Trials of Hypertension Prevention, phase 2. Ann. Intern. Med. 134, 1–11.

Stewart, A., Howard, P., 1992. Indications for long-term oxygen therapy. Resp. Physiol. 59, 8–13.

Stewart, S., Hart, C., Hole, D., McMurray, J., 2002. A population-based study of the long-term risks associated with atrial fibrillation: 20-year follow-up of the Renfrew/Paisley Study. Am. J. Med. 113, 359–364.

Strik, J., Denollet, J., Lousberg, R., Honig, A., 2003. Comparing symptoms of depression and anxiety as predictors of cardiac events and increased health care consumption after myocardial infarction. J. Am. Coll. Cardiol. 42, 1801–1807.

Strom, B., Abrutyn, E., Berlin, J., et al., 1998. Dental and cardiac risk factors for infective endocarditis: a population-based, case-control study. Ann. Intern. Med. 129, 761–769.

Sudlow, M., Rodgers, H., Kenny, R., Thomson, R., 1998. Identification of patients with atrial fibrillation in general practice: a study of screening methods. BMJ 317, 327–328.

Swenson, J., Clinch, J., 2000. Assessment of quality of life in patients with cardiac disease: the role of psychosomatic medicine. J. Psychosom. Res. 48, 405–415.

Thompson, R., Summerbell, C., Hooper, L., et al., 2004. Dietary advice given by a dietitian versus other health professional or self-help resources to reduce blood cholesterol (Cochrane Review). In: The Cochrane Library. John Wiley & Sons, Ltd, Chichester, UK, Issue 3.

Trichopoulou, A., Bamia, C., Trichopoulos, D., 2009. Anatomy of health effects of Mediterranean diet: Greek EPIC prospective cohort study. BMJ 339, 26–29.

Turnbull, F., Blood Pressure Lowering Treatment Trialists' Collaboration, 2003. Effects of different blood-pressure-lowering regimens on major cardiovascular events: results of prospectively-designed overviews of randomised trials. Lancet 362, 1527–1535.

United Kingdom Heart Attack Study (UKHAS) Collaborative Group, 1998. Effect of time from onset to coming under care on fatality of patients with acute myocardial infarction: effect of resuscitation and thrombolytic treatment. Heart 80, 114–120.

van den Born, B.J.H., Hulsman, C.A.A., Hoekstra, J.B.L., et al., 2005. Value of routine funduscopy in patients with hypertension: systematic review. BMJ 331, 73–76.

van Peski-Oosterbaan, A., Spinhoven, P., van Rood, Y., et al., 1999. Cognitive-behavioral therapy for noncardiac chest pain: a randomized trial. Am. J. Med. 106, 424–429.

van Walraven, C., Hart, R., Singer, D., et al., 2002. Oral anticoagulants vs aspirin in nonvalvular atrial fibrillation. JAMA 288, 2441–2448.

van Walraven, C., Hart, R., Wells, G., et al., 2003. A clinical prediction rule to identify patients with atrial fibrillation and a low risk for stroke while taking aspirin. Arch. Intern. Med. 163, 936–943.

van Weert, H., 2007. Diagnosing atrial fibrillation in general practice. BMJ 335, 355–356.

Vasan, R., 2003. Diastolic heart failure. BMJ 327, 1181–1182.

Vidaillet, H., Granada, J., Chyou, P.O., et al., 2002. A population-based study of mortality among patients with atrial fibrillation or flutter. Am. J. Med. 113, 365–370.

Wald, D., Law, M., Morris, J., et al., 2009. Combination therapy versus monotherapy in reducing blood pressure: meta-analysis on 11, 000 participants from 42 trials. Am. J. Med. 122, 290–300.

Wannamethee, S., Shaper, A., 1999. Type of alcoholic drink and risk of major coronary heart disease events and all-cause mortality. Am. J. Public Health 89, 685–690.

Wannamethee, S., Shaper, A., Walker, M., 1998. Changes in physical activity, mortality, and incidence of coronary heart disease in older men. Lancet 351, 1603–1608.

Whelton, S., Chin, A.V., Xin, X., He, J., 2002. Effect of aerobic exercise on blood pressure: a meta-analysis for randomised controlled trials. Ann. Intern. Med. 136, 493–503.

Wilber, J., Barrow, J., 1972. Hypertension: community problem. Am. J. Med. 52, 653–663.

Williams, B., Poulter, N., Brown, M., et al., 2004. British Hypertension Society guidelines for hypertension management 2004 (BHS-IV). J. Hum. Hypertens. 18, 139–185.

Wood, D., Durrington, P., Poulter, N., et al., 1998. Joint British recommendations on prevention of coronary heart disease in clinical practice. Heart 80 (Suppl. 2), S1–S29.

Wood, D., Wray, R., Poulter, N., et al., 2005. JBS2: joint British guidelines on prevention of cardiovascular disease in clinical practice. Heart 91 (Suppl. V), v1–v52.

Wright, S., Doughty, R., Pearl, A., et al., 2003. Plasma amino-terminal pro-brain natriuretic peptide and accuracy of heart-failure diagnosis in primary care. J. Am. Coll. Cardiol. 42, 1793–1800.

Writing Group of the PREMIER Collaborative Research Group, 2003. Effects of comprehensive lifestyle modification on blood pressure control. JAMA 289, 2083–2093.

Yip, G., Hart, R., Conway, D., 2002. Antithrombotic therapy for atrial fibrillation. BMJ 325, 1022–1025.

Yusuf, S., Peto, R., Lewis, S., et al., 1985. Beta-blockade during and after myocardial infarction: an overview of the randomized trials. Prog. Cardiovasc. Dis. 27, 355–371.

Yusuf, S., Sleight, P., Pogue, J., et al., 2000. Effects of an angiotensin-converting-enzyme inhibitor, ramipril, on cardiovascular events in high-risk patients. The Heart Outcomes Prevention Evaluation Study Investigators. N. Engl. J. Med. 342, 145–153.

Chapter 6

Respiratory problems

CHAPTER CONTENTS

ASTHMA

GUIDELINES

British Thoracic Society/Scottish Intercollegiate
Guideline Network. 2008. British guideline on the
management of asthma. Thorax 63 (Suppl IV),
iv1–iv121 This guideline is updated annually
and available on http://www.brit-thoracic.org.uk
and http://www.sign.ac.uk. See also
Appendices 11A–E

DIAGNOSIS

The probability of asthma is assessed from the history, supported by lung function tests and the diagnosis confirmed by response to treatment. The process should be clearly documented (British Thoracic Society/Scottish Intercollegiate Guideline Network 2008). For details of the diagnosis of asthma see *Evidence-based Diagnosis in Primary Care* by A. F. Polmear (editor) published by Butterworth-Heinemann, 2008.

1. **Typical history**
   (a) Variable symptoms of coughing, wheezing, chest tightness and shortness of breath.
   (b) Symptoms are often worse at night and are commonly triggered by viral infections, exercise and allergy.
   (c) A personal or family history of atopy supports the diagnosis.

DOI: 10.1016/B978-0-7020-3053-6.00006-4

2. **Lung function tests**

(a) *Evidence of airflow obstruction.* The presence and severity of airflow obstruction can be assessed by spirometry, though because asthma is a variable condition, a normal spirogram in an asymptomatic patient does not exclude asthma.

(b) *Objective evidence of variability.* Diurnal variation > 20% may conveniently be demonstrated by recording morning and evening peak flows over 2 weeks and demonstrating the typical 'saw tooth' pattern. A fall in peak flow > 20% when the patient next meets his or her trigger, or an increase > 20% in response to treatment may be noted as part of home charting. For 'normal' peak flow values see Appendix 8 (children) and 9 (adults), but note that a normal peak flow at a consultation does not exclude the diagnosis of asthma. Asthma is a dynamic condition and readings need to be taken over time in order to check for variability.

(c) A *formal reversibility test.* If the presenting lung function is low or the patient is symptomatic it may be possible to demonstrate a significant response to a single dose of a beta$_2$ agonist, a 6-week course of inhaled steroids or a 2-week course of oral steroids. An increase in forced expiratory volume in one second (FEV$_1$) greater than 400 ml, or an increase in peak flow > 20% suggests asthma.

3. **Probability of asthma and response to treatment. Based on the clinical presentation supported by lung function tests, assess the probability of asthma.**

(a) *High probability of asthma.* Commence a trial of treatment with a moderate dose of inhaled steroids and monitor the response, both symptomatically and with repeated measures of lung function. A good response confirms a diagnosis of asthma. A poor response, if inhaler technique and compliance are good, should lead to reconsideration of the diagnostic possibilities.

(b) *Low probability of asthma.* Investigate and treat for the more probable diagnosis, reconsidering asthma in those who do not respond.

(c) *Intermediate probability of asthma.* If the diagnosis is not clear, or the response to asthma treatment is poor, arrange further investigations. Spirometry is the pivotal test as the differential diagnosis and approach to management depends on whether the patient has airflow obstruction. Consider referral if the diagnosis remains unclear.

CHILDREN

The diagnosis of asthma in children follows a similar process of establishing probabilities and observing the response to a trial of treatment. There are, however, some specific caveats:

* Clarify what parents mean when they use the word 'wheeze' (Cane, Ranganathan and McKenzie 2000);
* Assess on the basis of symptoms supplemented by lung function tests (Sly, Cahill, Willet and Burton 1994). Children under 7 cannot reliably use a peak flow meter, though school age children can usually perform spirometry if encouraged by a skilled technician.

INFANTS

Wheezy infants present particular diagnostic difficulties and there is little evidence-based data to guide decisions (Cochran 1998; Bush 2000).

* *Exclude serious pathology,* e.g. cystic fibrosis, congenital heart defects, inhaled foreign body, oesophageal problems. Referral to a paediatrician is appropriate if the diagnosis is in doubt.
* *Distinguish between asthma and viral-associated wheeze* (Table 6.1). This can be a difficult distinction to make and the diagnosis may only be clear in retrospect, as children with viral-associated wheeze will usually lose that tendency after 2 or 3 years.

Table 6.1	Distinguishing between asthma and viral–associated wheeze	
SUGGESTIVE OF ASTHMA	**SUGGESTIVE OF VIRAL-ASSOCIATED WHEEZE**	
Family or personal history of atopy	Prematurity, small for dates Maternal smoking	
Cough and wheeze not associated with viral illness	Cough and wheeze only with viral infections	
Good response to treatment and relapse on cessation of treatment	Poor response to treatment	

(a) Consider risk factors and the clinical history.

(b) Record the presence of wheeze heard by a health professional.

(c) A carefully supervised trial of treatment may be helpful (Cochran 1998; Bush 2000), e.g. inhaled steroids for 8 weeks. Use up to beclometasone 1000 mcg daily, budesonide 800 mcg daily or fluticasone 500 mcg daily via a spacer ± mask, which may be needed to overcome practical problems with delivering inhaled therapy to very young children.

(d) A poor response to therapy makes asthma unlikely and treatment can be withdrawn.

(e) A good response to therapy should be confirmed by a withdrawal of treatment in order to exclude coincidental improvement.

MANAGEMENT

GENERAL MEASURES

* Advise on the avoidance of triggers:
  (a) Asthma UK produces useful information for patients about allergen avoidance;
  (b) common allergens include pets, especially cats, house-dust mite and pollen;
  (c) current chemical and physical measures for reducing house dust mite allergen have not been shown to be effective (Gøtzsche and Johansen 2008);
  (d) rhinitis is a common comorbidity and may be effectively treated with intranasal steroids (Scadding, Durham, Mirakian, *et al.* 2008; Taramarcaz and Gibson 2003);
  (e) adults in whom an occupational cause for their symptoms is suspected should be referred.
* Encourage smoking cessation. Both active and passive smoking status should be documented.
* Consider drug effects:
  (a) beta-blockers (systemic or topical eye drops) are contraindicated;
  (b) asthmatics sensitive to aspirin should not use non-steroidal anti-inflammatory drugs (NSAIDs).

THERAPEUTIC MANAGEMENT

Patients should start treatment at the step most appropriate to the severity at presentation (see Appendices 11A, B and C) (British Thoracic Society/Scottish Intercollegiate Guideline Network 2008).

Inhaled steroids are indicated for most symptomatic asthmatics. Regular treatment improves lung function, reduces symptoms, reduces use of rescue bronchodilation and reduces the risk of exacerbations (Adams, Bestall, Malouf, *et al.* 2005; Dennis, Solarte and FitzGerald 2008).

* Gain control by starting with a moderate dose (beclometasone or budesonide 400–800 mcg daily or fluticasone 250–500 mcg) and reduce to the lowest dose compatible with asthma control (British Thoracic Society/Scottish Intercollegiate Guideline Network 2008).

* Discuss attitudes to regular treatment. Compliance with inhaled steroid treatment is poor (van Staa, Cooper, Leufkens, *et al.* 2003), and may be improved by a simple once- or twice-daily regime (The British Thoracic Society/Scottish Intercollegiate Guideline Network 2008; Cochrane, Bala, Downs, *et al.* 2000).

* Explain ways of avoiding local side-effects. Candidiasis may be reduced by rinsing the mouth after administration or using a spacer device; dysphonia may be improved by reducing the dose.

* Reassure patients that important systemic side-effects are unlikely at moderate doses (beclometasone or budesonide < 800 mcg daily, fluticasone < 500 mcg daily) (British Thoracic Society/Scottish Intercollegiate Guideline Network 2008; Adams, Bestall, Malouf, *et al.* 2005). In children, despite an initial reduction in growth velocity, final height is not affected (Agertoft and Pedersen 2000; CAMP study 2000). High-dose inhaled steroids (beclometasone or budesonide > 1500 mcg daily, fluticasone > 750 mcg daily) have an increased risk of adrenal suppression, cataracts, reduced bone density and bruising (Lipworth 1999). Risks should be balanced against benefits and alternatives considered (see next page).

Beta$_2$ agonists provide symptomatic relief and should be prescribed on an 'as required' basis (British Thoracic Society/Scottish Intercollegiate Guideline Network 2008; Walters, Walters, Gibson and Jones 2003). They are less effective than inhaled steroids in the management of mild persistent asthma (Adams, Bestall, Malouf 2005; Haahtela, Jarvinen, Kava et al., 1991).

∗ Patients requiring relief medication more than three times a week, waking with asthma on more than one night a week or who have had an exacerbation in the last 2 years should be considered for regular prevention with inhaled steroids (British Thoracic Society/Scottish Intercollegiate Guideline Network 2008).

∗ Exercise-induced asthma which persists despite good asthma control with inhaled steroids may be prevented by using a beta$_2$ agonist prior to exercise (British Thoracic Society/Scottish Intercollegiate Guideline Network 2008).

Long-acting bronchodilators are given regularly twice a day as 'add-on therapy' to people whose asthma is not controlled on inhaled steroids. The addition of long-acting bronchodilators improves lung function, and symptom control compared with increasing the dose of inhaled steroids (British Thoracic Society/Scottish Intercollegiate Guideline Network 2008; Pauwels, Lofdahl, Postma, et al. 1997; Ni Chroinin, Greenstone and Ducharme 2004).

∗ In response to concerns about a very small increased risk in patients on long-acting beta$_2$ agonists of asthma deaths (Nelson, Weiss, Bleecker, et al. 2006), and serious adverse events (Cates, Cates and Lasserson 2008; Cates and Cates 2008), guidelines emphasize the importance of maintaining an adequate dose of inhaled steroids (British Thoracic Society/ Scottish Intercollegiate Guideline Network 2008). Patients should be counselled appropriately.

∗ Combination inhalers have the advantage of ensuring that patients cannot take long-acting bronchodilators without taking inhaled steroids, but with the disadvantage of reducing dosage flexibility of individual components.

∗ Flexible use of budesonide/formoterol combination as rescue medication in addition to regular use as preventer therapy is an effective treatment option for selected adult patients at step 2 (above beclometasone 400 mcg/day) or step 3 who are poorly controlled (British Thoracic Society/Scottish Intercollegiate Guideline Network 2008). Careful self-management education about this strategy is required.

Leukotriene antagonists are mediator antagonists which affect eosinophilic inflammation and are an option as 'add-on therapy' (British Thoracic Society/Scottish Intercollegiate Guideline Network 2008; Ducharme, Schwartz and Kakuma 2004). A recent review concluded that although they were less effective than long-acting beta$_2$ agonists in relieving symptoms over 12 weeks, the reduction in exacerbations over two years was similar, with some studies showing an improved safety profile (Joos, Miksch, Szecsenyi, et al. 2008). They are recommended as first line add-on therapy for children under 5 years (British Thoracic Society/ Scottish Intercollegiate Guideline Network 2008).

Other therapeutic options

∗ Sodium cromoglicate has a small overall treatment effect and should not be first line treatment for the prevention of asthma (Tasche, Uijen, Bernsen, et al. 2000).

∗ Theophyllines may be an option as 'add-on therapy' for a minority of patients (British Thoracic Society/Scottish Intercollegiate Guideline Network 2008).

∗ A short 'rescue' course of oral steroids may be needed at any time and at any step but consideration of maintenance therapy with oral steroids should prompt referral to a respiratory physician (British Thoracic Society/Scottish Intercollegiate Guideline Network 2008).

MANAGEMENT OF ADULTS AND CHILDREN 5 YEARS AND OVER NOT CONTROLLED ON A MODERATE DOSE OF INHALED STEROIDS (BRITISH THORACIC SOCIETY/SCOTTISH INTERCOLLEGIATE GUIDELINE NETWORK 2008)

■ Adult maximum daily maintenance dose: beclometasone 800 mcg, budesonide 800 mcg or fluticasone 400 mcg.

■ Children maximum daily maintenance dose: beclometasone 400 mcg daily, budesonide 400 mcg daily or fluticasone 200 mcg.

Assessment

(a) Is the diagnosis correct?

(b) Is the patient complying with the regular use of inhaled steroids?

(c) Can the patient use his or her inhaler device?

(d) Does the patient also have uncontrolled rhinitis?

(e) Are there any environmental factors?

1. Consider an objective trial of long-acting bronchodilators.
2. Monitor response with symptoms and peak flow charting.
3. If no response, stop the additional therapy and consider an alternative (e.g. leukotriene antagonists, increased dose of inhaled steroid).
4. If poor response to any of the options, consider the need for referral.

DEVICES

The effectiveness of inhaled therapy depends on inhaler technique and the particle size produced by the device. Inhaler devices should be selected for individual patients taking into consideration (Table 6.2):

(a) *The patient's ability to use a device.* This should always be checked before an inhaler is prescribed, and re-checked regularly (British Thoracic Society/Scottish Intercollegiate Guideline Network 2008). Only a minority of patients using a metered dose inhaler have adequate inhaler technique, with slightly better performance for other devices (Brocklebank, Ram, Wright, *et al.* 2001). Technique should be observed for:
   - the patient's inspirational flow rate compared to flow rate recommended by the manufacturer for efficient actuation and inhalation;
   - hand/breath coordination;
   - ability to follow the instructions for correct use.
(b) *The drug and dosage required.* High doses of inhaled steroid should be given by a spacer device.

(c) *NICE guidelines* recommend the use of spacers (with masks for infants) for children under the age of five (National Institute for Clinical Excellence 2000). Choice of spacer device should be guided by the information in the Summary of Product Characteristics (see www.nice.org.uk).
(d) *Patient preference* and lifestyle issues may be relevant.
(e) *Cost of the device.*

REGULAR REVIEW

Patients receiving treatment for asthma should be reviewed regularly by a GP or trained asthma nurse (British Thoracic Society/Scottish Intercollegiate Guideline Network 2008). Reviews in primary care, conducted face-to-face or by telephone (British Thoracic Society/Scottish Intercollegiate Guideline Network 2008; Pinnock, Bawden, Proctor, *et al.* 2003; Pinnock, Adlem, Gaskin, *et al.* 2007), should encompass the following three steps (Pinnock 2008):

1. Assessing control in order to target care appropriately

* *Specific morbidity questions.* Patients under-report symptoms (Haughney, Barnes, Partridge and Cleland 2004), and control should be assessed by asking standard morbidity questions at every asthma review consultation (British Thoracic Society/Scottish Intercollegiate Guideline Network 2008). The Royal College of Physicians' 'three questions' is an example of a suitable morbidity score (Pearson and Bucknall 1999).

Table 6.2	Choice of inhaler device for different age groups	
AGE	**DEVICES TO CONSIDER**	**COMMENTS**
Preschool	MDI+spacer (with a mask for infants)	NICE recommendation (National Institute for Clinical Excellence 2000)
School-age	MDI+spacer	Recommended for inhaled steroids because it reduces oral deposition (National Institute of Clinical Excellence 2002a)
	Dry powder devices	Once a child has adequate inspiration and can be relied on not to blow by mistake
	Breath actuated devices	Once inspiration is adequate
Adults	MDI	If technique is adequate. Should be used with a spacer to deliver high doses of inhaled steroid
	Breath-actuated devices	
	Dry powder devices	

MDI = metered-dose inhaler.

1. Have you had difficulty sleeping because of your asthma symptoms (including cough)?
2. Have you had your usual asthma symptoms during the day (cough, wheeze, tight chest or breathlessness)?
3. Has your asthma interfered with your usual activities (housework, work or school, etc.)?

* *Use of relief medication.* Good asthma control is associated with little or no need for short-acting beta$_2$ agonists (British Thoracic Society/Scottish Intercollegiate Guideline Network 2008). At the other extreme, use of two or more canisters a month is a marker for 'at-risk' asthma (British Thoracic Society/Scottish Intercollegiate Guideline Network 2008).

* *Frequency of acute attacks.* Acute attacks requiring a course of oral steroids are a marker of uncontrolled asthma (British Thoracic Society/Scottish Intercollegiate Guideline Network 2008).

2. Responding to that assessment by identifying reasons for poor control and adjusting management strategy accordingly

* *Review the diagnosis:* failure to respond to treatment may indicate an incorrect diagnosis, or the development of a comorbid cause for symptoms (British Thoracic Society/Scottish Intercollegiate Guideline Network 2008).

* *Check and correct inhaler technique.*

* *Assess and address adherence:* patients and their healthcare professionals both overestimate compliance with regular medication. Non-judgemental questioning and achieving concordance about treatment goals may improve compliance (British Thoracic Society/Scottish Intercollegiate Guideline Network 2008).

* *Ask about, and treat rhinitis:* three quarters of people with asthma have symptoms of rhinitis, which should be treated with nasal steroids (Scadding, Durham, Mirakian, *et al.* 2008; Thomas and Price 2008).

* *Assess smoking status and offer cessation advice:* smoking adversely affects asthma control. This may be because of a comorbid diagnosis of chronic obstructive pulmonary disease (COPD), or because smoking reduces the effectiveness of inhaled steroids (British Thoracic Society/Scottish Intercollegiate Guideline Network 2008; Haughney, Price, Kaplan, *et al.* 2008). Persistent smokers need relatively high doses of inhaled steroids (British Thoracic Society/Scottish Intercollegiate Guideline Network 2008).

* *Adjust therapy according to evidence-based guidelines.*

3. Exploring patients' ideas, concerns and expectations, and guiding self-management to facilitate on-going control

* *Education and self-management.* Every asthma consultation is an opportunity to review, reinforce and extend asthma knowledge and skills (British Thoracic Society/Scottish Intercollegiate Guideline Network 2008). Education should aim to empower patients to be in control of their asthma and should include the provision of written asthma action plans (Gibson, Powell, Wilson, *et al.* 2002).

PERSONAL ASTHMA ACTION PLANS

Education involving self-monitoring and written action plans reduces hospitalizations, emergency consultations, reduction in days off work or school, and nocturnal asthma (Gibson, Powell, Wilson, *et al.* 2002; Wolf, Guevara, Grum, *et al.* 2002).

* Offer all asthmatics a written asthma action plan which should (British Thoracic Society/Scottish Intercollegiate Guideline Network 2008; Gibson and Powell 2004):

(a) be tailored to the individual patient, taking into account his or her clinical condition and preference for autonomy;

(b) involve self-monitoring, based on peak flows and/or symptoms;

(c) provide information about features which would indicate that the patient's asthma is worsening;

(d) advise what action the patient should take, including information about increasing inhaled steroids and starting oral steroids.

An example can be found on the Asthma UK website: www.asthma.org.uk

INDICATIONS FOR OUTPATIENT REFERRAL

Referral to a respiratory physician or paediatrician should be considered if (British Thoracic Society/ Scottish Intercollegiate Guideline Network 2008):

(a) the diagnosis is not clear;

(b) the patient is not controlled with moderate doses of inhaled steroids ± add-on therapy and their inhaler technique is satisfactory;

(c) there is a possibility of occupational asthma;

(d) there is a history of life-threatening attacks or brittle asthma.

ACUTE ASTHMA

ACUTE ASTHMA IN ADULTS AND SCHOOLCHILDREN (see Appendices 11D and E)

Delay is the commonest factor identified as contributing to asthma deaths, often related to a failure on the part of the patient or the healthcare professional to appreciate the severity of the attack (British Thoracic Association 1982). The presence of psychosocial problems is an important risk factor for fatal asthma (British Thoracic Society/ Scottish Intercollegiate Guideline Network 2008; Mohan, Harrison, Badminton, *et al.* 1996).

* Assess and record the severity

(a) *General condition.* Inability to speak, exhaustion, cyanosis and a silent chest indicate life-threatening asthma.

(b) *Peak flow.* Peak flow (PF) at presentation should be compared with the patient's best (or predicted if best is not known) (British Thoracic Society/Scottish Intercollegiate Guideline Network 2008):

● PF < 75% of best = moderate asthma exacerbation;

● PF < 50% of best = acute severe asthma;

● PF < 33% of best = life-threatening asthma.

(c) *Respiratory rate (RR):* > 25/minute in adults, > 30/minute in children over 5 years indicates severe asthma.

(d) *Heart rate (HR):* > 110/minute in adults, > 125/minute in children over 5 years indicates severe asthma.

(e) *Oximetry:* Oxygen saturation < 92% should alert the clinician to the severity of the attack.

* Act promptly to provide relief

(a) *Bronchodilation:* Administer multiple (10–20) doses of a beta2 agonist through a large-volume spacer, or 5 mg salbutamol/10 mg terbutaline by oxygen-driven nebuliser (The British Thoracic Society/Scottish Intercollegiate Guideline Network 2008; Cates, Crilly and Rowe 2006). Nebulisers require flow rates of 6–8 litres a minute (O'Driscoll, Howard and Davison 2008). Consider adding ipratropium in severe or life-threatening asthma (British Thoracic Society/Scottish Intercollegiate Guideline Network 2008).

(b) *Oxygen:* give at high flow rates for severe or life-threatening asthma aiming to maintain oxygen saturation between 94 and 98% (British Thoracic Society/Scottish Intercollegiate Guideline Network 2008; O'Driscoll, Howard and Davison 2008).

(c) *Systemic steroids:* steroids reduce mortality, relapses, subsequent hospital admission and the requirement for beta$_2$ agonist therapy (British Thoracic Society/Scottish Intercollegiate Guideline Network 2008; Rowe, Spooner, Ducharme, *et al.* 2001; Rowe, Spooner, Ducharme, *et al.* 2007). Early administration improves outcomes; prednisolone 40–50 mg for adults, 30 mg for children should therefore be given at the consultation. The NNT to prevent one admission in patients with severe asthma is five (95%CI 4 to 7).

(d) *Assess response.*

Note: Infective triggers for acute asthma are usually viral. Routine prescribing of antibiotics is not appropriate (British Thoracic Society/Scottish Intercollegiate Guideline Network 2008).

* Arrange further care

1. Admit:

(a) patients with life-threatening asthma;

(b) patients with severe asthma who do not respond to emergency bronchodilation.

Other factors, e.g. the time of day, social situation, previous history of severe attacks, will influence the decision to admit (British Thoracic Society/ Scottish Intercollegiate Guideline Network 2008).

2. Instructions
   (a) Bronchodilation may be repeated 3 to 4 hourly. Ideally, progress should be monitored by peak flow.
   (b) Prednisolone 40–50 mg daily for at least 5 days or until recovery (adults); 30 mg daily for 3 days (children).
   (c) Increase (or recommence) inhaled steroids (beclometasone 800 mcg daily, budesonide 800 mcg daily or fluticasone 500 mcg) until full control is regained.
   (d) Ensure the patient knows when and how to call further medical help.

3. *Early follow-up:* arrange to assess progress within 24 hours (severe asthma) or 48 hours (uncontrolled asthma).

4. *Review:* arrange for a review of overall asthma control and revision of Personal Asthma Action Plan.

ACUTE ASTHMA IN PRESCHOOL CHILDREN
(See Appendices 11C and E)

* *Assess and record the severity:* exhaustion, agitation, drowsiness, too breathless to feed, use of accessory muscles, RR > 40/minute or HR > 140/minute are signs of severe or life-threatening asthma.
* *Act promptly to provide relief*
  1. *Bronchodilation:* 2.5 mg salbutamol or 5 mg terbutaline by nebulizer or multiple (10–20) doses through a large volume spacer ± mask.
  2. *Oxygen* should be given at high flow rates.
  3. *Systemic steroids:* soluble prednisolone 20 mg.
  4. *Assess response:* RR, HR and general condition.
* Arrange further care. Admit:
  (a) children with any features of severe or life-threatening asthma;
  (b) children who do not respond to bronchodilation or who relapse within 3 hours.
* Poor social circumstances or a previous history of a severe attack should lower the threshold for admission.

* Children not admitted should be given prednisolone 20 mg for 3 days and clear instructions for review.

PROFESSIONAL GROUPS

General Practice Airways Group (GPIAG): http://www.gpiag.org. Secretariat: GPIAG, Smithy House, Waterbeck, Lockerbie DG11 3EY, tel. 01461 600639; fax, 01361 331811; email, info@gpiag.org. The GPIAG is a group of primary care professionals with an interest in respiratory disease. They are active in lobbying, research, education and publish the *Primary Care Respiratory Journal.* Their website provides online access to the journal, opinion sheets, resources for practices.

International Primary Care Respiratory Group (IPCRG): http://www.theipcrg.org. Secretariat: IPCRG, Department of General Practice and Primary Care, Foresterhill Health Centre, Westburn Road, Aberdeen AB25 2AY, tel: 01224 552427. The IPCRG is an umbrella organization for national primary care respiratory interest groups. Its website includes practical guidance and resources for primary care, and links to websites of member countries

British Thoracic Society: http://www.brit-thoracic.org.uk. 17 Doughty Street, London WC1N 2PL, tel. 020 7831 8778; fax, 020 7831 8766; email, admin1@brit-thoracic.org.uk. The society for all professionals with an interest in respiratory disease. Their guidelines may be downloaded from their website. Also available are some information sheets for patients on a wide range of respiratory problems.

GUIDELINES

British Thoracic Society/Scottish Intercollegiate Guideline Network. The regularly updated British Guideline on the management of asthma and many web-based resources are available online from: www.brit-thoracic.org.uk and www.sign.ac.uk

The Global Initiative on Asthma. *Asthma Prevention and Management: A Practical Guide for Public Health Officials and Health Care Professionals.* Available: www.ginasthma.com

RESPIRATORY TRAINING

Education for Health: http://www.educationforhealth.org.uk/

The Athenaeum, 10 Church Street, Warwick CV34 4AB, tel. 01926 493313

Respiratory Education UK: http://www.respiratoryetc.com

University Hospital Aintree, Lower Lane, Liverpool L9 7AL, tel: 0151 529 2598 or 0151 529 3943.

PATIENT GROUPS

Asthma UK: http://www.asthma.org.uk Summit House, 70 Wilson Street, London EC2A 2DB; tel. 020 7786 4900. Helpline 0845 7010203. Asthma UK provides information leaflets about asthma for patients and resources such as asthma action plans which can be ordered or downloaded from their website. British Lung Foundation: www.lunguk.org 73-75 Goswell Road, London EC1V 7ER, tel. 020 7688 5555. Helpline 08458 50 50 20.

The BLF produces information for patients about a wide range of respiratory diseases which may be ordered or downloaded from their website. It runs local 'Breathe Easy' groups. Action on Smoking and Health: www.ash.org.uk ASH publishes information about smoking and provides information about smoking cessation with links to other useful sites. Quitline: 0800 00 22 00 Provides telephone support line for patients wanting to quit.

LOWER RESPIRATORY TRACT INFECTION

GUIDELINES

British Thoracic Society. 2001. Guidelines for the management of community acquired pneumonia in adults. Thorax 56 (IV), 1–64. [2004 update is available from www.brit-thoracic.org.uk]

Scottish Intercollegiate Guidelines Network. *Community Management of Lower Respiratory Tract Infection in Adults.* SIGN 59: Edinburgh 2002. Available: www.sign.ac.uk

National Institute for Health and Clinical Excellence. Prescribing of Antibiotics for self-limiting Respiratory Tract Infections in Adults and Children in Primary Care. NICE 2008. Available: www.nice.org.uk

- The majority of previously well patients who present to their GP with acute respiratory symptoms have a self-limiting illness (Macfarlane, Holmes, Gard, *et al.* 2001).
- Less than half have evidence of a bacterial infection (Macfarlane, Holmes, Gard, *et al.* 2001; Macfarlane, Colville, Guion, *et al.* 1993).
- Without a chest X-ray (CXR), identification of the 6% of patients with lower respiratory tract infection who have community-acquired pneumonia is imprecise, with no individual sign or symptom being reliably predictive (Macfarlane, Holmes, Gard, *et al.* 2001; Metlay, Kapoor and Fine 1997). For details of the diagnosis of acute respiratory infections see *Evidence-based Diagnosis in Primary Care* by A. F. Polmear (editor) published by Butterworth-Heinemann, 2008.

CLINICAL ASSESSMENT

The aim of the initial history and examination is to identify patients with, or at risk of developing, severe or complicated illness (Macfarlane, Holmes, Gard, *et al.* 2001; Macfarlane, Colville, Guion, *et al.* 1993; Metlay, Kapoor and Fine 1997).

* *Identify high-risk groups.* The risk of pneumonia increases with age and in institutionalized patients (Metlay, Kapoor and Fine 1997; Scottish Intercollegiate Guidelines Network 2002; British Thoracic Society 2001). Clinical features are less reliable in the elderly (Scottish Intercollegiate Guidelines Network 2002).

* *Ask about comorbidity.* Premorbid conditions which increase the risk of pneumonia include COPD, congestive heart failure (Scottish Intercollegiate Guidelines Network 2002; British Thoracic Society 2001; National Institute for Health and Clinical Excellence 2008; Farr, Woodhead, MacFarlane, *et al.* 2000) neurological disease, diabetes, alcoholism, and chronic renal or hepatic failure (Scottish Intercollegiate

Guidelines Network 2002; British Thoracic Society 2001; National Institute for Health and Clinical Excellence 2008).

* *Examine the chest.* The presence of localized chest signs is positively correlated with radiographic evidence of pneumonia, but their absence does not exclude the diagnosis (Macfarlane, Holmes, Gard, *et al.* 2001; Metlay, Kapoor and Fine 1997).

* *Assess severity.* Fever $> 40°C$, RR > 30/minute, BP $< 90/60$, pleuritic chest pain, or confusion indicate severe infection (Scottish Intercollegiate Guidelines Network 2002; British Thoracic Society 2001; National Institute for Health and Clinical Excellence 2008; Fine, Smith, Carson *et al.* 1996; Ewig, Schafer and Torres 2000) and should prompt referral.

* *Assess oximetry.* An oxygen saturation $< 92\%$ indicate significant hypoxia and should prompt referral.

INVESTIGATIONS

Investigations are rarely needed in primary care (Macfarlane, Holmes, Gard, *et al.* 2001; Scottish Intercollegiate Guidelines Network 2002; British Thoracic Society 2001).

(a) CXR may be indicated if there are focal chest signs and in high-risk patients or those with signs of severe disease even in the absence of focal chest signs (Scottish Intercollegiate Guidelines Network 2002; British Thoracic Society 2001). Persistence of systemic illness, the development of unexpected symptoms (e.g. haemoptysis or pleuritic pain) or failure of respiratory symptoms to resolve should prompt investigation.

(b) A raised C-reactive protein (CRP) (> 50mg/l) is positively correlated with radiographic evidence of pneumonia (Macfarlane, Holmes, Gard, *et al.* 2001; British Thoracic Society 2001), but is of no value in assessing severity.

(c) A raised blood urea (> 11 mmol/l) and a leukocytosis ($> 20,000$ white blood cells (WBC)/ml) or leukopenia (< 4000 WBC/ml) indicate severe infection and should prompt urgent referral (British Thoracic Society 2001; Fine, Smith, Carson *et al.* 1996; Ewig, Schafer and Torres 2000).

MANAGEMENT OF *WELL* PATIENTS WITH LOWER RESPIRATORY TRACT SYMPTOMS WITHOUT FOCAL CHEST SIGNS

* *Discuss the natural history of lower respiratory tract illness.* The provision of leaflets explaining the nature of a cough and the expected duration (up to 3 weeks) can reduce reconsultation rates (National Institute for Health and Clinical Excellence 2008; Macfarlane, Holmes and Macfarlane 1997). Advise that failure to improve as expected, deterioration or development of new symptoms should prompt reconsultation (see Appendix 12).

* *Provide advice on symptomatic treatment*:
  (a) Paracetamol, extra fluids, hot lemon and bed rest are commonly recommended in the acute phase, although there are no studies to validate these common remedies.
  (b) Zinc used within 24 hours of the onset of symptoms has been shown to significantly improve the resolution rate of upper respiratory tract symptoms (Mossad, Mackin, Medendorp and Mason 1996).
  (c) The use of vitamin C supplements to prevent or treat respiratory infection is unproven.
  (d) Cough medicines are often bought over the counter but there is no evidence to support effectiveness.

* *Avoid prescribing antibiotics in well patients with no additional risk factors.* Benefits from antibiotics are modest and, for most patients, will not outweigh the risk of adverse effects, the costs or the negative consequences of antibiotic resistance (National Institute for Health and Clinical Excellence 2008; Fahey, Smucny, Becker and Glazier 2004).
  (a) Antibiotics increase the resolution of symptoms by about half a day (National Institute for Health and Clinical Excellence 2008; Fahey, Smucny, Becker and Glazier 2004; Smucny, Becker, Glazier and McIsaac 1998; Bent, Saint, Vittinghof and Grady 1999).
  (b) The magnitude of benefit is similar to that of the detriment from adverse reactions (NNT=18, NNH=14) (Smucny, Becker, Glazier and McIsaac 1998).
  (c) Patients who also have the typical symptoms of URTI and have been ill for less than a week may be least likely to benefit from antibiotics (Fahey, Smucny, Becker and Glazier 2004).

(d) Prescribing antibiotics did not reduce the reconsultation rate in a UK primary care study (Holmes, Macfarlane, Macfarlane *et al.* 1997).

(e) Declining the request for antibiotics and educating patients on the limitations and disadvantages of treatment is effective in reducing antibiotic use (Gonzales, Steiner, Lum, Barrett Jr 1999).

* Use the opportunity to provide smoking cessation advice.

MANAGEMENT OF PATIENTS WITH LOWER RESPIRATORY TRACT SYMPTOMS WITH FOCAL CHEST SIGNS OR WHERE THE PATIENT IS AT HIGH RISK OF PNEUMONIA OR IS SYSTEMICALLY ILL

Community-acquired pneumonia is a potentially serious condition with a mortality of 5% (British Thoracic Society 2001; Farr, Woodhead, MacFarlane, *et al.* 2000).

* *Consider the need for a CXR* to confirm the diagnosis of pneumonia. An FBC and U&Es may help to assess severity (British Thoracic Society 2001).

* *Prescribe antibiotics* (Scottish Intercollegiate Guidelines Network 2002; British Thoracic Society 2001; National Institute for Health and Clinical Excellence 2008; Loeb 2008). Antibiotic treatment should not be delayed if a diagnosis of pneumonia is suspected. Use:

(a) Amoxicillin 500 mg–1 g t.d.s. for 5–7 days (British Thoracic Society 2001) (erythromycin 500 mg q.d.s. or clarithromycin 500 mg b.d. are alternatives).

(b) Erythromycin or clarithromycin are first choice for mycoplasma pneumonia.

(c) Local microbiologists can provide information about local resistance patterns.

* *Arrange follow-up* (Scottish Intercollegiate Guidelines Network 2002; British Thoracic Society 2001). Fever should settle within 2 days. Consider investigating or admitting patients who fail to respond. Some symptoms such as cough may persist after the antibiotics course has finished. If symptoms persist and the initial CXR was abnormal, it should be repeated 6 weeks later to exclude underlying malignancy, especially in patients who smoke.

* *Consider the need for admission* (Scottish Intercollegiate Guidelines Network 2002; British Thoracic Society 2001). Admission is recommended in the presence of:

(a) signs of severe disease (British Thoracic Society 2001; Farr, Woodhead, MacFarlane, *et al.* 2000; Fine, Smith, Carson, *et al.* 1996) (fever > 40°C, RR > 30/minute, BP < 90/60, pleuritic chest pain, confusion). These parameters may be combined in the CRB-65 score to inform the decision to admit (British Thoracic Society 2001) (see below)

(b) high-risk conditions, e.g. pneumonia associated with influenza, chicken pox;

(c) suspected complications (e.g. pleural effusion, malignancy);

(d) diagnostic uncertainty.

Factors which may contribute to the decision to admit are:

(a) comorbidity (British Thoracic Society 2001; Fine, Smith, Carson, *et al.* 1996) (COPD, CCF, diabetes, alcoholism, chronic renal or hepatic failure);

(b) unsatisfactory social circumstances;

(c) failure to respond to first line antibiotics.

CRB-65 SCORE

Score 1 point for each of the following parameters: Confusion, Respiratory rate > 30/minute, BP < 90/60, 65 years or older

CRB 0   Low risk.   Referral to hospital not indicated for clinical reasons

CRB 1 or 2   Increased risk.   Consider the need for hospital assessment

CRB 3 or 4   High risk of death.   Arrange urgent hospital admission

VACCINATION

● Influenza vaccination is recommended for patients in high-risk categories (British Thoracic Society 2001; British National Formulary 2008a):

(a) age over 65 years and institutionalized patients;

(b) patients with comorbidity: chronic respiratory disease, including asthma, chronic heart disease, neurological disease, diabetes, alcoholism, chronic renal or hepatic failure;

(c) asplenic and immunosuppressed patients.

● Pneumococcal vaccination is recommended for the last two of these three categories.

TUBERCULOSIS (TB)

GUIDELINE

National Collaborating Centre for Chronic Conditions. *Tuberculosis: Clinical Diagnosis and Management of Tuberculosis, and Measures for its Prevention and Control.* London: Royal College of Physicians, 2006. Available: www.nice.org.uk

Patients with TB should be managed by physicians or paediatricians with specialist expertise in the management of tuberculosis, supported by tuberculosis nurse specialists or health visitors (National Collaborating Centre for Chronic Conditions 2006). The role of primary care is to:

* *Be alert to the increasing incidence of TB* (Health Protection Agency for Infections 2008). This increase is greatest in urban areas (especially London), with 72% of notifications occurring in patients born outside the UK. New patient medicals may be an opportunity to check the BCG status of immigrants. Other high-risk groups include patients with impaired immunity (including HIV), patients on steroids, the homeless, and those dependent on alcohol or drugs.

* *Consider the diagnosis.* Symptoms of fever and night sweats, cough, weight loss and haemoptysis should prompt investigation (National Collaborating Centre for Chronic Conditions 2006). A CXR should be arranged and three sputum samples may be sent for microscopy, culture and sensitivity and should be marked as 'suspected TB'.

* *Ensure prompt referral.* Most patients can be treated as outpatients (National Collaborating Centre for Chronic Conditions 2006). Inpatient care may be considered because of clinical severity or to ensure compliance with treatment regimes.

* *Encourage compliance.* Treatment regimes will involve a combination of drugs and will continue for at least 6 months (National Collaborating Centre for Chronic Conditions 2006). Supervision will be arranged by the hospital clinic in accordance with local policy. 'Directly observed therapy' may be needed to ensure compliance.

* *Support the patient and their family.* Information for clinicians and answers to 'Frequently asked questions' in a range of languages are available on the British Lung Foundation website: http://www.lunguk.org/you-and-your-lungs/conditions-and-diseases/tuberculosis.htm

* *Be prepared for concerned enquiries from contacts.* Contact tracing is undertaken according to defined procedures usually by a respiratory nurse specialist (National Collaborating Centre for Chronic Conditions 2006). Close contacts are defined as people from the same household, close friends or frequent visitors to the household. Most other contacts are usually 'casual contacts' and are at considerably lower risk of infection. In the event of a local outbreak the local Consultant in Communicable Disease can provide advice.

CHRONIC OBSTRUCTIVE PULMONARY DISEASE (COPD)

For details of the diagnosis of COPD see *Evidence-based Diagnosis in Primary Care* by A. F. Polmear (editor) published by Butterworth-Heinemann, 2008.

GUIDELINES

National Institute for Clinical Excellence. 2004. National clinical guideline. Management of chronic obstructive pulmonary disease in adults primary and secondary care. Thorax 59 (Suppl. 1), S1–232. Available: www.nice.org.uk
   Global Initiative for Obstructive Lung Disease. *Global Strategy for the Diagnosis, Management and Prevention of Chronic Obstructive Pulmonary Disease;* NHLBI/WHO workshop report. Updated 2008. Available: www.goldcopd.com
   van Schayck OCP, Pinnock H, Ostrem A, Litt J for the IPCRG. 2008. IPCRG Consensus statement: tackling the smoking epidemic – practical guidance for primary care. Prim Care Respir J 17, 185–193

The aim of the management of patients with COPD is to make an objective diagnosis as early as possible in the course of the disease in order to encourage smoking cessation and prevent progression. Treatment is aimed at providing the best possible relief of symptoms and improving quality of life. As the disease progresses, treatment levels and professional support should be stepped up to provide adequate palliation (National Institute for Clinical Excellence 2004).

DIAGNOSIS

HISTORY

* *Ask about smoking.* Smoking history may be recorded as 'pack years' (i.e. one pack year = 20 cigarettes a day for 1 year). Note any occupational exposure (e.g. coal mining).
* *Ask about symptoms of cough, sputum production, wheeze and breathlessness* and their impact on lifestyle. These symptoms have an insidious onset, usually after the age of 35 years, and progress slowly with little variability. Suspect bronchial carcinoma if there is haemoptysis.
* *Use the MRC dyspnoea scale* to grade the degree of breathlessness (Table 6.3) (Fletcher, Elmes, Fairbairn, *et al.* 1959).
* *Examine the chest.* The chest will usually be clear in mild COPD; rhonchi develop during exacerbations and as the disease progresses. Localized signs may indicate an underlying carcinoma.
* *Record body mass index.* The normal range is between 20 and 25.

Table 6.3	MRC dyspnoea scale (Fletcher, Elmes, Fairbairn, *et al.* 1959)
GRADE	DEGREE OF BREATHLESSNESS RELATED TO ACTIVITIES
1	Not troubled by breathlessness except on strenuous exercise
2	Short of breath when hurrying or walking up a slight hill
3	Walks slower than contemporaries on level ground because of breathlessness or has to stop for breath when walking at own pace
4	Stops for breath after walking about 100 m or after a few minutes on ground level
5	Too breathless to leave the house, or breathless when dressing or undressing

* *Check for signs of chronic hypoxia.* Cyanosis and confusion can occur with the onset of respiratory failure; ankle oedema suggests cor pulmonale.

Investigations

* *Arrange spirometry.* The diagnosis should be confirmed by spirometry (National Institute for Clinical Excellence 2004). Peak flows do not accurately reflect the degree of airway obstruction in COPD. However, a peak flow chart may be useful to exclude asthma by confirming the absence of variability.
* *Consider the need for other investigations*:
  (a) A CXR should be considered at initial presentation to exclude other pathology.
  (b) The presence of polycythaemia, peripheral oedema or an oxygen saturation of $< 92\%$ suggests chronic hypoxia and should prompt referral for blood gas estimations (National Institute for Clinical Excellence 2004; Roberts, Bulger, Melchor, *et al.* 1993).

Spirometry should be undertaken when the patient is stable, i.e. at least 6 weeks should have elapsed since an exacerbation.

(a) Spirometry in COPD demonstrates an obstructive pattern (forced expiratory volume in 1 second (FEV_1) $< 80\%$ predicted and FEV_1/ forced vital capacity (FVC)$< 70\%$).

(b) Post-bronchodilator FEV_1 expressed as a percentage of predicted may be used to classify the severity of COPD (National Institute for Clinical Excellence 2004):

* mild COPD is defined as $FEV_1 < 80\%$ of predicted;
* moderate COPD is defined as $FEV_1 < 50\%$ of predicted;
* severe COPD is defined as $FEV_1 < 30\%$ of predicted.

In most cases the diagnosis of COPD will be suggested by the combination of clinical history, signs, and spirometry which does not return to normal with drug therapy. In order to exclude asthma, it will be important to confirm the lack of reversibility. This may be demonstrated by:

(a) serial peak flow measurements showing $< 20\%$ variability;

(b) a poor response (< 400 ml increase in FEV_1) to bronchodilators, inhaled or oral steroids. This may be undertaken as a therapeutic trial or as a formal reversibility test.

MANAGEMENT

* *Use every opportunity to encourage the patient to stop smoking* (see page 498). This is the only intervention that can prevent the accelerated decline in lung function that occurs in patients with COPD (Fletcher and Peto 1977; Anthonisen 1994). It is essential that patients understand the implications of continuing to smoke and the benefit of quitting – even with severe disease (National Institute for Clinical Excellence 2004; Global Initiative for Obstructive Lung Disease 2003). Combine pharmacotherapy with appropriate support to aid quit attempts (National Institute for Clinical Excellence 2002b; van Schayck, Pinnock, Ostrem and Litt 2008).

* *Encourage exercise.* Exercise is a key component of all pulmonary rehabilitation programmes which have been shown to improve exercise capacity and the quality of life (Lacasse, Guyatt and Goldstein 1997). Explain that breathlessness is uncomfortable but not dangerous.

* *Stress the importance of good nutrition in all patients.* Refer patients with an abnormal BMI for dietetic advice. Nutritional supplements may be recommended for underweight patients (National Institute for Clinical Excellence 2004; Global Initiative for Obstructive Lung Disease 2003).

* *Advise vaccination.* Influenza vaccination reduces the number of patients who experience an exacerbation (odds ratio (OR) 0.44 (95% CI -0.68 to -0.20) (Poole, Chacko, Wood-Baker and Cates 2006). Reactions to the vaccine are mild and transient. COPD patients are at increased risk of pneumonia and pneumococcal vaccination is recommended (British National Formulary 2008a).

* *Provide information.* The British Lung Foundation publishes patient information about COPD. (available from http://www.lunguk.org/you-and-your-lungs/conditions-and-diseases/copd.htm). They also run 'Breathe Easy' clubs in many areas.

DRUG MANAGEMENT

Bronchodilators

These are the cornerstone of treatment for symptomatic COPD (National Institute for Clinical Excellence 2004; Global Initiative for Obstructive Lung Disease 2003). They reduce breathlessness but have a only small effect on lung function (Sestini, Renzoni, Robinson, *et al.* 2002; Kerstjens, Postma and ten Hacken 2008).

* *Start with a short acting beta$_2$ agonist or anticholinergic.* Both are effective in COPD and there may be a small additive effect (Kerstjens, Postma and ten Hacken 2008). They should be prescribed on an 'as required' basis (National Institute for Clinical Excellence 2004; Global Initiative for Obstructive Lung Disease 2003).

* *Introduce a new drug as a therapeutic trial,* accepting improved lung function or subjective improvement, such as reduced breathlessness, improved exercise capacity or activities of daily living as end points (National Institute for Clinical Excellence 2004; Global Initiative for Obstructive Lung Disease 2003).

* *Add a long-acting bronchodilator* if still symptomatic. Long-acting beta$_2$ agonists or long-acting anticholinergics can produce a small increase in lung function, a reduction in breathlessness, symptom scores and improved quality of life (National Institute for Clinical Excellence 2004; Global Initiative for Obstructive Lung Disease 2003; Kerstjens, Postma and ten Hacken 2008).

* *Consider using a long-acting bronchodilator* in patients who have two or more exacerbations a year. Both long-acting beta$_2$ agonists and long-acting anticholinergics have been shown to reduce exacerbation rates (Appleton, Poole, Smith, et al. 2006; Calverley, Pauwals, Vestbo, *et al.* 2003; Barr, Bourbeau and Camargo 2005; Tashkin, Celli, Senn, *et al.* 2008).

* *Check inhaler technique* before prescribing an inhaler, choosing a device the patient is able to use (Brocklebank, Ram, Wright, *et al.* 2001).

* *Consider using a theophylline* if control is still poor, or in patients unable to use inhaled therapy. They have a modest effect on lung function and variable effect on symptoms and exercise capacity. Side-effects are frequent, limiting their value (National Institute for Clinical Excellence 2004; Global Initiative for Obstructive Lung Disease 2003).

Inhaled steroids

* Inhaled steroids do not reduce the underlying rate of decline in lung function (Burge, Calverley, Jones, *et al.* 2000; Pauwels, Lofdahl, Laitenen, *et al.* 1999).

- In patients with moderate or severe COPD ($FEV_1 < 50\%$ predicted) inhaled steroids have been shown to reduce the exacerbation rate by 25% (Burge, Calverley, Jones, *et al.* 2000).
- Bruising occurs more frequently in patients on inhaled steroids (Pauwels, Lofdahl, Laitenen, *et al.* 1999). There is a potential risk of osteoporosis in patients using high-dose inhaled steroids (National Institute for Clinical Excellence 2004).
- * Prescribe inhaled steroids for patients with moderate/severe COPD ($FEV_1 < 50\%$ predicted) who have two or more exacerbations a year (National Institute for Clinical Excellence 2004; Global Initiative for Obstructive Lung Disease 2003). Doses used in trials have varied (e.g. budesonide 400 mcg b.d. or fluticasone 500 mcg b.d.).

Combination therapy

* *Consider the potential advantages of combination inhalers* (e.g. beta$_2$ agonists + anticholinergics, or long-acting bronchodilators + inhaled steroids) in terms of convenience and cost for patients in whom both drugs are indicated (National Institute for Clinical Excellence 2004; Global Initiative for Obstructive Lung Disease 2003; Burge, Calverley, Jones, *et al.* 2000; Szafranski, Cukier, Ramirez, *et al.* 2003).

Mucolytic therapy

* *Consider mucolytic therapy* in patients with a chronic productive cough. Mucolytic therapy can improve symptoms and reduce exacerbations: the odds ratio for having no exacerbations was 2.13 (95%CI 1.86 to 2.42). Carbocisteine is now available in the UK (Poole and Black 2006).

MODERATE AND SEVERE COPD

Patients with COPD become progressively more disabled. Regular monitoring of symptoms (e.g. with the MRC dyspnoea score) and lung function should prompt increasingly aggressive therapy.

* *Consider referral to a pulmonary rehabilitation unit.* These offer a multidisciplinary, holistic approach to the care of patients with COPD. They are often hospital based, although some programmes are carried out in the community. They have been shown to increase exercise tolerance, relieve breathlessness and improve quality of life even though they do not improve lung function (Lacasse, Wong, Guyatt, *et al.* 1996). The decision to refer should be based on disability (e.g. MRC dyspnoea grade 3) rather than lung function (National Institute for Clinical Excellence 2004).

* *Consider the need for a high-dose bronchodilator* for symptomatic relief. This may conveniently be delivered by multiple doses through a spacer device. Assessment for a home nebulizer should follow the regime provided in the BTS guidelines for nebuliser therapy (British Thoracic Society 1997) and should normally be undertaken by a healthcare professional with a specialized interest in respiratory disease.

* *Consider referral for assessment for long-term oxygen therapy.* In patients who are chronically hypoxic, oxygen therapy for at least 15 hours a day has been shown to improve 5-year survival; OR 0.45 (95%CI 0.25 to 0.81) (Medical Research Council Working Group 1981; Cranston, Crockett, Moss and Alpers 2005). Patients with severe COPD ($FEV_1 < 30\%$ predicted), with oxygen saturation < 92%, with polycythaemia or peripheral oedema should be referred for assessment (National Institute for Clinical Excellence 2004). The criteria depend on lung function, blood gas estimations and the presence of complications. The evidence to support the use of short bursts of oxygen to relieve exercise-induced breathlessness is less clear (National Institute for Clinical Excellence 2004), although some severely dyspnoeic patients may benefit (Garrod, Paul and Wedzicha 2000; Killen and Corris 2000).

* *Look for depression.* It is common in COPD and may require treatment with antidepressants (Light, Merrill, Despars, *et al.* 1985).

* *Advise disabled patients that they may qualify for benefits* (National Institute for Clinical Excellence 2004). Advice may be obtained from the Benefits Agency.

* *Consider the need for practical help* (Gore, Brophy and Greenstone 2000). Provision of appliances such as walking aids, stair lifts, bath aids may be appropriate. Support with domestic care may be needed. A wheelchair and a disabled parking permit may prevent the COPD patient becoming housebound and day-care may provide a break for both the patient and the carer.

* *Remember that patients with severe COPD are severely disabled.* They may have disabling symptoms for many years but rarely receive support from specialist palliative care services (Gore, Brophy and Greenstone 2000).

* *Even though accurate prognosis is difficult, identify patients at risk of dying* (Murray, Pinnock and Sheikh 2006). Repeated hospital admissions, comorbidity, chronic hypoxia, low BMI, and being housebound are all indicators of poor prognosis. Such patients need the same attention to symptom control (especially relief of breathlessness) and support as patients dying of cancer. They may welcome the opportunity to be able to discuss their prognosis and to consider their preferences in the event of future exacerbations.

PALLIATIVE PRESCRIBING FOR PATIENTS WITH END-STAGE COPD (BRITISH NATIONAL FORMULARY 2008B)
(Table 6.4)

Note: Sedatives and cough suppressants are normally contraindicated in COPD. Their role is limited to palliative care where control of distressing symptoms is the priority.

INDICATIONS FOR REFERRAL FOR SPECIALIST ADVICE (NATIONAL INSTITUTE FOR CLINICAL EXCELLENCE 2004)

(a) For an objective diagnosis if spirometry is not available in primary care.
(b) If the diagnosis is not clear (e.g. apparent COPD in a non-smoker).
(c) Aged under 40 or rapid deterioration in symptoms of lung function.
(d) Frequent infective exacerbations.
(e) Onset of cor pulmonale.
(f) Assessment for long-term oxygen therapy or regular nebulizer use.
(g) Assessment for pulmonary rehabilitation
(h) The possibility of industrial disease, e.g. pneumoconiosis, or if there is possibility of an occupational cause for the COPD.

ACUTE EXACERBATIONS OF COPD

Although commonly due to infection, worsening of previously stable COPD may be due to the development of other pathology including lung cancer, left ventricular failure, pulmonary embolism, pneumothorax (National Institute for Clinical Excellence 2004; Global Initiative for Obstructive Lung Disease 2003).

Assessment

The history. Ask about:

(a) onset and duration of current exacerbation;
(b) increased volume and purulence of sputum;

Table 6.4	Palliative prescribing for patients with end-stage COPD	
SYMPTOM	ADVICE	SUGGESTED PRESCRIPTION
Dyspnoea	Opiates, titrating the dose to achieve relief of dyspnoea (Jennings, Davies, Higgins and Broadley 2001) Oxygen may have a small effect on dyspnoea Cool air, e.g. from a fan, sometimes increases comfort	Initial dose: morphine 5 mg 4 hourly
Cough	Opiates	Morphine 5 mg 4 hourly
Excess secretions	Anticholinergics (but take care to avoid the discomfort of a dry mouth)	s.c hyoscine: 400–600 mg 4–6 hourly
Anxiety	Benzodiazepines Note: high doses of beta-agonists can aggravate anxiety	Diazepam 5–10 mg daily
Confusion	Oxygen may reduce confusion due to hypoxia Chlorpromazine or haloperidol may ease confusion and restlessness	Chlorpromazine 25–50 mg 8 hourly Haloperidol 1–3 mg 8 hourly

(c) increased wheeze and shortness of breath;

(d) increasing confusion or decreasing conscious level;

(e) condition when stable, especially the need for long-term oxygen;

(f) severity of previous exacerbations and previous admissions.

The examination. Look for:

(a) cyanosis, confusion, exhaustion, level of activity;

(b) severity of breathlessness, use of accessory muscles, respiratory rate;

(c) peripheral oedema, right heart failure.

Consider:

(a) the patient's social circumstances;

(b) the possibility of other respiratory pathology (e.g. carcinoma or TB);

(c) the possibility of non-respiratory comorbidity. In one study, 40% of patients with an exacerbation of COPD were found to have other conditions (e.g. hypertension, CHD and diabetes); 14% had more than one condition (O'Brien, Guest, Hill, *et al.* 2000).

Initial treatment

* *Bronchodilators* to relieve airway obstruction (National Institute for Clinical Excellence 2004; Global Initiative for Obstructive Lung Disease 2003).

(a) Increase or add a beta$_2$ agonist and/or anticholinergic drugs (Sestini, Renzoni, Robinson, *et al.* 2002; McCrory and Brown 2003).

(b) Check inhaler technique (MDI + spacer may be easiest for the breathless patient).

(c) Consider nebulized therapy for the severely breathless.

* *Antibiotics* if there is increased volume of purulent sputum and increased breathlessness (National Institute for Clinical Excellence 2004; Global Initiative for Obstructive Lung Disease 2003; Anthonisen, Manfreda, Warren, *et al.* 1987; Saint, Bent, Vittinghoff and Grady 1995). Give amoxycillin, tetracycline or erythromycin (British National Formulary 2008c). Prescribers should take account of any guidance issued by local microbiologists (National Institute for Clinical Excellence 2004; Global Initiative for Obstructive Lung Disease 2003).

* *Oral steroids* increase the rate of lung function improvement over the first 72 hours of an exacerbation (Wood-Baker, Gibson, Hannay, *et al.* 2005; Niewoehner, Erbland, Deupree, *et al.* 1999). In general practice, patients with moderate or severe COPD (i.e. baseline FEV$_1$ < 50% predicted) who have a significant increase in breathlessness should be given prednisolone in a dose of 30 mg daily for 7–14 days for severe exacerbations unless contra-indicated (National Institute for Clinical Excellence 2004).

* *Diuretics* may be given for peripheral oedema due to cor pulmonale (see page 156).

Arrange further care

* Consider admission if there is:

(a) confusion, or deteriorating general condition; or

(b) cyanosis, SaO$_2$ < 90%, or the patient is already on long-term oxygen therapy; or

(c) severe breathlessness and poor response to treatment; or

(d) worsening peripheral oedema; or

(e) social circumstances are poor or there is an inability to cope at home.

* *Arrange follow-up* bearing in mind the following points:

(a) failure to make a recovery should prompt a CXR;

(b) smoking cessation should be encouraged and lifestyle advice given;

(c) regular treatment should be optimized.

Hospital at home. About one in four patients presenting to hospital emergency departments with acute exacerbations of COPD can be safely and successfully treated at home with support from respiratory nurses, sometimes called 'intermediate care'. Both patients and carers preferred this 'hospital at home' scheme to inpatient care (Ram, Wedzicha, Wright and Greenstone 2003).

References

Adams, N.P., Bestall, J.C., Malouf, R., et al., 2005. Beclomethasone versus placebo for chronic asthma. Cochrane Database Syst. Rev. (1), CD002738. DOI: 10.1002/14651858.CD002738.pub2.

Agertoft, L., Pedersen, S., 2000. Effect of long-term treatment with inhaled budesonide on adult height in children with asthma. N. Engl. J. Med. 343, 1064–1069.

Anthonisen, N.R., 1994. The Lung Health Study. Effects of smoking intervention and the use of an inhaled anticholinergic bronchodilator on the rate of decline of FEV_1. JAMA 272, 1497–1505.

Anthonisen, N.R., Manfreda, J., Warren, C.P.W., et al., 1987. Antibiotic therapy in exacerbations of chronic obstructive pulmonary disease. Ann. Intern. Med. 106, 196–204.

Appleton, S., Poole, P., Smith, B., et al., 2006. Long-acting beta2-agonists for poorly reversible chronic obstructive pulmonary disease. Cochrane Database Syst. Rev. (3), CD001104. DOI: 10.1002/14651858.CD001104.pub2.

Barr, R.G., Bourbeau, J., Camargo, C.A., 2005. Tiotropium for stable chronic obstructive pulmonary disease. Cochrane Database Syst. Rev. (2), CD002876. DOI: 10.1002/14651858.CD002876.pub2.

Bent, S., Saint, S., Vittinghof, E., Grady, D., 1999. Antibiotics in acute bronchitis: a meta analysis. Am. J. Med. 107, 62–67.

British National Formulary, 2008a. Immunological products and vaccines. British National Formulary September, 56, Section 14, 651–674.

British National Formulary, 2008b. Prescribing in palliative care. British National Formulary September 56, 15–19.

British National Formulary, 2008c. Summary of antibiotic therapy.

British National Formulary September 56, 283–288.

British Thoracic Association, 1982. Death from asthma in two regions of England. BMJ 285, 1251–1255.

British Thoracic Society, 1997. Current best practice for nebuliser treatment. Thorax 52 (S2), S1–106.

British Thoracic Society/Scottish Intercollegiate Guideline Network, 2008. British Guideline on the management of asthma. Thorax 63 (Suppl. 4), i1–i121. Annual updates available http://www.brit-thoracic.org.ukhttp://www.sign.ac.uk.

British Thoracic Society, 2001. Guidelines for the management of community acquired pneumonia in adults. Thorax 56, (IV), 1–64. [Update 2004 is available from www.brit-thoracic.org.uk]

Brocklebank, D., Ram, F., Wright, J., et al., 2001. Comparison of the effectiveness of inhaler devices in asthma and chronic obstructive airways disease: a systematic review of the literature. Health Technol. Assess. 5, 1–149.

Burge, P.S., Calverley, P.M.A., Jones, P.W., et al., on behalf of ISOLDE, 2000. Randomised, double blind, placebo controlled study of fluticasone propionate in patients with moderate to severe chronic obstructive pulmonary disease: the ISOLDE study. BMJ 320, 1297–1303.

Bush, A., 2000. Diagnosis of asthma in children under five. Asthma Gen. Pract. 8 (1), 4–6.

Calverley, P., Pauwals, R., Vestbo, J., et al., for the TRISTAN group, 2003. Combined salmeterol and fluticasone in the treatment of chronic obstructive pulmonary disease: a randomised controlled trial. Lancet 361, 449–456.

CAMP study, 2000. Long term effects of budesonide or nedocromil in children with asthma. The Childhood Asthma Management Program Research Group. N. Engl. J. Med. 343 (15), 1054–1063.

Cane, R.S., Ranganathan, S.C., McKenzie, S.A., 2000. What do parents of wheezy children understand by "wheeze"? Arch. Dis. Child. 82, 327–332.

Cates, C.J., Cates, M.J., 2008. Regular treatment with salmeterol for chronic asthma: serious adverse events. Cochrane Database Syst. Rev. (3), CD006363. DOI: 10.1002/14651858.CD006363.pub2.

Cates, C.J., Cates, M.J., Lasserson, T.J., 2008. Regular treatment with formoterol for chronic asthma: serious adverse events. Cochrane Database Syst. Rev. (4), CD006923. DOI: 10.1002/14651858.CD006923.pub2.

Cates, C.J., Crilly, J.A., Rowe, B.H., 2006. Holding chambers (spacers) versus nebulisers for beta-agonist treatment of acute asthma. Cochrane Database Syst. Rev. (2), CD000052. DOI: 10.1002/14651858.CD000052.pub2.

Cochran, D., 1998. Diagnosing and treating chesty infants. BMJ 316, 1546–1547.

Cochrane, M.G., Bala, M.V., Downs, K.E., et al., 2000. Inhaled corticosteroids for asthma therapy: patient compliance, devices and inhalation technique. Chest 117 (2), 542–550.

Cranston, J.M., Crockett, A., Moss, J., Alpers, J.H., 2005. Domiciliary oxygen for chronic obstructive pulmonary disease. Cochrane Database Syst. Rev. (4), CD001744. DOI: 10.1002/14651858.CD001744.pub2.

Dennis, R.J., Solarte, I., FitzGerald, M., 2008. Asthma in adults. Clinical Evidence. BMJ Publishing Group, London. Available from http://clinicalevidence.bmj.com.

Ducharme, F., Schwartz, Z., Kakuma, R., 2004. Addition of anti-leukotriene agents to inhaled corticosteroids for chronic asthma. Cochrane Database Syst. Rev. (1), CD003133. DOI: 10.1002/14651858.CD003133.pub2.

Ewig, S., Schafer, H., Torres, A., 2000. Severity assessment in community acquired pneumonia. Eur. Respir. J. 16, 1193–1201.

Fahey, T., Smucny, J., Becker, L., Glazier, R., 2004. Antibiotics for acute bronchitis. Cochrane Database Syst. Rev. (4), CD000245. DOI: 10.1002/14651858.CD000245.pub2.

Farr, B.M., Woodhead, M.A., MacFarlane, J.T., et al., 2000. Risk factors for community-acquired pneumonia diagnosed by general practitioners in the community. Respir. Med. 94, 422–427.

Fine, M.J., Smith, M.A., Carson, C.A., et al., 1996. Prognosis and outcome measures of patients with community acquired pneumonia: a meta analysis. JAMA 275, 134–141.

Fletcher, C.M., Elmes, P.C., Fairbairn, M.B., et al., 1959. The significance of respiratory symptoms and the diagnosis of chronic bronchitis in a working population. BMJ 2, 257–266.

Fletcher, C., Peto, R., 1977. The natural history of chronic airflow obstruction. BMJ 1, 1645–1648.

Garrod, R., Paul, E.A., Wedzicha, W., 2000. Supplemental oxygen during pulmonary rehabilitation in patients with COPD with exercise hypoxaemia. Thorax 55, 539–543.

Gibson, P.G., Powell, H., 2004. Written action plans for asthma: an evidence-based review of the key components. Thorax 59, 94–99.

Gibson, P.G., Powell, H., Wilson, A., et al., 2002. Self-management education and regular practitioner review for adults with asthma. The Cochrane Database Syst.

Rev. (3), CD001117. DOI: 10.1002/14651858.CD001117.

Global Initiative for Obstructive Lung Disease, 2003. Global strategy for the diagnosis, management and prevention of chronic obstructive pulmonary disease; NHLBI/WHO workshop report. Online. Available: www.goldcopd.com.

Gonzales, R., Steiner, J.F., Lum, A., Barrett Jr, P.H., 1999. Decreasing antibiotic use in ambulatory practice. Impact of a multidimensional intervention on the treatment of uncomplicated acute bronchitis in adults. JAMA 281, 1512–1519.

Gore, J.M., Brophy, C.J., Greenstone, M.A., 2000. How well do we care for patients with end stage chronic obstructive pulmonary disease (COPD)? A comparison of palliative care and quality of life in COPD and lung cancer. Thorax 55, 1000–1006.

Gøtzsche, P.C., Johansen, H.K., 2008. House dust mite control measures for asthma. Cochrane Database Syst. Rev. (2), CD001187. DOI: 10.1002/14651858.CD001187.pub3.

Haahtela, T., Jarvinen, M., Kava, T., et al., 1991. Comparison of a beta agonist, terbutaline, with an inhaled corticosteroid, budesonide, in newly detected asthma. N. Engl. J. Med. 325, 388–392.

Haughney, J., Barnes, G., Partridge, M., Cleland, J., 2004. The Living & Breathing study: a study of patients' views of asthma and its treatment. Prim. Care Respir. J. 13, 28–35.

Haughney, J., Price, D., Kaplan, A., et al., 2008. Achieving asthma control in practice: Understanding the reasons for poor control. Respir. Med. 102, 1681–1693.

Health Protection Agency for Infections, 2008. Tuberculosis in the UK: Annual report on tuberculosis surveillance in the UK 2008, London.

Holmes, W.F., Macfarlane, J.T., Macfarlane, R.M., et al., 1997. The

influence of antibiotics and other factors on reconsultation for acute lower respiratory tract illness in primary care. Br. J. Gen. Pract. 47, 815–818.

Jennings, A.L., Davies, A.N., Higgins, J.P.T., Broadley, K.E., 2001. Opioids for the palliation of breathlessness in terminal illness. Cochrane Database Syst. Rev. (3), CD002066. DOI: 10.1002/14651858.CD002066.

Joos, S., Miksch, A., Szecsenyi, J., et al., 2008. Montelukast as add-on therapy to inhaled corticosteroids in the treatment of mild to moderate asthma: a systematic review. Thorax 63, 453–462.

Kerstjens, H., Postma, D., Ten Hacken, N., 2008. COPD. Clinical Evidence, BMJ Publishing Group, London.

Killen, J.W.W., Corris, P.A., 2000. A pragmatic assessment of the placement of oxygen when given for exercise induced dyspnoea. Thorax 55, 544–546.

Lacasse, Y., Guyatt, G.H., Goldstein, R.S., 1997. The components of a respiratory rehabilitation program. A systematic overview. Chest 111, 1077–1088.

Lacasse, Y., Wong, E., Guyatt, G.H., et al., 1996. Meta analysis of respiratory rehabilitation in chronic obstructive pulmonary disease. Lancet 348, 1115–1119.

Light, R.W., Merrill, E.J., Despars, J.A., et al., 1985. Prevalence of depression and anxiety in patients with COPD: relationship to functional capacity. Chest 87, 35–38.

Lipworth, B.J., 1999. Systemic adverse effects of inhaled corticosteroid therapy: a systematic review and meta-analysis. Arch. Intern. Med. 159, 941–955.

Loeb, M., 2008. Community Acquired Pneumonia. Clinical Evidence. BMJ Publishing Group, London. Available: http://clinicalevidence.bmj.com.

McCrory, D.C., Brown, C.D., 2003. Anticholinergic bronchodilators versus beta2-sympathomimetic agents for acute exacerbations of chronic obstructive pulmonary disease. Cochrane Database Syst. Rev. (1), CD003900. DOI: 10.1002/14651858.CD0.

Macfarlane, J.T., Colville, A., Guion, A., et al., 1993. Prospective study of aetiology and outcome of adult lower-respiratory-tract infections in the community. Lancet 341, 511–514.

Macfarlane, J., Holmes, W., Gard, P., et al., 2001. Prospective study of the incidence, aetiology and outcome of adult lower respiratory tract illness in the community. Thorax 56, 109–114.

Macfarlane, J.T., Holmes, W.F., Macfarlane, R.M., 1997. Reducing reconsultations for acute lower respiratory illness with an information leaflet: a randomised controlled study of patients in primary care. Br. J. Gen. Pract. 47, 719–722.

Medical Research Council Working Group, 1981. Long term domiciliary oxygen therapy in chronic hypoxic cor pulmonale complicating chronic bronchitis and emphysema. Lancet I, 681–686.

Metlay, J.P., Kapoor, W.N., Fine, M.J., 1997. Does this patient have community acquired pneumonia? Diagnosing pneumonia by history and physical examination. JAMA 278, 1440–1445.

Mohan, G., Harrison, B.D., Badminton, R.M., et al., 1996. A confidential enquiry into deaths caused by asthma in an English health region: implications for general practice. Br. J. Gen. Pract. 46 (410), 529–532.

Mossad, S.B., Mackin, M.L., Medendorp, S.V., Mason, P., 1996. Zinc gluconate lozenges for treating the common cold. Ann. Intern. Med. 125, 81–88.

Murray, S., Pinnock, H., Sheikh, A., 2006. Palliative care for people with COPD: we need to meet the challenge. Prim. Care. Respir. J. 15, 362–364.

National Collaborating Centre for Chronic Conditions, 2006. Tuberculosis: Clinical Diagnosis and Management of Tuberculosis, and Measures for its Prevention and Control. Royal College of Physicians, London. Available: www.nice.org.uk.

National Institute for Clinical Excellence, 2000. Guidance on the use of inhaler systems (devices) in children under the age of 5 years with chronic asthma. Technology Appraisal Guidance No. 10 http://www.nice.org.uk.

National Institute for Clinical Excellence, 2002a. Inhaler devices for routine treatment of chronic asthma in older children (aged 5–15 years). Technology Appraisal Guidance No. 38 http://www.nice.org.uk.

National Institute for Clinical Excellence, 2002b. Guidance on the use of nicotine replacement therapy (NRT) and bupropion for smoking cessation. NICE Technology Appraisal Guidance No.39. 2002. National Institute for Clinical Excellence, London.

National Institute for Clinical Excellence, 2004. National clinical guideline management of chronic obstructive pulmonary disease in adults primary and secondary care. Thorax 59 (Suppl. 1), S1–S232.

National Institute for Health and Clinical Excellence, 2008. Prescribing of antibiotics for self-limiting respiratory tract infections in adults and children in primary care. Available from www.nice.org.uk.

Nelson, H.S., Weiss, S.T., Bleecker, E.R., et al., and the SMART study group, 2006. The salmeterol multicenter asthma research trial: a comparison of usual pharmacotherapy for asthma or usual pharmacotherapy plus salmeterol. Chest 129, 15–26.

Ni Chroinin, M., Greenstone, I.R., Ducharme, F.M., 2004. Addition of inhaled long-acting beta2-agonists to inhaled steroids as first line therapy for persistent asthma in steroid-naive adults. Cochrane Database Syst. Rev. (4), CD005307. DOI: 10.1002/14651858.CD005307.

Niewoehner, D.E., Erbland, M.L., Deupree, R.H., et al., 1999. Effect of systemic glucocorticoids on exacerbations of chronic obstructive pulmonary disease. N. Engl. J. Med. 340, 1941–1947.

O'Brien, C., Guest, P.J., Hill, S.L., et al., 2000. Physiological and radiological characterisation of patients diagnosed with chronic obstructive pulmonary disease in primary care. Thorax 55, 635–642.

O'Driscoll, B.R., Howard, L.S., Davison, A., on behalf of the British Thoracic Society, 2008. BTS guidelines for emergency oxygen use in adult patients. Thorax 63 (Suppl 4), vi1–vi73.

Pauwels, R.A., Lofdahl, C.G., Laitenen, L.A., et al., for EUROSCOP, 1999. Long term treatment with inhaled budesonide in persons with mild chronic obstructive pulmonary disease who continue smoking. N. Engl. J. Med. 340, 1948–1953.

Pauwels, R.A., Lofdahl, C.G., Postma, D.S., et al., 1997. (FACET) Effect of inhaled formoterol and budesonide on exacerbations of asthma. N. Engl. J. Med. 337, 1405–1411.

Pearson, M., Bucknall, C., 1999. Measuring Clinical Outcome in Asthma: A Patient Focussed Approach. R. Col. Physicians (July), London.

Pinnock, H., Adlem, L., Gaskin, S., et al., 2007. Accessibility, clinical effectiveness and practice costs of providing a telephone option for routine asthma reviews:

controlled implementation study. Br. J. Gen. Pract. 57, 714–722.

Pinnock, H., Bawden, R., Proctor, S., et al., 2003. Accessibility, acceptability, and effectiveness in primary care of routine telephone review of asthma: pragmatic, randomised controlled trial. BMJ 326, 477–479.

Pinnock, H., Fletcher, M., Holmes, S., et al., 2010. Setting the standard for routine asthma consultations: a discussion of the aims, process and outcomes of reviewing people with asthma in primary care. Prim Care Respir J 19, 75–83.

Poole, P., Black, P.N., 2006. Mucolytic agents for chronic bronchitis or chronic obstructive pulmonary disease. Cochrane Database Syst. Rev. (3), CD001287. DOI: 10.1002/14651858.CD001287.pub2.

Poole, P., Chacko, E.E., Wood-Baker, R., Cates, C.J., 2006. Influenza vaccine for patients with chronic obstructive pulmonary disease. Cochrane Database Syst. Rev. (1), CD002733. DOI: 10.1002/14651858.CD002733.pub2.

Ram, F.S.F., Wedzicha, J.A., Wright, J., Greenstone, M., 2003. Hospital at home for acute exacerbations of chronic obstructive pulmonary disease. Cochrane Database Syst. Rev. (4), CD003573. DOI: 10.1002/14651858.CD003573.

Roberts, C.M., Bulger, J.R., Melchor, R., et al., 1993. Value of pulse oximetry in screening for long term oxygen therapy requirement. Eur. Respir. J. 6, 559–562.

Rowe, B.H., Spooner, C., Ducharme, F., et al., 2001. Early emergency department treatment of acute asthma with systemic corticosteroids. Cochrane Database Syst. Rev. (1), CD002178. DOI: 10.1002/14651858.CD002178.

Rowe, B.H., Spooner, C., Ducharme, F., et al., 2007. Corticosteroids for preventing relapse following acute exacerbations of asthma. Cochrane Database Syst. Rev. (3), CD000195. DOI: 10.1002/14651858.CD000195.pub2.

Saint, S., Bent, S., Vittinghoff, E., Grady, D., 1995. Antibiotics in chronic obstructive pulmonary disease exacerbations: a meta-analysis. JAMA 274, 1131–1132.

Scadding, G.K., Durham, S.R., Mirakian, R., et al., 2008. BSACI guidelines for the management of allergic and non-allergic rhinitis. Clin. Exp. Allergy 38, 19–42.

Scottish Intercollegiate Guidelines Network, 2002. Community Management of Lower Respiratory Tract Infection in Adults. SIGN 59 Edinburgh. Available: www.sign.ac.uk.

Sestini, P., Renzoni, E., Robinson, S., et al., 2002. Short-acting beta2-agonists for stable chronic obstructive pulmonary disease. Cochrane Database Syst. Rev. (3), CD001495. DOI: 10.1002/14651858.CD001495.

Sly, P.D., Cahill, P., Willet, K., Burton, P., 1994. Accuracy of mini peak flow meters in indicating changes in lung function in children with asthma. BMJ 308, 572–574.

Smucny, J.J., Becker, L.A., Glazier, R.H., McIsaac, W., 1998. Are antibiotics effective treatment for acute bronchitis? A meta analysis. J. Fam. Pract. 47, 453–460.

Szafranski, W., Cukier, A., Ramirez, G., et al., 2003. Efficacy and safety of budesonide/formoterol in the management of chronic obstructive pulmonary disease. Eur. Respir. J. 21, 74–81.

Taramarcaz, P., Gibson, P.G., 2003. Intranasal corticosteroids for asthma control in people with coexisting asthma and rhinitis. Cochrane Database Syst. Rev. (3), CD003570. DOI: 10.1002/14651858.CD003570.

Tasche, M.J.A., Uijen, J.H.J.M., Bernsen, R.M.D., et al., 2000. Inhaled disodium cromoglycate (DSCG) as maintenance therapy in children with asthma: a systematic review. Thorax 55, 913–920.

Tashkin, D.P., Celli, B., Senn, S., et al., for the UPLIFT Study Investigators. 2008. A 4-year trial of tiotropium in chronic obstructive pulmonary disease. N. Engl. J. Med. 359, 1543–1554.

Thomas, M., Price, D., 2008. Impact of co-morbidities on asthma. Expert Rev. Clin. Immunol. 4, 731–742.

van Schayck, O.C.P., Pinnock, H., Ostrem, A., Litt, J., for the IPCRG. 2008. IPCRG Consensus statement: Tackling the smoking epidemic -practical guidance for primary care. Prim. Care. Respir. J. 17, 185–193.

van Staa, T.P., Cooper, C., Leufkens, H.G.M., et al., 2003. The use of inhaled corticosteroids in the United Kingdom and the Netherlands. Respir. Med. 97, 578–585.

Walters, E.H., Walters, J.A.E., Gibson, P.G., Jones, P., 2003. Inhaled short acting beta2-agonist use in chronic asthma: regular versus as needed treatment. Cochrane Database Syst. Rev. (1), CD001285. DOI: 10.1002/14651858.CD001285.

Wolf, F.M., Guevara, J.P., Grum, C.M., et al., 2002. Educational interventions for asthma in children. Cochrane Database Syst. Rev. (4), CD000326. DOI: 10.1002/14651858.CD000326.

Wood-Baker, R.R., Gibson, P.G., Hannay, M., et al., 2005. Systemic corticosteroids for acute exacerbations of chronic obstructive pulmonary disease. Cochrane Database Syst. Rev. (1), CD001288. DOI: 10.1002/14651858.CD001288.pub2.

Chapter 7

Gastroenterological problems

CHAPTER CONTENTS

DYSPEPSIA

For details of the diagnosis of dyspepsia see *Evidence-based Diagnosis in Primary Care* by A. F. Polmear (editor) published by Butterworth-Heinemann, 2008.

GUIDELINES AND REVIEWS

NICE Clinical Guideline. 2004. Dyspepsia - management of dyspepsia in adults in primary care, August 2004, http://www.nice.org.uk
    SIGN Dyspepsia. 2003. A National Clinical Guideline, March 2003, www.sign.ac.uk
    BSG. 2002. *Dyspepsia Management Guidelines.* British Society of Gastroenterology, January 2002
    Delaney BC, Innes MA, Deeks J, *et al.* 2001. Initial management strategies for dyspepsia (Cochrane Review). In: The Cochrane Library, Issue 3. Update Software, Oxford.
    Logan R, Delaney B. 2001. Implications of dyspepsia for the NHS. BMJ 323, 675–677
    DoH. 2000. *Guidelines for Urgent Referral of Patients with Suspected Cancer.* London: Department of Health. Online. Available: www.doh.gov.uk/cancer/referral.htm

WHICH PATIENTS SHOULD HAVE AN INITIAL ENDOSCOPY WHEN PRESENTING WITH DYSPEPSIA?

● Patients who consult with dyspepsia have no more symptoms than those with dyspepsia who do not consult; but they do have more 'life events' and are more likely to fear that they have a life-threatening condition (Logan and Delaney 2001).

- Clinical diagnosis without investigation is unreliable (Danish Dyspepsia Study Group 2001); even gastroenterologists are correct in less than half their cases. Division of patients with dyspepsia into subgroups according to symptoms does not predict pathology at endoscopy (Agreus and Talley 1997).
- Endoscopy is needed to make a clear diagnosis but resources are limited and must be reserved in the first instance for those most likely to have positive findings, e.g. carcinoma of the stomach or oesophagus, peptic ulcer, gastritis, duodenitis, oesophagitis or stricture.
- Gastric and oesophageal carcinomas are more common in those aged > 55. Peptic ulcer can occur at any age but when it occurs in older patients, especially those on NSAIDs, complications are more likely.
- 'Alarm features' have been shown to be sensitive, but not specific, in screening for upper GI carcinoma. In a UK study of 1852 patients referred to a rapid access upper GI cancer service, only dysphagia, weight loss, and age > 55 were independent significant predictors of cancer. Furthermore, age > 55 was only a significant predictor if at least one other alarm feature was present (anaemia, anorexia, vomiting, dysphagia, weight loss or 'high risk features'). Simple dyspepsia, even if new or continuous, was *inversely* correlated with the finding of cancer in these older patients (Kapoor, Bassi, Sturgess and Bodger 2004). Most patients with dyspepsia will respond to a therapy of acid suppression, *H. pylori* eradication and possibly use of prokinetic drugs. This removes the need, in responders, for a precise endoscopic diagnosis. Short-term response does not, however, remove the possibility of serious underlying disease. Even gastric carcinomas may be masked initially by treatment with a PPI (Bramble, Suvakovic and Hungin 2000).

CONTROVERSY OVER THE NEED FOR ENDOSCOPY IN PATIENTS > 55 YEARS OLD WITH DYSPEPSIA

In the UK GPs have guidance from three sources which conflict. They all recommend endoscopy for a patient with alarm features, regardless of age. They differ on the management of the patient aged 55 and over. They are:

1. The National Institute for Clinical Excellence, which recommends that patients without alarm features do not routinely need endoscopy but that referral to a specialist might be considered in patients > 55 whose symptoms persist despite acid suppression and eradication, if present, of *H. pylori*, but only if they also have one of the following: previous GU or surgery, continuing need for an NSAID, a raised risk of gastric carcinoma, or anxiety about cancer (NICE 2004).

2. The SIGN guideline, which recommends that patients > 55 with persistent or recurrent symptoms after acid suppression who are either *H. pylori* negative, or whose symptoms continue despite confirmed eradication of *H. pylori*, should be considered for referral (Scottish Intercollegiate Guidelines Network 2003).

3. A later NICE guideline (no. 27, Referral for Suspected Cancer, 2005) which recommends urgent referral for any patient aged 55 and over with unexplained and persistent recent-onset dyspepsia. Their recommendations for urgent referral of those with alarm symptoms are as given below.

INDICATIONS FOR ENDOSCOPY AT FIRST PRESENTATION (NICE 2004)

Refer for urgent endoscopy patients with 'alarm features':

- gastrointestinal bleeding (admit);
- progressive dysphagia (prior barium swallow is needed);
- unintentional weight loss;
- persistent vomiting;
- epigastric mass;
- suspicious barium meal;
- iron deficiency anaemia.

INDICATIONS FOR REFERRAL IF THE PATIENT FAILS TO RESPOND TO MEDICAL TREATMENT (DERIVED FROM ALL THREE GUIDELINES ABOVE)

- Aged 55 or over with:
  (a) a recent onset of dyspepsia, or with continuous symptoms or with a change in symptoms; or
  (b) other risk factors for cancer or anxiety about cancer.

■ Of any age with:

(a) risk factors for peptic ulcer, e.g. family history or NSAID use;

(b) with severe symptoms;

(c) with a past history of gastric ulcer or previous gastric surgery;

(d) with a family history of upper GI cancer in > two first degree relatives;

(e) with a history of Barrett's oesophagus;

(f) with pernicious anaemia; or

(g) with known dysplasia, atrophic gastritis or intestinal metaplasia.

✳ Check Hb in all the above.

✳ Give antacids while referral is proceeding. Try where at all possible not to give acid-suppression prior to endoscopy but if the endoscopy is likely to be delayed for more than 4 weeks, consider giving a course of acid suppression for 2–4 weeks but complete the course at least 4 weeks before the endoscopy to avoid masking the pathology.

✳ If endoscopy is negative and symptoms do not respond to acid suppression, consider alternative investigations: ultrasound of the gall bladder and pancreas, serum amylase or lipase, and LFTs during an exacerbation of pain. Consider other causes of abdominal pain.

PATIENTS WITHOUT ALARM SYMPTOMS

The key facts are:

● One third of the population in the Western world admits to dyspepsia. Of these only a quarter seek medical help and of these, in the UK, 10% are referred for investigation. Of those who are endoscoped only 2% will have a gastric cancer, although only 30% will have normal results and be diagnosed as having non-ulcer dyspepsia (NICE 2004).

● All causes of dyspepsia are likely to respond to antacids and acid suppression.

● *H. pylori* eradication is likely to be helpful in patients with DU, GU, gastritis, duodenitis and, marginally, in non-ulcer dyspepsia. In a 6-year follow-up, eradication of *H. pylori* was more effective than initial endoscopy in patients with dyspepsia, resulting in fewer endoscopies and less use of antisecretory medication (Lassen, Hallas and Schaffalitzky de Muckadell 2004).

NICE recommends a step-wise approach, starting with a review of lifestyle and medication, moving to the following, in order, if the patient fails to respond or relapses: full dose PPI for 4 weeks; testing for *H. pylori* and eradicating if positive; changing to an H_2 receptor antagonist or a prokinetic drug for 4 weeks; consideration of referral to a specialist.

THE MANAGEMENT OF UNINVESTIGATED DYSPEPSIA

Cover the first three points in all patients, then move through steps 1 to 5 in sequence, stopping when an adequate response is obtained. A UK trial has shown that empirical acid suppression and 'test and treat' are equally good first line strategies for undiagnosed dyspepsia (Delaney, Qume, Moayyedi, *et al.* 2008). Steps 2 and 3 below could, therefore, be reversed.

✳ Explore the patient's fears and reassure as far as is justified. Worry about the seriousness of symptoms is a significant factor in bringing patients with dyspepsia to their GP. The perspective of the patient and doctor may differ widely (Lydeard and Jones 1989).

✳ Advise the patient to take an antacid and to stop smoking, and reduce coffee and alcohol intake, if appropriate. There is little evidence supporting changes in lifestyle and relief from upper GI symptoms but it would seem sensible especially when there are other potential health gains.

✳ Check that the patient is not taking a drug that can cause dyspepsia: e.g. aspirin or an NSAID, a calcium antagonist, a nitrate, a theophylline, a bisphosphonate or a steroid.

1. When symptoms are mild, wait 2 weeks to judge the effect of the antacid.

2. If symptoms are more severe, or there has been no response to antacid, give a proton pump inhibitor in full dosage for 4 weeks. ('Empirical acid suppression')

3. Test for *H. pylori* and eradicate if positive. ('Test and treat')

4. Prescribe a prokinetic agent, e.g. metoclopramide or, especially in the younger female, domperidone, both of which will facilitate gastric emptying.

5. Consider a trial of an H_2 receptor antagonist.

6. Consider referral to a specialist for a precise diagnosis and for a decision about the long-term strategy.

PATIENTS WHO RESPOND TO ACID SUPPRESSION BUT THEN RELAPSE

- Review whether any change can be made in lifestyle or use of other medications.
- Prescribe the PPI at low dose and plan with the patient how it can be used. Many patients can reduce their PPI use by using it as required rather than regularly.

TESTING FOR *H. PYLORI*

* Use a breath test, or, if unavailable, a stool antigen test. The bedside dipstick test on whole blood is unreliable (Weijnen, de Wit, Numans, *et al.* 2001) and laboratory serology has a lower positive predictive value (64%) than breath testing (88%) and stool antigen tests (84%) (NICE 2004).
* Stop a proton pump inhibitor (PPI) 2 weeks before the breath test and any antibacterial drug 4 weeks before.
* Wait 4 weeks after eradication before repeating the breath test. Stool antigen and serology cannot be used to assess the response to eradication. Serology stays positive for 6–12 months.

Eradicating *H. pylori*

Give 1 week of:
(a) PPI at double the standard dose (in two divided doses); and
(b) amoxicillin 1 g b.d.; and
(c) clarithromycin 500 mg b.d.
If the patient is intolerant of clarithromycin or amoxicillin, either can be changed to metronidazole 400 mg b.d. Alternatively, metronidazole may be used in place of amoxicillin first line, provided the patient is not from an area of high metronidazole resistance (e.g. a developing country or a UK inner city with a large immigrant community).

PATIENTS IN WHOM THE DIAGNOSIS HAS BEEN ESTABLISHED

Duodenal ulcer

* Test for *H. pylori* and eradicate if positive (see above) Only continue the PPI If there has been bleeding from the ulcer or perforation, in which case continue full dose PPI for a second week at the same dosage.

* If *H. pylori* negative, continue full dose PPI for 1–2 months.
* If the ulcer occurred in a patient taking an NSAID or aspirin, continue full dose PPI for 2 months, then eradicate *H. pylori* if present.
* Only confirm that eradication is successful in complicated or refractory ulcers. An absence of dyspeptic symptoms has been shown to correlate well with *H. pylori* eradication (Phull, Halliday, Price and Jacyna 1996).
* *Patients who are still breath-test positive or who relapse after successful* H. pylori *eradication* may have an antibiotic-resistant organism or may need long-term acid suppression. Refer to a gastroenterologist.

Gastric ulcer

* Test for *H. pylori* and eradicate if positive (see box).
* If negative, or if the patient was taking an NSAID, continue the PPI for 2 months.
* Ensure that follow-up endoscopy is performed until the ulcer is healed, and that repeated *H. pylori* testing confirms eradication. If *H. pylori* is still present prescribe a different eradication regimen.
* If symptoms recur after the ulcer has been shown to be healed and *H. pylori* eradicated decide, according to the severity of the symptoms, whether to control them with low-dose acid suppression or whether to retest for *H. pylori* and re-endoscope.

NSAID–induced peptic ulcer

* Stop the NSAID and treat the ulcer as above (but with *H. pylori* eradication only if testing for *H. pylori* is positive); or
* Continue the NSAID in patients who cannot do without it, and prescribe a healing dose of a PPI followed by a maintenance dose for as long as the patient continues to take the NSAID. *H. pylori* testing and eradication is unlikely to benefit the patient, who would anyway remain on long-term acid suppression (Seager and Hawkey 2001). Alternatives for ulcer prevention are misoprostol 800 mg daily or an H_2-receptor antagonist at double dose (Rostom, Dube, Wells, *et al.* 2002).

* Consider use of a COX-2 selective inhibitor or another newer NSAID, which is less toxic to gastric mucosa. The National Institute for Clinical Excellence (NICE) warns that even COX-2 selective inhibitors should be used with caution in patients with a history of peptic ulcer, of GI bleeding or of perforation. NICE's recommendations for the use of COX-2 selective inhibitors are summarized in the box below.

RECOMMENDATIONS ON THE USE OF COX-2 SELECTIVE INHIBITORS (NICE 2001A)

Use them only in patients at high risk of serious adverse GI adverse effects:

(a) age 65 and over;

(b) on concomitant medication which increases the risk of upper GI adverse effects (but not low-dose aspirin);

(c) with serious comorbidity; or

(d) when prolonged use at maximum dosage is contemplated.

In a patient at high risk of peptic ulceration they should be combined with a gastroprotective agent.

Note: Rofecoxib was withdrawn by the manufacturer in September 2004 because of an increase in the rates of myocardial infarction and stroke in patients taking it for > 18 months in the APPROVe study. The possibility that the excess morbidity was due to the tendency of all COX-2s to increase platelet aggregation and vasoconstriction has raised serious doubts about the safety of all drugs of this class (FitzGerald 2004).

* Peptic ulcer in a patient requiring long-term prophylactic aspirin. Reduce the aspirin dose to 75 mg daily and add a PPI. This gives a lower risk of GI bleeding than clopidogrel.

* Erosive duodenitis is part of the spectrum of duodenal ulcer disease and should be treated in the same ways as duodenal ulcer. Non-erosive duodenitis and gastritis should be treated symptomatically without *H. pylori* eradication, even if they are *H. pylori* positive.

Patients on long-term acid suppression for a proven peptic ulcer

* Consider *H. pylori* eradication, without further investigation, as for newly diagnosed patients (Hippisley-Cox and Pringle 1997).

Established diagnosis of non-ulcer dyspepsia

● This is the final diagnosis in 90% of patients with dyspepsia under the age of 45 and 75% of such patients who are *H. pylori* positive (Briggs, Sculpher, Logan, *et al.* 1996).

● The benefit from acid suppression is modest (Redstone, Barrowman and Veldhuyzen Van Zanten 2001). PPIs are slightly more effective than H_2 antagonists (Talley, Phung and Kalantar 2001).

● The benefit from *H. pylori* eradication in those who are positive is small with a mere 9% (95% CI 4% to 40%) reduction in the number of patients still suffering after treatment (Briggs, Sculpher, Logan, *et al.* 1996). Meta-analysis has confirmed this small benefit (Moayyedi, Deeks, Talley, *et al.* 2003).

* Many patients with functional or non-ulcer dyspepsia may also have reflux symptoms. In part these symptoms may well be related to delayed gastric emptying. Many of them will also have other symptoms, especially bloating as well as classical symptoms of IBS (see below). It is worth spending time looking for such symptoms although inevitably a significant number may still be referred for investigation.

* Continue the general measures above, with extra attention to an explanation of the nature of the condition.

* Explore whether psychological factors are playing a part.

* Test for *H. pylori* and eradicate it if present.

* Give antacids for acid-like symptoms or a prokinetic agent for dysmotility-like symptoms.

* Control more severe symptoms with short courses of acid suppression. Before repeating or continuing acid suppression, remember that the placebo response in non-ulcer dyspepsia is marked (MeReC 1998). Consider an antidepressant, even in patients who are not clinically depressed.

* Consider referral for counselling or psychotherapy for those in whom the psychological component appears to be large (Soo, Moayyedi, Deeks, *et al.* 2001).

GASTRO-OESOPHAGEAL REFLUX DISEASE (GORD)

For details of the diagnosis of heartburn see *Evidence-based Diagnosis in Primary Care* by A. F. Polmear (editor) published by Butterworth-Heinemann, 2008.

- The diagnosis is made either by a classical history or by the finding of oesophagitis on endoscopy.
- A normal endoscopy does not exclude the diagnosis. As many as 50% of patients whose symptoms are due to reflux will have no visible oesophagitis.
- Occasionally patients with duodenal or pre-pyloric channel ulcers may present with predominantly reflux symptoms as a result of pylorospasm.
- Symptoms of reflux, in the absence of alarm symptoms, may be treated empirically without endoscopy.
- Endoscopy is, however, necessary for the diagnosis of Barrett's oesophagus and stricture. These patients need long-term acid suppression but the role of regular endoscopy in the management of Barrett's oesophagus is controversial. Otherwise, the aim in patients with or without oesophagitis is to control symptoms.
- GORD is the one type of dyspepsia which does not improve with *H. pylori* eradication. It does not, however, appear to worsen it, despite earlier fears based on observational studies (Delaney and Moayyedi 2004). There is a case for recommending eradication in a patient who is being managed without endoscopy in case the patient has coincidental peptic ulceration (Fox and Forgacs 2006).

* Advise the patient to:
  (a) elevate the bed head by 6 inches. Encourage the patient to sleep in the left lateral decubitus position;
  (b) stop smoking;
  (c) avoid fatty foods (which delay gastric emptying), salty foods, onions, peppermint, citrus fruits, tomatoes and other foods known to make symptoms worse. However, alcohol and tea are not associated with reflux and heavy coffee drinking is associated with less reflux; a result which may be due to confounding (Nilsson, Johnsen, Ye, *et al.* 2004).

  (d) lose weight if obese;
  (e) avoid aspirin and other NSAIDs;
  (f) avoid lying down with a full stomach, and preferably eat 4 hours before going to bed.
  Of these, only elevation of the head of the bed, left lateral decubitus position and weight loss, have evidence to show that they improve reflux symptoms (Kaltenbach, Crockett and Gerson 2006).

Mild symptoms:

* 'Step-up' treatment as follows, moving to the next step if the previous one fails to control symptoms:
  1. *Antacids and/or alginates* in adequate doses after meals and at night. Raft antacids cost about four times as much, but appear to give better relief of symptoms than antacids alone.
  2. *Acid suppression:* a full dose PPI daily for 4 weeks. This controls symptoms in 83% and heals oesophagitis in 78%, as opposed to 60% and 50% for H_2 antagonists. *Continuous* use of a PPI gives the best results in heartburn (Howden, Henning, Huang, *et al.* 2001) but is not recommended in the UK for mild–moderate symptoms for reasons of cost (see NICE guidance below). If there is an inadequate response, see 'Severe symptoms' below.
  3. *Prokinetic agents* (metoclopramide or domperidone) may be helpful in individual patients, either alone or in combination with a proton pump inhibitor.

Severe symptoms:

* 'Step-down' treatment, starting with a full dose PPI, and reducing the dose or the frequency, then reducing to an H_2 antagonist or antacid as symptoms resolve. Exactly how to do this depends on the response to the initial 4 weeks of PPI:

* *Good response*: stop the PPI, recommend antacids and advise the patient to return if symptoms return.

* *Good response followed by relapse:* full dose PPI for a further 4 weeks then either a PPI on demand, or a continuous PPI at the lowest effective dose.

* *Partial response:* 4 more weeks of full dose PPI, then either a PPI on demand, or a continuous PPI at the lowest effective dose.

* *Poor response:* 4 more weeks of PPI at double dose. If response is still poor refer for endoscopy.

REFERRAL FOR ENDOSCOPY

✱ Refer patients who do not respond to medical treatment and those with alarm symptoms or signs (Fox and Forgacs 2006):
  - GI bleeding;
  - iron deficiency anaemia;
  - unexplained weight loss;
  - dysphagia;
  - persistent vomiting;
  - epigastric mass.
✱ Refer more readily if the patient is older, e.g. > 55.
✱ Then give a PPI long term if endoscopy shows erosive oesophagitis, stricture, bleeding, Barrett's oesophagitis, or the patient is on an NSAID and needs to continue it.

SURGERY

✱ Refer those who fail to respond to a continuous PPI to a surgeon able to perform laparoscopic fundoplication. Consider referral for those who do respond but in whom symptoms return as soon as the PPI is discontinued. A UK study of 357 patients with symptoms of GORD for at least a year (the REFLUX trial) found that those allocated to surgery had better relief of symptoms and better quality of life, than those randomized to medical treatment (Grant, Wileman, Ramsay, *et al.* 2008a). After 12 months, 90% of those on medical treatment were still taking medication against 14% of those who had surgery. However, surgery is more expensive and may not be cost-effective in those who can be managed by continuous PPI treatment (Grant, Wileman, Ramsay, *et al.* 2008b).
✱ Also consider referral in those in whom reflux is associated with respiratory symptoms, and in those in whom a hiatus hernia is causing mechanical problems.

Barrett's oesophagus

This occurs as a consequence of GORD and carries a risk of oesophageal adenocarcinoma that is > 30 times that of the general population. However, even those with Barrett's oesophagus develop carcinoma at the rate of only 0.5% per year. In a study of 143 patients with Barrett's an annual endoscopy was performed for 10 years and only one carcinoma was detected (MacDonald, Wicks and Playford 2000). Such surveillance is probably not justified and referral of patients with chronic GORD specifically for the detection of Barrett's oesophagus certainly is not (Spechler 2003).

GUIDANCE ON THE USE OF PPIs FROM THE NATIONAL INSTITUTE FOR CLINICAL EXCELLENCE (NICE 2001B

PPIs are appropriate:
(a) When a patient on an NSAID must continue it and has a documented NSAID-induced ulcer. The dose should be stepped down for maintenance.
(b) As part of an *H. pylori* eradication programme.
(c) For GORD, either where symptoms are severe or with proven pathology (oesophageal ulceration or Barrett's oesophagus). The dose should be 'stepped down' except in cases of complicated oesphagitis (stricture, ulcer or haemorrhage).
(d) In other situations, including undiagnosed dyspepsia, a short course may be indicated where other symptomatic treatment has failed.

IRRITABLE BOWEL SYNDROME (IBS)

GUIDELINE

National Institute for Health and Clinical Excellence. *Irritable Bowel Syndrome in Adults: Diagnosis and Management of Irritable Bowel Syndrome in Primary Care: NICE Clinical Guideline 61, 2008. Available:* www.nice.org.uk

● Irritable bowel syndrome is a functional disorder of the whole GI tract characterized by abdominal pain and bloating with disturbed bowel function, and which may be associated with dysmotility of the upper GI tract. The GP can and should make a positive diagnosis of IBS, and so avoid the overinvestigation that tends to increase the patient's excessive concern about the symptoms. For details of the diagnosis of irritable bowel syndrome see *Evidence-based Diagnosis in Primary Care* by A. F. Polmear (editor) published by Butterworth-Heinemann, 2008.
● Symptoms of IBS are present in up to 20% of adults, although up to 75% of them never consult.

- IBS is often associated with symptoms from outside the GI tract: lethargy, backache, headache, dyspareunia and an irritable bladder.
- Anecdotal evidence suggests that an episode of infective diarrhoea may trigger the onset of symptoms.
- Anxiety and depression are more common in patients with IBS than in the normal population, although the symptoms are often masked. Even those without an affective disorder tend to show an excessive concern about their symptoms.

PATIENTS WHO CAN BE DIAGNOSED FROM THE HISTORY

In the majority of patients, a positive diagnosis can be made from the history, using the Rome III criteria (see below).

THE ROME III CRITERIA FOR THE DIAGNOSIS OF IBS

Abdominal discomfort or pain for at least 3 days a month in the last 3 months, with an onset at least 6 months ago and with at least two of the following features:

1. relieved by defecation;
2. onset of symptoms associated with a change in the frequency of the stool;
3. onset of symptoms associated with a change in the form of the stool.

The following support the diagnosis but are not necessary for it:

(a) abnormal stool frequency (> 3 a day or < 3 a week);
(b) abnormal stool form;
(c) abnormal passage of stool (straining, urgency or a feeling of incomplete defecation);
(d) mucus;
(e) a feeling of abdominal distension.

To confirm that the symptoms are not due to another disease, check (NICE 2008):

- FBC
- ESR
- C-reactive protein
- antibody tests for coeliac disease

- faecal calprotectin if available. Its specificity as a test for organic disease is poor but early studies suggest that its ability to exclude organic disease approaches 100% (Meucci, D'Inca, Maieron, *et al.* 2009).

PATIENTS IN WHOM ORGANIC DISEASE MUST BE EXCLUDED

* Refer those:
  (a) over 40 years of age with symptoms of recent onset;
  (b) with a change in symptoms;
  (c) with rectal bleeding;
  (d) with loss of appetite, loss of weight or anaemia;
  (e) who have abdominal pain and altered bowel habit not fulfilling the Rome criteria; for details of the diagnosis of altered bowel habit see *Evidence-based Diagnosis in Primary Care* by A. F. Polmear (editor) published by Butterworth-Heinemann, 2008;
  (f) who have an abdominal or rectal mass;
  (g) who have a family history of cancer of the colon, breast, ovary or uterus; or of inflammatory bowel disease;
  (h) who feel unable to accept the diagnosis of IBS after full explanation;
  (i) who have severe symptoms despite the management outlined below.

MANAGEMENT OF PATIENTS WITH A CLEAR DIAGNOSIS OF IBS

* The GP's attitude at the first consultation is important. Show that you are taking the symptoms seriously, and examine the abdomen before reassuring the patient that there is no organic disease.
* Ask about the patient's fears, and especially the fear of cancer.
* If some investigation seems necessary, if only to assist in the reassurance, restrict it to FBC, ESR and stool for occult blood and pathogens. Consider hypothyroidism in the older patient.
* Explain the nature of the condition, and explore with the patient whether stress or diet is playing a part.

* *Smoking*. Some patients report improvement after stopping smoking.

* *Diet:* food intolerance. Explain that in up to 50% of patients certain foods can precipitate attacks. Encourage patients to keep a diary to explore this. Alcohol, tea and coffee are common precipitants. A diet free of wheat, eggs and milk is occasionally helpful in those with diarrhoea. Some patients with flatulence and diarrhoea absorb fructose and fructans poorly. In an uncontrolled study of patients with IBS who were found to have fructose malabsorbtion on breath test, in which fructose-containing foods (e.g. sweet fruit, some soft drinks, wheat, pasta, onions, leeks and asparagus) were avoided, 74% reported positively with improvement in all symptoms (Shepherd and Gibson 2006). Other exclusion diets are unlikely to be helpful (McKee, Prior and Whorwell 1987). Those with distension should avoid flatus-producing foods, e.g. onions, beans, celery, carrots, Brussels sprouts and wheat germ.

* *Dietary fibre*. Most patients with IBS eat too much insoluble fibre (NICE 2008) and the single most effective therapy may be to ban all cereal fibre, e.g. brown bread and bran (Whorwell 2009).

* *Constipation*. For patients with constipation and only minor pain, recommend soluble fibre, e.g. oats. If this helps the constipation but increases the pain, recommend instead an increase in fruit, vegetables, wholemeal rice and pasta. Of the prescribable bulk laxatives the best evidence is for ispaghula (Jones 2008).

* *Diarrhoea*. Use codeine phosphate, loperamide, or co-phenotrope for acute exacerbations of the diarrhoea.

* *Pain*. A trial of several antispasmodics, one after another, is worthwhile. The best evidence is for hyoscine butylbromide and peppermint oil (Jones 2008), both of which can be bought over the counter in the UK.

* *If traditional antispasmodics fail*, consider using low doses of a tricyclic antidepressant (e.g. amitriptyline 10 mg at night) for its anticholinergic effect, with a warning about the potential adverse effects. SSRIs have also been shown to have some benefit on symptoms regardless of the presence or absence of depression (Tabas, Beaves, Wang, *et al.* 2004). They are used in full dosage, as for depression. A trial of fluoxetine 20 mg daily for 12 weeks found benefit after 2 weeks which lasted at least 4 weeks after cessation of treatment (Vahedi, Merat, Rashidioon, *et al.* 2005). Short courses of an SSRI, therefore, may be effective, given to cope with an exacerbation of symptoms.

* Upper GI tract dysmotility symptoms. See dyspepsia, page 203.

* Recommend the national charity for IBS: Gut Trust, Unit 5, 53 Mowbray Street, Sheffield S3 8EN, tel: 0114 2723253, www.theguttrust.org The trust has details of self-help groups and their own fact sheet about IBS. Self-help has been shown to reduce symptoms and consultations for IBS. A study from Manchester has shown that a self-help guidebook is the crucial intervention; membership of a self-help group added nothing to the benefits achieved with the book (Robinson, Lee, Kennedy, *et al.* 2006).

TREATMENT OF THE PSYCHOLOGICAL COMPONENT

* Explore the patient's mood and attitude to the condition in more detail.

* If the patient does not see the condition as one with a psychological component, consider an explanation as follows: IBS appears to be a condition of disordered bowel motility. Although the mind is not the cause of the problem, it can exert some influence over the bowel through its extensive nerve supply.

* Consider counselling or psychotherapy for those with an excessive concern with their symptoms. A meta-analysis of cognitive behavioural therapy (CBT) found that it reduced symptoms by 50% with an NNT of 2 (Hayee and Forgacs 2007).

* *Depression*. Make a choice about counselling/psychotherapy and antidepressant drugs (see above). If using an antidepressant, use a tricyclic for patients with diarrhoea and an SSRI for patients with constipation.

* *Hypnotherapy* may help those still distressed by symptoms. However, a systematic review found that only 10 out of 18 trials were favourable and concluded that hypnotherapy could not be generally recommended. A GP whose patient wishes to try hypnotherapy should contact the British Society of Clinical and Academic Hypnosis, 28 Dale Park Gardens, Cookridge, Leeds LS16 7PT, tel 0844 884 3116, www.bscah.com.

CONSTIPATION

For details of the diagnosis of constipation see *Evidence-based Diagnosis in Primary Care* by A. F. Polmear (editor), published by Butterworth-Heinemann, 2008.

SYSTEMATIC REVIEW

NHS Centre for Reviews and Dissemination. 2001. Effectiveness of laxatives in adults. Effective Health Care **7** (1).

- Constipation is defined by the Rome II criteria as present when two or more of the following have been present for at least 12 weeks in the last year (Thompson, Longstreth, Drossman, *et al.* 1999):
  (a) straining at stool at least a quarter of the time;
  (b) lumpy and/or hard stools at least a quarter of the time;
  (c) a sensation of incomplete evacuation at least a quarter of the time;
  (d) three or fewer bowel movements per week.
- 10% of the British population are regularly constipated (3% of young adults, 20% or more in the elderly). A further large number use laxatives regularly because of an unjustified expectation of regularity.
- The frequency of constipation largely relates to the intake of dietary fibre, which has declined from about 40 g/day 100 years ago to less than 15–20 g/day today. Fibre reduces transit time, and increases stool bulk and softness.
- Many patients who complain of constipation are suffering from irritable bowel syndrome (IBS) and have normal transit times. They can be distinguished by the fact that, however much difficulty they feel they have in opening their bowels, they do not pass the hard and often pellet-like motions which are diagnostic of constipation. High fibre is worth using (see above and page 690), but these patients should not be given laxatives.

HIGH–FIBRE DIET

- Encourage the patient to increase the fibre content of the diet slowly. This will minimize the likely side-effects of bloating and flatulence, which will tend to subside anyway over 1–2 months.
- Aim for 30 g of fibre and at least 2 litres of fluid per day. The fibre should be obtained from as many different sources as possible. 5 g is found in:
  (a) two wholewheat cereal biscuits;
  (b) two slices of wholemeal bread or three of brown;
  (c) two apples, oranges, pears or bananas;
  (d) one helping of wholemeal pasta;
  (e) one helping of baked beans, peas, swedes or sprouts;
  (f) two helpings of boiled or baked potatoes, in their skins;
  (g) two helpings of carrots or lentils;
  (h) half a helping of kidney beans; or
  (i) one and a half sachets of Fybogel or Regulan.
  Insoluble particulate fibre is most effective (e.g. wheat bran); small particle or soluble fibre is less effective. Porridge and muesli contain oat bran, which is soluble, and so has less laxative value.

ACUTE CONSTIPATION

- Acute constipation most commonly occurs in patients recently confined to bed, those on opiates or other constipating drugs, during the immediate postnatal period or when defecation is painful.
- Constipation as a new symptom where there is no obvious cause raises the possibility of colorectal carcinoma, and warrants abdominal and rectal examination (see page 217). Red flags for colorectal carcinoma (persistent unexplained change in bowel habit, abdominal pain, rectal bleeding, systemic illness, e.g. weight loss or anaemia, abdominal mass) warrant referral. In the absence of red flags, no investigations are likely to be helpful (Rao, Ozturk and Laine 2005).
  * Look for a cause of the constipation and remove it if possible.
  * Anticipate the constipation if possible and give a stimulant laxative prophylactically, e.g. two senna tablets at night.
  * Continue the stimulant and increase tablets to four or even eight at night if constipation does occur.

* As an alternative, give a single dose of a polyethylene glycol laxative. A small study found this achieved complete success, usually within 24 hours, with no adverse effects (Di Palma, Smith and Cleveland 2002).
* Disimpact if necessary.

Disimpaction

* Insert a suppository at the time of examination and prescribe a further supply.
* Prescribe a high dose of a polyethylene glycol laxative (e.g. Movicol 8 sachets dissolved in a litre of water and drunk within 6 hours) if the patient is able to drink the large amount of water that is needed. It may be repeated on 2 further days.
* Arrange for an enema to be administered or a manual removal to be performed.
  (a) *If a rapid response is needed* – use a sodium phosphate or sodium citrate enema.
  (b) *If a more gentle response is needed* – use an arachis oil enema.
  (c) *For hard faeces in the rectum* – use a 5 ml enema containing a faecal softener, e.g. Fletcher's Enemette or Micolette.

CHRONIC CONSTIPATION

Assessment

* Confirm from the history that the patient is really constipated and not suffering from the abnormal non-propulsive contractions of IBS.
* Check that the patient is not taking constipating drugs.
* Ask whether there is soiling (see Faecal incontinence, below). Patients rarely volunteer this information.
* Examine the abdomen and rectum.
* Be alert for disorders that present as constipation, especially carcinoma of the large bowel and hypothyroidism.

Treatment

* Explain that regular evacuation depends on a regular stool habit, a diet high in fibre, regular exercise and regular meals.

* *Fluid intake.* Encourage extra fluid intake in the elderly.
* *Time and privacy for defecation.* Time must be set aside; colonic activity peaks after breakfast.
* *Fibre.* Encourage increased dietary intake of fibre (see above). Systematic review of the literature does not show any fibre or laxative to be superior to any other (Tramonte, Brand, Mulrow, *et al.* 1997). Where dietary fibre is not well tolerated, consider prescribing ispaghula, sterculia or methyl cellulose. These must be taken with a full glass of water or, in the case of methyl cellulose, two glasses. Do not add fibre in patients with constipation due to opiates, nor where it is associated with a hugely distended colon, nor in impaction. Warn patients that they should not have unrealistic expectations of the benefit that is likely from fibre. The mean increase is only 1.4 extra movements per week (NHS Centre for Reviews and Dissemination 2001).
* *Laxatives.* If there is no improvement or improvement is not maintained, start a stimulant laxative (e.g. senna 2 to 8 tablets or bisacodyl 2 to 4 tablets) at night or an osmotic laxative, or both. Find the dose that produces a motion the next morning. Prescribe it once or twice a week only, explaining the dangers of habituation if it is used more frequently.

Poor responders

Poor responders may need a laxative from each group as well as fibre both dietary and prescribed:
(a) *a stimulant*, e.g. senna or bisacodyl, or dantron in the elderly or terminally ill;
(b) *a stool softener.* Docusate orally may be ineffective (NHS Centre for Reviews and Dissemination 2001). Liquid paraffin is too dangerous alone, but seems safe as liquid paraffin and magnesium hydroxide emulsion;
(c) *an osmotic agent.* Magnesium sulphate is effective in 2 hours, but should not be used more than once a week. Lactulose is more expensive, and has been shown to be less effective than a combination of senna and fibre (Passmore, Wilson-Davies and Stoker 1993). Macrogols appear to be more expensive than lactulose but they also appear to be more effective and one study suggests that makes them more cost-effective (Ramkumar and Rao 2005).

* Consider colchicine 500 mcg t.d.s. in patients refractory to all other treatment, although it is unlicensed for this use. In a small study of patients resistant to standard medical treatment it increased the number of bowel movements with the only adverse effect an increase in abdominal pain in the first 3 weeks (Verne, Davis, Robinson, *et al.* 2003).
* Consider referral of patients with intractable constipation for colorectal function studies. Surgery may be helpful in the most severe cases.

Stopping laxatives in chronic constipation

Current advice suggests that laxatives should be tailed off once bowel movements are normal (Clinical Knowledge Summaries 2009). Behind this advice lies a fear, for which there is no evidence, that laxatives in normal doses, especially stimulant laxatives, can cause structural and functional damage to the nervous supply and to the smooth muscle of the bowel. No evidence for this exists (Wald 2003). In practice most patients with chronic constipation relapse once their laxatives are withdrawn and it seems reasonable to restart them long term, at the lowest effective dose, provided the prescriber is satisfied that a change of diet or lifestyle will not achieve the desired result.

FAECAL INCONTINENCE

REVIEW

Kamm MA. 1998. Fortnightly review: faecal incontinence. BMJ 316, 528–532.

● Faecal incontinence is found in 25–35% of elderly people in institutions (Barrett 1992). 6% of the population over the age of 40 report some degree of faecal incontinence; in 1.4% it is a major problem.

Treatment should be related to the underlying cause:

* *Diarrhoea*. Treat with an antidiarrhoeal agent once overflow diarrhoea has been excluded.
* *Sphincter weakness or damage*. Make the stool firmer by reducing the fibre intake and stopping laxatives, and if necessary giving a constipating drug such as loperamide or codeine phosphate. Consider referral for surgical repair of the sphincter. Simple repair will cure 80% of women with a sphincter tear from obstetric trauma.
* *Anal sensory impairment*. Keep the stool firm, and organize planned defecation with suppositories or enemas.
* *Impaction with overflow*. See 'Constipation'.
* *Immobility*. Reorganize the toileting arrangements.
* *Loss of higher control*, e.g. dementia or after stroke. Organize planned evacuation.
* *Rectal prolapse*. Consider referral for surgery.
* *Loss of pelvic floor tone*. Consider referral to physiotherapy for pelvic floor exercises, surgery to restore the anorectal angle, or sacral nerve stimulation.

ADULT COELIAC DISEASE

GUIDELINES

British Society of Gastroenterology. *Guidelines for the Management of Patients with Coeliac Disease*. London: BSG, 1996, revised 2002. Online. Available: www.bsg.org.uk
    Primary Care Society for Gastroenterology. *The Management of Adults with Coeliac Disease in Primary Care*, 2006. Available: www.pcsg.org.uk
    British Society of Gastroenterology. *Guidelines for Osteoporosis in Coeliac Disease and Inflammatory Bowel Disease*. London: BSG, 2000. Online. Available: www.bsg.org.uk

● Coeliac disease is common, with a prevalence in the UK of 0.5–1% (Hopper, Hadjivassiliou, Butt, *et al.* 2007), of whom over two thirds are undiagnosed. The diagnosis in those who present as adults is often made years after the first presentation. For details of the diagnosis of coeliac disease see *Evidence-based Diagnosis in Primary Care* by A. F. Polmear (editor) published by Butterworth-Heinemann, 2008. The condition is much more common in adults than in children with a ratio of 9:1.
● The endomysial antibody (EMA) test is a reasonably sensitive and specific screening test

for untreated coeliac disease, although estimates of sensitivity range from 64% to 95% and of specificity from 64% to 100%. One reason for a false negative test is that it measures IgA and will be falsely negative in the 2% of the UK population who are IgA deficient. An alternative test, the tissue transglutaminase antibody test (tTGA), can be performed on IgA and IgG. Although overall it is no more sensitive or specific than the EMA, the combination of tTGA and EMA can reduce the number of false negatives.

● Between 45% and 87% of patients with an established diagnosis fail to adhere to a gluten-free diet.

* Suspect coeliac disease in an adult or child with any of the following:

  (a) *gastroenterological features:* chronic or intermittent diarrhoea, persistent GI symptoms including nausea or vomiting, abdominal pain or distension;

  (b) *non-gastroenterological features:* anaemia, fatigue, arthralgia, myalgia, weight loss or, in children, failure to thrive, unexpectedly bad dental decay, mouth ulcers or other nonspecific symptoms especially if they are multiple or persistent. Do not be put off by the absence of gastrointestinal symptoms. In adults they are the exception, not the rule (Hin, Bird, Fisher, *et al.* 1999).

* *Offer screening* to an adult or child with: autoimmune thyroid disease, dermatitis herpetiformis, irritable bowel syndrome, type 1 diabetes.

* *Offer screening* to anyone who has a first degree relative with coeliac disease. The prevalence is at least 4.5%.

* *Consider offering screening* to anyone with: Addison's disease, amenorrhoea, autoimmune liver or heart conditions, idiopathic thrombocytopenic purpura, Down's syndrome, epilepsy, osteoporosis, lymphoma, microscopic colitis, persistently raised liver enzymes with no known cause, polyneuropathy, recurrent miscarriage, sarcoidosis, Sjögren's syndrome, Turner's syndrome, unexplained alopecia, or unexplained subfertility (Richey, Howdle, Shaw, *et al.* 2009). Those with a second degree relative with the disease may also be tested (prevalence 2.6%).

* Check the EMA and/or tTGA, according to local availability. NICE recommends the tTGA as first line, with an EMA test if the tTGA is equivocal (Richey, Howdle, Shaw, *et al.* 2009). If the laboratory reports evidence that IgA may be low, check the IgA level formally. IgA deficiency gives false negative results in coeliac disease.

* Refer if the EMA or tTGA is positive, for intestinal biopsy, without which a diagnosis cannot be made.

* Refer for biopsy a patient in whom serology is negative but the clinical picture is very suggestive. Up to 9% of cases are seronegative (Hopper, Hadjivassiliou, Butt, *et al.* 2007).

Note: Serological and biopsy tests are only likely to be positive in patients taking gluten in their diet. Explain to the patient that, in the 6 weeks before the test, they must eat gluten in at least two meals a day. Gluten is found in bread, wheat-based cereal, chapattis, pasta, biscuits and cake.

DIET

* Explain that a gluten-free diet will be needed for life. The patient should not relax this even if symptoms do not return. Patients with coeliac disease who continue to take even small amounts of gluten have an increased risk of lymphoma of the small intestine, osteoporosis and infertility. The exception to this appears to be oats, which may not be harmful to adults, although they should not be recommended in children nor in those patients with severe disease. Care must be taken to use uncontaminated oat products and to keep quantities low, e.g. < 50 g oats per day or one reasonable serving. It is worth testing for EMA or tTGA should the patient become symptomatic again when taking oats and if they are positive withdraw oats from the diet.

* Prescribe adequate amounts of gluten-free products, marking the prescription 'ACBS'.

* Prescribe supplements of iron, folic acid, vitamin B_{12} and calcium at the time of diagnosis, and continue until the patient is well established on a gluten-free diet which usually takes three months. Reintroduce supplements if a relapse occurs.

* *Women planning a pregnancy* should receive folic acid 5 mg daily until the 12th week.

FOLLOW-UP

* Keep a record of all patients with coeliac disease and call them for review each year.
* Check the following annually:
  (a) symptoms;
  (b) weight;
  (c) Hb, B_{12}, folate, ferritin, albumin, calcium, alkaline phosphatase, TFTs, LFTs. A low red cell folate or ferritin is likely to be due to excellent adherence to the diet rather than the opposite. A gluten-free diet may well be low in these and supplements will be needed.
* *If compliance is in doubt,* check the EMA or tTGA. A positive result suggests that the patient is not adhering to the diet.
* Perform a dual energy X-ray absorptiometry (DEXA) scan for osteoporosis at diagnosis and again at the menopause in women, at age 55 in men, and at any age if a fragility fracture occurs.
* Offer immunization against pneumoccocal and *H. influenzae* type b infection once and against influenza annually. 30% of patients have some degree of splenic atrophy.
* Recommend that first degree relatives are tested serologically. Different studies have shown rate of 4–22.5% (Hopper, Hadjivassiliou, Butt, *et al.* 2007).

UNCONTROLLED SYMPTOMS

* Re-refer to the dieticians:
  (a) if there is diarrhoea or weight loss or nutritional deficiency. Small amounts of gluten can be ingested in an unsuspected form, e.g. in commercial gluten-free wheat products;
  (b) if constipation is the problem; it may be due to the low fibre nature of the diet.
* Re-refer to a specialist for reassessment of the diagnosis if dietary assessment fails to solve the problem or if there is abdominal pain or blood in the stool. Even if the original diagnosis was correct, the patient may have developed associated pathology: small bowel lymphoma or adenocarcinoma or ulcerative jejunoileitis.

INFLAMMATORY BOWEL DISEASE (IBD)

GUIDELINES

Carter MJ, Lobo AJ, Travis SPL. 2004. Guidelines for the management of inflammatory bowel disease in adults. Gut 53(Suppl V), v1–v16.
    MeReC. 1999. Inflammatory bowel disease. MeReC Bulletin 10(12), 45–48. Available: www.npc.co.uk

* Two reviews outline the patient's perspective and expectations with respect to the care they receive for their IBD (British Society of Gastroenterology 1996; Carter, Lobo and Travis 2004).
  (a) GPs seem to underestimate the severity of their symptoms and delay the original referral;
  (b) patients with IBD should be seen as an individual and not be defined by their illness;
  (c) many decisions about treatment require the patient to make a choice, and to do this they need information and time;
  (d) even if symptoms cannot be alleviated, patients appreciate the healthcare team that acknowledges their presence and recognizes some problems may be impossible to solve;
  (e) patients place a high value on sympathy, compassion and interest;
  (f) at the time of diagnosis patients value the offer of suitable written and audio-visual material. Information regarding patient support groups, and an opportunity to meet clinical nurse specialists or medical social workers familiar with IBD.
* Training in self-management can reduce consultations and reduce the delay before relapses are managed effectively (Robinson, Thompson, Wilkin, *et al.* 2001).

● The role of the GP lies in the original referral for diagnosis, in the support of the patient with continuing symptoms and in the prompt treatment of relapses.

INITIAL INVESTIGATIONS

(a) FBC;

(b) ESR or CRP;

(c) serum albumin;

(d) LFTs;

(e) stool culture and *Clostridium difficile* toxin if relevant;

(f) faecal calprotectin if there is doubt about whether the patient has organic disease. Its specificity as a test for organic disease is poor but early studies suggest that its ability to exclude organic disease approaches 100% (Meucci, D'Inca, Maieron, *et al.* 2009).

DIAGNOSIS

✻ Refer anyone with diarrhoea for 2 weeks which is not improving, provided there is no previous history to suggest irritable bowel syndrome and the stool culture is negative.

✻ Refer more urgently anyone who is systemically unwell, or whose diarrhoea is heavily blood stained.

✻ Refer anyone with blood and mucus per rectum and with urgency and bowel frequency, even if the stools are formed.

✻ Consider the possibility of IBD in anyone with persistent abdominal pain, especially if associated with perianal disease, weight loss or systemic disturbance.

✻ Remember the possibility of toxic dilatation in UC.

MANAGEMENT

✻ The psychological effects of chronic IBD may be worse than the physical symptoms, and it is easy for doctor and patient to focus mainly on the organic side of the condition. Broach the subject directly and recommend the patients' organizations in the box on this page.

✻ Use the IBD nurse specialist, if available, as key worker to liaise with all members of the multidisciplinary team, primary care and other agencies as well as to support patients and carers.

PATIENT ORGANIZATIONS

National Association for Colitis and Crohn's Disease, 4 Beaumont House, Sutton Road, St Albans, Herts AL1 5HH, tel. 01727 830038; information line 0845 130 2233; www.nacc.org.uk. As well as information and support, the association can provide a 'Can't Wait' card, which will allow the patient to use the toilet in major shops.

British Colostomy Association, 15 Station Road, Reading, Berks RG1 1LG, tel. 0118 939 1537; helpline 0800 328 4257; www.bcass.org.uk

For the specific management of IBD see below.

ULCERATIVE COLITIS

ASSESSMENT OF THE ACUTE ATTACK

The criteria of Truelove and Witts (Table 7.1) are useful in grading the severity of an attack (Truelove and Witts 1955). Patients can look misleadingly well.

Patients with severe disease require hospital admission whereas those with mild/moderate disease can generally be managed as outpatients.

MANAGEMENT OF THE ACUTE ATTACK

✻ Admit any patient who:

(a) has a severe attack according to the criteria above, especially any who show signs of toxic megacolon; the cardinal sign is rebound tenderness;

(b) fails to respond after 1 week of high dose prednisolone (see below).

Inpatient treatment of a severe attack of UC will be managed jointly by a gastroenterologist in conjunction

Table 7.1	Truelove and Witts criteria		
FEATURE	**MILD**	**MODERATE**	**SEVERE**
Bloody motions (no./day)	< 4	4–6	> 6
Temperature	Apyrexial	Intermediate	> 37.8 on 2/4 days
Pulse rate	Normal	Normal	> 90 bpm
Haemoglobin(g/dl)	Normal	Intermediate	< 10.5
ESR(mm/h)	< 30	< 30	> 30

with a colorectal surgeon. There is a 25–30% chance of needing a colectomy. A stool frequency of > 8/day or CRP> 45 mg/l at 3 days appears to predict the need for surgery in 85% of cases.

Home management

* Maintain fluid and carbohydrate intake.

Distal disease:

* If disease is confined to the rectum or rectosigmoid give corticosteroids, e.g. Colifoam, rectally twice a day until symptoms have settled.
* If this fails, give daily rectal enemas of mesalazine for 2–4 weeks, or mesalazine suppositories if disease is confined to the rectum (DTB 1994), or oral prednisolone, as below.
* *Constipation* may need a laxative.

More generalized disease:

* Give prednisolone 40 mg daily for 2 weeks then tail off over 8 weeks. Avoid enteric-coated preparations, which may not be absorbed because of rapid transit. Refer urgently if there is no response after 1 week. Refer, but less urgently, patients needing frequent courses of steroids; or
* Give a 5-ASA drug e.g. mesalazine 2–4 g daily. If the patient is already on an aminosalicylate increase to full dose for 1 month, then reduce to a maintenance dose.
* *Control diarrhoea* with codeine phosphate, but not in the ill patient for fear of precipitating toxic megacolon.
* *Rectal symptoms.* Use rectally administered steroids or mesalazine, as for distal disease, in addition to oral medication.
* *Nutrition.* Patients unable to tolerate a simple diet will benefit from a prescribable food product, e.g. Enrich or Ensure. The prescription should be endorsed 'ACBS'.

Note: All aminosalicylates can cause marrow suppression. Check FBC at the start of treatment and warn patients to report bruising, bleeding, sore throat, fever or malaise (Anon. 1994).

MAINTENANCE THERAPY

Lifelong maintenance therapy is recommended for all patients except those with distal disease who relapse less than once a year. Maintenance with mesalazine can reduce the risk of colorectal cancer (Eaden 2003).

* *Oral aminosalicylates* reduce the annual relapse rate from 80% to 20%. They are less helpful in inducing remission. They are all equally effective. Check the serum creatinine before starting; nephrotoxicity is more likely in patients with pre-existing renal disease. Give:
  (a) sulfasalazine at the minimum effective dose, usually q.d.s. The commonest side-effects are nausea and headache; or
  (b) mesalazine 400 mg t.d.s. or olsalazine 500 mg b.d. for patients intolerant of sulfasalazine or men who do not wish to suffer oligospermia. They are considerably more expensive than sulfasalazine.
* *Rectal preparations.* Rectal steroids or mesalazine may be useful, especially in patients with proctitis or distal colitis. The patient administers one dose each night during an acute attack, reducing to once or twice a week for maintenance.
* *Systemic corticosteroids* are of little value in remission maintenance.
* *Azathioprine* 2 mg/kg is occasionally used for remission maintenance. It should be reserved for those patients who frequently relapse despite adequate doses of aminosalicylates, or are intolerant of 5-ASA therapy. It should only be started by a specialist. Regular blood counts are needed. Before starting treatment the specialist will test for the enzyme thiopurine methyltransferase. A deficiency puts the patient at risk of bone marrow toxicity.
* Check the haemoglobin yearly. Anaemia can occur even in patients in remission.

THE RISK OF CARCINOMA

* Patients who have had pancolitis for more than 8–10 years should be reviewed by a specialist annually with a view to colonoscopy. The risk of carcinoma is 17 times that of the normal population. The risk of carcinoma in patients with localized disease is only four-fold, and the need for regular screening is less clear.
* Current guidelines recommend that those with extensive colitis opting for surveillance should have colonoscopies performed every 3 years in the second decade, every 2 years in the third decade, and annually in the fourth decade of the disease.

- Four random biopsies every 10 cm from the entire colon are needed plus additional samples of suspicious areas.
- If dysplasia is detected and confirmed by a second gastrointestinal pathologist then colectomy is usually advised.

CROHN'S DISEASE (CD)

Activity in Crohn's disease is harder to assess. However active disease is still determined by history and confirmed by raised inflammatory markers. It is important to note than Crohn's disease can affect any part of the small and large bowel and that causes other than active disease may account for symptoms. These include bacterial overgrowth, bile salt malabsorption, fibrotic strictures, dysmotility and gallstones.

ACTIVE ILEAL/ILEOCOLONIC/COLONIC DISEASE

- Diagnosis and initiation of treatment is the province of the gastroenterologist, who should always be consulted in the management of exacerbations.
- Treatment comprises high dose aminosalicylates, different corticosteroids, nutritional therapy, antibiotics, new biological agents or surgery.

Basic approaches:

* The usual first line drug is oral prednisolone 40 mg/day, reducing gradually according to severity and patient response over 8 weeks. Mesalazine, a previous first line drug, has been shown to be little or no better than placebo (Cummings, Keshav and Travis 2008).
* In mild to moderate left-sided colonic CD prednisolone may be given rectally.

Alternatives in special situations:

* Sulfasalazine 4 g daily is effective for active colonic disease, but with a high incidence of adverse effects.
* Metronidazole 10–20 mg/kg/day has a role in selected patients with colonic or treatment resistant disease, or in those wishing to avoid steroids, but adverse effects are common.
* In disease confined to the ileum and/or ascending colon, the specialist may recommend a modified-release budesonide.

* Azathioprine may be used in active CD as adjunctive therapy and as a steroid sparing agent. However, its slow onset of action precludes its use as a sole therapy. Check FBC and LFTs monthly.
* Surgery should be considered for those who have failed medical therapy and may be appropriate primary therapy in those with limited ileal or ileocaecal disease.

MAINTENANCE OF REMISSION

* Give smokers all possible help to stop (see page 498). Smoking cessation is probably the most important factor in maintaining remission.
* Explain to the patient that steroids are ineffective in maintaining remission as well as having unacceptable adverse effects in long-term use.
* If disease activity returns as steroids are reduced, the patient is a candidate for immunomodulation, using azathioprine, mercaptopurine, methotrexate, or infliximab infusion, a chimeric anti-TNF monoclonal antibody with potent anti-inflammatory properties. Several controlled trials have shown it to be effective in active and fistulating CD. NICE has produced guidelines for its use in CD (NICE 2002). It is best used as part of a treatment strategy, including immunomodulation, once other options such as surgery have been discussed with the patient.

Primary care issues in patients on immunomodulators or biological therapies

The GP must be aware that patients on these drugs are at risk of immunosuppression and opportunistic infection, including tuberculosis and aspergillosis. They should not be given live vaccines.

ADDITIONAL MEASURES

(a) *Diet*. A high-fibre diet is of value while in remission, unless strictures are present. During exacerbations stop all other food and give an elemental diet, e.g. Triosorbon six packets a day, tailing off as symptoms settle, provided other measures to control the inflammation are in place.

(b) *Diarrhoea* may be controlled by antidiarrhoeals, e.g. codeine phosphate. Diarrhoea caused by free bile acids in patients with ileal resection or dysfunction may be helped by a low-fat diet and colestyramine.

(c) *Perianal sepsis* may respond to metronidazole 400 mg b.d. and/or ciprofloxacin 500 mg b.d. which are appropriate first line treatments for simple perianal fistulae. Azathioprine and infliximab may also be effective.

(d) *Surgery* is likely to be needed by 70–80% of patients at some stage. This is likely to be for stricture, fistula, perianal disease and abdominal mass that does not respond to medical treatment.

(e) *Ileal CD or following ileal resection.* Check the vitamin B_{12} level annually.

* Re-refer patients in relapse who:

(a) are failing to respond to systemic steroids;

(b) are needing frequent courses of systemic steroids;

(c) have symptoms suggesting obstruction;

(d) have severe weight loss;

(e) have symptoms suspicious of carcinoma or other cause for concern.

PREGNANCY IN PATIENTS WITH IBD

Maintaining adequate disease control is essential for both maternal and fetal health.

- Advise the patient to try to conceive during remission and to take folate supplements from before conception.
- Flexible sigmoidoscopy may be used safely if necessary and if findings will alter management.
- On the whole, management should be as in the non-pregnant woman. The best interests of the fetus are served by controlling the disease rather than by avoiding possible risks from drugs or X-rays.
- Mode of delivery needs to be considered carefully. Patients with perianal CD or ileoanal pouch may be best served by having a Caesarean section to avoid damage to the anal sphincter.
- Azathioprine may be continued but babies may be lighter.
- Corticosteroids can be used for active disease.
- Methotrexate is absolutely contraindicated in pregnancy.

EXTRA-INTESTINAL DISEASE

- IBD may manifest itself in many organs remote from the bowel: especially eyes, mouth, skin and joints. In some patients these symptoms flare and remit with the bowel disease; in others they follow a more independent course. The former group appear to respond to the treatment given for the bowel. The latter group are more difficult to treat other than symptomatically.

- Patients with IBD are at risk of osteoporosis (Scott, Gaywood and Scott 2000). For CD the risk is increased by 1.3; for UC by 1.2 (British Society of Gastroenterology 2007). It is not clear whether the increased risk is due to known risk factors (inactivity, steroid use) or is due in some way to the disease itself. The thinner the patient the greater the risk (Carter, Lobo and Travis 2004).

Recommend:

* Weight-bearing exercise;

* Stopping smoking;

* Reducing excess alcohol intake;

* An intake of 1500 mg calcium daily and oral vitamin D_3 800 mg daily;

* Bone densitometry at the menopause, or, in men, at the age of 55, provided the disease presented well before then. Further densitometry 2 years later would allow an estimation of the rate of bone loss. Treatment should be as for osteoporosis of any cause (see page 280).

COLORECTAL CANCER

GUIDELINES

SIGN. 1997. *Colorectal Cancer: A National Guideline Recommended for Use in Scotland by the Scottish Intercollegiate Guidelines Network.* Scottish Intercollegiate Guidelines Network. Online. Available: www.sign.ac.uk

NICE 2005. Referral Guidelines for Suspected Cancer. National Institute for Health and Clinical Excellence, available on www.nice.org.uk

Effective Health Care. 2004. Management of colorectal cancers. Effective Health Care Bulletin 8 (3).

PCSG. 2003. *Prevention and Early Detection of Colorectal Cancer in Asymptomatic Patients.* Primary Care Society for Gastroenterology. www.pcsg.org.uk

✳ Refer patients for screening if they have a sufficiently strong family history (see page 218).

✳ Refer patients of any age urgently (to be seen within 2 weeks) (NICE 2005) who have a new occurrence of:
  ▪ a right-sided lower abdominal mass; or
  ▪ a rectal (not pelvic) mass. (A pelvic mass should be referred to gynaecologist or urologist); or
  ▪ iron deficiency anaemia without an obvious cause (Hb < 11g/dl in men or < 10g/dl in postmenopausal women).

✳ Refer patients aged ≥ 40 urgently who have a new occurrence of:
  ▪ rectal bleeding *and* a change in bowel habit to looser stools and/or increased frequency of defecation persistent for 6 weeks; or

✳ Refer patients aged ≥ 60 urgently who have a new occurrence of:
  ▪ persistent rectal bleeding without anal symptoms; or
  ▪ a change in bowel habit to looser stools and/or increased frequency of defecation persistent for 6 weeks without rectal bleeding.

✳ Refer patients with other colorectal symptoms, but with less urgency.

Note that it is only possible to decide that there is no grounds for urgent referral after performing abdominal and rectal examinations and sending blood for haemoglobin.

For details of the diagnosis of colorectal carcinoma see *Evidence-based Diagnosis in Primary Care* by A. F. Polmear (editor), published by Butterworth-Heinemann, 2008.

SCREENING FOR COLORECTAL CANCER (CRC)

● Screening faeces for occult blood and/or endoscopy can detect colorectal cancer early and reduce mortality (Atkin 2006).

● Whole population screening is recommended in the USA for those age 50 and over. In England the screening programme is currently (2009) being rolled out offering screening every two years initially to those aged 60–69. Those age 70 and over may request a screening kit. Those under 60 who are at high risk may be referred for assessment by the GP. In Scotland screening covers those aged 50–74 and in Wales from 2010, those aged 60–74.

● Whole population screening is likely to result in positive results in 2–4%, who will need colonoscopy. Of these, 50% will be normal, 40% will have a polyp and 10% will have carcinoma.

● In addition to screening of the older population, the onus is on the GP to discover the 3% of the UK population with a significant family history as well as those with a personal history which puts them at risk. In an Oxfordshire study, contacting patients who had had colorectal cancer diagnosed before the age of 65 revealed that 28% of them had moderate or high-risk family members (Rose, Murphy, Munafo, *et al.* 2004).

Family history (Table 7.2)

Screening should start 10 years before the age at which the relative developed the cancer. Total colonoscopy is required.

Personal history:

(a) a previous colorectal cancer, successfully removed;

(b) a previous adenomatous colonic polyp;

(c) longstanding widespread inflammatory bowel disease. UK national guidelines recommend that regular colonoscopies begin after 8–10 years in those with pancolitis, and after 15–20 years in those with left-sided disease (Ballinger and Anggiansah 2007).

Risk lowering measures:

(a) Stopping smoking;

(b) Reduced dietary fat and meat and increasing fruit and vegetables (Fung, Hu, Fuchs, *et al.* 2003);

(c) Drinking less than 15 units of alcohol per week;

(d) NSAIDs and aspirin. Aspirin 300 mg daily reduces the risk of adenomas which are precursors of CRC (Flossman and Rothwell 2007). NSAIDs may be superior, but with more adverse effects (Rostom, Dube, Lewin, *et al.* 2007).

Table 7.2 Risk stratification related to estimated lifetime risk of developing CRC		
FAMILY HISTORY	RISK	ACTION
Background lifetime risk	1:30 (1:50 risk of death)	General advice on risk lowering measures
One FDR > 60 years	1:17	General advice on risk lowering measures
One FDR age > 45 years	1:15	As above plus emphasize awareness of early symptoms
One FDR and one SDR	1:12	As above
One FDR age < 45 years	1:10	Refer for assessment
Both parents any age	1:8.5	Refer for assessment
Two FDRs	1:6	Refer for assessment
Hereditary non-polyposis colorectal cancer (HNPCC)	1:3	Refer for assessment
Three FDRs	1:2	Refer for assessment
One FDR with familial adenomatous polyposis (FAP)	1:2	Refer for assessment

FDR = first degree relative. SDR = second degree relative.
HNPCC exists when three or more relatives have CRC; and one of them is a FDR of one of the others; and at least two generations are affected; and one was diagnosed before the age of 50.
HNPCC and FAP are autosomal dominant conditions which may also be associated with an increased incidence of ovarian, breast and endometrial carcinoma.

POSTGASTRECTOMY

In 1965, there were an estimated 500,000 patients in the UK who had had a partial gastrectomy. Some will still be alive now. All need life-long follow-up.

* Check FBC yearly.
* *Iron deficiency.* 50% become iron deficient. Give prophylactic oral iron for life.
* *B_{12} and folate deficiency.* Iron deficiency may mask the typical macrocytosis. Check the B_{12} and folate in any patient whose anaemia does not respond totally to iron.
* *Carcinoma of the stomach.* The risk after 20 years is double, and after 45 years is seven-fold.

GASTROENTERITIS IN OLDER CHILDREN AND ADULTS

For the management of gastroenteritis in young children see page 107.

* Encourage the patient to eat and drink normally if they can; if not, encourage the use of milk drinks and soups.
* Prescribe oral rehydration salts for the frail elderly and any others at risk of dehydration.
* Consider prescribing an antidiarrhoeal agent, e.g. loperamide, but not in a child nor in anyone with severe symptoms; it may precipitate ileus or toxic megacolon.

* Send stool for culture if:
  (a) there is blood or mucus in the stool; or
  (b) the patient has recently been abroad; or
  (c) more than one member of the family or institution is affected; or
  (d) diarrhoea continues for more than one week; or
  (e) you suspect a cause for the diarrhoea other than gastroenteritis; for details of the diagnosis of diarrhoea see *Evidence-based Diagnosis in Primary Care* by A. F. Polmear (editor); published by Butterworth-Heinemann, 2008 or
  (f) there is systemic upset.
* Notify as suspected food poisoning if two or more people who have eaten the same food develop gastroenteritis at the same time. Otherwise, only notify if the stool sample is positive.
* Exclude the patient from school or work until the diarrhoea has stopped. Food handlers and possibly healthcare workers should stay away from work until free from diarrhoea for 48 hours (unless typhoid or pathogenic *E. coli* are isolated, in which case the advice of the consultant in communicable diseases should be sought).
* Stress the importance of handwashing.
* *Antibiotics.* Only prescribe antibiotics for the limited number of conditions in which they have been shown to be of benefit. Those endemic in the UK are:

(a) campylobacter: use a macrolide or a quinolone;

(b) shigella and salmonella: use trimethoprim or a quinolone and then only if there is systemic illness;

(c) giardia: use metronidazole or tinidazole;

(d) for any other patient with the clinical picture of acute dysentery and who is too unwell to wait for the stool result: use a quinolone. Admission would, however, usually be more appropriate for such a patient.

∗ *Referral*. Admit those who are systemically severely ill or who are clinically dehydrated and unable to tolerate rehydration orally. Also admit those with concomittant illness which could be destabilized by the gastroenteritis. Refer any whose diarrhoea becomes chronic. An arbitrary definition of chronic diarrhoea is where three or more loose stools are passed daily for more than 4 weeks (Thomas, Forbes, Green, *et al.* 2003).

∗ *Prevention of antibiotic-associated diarrhoea.* Drinking a commercially available yoghurt drink containing probiotic bacteria (Actimel) twice a day during the antibiotic course and for 1 week thereafter can reduce the incidence of diarrhoea with an adjusted odds ratio of 0.25 (95%CI 0.07 to 0.85) (Hickson, D'Souza, Muthu, *et al.* 2007). In this study of older inpatients the NNT for avoiding all diarrhoea was 5 and the NNT for avoiding diarrhoea caused by *C. difficile* was 6.

MANAGEMENT OF ANTIBIOTIC-ASSOCIATED DIARRHOEA

∗ Stop the antibiotic or change it to one less likely to disturb the bowel flora, e.g. trimethoprim. Ensure that the patient remains hydrated and admit any with severe symptoms.

∗ If symptoms have not resolved in 3 days, and no other diagnosis is more likely, send stool for detection of *C. difficile* toxins A and B after discussion with the laboratory.

∗ If present, give oral metronidazole 400 mg t.d.s. for 10 days. A second course will be needed in the 20% who relapse after the first course. If the patient is systemically ill or at high risk, discuss the need for admission to an isolation unit with the consultant in communicable diseases. High-risk patients are the old and those with

lowered immunity. In some outbreaks the mortality in the frail elderly has been 25% (Starr 2005).

∗ If kept at home explain to the family that other healthy family members are not at risk. However, they should pay special attention to hand washing and to disinfection of surfaces in kitchen and bathroom, in order to avoid passing the spores to someone else with lowered immunity. Children are not particularly at risk; the majority of very young children already have the organism in the bowel.

∗ If the stool is negative for toxins, refer as for chronic diarrhoea (above). Antibiotic associated diarrhoea may still be the diagnosis; stool toxins are negative in up to 20% with *C. difficile*-related diarrhoea (Barbut and Meynard 2002). Conversely, a culture of *C. difficile* does not prove the diagnosis of *C. difficile*-related diarrhoea; 3% of healthy adults carry *C. difficile* in the bowel.

GASTROINTESTINAL BLEEDING

∗ Admit patients with current haematemesis or melaena. However, do not be surprised if the patient is discharged without endoscopy and without admission. A recent Scottish study has shown that patients who score negative on the Glasgow-Blatchford Bleeding Score (GBS) can safely be discharged in this way. In this study this applied to 22% of patients seen in secondary care with GI bleeding. The patient needs to have normal values of the following: Hb, urea, systolic blood pressure, pulse, and to have no history of melaena, syncope, hepatic disease or cardiac failure (Stanley, Ashley, Dalton, *et al.* 2009).

∗ Refer:

(a) by telephone for urgent endoscopy if the stool has returned to normal colour, but the bleed was within the last 7 days. These patients are very likely to rebleed, and the risk of this happening can be determined at endoscopy;

(b) urgently by letter if the bleed was over 7 days before;

(c) less urgently if the patient is anaemic with positive occult bloods but without a history of overt bleeding. However, in the UK such patients should still be seen within 2 weeks under Department of Health Guidelines (see Appendix 32). Stop NSAIDs if they are being taken, but do not assume that they were the cause of the blood loss until other pathology has been excluded. Start oral iron once iron deficiency is proved.

PREVENTION OF DRUG–INDUCED GI BLEEDING

- Low-dose aspirin doubles the risk of GI bleeding. However, this still leaves major GI bleeding relatively rare with a number needed to harm of 833. That is, 833 patients need to take low-dose aspirin for a year for there to be one patient with a major GI bleed due to aspirin (Laine 2006).
- Certain factors increase that risk: a past history of peptic ulceration or GI bleeding, steroid use, anticoagulants, and concomitant use of an NSAID.
- * If giving low-dose aspirin for cardiovascular prophylaxis to a patient with a risk factor for GI bleeding, use 75 mg daily and add a proton pump inhibitor. This led in one trial to a much lower rate of bleeding than changing aspirin to clopidogrel (Chan, Ching, Hung, *et al.* 2005).
- * If use of an NSAID is considered essential in a patient at risk of GI bleeding, choose a traditional NSAID with a lower risk of GI bleeding, or a COX-2 inhibitor. Whichever is chosen add a proton pump inhibitor (see page 202).

JAUNDICE

URGENT REFERRAL OR ADMISSION

(a) Fever, especially if associated with right upper quadrant (RUQ) tenderness and rigors; this may be ascending cholangitis;

(b) hepatic pre-coma, i.e. any alteration in mental state;

(c) portal hypertension, especially if associated with GI bleeding;

(d) an acute exacerbation of chronic liver disease;

(e) suspected malignant obstructive jaundice;

(f) pain or other evidence of biliary obstruction, or a palpable gall bladder;

(g) jaundice in the pregnant patient. If acute and associated with abdominal pain plus malaise it may be acute fatty liver, which carries a 20% mortality rate.

THE PATIENT WELL ENOUGH TO BE KEPT AT HOME

- * Base the diagnosis on:
  - (a) the history, including the drug history (e.g. phenothiazines, sulphonylureas, combined oral contraceptive (COC), paracetamol, NSAIDs);
  - (b) the examination;
  - (c) diagnostic tests:
    - *first line tests:* LFTs, FBC, prothrombin time, hepatitis serology, urine for bilirubin and urobilinogen, and ultrasound scan (USS). Over half of patients with acute jaundice have biliary obstruction. Early detection leads to speedier recovery and shorter overall hospital stays (Mitchell, Hussaini, McGovern, *et al.* 2002);
    - *second line tests:* serology for glandular fever, CMV or leptospirosis, according to the results of the first line tests.
- * Refer the patient who is not improving or in whom the diagnosis is not clear. A rising prothrombin time, an initial INR > 1.5, or a falling albumin are grounds for urgent referral.

ABNORMAL LIVER FUNCTION TESTS IN A PATIENT WHO IS NOT JAUNDICED

- * Examine for an enlarged liver or spleen and refer if present.
- * Ask about alcohol intake, risk factors for hepatitis, family history (Gilbert's disease, Wilson's disease, haemochromatosis).
- * Assess for risk factors for non-alcoholic fatty liver disease: central obesity, hypertension, abnormal glucose tolerance and abnormal serum lipids.
- * Ask about drugs and herbal remedies taken in the last 3 months.
- * Repeat LFTs in 2–3 weeks. In a study from Nottingham 15% had returned to normal in that time (Sherwood, Lyburn, Brown and Ryder 2001).

Table 7.3 Chronic liver disease screening tests: a suggested initial screen

INVESTIGATION	DISEASE
Hepatitis B surface antigen	Chronic hepatitis B
Hepatitis C antibody by ELISA	Chronic hepatitis C
Serum ferritin (> 1000 mcg/l)	Haemochromatosis (but ferritin may be high in alcoholism or chronic inflammation)
Transferrin saturation (> 55%)	
Antimitochondrial antibody titre > 1:250	Primary biliary cirrhosis
Anti-smooth muscle antibodies > 1:80	Autoimmune hepatitis
Antinuclear antibody > 1:80	
Immunoglobulins	
IgG	Autoimmune hepatitis
IgM	Primary biliary cirrhosis
IgA	Alcoholic liver disease
Serum α1 antitrypsin < 0.2g/l	α1 antitrypsin deficiency
Also PiZZ phenotype on electrophoresis	
Low caeruloplasmin	Wilson's disease

* If still abnormal, perform part or all of the screening tests in Table 7.3, according to pointers from the history. Unless a benign cause is found the patient will need referral to a hepatologist.

INTERPRETATION

1. *Isolated elevation of bilirubin* is usually due to Gilbert's disease. This is the commonest congenital failure of conjugation, affecting up to 7% in the UK. Diagnosis is on the basis of:

   (a) a mildly raised bilirubin with no bilirubin in the urine;

   (b) normal liver enzymes;

   (c) normal FBC, film and reticulocyte count.

* Explain the nature of the condition and that symptomatic episodes may occur, especially during periods of relative starvation.

* Encourage the patient to warn any other doctor who is performing blood tests that the bilirubin may be raised and why. This should avoid unnecessary investigations.

2. *Elevated transaminase* (ALT and AST)

   (a) Alcohol. The rise in AST is usually greater than that in ALT. 70% of those with alcoholic liver disease have a ratio greater than 2. See page 486 for management.

   (b) Drugs and herbal remedies. Common culprits are paracetamol, statins, azathioprine, amiodarone, antituberculous drugs and the combined oral contraceptive pill. It is not necessarily appropriate to stop the drug. See pages 268 (azathioprine), 162 (amioderone) and 165 (statins).

   (c) Hepatitis. Transaminase levels are likely to be higher in acute hepatitis than in alcoholic liver disease or chronic hepatitis. Serology permits a definitive diagnosis (see page 39).

   (d) Non-alcoholic fatty liver disease occurs more often in those with type 2 diabetes, obesity, hypercholesterolaemia and polycystic ovary syndrome (Day 2002). It is the commonest cause of elevated liver enzymes in the industrialized world. The condition can progress to fibrosis, end-stage liver disease and hepatocellular carcinoma. Those without diabetes at diagnosis are at high risk of developing it.

3. *Elevated alkaline phosphatase* (ALP)

   * Review the drug history. It occurs with co-proxamol and co-amoxiclav.

   * Ask about abdominal pain. It suggests biliary obstruction and needs urgent imaging. The additional presence of weight loss and anorexia suggests pancreatic carcinoma or hepatic metastases.

   * Ask whether the patient is itching. It raises the possibility of primary biliary cirrhosis or primary sclerosing cholangitis.

4. *Raised gamma glutamyl transferase* (γGT).

   • γGT is produced by the bile ducts. If raised in the company of a raised ALP it confirms that the ALP is hepatic and not of bony origin.

   • It is not specific for alcohol misuse but it may be raised in mild alcoholic hepatitis while the transaminases are normal.

   • It is often raised by drugs, e.g. anticonvulsants and phenothiazides.

MANAGEMENT OF NON–ALCOHOLIC FATTY LIVER DISEASE IN PRIMARY CARE

* Explain that the problem is inflammation of the liver by excess fat, that there is a small risk of progression to fibrosis and cirrhosis (1–2% over 15 years for patients in the early stages of the

condition), and that this risk can be reduced by the measures below.

* *Lifestyle changes.* Start the patient on a supervised programme of weight loss, exercise, alcohol cessation and healthy eating, as for the prevention of the development of diabetes.

* Assess cardiovascular risk and treat blood pressure and lipids if abnormal.

STOMA CARE

Patients with a stoma will, in the UK, be in contact with a stoma nurse. However, the GP may become involved when problems occur and may be the person best placed to ask the patient about the psychological impact of having a stoma.

* *Excoriated skin around the stoma.* Look for a cause: is effluent leaking around the stoma edge? Is the stool too loose? Is the patient failing to observe routine stomal hygiene? If there is no obvious cause, prescribe a protective cream while waiting for advice from the stoma nurse.

* *Parastomal hernia.* Prescribe a support belt, after taking advice from the stoma nurse. Surgery is usually unsuccessful because, when it occurs, it is due to weak musculature in the abdominal wall.

* *Prolapse.* Refer to the surgeon for fixing of the bowel proximal to the stoma. Meanwhile liaise

with the stoma nurse to discuss whether a larger appliance would help.

* *Sport and sexual activity.* Check whether the patient is avoiding these unnecessarily. A stoma cap can allow those with regular bowel movements to exercise without a bag.

* *Travel.* The patient may be avoiding travel unnecessarily. Advice on how to travel with a stoma is available on www.cancerbacup.org.uk

* *Psychological adjustment.* Always ask, at some point, how the patient feels about having a stoma. The impact on a patient's body image, is likely to be huge. Consider referral for counselling or to a Patient Group (see below).

PATIENT GROUPS

British Colostomy Association, 15 Station Road, Reading, Berks RG1 1LG, tel: 0118 939 1537, www.bcass.org.uk

IA - the Ileostomy and Internal Pouch Support Group, Peverill House, 1-5 Mill Road, Ballyclare, Co. Antrim, BT39 9DR, tel 028 9334 4043 or 0800 0184 724, www.the-ia.org.uk

Urostomy Association, 18 Foxglove Avenue, Uttoxeter, Staffs ST14 8UN, tel 0870 7707931, www.uagbi.org

References

Agreus, L., Talley, N., 1997. Challenges in managing dyspepsia in general practice. BMJ 315, 1284–1288.

Anon, 1994. Curr. Prob. Pharmacovigil. 21, 5–6.

Atkin, W., 2006. Impending or pending? The national bowel cancer screening programme. BMJ 332, 742.

Ballinger, A., Anggiansah, C., 2007. Colorectal cancer. BMJ 335, 715–718.

Barbut, F., Meynard, J., 2002. Managing antibiotic associated diarrhoea. BMJ 324, 1345–1346.

Barrett, J., 1992. Colorectal disorders in elderly people. BMJ 305, 764–766.

Bramble, M., Suvakovic, Z., Hungin, A., 2000. Detection of

upper gastrointestinal cancer in patients taking antisecretory therapy prior to gastroscopy. Gut 46, 464–467.

Briggs, A., Sculpher, M., Logan, R., et al., 1996. Cost-effectiveness of screening for and eradication of *H. pylori* in the management of dyspeptic patients under 45 years of age. BMJ 312, 1321–1325.

British Society of Gastroenterology, 1996. Inflammatory Bowel Disease. Guidelines in Gastroenterology, London.

British Society of Gastroenterology, 2007. Guidelines for Osteoporosis in Inflammatory Bowel Disease. Available: www.bsg.org.uk.

Carter, M., Lobo, A., Travis, S., 2004. Guidelines for the management of

inflammatory bowel disease in adults. Gut 53 (Suppl. V), v1–v16.

Chan, F., Ching, J., Hung, L., et al., 2005. Clopidogrel versus aspirin and esomeprazole to prevent recurrent ulcer bleeding. N. Engl. J. Med. 352, 238–244.

Clinical Knowledge Summaries, 2009. Constipation: National Library for Health. Available: www.cks.library.uk search on Constipation.

Cummings, J., Keshav, S., Travis, S., 2008. Medical management of Crohn's disease. BMJ 336, 1062–1066.

Danish Dyspepsia Study Group, 2001. Value of the unaided clinical diagnosis in dyspeptic patients in primary care. Am. J. Gastroenterol. 96, 1417–1421.

Day, C., 2002. Non-alcoholic steatohepatitis (NASH): where are we now and where are we going? Gut 50, 585–588.

Delaney, B., Moayyedi, P., 2004. Eradicating H pylori. BMJ 328, 1388–1389.

Delaney, B., Qume, M., Moayyedi, P., et al., 2008. *Helicobacter pylori* test and treat versus proton pump inhibitor in initial management of dyspepsia in primary care: multicentre randomised controlled trial (MRC-CUBE trial). BMJ 336, 651–654.

Di Palma, J.A., Smith, J.R., Cleveland, M., 2002. Overnight efficacy of polyethylene glycol laxative. Am. J. Gastroenterol. 97, 1776–1779.

DOH, 2000. Guidelines for the Urgent Referral of Patients with Suspected Cancer. Department of Health, London. Available: www.dh.gov.uk/cancer/referral.htm.

DTB, 1994. A mesalazine enema for ulcerative colitis. Drug Ther. Bull. 32, 38–39.

Eaden, J., 2003. Review article: the data supporting a role for aminosalicylates in chemoprevention of colorectal cancer in patients with inflammatory bowel disease. Aliment. Pharmacol. Ther. 18 (Suppl. 2), 15–21.

FitzGerald, G., 2004. Coxibs and cardiovascular disease. NEJM 351, 1709–1711.

Flossman, E., Rothwell, P., 2007. Effect of aspirin on long-term risk of colorectal cancer: consistent evidence from randomised and observational studies. Lancet 369, 1603–1613.

Fox, M., Forgacs, I., 2006. Gastro-oesophageal reflux disease. BMJ 332, 88–93.

Fung, T., Hu, F., Fuchs, C., et al., 2003. Major dietary patterns and the risk of colorectal cancer in women. Arch. Intern. Med. 163, 309–314.

Grant, A., Wileman, S., Ramsay, C., et al., 2008a. Minimal access surgery compared with medical management for chronic gastro-oesophageal reflux disease: UK collaborative randomised trial. BMJ 337.

Grant, A., Wileman, S., Ramsay, C., et al., 2008b. The effectiveness and cost-effectiveness of minimal access surgery amongst people with gastro-oesophageal reflux disease - a UK collaborative study. The REFLUX trial. Health Technol. Assess. 12 (31), 1–12.

Hayee, B., Forgacs, I., 2007. Psychological approach to managing irritable bowel syndrome. BMJ 334, 1105–1109.

Hickson, M., D'Souza, A., Muthu, N., et al., 2007. Use of probiotic *Lactobacillus* preparation to prevent diarrhoea associated with antibiotics: randomised double blind placebo controlled trial. BMJ 335, 80–83.

Hin, H., Bird, G., Fisher, P., et al., 1999. Coeliac disease in primary care: case finding study. BMJ 318, 164–167.

Hippisley-Cox, J., Pringle, M., 1997. A pilot study of a randomised controlled trial of pragmatic eradication of *H. pylori* in primary care. Br. J. Gen. Pract. 47, 375–377.

Hopper, A., Hadjivassiliou, M., Butt, S., et al., 2007. Adult coeliac disease. BMJ 335, 558–562.

Howden, C., Henning, J., Huang, B., et al., 2001. Management of heartburn in a large, randomized, community-based study: comparison of four therapeutic strategies. Am. J. Gastroenterol. 96, 1704–1710.

Jones, R., 2008. Treatment of irritable bowel syndrome in primary care. BMJ 337, 1361–1362.

Kaltenbach, T., Crockett, S., Gerson, L., 2006. Are lifestyle measures effective in patients with gastroesophageal reflux disease? Arch. Int. Med. 166, 965–971.

Kapoor, N., Bassi, A., Sturgess, R., Bodger, K., 2004. Predictive value of alarm features in a rapid access upper gastrointestinal cancer service. Gut 54, 40–45.

Laine, L., 2006. Review article: gastrointestinal bleeding with low-dose aspirin - what's the risk? Aliment. Pharmacol. Ther. 24, 897–908.

Lassen, A., Hallas, J., Schaffalitzky de Muckadell, O., 2004. *Helicobacter pylori* test and eradication versus prompt endoscopy for management of dyspeptic patients: 6.7 year follow up of a randomised trial. Gut 53, 1758–1763.

Logan, R., Delaney, B., 2001. Implications of dyspepsia for the NHS. BMJ 323, 675–677.

Lydeard, S., Jones, R., 1989. Factors affecting the decision to consult with dyspepsia: comparison of consulters and non-consulters. J. R. Coll. Gen. Pract. 39, 495–498.

MacDonald, C., Wicks, A., Playford, R., 2000. Final results from 10 year cohort of patients undergoing surveillance for Barratt's oesophagus: observational study. BMJ 321, 1252–1255.

McKee, A., Prior, A., Whorwell, P., 1987. Exclusion diets in irritable bowel syndrome: are they worthwhile? J. Clin. Gastroenterol. 9, 526–528.

MeReC, 1998. Proton pump inhibitors: their role in dyspepsia. MeReC Bulletin 11.

Meucci, G., D'Inca, R., Maieron, R., et al., 2009. Diagnostic value of faecal calprotectin in unselected outpatients referred for colonoscopy: a multicenter prospective study. Dig. Liver Dis. Aug 18 (epub).

Mitchell, J., Hussaini, H., McGovern, D., et al., 2002. The

'jaundice hotline' for the rapid assessment of patients with jaundice. BMJ 325, 213–215.

Moayyedi, P., Deeks, J., Talley, N., et al., 2003. An update of the Cochrane Systematic Review of *Helicobacter pylori* eradication therapy in nonulcer dyspepsia: resolving the discrepancy between systematic reviews. Am. J. Gastroenterol. 98, 2621–2626.

NICE, 2008. Irritable Bowel Syndrome in Adults: Diagnosis and Management of Irritable Bowel Syndrome in Primary Care: NICE Clinical Guideline 61. Available: www. nice.org.uk.

NHS Centre for Reviews and Dissemination, 2001. Effectiveness of laxatives in adults. Eff. Health Care 7 (1).

NICE, 2001a. Guidance on the use of COX II Selective Inhibitors for Osteoarthritis and Rheumatoid Arthritis: National Institute for Clinical Excellence Technology Appraisal No. 27. Available: www.nice.org.uk.

NICE, 2001b. Guidance on the Use of Proton Pump Inhibitors in the Treatment of Dyspepsia. London: NICE. Available: www.nice.org.uk.

NICE, 2002. Guidance on the use of Infliximab for Crohn's Disease: National Institute for Clinical Excellence. Available: www.nice. org.uk.

NICE, 2004. Dyspepsia: Managing Dyspepsia in Adults in Primary Care: National Institute for Clinical Evidence. Available: www.nice.org.uk choose 'Guidelines'.

NICE, 2005. Referral Guidelines for Suspected Cancer. London: National Institute for Health and Clinical Excellence. Available: www.nice.org.uk.

Nilsson, M., Johnsen, R., Ye, W., et al., 2004. Lifestyle related risk factors in the aetiology of gastro-oesophageal reflux. Gut 53, 1730–1735.

Passmore, A.P., Wilson-Davies, K., Stoker, A., 1993. Chronic constipation in long-stay elderly patients: a comparison of lactulose and a senna-fibre combination. BMJ 307, 769–771.

Phull, P., Halliday, D., Price, A., Jacyna, M., 1996. Absence of dyspeptic symptoms as a test for *Helicobacter* eradication. BMJ 312, 349–350.

Ramkumar, D., Rao, S., 2005. Efficacy and safety of traditional medical therapies for chronic constipation: systematic review. Am. J. Gastroenterol. 100, 936–971.

Rao, S., Ozturk, R., Laine, L., 2005. Clinical utility of diagnostic tests for constipation in adults: a systematic review. Am. J. Gastroenterol. 100, 1605–1615.

Redstone, H., Barrowman, N., Veldhuyzen Van Zanten, S., 2001. H2 receptor antagonists in the treatment of functional (nonulcer) dyspepsia: a meta-analysis of randomised controlled clinical trials. Aliment. Pharmacol. Ther. 15, 1291–1299.

Richey, R., Howdle, P., Shaw, E., et al., 2009. Recognition and assessment of coeliac disease in children and adults: summary of NICE guidance. BMJ 338, 1386–1388.

Robinson, A., Lee, V., Kennedy, A., et al., 2006. A randomised controlled trial of self-help interventions in patients with a primary care diagnosis of irritable bowel syndrome. Gut 55, 643–648.

Robinson, A., Thompson, D., Wilkin, D., et al., 2001. Guided self-management and patient-directed follow-up of ulcerative colitis: a randomized trial. Lancet 358, 976–981.

Rose, P., Murphy, M., Munafo, M., et al., 2004. Improving the ascertainment of families at high risk of colorectal cancer: a prospective GP register study. Br. J. Gen. Pract. 54, 267–271.

Rostom, A., Dube, C., Lewin, G., et al., 2007. Nonsteroidal anti-inflammatory drugs and cyclooxygenase-2 inhibitors for primary prevention of colorectal cancer: a systematic review prepared for the U.S. Preventive Services Task Force. Ann. Intern. Med. 146, 376–389.

Rostom, A., Dube, C., Wells, G., et al., 2002. Prevention of NSAID-induced gastroduodenal ulcers (Cochrane Review). The Cochrane Library. Available: www.nelh.nhs. uk.

Scott, E., Gaywood, I., Scott, B., for the British Society of Gastroenterology, 2000. Guidelines for Osteoporosis in Coeliac Disease and Inflammatory Bowel Disease. British Society of Gastroenterology. Available: www.bsg.org.uk.

Scottish Intercollegiate Guidelines Network, 2003. Dyspepsia: SIGN. Available: www.sign.ac.uk choose 'Guidelines'.

Seager, J., Hawkey, C., 2001. Indigestion and non-steroidal anti-inflammatory drugs. BMJ 323, 1236–1238.

Shepherd, S., Gibson, P., 2006. Fructose malabsorption and symptoms of irritable bowel syndrome: guidelines for effective dietary management. J. Am. Diet. Assoc. 106, 1631–1639.

Sherwood, P., Lyburn, I., Brown, S., Ryder, S., 2001. How are abnormal results for liver function tests dealt with in primary care? BMJ 50, 585–588.

Soo, S., Moayyedi, P., Deeks, J., et al., 2001. Psychological interventions for non-ulcer dyspepsia (Cochrane Review). In: The Cochrane Library. Issue 4. Update Software, Oxford.

Spechler, S., 2003. Managing Barratt's oesophagus. BMJ 326, 892–894.

Stanley, A., Ashley, D., Dalton, H., et al., 2009. Outpatient management of patients with low-risk upper-gastrointestinal haemorrhage: multicentre validation and prospective evaluation. Lancet 373, 42–47.

Starr, J., 2005. *Clostridium difficile* associated diarrhoea: diagnosis and treatment. BMJ 331, 498–501.

Tabas, G., Beaves, M., Wang, J., et al., 2004. Paroxetine to treat irritable bowel syndrome not responding to high-fibre diet: a double-blind, placebo-controlled trial. Am. J. Gastroenter. 99, 914–920.

Talley, N., Phung, N., Kalantar, J., 2001. Indigestion; when is it functional? BMJ 323, 1294.

Thomas, P., Forbes, A., Green, J., et al., 2003. Guidelines for the investigation of chronic diarrhoea, second ed. Gut 52 (Suppl. V), v1–v15.

Thompson, W., Longstreth, G., Drossman, D., et al., 1999. Functional bowel disorders and functional abdominal pain. Gut 45 (Suppl. II), II 43–II 47.

Tramonte, S., Brand, M., Mulrow, C., et al., 1997. The treatment of chronic constipation in adults. J. Gen. Intern. Med. 12, 15–24.

Truelove, S., Witts, L., 1955. Cortisone in ulcerative colitis. Final report on a therapeutic trial. BMJ 4947, 1041–1048.

Vahedi, H., Merat, S., Rashidioon, A., et al., 2005. The effect of fluoxetine in patients with pain and constipation-predominant irritable bowel syndrome: a double-blind randomized-controlled study. Aliment. Pharmacol. Ther. 22, 381–385.

Verne, G., Davis, R., Robinson, M., et al., 2003. Treatment of chronic constipation with colchicine: randomized, double-blind, placebo-controlled crossover trial. Am. J. Gastroenterol. 98, 1112–1116.

Wald, A., 2003. Is chronic use of stimulant laxatives harmful to the colon? J. Clin. Gastroenterol. 36, 386–389.

Weijnen, C., de Wit, N., Numans, M., et al., 2001. *Helicobacter pylori* testing in the primary care setting: which diagnostic test should be used? Aliment. Pharmacol. Ther. 15, 1205–1210.

Whorwell, P., 2009. The problem of insoluble fibre in irritable bowel syndrome. BMJ 338, 123.

Chapter 8

Endocrine problems

CHAPTER CONTENTS

DIABETES MELLITUS

GUIDELINES

Diabetes UK. *Recommendations for the Management of Diabetes in Primary Care.* 2nd edition, 2000. www.diabetes.org.uk, search on 'Diabetes in primary care'.
   Scottish Intercollegiate Guidelines Network. Management of Diabetes 2001. http://www.sign.ac.uk
   Department of Health. *Diabetes National Service Framework.* www.doh.gov.uk and search on 'Diabetes NSF'
   National Institute for Health and Clinical Excellence. *Type 2 Diabetes: National Clinical Guideline for Management in Primary and Secondary care.* CG 66; 2008. Partial update on 'Newer agents': CG 87. 2009. www.nice.org.uk

INTRODUCTION

UK estimates suggest that 2.5% of patients have known diabetes (8–10% of those over 65) and there are probably another 1–2% with undiagnosed diabetes. More recent data from the US suggest that, despite the UK's different ethnic mix, these figures may be underestimates (MMWR 2005).

The aim of treatment of both types 1 and 2 diabetes is to prevent the known complications occurring.

- Risks of microvascular complications are reduced by maintaining blood glucose levels as close as possible to normal. Macrovascular complications are reduced by blood sugar control and by tackling known risk factors

DOI: 10.1016/B978-0-7020-3053-6.00008-8

such as smoking, hypertension and hypercholesterolaemia.

- Structured care in general practice leads to outcomes that are at least as good as hospital care. This means a register of patients with diabetes, a recall system, a review at least annually and regular audit of the practice's performance (Griffin and Kinmonth 2000).
- The management of type 1 diabetes is, in the UK, carried out in secondary care or in primary care by GPs and nurses with a special interest in the condition. This section will focus on the management of type 2 diabetes.

AIMS (NATIONAL CHOLESTEROL EDUCATION PROGRAM (NCEP) EXPERT PANEL 2001)

- To prevent where possible new cases of type 2 diabetes.
- To identify all cases of diabetes in the practice.
- To provide a service, which supports patients in managing their diabetes and helps them adopt a healthy lifestyle.
- To provide high quality healthcare for people with diabetes in order to prevent the development of complications.
- To determine the development of complications and manage them appropriately to reduce the risk of disability and premature death.
- To optimize the outcome of pregnancies in women with diabetes.
- To help people with diabetes lead a full and satisfying life.

PREVENTION

- Both type 1 and type 2 diabetes are becoming increasingly common. In type 2 diabetes this is associated, in children as well as adults, with increasing obesity, a diet increasingly rich in fat, and a reduction in exercise. The term 'metabolic syndrome' is used for the phenomenon of insulin resistance where at least three of the following are present: central obesity, BP > 130/85, raised triglyceride, low HDL-cholesterol, and fasting blood glucose > 6.6 mmol/l (National Cholesterol Education Program (NCEP) expert panel 2001).
- The risk of developing diabetes can be reduced. A Finnish trial showed that a lifestyle intervention in middle-aged people with impaired glucose tolerance who were overweight reduced their risk of developing diabetes in the next 4 years from 23% to 11% (Tuomilheto, Lindstrom, Eriksson, et al. 2001). Another study showed that a lifestyle intervention in high-risk Americans prevented one case of diabetes for every seven people receiving the intervention for 3 years (Imperatore, Benjamin and Engelgau 2002). The benefits in lower risk UK populations may be less dramatic.

- Also at increased risk are those from ethnic minorities, women who have developed gestational diabetes, and women with polycystic ovary syndrome (PCOS) see page 328.

* Screen patients at high risk for diabetes (see below) and explain how diet and exercise can halve their risk. Draw up a plan for lifestyle change and arrange for them to be supported through it.

DIAGNOSIS

The WHO diagnostic criteria for diabetes are:

(a) fasting venous plasma glucose 7 mmol/l or above: or

(b) a random or 2-hour plasma glucose 11.1 mmol/l or above.

If the patient is asymptomatic then the diagnosis should be confirmed by a second test. An oral glucose tolerance test is not always necessary.

Impaired fasting glucose (IFG): a fasting plasma glucose of 6.1–6.9 mmol/l and a 2-hour glucose < 7.8 mmol/l.

Impaired glucose tolerance (IGT): a fasting plasma glucose less than 7.0 and a 2-hour glucose of 7.8–11.0 mmol/l (see page 230).

Gestational diabetes: the WHO definition is a fasting glucose of 7 mmol/l or above or a 2-hour glucose of 7.8 mmol/l or above (see page 396) although UK practice varies from Unit to Unit (American Diabetes Association 2000).

MEASURING THE 2-HOUR GLUCOSE IN PRIMARY CARE

1. Take fasting blood glucose. The patient should have been fasting overnight and on a normal diet for the 3 days before the test. The patient should not smoke on the day of the test.

2. Give 75 g anhydrous glucose. This can be given as Lucozade 394 ml (using the new 73 kcal/100 ml formulation). It should be drunk over no more than 5 minutes.

3. Take blood 2 hours later.

UNDIAGNOSED DIABETES

- Studies have shown that it takes, on average, 7–10 years before a patient with type 2 diabetes is diagnosed. At any one time 50% of patients with type 2 diabetes are undiagnosed.

- Up to 35% of newly diagnosed patients will have already suffered complications of diabetes (UKPDS 6 1990). It is therefore worthwhile identifying patients earlier as intervention has been shown to reduce the risk of subsequent complications.

- The UK National Screening Committee (July 2006) does not support universal screening for diabetes but advises that there might be a benefit from the screening of selected groups. It is still (August 2009) considering how best this might be done.

- Fasting plasma glucose alone is a poor screening test for impaired glucose regulation. An Australian study found that, if a cut-off of 6 mmol/l is used, 66% with IGT or IFG, and 36% with diabetes, will be missed. If a cut-off of 5.5 mmol/l is used, 50% with IGT or IFG, and 20% with diabetes, will be missed (UK National Screening Committee 2008). Adding the assessment of HbA_{1c} with a cut-off of 5.3% (34 mmol/mol) improves those figures but only modestly. Using an oral glucose tolerance test hugely improves detection but is too time consuming to be used as a first line screening test.

- The best approach is likely to be a combination of:
  - (a) identification that an individual belongs to a high-risk group, and, if so,
  - (b) a fasting plasma glucose with a cut-off of 5.5 mmol/l and an oral glucose tolerance test in those found to be positive.

- At the time of writing the most promising assessment of risk seems to be that provided by a diabetes risk score developed in Finland (FINDRISC) (Lindstrom and Tuomilehto 2003). The assessment form can be found on page 33 of the Handbook for Vascular Risk Assessment, Risk Reduction and Risk Management. www.screening.nhs.uk (choose 'all UK NSC policies' then 'adult policies' then 'vascular risk'). Points are awarded for age ≥ 45, BMI ≥ 25, waist circumference ≥ 94 cm in men or ≥ 80 cm in women, lack of exercise, diet low in vegetables, fruit and berries, taking medication for hypertension, a previous high blood glucose and a family history of diabetes. Up to 5 points may be awarded for one risk factor according to severity. A score of 12–14 gives a moderate risk of developing type 2 diabetes in the following 10 years (1 in 6), a score of 15–20 is high risk (1 in 3) and > 20 is very high (1 in 2). A UK alternative is the QDScore (Hippisley-Cox, Coupland, Robson, et al. 2009).

- General practices should consider screening those patients who are at high risk of having, or of developing, diabetes. Testing Caucasians from the West Country of England who were over 50 years old with a BMI over 26 and not known to be diabetic detected 2.6% who were diabetic and 5.2% with impaired fasting glycaemia: a number needed to test of 13 (Greaves, Stead, Hattersley, et al. 2004).

* Check from the practice electronic records whether there are any patients with abnormal plasma glucose results in whom the diagnosis of diabetes or impaired glucose regulation has neither been made nor excluded. A UK study of over 3 million records found that almost 1% of that population had a latest glucose reading (fasting or random) that was ≥ 7 mmol/l that had not been followed up (Holt, Stables, Hippisley-Cox, et al. 2008). 0.1% had a fasting level ≥ 7 mmol/ or a random level ≥ 11.1 mmol/l. Only 1 practice out of 480 had no such patients.

* Consider screening, with a fasting glucose, patients at moderate or high risk of having, or developing, diabetes (see next page and the FINDRISC score). If the fasting value is greater than 7 mmol/l repeat the test. A second value > 7 mmol/l confirms diabetes.

* If the fasting value is between 5 and 7 mmol/l check the 2-hour glucose.

* Repeat the screening every 5 years, or more frequently in those with multiple risk factors or with IGT or IFG.

- White Europeans aged > 40.
- Obesity (BMI > 30) or overweight with a sedentary lifestyle.
- Hypertension (140/90 or over).
- Cardiovascular disease.
- First degree family history of diabetes.
- Certain ethnic groups (Chinese, African Caribbean, Indian, Pakistani and Bangladeshi). Use cut-offs of BMI 23 and 27.5 instead of 25 and 30 to define overweight and obesity respectively.
- History of gestational diabetes, IGT or IFG.
- Polycystic ovary syndrome.
- Hypertriglyceridaemia.

IMPAIRED GLUCOSE TOLERANCE

Even if they do not develop diabetes, patients with IGT are at increased risk of cardiovascular disease: ischaemic heart disease, stroke and peripheral vascular disease. One in three will develop diabetes within 10 years, a rate which can be halved with appropriate lifestyle changes.

Management:

* Provide an intensive programme of weight loss, healthy eating, exercise, with management of blood pressure, lipids, and smoking as appropriate.
* Check the fasting glucose every 3 years or annually if there are multiple risk factors.
* Consider treatment with acarbose 100 mg daily in those at high risk of CVD. In an international study it halved the risk of major cardiovascular events or of developing hypertension over 3.3 years (NNT = 40) (Chiasson, Josse, Gomis, et al. 2003). Metformin and glitazones will also prevent the progression from IGT to diabetes but have yet to be shown to reduce the risk of CVD (Davies 2003). At the time of writing there is no national guidance in the UK or the US on whether the use of these agents is considered cost-effective. Medical treatment should not detract attention from the more important lifestyle changes above.

MANAGEMENT OF DIABETES

* Distinguish between type 1 and type 2 diabetes. Younger patients who present with acute illness, weight loss and ketonuria are type 1. However,

there are increasing numbers of younger patients who develop type 2 diabetes and are managed with diet only or with oral hypoglycaemics. Conversely, some patients with type 2 diabetes require insulin because of poor control with diet and oral agents but they retain the clinical features of a type 2 patient.

* Consider checking insulin autoantibodies and c-peptide status of patients in whom the type of diabetes is not clear. The presence of insulin auto antibodies in newly diagnosed patients supports the diagnosis of type 1 as does an absence of c-peptide.

INITIAL MANAGEMENT

● Newly diagnosed patients with ketosis, a blood glucose > 30 mmol/l, or who appear to have type 1 diabetes should be referred immediately for assessment and usually admission to hospital for treatment. This applies also to children, pregnant women and those with serious medical conditions (e.g. liver, renal and cardiac disease).
● Those with uncomplicated type 2 diabetes can be managed initially in general practice.

Examination: weight, height and girth, blood pressure, a cardiovascular assessment, examination for peripheral neuropathy, visual acuity and referral for retinal eye screening.

Blood tests: FBC, U&Es, glucose, HbA_{1c}, serum creatinine, thyroid function, LFTs, fasting cholesterol, HDL and triglycerides.

Urine: glucose, ketones and proteinuria.

* Take a history, including family history, past serious illnesses, current medication and lifestyle questions including smoking, alcohol, exercise and employment.
* Explain the nature of diabetes and give appropriate supporting literature.
* Explain the importance of diet, exercise and attention to glycaemic control.
* Refer every patient to a dietician and to a local diabetes educational programme if available.
* Explain the problems of the complications of diabetes and the importance of regular eye checks, foot care, and, where appropriate, blood pressure and cholesterol management. Half of

all patients with type 2 diabetes are hypertensive and require treatment to reduce their blood pressure to normal levels.

* Sign form FP92A if prescribing oral drugs or insulin to exempt patients from prescription charges.

* Explain to drivers that they need to notify the DVLA if prescribed oral drugs or insulin at any stage.

* Decide with the patient what form of home glucose monitoring is appropriate. Blood testing has the advantage of demonstrating hypoglycaemia, and of greater sensitivity. NICE (2008) comments that it is especially suitable for those on insulin or on glucose-lowering drugs; for those currently changing medication or lifestyle; during illness; and when a patient needs to check that there is no risk of hypoglycaemia during a potentially dangerous activity, such as driving. Urine testing is adequate for stable patients with type 2 diabetes managed on diet alone, if they prefer it. The mere provision of self-monitoring equipment is not enough. The patient must be taught how and when to use it and what action to take according to the results.

* However, this advice is not well supported by the evidence. A UK randomized trial in primary care found that self-monitoring of blood glucose over a 3-year period did not improve glycaemic control compared to controls (Farmer, Wade, Goyder, et al. 2007). Indeed, recent trials have failed to show any improvement of HbA$_{1c}$ in patients randomised to self-monitoring of blood glucose but they have shown that self-monitoring is associated with depression and a worse quality of life (Gulliford 2008).

* Attempt, in asymptomatic patients, to achieve control with the above measures for at least 3 months before giving oral hypoglycaemic agents. However, start drugs immediately if there are symptoms of hyperglycaemia or the fasting glucose is > 15 mmol/l.

HOME URINE TESTS FOR GLUCOSE

■ Test daily until the targets are reached then test twice weekly. Resume daily testing during intercurrent illness and if results on twice weekly testing fail to meet the targets.

■ Stress to the patient that urine testing is too crude for it to be used to assess excellence of blood sugar

control. It is more valuable in detecting serious glycaemic disturbance, as in intercurrent illness. Patients who want to use home testing to ensure tight glycaemic control need to test blood sugars using a meter.

When to test the urine	Target
Before breakfast	Negative
2 hours after the main meal	< 1/4%

HOME BLOOD TESTS FOR GLUCOSE IN NON-INSULIN TREATED DIABETES

* Choose a regimen that suits the patient. Typical options are:
  (a) Testing before each meal and before going to bed, on one day a week; or
  (b) Testing before bed every night plus one other test at a different time each day.
* Change to testing 4 times a day during intercurrent illness and if results on less intensive testing fail to meet the target (Table 8.1).

| Table 8.1 | Target values to be achieved when treating patients with diabetes in primary care. Adapted from a table first published by Diabetes UK |

TESTS	GOOD	BORDERLINE	POOR
Fasting blood glucose (mmol/l)	4.0–7.0	7.1–7.8	> 7.8
HbA$_{1c}$	< 6.5%	6.5–10.0	> 10.0
HbA$_{1c}$ (mmol/mol)	< 48	48–86	> 86
Serum cholesterol (mmol/l)			
Total	< 5.0	5.0–6.5	> 6.5
HDL	> 1.1	0.9–1.1	< 0.9
Fasting triglycerides (mmol/l)	< 1.7	1.7–2.2	> 2.2
BMI (kg/m^2)	< 25	25–27	> 27
Blood pressure	< 130/80	130/80–140/80	> 140/80
Albuminuria	< 20 mg/L	20–200mg/l	> 200 mg/l

GLYCAEMIC CONTROL

● Prolonged high blood sugar levels are associated with increased macrovascular and microvascular disease. Intensive treatment to reduce blood sugar levels and HbA$_{1C}$ has been shown to be effective in reducing the risk of vascular disease in both type 1 (Diabetes Control and Complications Trial Research Group 1993) and type 2 diabetes (UKPDS Group 1998a). However, two recent studies have suggested that intensive blood sugar lowering may not reduce cardiovascular complications and may even increase them (Sherifali 2009). A review of all recent major trials suggests that intensive control is of cardiovascular benefit long-term, but that patients at high cardiovascular risk should achieve glycaemic control gently, not aggressively (Sherifali 2009). Furthermore, ideal levels may not be achievable in some patients. A target should be set for each individual that takes into account age, other illnesses and other risk factors.

- Type 2 diabetes deteriorates with time. Glycaemic control can usually only be maintained by increasing doses of tablets, sometimes followed by a move to insulin.
- In the UK Prospective Diabetes Study (UKPDS) almost 80% required insulin after 9 years of oral treatment. Patients often resist the move but, if they can be persuaded to make it, they can expect better protection against micro- and macrovascular complications.

Type 2 diabetes

If good control is not achieved with diet and increasing physical activity add an oral agent. Allow 4 months between increments. The NICE 2009 guideline's quick reference guide includes a helpful flow-chart for the management of blood sugar control.

- *Prescribe metformin*. Early use of metformin reduces the risk of death or developing diabetes related complications (UKPDS Group 1998b).
- Do not use in patients with impairment of renal or liver function or in severe cardiac failure.
- Start with 500 mg daily and increase up to a maximum of 2–3 g per day.
- If the patient develops G-I adverse effects, consider a modified-release version.
- *Consider a sulphonylurea* instead if a rapid response is needed to control symptoms of hyperglycaemia; or the patient is not overweight; or metformin is contraindicated.
- If using a sulphonylurea, choose a shorter acting agent, e.g. gliclazide or tolbutamide. The longer

acting glibenclamide can be considered but is more likely to cause hypoglycaemia and should be avoided in those over 65 or those with impaired renal or hepatic function. On the other hand, its once-daily dosage may help when adherence is a problem.

- If good glycaemic control is not achieved by metformin at maximum dose, add a sulphonylurea.
- If one of them is not tolerated use the other plus a thiazolidinedione (pioglitazone or rosiglitazone) or a DPP-4 inhibitor (sitagliptin or vildagliptin).
- If control is not achieved, with the HbA1c $\geq 7.5\%$ (58 mmol/mol), add insulin to metformin and a sulfonylurea. However, NICE (2009) recommends the use of triple therapy (metformin, a sulphonylurea and a thiazolidinedione or sitagliptin) instead in patients who are unwilling to accept insulin or who are obese or have the metabolic syndrome.
- An intermediate-acting insulin, e.g. human isophane insulin, given once or twice a day, is a convenient starting point. Because of the detailed patient education required it should be initiated by those experienced in diabetes, whether in primary or secondary care. NICE recommends that insulin glargine, convenient though its once-daily regimen is, should be confined, in type 2 diabetes, to those who would otherwise need twice daily injections, or who are restricted by recurrent hypoglycaemia, or who need assistance to take their insulin (McIntosh, Hutchinson, Home, *et al.* 2002).
- If control on insulin (+/−oral agents) is poor, options are: pre-mixed insulin (biphasic insulin); and pre-prandial injections in addition to a basal regimen.

WARNINGS ON THE USE OF THIAZOLIDINEDIONES

- Take LFTs before starting and 2 months after starting. Stop the thiazolidinedione if the ALT exceeds 2.5 times the upper limit of normal.
- Do not use in the presence of heart failure. They cause fluid retention.
- Do not combine rosiglitazone with insulin; pioglitazone may be combined with insulin if it has been effective previously.

Alternative therapies

- *Repaglinide and nateglinide* are secretagogues which are no more effective than a sulphonylurea but may be useful in sulphonylurea intolerance.
- *Exenatide* is recommended by NICE (2009), in addition to metformin and a sulphonylurea for:
  - those with a BMI > 35 kg/m^2 (for someone of European origin) whose weight is causing problems and whose HbA_{1C} is $\geq 7.5\%$ (58 mmol/mol) on dual therapy. Only continue it if it shows benefit (at least a 1% reduction in HbA_{1C} after 6 months and at least 5% weight loss after a year); or
  - those with a BMI < 35 kg/m^2 who cannot accept the use of insulin or in whom weight loss would benefit other comorbidities.
  - Only continue exenatide if the HbA_{1C} has fallen by at least 1 percentage point and the initial body weight by at least 3% in 6 months.
- *Acarbose* delays the absorption of starch in the gut and can be used alone or as an adjunctive to other oral therapies. A systematic review has estimated that acarbose will reduce HbA_{1C} by between 0.5 and 0.9% (Campbell, White and Campbell 1996). NICE (2008) only recommends it for someone unable to use other oral agents.

ASSESSMENT OF GLYCAEMIC CONTROL

* Check glycated haemoglobin (HbA_{1C}) 2 monthly at first, then 6 monthly once stable. It is the most reliable method of estimating glycaemic control. Aim for an HbA_{1C} of less than 6.5% (52 mmol/mol). These lower levels offer greater protection against vascular complications; the UKPDS found the following risk reductions for every 1% reduction in HbA_{1C}: diabetes-related death 21%; myocardial infarction 14%, microvascular complications 37%. However, be ready to choose a higher target if the patient wishes it, despite understanding the above. Fear of hypoglycaemia or unacceptable lifestyle changes may cause the patient to choose a higher figure.

* Encourage blood glucose monitoring over urine testing (see above) but remain sensitive to the patient's preferences. At the annual review, ask how often monitoring was done, what benefit ensued, and check the patient's technique.

POINTS ABOUT GLYCATED HAEMOGLOBINS

- They represent an average of blood sugar control over the previous 6–8 weeks. They may be normal in patients with fluctuating sugar levels if the fluctuations are above and below the target, and should therefore be interpreted alongside the blood sugar tests.
- A falsely high HbA_1 occurs in alcohol abuse, uraemia and high levels of haemoglobin. HbA_{1c} is specific for blood glucose, with fewer false positives.
- Different laboratories may have different reference ranges although standardization is occurring rapidly.
- Check that there is no discrepancy between HbA_{1c} and self-monitored blood sugar levels. A patient with good pre-meal blood glucose levels but a high HbA_{1C} may have postprandial hyperglycaemia (> 8.5 mmol/l). If self-monitoring shows this, consider giving preprandial insulin.
- If discrepancy remains between HbA_{1c} and blood glucose levels, seek expert advice.

BLOOD PRESSURE

- Good control of blood pressure is important in reducing the risk of cardiovascular events (UKPDS Group 1998c; Hansson, Zanchetti, Carruthers, *et al.* 1998). Thus a reduction of 10 mmHg systolic blood pressure and 5 mmHg diastolic results in a 24% reduction in diabetic related end points after 9 years – a NNT of 60. The threshold for treatment is a sustained pressure of 140/80 or above.
- Various studies have used different target blood pressures. There are therefore different target blood pressures that are suggested by different guidelines. The British Hypertension Guidelines recommend that for patients with diabetes the aim should be for a diastolic below 80 mmHg and a systolic below 130 mmHg (Williams, Poulter, Brown, *et al.* 2004). However, the NICE guideline (2009) recommends $< 130/80$ for those with kidney, eye or cerebrovascular damage; otherwise $< 140/80$.

Note: The Clinical Quality Indicators suggest a target of 145/85 for *audit* purposes (Kenny 2004).

* Check BP annually if not hypertensive. Start treatment (see page 137) if the BP remains above

the threshold for treatment after 2 months (or after 1 month if > 150/90).

* Begin with an ACE inhibitor, or in a person of African-Caribbean origin, an ACE inhibitor plus a thiazide or calcium-channel blocker. Then proceed as for a non-diabetic hypertensive (see page 137).

LIPIDS

● There is good evidence that lipid lowering is worthwhile in reducing cardiovascular risk in high-risk patients (Pyorala, Pedersen, Kjekshus, *et al.* 1997). Sub-group analyses of diabetic patients in large primary prevention studies (Downs, Clearfield, Weiss, *et al.* 1998; Koskinen, Manttari, Manninen, *et al.* 1992) and the CARDS study in patients with type 2 diabetes (Colhoun, Betteridge, Durrington, *et al.* 2004) also suggest that lipid lowering is worthwhile in diabetic patients without CHD. The NNT in preventing one major cardiovascular event was 27 after 4 years of treatment.

● The 2004 British Hypertension Society Guidelines recommended that statins be given to all with type 2 diabetes. Current advice from NICE (2008) is that those with type 2 diabetes should be assessed using a 'risk engine' that calculates CVD risk using data from the UKPDS. The programme can be downloaded from www.dtu.ox.ac.uk/index.php?maindoc=/riskengine/. Using it, most, but not all, with type 2 diabetes will qualify for a statin because of a CVD risk of at least 20% over 10 years.

* If prescribing a statin, e.g. simvastatin 40 mg daily, check lipid profile 3 months later. Aim for a total cholesterol < 4 mmol/l; or an LDL-cholesterol < 2 mmol/l. If the target has not been reached, increase to 80 mg daily. If control is still not achieved consider adding ezetimibe, especially if the patient has cardiovascular disease or an increased albumin excretion rate.

* *Raised serum triglyceride.* Look for a treatable cause, especially poor glycaemic control. If the serum triglyceride remains > 4.5 mmol/l give a fibrate in addition to a statin. If that fails to bring the triglyceride below 4.5 mmol/l consider prescribing omega-3 marine triglycerides. Specialist advice would be wise at this point. In patients who already have CVD start a fibrate if the triglyceride is ≥ 2.3 mmol/l.

SMOKING

Although only around 15% of patients with diabetes are smokers it is important to identify these patients and make every effort to encourage them to give up.

* Consider nicotine replacement therapy or referral to specialist smoking cessation classes (see page 498).

EXERCISE

* Advise all sedentary patients with diabetes to increase their levels of exercise. Recommend aerobic exercise such as walking, jogging or swimming for at least 4 hours per week (Tuomilheto, Lindstrom, Eriksson, *et al.* 2001). Exercise lowers blood sugar, improves control and reduces the risk of macrovascular events.

* Give advice on footwear for those with peripheral neuropathy.

* Instruct patients on insulin or sulphonylureas to monitor their blood glucose before and after vigorous and prolonged exercise.

ANTI-THROMBOTIC TREATMENT

* *Aspirin.* In addition to the changes already mentioned, prescribe, or recommend, aspirin 75 mg daily for those with diabetes who are aged at least 50 and who are normotensive; and for those aged < 50 who have other risk factors for CVD. If aspirin is not tolerated use clopidogrel.

RENAL DISEASE (NATIONAL INSTITUTE FOR HEALTH AND CLINICAL EXCELLENCE 2008)

● The commonest cause of end-stage renal failure in adults is diabetes. Persistent hyperglycaemia can lead to microvascular damage of the kidneys. Hypertension in patients with diabetes also causes renal damage.

● Early identification and treatment can reduce the risks of end-stage renal failure or cardiovascular mortality. (NHS Centre for Reviews and Dissemination 2000).

● Spot tests for microalbuminuria have poor sensitivity and specificity because they vary according to the patient's fluid output. The albumin/creatinine ratio (ACR) is more reliable. It is also more sensitive than the protein/creatinine ratio (PCR).

∗ Test annually for:
  - proteinuria and, if negative, the urinary albumin/creatinine ratio
  - serum creatinine and calculate the GFR (see page 425).

Proteinuria

∗ If proteinuria is present check for infection with an MSU and repeat.
∗ If proteinuria persists refer to a diabetologist.
∗ If the eGFR is < 30 ml/min/1.73 m^2 refer to a consultant nephrologist.

MICROALBUMINURIA

- 25% of patients with type 2 diabetes have microalbuminuria and these patients have double the risk of death compared with those without. This risk can be reduced by treatment.
- In diabetes, microalbuminuria is clinically significant if the ACR is > 2.5mg/mmol in a man or > 3.5 mg/mmol in a woman.

∗ Repeat a positive test twice over the next 3–4 months on the first morning specimen, to exclude orthostatic proteinuria. If at least one of those tests confirms microalbuminuria, consider that a positive result. However, if a test on a single early morning sample is unequivocally abnormal (ACR ≥ 70 mg/mmol) further confirmation is not needed. Repeat negative tests annually (NHS Centre for Reviews and Dissemination 2000).

If microalbuminuria is confirmed:

∗ Control the blood pressure to a systolic of 120–129 and a diastolic < 80 mmHg.
∗ Control the blood sugar of patients even more intensively.
∗ Give an ACE inhibitor or ARB, even in those with normal blood pressure (NHS Centre for Reviews and Dissemination 2000). Titrate up to the maximum recommended dose.

FOOT CARE

- 15% of people with diabetes will develop foot ulcers associated with neuropathy and/or peripheral ischaemia. This can lead to joint involvement and may require amputation.

- All patients at their annual review should have their feet checked for ulcers, their peripheral pulses checked and their sensation tested. This is best done with monofilaments – plastic filaments of different thickness which can be used to test sensation more accurately.
- It is particularly important that those patients with sensory loss are given information about foot care as intensive management can reduce the risk of amputation by two thirds. This intervention includes care from a podiatrist.
- All patients with ulcers should be referred to a podiatrist for treatment.
- For the management of neuropathic pain see page 677. Briefly, NICE recommends a tricyclic, followed by the cheapest of duloxetine, gabapentin or pregabalin. If pain is still uncontrolled, further options are opiate analgesia and referral to the chronic pain management team.

EYE CARE

- The commonest cause of blindness in the working population is diabetes. This is aggravated by poor control of blood glucose.
- All patients with diabetes should have an annual review that includes an assessment of visual acuity and examination of the retina (NHS Centre for Reviews and Dissemination 1999).
- The best method of retinal screening is by retinal photography using a digital camera. An alternative is to use slit lamp microscopy. Local arrangements to provide this service are usually available through diabetes clinics in acute trusts but alternative sources of the service may be available. Direct ophthalmoscopy alone, especially if carried out by a general practitioner, is not sensitive or specific enough for routine use (NHS Centre for Reviews and Dissemination 1999; British Diabetic Association 1997).

∗ Refer to an ophthalmologist if proliferative, pre-proliferative or exudative retinopathy, or cataract, are detected, but not if only background retinopathy is present, unless it is at the macula and associated with a visual acuity of 6/12 or worse. Proliferative retinopathy warrants rapid referral. Refer too if there is visual deterioration which cannot be corrected with glasses.

OVERWEIGHT AND OBESITY

- Obesity is difficult to influence and indeed patients with type 2 diabetes who have been switched to insulin therapy often improve their glycaemic control whilst at the same time gaining weight. Despite this it is important to encourage patients to exercise and eat a healthy diet and to try to lose weight.
- Obese patients who have IFG or IGT need to lose weight in order to reduce their risk of developing diabetes.
- The mainstay of treatment includes a weight reducing diet and an increase in physical activity.
- * Agree with the patient an initial target of weight loss that is not too daunting, e.g. a loss of only 5–10% of the present weight. Stress that weight loss of even less than that is of benefit.
- * Consider the use of weight reducing drugs for those with a BMI over 27 kg/m^2 (for sibutramine) or over 28 kg/m^2 (for orlistat) (National Institute for Health and Clinical Excellence 2006). The drug should only be continued for > 3 months if weight loss of at least 5% has been achieved (see page 508).
- * Consider surgery for obesity if the BMI is ≥ 35 kg/m^2 and all other methods have failed over a 6 month trial. NICE recommends that surgery should be considered first line if the BMI is ≥ 50 kg/m^2 (National Institute for Health and Clinical Excellence 2006). Surgery should only be considered if combined with intensive therapy in a specialist obesity service, and the patient commits to long-term follow-up.

ERECTILE DYSFUNCTION

Approximately 40% of males with diabetes suffer from impotence. Many patients are reluctant to raise this but are pleased that the clinician does so.

- * Check for an underlying vascular cause.
- * Check that it is not the side effect of medication, e.g. antihypertensives.
- * Consider treatment with a phosphodiesterase type-5 inhibitor e.g. sildenafil (see page 372). These drugs have made the treatment of impotence acceptable to many more patients and are effective in men with both type 1 and type 2 diabetes (Rendell 1999).

DEPRESSION

Mental disorders are common in patients with diabetes, especially depression.

- * Check for depression using the screening questions on page 452.

DIABETES IN PREGNANCY

- Approximately 3 in 1000 pregnancies occur in women with type 1 diabetes. These patients should be referred for specialist care as optimum glycaemic control is essential to ensure the best outcome for mother and child (Scottish Intercollegiate Guidelines Network 2001) (see page 396).
- Depending on the criteria for diagnosis, between 1 and 4% of women will develop gestational diabetes, which is associated with increased complications for the mother, and poorer fetal outcomes. Moreover, 30% of women with gestational diabetes will develop established diabetes later in life (see page 372).
- Women with gestational diabetes are at higher risk of developing eclampsia, having a Caesarean section and having a large baby.

THE ANNUAL REVIEW

All patients with diabetes should be on a register and have an annual review.

The review should include an opportunity to offer education where this is lacking. Some practices offer all but the eye check on a 6 monthly rather than on an annual basis. An annual check should be regarded as the minimum monitoring that patients with uncomplicated diabetes receive.

ANNUAL CHECKS

(a) Weight and waist circumference.

(b) Blood pressure.

(c) Urinalysis for protein. If positive (i.e. more than a trace), urine microscopy and culture. Repeat the urinalysis. If proteinuria persists refer for investigation.

(d) If no proteinuria, send urine for albumin/creatinine ratio (ACR).

(e) Feet. Refer any problems to a chiropodist.

(f) Eye check – visual acuity and fundi, preferably by digital photography.

(g) Check the patient's glucose self-monitoring technique.

(h) Random blood sugar, preferably obtaining an immediate result by using a reflectance meter.

(i) HbA$_{1C}$.

(j) Total cholesterol, HDL-cholesterol and triglycerides.

(k) Serum creatinine and estimate GFR.

EDUCATION

● Education is the mainstay of the management of diabetes. Patients who understand the disease are most likely to adhere to their management although there is little evidence that they are less likely to suffer complications.

● All new patients should receive structured education about the nature of diabetes, its day to day management, the handling of special problems such as hypoglycaemia and advice on living with diabetes. This should be reinforced at least annually.

● Belonging to Diabetes UK provides an alternative source of information and supports patients in managing their diabetes.

THE DIABETIC DIET

Despite having seen a dietician and/or a specialist nurse, patients will still ask the GP about their diet. The modern diabetic diet is one that stresses the positive rather than the negative, and which aims as much at the prevention of CVD as at the reduction of carbohydrate. The basis is:

■ *fruit and vegetables*: eat ≥ five portions a day;

■ *bread, whole-grain cereals, potatoes, pasta, rice*: eat five portions a day;

■ *beans and lentils*: eat regularly;

■ *oily fish*: eat at least two portions a week;

■ *fatty or sugary foods, saturated fat (e.g. butter, margarine, cheese, fatty meat) and alcohol*: eat as little as possible.

HYPOGLYCAEMIA

● Patients on insulin or long-acting oral hypoglycaemics if they are well controlled with an HbA$_{1C}$ below 7.5% (58 mmol/mol) are likely to experience occasional hypoglycaemic attacks.

✳ Teach patients how to prevent a hypoglycaemic attack. Explain the importance of always having a

source of glucose with them and suggest they wear an alert bracelet (see page 590).

✳ Consider training a spouse or another family member to give glucagon parenterally particularly with patients who have experienced severe hypoglycaemic episodes.

The management of a hypoglycaemic attack

✳ Give oral glucose.

✳ If the patient is unconscious, give glucagon 1 mg i.v., i.m. or s.c. Once the patient is conscious, give oral glucose; the benefit of glucagon is shortlived.

✳ Alternatively, give 50 ml of 20% glucose intravenously.

REFERRAL FOR SPECIALIST CARE

Referral criteria for secondary care should be agreed with the local consultants. In general this should include:

(a) all newly diagnosed patients with type 1 diabetes or with ketosis;

(b) all children;

(c) all pregnant women;

(d) all patients with serious complications such as ischaemic heart disease, renal impairment, retinopathy or neuropathy;

(e) patients in whom optimum control of blood sugars or blood pressure cannot be achieved.

DRIVING

Insulin treated patients are barred from driving HGV or PCV vehicles. They may drive a car but must notify the DVLA and their car insurance company and should stop driving if experiencing disabling hypoglycaemia.

Patients on oral hypoglycaemics or with diabetic complications should also inform the DVLA. Those with no complications and controlled by diet alone do not need to inform the DVLA (DVLA 2001).

PNEUMOCCOCCAL VACCINE AND FLU VACCINE

All patients with diabetes should be offered an annual flu vaccine and a pneumoccocal vaccine every 5 years.

DIABETES UK

Diabetes UK is the largest organization in the UK specifically aimed at supporting patients with diabetes. They produce excellent advice for patients with diabetes, support the formation and running of local support groups and run regular educational events for people with diabetes. All newly diagnosed patients should be advised of their existence. Their address is Diabetes UK, 10 Parkway, London NW1 7AA, tel. 020 7424 1000, www.diabetes.org.uk.

MANAGING INTERCURRENT ILLNESS ('SICK DAY RULES')

When managing intercurrent illness in a diabetic patient check that the patient knows to do the following:

* Test blood (or urine) for glucose more often. Testing 4 hourly may be necessary in type 1 diabetes. Call if the urine sugar shows 2%.
* Test capillary blood or urine for ketones if on insulin. Call if more than a trace of ketosis appears.
* Continue to take the prescribed tablets or insulin. Call if unable to do so.
* Eat a normal diet or take equivalent carbohydrate-containing drinks.
* Drink plenty of fluid.

Adherence to these rules will reduce the need to increase the patient's insulin. However, if glycaemic control is slipping or mild ketosis appears, increase the current insulin by small increments.

Admit a patient with more marked ketosis or hyperglycaemia or who is unable to eat and take medication.

THYROID DISEASE

REVIEWS AND GUIDELINES

Topliss DJ, Eastman CJ. 2004. Diagnosis and management of hyperthyroidism and hypothyroidism. Med J Australia 180, 186–193
   Royal College of Physicians, *et al.* 2008. *The Diagnosis and Management of Primary Hypothyroidism.* London. Available: www.rcplondon.ac.uk

HYPERTHYROIDISM

* Confirm the diagnosis by checking circulating free thyroxine (FT_4), free tri-iodothyronine (FT_3) and thyroid stimulating hormone (TSH) – either FT_4 or FT_3 or both will be raised. The TSH is usually depressed.
* Beware of diagnosing hyperthyroidism solely on a low TSH; it can be low in patients ill with other conditions.
* Consider the diagnosis of pituitary adenoma if the FT_4 is raised and the TSH is normal or raised.
* Check the WBC before treatment is started. Agranulocytosis occurs in 0.3% of patients treated with antithyroid drugs. A baseline WBC allows the neutropenia associated with thyrotoxicosis to be distinguished from drug-induced agranulocytosis (Singer, Cooper, Levy, *et al.* 1995).

TREATMENT

● The definitive treatment of Graves' hyperthyroidism includes antithyroid drugs, radioactive iodine (I^{131}) or thyroid surgery.
* Repeat the FT_4, FT_3 and TSH before starting antithyroid drugs. Specific treatment should usually be withheld until a firm biochemical diagnosis has been made.
* Prescribe a beta-blocker for those with tremor or tachycardia who need symptomatic relief (e.g. long-acting propranolol 160 mg/day or nadolol 80 mg/day). For the management of atrial fibrillation in thyrotoxicosis see page 160.
* Refer all patients with thyrotoxicosis to a specialist. Usual antithyroid drugs include carbimazole and propylthiouracil. A policy should be agreed with the local hospital as to whether antithyroid treatment should be started by the general practitioner before the patient is seen by the specialist. Antithyroid drugs should not be given in thyroiditis but symptoms can be relieved with a beta-blocker.
* If treating in primary care, start with carbimazole 15–40 mg/day maintained for 4–8 weeks until the patient is euthyroid. Thereafter, titrate the dosage against the TSH. It can usually be reduced to a daily dose of 5–15 mg and should be continued for 12–18 months.

* If the patient develops a rash or pruritus change to propylthiouracil propylthiouracil 200–400 mg daily not all patients will be sensitive to both drugs. Again the dosage will subsequently be reduced to a maintenance dose, usually 50–150 mg daily.

* Alternatively, give higher doses of antithyroid drugs with levothyroxine sodium: the 'block and replace regimen'. The hope was that this would reduce the incidence of iatrogenic hypothyroidism but this is not supported by the evidence (Abraham, Avenell, Watson, *et al.* 2005).

* *Agranulocytosis.* Warn all patients on carbimazole or propylthiouracil to seek attention promptly if they develop a sore throat, a rash or unusual itching.

* *Follow-up.* See patients 4 weekly until euthyroid and then every 3 months. At follow-up appointments check the weight, pulse and blood pressure and a blood test for FT_4, FT_3 and TSH.

* *Duration of treatment.* In Graves' disease, give antithyroid drugs for 12–18 months; even then there is a 50% relapse rate after stopping the drugs. Check the FT_4 and TSH at 2 months and at 1 year after treatment has been stopped. Patients that relapse require definitive ablation of the gland either with I^{131} or with thyroid surgery. Definitive treatment is always needed in toxic nodular goitre, though there is likely to be a response to antithyroid drugs while they are taken.

* *Pregnancy.* Patients who are being treated for thyrotoxicosis and become pregnant have an increased risk of miscarriage, pre-eclampsia and other problems, and should be referred back to a specialist. Hyperthyroidism arising in pregnancy is probably transient gestational hyperthyroidism, especially in South Asian women, but Graves' disease does occur and needs careful treatment to reduce maternal and fetal adverse outcomes.

* *Subclinical hyperthyroidism* is diagnosed by the finding of a low TSH but a normal FT_3 and FT_4. Even if the TSH is < 0.1 mIU/l the risk of progression to overt hyperthyroidism is only 1–2% per year (Surks, Ortiz, Daniels, *et al.* 2004). However, subclinical hyperthyroidism is associated with a three-fold increased risk of atrial fibrillation and such patients with AF should be referred for consideration of treatment, as should any with osteoporosis or symptoms of hyperthyroidism. Treatment is usually only given to those with a serum TSH < 0.1 mU/l, with the aim of getting the TSH into the normal range (Pearce 2006). If not treating, repeat TFTs yearly (Col, Surks and Daniels 2004).

Table 8.2	Summary of laboratory tests in patients treated for hyperthyroidism		
	FT_4	FT_3	TSH
Overtreated	Low	Low	High
Adequate	N	N	N
Undertreated	High	High	Low

GOITRE IN A EUTHYROID PATIENT

* *A solitary thyroid nodule* may be malignant. Refer to medical or surgical outpatients urgently, according to the local expertise.

* *A generalized multinodular goitre* should also be referred for a decision about management but not urgently, although certain features would make malignancy more likely:
  (a) onset under age 20 or over 60;
  (b) male sex;
  (c) a history of radiation;
  (d) a short history;
  (e) lymphadenopathy.

* *A small diffuse goitre* need not be investigated, especially if it occurs at puberty.

AFTER RADIOTHERAPY OR PARTIAL THYROIDECTOMY

● Those who have had ablative radiotherapy will have been put on replacement levothyroxine sodium. This should be monitored clinically and a TSH should be measured yearly.

● Patients treated with I^{131} or surgery should be placed on a practice register and have their TFTs checked annually. 50% become hypothyroid and will require thyroxine supplementation (Vanderpump, Ahlquist, Franklyn, *et al.* 1996).

ADULT HYPOTHYROIDISM

- The clinical diagnosis of hypothyroidism is notoriously difficult in the early stages.
- In the elderly patient consider hypothyroidism in patients with non-specific illness, e.g. falling or mental deterioration. Only a third of elderly hypothyroid patients have classical signs (Roberts and Ladenson 2004).
- Overt hypothyroidism presents with cold intolerance, weight gain, constipation, dry skin, bradycardia, hoarseness and slowing of mental processing.
- The majority of adults with hypothyroidism are diagnosed and managed successfully in primary care (Royal College of Physicians 2008).

DIAGNOSIS

- Diagnosis depends on identifying a low level of FT_4 with a raised level of TSH.
- FT_3 is an unreliable indicator of hypothyroidism (Lindsay and Toft 1997). 5% of patients over 60 have a low FT_3, but in as many as 80% of these it is due to non-thyroid conditions rather than hypothyroidism. If it occurs alone, a low FT_3 is probably due to a partial failure of conversion of FT_4 to FT_3 in a euthyroid patient. This 'sick euthyroid' syndrome occurs in intercurrent illness and old age, or may be due to drugs; lithium, amiodarone, non-selective beta-blockers in high dosage and corticosteroids.

ATYPICAL TESTS

- * If the TSH is not raised in hypothyroidism, consider hypopituitarism. However, older people may fail to raise their TSH in the face of mild hypothyroidism and may even have a slightly low FT_4 and TSH as part of normal aging.
- * *Subclinical hypothyroidism.* If the TSH is raised but the FT_4 is normal and the patient is well, the patient has subclinical hypothyroidism. Whether these patients should be treated is controversial (Gussekloo, van Exel, de Craen, *et al.* 2004) (see below).
- * *Postpartum thyroiditis* is common (estimates range from 4 to 17%). It occurs within 6 months of pregnancy. All pregnant and postpartum

cases of hypothyroidism should be referred to a specialist.

- * Give levothyroxine sodium if the patient has symptoms, but prepare to be able to withdraw it after a few months.
- * If her antithyroid antibodies are positive, she will need annual TFTs for life.

Refer

(a) Younger patients to outpatients. They merit an endocrinological assessment for a condition that will probably be lifelong.

(b) Pregnant or postpartum women.

(c) Patients with evidence of pituitary disease.

(d) Patients with ischaemic heart disease.

(e) Patients on amiodarone or lithium.

(f) Admit anyone who is severely hypothyroid, e.g. who is unable to leave the house because of the hypothyroidism, who is at risk of hypothermia or who develops angina, arrhythmias or heart failure on treatment.

MANAGEMENT

Treat, without referral, older patients who are not severely ill.
  Check for:

(a) auto-antibodies (also be aware of the increased incidence of pernicious anaemia, hypoparathyroidism, Addison's disease and diabetes in those with antithyroid antibodies);

(b) lipids;

(c) coronary heart disease, including an ECG.

Younger patients without evidence of heart disease

- * Give levothyroxine sodium at a dose of 50–100 mcg daily with increments of 50 mcg per day every 4–6 weeks. This regimen will restore biochemical normality faster than the more cautious approach for older patients advocated below, but the clinical improvement will be no faster (Roos, Linn-Rasker, van Domburg, *et al.* 2005).
- * Review the patient regularly until the TSH is normal and the patient is clinically euthyroid. Monitoring can then be reduced to 6 monthly.

✻ Warn all patients that they will not feel the benefits of treatment immediately. After 3 months they should notice the difference, but complete recovery can take up to a year.

Patients over 60 or with IHD, with a long history, or more severely hypothyroid

1. Start levothyroxine sodium 25 mcg daily.
2. Increase by 25 mcg each month until 100 mcg a day is reached. Most patients are controlled by 100–150 mcg. Children need more, and old people often less.
3. 6 weeks later: check TFTs. Aim for an FT_4 that is normal or raised and an FT_3 that is low normal. The TSH should be suppressed into the normal range. If it is not, consider the possibility that the patient is not taking the tablets. However, in longstanding hypothyroidism there may be pituitary hyperplasia and the TSH may take 3–6 months to fall to normal.
4. Increase by a further 25 mcg daily to 150 mcg daily if the TSH is still raised. Very few patients need higher doses than this. Wait 4–6 weeks after each dose change before checking the TSH; it takes this long to readjust. Levothyroxine sodium given twice a week is as effective as once a day. This can be helpful when someone else has to administer it. Ensure that the total dose per week is equivalent (Taylor, Williams, Frater, et al. 1994).

Table 8.3	Summary of tests in the treatment of hypothyroidism		
	FT_4	FT_3	TSH
Adequate	Normal/high	Low normal	Normal/low
Overtreated	High	High or high normal	Low
Undertreated	Normal/low	Low	High

General points

● UK guidelines recommend that all patients on thyroxine replacement should have a yearly clinical assessment and check of thyroid function tests (Association for Clinical Biochemistry 2006).

● Some doubt the value of the biochemical check in monitoring the dose of levothyroxine sodium. One study found that routine monitoring was unreliable in detecting over- and underdosage, compared to clinical assessment (Fraser, Biggart, O'Reilly, et al. 1986).
● Studies have failed to substantiate the idea that biochemical 'over-treatment' (i.e. treatment leading to a suppressed TSH) is harmful (Leese, Jung, Gutherie, et al. 1992).
● The best compromise seems to be to increase the dose of levothyroxine until the TSH is in the normal range and to be prepared to wait up to a year for the clinical state to improve. In support of this is a recent randomized trial which found that, provided the TSH was between 0.1 and 4.8 mU/l, further adjustment had no effect on symptoms (Walsh, Ward, Burke, et al. 2006).
● Patients who are taking levothyroxine sodium to suppress a thyroid carcinoma are usually on doses of 200 mcg or over. Their TSH should be undetectable.

Subclinical hypothyroidism

● Between 3% and 8% of the US population has subclinical hypothyroidism, as defined above (Fatourechi 2009). The frequency increases with age.
● There is no clear evidence of benefit for the treatment of the condition but this may be due to the lack of large-scale randomized controlled trials that examine the cardiovascular benefits of treatment (Villar, Saconato, Valente, et al. 2007). What is clear is the danger of progression to clinical hypothyroidism. If the TSH is raised and antithyroid antibodies are present, 5% will become overtly hypothyroid each year (Vanderpump, Tunbridge, French, et al. 1995).
✻ Given the doubt about the benefit of treatment, consider it if:
  ■ there is a goitre, or
  ■ antithyroid antibodies are positive, or
  ■ the TSH is more than 10 mU/l, or
  ■ repeat TFTs after 6 months show a deterioration, or
  ■ the patient has a low HDL or a high LDL cholesterol.
✻ If not treating, check TFTs yearly.

Patients who may no longer need levothyroxine sodium

● Up to 28% of patients may be taking levothyroxine sodium inappropriately (Swansea Vocational Training Scheme 1985).

∗ Do not accept uncritically the diagnosis of hypothyroidism where there is no confirmation of the diagnosis from thyroid function tests (TFTs). Too often thyroid replacement therapy is started because of a complaint of tiredness or because the patient wanted to lose weight. The patient then passes to the care of another practitioner with an apparent diagnosis of hypothyroidism. Less commonly the patient suffered from transient hypothyroidism, confirmed by TFTs, but has been kept on thyroxine replacement after the need for it has passed.

∗ Attempt to withdraw levothyroxine sodium in patients without clear evidence of irreversible hypothyroidism. Reduce the dose to half, and repeat the TSH after 2 months. If it is not raised, stop levothyroxine sodium and repeat the TSH after a further 2 months. If it is still not raised, the patient does not need thyroxine replacement, but does need a yearly check.

ADDISON'S DISEASE

REVIEWS AND GUIDANCE

Ten S, New M, Maclaren N. 2001. Clinical review 130: Addison's disease. Clinical Endocrino l Metab, 6, 2909–2922

   Axford J, O'Callaghan C. 2004. Medicine, 2nd edition. Blackwells, Oxford

● Primary Addison's disease is due to disease/destruction of the adrenal glands usually through an autoimmune reaction or more rarely due to tuberculosis or malignancy.

● Secondary Addison's disease is very rare and due to a reduction in ACTH secretion by the pituitary gland.

● Approximately 1 in 10,000 patients will have Addison's disease. The incidence is approximately 1 in 180,000 per annum.

● It presents insidiously with tiredness, muscle weakness, anorexia, weight loss, increased pigmentation (gums, skin creases, scars) and low blood pressure. 25% are first diagnosed following an Addisonian crisis caused by an intercurrent infection or illness. This presents with abdominal or back pain, vomiting, dehydration, low blood pressure, confusion and coma. This is a medical emergency.

∗ Diagnosis is made through measuring serum cortisol levels and following a synacthen test. Patients may have hyperkalaemia and hyponatraemia.

∗ Refer those with a clinical suspicion to an endocrinologist for investigation.

TREATMENT

Treatment is with replacement of cortisol with hydrocortisone in divided doses throughout the day, and replacement of aldosterone with a daily dose of fludrocortisone.

∗ Check that the patient is wearing an alert bracelet and carrying a card listing their medication.

∗ Check that they know not to stop their medication and that if they suffer an intercurrent infection they need to increase their hydrocortisone. As a rule of thumb suggest that the patient:
   (a) doubles the daily dose of hydrocortisone for mild fevers and trebles it for high fevers;
   (b) maintains this dose until well, with no alteration in fludrocortisone;
   (c) reduces the dose according to how long they have been ill. If the illness has only been a few days this can be dropped down immediately to the maintenance dose. For longer illnesses the reduction should be reduced slower. Discuss with the local specialist.

∗ *Self-injection kits*. Prescribe hydrocortisone 100 mg (two vials) for the patient to keep at home, preferably in the fridge (with syringe and needles) for use in emergencies. They should be advised to give this themselves, intramuscularly, if they detect they are becoming seriously ill and there is likely to be any delay in obtaining medical help.

* *Addisonian crisis*. Patients who become ill with an Addisonian crisis should be given 100 mg hydrocortisone i.v. and referred urgently to hospital.

PATIENT ORGANIZATION

Addison's Disease Self Help Group. www.adshg.org.uk. The website includes an Addison's Owner's Manual (a self-help guide for patients), a credit card sized Emergency Card and an Emergency Crisis Letter, which the GP can complete for the patient to present at A&E in a crisis, so that the correct treatment is given promptly.

HYPERCALCAEMIA

REVIEW

Carroll MF, Schade DS. 2003. A practical approach to hypercalcaemia. Am Fam Physician 67, 1959–1966

Guideline

Department of Health. 2008. *Suspected Hypercalcaemia*. Map of Medicine Healthguides. Available: http://healthguides.mapofmedicine.com/choices/map/hypercalcaemia1.html

---

WHEN HYPERCALCAEMIA IS FOUND, ASK:

Is the patient symptomatic and how high is the serum level?

- *Mild hypercalcaemia* (serum Ca^{++} 2.65–2.9 mmol/l). If symptoms are present they will be polyuria, polydipsia, dyspepsia, depression and mild cognitive impairment. There is time for further investigation before referral.
- *Moderate hypercalcaemia* (serum Ca^{++} 3.0–3.4 mmol/l). Symptoms will be present, as above, plus muscle weakness, constipation, anorexia and nausea, fatigue. Refer urgently.
- *Hypercalcaemic crisis* (serum Ca^{++} 3.5 mmol/l and above). All of the above will be present plus abdominal pain, vomiting, dehydration, lethargy. Admit urgently.

If urgent referral is not required

1. Recommend that the patient stay well hydrated and mobile.
2. Repeat the blood test with a serum albumin estimation (see below), taking blood from an uncuffed arm.
3. Check the patient's medication: thiazides, lithium, self-medication with high doses of vitamin A or D or with calcium-containing antacids can cause hypercalcaemia. However, follow-up the serum calcium after stopping the drug to make sure it returns to normal. A thiazide may have unmasked an underlying primary hyperparathyroidism.
4. Check the family history for evidence of familial hypocalciuric hypercalcaemia.
5. If the calcium is still raised check the FBC, creatinine, phosphate, alkaline phosphatase parathyroid hormone (PTH) and thyroid function.
6. If the PTH is raised and the phosphate low, this is probably primary hyperparathyroidism, due to a parathyroid adenoma. This affects 2/1000 women and 1/1000 men, over the age of 60. 3% will be malignant. Refer to an endocrinologist.
7. If the PTH is normal or low, this is probably malignancy, the mechanism being either humoral hypercalcaemia of malignancy (found especially in cancer of the lung, kidney, ovary, head and neck) or bony metastases. In the latter the alkaline phosphatase is usually very high. Look for the site of the tumour and refer appropriately.
8. If the cause is unclear but the hypercalcaemia is sustained, refer to an endocrinologist.

CORRECTING THE SERUM CA^{++} RESULT

Half of serum calcium is free and 'active' or 'ionized'; the other half is bound to albumin. A low albumin will result in a calcium level that underestimates the severity of the condition, while a raised albumin overestimates its severity: indeed the free calcium may be normal.

Correct the serum calcium result as follows (unless the laboratory has already corrected it):

- assume that the normal serum albumin is 40 g/l;
- add 0.02 mmol/l for every 1.0 g/l that the serum albumin is below 40 g/l;
- subtract 0.02 mmol/l for every 1.0 g/l that the serum albumin is above 40 g/l.

HIRSUTISM

REVIEWS

Koulouri O, Conway GS. 2009. Management of hirsutism. BMJ 338, 823–826
  Sathyapalan T, Atkin SL. 2009. Rational testing: investigating hirsutism. BMJ 338,1070–1072

● Hirsutism in young women is a common problem with up to 10% of young women having a significant degree of excess hair.

● In many the problem is genetically determined and is related to ethnic origin or family history. In a proportion there will be an underlying endocrinological cause that will benefit from treatment (Michelmore, Balen, Dunger, et al. 1999). A common cause is polycystic ovary syndrome (72%) (PCOS). Other causes include idiopathic hyperandrogenism (23%), non-classic adrenal hyperplasia (4.3%), Cushing's disease, a pituitary dysfunction or, very rarely, an androgen-secreting tumour of the ovary or adrenal glands (0.2%) (Sathyapalan and Atkin 2009). Hirsutism after the menopause may be due to a normal level of testosterone, now unopposed by sufficient oestrogen.

● Diagnosis has in the past been difficult because of the variable reliability of the total serum testosterone as a measure of androgen excess. Much of this variability is due to variations in sex hormone binding globulin. Measurement of the free androgen index (total testosterone over the sex hormone binding globulin) overcomes this problem.

● Hirsutism is characterized by darker terminal hair in the male pattern and should be distinguished from hypertrichosis where fine downy vellus hair occurs in a distribution unrelated to gender (Al-Khawajah and Fouda Neel 1997).

∗ Ask about a family history, ethnic origin including the Mediterranean countries, and menstrual history. Menstrual irregularity suggests PCOS (see page 328).

∗ Ask about age of onset. Rapidly progressive hair growth of recent onset raises the possibility of abnormal androgen secretion. An onset of mild

hirsutism at the time of, or shortly after, the menarche is typical of PCOS.

∗ Examine:
  (a) *Is the excess hair all over (hypertrichosis)?* This suggests a general endocrine disturbance, e.g. Cushing's disease, acromegaly or hypothyroidism, or a drug cause or anorexia nervosa.
  (b) *Is the excess hair in the male pattern (hirsutism)?* Look specifically for signs of virilism, e.g. male pattern hair growth, increased muscle bulk and clitoromegaly. This suggests an excess of androgenic hormones.
  (c) *Is there ovarian enlargement on vaginal examination?*
  (d) *Is the patient cushingoid?*

Consider the diagnosis of PCOS if two of the following three criteria are met:

(a) Polycystic ovaries on USS (either 12 or more follicles in at least one ovary or increased ovarian volume ($> 10cm^3$).
(b) Oligo- or anovulation: as suggested by menstrual cycles longer than 35 days or < 10 periods a year.
(c) Clinical and/or biochemical signs of hyperandrogenism. Clinical signs include acne, hirsutism and androgenic alopecia. The biochemical confirmation required is a raised free testosterone. A raised LH/FSH ratio is no longer considered useful in the diagnosis because of its inconsistency.

∗ Exclude an iatrogenic cause, e.g. androgenic oral contraceptives, steroids, antiepileptic medication, diazoxide and minoxidil.

∗ Take blood for free testosterone (or free androgen index), LH and FSH at 9.00 am on day 2 of the cycle.

(a) A free testosterone level up to twice that of normal is consistent with a diagnosis of PCOS. Total testosterone levels > 4.8 nmol/l may indicate a tumour or adrenal hyperplasia, especially in those with a rapid history of excessive hair growth.
(b) A LH/FSH ratio of > 2.5 is suggestive of PCOS (see page 329) although a ratio < 2.5 does not exclude it. The test has been superseded by the free testosterone.

∗ If the blood results or the clinical picture suggest PCOS, order an ovarian ultrasound scan. However, do not order a scan if they are not suggestive: 1/3 women in the UK have polycystic ovaries on scan and, of them, only 1/3 have PCOS. A positive scan in a woman with no other evidence of PCOS is likely to be a false positive.

* *Menstrual irregularities.* Consider checking prolactin and TSH, in addition to the above.

TREATMENT

* Advise on cosmetic methods: shaving, bleaching agents, depilatory creams, plucking.
* Discuss the expensive options of electrolysis or laser treatment. Treatment should reduce hair by 50% over 6 months.
* Warn those planning to seek either of the last two options to check that the practitioner is a member of the appropriate professional body, e.g. the Institute of Electrolysis or the British Medical Laser Association. Discourage the use of self-administered electrolysis at home.
* Consider prescribing eflornithine cream. It inhibits hair growth and may be useful after hair has been removed by other methods. One study found a 26% reduction in hair after 24 weeks treatment.
* Recommend weight loss if appropriate. It can reduce androgen levels and may be helpful although in women with insulin resistance and impaired adipocyte lipolysis, weight loss will be more difficult to achieve.
* Attend to the emotional effect of being hirsute. Hirsute women often have high levels of anxiety and psychological support may be required (Sonino, Fava, Mani, *et al.* 1993).
* Women with PCOS are insulin resistant (Unluhizarci, Karababa, Bayram, *et al.* 2004) and at increased risk of developing diabetes and cardiovascular disease and may experience problems with fertility. Regular follow-up of such women is recommended (Lobo and Carmina 2000; Wild, Pierpoint, McKeigue, *et al.* 2000). Careful consideration should be given to the impact such a diagnosis may have on a woman's sense of well-being.

MEDICAL THERAPIES

Women with normal blood tests and no other abnormalities on history or examination can be treated in primary care.

* Explain that medical treatments are unlikely to produce any effect in the first 6 months; and that any benefit will be lost when the treatment is stopped. Furthermore, even the more effective treatments are unlikely to reduce hair growth by more than 30%.
* *Use a combined oral contraceptive* to suppress ovarian androgens. COCs with low androgenic progestogens are preferred (e.g. desogestrel-containing formulations such as Marvelon® and Mercilon®).
* *cyproterone.* In severe cases or those with accompanying acne use co-cyprindiol (a combination of the anti-androgen cyproterone acetate 2 mg and ethinylestradiol and specifically licensed for the treatment of hirsutism and severe acne). Both desogestrel-containing COCs and co-cyprindiol have demonstrated clinical benefit (Porcile and Gallardo 1991). Some women will be intolerant of COCs, but there is sparse evidence to support the use of cyproterone acetate alone or in higher doses than 2 mg (van der Spuy, Le Roux, Matjila 2003). Its use without adequate contraceptive cover is strongly opposed because of the risk of fetal feminization after exposure *in utero.* Co-cyprindiol is associated with a higher risk of venous thromboembolism than low-dose COCs (Seaman, de Vries and Farmer 2004).
* *Spironolactone.* A recent systematic review of spironolactone 50–200 mg daily has suggested that it produces a significant reduction of hair growth (Farquhar, Lee, Toomath, *et al.* 2003).
* *Metformin, the thiazolidinediones, finasteride, and flutamide* have all been shown to be useful but are unlicensed for hirsutism. They have their own problems, especially flutamide, with its high risk of liver toxicity.
* Refer to a specialist any patients who have failed on other therapies and want a second opinion.

Simple guide to the choice of medical therapy (Koulouri and Conway 2009)

● *Lean young women*: an oral contraceptive containing cyproterone acetate or drospienone, possibly with topical eflornithene for the first 12 weeks to obtain a faster response.
● *Obese women with polycystic ovary syndrome*: weight loss above all. If drugs are needed use metformin and spironolactone.

● *Hirsutism at and after the menopause:* oestrogen replacement (HRT). If that alone is insufficient, add drospienone to the oestrogen; it is an antiandrogen. In addition, use spironolactone. If HRT is contraindicated use topical eflornithine, or spironolactone or cyproterone acetate.

REFERRAL

Refer anyone with abnormal blood tests, rapid onset, virilism, galactorrhoea or menstrual disturbance:

(a) to a gynaecologist if the clinical picture is predominantly that of PCOS (a woman age 18–35 with menstrual disturbance, infertility or a raised free testosterone), or (at any age) a pelvic mass; or

(b) to an endocrinologist if the picture is more one of rapid onset of hirsutism with virilism and a very high serum testosterone, especially if these occur outside the age range of 18–35.

PATIENT INFORMATION

British Association of Dermatology. 2006. *Hirsutism.* Patient Information Leaflet, January. Available: http://bad.org.uk

GYNAECOMASTIA

Gynaecomastia is common especially in adolescents and in older men. It is uncommon to find a secondary cause.

* Check that it is not a carcinoma. These are usually unilateral, off centre and often tethered to skin or underlying tissues.

* Ask about alcohol use.

* Check for a drug cause, e.g. oestrogens, cimetidine, spironolactone.

* Check the testes for tumour and order LFTs if there is any reason to suspect liver dysfunction.

* Refer adult men to the breast unit for further investigation, even if no cause is found.

If the patient is adolescent and no cause is found

* Check what aspect bothers the patient. Many are satisfied with the explanation that the balance between oestradiol and testosterone seems to be disturbed, and that, in adolescents at least, it will resolve.

* If the patient wants treatment, offer tamoxifen 10–20 mg daily for 2 months (Khan and Blamey 2003). From the small studies so far performed it seems effective and safe. Evidence for clomifene and danazol is less strong. Surgery is rarely justified and may not be cosmetically successful.

HYPOGONADISM IN ADULT MEN

REVIEWS

DTB. 1999. Replacing testosterone in men. Drug Ther Bull 37, 3–6.
    Jones TH. 2009. Late onset hypogonadism. BMJ 338, 785–786.

● 1 in 200 men have hypogonadism, with abnormally low testosterone levels and a raised FSH. In the age group 50 to 79 up to 8.4% may be affected.

● Symptoms, if present, are: reduced facial, body and pubic hair growth; loss of libido and/or impotence; tiredness; gynaecomastia. Other patients will be asymptomatic and present because of a low testosterone level found as part of the work-up for osteoporosis.

● Older men may have slightly low testosterone levels without a raised FSH and without apparent ill effects. One study found that 20% of men > 60 years old had total serum testosterone concentrations that were below the normal range for young men (Snyder 2004).

● Men with definitely low testosterone levels have been shown to experience improvements, with testosterone replacement, in bone density, libido and erectile function, self-perceived functioning, and exercise-induced coronary ischaemia (Gruenewald and Matsumoto 2003).

* Check blood for total serum testosterone level at 9.00 am when testosterone production is at its peak. In obese patients also check free testosterone and SHBG.

* If the level is low, repeat it and check prolactin, LH, FSH and TFTs.

* Ask about mumps and other illnesses or accidents that could have affected the testicles.

* Ask about drugs that interfere with testicular function: alcohol, cimetidine, cyproterone

Table 8.4	Test results in primary and secondary hypogonadism					
CONDITION	TESTOSTERONE	FSH	LH	PROLACTIN	TFTs
Primary hypogonadism	Low	Raised	Raised	Normal	Normal
Secondary hypogonadism	Low	Normal or low	Normal or low	Raised in prolactinoma	Secondary hypothyroidism

acetate, flutamide, ketoconazole and spironolactone.

* Check the size of the testicles and the development of secondary sexual characteristics. Congenital causes, e.g. Klinefelter's syndrome, may only be detected in adult life.

* Order a bone density scan.

* Refer, to an endocrinologist, patients with symptoms, with osteopenia or osteoporosis, with evidence of pituitary failure or with markedly low testosterone levels from primary testicular failure. Further investigations and a decision about testosterone replacement

therapy, usually with implants or patches, are needed.

* Explain to older men who come into none of the above categories, that hormone replacement is of uncertain benefit, that there are potential hazards (e.g. mood alteration and, in theory, prostatic hypertrophy and carcinoma) and that 6-monthly testosterone levels are a better option, with the possibility of treatment if there is a progressive fall. Guidance from the US is that replacement should be considered if the total testosterone level is < 200 ng/dl (6.9 nmol/l) on three occasions (Snyder 2004).

References

Abraham, P., Avenell, A., Watson, W., et al., 2005. Antithyroid drug regimen for treating Graves' hyperthyroidism. Cochrane Database Syst. Rev. (2) CD003420.

Al-Khawajah, M., Fouda Neel, M., 1997. Women with clinically significant hirsutism always have detectable endocrinological abnormalities. J. Eur. Acad. Dermatol. Venereol. 9, 226–231.

American Diabetes Association, 2000. Report of the Expert Committee on the Diagnosis and Classification of Diabetes Mellitus. Diabetes Care 23 (Suppl. 1), S4–S19.

Association for Clinical Biochemistry, 2006. UK Guidelines for the use of Thyroid Function Tests.

British Diabetic Association, 1997. Retinal Photographic Screening for Diabetic Eye Disease. BDA, London.

Campbell, L., White, J., Campbell, R., 1996. Acarbose: its role in the treatment of diabetes mellitus. Ann. Pharmacother. 30, 1255–1262.

Chiasson, J., Josse, R., Gomis, R., et al., 2003. Acarbose treatment and the risk of cardiovascular disease and hypertension in patients with impaired glucose tolerance: the STOP-NIDDM trial. JAMA 290, 486–494.

Col, N., Surks, M., Daniels, G., 2004. Subclinical thyroid disease: clinical applications. JAMA 291, 239–243.

Colhoun, H., Betteridge, D., Durrington, P., et al., 2004. Primary prevention of cardiovascular disease with atorvastatin in type 2 diabetes in the Collaborative Atorvastatin Diabetes Study (CARDS): multicentre randomised placebo-controlled trial. Lancet 364, 685–696.

Davies, M., 2003. The prevention of type 2 diabetes mellitus. Clin. Med. 3, 470–474.

Diabetes Control and Complications Trial Research Group, 1993. The effect of intensive treatment on the development and progression of

long-term complications in insulin-dependent diabetes mellitus. N. Engl. J. Med. 329, 977–986.

Downs, J., Clearfield, M., Weiss, S., et al., 1998. Primary prevention of acute coronary events with lovastatin in men and women with average cholesterol levels: results of AFCAPS/TexCAPS Prevention Study. JAMA 279, 1615–1622.

DVLA, 2001. Guide to the Current Medical Standards of Fitness to Drive. Drivers Medical Unit, DVLA, Swansea.

Farmer, A., Wade, A., Goyder, E., et al., 2007. Impact of self monitoring of blood glucose in the management of patients with non-insulin treated diabetes: open parallel group randomised trial. BMJ 335, 132–139.

Farquhar, C., Lee, O., Toomath, R., et al., 2003. Spironolactone versus placebo or in combination with steroids for hirsutism and/or acne (Cochrane Review). Cochrane Database Syst. Rev. (4).

Fatourechi, V., 2009. Subclinical hypothyroidism: an update for primary care physicians. Mayo Clin. Proc. 84, 65–71.

Fraser, W., Biggart, E., O'Reilly, D., et al., 1986. Are biochemical tests of thyroid function of any value in monitoring patients receiving thyroxine replacement? BMJ 293, 808–810.

Greaves, C., Stead, J., Hattersley, A., et al., 2004. A simple pragmatic system for detecting new cases of type 2 diabetes and impaired fasting glycaemia in primary care. Fam. Pract. 21, 57–62.

Griffin, S., Kinmonth, A., 2000. Diabetes care: the effectiveness of systems for routine surveillance for people with diabetes. Cochrane Database Syst. Rev. 2, CD000541.

Gruenewald, D., Matsumoto, A., 2003. Testosterone supplementation therapy for older men: potential benefits and risks. J. Am. Geriatr. Soc. 51, 101–115.

Gulliford, M., 2008. Self monitoring of blood glucose in type 2 diabetes. BMJ 336, 1139–1140.

Gussekloo, J., van Exel, E., de Craen, A., et al., 2004. Thyroid status, disability and cognitive function, and survival in old age. JAMA 292, 2591–2599.

Hansson, l., Zanchetti, A., Carruthers, S., et al., 1998. Effects of intensive blood pressure lowering and low-dose aspirin in patients with hypertension: principal results of the Hypertension Optimal Treatment (HOT) randomised trial. Lancet 351, 1755–1762.

Hippisley-Cox, J., Coupland, C., Robson, J., et al., 2009. Predicting risk of type 2 diabetes in England and Wales: prospective derivation and validation of QDScore. BMJ 338, b880.

Holt, T., Stables, D., Hippisley-Cox, J., et al., 2008. Identifying undiagnosed diabetes: cross-sectional survey of 3.6 million patients' electronic records. Brit. J. Gen. Pract. 58, 192–196.

Imperatore, G., Benjamin, S., Engelgau, M., 2002. Targeting people with pre-diabetes. BMJ 325, 403–404.

Kenny, C., 2004. Diabetes and the new GMS contract: explaining the possibilities. Diabetes Primary Care 6, 140–144.

Khan, H., Blamey, R., 2003. Endocrine treatment of physiological gynaecomastia. BMJ 327, 301–302.

Koskinen, P., Manttari, M., Manninen, V., et al., 1992. Coronary heart disease incidence in NIDDM patients in the Helsinki Heart Study. Diabetes Care 15, 820–825.

Koulouri, O., Conway, G., 2009. Management of hirsutism. BMJ 338, 823–826.

Leese, G., Jung, R., Gutherie, C., et al., 1992. Morbidity in patients on L-thyroxine: a comparison of those with a normal TSH to those with a suppressed TSH. Clin. Endocrinol. 37, 500–503.

Lindsay, R., Toft, A., 1997. Hypothyroidism. Lancet 349, 413–417.

Lindstrom, J., Tuomilehto, J., 2003. The Diabetes Risk Score. Diabetes Care 26, 725–731.

Lobo, R., Carmina, C., 2000. The importance of diagnosing the polycystic ovary syndrome. Ann. Int. Med. 132, 989–993.

McIntosh, A., Hutchinson, A., Home, P., et al., 2002. Clinical guidelines for type 2 diabetes: management of blood sugar. NICE inherited guideline available: www.nice.org.uk.

Michelmore, K., Balen, A., Dunger, D., et al., 1999. Polycystic ovaries and associated clinical and biochemical features in young women. Clin. Endocrinol. 51, 779–786.

MMWR, 2005. Prevalence of diabetes and impaired fasting glucose in adults - United States, 1999–2000: Centre for Disease Control and Prevention. Available: www.cdc.gov (search on 'impaired fasting glucose').

National Cholesterol Education Program (NCEP) expert panel, 2001. Executive Summary of the third report of the National Cholesterol Education Program (NCEP) expert panel on detection, evaluation and treatment of high blood cholesterol in adults (Adult Treatment Panel III). JAMA 285, 2486–2497.

National Institute for Health and Clinical Excellence, 2006. Obesity: guidance on the prevention, identification, assessment and management of overweight and obesity in adults. NICE Clinical Guideline 43. Available: www.nice.org.uk.

National Institute for Health and Clinical Excellence, 2008. Chronic kidney disease. Clinical Guideline 73www.nice.org.uk.

NHS Centre for Reviews and Dissemination, 1999. Complications of diabetes: screening for retinopathy. Eff. Health Care 5 (4).

NHS Centre for Reviews and Dissemination, 2000. Complications of diabetes: renal disease and promotion of self management. Eff. Health Care 6 (1).

Pearce, E., 2006. Diagnosis and management of thyrotoxicosis. BMJ 332, 1369–1373.

Porcile, A., Gallardo, E., 1991. Long term treatment of hirsutism: desogestrel compared with cyproterone acetate in oral contraceptives. Fertil. Steril. 55, 877–881.

Pyorala, K., Pedersen, T., Kjekshus, J., et al., 1997. Cholesterol lowering with simvastatin improves prognosis of diabetic patients with coronary heart disease. A sub group analysis of the Scandanavian Simvastatin

Survival Study (4S). Diabetes Care 20, 614–620.

Rendell, M., 1999. Sildenafil for the treatment of erectile dysfunction in men with diabetes. JAMA 281, 421–426.

Roberts, C., Ladenson, P., 2004. Hypothyroidism. Lancet 363, 793–803.

Roos, A., Linn-Rasker, S., van Domburg, R., et al., 2005. The starting dose of levothyroxine in primary hypothyroidism treatment: a prospective, randomized, double-blind trial. Arch. Intern. Med. 165, 1714–1720.

Royal College of Physicians, 2008. The diagnosis and management of primary hypothyroidism. Available:www.rcplondon.ac.uk.

Sathyapalan, T., Atkin, S., 2009. Rational Testing: investigating hirsutism. BMJ 338, 1070–1072.

Scottish Intercollegiate Guidelines Network, 2001. Management of Diabetes. SIGN. Available:www.sign.ac.uk.

Seaman, H., de Vries, C., Farmer, R., 2004. Venous thromboembolism associated with cyproterone acetate in combination with ethinyloestradiol (Dianette): observational studies using the UK General Practice Research Database. Pharmacoepidemiol. Drug Saf. 13, 427–436.

Sherifali, D., 2009. To lower or not to lower? Making sense of the latest research on intensive glycaemic control and cardiovascular outcomes. Evid. Based. Med. 14 (2), 34–37.

Singer, P., Cooper, D., Levy, E., et al., 1995. Treatment guidelines for patients with hyperthyroidism and hypothyroidism. JAMA 273, 808–812.

Snyder, P., 2004. Hypogonadism in elderly men–what to do until the evidence comes. N. Engl. J. Med. 350, 440–442.

Sonino, N., Fava, G., Mani, E., et al., 1993. Quality of life of hirsute women. Postgrad. Med. J. 69, 186–189.

Surks, M., Ortiz, E., Daniels, G., et al., 2004. Subclinical thyroid disease: scientific review and guidelines for diagnosis and management. JAMA 291, 228–238.

Swansea Vocational Training Scheme, 1985. Evaluation of long-term thyroid replacement treatment. BMJ 291, 1476–1478.

Taylor, J., Williams, B., Frater, J., et al., 1994. Twice-weekly dosing for thyroxine replacement in elderly patients with primary hypothyroidism. J. Int. Med. Res. 22, 273–277.

Tuomilheto, J., Lindstrom, J., Eriksson, J., et al., 2001. Prevention of type 2 diabetes mellitus by changes in lifestyle among subjects with impaired glucose tolerance. N. Engl. J. Med. 344, 1343–1349.

UK National Screening Committee, 2008. The Handbook for Vascular Risk Assessment, Risk Reduction and Risk Management. www.screening.nhs.uk (choose 'All UK NSC policies' then 'Adult policies' then 'Vascular risk').

UKPDS 6, 1990. Complications in newly diagnosed type 2 diabetic patients and their association with different clinical and biochemical risk factors. Diabetes Res. 13, 1–11.

UKPDS Group, 1998a. Intensive blood-glucose control with sulphonylureas or insulin compared with conventional treatment and risk of complications in patients with type 2 diabetes (UKPDS 33). Lancet 352, 837–853.

UKPDS Group, 1998b. Effect of intensive blood-glucose control with metformin on complications in overweight patients with type 2 diabetes (UKPDS 34). Lancet 352, 854–865.

UKPDS Group, 1998c. Tight blood pressure control and risk of macrovascular and microvascular complications in type 2 diabetes: UKPDS 38. BMJ 317.

Unluhizarci, K., Karababa, Y., Bayram, F., et al., 2004. The investigation of insulin resistance in patients with idiopathic hirsutism. J. Clin. Endocrinol. Metab. 89, 2741–2744.

Vanderpump, M., Ahlquist, J., Franklyn, J., et al., 1996. Consensus statement for good practice and audit measures in the management of hypothyroidism and hyperthyroidism. BMJ 313, 539–544.

van der Spuy, Z., Le Roux, P., Matjila, M., 2003. Cyproterone acetate for hirsutism. Cochrane Database Syst. Rev.

Vanderpump, M., Tunbridge, W., French, J., et al., 1995. The incidence of thyroid disorders in the community: a twenty-year follow-up of the Whickham Survey. Clin. Endocrinol. 43, 55–68.

Villar, H., Saconato, H., Valente, O., et al., 2007. Thyroid hormone replacement for subclinical hypothyroidism (Review). Cochrane Database Syst. Rev. 18, CD003419.

Walsh, J., Ward, L., Burke, V., et al., 2006. Small changes in thyroxine dosage do not produce measurable changes in hypothyroid symptoms, well-being, or quality of life: results of a double-blind, randomized clinical trial. J. Clin. Endocrinol. Metab. 91, 2624–2630.

Wild, S., Pierpoint, T., McKeigue, P., et al., 2000. Cardiovascular disease in women with polycystic ovary syndrome at long term follow up: a retrospective cohort study. Clin. Endocrinol. 52, 595–600.

Williams, B., Poulter, N., Brown, M., et al., 2004. British Hypertension Society guidelines for hypertension management 2004 (BHS-IV). J. Hum. Hypertens. 18, 139–185.

Chapter 9

Rheumatological problems

CHAPTER CONTENTS

© 2011 Elsevier Ltd.
DOI: 10.1016/B978-0-7020-3053-6.00009-X

OSTEOARTHRITIS

CLINICAL REVIEW

Walker-Bone K, Javaid K, Arden N, Cooper C. 2000. Regular review: medical management of osteoarthritis. BMJ 321, 936–940. http://www.bmj.com/cgi/content/full/321/7266/936

Guideline

National Institute for Health and Clinical Excellence. 2008. *Osteoarthritis: The Care and Management of Osteoarthritis in Adults*. NICE clinical guideline 59, February. Available: http://www.nice.org.uk/Guidance/CG59

The aims of management are to:

- empower the patient in self-management;
- control symptoms: mainly pain and stiffness;
- prevent progression of joint damage;
- reduce disability and improve function.

MANAGEMENT STRATEGY

* Make a holistic assessment of the impact of osteoarthritis on the patient in terms of:
  - function, occupation, leisure activities;
  - quality of life;
  - mood and sleep;
  - relationships;
  - comorbidities.
* Elicit the patient's understanding of the illness and concerns.
* Discuss the risks and benefits of treatment options.
* Formulate a management plan with the patient on the basis of the above and taking account of the patient's values and preferences.
* Screen for depression which is commoner in patients with long term disability.

Management can be divided into three domains (Table 9.1):

EDUCATION AND SELF-MANAGEMENT

Education

* Address concerns and counter any misconceptions, for example, that the disease inevitably progresses to joint replacement.

Table 9.1	Management of osteoarthritis	
Core treatment	These should be considered for all patients	Education Exercise Weight loss for the overweight
Relatively safe pharmaceutical options	These should be considered before adjunctive treatments	Paracetamol Topical NSAIDs
Adjunctive treatments	This refers to treatments which have less proof of efficacy or involve more risk to the patient	Pharmaceutical • NSAIDs • Opioids • Intra-articular steroids • Capsaicin Self-management • Local heat and cold • Assistive devices Other non-pharmacological • Supports and braces • Shock absorbing shoes and insoles • TENS • Manual therapy • Surgery

Patient-centred consultations result in better outcomes and better use of resources (such as fewer unhelpful investigations).

* Explain the disease in appropriate language and back this up with an offer of written information.

PATIENT INFORMATION

Arthritis Research UK. Osteoarthritis: an information booklet. Online: www.arthritisresearchuk.org
   Arthritis Care: Living with Osteoarthritis. http://www.arthritiscare.org.uk/PublicationsandResources/Listedbytype/Booklets

Exercise

* Encourage exercise:
  - local muscle strengthening;
  - general aerobic exercise.

Exercise advice can be found on the Arthritis Care website: www.arthritiscare.org.uk/PublicationsandResources/Listedbytype/Booklets

* Refer to physiotherapy for exercise according to local policies.

Weight loss

* Encourage weight loss in the overweight. This improves function though whether it reduces pain is not certain.

RELATIVELY SAFE PHARMACEUTICAL OPTIONS

* Recommend paracetamol. Regular doses, namely 1 g four times daily, might be better than taking a dose 'as required'.
* For some joints, such as the knee, recommend topical NSAIDs before progressing to adjunctive drugs with their associated risks.

ADJUNCTIVE NON–PHARMACOLOGICAL, NON–SURGICAL MANAGEMENT

* Consider the following for pain relief:
  (a) local application of heat or cold;
  (b) referral for manipulation or stretching;
  (c) transcutaneous electrical nerve stimulation.
* Refer to the most appropriate agency according to local policies, (for example, physiotherapy or occupational therapy) for:
  (a) assessment for bracing, joint supports, or insoles in those with biomechanical joint pain or instability;
  (b) assistive devices such as walking sticks.
* Advise on footwear. Shock absorbing shoes (trainers) and insoles (which can be purchased from pharmacies) may help weight bearing joints.
* Advise the patient to keep active and to pace himself/herself, that is to say, take planned rest periods and avoid bursts of overactivity.
* Look out for depression. If present, treating it not only improves mood but results in less pain and improved function at 12 months (Lin, Katon, Von Korff, et al. 2003).
* Recommend tricyclic antidepressants if sleep or mood disturbance are present.
* Do not recommend electroacupuncture. Consider the use of acupuncture when there are few options left.

ADJUNCTIVE PHARMACOLOGICAL MANAGEMENT

* Prescribe either a weak opioid or an oral NSAID (see NSAID section) depending on patient preferences and comorbidities.
* Educate the patient in the self-management of analgesics so that he/she can step up or down the scale of treatment:
  (a) recommend that NSAIDs be used for the shortest period possible;
  (b) explain that paracetamol *or* co-codamol can be used with ibuprofen, but that co-codamol should *never* be taken with paracetamol because it contains the same drug;
  (c) make sure the patient is not on more than one NSAID, including OTC preparations, e.g. aspirin.
* Consider intra-articular steroid injections.
* Consider topical capsaicin.
* Do not prescribe glucosamine or chondroitin (Towheed, Maxwell, Anastassiades, *et al.* 2005).

LOCAL INJECTIONS

● Intra-articular corticosteroid injections provide short term pain relief and may give patients the opportunity to begin other interventions such as exercise.
● Intra-articular hyaluronic acid injections have been shown to have only a weak effect.
* Consider a steroid injection for moderate to severe pain and for flare-ups.
* Do not refer for intra-articular hyaluronic acid injections for knees.

DISABILITY

* Consider the patient's need for aids, e.g. bath aids, and refer as appropriate.
* Consider eligibility for benefits, e.g. Attendance Allowance, or a disabled driver's badge, and refer to the appropriate agency for advice.
* Consider the need for support and rehabilitation. Refer, according to local circumstances, to social services or a rehabilitation team or to a hospital-based multidisciplinary team.

X-RAYS

Plain X-rays are not routinely indicated. They cannot confirm the diagnosis because degenerative changes in several joints, e.g. spine and knees, start in middle age and X-ray appearances correlate poorly with the symptoms (Royal College of Radiologists 2003). Diagnosis is mainly clinical in many syndromes and plain X-rays do not differentiate between disease and non-disease, e.g. shoulder impingement syndrome.

* Refer for X-ray when:
  (a) soft tissue calcification is suspected, e.g. shoulder, and when the result might inform the choice to use an NSAID or steroid injection;
  (b) referral for joint replacement is being considered;
  (c) there is knee pain with locking: X-ray may show radio-opaque loose bodies;
  (d) there is diagnostic doubt.

REFERRALS TO A SPECIALIST

* Consider referral for joint replacement surgery when a patient experiences joint symptoms, whether pain, stiffness, or reduced function, that impact substantially on their quality of life and have not responded to core and adjunctive treatments. Referral is best made before prolonged functional limitation and severe pain become established.
* Follow local referral thresholds, which vary, but age, gender, smoking, obesity and comorbidities should not be barriers to referral.

POSTOPERATIVE CARE

Patients will occasionally ask their GP about their return to normal activities.

* Advise the patient who has had a hip replacement not to cross the legs or drive for 6 weeks. The danger of dislocation is greatest in the first 6 weeks and occurs when the hip is flexed, especially if internally rotated and adducted.
* Advise patients that they may resume activities, including walking, swimming, bicycling and tennis, *after 6 weeks*, provided they take care not to fall. Contact sports and ladders are not advised.

Recurrence of pain

* Arrange for an X-ray, ESR and WBC in any patient with a hip prosthesis who develops pain. This may show loosening, infection, stress fracture or dislocation. Refer any of these to the surgeon urgently. Refer anyway if the pain does not settle with rest. Any of the above may be present despite a normal X-ray.

Antibiotic prophylaxis

Patients with prosthetic joint implants including total hip replacements do not need antibiotic prophylaxis for dental treatment (Uçkay 2008).

LOW BACK PAIN (LBP)

GUIDELINE

National Institute for Health and Clinical Excellence. 2009. *Low Back Pain: Early Management of Persistent Non-Specific Low Back Pain*. NICE clinical guideline 88. Available www.nice.org.uk

DEFINITIONS OF LOW BACK PAIN (NACHEMSON AND JONSSON 2000)

- Acute LBP: ≤ 6 weeks.
- Subacute LBP: 6–12 weeks.
- Chronic LBP: ≥ 3 months.

LBP is extremely common. At any one time, 15% of adults have it and 60% will have it some time in their lives (Mason 1994). Back pain is the commonest cause of long-term sickness: 52 million working days are lost each year from back pain. Mechanical LBP is self-limiting: 80–90% of patients recover spontaneously within 3 months.

For details of the diagnosis of the causes of back pain see *Evidence-based Diagnosis in Primary Care* by A. F. Polmear (editor) published by Butterworth-Heinemann, 2008.

AIMS OF MANAGEMENT

● Reduce pain and the length of sickness in mechanical back pain.

- Identify early the small minority with serious pathology needing immediate or urgent attention.
- Prevent acute back pain becoming chronic.

MANAGEMENT OF ACUTE LBP

At presentation:

* Triage patients into one of the three following groups on the basis of history and examination:
  (a) mechanical back pain;
  (b) nerve root compression;
  (c) possible serious spinal pathology – look for *Red Flags* (see page 257) and act accordingly.
* Note any psychological or social influences that might retard recovery: so-called *Yellow Flags*.

MANAGING ACUTE MECHANICAL LBP

FEATURES OF MECHANICAL BACK PAIN

(a) Presentation at age 20–55.
(b) Pain felt over lumbosacral area, buttocks or thighs.
(c) 'Mechanical' pain, i.e. alters with posture and activity.
(d) The patient is well.

AT PRESENTATION

* Take time to listen and examine, explain and reassure. This has a beneficial effect on pain and on anxiety.
* Encourage continued activity, including work if appropriate. Bed rest worsens outcome and should only be taken if pain is severe, and then for no more than necessary (Waddell, Feder and Lewis 1997).
* Prescribe analgesics or NSAIDs.
* Avoid prescribing muscle relaxants, e.g. diazepam. They control pain but the abuse potential and the availability of other analgesic options means that it should not be common practice.
* Ensure the patient has a medium-firm mattress (5 on the European Committee for Standardisation scale). This has been shown to be more effective than a firm one (Kovacs, Abraira, Pena, *et al.* 2003).

* Demonstrate stretching exercises or give written instructions (e.g. ARC booklet on www.arc.org.uk search on 'Back Pain'). Many exercises are available and some have fanatical supporters but there is no evidence that any specific type of exercise is best (Tulder, Malmivaara, Esmail, *et al.* 2000).

FOLLOW-UP CONSULTATIONS (2–6 WEEKS)

* If activity and function are improving, encourage return to normal activities even if pain is still present. Stress that activity will not damage the back.
* If not improving, advise graded return to normal activity and set a return date to work.
* If not improving, also consider referral to another health professional with expertise in LBP, usually a physiotherapist, or possibly a manipulative therapist.
* Reassess for *Red Flags* (see page 257).
* Reassess for *Yellow Flags* (see below). If present, be positive, schedule regular reviews, encourage a programme of activity. Consider early referral.

PSYCHOSOCIAL BLOCKS TO RECOVERY
Yellow Flags

The patient has:

(a) a belief that back pain is harmful or potentially disabling;
(b) fear-avoidance behaviour (avoiding a movement or activity due to misplaced anticipation of pain) and reduced activity levels;
(c) a tendency to low mood and withdrawal from social interaction; an expectation that passive treatments rather than active participation will help; awaiting compensation;
(d) a history of absence from work for back pain or other problems;
(e) poor job satisfaction, long hours, heavy work;
(f) an overprotective family or a lack of support at home.

Note that these Yellow Flags should not be used pejoratively. They are a guide to those patients in whom early intervention and early return to work are especially important.

FAILURE TO PROGRESS AFTER 6 WEEKS

* Continue and intensify current management; and
* consider referral to specialist services.

MANAGEMENT OF CHRONIC LBP

The prevalence of LBP is not increasing but the level of disability and claims for long-term sickness benefits are. The management of chronic LBP therefore encompasses several approaches:

(a) appropriate referral for physical treatments (see below);
(b) principles of chronic pain management;
(c) attention to psychosocial issues.

* Recommend regular physical exercise. This should start as soon as possible in the course of the illness. A light mobilization programme for patients who have had back pain for 8–12 weeks has been shown to improve outcomes initially and at 3 years (Hagen, Eriksen and Ursin 2000).
* Treat underlying anxiety or depression if present.
* Consider prescribing a tricyclic antidepressant at low doses, even if depression is not present (Staiger, Gaster, Sullivan, *et al.* 2003).
* Explore work-related issues. If return to former employment is unlikely, advise the patient to see the disability employment adviser at the job centre.
* Consider referral to a multidisciplinary team; this can be effective in resistant cases (Guzmán, Esmail, Karjalainen, *et al.* 2001).

NERVE ROOT COMPRESSION

● Mechanical back pain can be referred down the leg so not all sciatica arises from a prolapsed disc; nerve root compression is more likely if pain extends down to the foot. Conversely, not all prolapsed discs cause sciatica since they can be demonstrated in 50% of asymptomatic adults.
● Sciatica arising from a prolapsed disc that causes significant disability has a lifetime prevalence of 5%.
● Recognizing nerve root compression is important because surgery leads to quicker

recovery than natural resolution, although there may be no difference in long-term outcomes (Peul, van Houwelingen, van den Hout, *et al.* 2007).
● Chymopapain discolysis is also effective but not widely used in the UK.
* At presentation, test for limitation of straight leg raising (see below).
* Look for neurological deficit from L5/S1 compression: loss of sensation over the lateral border of the lower leg and foot, weakness of dorsi- and plantar flexion of foot, and impairment of the ankle reflex. In L3/4 compression the knee reflex may be impaired.
* Manage sciatica as you would acute LBP.
* Refer patients whose pain is not settling (the timescale will depend on local circumstances) or where there is increasing neurological deficit.

DIAGNOSING NERVE ROOT COMPRESSION (VROOMEN, DE KROM AND KNOTTERUS 1999)

The vast majority of cases involve the L5/S1 nerve roots.

● *Symptoms:* pain radiating below the knee.
● *Signs:*
    (a) limitation of SLR is a very sensitive finding; its absence makes nerve root compression very unlikely (sensitivity 0.88 to 1);
    (b) crossed SLR is a fairly specific test; its presence makes nerve root compression very likely (specificity 0.84 to 0.95).

REFERRALS

Whom to refer to will depend on local availability and agreed care pathways: physiotherapist, pain clinic, multidisciplinary team, orthopaedic physicians or orthopaedic surgeons.

FAILURE TO PROGRESS IN ACUTE LBP

All guidelines are consistent in recommending early referral (2 weeks or less) for physiotherapy or manipulation in order to prevent acute LBP becoming chronic. However, there is conflicting evidence about whether this makes a difference to long-term outcome, although a large UK trial shows evidence of modest benefit at 3 and 12 months from manipulation (UK BEAM Trial Team 2004). This held whether the manipulation was in NHS or private facilities. Conversely, it is now clear that, even in sciatica, epidural corticosteroid injection offers no long-term benefit, although there may be transient benefit at 3 weeks (Arden, Price, Reading, *et al.* 2005).

* Be prepared (Hazard, Haugh, Reid, *et al.* 1997) to discuss manipulation; many patients take themselves to osteopaths or chiropractors and many physiotherapists practice a related treatment, mobilization. The evidence for manipulation is of low quality but it may lead to quicker recovery in the first few weeks without making any difference to long-term outcomes (Koes, Assendelft, van der Heijden, *et al.* 1996).
* There is insufficient evidence for physical agents and passive modalities, e.g. ice, heat, short-wave diathermy, massage, ultrasound, transcutaneous electrical stimulation and acupuncture but they remain popular.

FAILURE TO PROGRESS WITH NEUROLOGICAL SYMPTOMS OR SIGNS, AND OTHER SERIOUS SITUATIONS

Evidence of benefit from discectomy, which may be long term, is accumulating for patients with disc herniation, spinal stenosis and spondylolisthesis (Gibson 2007).

* *Sciatica*. The ideal timing of referral to an orthopaedic surgeon of patients with sciatica which is not improving is not clear. A BMJ leading article suggests 8 weeks (Fairbank 2008); patients with severe pain will be referred earlier.
* *Cauda equina syndrome* (see below): refer immediately to an orthopaedic surgeon.
* *Other Red Flags* – refer urgently where appropriate and, if a malignancy is suspected, refer urgently according to the recommendations of the Department of Health (DOH 2000).

X-RAYS

* Explain to patients with mechanical LBP why X-rays are unhelpful: degenerative changes are common, most disorders are of soft-tissue which cannot be shown on X-ray and the dose of radiation is high (60 times that of a chest X-ray) (Royal College of Radiologists 2003).

* Consider X-rays in the presence of Red Flags, alongside urgent referral.

POSSIBLE SERIOUS SPINAL PATHOLOGY
Red Flags

(a) Cauda equina syndrome (features include urinary retention, bilateral neurological symptoms and signs, saddle anaesthesia – urgent referral is indicated).
(b) Significant trauma (risk of fracture).
(c) Weight loss (suggestive of cancer).
(d) History of cancer (suggestive of metastases).
(e) Fever (suggestive of infection).
(f) Intravenous drug use (suggestive of infection).
(g) Steroid use (risk of osteoporotic collapse).
(h) Patient aged over 50 years (cancer unlikely below this age).
(i) Severe, unremitting night-time pain (suggestive of cancer).
(j) Pain that gets worse when patient is lying down (suggestive of cancer).

THE ELDERLY WITH ACUTE BACK PAIN

These patients are a special case because osteoporotic collapse and malignancy are more likely and they need an early X-ray. Half will have definite abnormality, and 10% will have a malignancy (Frank 1993).

ADVICE/EXERCISES FOR LBP

The following is taken from the BackCare leaflet: *Exercise for a Better Back*; and from the ARC leaflet: *Back Pain*, see below.

* Pay attention to sitting, lifting and bending to avoid aggravating pain and to prevent recurrence.
  (a) *Sitting*: avoid prolonged sitting. A rolled towel in the small of the back may ease pain.
  (b) *Lifting*: always lift with a straight back and bent knees.
  (c) *Bending*: avoid spending too long at a job that requires bending, e.g. ironing.
* Exercise regularly.
  (a) Stretching exercises to maintain flexibility – daily. You may start these early on in an attack and should keep them up long term.

(b) Muscle strengthening exercises – daily. You should start these as your pain improves and should keep them up long term.

(c) Take up aerobic exercise for general fitness, e.g. swimming.

Suitable exercises (there are many others):

Starting position: on all fours with hands shoulder width apart, arms and thighs vertical.

1. Arch the back and look down. Then lower the stomach towards the floor, hollowing the back.
2. Slowly walk the hands around to one side, back to the starting position, then around to the other side.
3. Raise one hand off the floor, reach underneath your body as far as you can. On the return, swing the arm out to the side as far as you can then return to the starting position. Follow the moving hand with the eyes. Repeat with the other arm.
4. Draw alternate knees to the opposite elbow.
5. Stretch one arm forward in front, at the same time stretching the opposite leg out behind. Repeat on the other side.
6. Swing the seat from side to side.

All exercises should be repeated 10 times. Exercises that hurt should be set aside and returned to with fewer repetitions on another occasion.

PATIENT INFORMATION

ARC. Back Pain. Online. Available: www.arc.org.uk (search on 'Back pain').

BackCare 16 Elmtree Road, Teddington, Middlesex, TW11 8ST, tel. 020 8977 5474. Has several leaflets on aspects of neck and back pain, e.g. surgery, exercises, which are also available for download from www.backcare.org.uk (Choose 'About Back Pain').

NECK PAIN

REVIEW

Ray A, Cowie R. 2005. What should be done for the patient with neck pain (X-rays show cervical spondylosis)? Collected reports on the rheumatic diseases, series 4 (revised) http://www.arc.org.uk/arthinfo/documents/6507.pdf

---

Guideline

National Library for Health. *Neck Pain Management.* Clinical Knowledge Summaries. http://cks.library.nhs.uk/neck_pain/management/detailed_answers

---

For details of the diagnosis of neck pain see *Evidence-based Diagnosis in Primary Care* by A. F. Polmear (editor), published by Butterworth-Heinemann, 2008.

The principles of management of low back pain apply to neck pain (Nachemson and Jonsson 2000).

- Triage neck pain into mechanical, nerve root compression (often termed radiculopathy) and potential serious pathology (*Red Flags*).
- In mechanical neck pain, keeping active is more effective than immobilization.
- Similar medication may be prescribed.
- Psychosocial factors are important (see page 255).
- Imaging is not routinely indicated.
- Manipulation or mobilization may be effective in the short term (Gross, Hoving, Haines, *et al.* 2004).
- Acupuncture is not effective (Trinh, Graham, Gross, *et al.* 2006).

MECHANICAL PAIN

---

* Recognize by:
  (a) aged 18–55;
  (b) absence of signs of radiculopathy or Red Flags;
  (c) made worse by posture/activity.
* Advise the patient to stay active (Aker, Gross, Goldsmith, *et al.* 1996). Collars should only be worn for a limited period.
* Give regular analgesia.
* Advise or refer for exercises (Kay, Gross, Goldsmith, *et al.* 2005).
* Treat hyperextension injuries (including whiplash injuries) in the same way but avoid a collar as this prolongs symptoms.

DAILY STRETCHING AND STRENGTHENING EXERCISES

(Based on the ARC information leaflet *Pain in the Neck.*)

Advise the patient to hold the neck for 10 seconds in each of the six positions (right and left lateral flexion and rotation, flexion and extension) within the pain free range. Repeat 10 times.

RADICULOPATHY

* Distinguish radiculopathy from neck pain that is referred to the shoulder and arm.
* Look for the following signs, though their sensitivity and specificity has not been adequately assessed:
  (a) diminished reflexes (triceps, biceps, supinator);
  (b) diminished power;
  (c) diminished sensation along dermatomes;
  (d) the axial compression test: extend the neck and rotate the head to the side of the pain, then apply pressure to the head. Reproducing pain or paraesthesiae in the arm signifies likely radiculopathy.
* Treat as for mechanical neck pain but refer if there is no improvement after 4 weeks. Refer earlier if there is loss of power, and refer immediately if deterioration is rapid. However, warn the patient that surgery is no better than conservative treatment except in severe cases (Kadanka, Mares, Bednarik, *et al.* 2002).

RED FLAGS

Red Flags for malignancy, infection and inflammation are as for LBP.

A Red Flag specific for neck pain is evidence of cervical myelopathy (the equivalent of the cauda equina syndrome). Neck pain may be absent but the syndrome should be suspected when any of the following features are present:

(a) sensory disturbances in upper and lower limbs;
(b) weakness in upper and lower limbs;
(c) clumsiness and gait disturbance;
(d) spasticity of lower limbs (upper limbs may be normal, spastic or flaccid);
(e) increased tendon reflexes;
(f) Lhermitte's sign: paraesthesiae in limbs on neck flexion indicates neck instability and warrants *immediate* admission.

* Refer patients with one or more Red Flags urgently for a specialist opinion.

REGIONAL PROBLEMS

REVIEWS

Arthritis Research UK. Rheumatic disease in practice, practical advice on management of rheumatic diseases. Online: www.arthritisresearchuk.org (choose 'Arthritis info' then 'Publications for medical professionals').
   Silver, T. 1999. *Joint and Soft Tissue Injection. Injecting with Confidence*, 2nd edition. Radcliffe Medical Press, London.

Patient information

Arthritis Research UK. Copeman House, St Mary's Court, St Mary's Gate, Chesterfield, Derbyshire S41 7TD, tel: 0870 850 5000, www.arthritisresearchuk.org (choose 'Arthritis info' then 'Publications for people with arthritis')

PROBLEMS WITH THE UPPER LIMBS

ACUTE SHOULDER PAIN

REVIEW

Mitchell C, Adebajo A, Hay E, Carr A. 2005. Shoulder pain: diagnosis and management in primary care. BMJ 331, 1124–1128

Acute onset with injury

* Clinical fracture or dislocation: send to the emergency department. If not:
* X-ray and send to the emergency department if fracture or dislocation shown.
* If the X-ray is normal: control pain for 3 weeks with analgesia and a sling.
* If pain or loss of movement continues beyond 3 weeks: perform L.A. test (see below).

(a) If pain and movement are both improved refer for physiotherapy.

(b) If pain is improved but not movement refer urgently to an upper limb specialist (fracture clinic) as suspected rotator cuff tear. Repair, if needed, should be performed within 6–8 weeks of the injury.

The L.A. test helps to distinguish pain from a tear as the cause of an inability to raise the arm.

Instil 2 ml of local anaesthetic (LA) e.g. I% lidocaine, anterolaterally into the subacromial bursa. Pain should be relieved within 5 minutes. If indicated, steroid can be given through the same needle, e.g. 40–80 mg Depo-Medrone.

Acute onset without injury

Sudden onset of desperate pain

* Refer to A&E. This may indicate acute de-calcification of an area of calcification in the rotator cuff which would need urgent decompression.
* If the situation is less desperate: X-ray:
  (a) if normal, give local anaesthetic and steroid injection and advice on cuff strengthening exercises. If that fails, refer to OPD. If it helps substantially but is followed by relapse give further injections with a maximum of 3 per year;
  (b) if abnormal, refer according to diagnosis (see below).

Arthritis of ACJ or GHJ

* *Mild symptoms.* Give analgesia, an NSAID, heat, shoulder exercises or refer to physiotherapy.
* *More severe symptoms.* Support as above and refer to OPD.

Calcification in the rotator cuff

* Refer to OPD. They are more likely to need surgery at some stage. They may benefit from a subacromial injection of local anaesthetic and steroid meanwhile.

Red Flags for systemic disease

* Investigate further if the patient is systemically unwell (e.g. with fever or weight loss), has a history of cancer, has arthritis elsewhere, has a mass or neurological symptoms or signs in that arm.

Chronic shoulder pain

Is it ACJ pain?

Characteristics: pain is localized to the ACJ, the joint may be swollen and tender with crepitus, and abduction is painful in the final 20 degrees).

* Inject local anaesthetic and steroid and give analgesia. If not better in 2 weeks, refer to physiotherapy. If still no better, check the diagnosis and refer.

Is it a rotator cuff lesion?

Characteristics: pain is usually felt at the deltoid insertion. Any or all movements are painful; active movements are more painful than passive movements and pain is felt on resisted active elevation. This is the impingement sign.

(a) *Mild pain:* give analgesia and advice on cuff strengthening exercises. If no improvement after 3 weeks refer to physiotherapy (Green, Buchbinder and Hetrick 2003). If physiotherapy is unhelpful give a subacromial injection of L.A. Subacromial injection of steroid has been shown to be no better than the same injection into the buttock (Koes 2009).

(b) *Moderate or severe pain:* perform the L.A. test.

  * If the pain is improved and power is full, refer to physio. If still unresolved, refer.
  * If pain is improved but there is weakness, refer urgently as a suspected rotator cuff tear.
  * If pain is not improved, refer.
  * If pain and power improve substantially but return, give further injections up to a maximum of 3 per year.

Is it chronic capsulitis (frozen shoulder)?

Characteristics: there is tenderness anteriorly between the coracoid process and the head of the humerus, all movements are painful and restricted, whether active or passive, but there is less pain on resisted active movement, when the joint does not move. Characteristically, the loss of external rotation is the most marked, there is no crepitus, and no arthritis elsewhere.

* Explain the nature of the condition and the fact that spontaneous resolution can be expected, with a mean duration of 30 months. However, explain that some long-term restriction of movement is usual (Dias, Cutts and Massoud 2005).
* Order mobilization physiotherapy, designed to keep the shoulder mobile within the limits of pain (Green, Buchbinder and Hetrick 2003).

✳ At the same time, give a single steroid injection into the glenohumeral joint. The earlier the injection is given, the more effective it is (Dias, Cutts and Massoud 2005).

✳ Refer refractory cases which have not resolved after 30 months for consideration of manipulation under anaesthesia or arthroscopic release.

Is it GHJ arthrosis?

The characteristics are the same as in chronic capsulitis but crepitus may be felt and there may be arthritis elsewhere.

✳ Confirm with an X-ray. Management depends on both the degree of pain and functional loss:

  (a) If mild, give analgesia and advice on exercises.

  (b) If moderate or severe, refer with a view to replacement surgery.

Is the GHJ joint unstable?

Characteristics: there may be a history of subluxation or dislocation. There are two tests for this:

1. Fix the shoulder girdle with one hand and, with the other, try to rock the head of the humerus backwards and forwards in the glenoid fossa.

2. Hold the arm abducted to 90° with the upper arm pointing forwards. Does external rotation cause apprehension and pain?

✳ Refer for consideration of specialist physiotherapy or surgery.

Note: Nerve root compression in the neck frequently presents as shoulder pain, co-exists with it and can cause it!

  Note: Young sports people with shoulder pain frequently have occult instability; refer them readily.

  ACJ = Acromioclavicular joint; GHJ = glenohumeral joint

THE FOLLOWING SIMPLIFIED GUIDE WILL COVER MOST CASES OF SHOULDER PAIN

✳ If the patient is unwell or has other disorders that could cause shoulder pain, investigate further.

✳ If the pain is acute and the patient cannot raise the arm actively but you can raise it passively, refer urgently as a suspected rotator cuff tear.

✳ If there is a history of partial or complete dislocation, refer for assessment of instability.

✳ Otherwise, decide between:

  (a) acromioclavicular joint pain (tender over the AC joint with restriction of moving the arm across the front of the chest)

  (b) glenohumeral joint pain (active and passive movements of the shoulder painful and restricted).

✳ In both those conditions recommend:

  (a) analgesia and rest until the acute pain eases

  (b) exercises within the limits of pain to keep the joint mobile;

  (c) the ARC booklet (see below) and explain the likely outcome; and possibly steroid/local anaesthetic injection into the appropriate joint.

EXERCISES FOR THE SHOULDER

Flexibility. Demonstrate pendular exercises:

  (a) Stand up and lean forward with arm of affected side hanging perpendicularly.

  (b) Sweep the arm around in a circle within the pain-free range. Do this 20–30 times.

  (c) As time goes on, increase the range of the movement and length of time.

Strengthening the rotator cuff:

  (a) Hold your arm outstretched at shoulder height and out to the side.

  (b) Bring your arm forward then up, push to the back then down to the starting position.

  (c) Repeat 10 times. As time goes on, build up to doing three sets of 10 repetitions.

PATIENT INFORMATION

Arthritis Research UK. *The painful shoulder.* Online: www.arthritisresearchuk.org

---

TENNIS ELBOW (LATERAL EPICONDYLITIS)

Smidt N, van der Windt D. 2006. Tennis elbow in primary care. BMJ 333, 927–928

A randomized trial has now clarified the benefits of therapy (Bisset, Beller, Jull, *et al.* 2006).

✳ Recommend that the patient avoid or reduce the provoking action. They should not be tempted to resume the activity until the pain has gone.

✳ Recommend an analgesic or an NSAID either topically or orally. There is evidence for short-term but not long-term benefit.

✳ *Explain that waiting for recovery* is as effective as any other approach, with 89% of patients recovered within 1 year. Refer for a brace if the pain is troublesome enough to warrant it.

* *Consider referral to physiotherapy* for manipulation and exercises: in the short term it is superior to a wait-and-see approach although at one year it shows no benefit.

* *Do not offer corticosteroid injection.* Despite some benefit at 6 weeks the relapse rate is high (72%) and the results at 1 year are worse than physiotherapy and worse even than a wait-and-see approach.

* *Consider referral for surgery* if the patient's life is sufficiently disturbed one year after onset. There is some evidence for benefit (Verhaar, Walenkamp, Kester, *et al.* 1993).

CARPAL TUNNEL SYNDROME

Ashworth N. Carpal tunnel syndrome. *Clinical Evidence* 2007 www.clinicalevidence.com (search on 'carpal tunnel')

* Advise the patient to rest the joint if possible and avoid provoking activities.

* Advise the patient to try a night splint (Futuro, Ace) to reduce the flexion of the joint.

* Do not give diuretics. Although commonly prescribed, there is no evidence that they are of value.

* Refer for steroid injection or surgical treatment, if:
  (a) there is thenar wasting or constant sensory impairment; or
  (b) symptoms are severe; or
  (c) there has been no improvement after 3 months. Surgical decompression is more effective than splinting (Verdugo, Salinas, Castillo, *et al.* 2003).

* Consider oral steroids while waiting for the appointment. There is evidence of benefit after 2 weeks.

DE QUERVAIN'S TENOSYNOVITIS

* Consider injection of steroid into the tendon sheath, although accurate placing of the needle is difficult.

GANGLION

* Explain to the patient that the lesion is harmless, that 40% resolve spontaneously and that surgery has its problems: excision does not always relieve pain; recurrence after surgery is common; and the scar may be unsightly.

* Consider aspiration with a wide bore needle under local anaesthesia.

* Refer the following if they are painful:
  (a) dorsal wrist ganglia (over the scapholunate ligament). Recurrence after surgery is 5–10%;
  (b) palmar digital ganglia (from the flexor tendon sheath at the base of the finger). Recurrence after surgery is rare.

* Try to avoid referring palmar wrist ganglia. Recurrence after surgery is 45%.

PROBLEMS WITH THE LOWER LIMBS

ACUTE KNEE INJURY

● The 'Ottawa Knee Rules', reduce the need for an X-ray after acute knee injury by 26%. They are as reliable in children as in adults (Bulloch, Neto, Plint, *et al.* 2003). Patients with major trauma are not suitable candidates for the use of the decision rule.

● The economic impact of adopting this approach could be a cost saving to the NHS of nearly £2 million (Nichols, Stiell, Wells, *et al.* 1999).

● The rules state that a **knee X-ray series** is only required for knee injury patients with **any** of these findings:
  (a) age 55 or older;
  (b) isolated tenderness of the patella (that is, no bone tenderness of the knee other than the patella);
  (c) tenderness at the head of the fibula;
  (d) inability to flex to 90°
  (e) inability to bear weight both immediately and when examined (they should be able to take four steps, i.e. take their weight on each leg twice even if they limp).

If there is no fracture:

* mobilize as soon as pain permits;
* encourage quadriceps exercises (see below);
* provide suitable analgesia.

ANTERIOR KNEE PAIN

Where there is a past history of injury

* Refer to the next fracture clinic if pain and effusion have persisted for > 2 weeks.
* If no grounds for immediate referral, arrange an x-ray. Request AP, lateral and skyline views.
* *If the X-ray is abnormal*, refer to the next fracture clinic. This applies whether the fracture is of the patella or a flake of bone from an osteochondral fracture.
* *If the X-ray is normal*, refer to orthopaedic outpatients if there is a good history of patella dislocation or the patella is unstable on examination.
* If neither of these applies, give advice (see below) and review after 8 weeks. Most young patients with anterior knee pain will have improved spontaneously in that time (Heintjes, Berger, Bierma-Zeinstra, *et al.* 2003a).

Where there is no history of injury

* Examine for gross abnormalities which might warrant immediate attention.
* Reassure the patient if it is Osgood-Schlatter disease (see page 127). Otherwise advise as below.

Patients still in pain after 8 weeks (with or without a history of injury)

* Arrange an X-ray, if not already done.
  (a) *If abnormal*, refer to OPD for assessment.
  (b) *If normal*, refer for physiotherapy. If still no progress, refer to OPD for assessment. Advise the patient that it may mean specialist physiotherapy or a brace rather than surgery.

General advice for patello–femoral pain

1. Avoid provoking activities (e.g. stairs, walking up and down hill, the breast-stroke kick, skiing, cycling, exercise bikes, and high impact aerobics).
2. Recommend quads exercises (see below) and hamstring stretching exercises. There is some evidence that exercise may reduce anterior knee pain (Heintjes, Berger, Bierma-Zeinstra, *et al.* 2003b).
3. Recommend simple analgesics. NSAIDs may reduce pain in the short term but not after 3 months.
4. Recommend a support bandage.

Knee exercises

(a) Stretching the hamstrings
  1. Stand up with the affected leg slightly in front.
  2. Place both palms over the knee cap and push towards the ground. Keep this position for 30 seconds.
  3. Repeat four times. As time goes on, try to increase the stretch by pointing your toes upwards.
(b) Strengthening the quadriceps
  1. Lying down on your back, lift the leg with the knee straight to a position about 45° off the horizontal.
  2. Hold this position for a count of 10 seconds.
  3. Lower the leg, and rest.
  4. Repeat 10 times. As time goes on, build up to doing three sets of ten repetitions.

Steroid injections at the knee

* Consider injections for:
  (a) anserine bursitis;
  (b) the knee joint;
  (c) the medial ligament of the knee.
Protection. Recommend impact-cushioning soles.

ACUTE ANKLE INJURY

The Ottawa Ankle Rule reduces the need for X-rays following ankle injury by 30–40% (see Table 9.2) (Bachmann, Kolb, Koller, *et al.* 2003). Note that the rule is very good at identifying patients who do not need an X-ray (high sensitivity). It is poor at identifying those who have a fracture (low specificity).

An *ankle x-ray* is required if there is any pain in the malleolar zone and:

(a) there is bone tenderness at the posterior edge or tip of the lateral malleolus; or
(b) there is bone tenderness at the posterior edge of the medial malleolus; or

Table 9.2	Reliability of the Ottawa Ankle Rules for identifying ankle and foot fractures or avulsion fractures		
PATIENT GROUPS	SENSITIVITY (95% CI)	SPECIFICITY (INTERQUARTILE RANGE)	LR−
All patients	96% (94 to 99%)	26% (19 to34%)	0.10
Ankle injuries	98% (96 to 99%)	40% (30 to 48%)	0.08
Midfoot injuries	99% (97 to 100%)	38% (25 to70%)	0.08

LR− is the likelihood ratio for a negative result.

(c) the patient is unable to weight bear both at injury and when seen.

A *foot X-ray* is required if there is pain in the midfoot zone and:

(a) there is bone tenderness at the navicular; or

(b) there is bone tenderness at the base of the 5th metatarsal; or

(c) the patient is unable to weight bear both at injury and when seen.

The immediate treatment of an ankle sprain (as for any injured joint or limb) is RICE (rest, ice, compression, elevation). Of these, compression appears to be the most important and, with elevation, must be maintained for at least 48 hours (Smith 2003). Ice should be applied no more than 20 minutes at a time, three times a day and the skin should be separated from the ice by a wet towel (Institute for Clinical Systems Improvement (ICSI) 2003). It is an approach based on experience rather than evidence.

* Analgesia, support with mobilization, immobilization and surgical repair are all used in inversion injuries of the ankle. There is no robust evidence to guide the clinician in their use although the use of support and early mobilization seems to result in faster recovery and better long-term outcomes (Kerkhoffs, Rowe, Assendelft, *et al.* 2002).

Rehabilitation after ankle injuries

* Recommend active mobilization to restore proprioception. This can be achieved by regular exercises:

(a) imagine writing the alphabet with the foot, first capitals then small letters;

(b) balance on the injured leg while moving the free leg forward and backward and side-to-side; initially with eyes open then with eyes shut;

(c) use a wobble board.

HEEL PAIN

GUIDELINE

Thomas JL, Christensen JC, Kravitz SR, *et al.* 2001. The diagnosis and treatment of heel pain; clinical practice guideline. J Foot Ankle Surg 40, 329–340. www.acfas.org/ (search on 'Heel pain')

Plantar fasciitis

Characteristics: isolated plantar heel pain on initiation of weight bearing either in the morning on rising or after a period of sitting. The pain tends to decrease after a while but increases as time on the feet increases.

* Examine to confirm heel tenderness and to check the range of movements. There may be associated tightness of the Achilles tendon.

* Do not X-ray. The presence of a calcaneal spur does not alter treatment.

* Advise the patient about weight reduction, if appropriate, and the use of cushioned shoes.

* Give analgesics. There is no evidence that NSAIDs are more effective than simple analgesics.

* Advise the patient about stretching exercises (plantar fascia and Achilles tendon) although there is no evidence of effectiveness (Digiovanni, Nawoczenski, Lintal, *et al.* 2003).

* Refer to a podiatrist if there is no improvement after 6 weeks.

● The benefit of steroid injection is likely to be temporary, if any, and not worth the possible harms (Crawford 2004). There is evidence of benefit from shock wave application if it is available (Rompe, Decking, Schoellner, *et al.* 2003).

1. Sit with the affected foot crossed over the other knee.
2. Grasp the toes and pull towards the shin until the plantar fascia is stretched.
3. Hold each stretch for a count of 10 and repeat 10 times, three times a day, for 8 weeks.

Achilles tendonopathy

Characteristics: an insidious onset leading to chronic posterior heel pain and swelling. The pain is worse with activity and pressure from shoes. There may be swelling medially and laterally to the insertion of the Achilles tendon.

There is insufficient evidence to determine which treatment is most appropriate. However, the following are commonly tried:

(a) open backed footwear;
(b) stretching exercises to lengthen the Achilles tendon;
(c) simple analgesia. The condition is not one of inflammation and there is no reason to prefer an NSAID (Khan, Cook, Kannus, *et al.* 2002).

Achilles tendon rupture

There may be a history of a sharp snap felt in the tendon on exertion or on injury, e.g. slipping off a ladder.
Up to 20% of ruptures are missed (Maffulli 1999).

* Consider the possibility of rupture in those with an acute history (as above) and all those who have a longer standing Achilles swelling or ankle injury that is slow to resolve.
* Diagnose rupture by lying the patient face down with the feet over the end of the couch. Squeeze the calf firmly. If the tendon is intact this will cause plantar flexion of the foot. If the tendon is ruptured there will be, at most, a small flicker of the foot (Thompson's test).
* Refer any patient with a suspected rupture to be seen within 24 hours.

PROBLEMS WITH THE FEET

BUNIONS

Although a percentage of bunions are inherited by an autosomal dominant gene this is of variable penetrance and hence not a reason for early referral or assessment.

* Examine to exclude heel valgus deformity and flatfoot and refer to a podiatrist if either is found. Orthoses may help reduce pain (Ferrari 2003). While awaiting the appointment teach the patient calf and foot exercises.
* Refer only those whose lives are severely affected by the bunion. They should be aware that:
  (a) after the operation they will not be able to wear a shoe for 8 weeks; and
  (b) recovery of function will take at least 6 months.

HALLUX RIGIDUS

* Advise the patient to wear a shoe with a rigid sole or to insert a rigid insole into the shoe.
* Refer if pain is interfering with work or sleep. Advise the patient that surgery is similar to bunion surgery as is the recovery time.

METATARSALGIA

Examine for a high arch and the presence of corns or calluses beneath the metatarsal heads.

* Refer to a podiatrist.
* Advise the patient to wear a metatarsal pad on the foot (just behind the site of the pain) or an adhesive pad inserted into the shoe to relieve the pressure on the metatarsal heads.
* Refer those not responding and patients with severe lancinating pain radiating down the cleft between two toes (Morton's neuroma).

STEROID INJECTIONS IN SOFT TISSUE LESIONS

BENEFITS

The poor quality of many studies means that evidence of long-term benefit is lacking. However, it is used because clinical experience demonstrates at least short-term relief, for which there is evidence (Speed 2001).

HARMS (SPEED AND HAZELMAN 2001)

The following are found in injections of the shoulder and similar figures will apply to injections in other sites:

(a) infection in one in 14,000–50,000 injections;
(b) tendon rupture in less than 1%;

(c) local scarring in less than 1%.

* Discuss with the patient the benefits and harms.
* Familiarize yourself with the common techniques (Silver 1999).

INDICATIONS

(a) Intensive use of other approaches for at least 2 months has failed; or
(b) rehabilitation is inhibited by symptoms.

GOOD PRACTICE

- Obtain the patient's consent.
- Check that you can define the local anatomy.
- Select the finest needle that will reach the lesion.
- Clean your hands and the patient's skin.
- Use a no-touch technique.
- Use short- or medium-acting corticosteroid preparations in most cases, with local anaesthetic.
- Injection should be peritendinous; avoid injection into tendon substance.
- Minimum interval between injections should be 6 weeks.
- Use a maximum of three injections at one site.
- Soluble preparations may be useful in those patients who have had hypersensitivity/local reaction to a previous injection.
- Record details of the injection.
- Do not repeat if two injections do not provide at least 4 weeks relief.

POST-INJECTION ADVICE

Warn the patient of early post-injection local anaesthesia and to avoid initial overuse. Advise resting for at least 2 weeks after injection and avoid heavy loading for 6 weeks. The patient should inform the doctor if there is any suggestion of infection or other serious adverse event.

CONTRAINDICATIONS TO CORTICOSTEROID INJECTION IN SOFT TISSUE LESIONS

(a) If pain relief and anti-inflammatory effects can be achieved by other methods.
(b) Local or systemic infection.
(c) Coagulopathy.
(d) Tendon tear.
(e) Young patients.

ORAL NON-STEROIDAL ANTI-INFLAMMATORY DRUGS

REVIEW

National Prescribing Centre. 2007. Cardiovascular and gastrointestinal safety of NSAIDs. MeReC Extra Issue No 30, November.
    http://www.npc.co.uk/MeReC_Extra/2008/no30_2007.html

ROLE OF NSAIDs IN MUSCULOSKELETAL DISORDERS

- NSAIDs have good analgesic action but many patients with acute or chronic pain can be managed with paracetamol or weak opioids such as codeine.
- NSAIDs taken *regularly at full dosage* have an anti-inflammatory action which is beneficial in controlling swelling and stiffness, as well as pain, in inflammatory diseases such as rheumatoid arthritis (RA) and the spondyloarthropathies (SpA) and in some cases of advanced osteoarthritis.
- Unlike opioids, they do not cause constipation, drowsiness or dependence. Against this must be set serious cardiovascular and gastrointestinal risks, particularly in the elderly.

WHICH ORAL NSAID?

- The clinical effects of NSAIDs vary from patient to patient. There are important differences between NSAIDs in their relative cardiovascular and gastrointestinal toxicity.
- Selective cyclo-oxygenase 2 (coxibs) have a lower risk of serious gastrointestinal effects than traditional NSAIDs. However, this advantage may be lost if prophylactic low-dose aspirin is also prescribed.

- Of the traditional NSAIDs, low dose ibuprofen (1.2 g daily) has the lowest gastrointestinal toxicity.
- Coxibs increase the risk of thrombotic events and are therefore contraindicated in established cardiovascular disease. Diclofenac has the same thrombotic risk as coxibs.
- Low-dose ibuprofen and naproxen 1000 mg daily have the lowest risk of thrombotic events.
- The choice of NSAID, therefore, should take account of the individual's risk profile.
- The Committee on the Safety of Medicines has restricted the use of azapropazone to inflammatory arthritis when other NSAIDs have failed and the Committee for Medicinal Products for Human Use (CHMP) has recommended similar caution with piroxicam. This does not apply to topical piroxicam formulations.

ADVERSE DRUG REACTIONS

(a) Upper GI disease: peptic ulceration, bleeding, non-ulcer dyspepsia.
(b) Fluid retention, leading to aggravation of heart failure.
(c) Renal failure, precipitated in pre-existing renal impairment.
(d) Hypersensitivity.
(e) Worsening of hypertension control.

CONTRAINDICATIONS AND CAUTIONS
Absolute contraindications to all NSAIDs

(a) Active peptic ulceration.
(b) Hypersensitivity (rhinoconjunctivitis, bronchospasm, urticaria, angioedema, and laryngeal oedema) to aspirin or another NSAID. Avoidance is essential to prevent life-threatening reactions.
(c) Pregnancy – third trimester.
(d) Severe heart failure.

Absolute contraindications to coxibs

(a) Ischaemic heart disease.
(b) Cerebrovascular disease.
(c) Peripheral arterial disease.
(d) Moderate heart failure.

Cautions for all NSAIDs

(a) Breastfeeding – largely due to manufacturers' warnings. The BNF states the amounts in breast milk for most NSAIDs are insignificant. See individual NSAIDs in Appendix 3 of the BNF.
(b) Renal, cardiac or liver failure – renal failure may worsen. Monitor U&Es.
(c) Asthma – worsening of asthma may be due to prescribed or OTC NSAIDs.
(d) Coagulation defects – including anticoagulation therapy.
(e) The elderly.
(f) Previous peptic ulceration.
(g) Concomitant use of medications that increase GI risk, e.g. steroid therapy or anticoagulants.

Cautions for the use of coxibs

(a) Left ventricular dysfunction.
(b) Hypertension.
(c) Oedema for any other reason.
(d) Patients with risk factors for heart disease.

PRESCRIBING PRACTICE

* Before prescribing an oral NSAID, consider using a topical NSAID.
* Weigh up the risks and benefits (see Table 9.3) for the individual and involve the patient in the decision.
* Prescribe the lowest effective dose for the shortest period to control symptoms.
* If the patient has not responded after 3 weeks, consider changing to an NSAID from another class.
* Advise patients to take their tablets with meals and to report dyspepsia immediately.
* For patients at high risk of developing GI complications, whether prescribing a traditional NSAID or a coxib, co-prescribe a gastroprotective drug. Use a proton pump inhibitor (PPI) though side-effects (colic and diarrhoea) may limit its use. Misoprostol is an alternative. Old age is one such high risk factor. Indeed NICE guidance on osteoarthritis recommends the routine prescription of a PPI for all patients on

Table 9.3   Comparative risks of traditional NSAIDs and coxibs (National Prescribing Centre 2007)

	TRADITIONAL NSAID	COXIBS
Thrombotic Risk	Relative risks (RR) compared to placebo are: diclofenac 1.63* (equivalent to a coxib) low-dose ibuprofen 1.51 (not statistically significant) naproxen 0.92 (not statistically significant)	Relative risk 1.42 NNH** compared to placebo = 300 per annum The risk remains constant for the period of use
GI risk	RRs compared to placebo (from RCTs) are: diclofenac 1.7 ibuprofen 1.2 naproxen 1.8 The risk is highest during first week	RR compared to traditional NSAIDs: 0.39 However, coxibs still carry some GI risk, probably equivalent to low-dose ibuprofen

*Meaning that diclofenac increases the risk of a thrombotic event by 63%. The absolute increase in risk depends on the baseline risk.
**NNH = Number Needed to Harm = the number who need to take the drug for one of them to have an excess adverse effect.

oral NSAIDs or coxibs (National Institute for Health and Clinical Excellence 2008a).

* Review the patient's continued need for NSAIDs regularly.

MANAGING NSAID-INDUCED GASTROINTESTINAL COMPLICATIONS (NEW ZEALAND GUIDELINE GROUP 2004)

Uninvestigated dyspepsia (Group NZG 2004)

* Review risk factors for NSAID-induced ulcer. These are:
   ■ past history of proven peptic ulcer disease or serious GI complications;
   ■ on medications likely to increase GI complications such as steroids or anticoagulants or bisphosphonates;
   ■ patients with significant comorbidity, such as heart failure;
   ■ H. pylori infection;
   ■ previous NSAID gastropathy;
   ■ high dose of NSAID or taking an NSAID plus aspirin.
* Consider as being at increased risk patients who are:
   ■ aged over 65 years plus one risk factor;
   ■ aged under 65 years plus two risk factors.

If at increased risk

* Refer patients for endoscopy if risk factor for ulcer present. Stop the NSAID pending the outcome (NICE 2004); and
* test and treat for H. pylori if positive.

If not at increased risk

* Stop the NSAID if possible, or reduce the dose, or change to a less toxic NSAID or to a coxib.
* If there is a need to continue an NSAID, prescribe a PPI. Misoprostol is an alternative.
* Proceed to endoscopy and testing for H. pylori as above only if there is no improvement.

Proven peptic ulcer

If *NSAID treatment needs to be continued after ulcer healing:*

* co-prescribe a PPI or misoprostol; and
* consider switching to a coxib.

Classes of NSAIDs

■ Salicylates: aspirin, diflunisal, benorylate.
■ Acetic acids: diclofenac, etodolac, indometacin, sulindac, tolmetin.
■ Propionic acids: fenbufen, fenoprofen, flurbiprofen, ketoprofen, ibuprofen, naproxen, tiaprofenic acid.
■ Fenamic acids: flufenamic, mefenamic.
■ Enolic acids: piroxicam, tenoxicam.
■ Non-acidic acids: nabumetone.
■ Selective COX-2 inhibitors: celecoxib, etoricoxib.

MONITORING PATIENTS TAKING DISEASE MODIFYING ANTIRHEUMATIC DRUGS (DMARDS)

See page 274 and Appendix 13.

BIOLOGIC THERAPY MONITORING

THE GP's ROLE IN MANAGING THE PATIENT ON INFLIXIMAB AND OTHER CYTOKINE MODULATORS

GUIDELINES

Kyle S, Chandler D, Griffiths CF, *et al.* 2005. Guideline for anti-TNF-α therapy in psoriatic arthritis. Rheumatology 44, 390–397, http://rheumatology.oxfordjournals.org

Keat A, Barkham A, Bhalla A, *et al.* 2005. BSR guidelines for prescribing TNF-α blockers in patients with ankylosing spondylitis. Rheumatology 44, 939–947, http://rheumatology.oxfordjournals.org

Royal College of Nursing. 2003. *Guidelines on Assessing, Managing and Monitoring Biologic Therapies for Inflammatory Arthritis,* http://www.rheumatology.org.uk. Choose 'Guidelines', then 'Other guidelines'

- Patients receiving biologicals will be monitored in secondary care. DMARDs may be co-prescribed; if so, monitoring should be in line with the recommendation for the DMARDs.
- Patients receiving biologicals are at increased risk of serious infections. They also have an increased risk of malignancies and possibly auto-immune diseases, including demyelinating and lupus like syndromes.
- Therefore, for GPs it is more important to be alert for the appearance of symptoms suggestive of these complications than to rely on routine monitoring.
- * Warn patients of the risk of infection and advise them to report symptoms other than minor illnesses.
- * Pay particular attention to the risk of tuberculosis. If the patient develops a productive cough or haemoptysis, weight loss and fever, stop treatment and send a sputum sample to be tested for acid fast bacilli.
- * Warn patients who are not immune to varicella of the need to avoid contact with chicken pox and shingles, and of the need to report any inadvertent contact (see page 52)
- * Ensure that the patient has had a single immunization against pneumococcus and annual influenza vaccine (see page 43).
- * If the patient develops a lupus like rash, take blood for antinuclear antibodies (ANA) and double stranded DNA binding (dsDNA) and inform the rheumatologist.

GOUT

REVIEW

Jordan KM. *An update on gout.* Arthritis Research UK. www.arthritisresearchuk.org

Guideline

Jordan KM, Cameron JS, Snaith M, *et al.* 2007. British Society for Rheumatology and British Health Professionals in Rheumatology guideline for the management of gout. Rheumatology 46, 1372–1374. Available: http://rheumatology.oxfordjournals.org/cgi/reprint/kem056av1

AIMS OF MANAGEMENT

- ■ To terminate an attack.
- ■ To prevent recurrent attacks.
- ■ To prevent complications.

TREATMENT OF THE ACUTE ATTACK

- * Consider the possibility of septic arthritis and refer urgently if this is suspected.

Non-pharmacological:

- * advise resting of the affected joint(s);
- * advise the application of a cold pack.

Pharmacological:

- * prescribe a fast-acting NSAID at maximum dose providing there are no contraindications;
- * advise that the NSAID should be continued until symptoms subside and for 1–2 weeks thereafter;
- * prescribe additional analgesia in the form of opiates, if needed for severe pain.

Patients with comorbidity

* For patients at increased risk of GI complications: follow advice under NSAID section or consider an alternative.
* For patients on a diuretic for hypertension consider changing to another hypertensive.
* For patients with heart failure, do not stop the diuretic.
* For patients with heart failure or renal failure, limit the use of NSAID or consider an alternative.

Alternatives to an NSAID

* Prescribe colchicine at a dose of 500 mcg b.d.–q.d.s. Do not use higher doses because of the risk of adverse effects (vomiting, diarrhoea and abdominal cramps). The drug should be stopped when the attack abates or if side-effects outweigh the benefit. Caution is urged in breastfeeding, the elderly, in hepatic and renal impairment and in GI and cardiac disease; or
* Prescribe prednisolone 35 mg daily until the attack is settling, then reduce to zero so that the total course is 7–10 days (Janssens, Janssen, van de Lisdonk, *et al.* 2008).

Patients not responding to the above:

* Consider an intra-articular injection of methylprednisolone (40 mg or 10 mg for a small joint) as a single dose.

MANAGEMENT AFTER AN ATTACK

* Review the patient at 4–6 weeks.
* Educate the patient regarding self-management. Advise the patient to start treatment *as soon as possible* after the onset of any future attacks and to have a standby supply of NSAID or alternative.
* Assess all patients for conditions associated with hyperuricaemia:
  (a) obesity;
  (b) alcohol consumption;
  (c) blood pressure;
  (d) hyperlipidaemia;
  (e) diabetes;
  (f) renal failure.

Investigations

■ Uric acid – check this after the attack has settled because it may be lowered during an attack. A raised level does not prove the diagnosis nor does a low level exclude it. The main value is in determining and monitoring prevention.
■ Blood tests: renal function, serum glucose and cholesterol.
■ Consider joint aspiration when the diagnosis is in doubt, e.g. knee monoarthritis when the differential diagnosis may be gout or pseudogout (urate crystals and calcium pyrophosphate dihydrate crystals seen respectively on microscopy). Send the aspirate immediately in a plain glass bottle for polarising microscopy (by prior arrangement).
■ X-rays are rarely helpful but can sometimes confirm pseudogout (chondrocalcinosis seen on plain films) or demonstrate joint damage from chronic gout, which is more likely to happen as an insidious process in the elderly.

PREVENTION OF RECURRENCE AND COMPLICATIONS

Lifestyle

Advise patients to:

■ lose weight if obese but to avoid rapid weight loss, which can precipitate an attack;
■ restrict alcohol to recommended limits, have three alcohol free days each week and to avoid beer and fortified wines;
■ avoid excessive amounts of purine-rich foods, e.g. offal, red meat, yeast extract, oily fish and shellfish;
■ take skimmed milk, low fat dairy products e.g. yoghourt, and vegetable sources of protein such as beans and cherries.
■ maintain a fluid intake > 2l/day.

Review medication

* Consider stopping drugs which reduce uric acid excretion, or reduce them to the lowest effective dose. They are aspirin (though not low dose aspirin used in cardiovascular protection), thiazides and loop diuretics.

Drug prophylaxis

Indications for drug prophylaxis:

(a) if a second or further attacks occur within a year;

(b) polyarticular gout;

(c) the presence of tophi;

(d) clinical or radiological signs of chronic gouty arthritis;

(e) prophylaxis when cytotoxic therapy is given for haematological malignancy;

(f) recurrent uric acid renal stones.

Asymptomatic hyperuricaemia is not considered an indication for drug prophylaxis.

Note: Wait until the acute attack has subsided for at least 2 weeks before starting prophylaxis, otherwise the attack may be prolonged.

PROPHYLACTIC DRUGS

Allopurinol

* Prescribe allopurinol as the first choice because it is effective and does not increase the risk of uric acid stone formation (unlike uricosurics below).

* Prescribe allopurinol starting at 50–100 mg daily, increasing by 50–100 mg every few weeks until the serum uric acid is below 300 μmol/l. The maximum dose is 900 mg/day. Doses above 300 mg daily should be divided.

* Check uric acid and creatinine yearly.

* If minor side-effects occur, e.g. rash, stop allopurinol and then reintroduce it at as low a dose as the patient can cut from a 100 mg tablet, e.g. 10 mg. If this is tolerated, increase the dose slowly.

* Do not restart if the rash was exfoliative dermatitis or if it was associated with fever or involvement of another organ.

* Give colchicine or an NSAID for the first 3–6 months; attacks may be precipitated in the early stages of allopurinol treatment. Use colchicine 500 mcg b.d. for the first 3–6 months or a standard dose of an NSAID for up to 6 weeks.

* If an attack occurs during prophylaxis, continue to use allopurinol at the same dose and treat the attack in its own right.

If allopurinal fails:

* Check compliance and review lifestyle, e.g. alcohol consumption.

* Consider referral for uricosuric drugs.

INDICATIONS FOR REFERRAL (NATIONAL LIBRARY FOR HEALTH 2008)

■ Septic arthritis is suspected: referral is urgent.

■ The diagnosis is uncertain.

■ There is a suspicion of an underlying systemic illness (e.g. rheumatoid arthritis or connective tissue disorder).

■ Gout occurs during pregnancy or in a young person (under 25 years of age).

■ Allopurinol is contraindicated or not tolerated, or is being started but NSAIDs and colchicine are contraindicated or not tolerated.

■ Allopurinol at maximum dose has been ineffective.

■ A person has persistent symptoms during an acute attack despite maximum doses of anti-inflammatory medication (alone or in combination).

■ An intra-articular steroid injection is indicated but the facilities or expertise are not available.

■ Complications are present, including urate kidney stones, or urate nephropathy.

PATIENT EDUCATION

Arthritis Research UK. Gout: *An Information Booklet.*
www.arthritisresearchuk.org

RHEUMATOID ARTHRITIS

REVIEWS

Walker DJ. 2007. *Diagnosing Inflammatory Disorders,* in Reports on the Rheumatic Diseases Series 5, Hands on. June. http://www.arc.org.uk/arthinfo/medpubs/6532/6532.asp#future
   Smith HR. Rheumatoid arthritis. *Emedicine.* Article Last Updated: 19 November, 2008;
   http://www.emedicine.com/med/topic2024.htm

Guidelines

Luqmani R, Hennell S, Estrach C, *et al.* 2006. British Society for Rheumatology and British Health Professionals in Rheumatology Guideline for the management of rheumatoid arthritis (the first 2 years). Rheumatology 45, 1167–1169

National Institute for Health and Clinical Excellence. 2009. *Rheumatoid Arthritis: The Management of Rheumatoid Arthritis in Adults.* NICE clinical guideline 79. Available: www.nice.org.uk

AIMS OF MANAGEMENT

(a) To suppress or minimize disease progression.
(b) To control symptoms: pain and stiffness.
(c) To preserve function.
(d) To minimize drug side-effects.
(e) To promote independence and quality of life.

GENERAL

- The impact of early intensive treatment with disease modifying antirheumatic drugs (DMARDs) has raised hopes that they may suppress rheumatoid disease. However, complete disease suppression is limited by side-effects.
- Treatment needs to be started as soon as possible before joint damage occurs. This 'window of opportunity' is within 3 months of the onset of symptoms. Yet early diagnosis is difficult even for specialists.
- Therefore, the GP has a vital role in referring patients as soon as the suspicion of RA arises, when they have *undifferentiated inflammatory arthritis* and before the diagnosis is confirmed. 12–15% of such patients will eventually turn out to have RA.
- The GP has a continuing role in managing the patient in the long term, within protocols shared with secondary care. The GP also has a role in managing the illnesses that accompany RA.
- Patients with RA have an increased risk of cardiovascular disease and mortality.

MODEL OF CARE

- Early referral from primary care for suspected RA for early diagnosis.
- Early intervention with DMARDs in the 'window of opportunity' before joint erosion occurs.
- Intense initial secondary care management and patient education.

- Patient access and primary care management when the disease is stabilized.
- Regular review by a specialist nurse in secondary care.

PATIENT ASSESSMENT

* Assess the impact on the patient's mental health, sleep, fatigue, acts of daily living and social function.
* Screen for and treat cardiovascular risk factors.
* Check for extra-articular manifestations including constitutional upset.

REFERRAL

* Refer whenever any of the following are present for over 6 weeks (Scottish Intercollegiate Guidelines Network 2000):
   (a) three or more joints are swollen;
   (b) the metacarpophalangeal or metatarsophalangeal joints are involved;
   (c) early morning stiffness lasts longer than 30 minutes.

The secondary care service should provide:

(a) formal assessment of the severity of disease as baseline for monitoring;
(b) a range of responses from a multidisciplinary team of nurses, physiotherapists, occupational therapist, social workers, dieticians, orthopaedic surgeons and podiatrists;
(c) a specialist nurse to review patients and to provide a telephone helpline. Secondary care may provide an educational programme.

PRE-REFERRAL INVESTIGATIONS

* Follow local protocols and in accordance with the availability of tests at the local laboratory
* Consider ordering the following with results to accompany the referral:
   - ESR and C-reactive protein (CRP), as an indication of disease activity.
   - Rheumatoid factor – do this because a positive result early in the disease has prognostic significance. However, the sensitivity and specificity are not sufficiently high to make a diagnosis.
   - The anti-cyclic citrullinated peptide (anti-CCP) (Maddison and Huey 2006). It is highly

specific (> 95%) for rheumatoid at all stages of the disease. This means that a positive finding makes the diagnosis almost certain. However, the sensitivity is not sufficiently high in early disease (45–60%) to rule out disease so, if it is negative, referral should still be made on clinical grounds.

- FBC, because the anaemia of chronic disease is common and to get a baseline because some DMARDs and biologicals affect the blood count.
- LFTs – some DMARDs and biologicals affect the liver.
- U&Es and dip testing of urine because some DMARDs and biologicals affect renal function.
- Viral serology if recent illness suggests a viral arthritis.
- Consider X-ray of affected joints and of the hands and feet because rheumatologists usually request them as a baseline for future progression. However, X-rays are unlikely to be helpful in diagnosis because erosive changes are not usually apparent early in the disease (Royal College of Radiologists 2003).

PATIENTS WITH POOR PROGNOSIS

The following carry a poor prognosis if present early in the disease:

(a) persistent synovitis;
(b) high ESR or C-reactive protein;
(c) positive rheumatoid factor;
(d) male sex.

SHARED CARE: PHARMACOLOGICAL TREATMENT

PAIN CONTROL

* Recommend paracetamol as a first line analgesic. It is effective and safe.
* Weigh up and discuss the risks and benefits of additional strategies for controlling pain: NSAIDs and opiates.
  - NSAIDs. The benefits: superior to paracetamol in controlling stiffness and swelling. The risks: GI, renal and cardiovascular effects (see page 267).

* Choose an NSAID or coxib according to the patient's risk and comorbidities. It is customary to try a patient on one NSAID or coxib for a period of several weeks and then to switch to an alternative if it is ineffective.
* If NSAIDs or coxibs are needed for the long term, prescribe the lowest effective dose.
* Start with a weak opiate such as codeine.
* If necessary, prescribe stronger opiates.
* Bear in mind the effects of pain and of side-effects on the individual's lifestyle.

STEROIDS

* Consider using systemic steroids in the following situations:
  (a) bridging disease control between different DMARD therapies;
  (b) to achieve rapid control of symptoms but only once the diagnosis has been established;
* Recommend local steroid injections for localized flare-ups.

Note: Caution is required in long-term steroid use: see steroids in sections Polymyalgia and Temporal arteritis and section on Osteoporosis.

DMARDS

- They include antimetabolites, antimalarials, and biologic agents (Table 9.4).
- The choice of DMARD will be made by the patient and consultant.
- Methotrexate has emerged as the most commonly prescribed DMARD closely followed by sulfasalazine.
- Cytokine modulators (anti-TNF drugs) are indicated in patients who have failed to respond to at least two DMARDs, including methotrexate (unless contraindicated).

The GP's role

* Support patients during the initiation of therapy. There may be no benefit for 2–6 months.
* Counsel patient to report potential adverse effects promptly (see Table 9.4).

Table 9.4	DMARDs, usual dose and selected toxicity (see BNF for full list of adverse effects)	
DRUG	USUAL MAINTENANCE DOSE	TOXICITY
Methotrexate	7.5–15 mg per week	GI symptoms, stomatitis, rash, alopecia, infrequent myelosuppression, hepatotoxicity, rare but serious (even life-threatening) pulmonary toxicity
Sulfasalazine	1000 mg twice or three times daily	Rash, myelosuppression (infrequent), GI intolerance
Leflunomide	Maintenance, 10–20 mg once daily	Hepatotoxicity, myelosuppression. GI symptoms, rashes including Stevens-Johnson syndrome, toxic epidermal necrolysis
Cytokine modulators, Anti-TNF drugs: (etanercerpt, adalimumab, infliximab)	Etanercerpt, weekly or fortnightly s.c. injection Infliximab i.v. infusion every 8 weeks Adalimumab fortnightly s.c. injection	Infections, sometimes severe, including tuberculosis, septicaemia, and hepatitis B reactivation. Hypersensitivity reactions, including lupus erythematosus-like syndrome, pruritus, injection-site reactions, and blood disorders myelosuppression. Worsening heart failure
Hydroxychloroquine	200 mg twice daily	Rash (infrequent), diarrhoea, retinal toxicity (rare)
Injectable gold salts	25–50 mg i.m. every 2–4 weeks	Rash, stomatitis, myelosuppression, thrombocytopenia, proteinuria
Oral gold	3 mg daily or twice daily	Same as injectable gold but less frequent, plus frequent diarrhoea
Azathioprine	50–150 mg daily	Myelosuppression, hepatotoxicity (infrequent), early flu-like illness with fever, GI symptoms, elevated LFTs
Penicillamine	250–750 mg daily	Rash, stomatitis, loss of taste, proteinuria, myelosuppression, infrequent but serious autoimmune disease

* Ensure patients know about the dangers to conception:
  ■ several DMARDs are contraindicated in pregnancy;
  ■ both male and female patients may need to delay conception until a period has elapsed after stopping cytotoxics. The period depends on the DMARD, e.g., 3 months for MTX, 2 years for women on leflunomide.
* Follow local protocols for monitoring the adverse effect of these drugs, as protocols vary between institutions. See Appendix 13 for a proposed protocol.

Methotrexate

The National Patient Safety Agency reports errors in prescribing and dispensing.

* State clearly on prescriptions for methotrexate that the dose is to be taken *weekly.*
* Prescribe *only one strength* (usually 2.5 mg).
* Prescribe folic acid 5 mg to be taken on a separate day of the week to reduce nausea.

ANTIDEPRESSANTS

* Ask about sleep disturbance and fatigue.
* Prescribe an antidepressant to aid sleep and reduce pain as well as to treat depression, if present.

NON-DRUG MANAGEMENT

Education, physiotherapy and related interventions remain at the centre of care.

* Constantly review patients not under the care of the multidisciplinary hospital team for the need for referral to any of the following:
  (a) physiotherapists – for education, exercise programmes and splints;
  (b) occupational therapists – for mobility and daily living aids;
  (c) nurse specialists;
  (d) orthotic and prosthetic departments;
  (e) chiropodists;
  (f) orthopaedic surgeon.

EDUCATION

Education improves knowledge, symptom control, adherence and self-management.

* Consider every consultation an opportunity to educate the patient.
* Provide information leaflets (see box).

PATIENT INFORMATION

National Rheumatoid Arthritis Society. www.rheumatoid.org.uk and choose 'About rheumatoid arthritis'. Helpline 0800 298 7650

Arthritis Research UK. *Rheumatoid Arthritis: An Information Booklet.* Online: www.arthritisresearchuk.org

Arthritis Care. *Rheumatoid Arthritis.* http://www.arthritiscare.org.uk/AboutArthritis/Conditions/Rheumatoidarthritis

EXERCISE

* Advise patients to keep active and exercise. This improves mood and encourages self-sufficiency.
* Advise the patient to pace activities to a realistic level.
* Explain the benefits of the different forms of exercise:
  (a) range of movement or stretching exercises relieve stiffness and maintain flexibility;
  (b) strengthening exercises maintain muscle strength, needed for function and joint support;
  (c) aerobic exercise improves cardiovascular risk, aids weight control and overall function.

TENS, HEAT AND COLD APPLICATIONS

There is no evidence that they do harm, though cold rather than heat application is usually recommended for actively inflamed joints. There is evidence they may provide short-term relief.

SURGERY

Surgery can be highly effective in selected cases (Scott, Shipley, Dawson, *et al.* 1998) and covers tendon transfers, arthroplasties (including upper limb and small joints), and arthrodeses.

OSTEOPOROSIS

Patients with RA are at an increased risk of osteoporosis.

* Calculate the patient's fracture risk, see page 280.

ALTERNATIVE THERAPIES/DIET

60% of RA patients have tried alternative therapies and diets. Be prepared to discuss alternative and complementary strategies.

Complementary therapies that may help but require further research:

■ Gamma-linolenic acid (GLA) containing plant oils, such as evening primrose, borage and blackcurrant. GLA may relieve pain and morning stiffness. Side-effects include flatulence, nausea, and diarrhoea. Some plant oils can cause liver damage or interact with medications.

■ Fish oils containing eicosapentaenoic acid (EPA) or docosahexaenoic acid (DHA). EPA and DHA may reduce pain and stiffness. Side-effects include flatulence and nausea. Fish oil can interact with medication (Mayo Clinic 2008).

■ *Acupuncture.* Electroacupuncture may relieve pain but acupuncture has no effect on symptoms, function, or quality of life (Casimiro, Barnsley, Brosseau, *et al.* 2005).

Recommend the ARC information booklet *Complementary and Alternative Medicine for Arthritis* available on www.arc.org.uk and search on 'Complementary'.

DISABILITY

Historically, over 80% of patients would have been at least moderately disabled after 20 years. This may change with the use of DMARDs.

* Manage the disability according to the guidance on page 619.

SPONDYLOARTHROPATHIES

REVIEWS

Kataria RK, Brent LH. 2004. Spondyloarthropathies. Am Fam Physician 69, 2853–2860, http://www.aafp.org/afp/20040615/2853.html

Brent LH, Kalagate R. 2006. Ankylosing spondylitis and undifferentiated spondyloarthropathy. emedicine. http://www.emedicine.com/med/TOPIC2700.HTM#table4

Guideline

Zochling J, van der Heijde D, Burgos-Vargas R, *et al.* 2006. ASAS/EULAR recommendations for the management of ankylosing spondylitis. Ann Rheum Dis 65, 442–452

The spondyloarthropathies (SpA) are a group of conditions characterized by inflammatory spinal pain and enthesitis. They are associated with the HLA-B27 tissue type. The category includes:

(a) ankylosing spondylitis (AS);
(b) reactive arthritis (following an infection, usually bowel or genitourinary, the latter often termed Reiter's syndrome);
(c) psoriatic arthritis;
(d) inflammatory bowel disease associated arthritis;
(e) undifferentiated spondyloarthropathy.

AIMS OF MANAGEMENT

* Control symptoms: pain, stiffness and disability
* Prevent deformity and disability
* Manage non-skeletal complications: fatigue, anterior uveitis, pulmonary and thoracic restriction (AS), aortic incompetence (AS), and inflammatory bowel disease.

DIAGNOSIS OF AS

● Early diagnosis is important to establish an exercise programme and to start effective pharmacotherapy to prevent deformity. The average delay in diagnosis is 5–7 years.
● A history suggestive of inflammatory back pain (see below) has both a sensitivity and specificity of about 75% for AS.

FEATURES OF INFLAMMATORY BACK PAIN (SIEPER AND RUDWALEIT 2005)

■ Morning stiffness of > 30 minutes' duration.
■ Improvement in back pain with exercise.
■ Pain at night or on early wakening.
■ Good response to NSAIDs.

DIAGNOSIS OF OTHER SPONDYLOARTHROPATHIES

* Search for clues in the personal and family histories and on examination for diseases of bowel and skin and sexually transmitted disease.

INVESTIGATIONS

● CRP and ESR are frequently raised but may be normal.
● HLA-B27 does not confirm the diagnosis since the background incidence is 6–8% in the general population. However, a negative result makes the diagnosis unlikely because 95% of AS sufferers are positive.
● X-rays of the sacroiliac joints (SIJs) give a high dose of radiation with little benefit, because diagnostic changes take years to develop. MRIs are more accurate than X-rays.
* Ask for CRP and ESR to assess inflammation.
* Check FBC for the anaemia of chronic disease.
* Check U&Es and LFTs if referring as DMARD or anti-TNF therapy may be considered.
* Explain why a plain X-ray is unlikely to help early in the disease. Consider X-ray of the sacroiliac joints if symptoms have been present for several years. Consider referral for diagnosis.

MANAGEMENT

* Prescribe an NSAID at full dose. Choose one with a long half-life to ease morning stiffness, e.g. naproxen. Prescribe an alternative NSAID if response after 4–6 weeks is insufficient.
* Prescribe or advise over-the-counter analgesics for use as needed.
* Explain the need for regular, daily exercise: it helps to control pain, prevents increasing stiffness and prevents deformity (Elyan and Khan 2008). Swimming is a good all-round exercise but specific daily exercises have been developed for maintenance of posture.
* Refer to physiotherapy for exercises or to the local NASS group (see box below), or both.
* During flare-ups, advise patients to continue exercises within the limits of pain.
* Advise patient to lie on floor prone or supine for 20 minutes each day.
* Prescribe low-dose antidepressants for nocturnal pain and fatigue (Koh, Pande, Samuels, et al. 1997).
* Advise the patient to stop smoking. Limitation of chest expansion occurs over time.
* Prescribe or advise hypromellose eye drops for conjunctival disease (dry gritty eyes).
* Watch out for and warn the patient of the symptoms of acute iritis.

* Consider local steroid injections for peripheral joint disease or enthesitis for short-term relief during flare-ups.

REFERRALS

To a rheumatologist

* Refer suspected new cases:
  (a) Age under 45 years at onset; AND
  (b) Pain present for over 3 months; AND
  (c) Inflammatory back pain features or sacroiliitis shown on X-ray or MRI (Sieper and Rudwaleit 2005).
* Refer if flare-ups fail to settle.
* Refer established patients if NSAIDs alone are insufficient. Options which can be initiated in secondary care include DMARDs (methotrexate and sulfasalazine) and biologicals (adalimumab and etanercept).

To other specialities

* Refer immediately for an ophthalmological opinion if you suspect acute iritis.
* Refer to a gastroenterologist in presence of symptoms of inflammatory bowel disease (National Institute for Health and Clinical Excellence 2008b).

PATIENT INFORMATION

National Ankylosing Spondylitis Society (NASS), Unit 0.2, 1 Victoria Villas, Richmond, Surrey TW9 2GW. Tel: 020 8948 9117. *Guidebook for patients: A Positive Response to Ankylosing Spondylitis*, Available: www. nass.co.uk (click on 'Download guidebook' in the Welcome Message)

CONNECTIVE TISSUE DISEASES

REVIEWS

Ahmad Y, Bruce I. 2000. Connective tissue disease and the role of the general practitioner. Arthritis Research UK. Rheumatic disease in practice, Number 3. www. arthritisresearchuk.org

---

Davenport G. 2008. Connective tissue disease in primary care. ARC. Rheumatic Disease in Practice, Number 3. http://www.arc.org.uk/arthinfo/medpubs/6529/6529.asp

---

The connective tissue diseases

Systemic lupus erythematosus.
Systemic sclerosis.
Polymyositis.
Dermatomyositis.
Sjögren's syndrome.
Raynaud's disease.
Mixed connective tissue disorder.

* The term connective tissue diseases (CTDs) covers a group of inflammatory diseases affecting multiple systems which have a variable presentation and course and whose features overlap. They are strongly associated with several autoantibodies.
* Complications can be serious and fatal, e.g. lung fibrosis, renal failure, gangrene.
* Many features, especially early in the disease, are non-specific.
* A group practice with 8000 patients may have 50–80 patients with Sjögren's syndrome, four with systemic lupus erythematosus (SLE), and four to eight with other CTDs. They are uncommon but the GP has a special role in both diagnosis and treatment because of their multisystem and chronic nature.
* Evidence-based guidelines are not available for CTDs in general. However, many of the management issues overlap with those of other inflammatory rheumatic conditions already mentioned.

DIAGNOSIS

* Most present with either arthralgia or Raynaud's phenomenon.
* Suspect a CTD when:
  (a) there is arthralgia but no evidence of clinical synovitis;
  (b) a rash is present (malar rash of SLE spares the nasolabial fold, the rash of dermatomyositis affects face and hands);

(c) muscle weakness, rather than the stiffness of PMR, is present;

(d) symptoms suggest multiple system involvement. The more suggestive features there are, the greater is the likelihood of disease being present, especially if combined with non-specific features.

* Review the medical history for salient features which may have been overlooked in the past, e.g. miscarriages.

* Order the following tests:

(a) FBC: leucopenia, lymphopenia, thrombocytopenia or haemolysis suggest a CTD;

(b) urine dipstick and U&Es to screen for renal disease;

(c) creatine kinase;

(d) ESR/CRP: they are usually raised in a CTD (but note that the CRP is often normal in SLE in the absence of infection);

(e) serum ANA: it is positive in over 90% of many CTDs. However, it should *not* be relied on as a diagnostic test in the absence of clinical features as it is positive in 5% of the general population and > 30% of people with rheumatoid arthritis.

MANAGEMENT

* Refer suspected cases early to a rheumatologist for diagnosis and a management plan.

* Share care for monitoring progress and therapy with the hospital specialist (as for RA).

* Screen for and manage other cardiovascular risk factors, e.g. hypertension (especially when renal disease is present or high dose steroid therapy used).

* *Women's health:* consider the increased risk of thromboses and drug therapy (e.g. cytotoxics) for CTD in preconception counselling, contraception, pregnancy and hormone replacement therapy (HRT).

* Treat infections promptly in SLE as they may lead to flare-ups. Consider the possibility of atypical organisms in the immunocompromised.

* Maintain a high index of suspicion for malignancy which may underlie the disease, complicate the disease or complicate immunosuppressive treatment.

PATIENT INFORMATION

The British Sjögren's Syndrome Association, PO Box 10867, Birmingham B16 0ZW, tel. 0121 455 6532, helpline 0121 455 6549, www.bssa.uk.net

Lupus UK, St James House, Eastern Road, Romford, Essex RM1 3NH, tel. 01708 731 251, www.lupusuk.com

The Raynaud's and Scleroderma Association, 112 Crewe Road, Alsager, Cheshire ST7 2JA, tel. 01270 872 776, www.raynauds.org.uk

Arthritis Research UK:

Lupus (SLE): An Information Booklet.

Polymyositis and Dermatomyositis: An Information Booklet.

Raynaud's Phenomenon: An Information Booklet. www.arthritisresearchuk.org

OSTEOPOROSIS

REVIEW

Jacobs-Kosmin D. *Osteoporosis.* Emedicine 2008. http://www.emedicine.com/MED/topic1693.htm

Guidelines

National Osteoporosis Guideline Group (NOGG). *Guideline for the Diagnosis and Management of Osteoporosis in Postmenopausal Women and Men from the Age of 50 Years in the UK,* 2008. http://www.shef.ac.uk/NOGG/downloads.html

National Institute for Health and Clinical Excellence (NICE). *Osteoporosis: Primary Prevention,* and *Osteoporosis: Secondary Prevention including Strontium Ranelate,* 2008. Available: www.nice.org.uk

The NOGG guidelines have been used in this section because:

■ They cover both men and women.

■ They include corticosteroid induced osteoporosis.

■ They give explicit guidance on risk calculation.

BACKGROUND

● Osteoporosis is a disorder of diminished bone density and degenerate microarchitecture leading to fragility and increasing the risk of fracture.

- Osteoporosis causes over 200,000 fractures each year in the UK.
- Most fractures occur in the larger group with lesser degrees of demineralization (osteopenia) through interaction with other risk factors (see below).
- A fragility fracture is a fracture occurring on minimal trauma (e.g. falling when standing on the ground) after the age of 40, in a typical site, including the vertebral bodies, distal radius, proximal femur and the proximal humerus.

DEFINITIONS OF OSTEOPENIA AND OSTEOPOROSIS

These conditions are defined by the result of DXA (dual energy X-ray absorptiometry) measurements of bone mineral density (BMD).

- T score below -2.5 = *osteoporosis*. The BMD is > 2.5 standard deviations below the young adult mean.
- T score between -1 and -2.5 = *osteopenia*. The BMD is between 1 and 2.5 standard deviations below the young adult mean.
- T score above -1 = *normal*.

Where more than one site is scanned, the lowest score is used.

GENERAL PRINCIPLES

- Diagnosis is based on case-finding, namely, identifying those likely to be at risk because of either:
  - (a) a previous fragility fracture; or
  - (b) the presence of significant clinical risk factors in postmenopausal women or men over the age of 50.
- The risk of future fracture is used as a *guide* to further management. Clinical judgment still has a place. Calculators do not take account of a tendency to falls, the greater prognostic risk attached to vertebral relative to other fractures, or the greater risk after more than one fragility fracture.
- There is geographical variation in how services are organized and which speciality leads them. *The GP's role, referral routes and pre-referral work-up will vary accordingly and local protocols need to be observed.*

- Assessment in general practice includes the search for a possible cause of secondary osteoporosis and a differential diagnosis, according to the individual's age, sex and clinical features.
- ✱ Take a history, perform an examination and order investigations appropriate to the individual's clinical picture (see box).
- ✱ Refer younger men with osteoporosis for further investigation since there is a greater chance of secondary osteoporosis in this group.

PROCEDURES PROPOSED IN THE INVESTIGATION OF OSTEOPOROSIS

Routine

- History and physical examination.
- Blood cell count, sedimentation rate or C-reactive protein, serum calcium, albumin, creatinine, phosphate, alkaline phosphatase and liver transaminases.
- Thyroid function tests.
- Bone densitometry (DXA).

Other procedures, if indicated

- Lateral radiographs of lumbar and thoracic spine/ DXA-based vertebral imaging.
- Protein immunoelectrophoresis and urinary Bence Jones proteins.
- Serum testosterone, SHBG (sex-hormone binding globulin), FSH (follicle stimulating hormone), LH luteinizing hormone (in men).
- Serum prolactin.
- Screening tests for coeliac (see page 211).

APPROACH TO PROGNOSIS AND INTERVENTION

- ✱ Be alert to patients at risk with a previous fragility fracture or significant clinical risk factors (CRF), see box.
- ✱ Consider pharmacological intervention in post-menopausal women with a fragility fracture without performing a DXA scan (NICE recommendations differ, suggesting this strategy for women over 75).
- ✱ For all other cases, use the FRAX tool to assess the patient's 10-year probability of a major

osteoporotic fracture, http://www.sheffield.ac.uk/FRAX/index.htm. The tool will place the patient in one of three bands: *low, intermediate or high risk.*

* If the risk is intermediate, arrange for a DXA scan because the results may alter management. Recalculate the risk using the FRAX tool and the result of the DXA. The tool will now place the patient in one of two bands: *low or high risk.*
* *Low risk.* Give general advice (see below).
* *High risk.* Offer pharmacological intervention (see below).

CLINICAL RISK FACTORS (CRFS) FOR OSTEOPOROSIS

- Age
- Sex
- Low body mass index ($\leq$ 19 kg/m2)
- Previous fragility fracture, particularly of the hip, wrist and spine including morphometric vertebral fracture
- Parental history of hip fracture
- Current glucocorticoid treatment (any dose, by mouth for 3 months or more)
- Current smoking
- Alcohol. Dose dependent, risks starts at daily intake of 3 or more units
- Causes of secondary osteoporosis including:
  (a) rheumatoid arthritis
  (b) untreated hypogonadism in men and women
  (c) prolonged immobility
  (d) organ transplantation
  (e) type I diabetes
  (f) hyperthyroidism
  (g) gastrointestinal disease
  (h) chronic liver disease
  (i) chronic obstructive pulmonary disease
- Falls*

* This CRF is the only one not used in the FRAX calculation.

GENERAL MANAGEMENT

* Assess the risk of falls and refer to local the falls prevention services as appropriate.
* Encourage exercise: resistance exercises (lifting weights) and weight bearing impact exercise (skipping, dancing) (Scottish Intercollegiate Guidelines Network 2003).
* Advise a diet that provides a daily intake of 1000 mg calcium and 800 IU of vitamin D_3. The recommended calcium intake can be achieved with one pint of semi-skimmed milk plus one of: 3 oz hard cheese, three slices of white bread (or six of wholemeal bread), one small pot of yoghourt or 3 oz of canned sardines. The National Osteoporosis Society has a list of calcium and vitamin D contents which can be useful for vegans and religious observances.
* Give the same dietary advice to those receiving pharmacological intervention.
* Prescribe calcium and ergocalciferol 1 tablet twice daily to the housebound elderly.

PHARMACOLOGICAL INTERVENTION

Prevention and treatment relate to the prevention of osteoporosis and treatment of established osteoporosis, not the prevention and treatment of fractures.

First line

* Prescribe alendronate as a first line agent because of a good evidence base for the prevention of fractures at several sites and its cost-effectiveness. It is suitable in both men and women for the:
  - treatment of postmenopausal osteoporosis, 10 mg daily or 70 mg once weekly;
  - treatment of osteoporosis in men, 10 mg daily;
  - prevention of postmenopausal osteoporosis, 5 mg daily;
  - prevention and treatment of corticosteroid-induced osteoporosis, 5 mg daily but for postmenopausal women not receiving hormone replacement therapy, 10 mg daily.

The practicalities of prescribing bisphosphonates

* Advise the patient to swallow the tablets whole with plenty of water, half an hour before breakfast and to remain upright for half an hour afterwards.
* Correct disturbances of calcium and mineral metabolism (e.g. vitamin D deficiency, hypocalcaemia) before starting. Monitor serum calcium concentration during treatment.

* Advise the patient on good dental hygiene during and after treatment to avoid the rare complication of osteonecrosis of the jaw. If remedial dental treatment is needed, advise the patient to consider having it done before starting alendronate.

* If alendronate is not tolerated or contraindicated, consider an alternative bisphosphonate, strontium ranelate or raloxifene. The bisphosphonates have similar contraindications and side-effects. If GI side-effects are prominent, a weekly formulation (alendronate 70 mg or risedronate 35 mg) may be tried.

CONTRAINDICATIONS

- Abnormalities of the oesophagus which delay emptying (alendronate, risedronate);
- inability to stand or sit upright for at least 30 minutes;
- hypocalcaemia;
- pregnancy;
- breastfeeding.

Cautions

- Other upper GI problems;
- significant renal failure (creatinine clearance < 30 mL/minute)

Alternative interventions to bisphosphonates

The effectiveness of some drugs in the prevention of certain fractures or in men has not been adequately evaluated making them less suitable as first line agents.

* Consider prescribing raloxifene for postmenopausal osteoporosis. Advise the patient it does not reduce menopausal vasomotor symptoms.

* Consider referring for strontium ranelate, intravenous bisphosphonates (ibandronic acid or zoledronic acid, quarterly or annually respectively) or parathyroid hormone or peptide (teriparatide).

CORTICOSTEROID–INDUCED OSTEOPOROSIS

* Keep doses of oral corticosteroids as low as possible and courses as short as possible.

* Consider the risk of osteoporosis in patients with cumulative doses from intermittent courses. Long-term use of high-dose inhaled corticosteroids may also carry a risk.

PATIENT INFORMATION

Arthritis Research Campaign (ARC). *Osteoporosis: An Information Leaflet.* http://www.arc.org.uk/arthinfo/patpubs/6028/6028.asp

National Osteoporosis Society. www.org.uk. Click on the 'Osteoporosis' tab and follow the links, or go to the leaflets link: http://www.nos.org.uk/NetCommunity/Page.aspx?pid=466&srcid=234

POLYMYALGIA RHEUMATICA (PMR)

MANAGEMENT OBJECTIVES

- To control symptoms of stiffness and pain (plus associated constitutional symptoms, e.g. fatigue, weight loss).
- To reduce the risk of the complication of temporal arteritis.
- To minimize the risks of steroid therapy.

DIAGNOSIS

- The patient is being committed to at least 2 years of steroid therapy. As no single test reliably confirms the diagnosis, the history is important.
- The typical history in PMR is of pain, stiffness, or both, affecting the upper arms and upper legs with diurnal variation, that is to say, worse in the mornings. This history is present in 95% of cases (Bahlas, Ramos-Remos and Davis 1998).
- Confidently diagnose PMR if three or more of the diagnostic criteria (see box) are present or if one criterion is associated with a clinical or pathological abnormality of the temporal artery. The sensitivity for this criterion-based test is 92% (i.e. it will correctly identify 92% of all cases) and the specificity is 80% (i.e. it will correctly exclude 80% of normals) (Bird, Esselinckx, Dixon, *et al.* 1979).

FEATURES OF POLYMYALGIA RHEUMATICA

- Bilateral shoulder pain or stiffness.
- Onset of illness < 2 weeks duration.
- Initial ESR > 40 mm/h.
- Age 65 years or more.
- Depression and/or weight loss.
- Bilateral tenderness in the upper arms.

INVESTIGATIONS

* Check ESR or CRP. Note that the ESR may be normal in 20% of cases.
* Consider tests to rule out alternative diagnoses as appropriate:
  (a) TFTs for hypothyroidism;
  (b) creatinine kinase for polymyositis and statin-induced myositis;
  (c) CXR. Malignancy, especially lung cancer, can cause polymyalgia;
  (d) protein electrophoresis to exclude multiple myeloma.

INITIAL MANAGEMENT

* Check FBC; a normocytic normochromic anaemia is common.
* Measure weight, BP and check serum glucose before starting steroids.
* Prescribe prednisolone 15 mg daily. Higher starting doses are rarely needed and are more likely to cause adverse effects (Kyle and Hazleman 1989a).
* Review within a fortnight. Expect a dramatic response within days.
* If there is no response to steroids, review alternative diagnoses as above plus:
  (a) cervical spondylosis (the commonest differential diagnosis);
  (b) rheumatoid arthritis.
* Raise the dose of prednisolone to 30 mg daily if you have confidently excluded other diagnoses.

MAINTENANCE STEROID THERAPY

- The risk of relapse is highest early on in treatment and at doses below prednisolone 10 mg. Temporal arteritis is more likely to develop at doses below 10 mg daily.
- Treatment needs to be maintained for at least 2 years. Even then, only a quarter of patients can stop steroids after this time (Kyle and Hazleman 1993).
- Over half of patients with PMR (and GCA) will develop complications of steroids, the commonest being weight gain (Kyle and Hazleman 1989b).

The principle: reduce the prednisolone dose to the lowest possible to maintain control.

A suggested routine is as follows (Clinical Knowledge Summaries 2009):

* Prescribe 15 mg daily for the first month. Check inflammatory markers after 2–6 weeks.
* Reduce by 2.5 mg each fortnight until 10 mg daily is reached, providing there is no relapse of symptoms or rise in inflammatory markers.
* Review the patient 1 week after each dose reduction.
* Reduce the daily dose by 1 mg every 6 weeks until 5–7 mg daily is reached.
* Maintenance dose: 5–7 mg for 12 months providing there is no relapse of symptoms or inflammatory markers.
* Final reduction: reduce the daily dose by 1 mg every 6–8 weeks, until 3 mg daily is reached, then by 1 mg every 12 weeks, providing symptoms and (less importantly) inflammatory markers remain controlled.
* If symptoms suggest continuing disease in the presence of normal inflammatory markers, give more weight to the former.
* Warn patients that symptoms may return and advise early consultation. A return of symptoms is a more reliable early indication of relapse than inflammatory markers.

REFERRAL

Refer patients when:

(a) Symptom control requires a high maintenance dose of steroids or the patient develops significant adverse steroid effects on lower doses (steroid sparing drugs may be considered).

(b) There is doubt about the diagnosis, particularly when there is synovitis and anaemia suggestive of rheumatoid arthritis.

PATIENT EDUCATION

* Advise patients to seek urgent attention if they develop symptoms suggestive of GCA: a unilateral headache, tenderness in the scalp or jaw claudication (facial pain on chewing).
* Advise patients about the risks of steroids (see below) and precautions to take.
* Offer the ARC booklet, available: www.arc.org. uk (choose 'Index' then 'P' for polymyalgia rheumatica).

TEMPORAL ARTERITIS (TA)

● TA is the commonest form of giant cell arteritis (GCA). but other arteries may be involved. After headache or pain in the temple, the next most common syndrome is jaw claudication.
● It is almost exclusively a disease of white people.
● A normal ESR, CRP or negative temporal artery biopsy do not rule out the disease. The chance of obtaining a positive biopsy after 1 week of steroid therapy falls to 10% (Pountain and Hazleman 1995).
● Steroid therapy should not be delayed pending the results of investigations because untreated GCA carries a risk of visual loss in 40% of patients.

DIAGNOSTIC CRITERIA: AMERICAN COLLEGE OF RHEUMATOLOGY (ACR) (HTTP://WWW. RHEUMATOLOGY.ORG/PUBLICATIONS/ CLASSIFICATION/TCA.ASP)

The presence of three of the following has a sensitivity and specificity greater than 90%.
■ Age at onset over 50 years.
■ New type of headache.
■ Clinically abnormal temporal artery; thickened, tender, or nodular with decreased pulsation.
■ ESR greater than 50 mm/hour.
■ Positive arterial biopsy.

For more details of the diagnosis of giant cell arteritis see *Evidence-based Diagnosis in Primary Care* by A. F. Polmear (editor), published by Butterworth-Heinemann 2008.

INITIAL MANAGEMENT (POUNTAIN AND HAZLEMAN 1995)

* *Likely clinical diagnosis according to ACR criteria with visual loss:* if vision is impaired, give prednisolone up to 80 mg immediately and make an urgent referral to an ophthalmologist. If there is likely to be a delay, continue that dose daily.
* *Likely clinical diagnosis according to ACR criteria without visual loss:*
  (a) Take blood for an ESR, CRP and FBC;
  (b) Start prednisolone 40 mg daily;
  (c) See the patient after 48 hours:
* If there is no response, review the diagnosis.
* *Suspected diagnosis:* Check ESR or CRP, start steroids 40 mg daily and arrange for the patient to be seen within 48 hours by a rheumatologist/ophthalmologist.

REFERRAL

Opinion varies on the use of routine temporal artery biopsy. Follow local guidance.

MAINTENANCE TREATMENT

* Reduce the dose by 5 mg every 4 weeks down to 10 mg daily, then as for polymyalgia rheumatica.
* If long-term maintenance is needed, keep the dose as low as possible, e.g. about 3 mg daily.

Steroids

Adverse effects will develop in up to 50% of patients. The risk is positively associated with the dose.
* Educate the patient about the risks:
  (a) weight gain;
  (b) hypertension;
  (c) osteoporosis;
  (d) development of diabetes/worsening of diabetic control;
  (e) infection risk;
  (f) risk of GI perforation in combination with NSAIDs;
  (g) adrenal suppression.
* Ensure the patient has an up-to-date steroid card.

✳ Follow guidance on steroid induced osteoporosis on page 281.

✳ Advise the patient not to stop steroids suddenly.

✳ Advise the patient that it may be necessary to increase the dose of steroids during intercurrent illness and to seek medical advice.

✳ Warn the patient to avoid contagious contacts with chicken pox and shingles (there is a risk of fatal disseminated chickenpox if not immune). Advise them to seek urgent medical advice if they are exposed. Obtain specialist advice if such exposure occurs (see page 52).

✳ Consider testing immune status for chickenpox when commencing steroid therapy.

✳ Check weight, BP and urine (or blood) for glucose every 3 months.

✳ Patients are likely to be on 7.5 mg or more prednisolone daily for 6 months so should be started on prophylaxis against osteoporosis (see Osteoporosis, above).

✳ Recommend pneumococcal and flu vaccination.

FIBROMYALGIA

REVIEW

Perrot S, Dickenson AH, Bennett RM. 2008. Fibromyalgia: harmonizing science with clinical practice considerations. Pain Pract 8, 177–189

Guideline

Carville SF, Arendt-Nielsen S, Bliddal H, *et al.* 2008. EULAR evidence based recommendations for the management of fibromyalgia syndrome. Ann Rheum Dis 67, 536–541. Available: www.eular.org (choose 'Recommendations')

For details of the diagnosis of fibromyalgia see *Evidence-based Diagnosis in Primary Care* by A. F. Polmear (editor) published by Butterworth-Heinemann, 2008.

GENERAL

● This is a distinct syndrome of widespread, chronic pain. The mechanism for the pain is thought to be driven primarily by central sensitization. The criteria for diagnosis are (Wolfe, Smythe, Yunus, *et al.* 1990):

1. a history of widespread pain: pain must be present in all four quadrants of the body and in the spine;

2. pain should be elicited in at least 11 of 18 specified tender point sites on digital palpation. These are:
   - *occiput:* suboccipital muscle insertions.
   - *low cervical:* anterior aspects of the intertransverse spaces at C5–C7.
   - *trapezius:* midpoint of the upper border.
   - *supraspinatus:* origins, above the scapula spine near the medial border.
   - *second rib:* at the second costochondral junctions, just lateral to the junctions on upper surfaces.
   - *lateral epicondyle:* 2 cm distal to the epicondyles.
   - *gluteal:* in upper outer quadrants of buttocks in anterior fold of muscle.
   - *greater trochanter:* posterior to the trochanteric prominence.
   - *knee:* the medial fat pad proximal to the joint line.

3. symptoms have been present for over 3 months.

MANAGEMENT

✳ Find out the patient's concerns and worries and answer appropriately. A patient-centred approach has been found to be associated with less pain and less distress 1 year later (Alamo, Moral and de Torres 2002).

✳ Explain that there is no serious pathology and that pain arises from abnormal processing of pain signals.

✳ Prescribe simple analgesics and weak opiates. Do not prescribe steroids or strong opiates.

✳ Refer for heated pool treatment with or without exercise if available.

✳ Advise gradually increasing aerobic exercise of the sort recommended for cardiovascular fitness (Busch, Schachter, Peloso, *et al.* 2007).

✳ Explain the value of antidepressants in raising the pain threshold and improving sleep and function.

✳ Prescribe low dose amitriptyline 25 mg o.n. and increase according to the response (O'Malley,

Balden, Tomkins, *et al.* 2000). There is no evidence that any one antidepressant is better than any other.

* In severe unremitting cases, consider referral to a multidisciplinary team. The EULAR guideline recommendations recommend a multidisciplinary approach on the basis of expert opinion; there is no evidence that it is better in the majority of cases (Karjalainen, Malmivaara, van Tulder, *et al.* 2000).

* Consider referral for cognitive behavioural therapy.

Complementary and alternative remedies are often tried. The one systematic review was not of sufficient quality to draw conclusions (Holdcraft, Assefi, Buchwald, *et al.* 2003).

References

Aker, P., Gross, A., Goldsmith, C., et al., 1996. Conservative management of mechanical neck pain: systematic overview and meta-analysis. BMJ 313, 1291–1296.

Alamo, M., Moral, R., de Torres, L., 2002. Evaluation of a patient-centred approach in generalised musculoskeletal chronic pain/fibromyalgia patients in primary care. Patient Educ. Couns. 48, 23–31.

Arden, N., Price, C., Reading, I., et al., 2005. A multicentre randomized controlled trial of epidural corticosteroid injections for sciatica: the WEST study. Rheumatol. 44, 1399–1406.

Bachmann, L., Kolb, E., Koller, M., et al., 2003. Accuracy of Ottawa ankle rules to exclude fractures of the ankle and mid-foot: systematic review. BMJ 326, 417–419.

Bahlas, A., Ramos-Remos, C., Davis, P., 1998. Clinical outcome of 149 patients with polymyalgia rheumatica and giant cell arteritis. J. Rheumatol. 25, 99–104.

Bird, H., Esselinckx, W., Dixon, A., et al., 1979. An evaluation of criteria for polymyalgia rheumatica. Ann. Rheum. Dis. 38, 434–439.

Bisset, L., Beller, E., Jull, G., et al., 2006. Mobilisation with movement and exercise, corticosteroid injection, or wait and see for tennis elbow: randomised trial. BMJ 333, 939–941.

Bulloch, B., Neto, G., Plint, A., et al., 2003. Validation of the Ottawa knee rule in children: a multicenter study. Ann. Emerg. Med. 42, 48–52.

Busch, A., Schachter, C., Peloso, P., et al., 2007. Exercise for treating fibromyalgia syndrome. Cochrane Database Syst. Rev (4): CD003786.

Casimiro, L., Barnsley, L., Brosseau, L., et al., 2005. Acupuncture and electroacupuncture for the treatment of rheumatoid arthritis. Cochrane Database Syst. Rev. (4) CD003788. DOI: 10.1002/14651858.CD003788.pub2.

Clinical Knowledge Summaries, 2009. How do I treat someone with polymyalgia rheumatica? National Library for Health. Availablewww.cks.library.uk search on polymyalgia.

Crawford, F., 2004. Plantar Heel Pain (Including Plantar Fasciitis). Clinical Evidence. BMJ Publishing Group. Available: www.clinicalevidence.com.

Dias, R., Cutts, S., Massoud, S., 2005. Frozen shoulder. BMJ 331, 1453–1456.

Digiovanni, B., Nawoczenski, D., Lintal, M., et al., 2003. Tissuespecific plantar fascia-stretching exercise enhances outcomes in patients with chronic heel pain. J. Bone Joint Surg. Br. 85, 1270–1277.

DOH, 2000. Guidelines for the urgent referral of patients with suspected cancer. Department of Health, London. Available: www.dh.gov.uk/cancer/referral.htm.

Elyan, M., Khan, M., 2008. Does physical therapy still have a place in the treatment of ankylosing spondylitis? Curr. Opin. Rheumatol. 20, 282–286.

Fairbank, J., 2008. Prolapsed intervertebral disc. BMJ 336, 1317–1318.

Ferrari, J., 2003. Bunions: Clinical Evidence. www.clinicalevidence.com.

Frank, A., 1993. Low back pain. BMJ 306, 90.

Gibson, J., 2007. Surgery for disc disease. BMJ 335, 949.

Green, S., Buchbinder, R., Hetrick, S., 2003. Physiotherapy interventions for shoulder pain. Cochrane

Database Syst. Rev. www. thecochranelibrary. com.

Gross, A., Hoving, J., Haines, T., et al., 2004. Manipulation and mobilisation for mechanical neck disorders. Cochrane Database Syst. Rev. 1, CD004249.

Group NZG, 2004. Management of Dyspepsia and Heartburn. Available: http://www.nzgg.org. nz/guidelines/dsp_guideline_ popup.cfm?guidelineCatID= 40&guidelineID=77.

Guzmán, J., Esmail, R., Karjalainen, K., et al., 2001. Multidisciplinary rehabilitation for chronic low back pain: systematic review. BMJ 322, 1511–1516.

Hagen, E., Eriksen, H., Ursin, H., 2000. Does early intervention with a light mobilization program reduce long-term sick leave for low back pain? Spine 28, 2309–2316.

Hazard, R., Haugh, L., Reid, S., et al., 1997. Early physician notification of patient disability risk and clinical guidelines after low back injury: a randomized, controlled trial. Spine 22, 2951–2958.

Heintjes, E., Berger, M., Bierma-Zeinstra, S., et al., 2003a. Pharmacotherapy for patellofemoral pain syndrome. Cochrane Database Syst. Rev www.thecochranelibrary.com.

Heintjes, E., Berger, M., Bierma-Zeinstra, S., et al., 2003b. Exercise therapy for patellofemoral pain syndrome. Cochrane Database Syst. Rev. www. thecochranelibrary.com.

Holdcraft, L., Assefi, N., Buchwald, D., et al., 2003. Complementary and alternative medicine in fibromyalgia and related syndromes. Best Pract. Res. Clin. Rheumatol. 7, 667–683.

Institute for Clinical Systems Improvement (ICSI), 2003. Ankle sprain: Bloomington (MN). Available: www.ngc.gov (search on 'Ankle sprain').

Janssens, H., Janssen, M., van de Lisdonk, E., et al., 2008. Use of oral prednisolone or naproxen for the treatment of gout arthritis: a double-blind, randomised equivalence trial. Lancet 371, 1854–1860.

Kadanka, Z., Mares, M., Bednarik, J., et al., 2002. Approaches to spondylotic cervical myelopathy. Spine 27, 2205–2211.

Karjalainen, K., Malmivaara, A., Van Tulder, M., et al., 2000. Multidisciplinary rehabilitation for fibromyalgia and musculoskeletal pain in working age adults. Cochrane Database Syst. Rev. 2, CD001984.

Kay, T., Gross, A., Goldsmith, C., et al., 2005. Exercises for mechanical neck disorders. Cochrane Database Syst. Rev. 3, CD004250.

Kerkhoffs, G., Rowe, B., Assendelft, W., et al., 2002. Immobilisation and functional treatment for acute lateral ankle ligament injuries in adults. Cochrane Database Syst. Rev. 3, .

Khan, K.M., Cook, J.L., Kannus, P., et al., 2002. Time to abandon the 'tendinitis' myth. BMJ 324, 626–627.

Koes, B., 2009. Corticosteroid injection for rotator cuff disease. BMJ 338, 245–246.

Koes, B., Assendelft, W., van der Heijden, G., et al., 1996. Spinal manipulation for low back pain: an updated systematic review of randomized clinical trials. Spine 21, 2860–2871.

Koh, W., Pande, I., Samuels, A., et al., 1997. Low dose amitriptyline in ankylosing spondylitis: a short term, double blind, placebo controlled study. J Rheumatol. 24, 2158–2161.

Kovacs, F., Abraira, V., Pena, A., et al., 2003. Effect of firmness of mattress on chronic non-specific low-back pain: randomised, double-blind, controlled, multicentre trial. Lancet 362, 1599–1604.

Kyle, V., Hazleman, B., 1989a. Treatment of polymyalgia rheumatica and giant cell arteritis. I. Steroid regimens in the first two months. Ann. Rheum. Dis. 48, 658–661.

Kyle, V., Hazleman, B., 1989b. Treatment of polymyalgia rheumatica and giant cell arteritis. II. Relation between steroid dose and steroid-associated side effects. Ann. Rheum. Dis. 48, 662–666.

Kyle, V., Hazleman, B., 1993. Clinical and laboratory course of polymyalgia rheumatica/giant cell arteritis after the first two months of treatment. Ann. Rheum. Dis. 52, 847–850.

Lin, E., Katon, W., Von Korff, M., et al., 2003. Effect of improving depression care on pain and functional outcomes among older adults with arthritis: a randomized controlled trial. JAMA 290, 2428–2429.

Maddison, P., Huey, P., 2006. Rheumatic diseases: serological aids to early diagnosis: Arthritis Research Campaign: reports on the rheumatic diseases series 5: topical reviews. www.arc.org.uk.

Maffulli, N., 1999. Rupture of the Achilles tendon. J. Bone Joint Surg. Am. 7, 1019–1036.

Mason, V., 1994. The Prevalence of Back Pain in Great Britain. OPCS HMSO, London.

Mayo Clinic, 2008. Rheumatoid Arthritis. http://www. mayoclinic.com/health/ rheumatoid-arthritis/DS00020/ DSECTION=11.

Nachemson, A., Jonsson, E. (eds.), 2000. Neck and Back Pain. Lippincott Williams & Wilkins, Philadelphia.

National Institute for Health and Clinical Excellence, 2008a. Osteoarthritis: The Care and Management of Osteoarthritis in Adults. NICE clinical guideline 59. Available: http://www.nice.org. uk/Guidance/CG59.

National Institute for Health and Clinical Excellence (NICE), 2008b. Adalimumab, Etanercept and Infliximab for Ankylosing Spondylitis. London: Technology Appraisal Guidance; no. 143.

National Library for Health, 2008. Clinical Knowledge Summaries: Gout Management. http://cks.library.nhs.uk/gout/management/detailed_answers/when_to_refer.

National Prescribing Centre, 2007. Cardiovascular and gastrointestinal safety of NSAIDs. MeReC Extra Issue No 30. Available: http://www.npc.co.uk/MeReC_Extra/2008/no30_2007.html.

New Zealand Guideline Group, 2004. Management of dyspepsia and heartburn. Available: www.nzgg.org.nz.

NICE, 2004. Dyspepsia: Managing Dyspepsia in Adults in Primary Care: National Institute for Clinical Excellence. Available: www.nice.org.uk choose 'Guidelines'.

Nichols, G., Stiell, I., Wells, G., et al., 1999. An economic analysis of the Ottowa knee rule. Ann. Emerg. Med. 34, 438–447.

O'Malley, P., Balden, E., Tomkins, G., et al., 2000. Treatment of fibromyalgia with antidepressants: a meta-analysis. J. Gen. Int. Med. 15, 659–666.

Peul, W., van Houwelingen, H., van den Hout, W., et al., 2007. Surgery versus prolonged conservative treatment for sciatica. NEJM 356, 2245–2256.

Pountain, G., Hazleman, B., 1995. Polymyalgia rheumatica and giant cell arteritis. BMJ 310, 1057–1059.

Rompe, J., Decking, J., Schoellner, C., et al., 2003. Shock wave application for chronic plantar fasciitis in running athletes. Am. J. Sports Med. 31, 268–275.

Royal College of Radiologists, 2003. Making the Best Use of a Department of Clinical Radiology, 5th ed. RCR, London.

Scott, D., Shipley, M., Dawson, A., et al., 1998. The clinical management of rheumatoid arthritis and osteoarthritis: strategies for improving clinical effectiveness. Br. J. Rheumatol. 37, 546–554.

Scottish Intercollegiate Guidelines Network, 2000. Management of Early Rheumatoid Arthritis. Guideline No 48.

Scottish Intercollegiate Guidelines Network, 2003. Management of Osteoporosis: Guideline No. 71. www.sign.ac.uk.

Sieper, J., Rudwaleit, M., 2005. Early referral recommendations for ankylosing spondylitis (including pre-radiographic and radiographic forms) in primary care. Ann. Rheum. Dis. 64, 659–663.

Silver, T., 1999. Joint and Soft Tissue Injection, Injecting with Confidence, 2nd ed. Radcliffe Medical Press, London.

Smith, G., 2003. Sprains and soft tissues injuries: do you know the latest priorities? The New Generalist 1 (4), 21–22.

Speed, C., 2001. Corticosteroid injections in tendon lesions. BMJ 323, 382–386.

Speed, C., Hazelman, B., 2001. Shoulder pain. Clin. Evid. (5) BMJ Publishing Group London.

Staiger, T., Gaster, B., Sullivan, M., et al., 2003. Systematic review of antidepressants in the treatment of chronic low back pain. Spine 28, 2540–2545.

Towheed, T., Maxwell, L., Anastassiades, T., et al., 2005. Glucosamine therapy for treating osteoarthritis. Cochrane Database Syst. Rev. 2, CD002946. DOI: 10.1002/14651858.CD002946.pub2.

Trinh, K., Graham, N., Gross, A., et al., 2006. Acupuncture for neck disorders. Cochrane Database Syst. Rev. 3, CD004870.

Tulder, M., Malmivaara, A., Esmail, R., et al., 2000. Exercise therapy for low back pain (Cochrane Review). In: The Cochrane Library. Issue 2. Update Software, Oxford.

Uçkay, I., 2008. Antibiotic prophylaxis before invasive dental procedures in patients with arthroplasties of the hip and knee. J. Bone Joint Surg. Br. 90, 833–838.

UK BEAM Trial Team, 2004. United Kingdom back pain exercise and manipulation (UK BEAM) randomised trial: effectiveness of physical treatments for back pain in primary care. BMJ 329, 1377–1381.

Verdugo, R., Salinas, R., Castillo, J., et al., 2003. Surgical versus non-surgical treatment for carpal tunnel syndrome. The Cochrane Database of Systematic Reviews. Online; www.thecochranelibrary.com.

Verhaar, J., Walenkamp, G., Kester, A., et al., 1993. Lateral extensor release for tennis elbow. J. Bone Joint Surg. 75A, 1034–1043.

Vroomen, P., de Krom, M., Knotterus, J., 1999. Diagnostic value of history and physical examination in patients suspected of sciatica due to disc herniation: a systematic review. J. Neurol. 246, 899–906.

Waddell, G., Feder, G., Lewis, M., 1997. Systematic reviews of bed rest and advice to stay active for acute low back pain. Br. J. Gen. Pract. 47, 647–652.

Wolfe, F., Smythe, H., Yunus, M., et al., 1990. The American College of Rheumatology 1990 criteria for the classification of fibromyalgia: report of the multicenter criteria committee. Arthritis Rheum. 33, 160–172.

Chapter 10

Neurological problems

CHAPTER CONTENTS

HEADACHE

For details of the diagnosis of headache see *Evidence-based Diagnosis in Primary Care* by A. F. Polmear (editor), published by Butterworth-Heinemann, 2008.

GUIDELINES

British Association for the Study of Headache (BASH). 2007. Guidelines for all healthcare professionals in the diagnosis and management of migraine, tension-type, cluster and medication-overuse headache. April. Available: www.bash.org.uk

   Scottish Intercollegiate Guidelines Network. 2008. *The Diagnosis and Management of Headache in Adults.* (Guideline No. 107). SIGN, Edinburgh. Available: www.sign.ac.uk

MIGRAINE

- The current management of migraine in primary care is far from satisfactory. Studies from Europe and North America show a similar picture: only about 50% of sufferers currently consult their doctor; half of those consulting are not correctly diagnosed; and many of those who are diagnosed are not being given effective treatment (Edmeads, Lainez, Brandes, *et al.* 2001). All available pharmacological treatments, with the exception of paracetamol given alone, have good evidence for benefit in large enough groups, but any one treatment will probably be

DOI: 10.1016/B978-0-7020-3053-6.00010-6

no better than placebo in any one patient (i.e. the NNT is at least 2).

- Guidelines, including the BASH guideline above, usually recommend some form of stepped care, starting with simple analgesics and only moving up if they fail. A large randomized trial has shown that stratified care, in which treatment is tailored to the individual patient according to the severity of the migraine, is more effective, although at the expense of more adverse effects (Lipton, Stewart, Stone, *et al.* 2000). That approach is chosen here, because of the importance of getting the treatment right as soon as possible, and so keeping the patient's confidence, and because of the reduction in physician time that is likely to ensue.

ONCE THE DIAGNOSIS IS MADE

* Explain the nature of migraine, supplemented with a leaflet and details of the Migraine Action Association (see below).
* Explain that the large majority of patients can be successfully treated but finding the best treatment can take time.
* Assess the severity of the migraine and plan the drug treatment (see below).
* Check that another type of headache is not also present: either analgesic overuse headache in a patient taking analgesics on at least 10 days a month, or tension-type headache.
* Discuss lifestyle changes that might make a difference (see below).
* Discuss the possibility of non-drug therapies (see below).
* Make a follow-up appointment at a time calculated to give the patient a chance to have had three or four further attacks.

DRUG TREATMENT

- Of the various symptoms of migraine only the headache and nausea respond to drug treatment. Acute use of drugs has therefore nothing to offer the patient who is most troubled by the aura.
- Aspirin, paracetamol, an NSAID and sumatriptan 50 mg have similar efficacy in moderate or severe migraine, with roughly 50% of patients

experiencing relief at 2 hours against 30% with placebo. Those taking sumatriptan are more likely to be *free* from pain at 2 hours than those taking an analgesic.

- Many patients will not achieve satisfactory relief with monotherapy. Be prepared to offer two or three drugs for use during the attack, provided each has been found to be useful by that patient (Krymchantowski 2004).

Mild to moderate attacks

* Explain that, whatever drug is used, other than a triptan, it appears to be more effective the earlier it is taken in the attack.

Give:

(a) dispersible aspirin 900 mg. About half of patients report relief at 2 hours (Scottish Intercollegiate Guidelines Network 2008); or

(b) paracetamol 1000 mg. One trial found it equivalent to aspirin despite the tradition that aspirin is more effective (Scottish Intercollegiate Guidelines Network 2008); or

(c) an NSAID, e.g. ibuprofen 200 mg. A large RCT found it was as effective as 400 mg (Codispoti, Prior, Fu, *et al.* 2001);

(d) add metoclopramide 10 mg, or domperidone 10 mg orally or a 30 mg suppository, or a buccal tablet of prochlorperazine 3–6 mg, to any of the above. This may reduce nausea and lead to quicker absorption of the analgesic (Oldman, Smith, McQuay *et al.* 2002). In addition, when the patient is vomiting, the NSAID may be given as a suppository, e.g. diclofenac 100 mg.

Do not use codeine or other opioids: they tend to worsen nausea and are more prone to lead to medication-overuse headache.

Moderate to severe attacks (or mild attacks that do not respond to analgesics)

* Give an oral 5-HT$_1$ agonist (a triptan), see below. The triptans work at whatever stage of the headache they are given (Ryan, Elkind, Baker, *et al.* 1997), but they have no effect on an aura (Bates, Ashford, Dawson, *et al.* 1994) and may be less effective if taken then (British Association for the Study of Headache 2004). If one triptan fails or causes side-effects, consider a trial of another. A second dose of triptan may be taken

2 hours after the first but only if the first was initially successful. Observe the contraindication of cardiovascular disease (CVD), and even of high risk of CVD.

* In addition, give rescue medication in the form of a simple analgesic from the list above, with or without an antiemetic.
* For those with severe nausea or vomiting give diclofenac 100 mg suppositories and domperidone 30 mg suppositories.
* Hold ergotamine in reserve for use only if the above fail and observe the restrictions on its use listed in the *BNF*. Oral ergotamine is ineffective, being almost entirely removed by first-pass metabolism. The benefits of ergotamine are usually outweighed by its problems: side-effects are common (20%), especially nausea and abdominal pain; overuse leads to headache, which is only relieved by taking further ergotamine; it should not be used in those with vascular disease, nor in those on propranolol or methysergide, nor if sumatriptan has been taken in the previous 6 hours. SIGN does not recommend its use in acute migraine.

CHOICE OF TRIPTAN

The different triptans have similar NNTs although comparisons are difficult because different preparations have different strengths. The SIGN guideline recommends almotriptan 12.5 mg, eletriptan 40–80 mg, or rizatriptan 12.5 mg. A tablet is the most convenient formulation for most patients although a few will favour the nasal spray for its speed of onset and others the injection for its greater effectiveness (NNT for relief at 2 hours 2.0 (1.8 to 2.2)). Do not use the nasal spray in the vomiting patient in the hope that it will be absorbed from the nasopharynx. It is swallowed and absorbed from the gastrointestinal tract.

Patients who respond and then relapse

* Repeat the medication that worked earlier provided that doing so does not exceed dosage limits. 20–50% of those given a triptan are likely to relapse. Be aware that a rebound phenomenon has been described with triptans; do not continue to repeat them for repeated relapses.

* In those who can be predicted to relapse, give sumatriptan 50–100 mg plus naproxen 500 mg. If that fails, change to naratriptan on theoretical grounds because of its longer half-life (British Association for the Study of Headache 2004).

If the doctor is called

* Administer either a triptan (e.g. sumatriptan s.c) unless two injections have already been given in the last 24 hours or one dose in the last hour; or diclofenac 75 mg i.m. plus metoclopramide 10 mg i.m. Parenteral metoclopramide relieves the pain of migraine in its own right as well as reducing nausea and vomiting (Colman, Brown, Innes, *et al.* 2004).
* Avoid giving an opiate. It is likely to worsen nausea and its addictive potential makes it difficult to decide what is happening in the patient who presents frequently, saying that only an opiate helps.
* Admit the patient with a prolonged attack who is becoming dehydrated.

PREVENTION

* Encourage the patient to discover the triggers of an attack and see how they can be altered, e.g. stress, excitement, certain foods, alcohol, hunger, fatigue, exertion, oversleeping, menstruation and coitus. However, food may be unfairly blamed as a migraine trigger. Only accept the suggestion if attacks occur within 6 hours of ingestion, the association is repeated and avoiding that food reduces the frequency of attacks.
* Encourage physical fitness, provided exercise does not trigger attacks. Fitness can reduce the frequency of attacks.
* Stop combined oral contraceptives (COCs) in a woman whose migraine starts or worsens when taking them, especially if focal symptoms develop. Their use is associated with an increased risk of cerebral thrombosis. If stopping the COC is unacceptable, give low-dose aspirin daily, and use the lowest oestrogen pill acceptable.
* Discuss non-drug therapies, even though most are not available on the NHS. Evidence of

benefit exist for relaxation therapy, stress reduction, biofeedback, chiropractic, and acupuncture. Acupuncture has been shown to reduce the number of attacks with a 15% reduction in medication used, a 25% reduction in visits to the GP and a 15% reduction in days lost to work (Vickers, Rees, Zollman, *et al.* 2004). It is, however, more expensive than usual care (Wonderling, Vickers, Grieve and McCarney 2004) and a Cochrane review found that, when the evidence from all trials was considered, the evidence of benefit was unconvincing (Melchart, Linde, Berman, *et al.* 2001). Reflexology and homeopathy appear to have no more than a placebo effect.

* Reconsider the diagnosis in a patient who uses rescue medication more than once a week.
* Consider drug prophylaxis in anyone whose life is sufficiently disturbed by attacks.

DRUG PROPHYLAXIS

Two or more attacks per month is the usual criterion for prophylaxis, but a patient with severe attacks may choose prophylaxis with fewer than that.

* Explain that most of the prophylactic drugs have the same efficacy, reducing the frequency or severity of attacks by about one third (Tronvik, Stovner, Helde, *et al.* 2003), but that individual patients respond to some and not others so a trial of drugs will be necessary.
* Choose between a beta-blocker, a tricyclic antidepressant and an anticonvulsant. In choosing between these, be guided by the existence of other conditions or lifestyle considerations the patient may have.
* Titrate each drug up to an effective dose, or to the maximum recommended dose.
* Try each for 4–6 weeks at full dose before abandoning it. Ask the patient to monitor attacks with a diary.
* Continue a drug that is effective for 6–12 months, and tail off over 2–3 weeks (except methysergide, see below). The migraine may be in remission.
* Use only one prophylactic drug at a time, except as an extreme measure, although the combination of a beta-blocker and amitriptyline may be useful in a patient who also has tension-type headaches.

(a) *Beta-blockers without intrinsic sympathomimetic activity (ISA)*. Propranolol, atenolol, metoprolol, nadolol and timolol. Start at a low dose, e.g. propranolol 80 mg daily or atenolol 25 mg b.d., and increase monthly. A patient may fail to respond to one beta-blocker but respond to another.

(b) *Tricyclic antidepressants*. The drug most studied is amitriptyline 10–150 mg at night. The NNT for global improvement is 3.2 (95%CI 2.5 to 4.3) (Anon. 2001). They are likely to be especially helpful in patients with a combination of migraine and tension headaches. Venlafaxine is an alternative. To avoid misunderstanding, explain that you are not giving them for their antidepressant effect.

(c) *Anticonvulsants,* of which sodium valproate is the best studied, are helpful both in migraine and tension-type headache. Sodium valproate has an NNT of 3.8 (95% CI 3.2 to 4.6) for reducing migraine frequency by at least 50% compared to placebo (Chronicle and Mulleners 2004). These results were based on low starting doses (200 mg b.d.) with upward titration until a response was seen or a dose of 1500 mg/day was reached. Nausea was the most common adverse effect with a number needed to harm (NNH) of 3.1 (Anon. 2000). The best alternative is topiramate but it is recommended for specialist supervision only (Scottish Intercollegiate Guidelines Network 2008). However, once topiramate is started, ongoing care is usually the responsibility of the GP. Side-effects are common. The drug should not be stopped rapidly. If the patient suffers from any visual problems reduce and stop the drug as rapidly as possible while seeking urgent advice from an ophthalmologist; acute myopia and secondary angle-closure glaucoma can occur.

Other possibilities in unresponsive patients

(a) *Aspirin* 75–500 mg daily helps up to 30% of patients (Nelson-Piercy and De Swiet 1996), but in many studies so does placebo.

(b) *Pizotifen* helps 60% of patients (Anon 2001), but side-effects of sleepiness and weight gain are common. Start at 1.5 mg at night. If tolerance develops, increase the dose.

(c) *Methysergide* still has a role where all other prophylaxis has failed, but it should be given under specialist supervision for 4 months at a time with 1 month between courses to reduce the risk of retroperitoneal fibrosis.

(d) *Feverfew* 200 mg daily. Despite five trials, a Cochrane review found the evidence mixed and unconvincing (Pittler and Ernst 2004). It is not prescribable. If used, patients should always buy the same product, because the constituents are not standardized. The BASH guideline warns that it contains potential carcinogens.

(e) *Calcium-channel blockers.* Nifedipine, verapamil and diltiazem are thought to be effective in conventional doses, but there is a lack of evidence.

MIGRAINE IN WOMEN OF REPRODUCTIVE AGE

MENSTRUAL MIGRAINE

If symptomatic treatment fails to provide adequate relief, consider intermittent prophylaxis:

* *an NSAID*, traditionally mefenamic acid 500 mg t.d.s., starting 2 days before the migraine is expected, and ending after the risk has passed, usually 2–3 days after the onset of menses; or

* *a triptan* with the same timing (Silberstein 2001) e.g. frovatriptan 5 mg b.d. on the first day then 2.5 mg b.d. on days 2 to 6. Warn the patient that she may experience rebound headache after stopping the triptan.

* *Percutaneous oestrogen* is most likely to help those with true menstrual migraine (migraine which only occurs in relation to the menses) (MacGregor, Chia, Vohrah and Wilkinson 1990). A convenient method is to use a single patch, e.g. Estraderm TTS patch (an unlicensed use) applied 3 days before the migraine is likely to start and left on for 7 days. Start with the 50 mcg patch and adjust the strength up or down according to the response. Warn the patient about the possibility of rebound headache on stopping the oestrogen. Do not use oestrogens in women who have ever had migraine with aura because of the risk of stroke.

* *Women already on the COC*. Consider the tricycle regimen (see page 354) to reduce the frequency of menstruation to once every 10 weeks. Consider a change to an ultra-low-dose oestrogen. If necessary, oestrogen, without progestogen, can be given in the pill-free interval.

MIGRAINE AND ORAL OESTROGENS

* *Migraine with aura*. The International Headache Society Task Force recommends that the combined oral contraceptive should not be used by women with aura. It is more likely to worsen the migraine than in women without aura (Granella, Sances, Pucci, *et al.* 2000). Furthermore, they have double the risk of ischaemic stroke and myocardial infarction (Kurth, Schurks, Logroscino, *et al.* 2008), which is worsened by the COC (possibly doubled again) (Silberstein 2001). A more recent authoritative study has confirmed the risk of ischaemic stroke in women with migraine with aura but failed to find an increase in this risk with the COC (Donaghy, Chang and Poulter 2002). At the time of writing the BNF (Issue 56) continues to list migraine with focal aura as a contraindication. Only prescribe it after a full, documented, discussion with the patient. Progestogen-only contraception is probably safe.

* *Migraine without aura*. Use the COC up to the age of 35, provided there are no other risk factors for stroke, and the patient is not using ergotamine. The US Women's Health Study found no evidence of an increase in stroke risk in women without aura (Kurth, Schurks, Logroscino, *et al.* 2008).

* *The menopause*. Use HRT if indicated. There is no evidence that its use in migaineurs increases stroke risk (Silberstein 2001) although the migraine itself may be exacerbated. If so, change the type of oestrogen and/or progestogen.

MIGRAINE IN PREGNANCY AND LACTATION

Most women find that their migraine improves in pregnancy. In those still troubled by attacks, the treatment options are limited. Triptan pregnancy registers have so far failed to demonstrate an increased risk of fetal abnormality but one may yet emerge. It seems that sumatriptan increases the risk of preterm delivery (OR 6.3, 95%CI 1.2 to 32.0) (Silberstein 2001).

* Use paracetamol for acute relief, or aspirin or an NSAID, plus metoclopramine or domperidone, in the first or second trimester.
* Give low-dose propranolol or amitriptyline prophylactically in those with frequent attacks (Welch 1994).
* Be wary of making a new diagnosis of migraine in a pregnant woman. Cerebral venous thrombosis may mimic migraine.
* In lactating women use paracetamol, ibuprofen, diclofenac, and/or domperidone. Sumatriptan is probably safe.

CLUSTER HEADACHES (MIGRAINOUS NEURALGIA)

ACUTE TREATMENT

* *A triptan, given parenterally,* e.g. sumatriptan 6 mg s.c., will abolish or reduce to mild pain 46% of attacks within 15 minutes, compared to placebo (NNT approximately 2) (Sumatriptan Cluster Headache Study Group 1991). Intranasal sumatriptan is almost as effective with an NNT of 3 at 30 minutes (van Vliet, Bahra, Martin, *et al.* 2003). There is no place for oral preparations because of the short-lived nature of the attacks.
* *100% oxygen* at 15 l/minute through a non-rebreathing mask for 10–20 minutes aborts an attack in some people. If found to be useful in A&E, oxygen can be ordered for home use on the Home Oxygen Order Form.

PREVENTION

* Attacks are so devastating that prevention is needed in most cases. BASH recommends specialist referral but the GP is likely to be involved in initiating or changing treatment before or between specialist appointments.
* Prophylaxis should be continued for 2 weeks after the last attack then tailed off.
* Trial evidence for the treatments below is scanty; it is probably best for verapamil.

Give:
* *verapamil 80 mg* t.d.s. increasing as high as 320 mg t.d.s. It will stop two thirds of episodes once attacks begin;
* an antiepileptic, e.g. topiramate or gabapentin. Valproate seems to be ineffective;
* *lithium carbonate* is probably beneficial, and should be used as for manic–depressive illness (see page 479);
* *prednisolone* 60–100 mg daily for 5 days then tailed off over 2 weeks is justified if other prophylactic treatments fail. It can be given as well as other prophylactic treatments and may be the GP's best initial drug while waiting for specialist assessment;
* *ergotamine* (see page 291) taken half an hour before an attack is due may prevent some attacks. It is useless as treatment once the attack has started.

PATIENT ORGANIZATION

Organisation for the Understanding of Cluster Headache (OUCH), OUCH (UK), 74 Abbotsbury Road, Broadstone, Dorset BH18 9DD. Tel. 01646 651979; www.ouchuk.org

NON-MIGRAINOUS HEADACHE

* A history and simple examination (BP, fundi and a search for focal neurological signs) permit a clinical diagnosis in most patients. An ESR may be needed in patients over 50 to exclude giant cell arteritis. Cervical spondylosis, sinusitis, intracranial haemorrhage and other conditions of which headache is a symptom will need treatment in their own right.
* *Analgesic headache* may complicate management, and is most likely to occur in patients taking analgesics combined with benzodiazepines or opioids. Analgesics for headaches should not be taken on more than 15 days per month (Olesen 1995).

TENSION–TYPE HEADACHE

* Exclude conditions which can be associated with tension-type headache, e.g. cervical spondylosis, poor neck posture, temporomandibular (TM)

joint dysfunction, sinus pain or eye muscle disorders.

* Explain that the condition is real and benign and that treatment aims at reducing the frequency and severity of symptoms rather than cure.
* Explore the tensions in the patient's life.
* Advise relaxation techniques: yoga, massage, 'time out' from a stressful day or more formal stress management (Holroyd, O'Donnell, Stensland, *et al.* 2001).
* Assess whether depression is present.
* Check whether medication overuse is contributing to the headache.
* Recommend paracetamol or aspirin over the counter.
* Prescribe, as acute treatment: *an NSAID*, e.g. ibuprofen 400 mg t.d.s. if needed, but for no more than 3 days per week;
* Prescribe as prophylaxis, in those whose attacks are sufficiently severe and frequent:
  ■ *a tricyclic antidepressant*, e.g. amitriptyline 25–150 mg at night. Explain that it is not being given for its antidepressant effect. Venlafaxine is an alternative; or
  ■ *sodium valproate*. Start at 200 mg b.d.; or
  ■ *a regular NSAID*, e.g. naproxen 250–500 mg b.d., for 3 weeks to break a pattern of particularly troublesome and frequent attacks.
* Aim to tail off prophylactic treatment after 4–6 months if remission has occurred.
* Refer to a headache clinic where cognitive behavioural therapy and acupuncture may be available.

MEDICATION–OVERUSE HEADACHE

* Establish the diagnosis. Headache may be daily or at least 15 days/month. It is usually bilateral and/or pressing/tightening in nature and/or mild to moderate in intensity. Consider it in a patient who has taken simple analgesics on ≥ 15 days/month for at least 3 months, or who has taken a triptan, ergotamine, opioids or combination analgesics for ≥ 10 days/month for at least 3 months. It may exist in conjunction with another type of headache, usually tension-type headache but also migraine.

* Explain the diagnosis to the patient. Patients are often hard to convince, especially the minority whose headache takes up to 2 months without analgesics to resolve.
* Stop simple analgesics and triptans abruptly. The headache will worsen initially but 97% of patients will notice improvement within 2 weeks (Scottish Intercollegiate Guidelines Network 2008).
* Wean the patient off any opioid analgesics more slowly.
* Ascertain whether the patient can distinguish the medication-overuse headache from the original headache (e.g. tension-type headache) for which the medication was originally taken. If the patient can, plan treatment for the later with explanation that the patient should not take the medication if he or she starts to approach the limit of medication on 15 days a month. Half the patients who stop their medication overuse because of a diagnosis of medication-overuse headache relapse within a year (Scottish Intercollegiate Guidelines Network 2008).

CHRONIC DAILY HEADACHE

This is said to exist when headache lasts for at least 4 hours and occurs at least 15 times a month. Most patients are suffering from one or more of the following: migraine, tension-type headache, and analgesic-overuse headache. Management is of the underlying cause. If analgesic-overuse headache is present, tackle that first.

CHRONIC PAROXYSMAL HEMICRANIA

These are repeated attacks of unilateral headache lasting less than 45 minutes.

* Indometacin 25–75 mg t.d.s. reducing to 25 mg daily, should prevent attacks. Indeed, If it does not, reconsider the diagnosis.

EXERTIONAL AND COITAL HEADACHE

* Give an NSAID or propranolol before attacks once a pattern is established.

SEVERE HEADACHE OF SUDDEN ONSET

* Refer urgently if the first attack is sufficiently severe to present acutely. It may be a subarachnoid haemorrhage, presaging a more severe bleed (Linn, Wijdicks, van der Graaf, *et al.* 1994).

RAISED INTRACRANIAL PRESSURE

This is rarely the cause of headache in a patient without vomiting, papilloedema or neurological signs. However, exceptions occur.

* Refer patients with a short history of headache (less than 4 months), especially if it is localized, worse on waking, worse on coughing or straining, and especially in the older patient (Clough 1989).

EPILEPSY

GUIDELINES

National Institute for Health and Clinical Excellence. 2004. *The Epilepsies: The Diagnosis and Management of the Epilepsies in Adults and Children in Primary and Secondary Care.* NICE Clinical Guideline 24. Available: on www.nice.org.uk

Scottish Intercollegiate Guidelines Network. 2003. *Diagnosis and Management of Epilepsy in Adults.* SIGN Guideline No. 70, April. Available: www.sign.ac.uk

Stokes T, Shaw EJ, Juarez-Garcia A, *et al.* 2004. *Clinical Guidelines and Evidence Review for the Epilepsies: Diagnosis and Management in Adults and Children in Primary and Secondary Care.* Royal College of General Practitioners, London.

MANAGEMENT OF A MAJOR FIT

1. Turn the patient into the coma position and ensure that the airway is not obstructed.
2. Prevent onlookers from restraining the fitting patient.
3. Do not give drugs initially – the fit is likely to have stopped before they can act. Give drugs if the fit is continuing without signs of abating after 5 minutes or if three seizures occur within 1 hour.

4. Check the patient's cardiovascular and neurological status.
5. Admit any patient with a fit if there is suspicion that the fit is secondary to other illness; if the patient fails to recover completely after the fit (other than feeling sleepy); or if there is status epilepticus.

Status epilepticus exists if more than one seizure occurs without the patient regaining consciousness, or if the fitting continues for over 30 minutes; 5 minutes of fitting is a more reasonable guide to when drugs should be given.

1. Give diazepam 10 mg rectally and repeat it after 30 minutes if the seizure continues and the ambulance has not arrived. Monitor the patient's cardiac and respiratory status. An alternative is buccal midazolam but it is unlicensed and the RCGP warns that it should only be used according to a protocol agreed with a specialist and administered by those trained in its use. Another option is lorazepam 4 mg i.v. slowly. It is slightly more effective than diazepam (Alldredge, Gelb, Isaacs, *et al.* 2001) but needs to be kept in the refrigerator. Intravenous administration by paramedics (using half that dose) can reduce respiratory or circulatory complications from 20%, with placebo, to 10% with the benzodiazepine.
2. Check the blood glucose with a test strip.
3. Arrange immediate admission even if the fits are controlled – the patient may need other measures to prevent cerebral oedema.

SUBSEQUENT MANAGEMENT

- *A single fit* is not necessarily epilepsy. It is only followed by recurrence in 40% of patients over 15. If the EEG is normal, the chance of further fits is between 13% and 40% and does not warrant anticonvulsants (Scottish Intercollegiate Guidelines Network, 2003). For details of the diagnosis of convulsions in adults see *Evidence-based Diagnosis in Primary Care* by A. F. Polmear (editor), published by Butterworth-Heinemann, 2008.
- Refer for neurological assessment, to be seen, if possible, within 2 weeks, because of the need to exclude an underlying cause and because of the implications for work and driving. Refer more urgently if there are multiple seizures or focal neurological signs. The only patient who need

not be referred is a child aged 18 months to 5 years who has recovered promptly from a febrile convulsion.

- The NICE guideline recommends that referral without drug treatment should be the norm. Discuss with the specialist the need to start an antiepileptic drug before the patient has been seen if there has been a previous fit in the preceding 12 months or if the waiting list is longer than 4 weeks. Patients with a congenital neurological deficit are also candidates for drugs at this stage (Scottish Intercollegiate Guidelines Network 2003) as is a patient who does not wish to take the chance of another seizure before the neurological assessment.

- Once the diagnosis of epilepsy has been made and a decision taken about drug treatment, the role of the GP depends on who else is in the team. An epilepsy nurse specialist may be best suited to act as key worker but the GP is best placed to see the epilepsy in the context of the patient's other medical needs, and will be the only professional in the community available out of hours. Whoever undertakes it, follow-up must be structured, with a review at least annually, and defaulters sought out. Repeat prescriptions of drugs and a policy of waiting until a patient complains of problems are inadequate. The NICE guideline recommends that the care plan be in writing, that it should be agreed by professionals, patient and carers, and that it should include details of how to access care, about drug treatment including benefits and possible adverse effects, and lifestyle issues such as employment, driving and swimming.

- Re-referral is needed where:
  (a) control is poor or the drugs are causing side-effects;
  (b) seizures have continued for 5 years;
  (c) there are pointers to a previously unsuspected cause for the fits;
  (d) concurrent illness complicates management; or
  (e) the patient needs preconceptual advice.

INITIAL MANAGEMENT

* Find out how much the patient and his or her family understand about epilepsy, and answer their questions. Issues to discuss are:

(a) *heredity*. If one parent has generalized epilepsy the risk for a child is increased from 0.5–1% to 4% (although this risk seems to be mainly if the mother is the one with epilepsy). If both parents have epilepsy the risk increases to 15–20% (O'Brien and Gilmour-White 1993). With symptomatic focal epilepsy the risk does not appear to be hereditary;

(b) *underlying pathology*. It is not usually evidence of a brain tumour. Only 5% of those having their first fit over 21 years old have cerebral pathology. For those aged 45–55 it is still only 10%;

(c) *prognosis*. In 80% of patients with epilepsy, fits can be controlled by drug treatment and most of those patients need drug treatment for less than 5 years (Anon. 1990).

* Acknowledge the distress and anger the patient and family feel at the disruption this diagnosis has brought to their lives.

* *Driving*. Advise the patient of the need to notify the DVLA and the insurance company of any seizure, however minor. Document this advice. A licence is likely to be withdrawn until:
  (a) free from fits for 1 year; or
  (b) if the patient's fits in the last year have been while asleep *and* the patient has had fits while asleep for > 3 years with no fits while awake in that time (see page 10). Fits at the time of waking or falling asleep count as 'daytime' fits.

* *Employment*. Advise the patient not to work at heights or near dangerous machinery. An HGV or PSV licence will be lost until fit-free for 10 years.

* *Lifestyle*. Stress the positive side of how few changes there need to be. Swimming is possible provided someone else is present who could lifesave if necessary, provided the patient is not in one of the higher risk categories (see box). Cycling in traffic is probably unwise. Counsel the patient about disclosing the diagnosis to friends and employers. It appears that more than half do not tell their fiancées.

SELF-HELP GROUPS

Epilepsy Action, New Anstey House, Gate Way Drive, Yeadon, Leeds LS19 7XY, www.epilepsy.org.uk, helpline 0808 800 5050

National Society for Epilepsy, Chesham Lane, Chalfont St Peter, Bucks SL9 ORJ, helpline 01494 601400 for details of local groups and also as an excellent source of information. www.epilepsynse.org.uk

The Joint Epilepsy Council website has links to all the UK and Irish patient organizations: http://www.jointepilepsycouncil.org.uk

THE DANGER OF SWIMMING (BELL, GAITATZIS, BELL, *ET AL*. 2008)

The danger of swimming for a patient with epilepsy varies according to clinical situation, as follows, compared to the general population:

- All types of epilepsy: ×15.
- Prevalent epilepsy: ×18.
- Epilepsy and learning disability: × 26.
- Temporal lobe excision performed: × 41.
- Epilepsy and in institutional care: × 97.

DRUG TREATMENT

- Prescribe by brand name because of evidence that generic prescribing leads to patients being switched between brands, and this carries a 10% risk of a worsening of seizure control (Crawford, Hall, Chappell, et al. 1996).
- Five drugs are effective in partial and generalized tonic-clonic seizures: sodium valproate, carbamazepine, phenytoin, lamotrigine and oxcarbazepine. The recent SANAD study suggests that sodium valproate is the first choice for generalized seizures (Marson, Al-Kharusi, Alwaidh, *et al.* 2007a) while lamotrigine is best for partial seizures (Marson, Al-Kharusi, Alwaidh, *et al.* 2007b). Individual patient characteristics might affect this choice. Lamotrigine is especially suitable in the elderly because it has little effect on behaviour and cognition. It does not cause weight gain and is appropriate for women taking the combined oral contraceptive pill. Sodium valproate is first choice in absence and myoclonic seizures although ethosuximide has been used for decades in children with absence seizures.
- Phenytoin is probably the last choice because of its narrow therapeutic window and the frequency of side-effects (DTB 1994).

Phenobarbital is rarely used because adverse effects are greater (Taylor, Tudur Smith, Williamson, *et al.* 2001).

- Only if control is not achieved with any first line drug should an add-on drug be given as well.

Procedure

1. Start at a low dose as follows, and increase until fits are controlled or side-effects occur:
   (a) *carbamazepine* 100 mg daily, increasing every week by 100 mg daily to a maximum of 600 mg b.d. Doses up to 2000 mg a day can be used with consultant advice;
   (b) *sodium valproate* 300 mg b.d. increasing by 200 mg daily every 3 days to 1 g b.d. Doses up to 2500 mg daily can be used with consultant advice;
   (c) *phenytoin* 200 mg daily, increasing every week by 100 mg daily to 600 mg a day. It was customary to recommend that a blood level be performed 1 week after each change of dose once 300 mg a day has been reached because of the narrow therapeutic window. However, the SIGN guideline points out that it is not possible to define a target range, and even for phenytoin drug level monitoring is best left to a specialist to be performed in situations where there is special concern;
   (d) *lamotrigine* 25 mg daily, if used as monotherapy, increasing fortnightly to 100–200 mg daily;
   (e) *oxcarbazepine* 300 mg b.d., increasing weekly to up to 2.4 g daily.
2. *If the control of fits is unsatisfactory* despite the prescription of adequate doses: check compliance. If there is reason to suspect it, performance of drug blood levels may be helpful, in consultation with the epilepsy specialist and/or chemical pathologist.
3. Abandon a drug if control is poor despite maximum dosage, but only after a sufficiently long trial (e.g. 2 months at full dosage), or, if fits are infrequent, the time in which three to five fits would be expected to occur (Shorvon 1991).
4. Tail off one drug only when the patient is established on the next. However, if two drugs are being taken, tail off one of them before adding a third.

5. Only if some, but not enough, benefit has been obtained from the first drug should it be continued as well as the second. Even then a single first line drug plus a newer add-on drug is probably better (NICE 2004).

Practical points

* Phenytoin can be given once daily, other drugs (unless given in the slow-release form) twice a day, except gabapentin which should be given three times a day.

* *Adverse effects.* Before starting a new drug note the adverse effects listed, for instance, in the BNF and discuss them with the patient.

* *Compliance.* Explain the importance of not missing doses and, especially, of not stopping treatment abruptly. Poor compliance may be a sign that the patient does not fully accept the diagnosis.

* *Alcohol.* Explain that moderate drinking of 1–3.5 units per day twice a week has no effect on seizure control. 1–2 units a day is probably safe. Heavier drinking may induce a fit as well as interact with antiepileptic drugs.

* *Drugs bought over the counter*
  (a) *Aspirin.* Warn patients taking sodium valproate against taking intermittent aspirin. It displaces valproate from protein-binding sites and so potentiates it. If regular aspirin is needed, the dose of valproate may need to be reduced to allow for this.
  (b) *St John's wort.* It reduces plasma concentrations of carbamazepine and phenytoin.

* Pregnancy
  (a) Warn women of child-bearing age to seek advice about the use of their drugs before trying to become pregnant. No drug can be said to be free of adverse effects. Taking an anticonvulsant appears to increase the risk of a major fetal abnormality from 2% to 4–6%. The risk is higher in women on multiple antiepileptic drugs. Sodium valproate seems to have the highest risk of major congenital malformation and carbamazepine the lowest (Breen and Davenport 2006). The principle is to maintain a woman who needs drugs on a single drug at the lowest effective dose. Dose adjustment may be needed; absorption may be poor and the drug will be diluted by the increased blood volume (see page 382). If a

woman gets pregnant unintentionally, **she should not stop treatment**. Any damage will already have been done, and she merely risks the hazards of uncontrolled fits.
  (b) Women taking sodium valproate or carbamazepine should be offered mid-trimester screening for neural tube defects.
  (c) Advise women to take folic acid 5 mg daily *before trying to conceive* and until the end of the first trimester.
  (d) Give oral vitamin K (phytomenadione 10 mg daily) in the last month of pregnancy and vitamin K_1 10 mg i.m. to the newborn. Antiepileptic drugs can increase the risk of haemorrhagic disease of the newborn.

* *Contraception.* Women taking hepatic enzyme-inducing drugs (phenytoin, phenobarbital, carbamazepine, oxcarbazepine or topiramate) should be advised as follows:
  (a) if requiring a COC, either increase the oestrogen dosage (see page 350) or change to a drug that does not induce hepatic enzymes. If increasing the oestrogen dose, measure the blood progesterone on day 21 to confirm that ovulation has been suppressed. Doses of oestrogen of up to 100 mcg may be needed. Three packs may be run into one, followed by a break of only 4 days (*tricycling*);
  (b) if the patient is using the progestogen-only pill, the method should be changed. If levonorgestrel is used for emergency contraception give 1.5 mg followed by another 1.5 mg 12 hours later.

* *Short-lived exacerbations of epilepsy.* Clobazam is useful to tide patients over times when fits are more likely, e.g. menstruation and tiredness. It can be used to control fits occurring in clusters. Tolerance prohibits longer term use.

* *Add-on drugs.* Vigabatrin, gabapentin, tiagabine, topiramate, and levetiracetam may be initiated by a specialist. They seem to be equally effective (Marson, Kadir, Chadwick, *et al.* 1996). The GP needs to know that:
  (a) vigabatrin, gabapentin, tiagabine, and levetiracetam do not interfere with oral contraceptives;
  (b) their half-life may be affected by other anticonvulsants, e.g. sodium valproate prolongs the half-life of lamotrigine. Conversely, lamotrigine can precipitate carbamazepine toxicity, topiramate can

precipitate phenytoin toxicity, while vigabatrin can lower phenytoin concentrations. These interactions are complex and unpredictable (see BNF section 4.8.1 *Control of epilepsy*).

FOLLOW-UP

(a) Review any fits (preferably recorded on a chart) and their precipitating causes. Almost half of people on anti-epileptic drugs in the UK still have seizures (Dobson 2004).

(b) Review the patient's attitude to the epilepsy and any social problems that have arisen. Encourage the family to attend, whether the patient is an adult or a child. The epilepsy may put other members of the family under considerable stress.

(c) Review drug compliance, by checking the frequency of repeat prescriptions.

(d) Review side-effects (see below).

(e) *Anticonvulsant levels.* Do not check anticonvulsant serum levels routinely (Scottish Intercollegiate Guidelines Network 2003). The serum level should not determine the anticonvulsant dose; the correct dose is the smallest dose that controls the seizures. Only check serum levels when control is poor, there is concern about toxicity, higher than usual doses are being considered, compliance is in doubt, or in renal or hepatic impairment (Chadwick 1987). The exception to this is phenytoin. A blood level is justified, because of phenytoin's narrow therapeutic window, when adjusting the dose.

(f) *Blood tests.* The RCGP and NICE guidelines make a case for some blood tests (FBC, U&Es, LFTs, vitamin D, calcium and alkaline phosphatase) every 2–5 years in those on enzyme inducing drugs, and a clotting screen in patients on valproate who are due for surgery. The SIGN guideline counsels against routine tests. SIGN's argument is as follows: most abnormalities are minor and would not affect treatment. Mild leucopenia and thrombocytopenia are not uncommon and require no action. Tests of serum electrolytes in patients on carbamazepine or oxcarbazepine in order to detect hyponatraemia may be worthwhile (Gandelman 1994). 20% have serum sodiums < 135 mmol/l but levels rarely fall below 125 mmol/l and symptoms are uncommon. The one potentially fatal hepatic side-effect, hepatotoxity due to sodium valproate, occurs in only 1 in 10,000, mainly in mentally handicapped children under 3 years old, and routine testing would not predict it anyway. Similarly, routine testing is unlikely to detect the rare case of severe blood dyscrasia.

ADVERSE EFFECTS OF ANTICONVULSANT DRUGS

Acute: Rash (usually seen shortly after starting the drug). Tail off the drug. If combined with fever and lymphadenophy the rash may represent a severe hypersensitivity syndrome. Multiple organ failure can occur. If the patient is systemically ill, admit. Discuss the possibility of substituting, in the acute stage, a drug that rarely causes rash (e.g. gabapentin or levetiracetam) with the relevant specialist (Browne and Holmes 2001).

Chronic: weight gain and sedation are the adverse effects most commonly complained of. Check that the patient is taking the lowest effective dose of as few drugs as possible. There is some evidence that the quality of life is better on the newer drugs but the NICE review did not consider the evidence to be strong. What is clear is that each drug has a different side-effect profile and individuals respond to a drug in different ways.

AVOIDING SUDEP (SUDDEN UNEXPECTED DEATH IN EPILEPSY) (HANNA, BLACK, SANDER, *ET AL.* 2002)

- The deaths of 500 people a year in the UK are attributed to SUDEP.
- One of the commonest factors associated with these deaths is uncontrolled epilepsy.
- Many of these cases are associated with suboptimal doses of anti-epileptics, and discontinuation of drugs without adequate substitution.

In order to reduce this risk, observe the following rules:

∗ titrate a drug up to the maximum tolerated dose, or until seizures are controlled;

∗ when discontinuing a drug, titrate a new drug up to an effective dose first and then tail the old drug off slowly. The only exception to this is the patient having a life-threatening reaction to a drug, in which case abrupt cessation (with immediate introduction of a new drug) is justified.

STOPPING TREATMENT

- Specialist advice is wise before withdrawing drugs in a patient who has been free from fits for a number of years. Ultimately it is the patient who must make the decision, weighing the problems of drug-taking against the upset of a further fit with its implications for driving, employment and family distress. Patients who stop their drugs and remain fit-free have higher morale than those who are fit-free on drugs (Jacoby, Johnson and Chadwick 1992).
- Withdrawal may be considered in generalized tonic-clonic seizures when the patient has been free of fits for 2 years, although there is no evidence on which to base this (Sirven, Sperling, Wingerchuk, *et al.* 2001). It is likely to be followed by relapse in half of adults and 20% of children in the first year, against a recurrence rate of 33% for adults who remained on medication. Recurrence does not worsen the overall prognosis (Chadwick, Taylor and Johnson 1996).
- Withdrawal is most likely to be successful in patients with:
  - (a) primary generalized epilepsy;
  - (b) epilepsy controlled on a single drug with no seizures on treatment;
  - (c) a normal EEG;
  - (d) a few seizures over a short space of time;
  - (e) childhood or teenage onset;
  - (f) no family history of mental retardation or cerebral pathology (Medical Research Council Antiepileptic Drug Withdrawal Study Group 1993).
- *Maximum dose reduction.* In adults the maximum reduction each time should be: carbamazepine 200 mg; phenytoin 50 mg; sodium valproate 200 mg; phenobarbitone 30 mg; primidone 125 mg.
- *Speed of withdrawal.* Withdrawal should take at least 3 months, or 6 if the patient is taking a barbiturate or a benzodiazepine. Withdraw one drug at a time and make sure the patient knows that, if a seizure occurs, the dose should be increased by one step back. If a drug is being withdrawn and being replaced by another it can be withdrawn faster, but in steps not shorter than one every 3 weeks.
- *Driving when stopping medication.* The DVLA recommends that patients should be advised not to drive during withdrawal and for 6 months after cessation of treatment. It does not, however, remove their licence during this time and the patient does not have to notify them that withdrawal is taking place.

PARKINSON'S DISEASE

GUIDELINES

National Institute for Health and Clinical Excellence. *Parkinson's Disease: Diagnosis and Management in Primary and Secondary Care.* NICE clinical guideline 35; 2006. Available: www.nice.org.uk
   Primary Care Task Force of the Parkinson's Disease Society (UK). *Parkinson's Aware in Primary Care.* 3rd edition 2003. Available: www.parkinsons.org.uk

- The disease should be confirmed by a specialist in all cases. A study in London found that at least 15% of patients with a diagnosis of Parkinson's disease did not have it and 20% who were under the care of their GP with symptoms of Parkinson's disease had not had the diagnosis made (Schrag, Ben-Shlomo and Quinn 2002). The NICE guideline group recommends that the new patient with mild disease should be seen within 6 weeks.
- Because the diagnosis is a clinical one, the possibility that another disease is causing the symptoms should always be borne in mind. A patient responding poorly to antiparkinsonian drugs should be reviewed by a neurologist and that review should include a review of the diagnosis.
- 'Parkinsonism', whether due to drugs, multiple small strokes or other causes, does not respond to treatment with levodopa and must not be confused with Parkinson's disease.
- It is impossible to give a patient a prognosis. In one Australian study of 126 patients, after 10 years 13 remained without significant disturbance of function, and of the 113 with significant disability, only 9 were confined to bed or a wheelchair. Patients with more severe disability at presentation appear to do worse, as do older patients and those who present with rigidity and bradykinesia rather than tremor (Marras, Rochon and Lang 2002).

MANAGEMENT

The diagnosis of Parkinson's disease has huge medical, psychological and social implications for the patient and family. The key worker, who may be a GP, specialist nurse or consultant, is needed to coordinate the professionals involved. The medical aspects of care will be shared between specialist and GP. While the specialist will initiate treatment, the GP or Parkinson's disease specialist nurse is often responsible for coping with adverse effects, with altering drug doses, with supporting the patient and family between hospital appointments and with end-of-life care.

* Find out what specific problems the patient has. Treatment should be individually tailored to these problems.
* Explain the diagnosis and the management plan. Stress that almost everybody enjoys prolonged benefit from treatment.
* Explain the problem that lies at the heart of drug treatment: that levodopa is the most effective drug for the relief of disability but that prolonged use leads to the problems described below. Delaying its use and keeping its dose low may mean that it will remain effective later in the disease: hence the use of other agents early, and of levodopa-sparing agents later.
* *Depression.* Use antidepressants as you would in other depressed patients. Depression occurs in almost half of patients and is part of the disease, not merely a reaction to the disability.
* *Dementia* occurs in 30% (Rascol, Goetz, Koller, *et al.* 2002) and is likely to be missed unless specifically tested for. Its discovery has important implications in planning treatment (see page 602).
* *Sleep disturbance.* Discover the type of disturbance and its cause: e.g. daytime sleepiness, restless legs syndrome, nocturnal akinesia
* *Constipation* should be treated by encouraging mobility, a high-fibre diet if the patient can swallow it, and laxatives.
* *Orthostatic hypotension* occurs in 15–20% as part of the autonomic dysfunction that is a feature of the disease. No evidence exists for any beneficial treatment (Rascol, Goetz, Koller, *et al.* 2002).
* *Physiotherapy.* There is a strong clinical impression that it may be helpful though the evidence is sparse (Deane, Jones, Playford, *et al.* 2001). One meta-analysis found that physiotherapy could improve walking speed and the activities of daily living (de Goede, Keus, Kwakkel, *et al.* 2001). NICE strongly recommends access to physiotherapy re: gait, enhancement of aerobic capacity, improvement in movement initiation and improvement in functional independence.
* *Occupational therapy* can help with difficulties with feeding and dressing, and provide alterations to the bed, chair and bath., Again, there is a strong clinical impression of benefit although the evidence is sparse (Deane, Ellis-Hill, Playford, *et al.* 2001).
* *Difficulties with speech and swallowing.* Referral to speech therapy may help to make the voice more forceful (Deane, Whurr, Playford, *et al.* 2004). There is no evidence either way on benefit for dysphagia (Deane, Whurr, Clarke, *et al.* 2004).
* Consider whether referral to the district nurse, dietician, continence adviser, or chiropodist would help.
* *Financial benefits.* Many patients are eligible for benefits for the disabled (see page 6).
* *Carers.* Assess, and reassess, the ability of the carer to cope.
* *Driving.* Advise drivers to notify the DVLA and their insurance company.
* *Surgery.* A few patients will be candidates for pallidotomy or deep brain stimulation. They are likely to be those under 70, with no other cerebral disease, who have severe unilateral tremor or dyskinesia.

SELF–HELP GROUP

The Parkinson's Disease Society, 215 Vauxhall Bridge Road, London SW1V 1EJ, tel. 020 7931 8080, has information for patients and carers and organizes local groups. Helpline: 0808 800 0303; www.parkinsons.org.uk

DRUG TREATMENT

● Choice and timing of drug therapy depends on the age of the patient, because of the limited time for which levodopa is likely to be effective. Its benefit starts to wear off after 4–5 years, although this may be delayed if low doses (< 500 mg/day) are used. As higher doses are needed adverse effects become more problematic.

- NICE recommends that the choice of medication is for the specialist and that the new patient be referred untreated.
- No drugs have been shown to be truly neuroprotective. However, dopamine agonists, MAO-B inhibitors and COMT inhibitors are 'levodopa-sparing'; that is, they delay the need to start levodopa itself, or they allow it to be given at a lower dose, thus enabling the patient to use levodopa with benefit until later on in the disease than if the 'levodopa-sparing' drug had not been used.
- Note that those drugs which need to be increased slowly should also be withdrawn slowly, even if they appear to have been ineffective. The old practice of 'drug holidays' is contraindicated because sudden cessation may give rise to acute akinesia or to neuroleptic malignant syndrome.

Starting drugs for Parkinson's disease

Drugs should be started only when they are needed for symptom control. Options are:

(a) *Dopamine agonists:* bromocriptine, cabergoline, pergolide, pramipexole, ropinirole and rotigotine can all relieve symptoms. Initial treatment with bromocriptine rather than levodopa appears to be slightly less effective in reducing disability with fewer motor complications (Lees, Katzenschlager, Head, *et al.* 2001) but greater risk of neuropsychiatric side-effects.

Adverse effects:
- Dopamine agonists are very likely to cause initial nausea or vomiting and domperidone may be needed.
- Bromocriptine, cabergoline, and pergolide carry the risk of pulmonary, retroperitoneal and pericardial fibrosis. Check the CXR, ESR and serum creatinine before starting the drugs, then annually, and be alert for suggestive symptoms (e.g. cough, dyspnoea, abdominal pain).
- Pergolide has been associated with the development of cardiac valvulopathy which makes it an even less attractive option. Pramipexole, ropinirole and rotigotine are therefore the dopamine agonists of first choice.

- Dopamine agonists can also cause sleepiness and sudden onset of sleep. Warn all patients about this, especially those who drive, operate machinery or put themselves in dangerous situations (e.g. hill walking).

(b) *MAO-B inhibitors*, e.g. selegiline, may be used in a patient not yet affected enough to start levodopa or as an adjunct to levodopa to reduce 'end-of-dose' deterioration.

(c) *Levodopa* which should be started when symptoms interfere sufficiently with the patient's life, despite the above.

- Warn patients about the immediate side-effects, e.g. nausea, postural hypotension and sleepiness. Give the tablets after food to avoid nausea. Be aware, however, that a protein meal can compete with levodopa for absorption. If an antiemetic is needed, use domperidone. Check the standing blood pressure before and after starting the drug.
- Use a preparation that combines levodopa with a decarboxylase inhibitor.
- Agree on a specific goal that treatment should achieve, e.g. being able to walk to the shops.
- Start with a low dose, containing levodopa 50 mg t.d.s., and increase by 50 mg a week until the goal has been achieved.
- Monitor the response. As well as asking about the benefit, set the patient a task (e.g. unbuttoning a coat or walking to the door) and time it for an objective assessment.
- Stop increasing the dose as soon as sufficient benefit has been achieved.

Other drugs available if needed are:

(d) *Amantadine* at a dose of 100 mg b.d. is thought to be of modest benefit but this may be lost after the first few months. There is no reliable trial evidence for it (Crosby, Deane and Clarke 2004).

(e) *Entacapone* inhibits levodopa breakdown and, when added to levodopa, can smooth out fluctuations and permit a reduction of 10–30% in the levodopa dose.

(f) *Anticholinergics*, which are traditionally given for tremor in younger patients, although no evidence exists that they are more effective for one symptom than for another (Katzenschlager, Sampaio, Costa and Lees 2004). They are very prone to cause confusion in the elderly, and in these patients the only strong indication for them is excessive salivation. A convenient choice is trihexyphenidyl 2 mg daily, increasing up to a maximum of 5 mg t.d.s., or orphenadrine 50 mg t.d.s. increasing to a maximum of 400 mg daily.

- If the main side-effect is a dry mouth, take before food;
- If the main side-effect is nausea, take after food.

Later problems with levodopa

These may not begin for 5–10 years after the drug is started:

(a) end-of-dose deterioration;

(b) dyskinesia, usually at peaks of levodopa levels but also as the dose wears off;

(c) on–off motor fluctuations unrelated to levodopa dose;

(d) nausea and vomiting;

(e) psychiatric side-effects and acute confusion (see Psychiatric problems, below).

Management of motor complications:

(a) Give a smaller amount more often to avoid the peaks and troughs of drug levels. In extreme cases, 2-hourly doses may be needed. Alternatively, change to a modified-release preparation. They are less well absorbed; a 20–30% increase in dose is likely to be needed. Continue to give a standard preparation for the first dose in the morning, for the sake of its quicker onset. Dispersible co-beneldopa is especially suitable for this purpose. NICE is sufficiently concerned about the problem of poor absorption that it recommends that, if they are used, they be combined with an immediate-release preparation. Giving frequent and accurately timed doses can be difficult. Automatic pill dispensers may be available from local services. One manufacturer is Pivotell; www.pivotell.co.uk.

(b) Add a dopamine agonist (see above), increasing the dose slowly as detailed in the BNF. Reduce the dose of levodopa by one third. Confusion and postural hypotension often limit the value of these drugs. One of the newer dopamine agonists may suit an individual patient better.

(c) Add an MAO-B inhibitor, e.g. selegiline, which will improve end-of-dose deterioration in 50% of patients and permit a reduction in levodopa dose.

(d) Add a COMT inhibitor, namely entacapone. It can smooth out motor fluctuations and allow a reduction in levodopa dose. It can be combined with levodopa and carbidopa. Warn the patient about the change in urine colour to reddish brown.

(e) Add amantidine to reduce dyskinesia.

(f) Arrange for admission for initiation of apomorphine injections which the patient or carer can then give at home. Apomorphine is useful in patients with fluctuating motor responses, on–off oscillations and dyskinesias. It works within 20 minutes, but benefit only lasts for about an hour (Choudhury and Clough 1998). However, NICE recommends that it only be initiated by expert units with access to a trained professional who can monitor its use at home.

Nausea and vomiting:

(a) Ensure that doses are taken after meals.

(b) Decrease the dose of levodopa while increasing the dose of decarboxylase inhibitor. The intention is to lower the extracerebral level of levodopa without lowering the intracerebral level.

(c) Add domperidone.

Psychiatric problems

In addition to the difficulty that a patient is likely to have in adjusting to the condition, Parkinson's disease and its treatment cause a whole range of psychiatric disorders.

- *Levodopa* can cause anxiety, agitation, elation, depression, insomnia, paranoia, hallucinations and delusions. Dose reduction is more effective than trying to treat the reaction with further drugs.
- *Depression* may be part of the disease rather than a reaction to the disease. It responds to antidepressants. Choose a first generation tricyclic if anticholinergic action is required as well, e.g. in excessive salivation. If constipation is already a problem or the patient is already on an anticholinergic drug, choose one with less anticholinergic activity such as lofepramine or a selective serotonin reuptake inhibitor (SSRI).
- *Psychosis* may be due to Parkinson's disease or to the medication. Withdraw the latter in the manner outlined below. If part of the disease, neuroleptics may be needed despite the detrimental effect they are likely to have on

the parkinsonism. Clozapine is least likely to cause extrapyramidal side-effects.

- *Organic confusion* is likely to be due to the medication. Stop the drug most recently added. If there has been no recent change, stop drugs in the following order: anticholinergics, selegiline, amantadine and dopamine agonists. Levodopa is the drug least likely to cause confusion, but its dose may need to be altered.
- *Dopamine dysregulation syndrome* is described in which dopaminergic medication is misused in association with various abnormal behaviours, e.g. hypersexuality, pathological gambling and stereotypic acts.

Coping with cognitive problems in Parkinson's disease

> **PATIENT INFORMATION**
>
> Dementia and Parkinson's. PDS information sheet 58, 2004. Available: www.parkinsons.org.uk (choose 'About Parkinson's' then 'Information and resources' then 'Dementia'

Patients with Parkinson's disease may suffer a number of cognitive problems:

(a) dementia;

(b) communication problems;

(c) confusion, both secondary to the disease and drug related.

Dementia may affect:

(a) concentration;

(b) short-term memory with inability to remember names, recent events and how to perform simple tasks;

(c) slowness of thought processes which may be a feature of PD without dementia;

(d) language, particularly difficulty in finding words and understanding what is being said;

(e) the ability to recognize faces and objects;

(f) the ability to make decisions, to reason, to cope with new things.

Communication problems are common and more severe in those who have dementia, as communication is affected in both. Specific to PD are:

(a) the lack of facial expression and body language, which add to the difficulties in communicating;

(b) slowness of thought (bradyphrenia) but with correct answering after a delay. The same can occur in depression which is also common in PD.

✳ Explain to the carer, at an appropriate time in the illness, that communication can be affected as follows:

(a) words: inability to find the right word, restricting communication to everyday words and later difficulties in pronouncing letters and words;

(b) sentences may be affected later in the disease;

(c) responses give the impression that the person is not interested in what others are saying;

(d) humour, sarcasm or subtlety are missed. Conversation is restricted and becomes dull. The patient may be unable to sustain a logical flow of ideas;

(e) in later stages the person may hardly communicate while automatic responses, e.g. 'hello', may be preserved and short phrases repeated.

✳ Advise the carer to follow the general principles of coping with a person with cognitive impairment (see page 603).

Palliative care of the terminal patient

A time will come when no further alteration in drugs will be helpful, and the patient and family will need an increased amount of support. Check that the patient and family have been given a chance to state how they want this stage of the patient's life to be managed. Adequate analgesia and sedation of the patient will be needed, as in any palliative situation.

> **MAIN DRUGS TO AVOID IN PARKINSON'S DISEASE**
>
> - *Antipsychotics:* e.g. chlorpromazine, haloperidol, thioridazine. Use clozapine carefully in even lower doses than usual.
> - *Antiemetics:* e.g. metoclopramide, prochlorperazine. Use domperidone.
> - *MAOIs:* they may provoke adverse effects from any levodopa that is being taken. Hypertensive crises have been reported.

- *Hypotensives*. Hypotension is an adverse effect of the disease.
- *Baclofen* may cause agitation and confusion.
- *Pyroxidine* can antagonize the action of levodopa.

STROKE

GUIDELINES

National Collaborating Centre for Chronic Conditions. 2008. *Stroke: National Clinical Guideline for Diagnosis and Initial Management of Acute Stroke and Transient Ischaemic Attack (TIA)*. NICE guideline. Royal College of Physicians, London
   Intercollegiate Working Party on Stroke. 2004. *National Clinical Guidelines for Stroke, 2nd edition*. The Royal College of Physicians, London, available on www.rcplondon.ac.uk
   Scottish Intercollegiate Guidelines Network (SIGN). *Management of Patients with Stroke*; Parts 1–4. Available: www.sign.ac.uk/guidelines
   The National Service Framework for Older People. 2001. Department of Health, London. Available: www.doh.gov.uk/nsf/olderpeople.htm

- Management of stroke patients in a stroke unit is associated with a sustained reduction in death and dependency compared to usual care with an odds ratio at one year of 0.78 (95%CI 0.68 to 0.89) (Stroke Unit Trialists' Collaboration 2004). The guidance below is based on the assumption that patients will be admitted to a stroke unit.
- Rehabilitation, physiotherapy, occupational therapy and psychological support are all part of well-organized stroke care. 7% of patients should be spared a poor outcome as a result of the care of such a team (Outpatient Service Trialists 2003).
- Brain imaging by CT or MRI scanning should be undertaken to detect intracerebral or subarachnoid haemorrhage, and to exclude other causes of the stroke syndrome, in all patients within 24 hours of onset unless there are good clinical reasons for not doing so (Intercollegiate Working Party for Stroke 2004). Patients who are candidates for thrombolysis, or who have complicating clinical features, need imaging within 1 hour of the onset of symptoms.

- Thrombolysis in selected patients reduces the risk of death or dependency at 3–6 months after a stroke with an odds ratio of 0.66 (95%CI 0.53 to 0.83) (NNT = 7) if given in the first 3 hours and 0.84 (95%CI 0.75 to 0.95) if given in the first 6 hours (Wardlaw, del Zoppo, Yamaguchi and Berge 2004). It is only suitable for patients who can be admitted to a specialist unit with experience of thrombolysis within 3 hours of the onset of the stroke (Intercollegiate Working Party on Stroke 2002).

ACUTE STROKE

* Admit all patients to an acute stroke unit unless there is a reason why that would be inappropriate, for instance the patient is already in the terminal stage of another illness.
* Admit by dialling 999, without seeing the patient if necessary. This will trigger the local protocol for the management of acute stroke. Assessment of the patient by paramedics using FAST (see box) has been found, in Newcastle, to be as accurate as assessment by general practitioners (Harbison, Hossain, Jenkinson, *et al.* 2003). Patients who are candidates for brain imaging within hour of the onset of symptoms are:
   - those who are candidates for thrombolysis (i.e. they are within 3 hours of the start of symptoms);
   - patients on anticoagulants or with a bleeding tendency;
   - those with a depressed level of consciousness (Glasgow Coma Score < 13);
   - those with progressive or fluctuating symptoms;
   - those with signs of alternative pathology: neck stiffness, papilloedema, fever;
   - those whose stroke begins with severe headache of sudden onset (National Collaborating Centre for Chronic Conditions 2008).
* Admit to the stroke unit less urgently, but still that day, those who fall outside these categories, usually because they have delayed their presentation. They need imaging within 24 hours of the onset of symptoms (National Collaborating Centre for Chronic Conditions 2008).

FAST (FACE ARM SPEECH TEST)

Paramedics are taught to look for:

■ a new asymmetry of the mouth;

■ a new inability to hold one arm out for 5 seconds compared to the other arm;

■ new slurred speech or new inability to understand or say words.

The patient has a suspected stroke if an abnormality is found in any of these. The positive predictive value for stroke is 78% (Harbison, Hossain, Jenkinson, *et al.* 2003).

LONGER TERM MANAGEMENT

● Early discharge is appropriate once the patient can transfer from bed to chair and provided a specialist community stroke rehabilitation team is available. If so, early discharge may improve outcomes (Mayo, Wood-Dauphinee, Cote, *et al.* 2000) but at the risk of worsening the mental health of the carers (Anderson, Mhurchu, Rubenach, *et al.* 2000).

∗ Refer to the community rehabilitation team, if they are not already involved. This team will manage the rehabilitation process but may need support from the GP.

∗ Check that a multidisciplinary assessment has been performed, including assessment of consciousness level, swallowing, speech, pressure sore risk, nutritional status, cognitive impairment, movement and handling needs.

∗ Check for faecal incontinence. It is present initially in 30% and in 15% at 3 years (Harari, Coshall, Rudd, *et al.* 2003). Avoidance of constipation and easy access to the toilet may help.

∗ Check that carers and family have been involved closely with the planning of discharge from inpatient care. Giving carers information and support, as well as training in basic nursing skills, improves the quality of life for carers and for their patients with an overall reduction in costs (Hankey 2004).

∗ *Spasticity.* Local spasticity that is interfering with function may benefit from physiotherapy. The family can help with stretching exercises. In addition, use antispasmodics if the spasticity is widespread, e.g. baclofen 5 mg t.d.s. doubling the dose every 2 weeks, up to 100 mg daily, or until benefit, or adverse effects, are seen. If stopping the drug, tail off slowly. An alternative is diazepam 2–10 mg three times daily, but other drugs which have fewer central adverse effects are dantrolene and tizanidine (which requires monitoring of the LFTs) (Ward, Begg, Kent, *et al.* 2004). Refer a patient who is still held back by spasticity despite the above measures, for consideration of botulinum toxin injections or intrathecal baclofen.

∗ *Depression.* Monitor for depression with a screening questionnaire (see page 452). Depression has been found in a third of patients in the first year after a stroke (Aben, Denollet, Lousberg, *et al.* 2002). The prevalence in carers is almost as high (Kotila, Numminen, Waltimo, *et al.* 1998). A further 20% of patients with stroke suffer from post stroke emotional lability (Brown, Sloan and Pentland 1998). Give information and advice, and consider antidepressant drug treatment (see page 454) if depression lasts at least 4 weeks. Continue, if effective, for at least 6 months. Tricyclic antidepressants and SSRIs are effective in major depression (Wiart, Petit, Joseph, *et al.* 2000) and in emotional lability (Brown, Sloan and Pentland 1998).

SECONDARY PREVENTION

The risk of recurrence is 8% per year (Lees, Bath and Naylor 2000) with the additional risk of other manifestations of cardiovascular disease.

∗ Set up a cardiovascular disease register. Identify patients who have had a stroke or TIA by searching for patients on antithrombotic therapy. To save time, exclude those with CHD or diabetes and examine the records of the rest. Ask patients with CHD or diabetes when they attend their respective clinics whether they have ever had a stroke or TIA. This will detect 1% of the population as having had a stroke, compared to 1.2% if the records of every patient on antithrombotic drugs is examined (Willoughby, Thomson and Chopra 2004).

∗ Set up a dedicated clinic with an agreed protocol. Call and recall patients to it annually.

∗ *Lifestyle changes.* Assist smokers to stop (see page 498) and urge weight reduction, dietary change, reduction of alcohol intake to within sensible limits, and exercise where appropriate (see page 689).

* *Aspirin*. Prescribe 300 mg daily unless the stroke is likely to have been haemorrhagic. If aspirin is not tolerated use clopidogrel or modified release dipyridamole 200 mg b.d. In patients with a previous ischaemic stroke, aspirin will prevent 39 events per 10,000 patients over a mean of 37 months but at the expense of 12 haemorrhagic strokes (He, Whelton, Vu, *et al.* 1998). The addition of dipyridamole adds significant benefit to aspirin alone (OR 0.78, 95%CI 0.65 to 0.93) (Leonardi-Bee, Bath, Bousser, *et al.* 2005). If the stroke occurs in a patient already taking aspirin 75 mg, increase to 300 mg daily, then to a dipyridamole/aspirin combination/ then to clopidogrel.

* *Blood pressure*. Once the initial phase of the stroke is over (usually about 2 weeks), control any hypertension to < 149/85 or < 130/80 in patients with diabetes (Williams, Poulter, Brown, *et al.* 2004) (see page 137). Treatment with perindopril 4 mg daily ± a thiazide reduces the risk of further stroke by 28% (95%CI 17 to 38%) whether or not the patient is hypertensive (PROGRESS Collaborative Group 2001). This finding has not, however, been translated into advice to treat non-hypertensives with an ACE inhibitor and thiazide.

* *ACE inhibition*. Give an ACE inhibitor (e.g. ramipril 2.5 mg daily increasing to 10 mg daily) unless the patient is already on an ACE inhibitor for hypertension. It can reduce the risk of future stroke by 32% independent of its effect on BP (Bosch, Yusuk, Pogue, *et al.* 2002).

* *Atrial fibrillation*. Arrange anticoagulation with warfarin whether valvular disease is present or not. Warfarin will halve the risk of serious vascular events compared to aspirin with an odds ratio of 0.55 (95%CI 0.36 to 0.83) (Koudstaal 2004).

* *Co-incidental cardiac disease*. Either:
  (a) arrange echocardiography in patients with stroke and cardiac disease (other than atrial fibrillation). Almost 20% will be found to have an intracardiac source of an embolus (He, Whelton, Vu, *et al.* 1998). However, interpretation of the significance of the echo may be difficult. A cardiac lesion may, or may not, be the cause of the stroke (Meenan, Saha, Chou, *et al.* 2002); or

  (b) anticoagulate, regardless of whether echo confirms the lesion as the cause of the stroke, if the patient has mitral valve disease, a prosthetic valve, left atrial enlargement or a myocardial infarction in the last 3 months (Intercollegiate Working Party for Stroke 2004).

* *Raised cholesterol*. Use a statin and diet to lower cholesterol as recommended in the prevention of coronary heart disease (see page 165). This will not only reduce the risk of stroke but will reduce the risk of all cardiovascular events by 17% (NNT 20 over 5 years).

* *Carotid artery surgery*. Check that the patient has been considered for carotid endarterectomy or angioplasty, if the stroke was in the appropriate carotid artery territory and a good recovery from the stroke is likely. Surgery in those with an occlusion ≥ 70% gives a 21% reduction in the risk of a further stroke in the next 5 years, provided the artery does not show 'near-occlusion' (Rothwell, Gutnikov, Warlow, *et al.* 2003). Men, though not women, with at least 50% occlusion show some, though less, benefit. Benefit is greatest in patients > 75 years old and least in those < 65. Benefit is greatest if the operation is performed in the 2 weeks after the last symptomatic event (Rothwell, Eliasziw, Gutnikov, *et al.* 2004).

Other routine matters

* Explain the prognosis if requested. 65% are likely to achieve independence but the GP can modify this figure according to the individual patient's clinical state. Those with a better prognosis are those who are continent, who have regained power on the affected side within 1 month and who are progressing towards walking within 6 weeks. Improvement is likely to continue for some months.

* *Driving*. Explain that the patient should not drive for at least 1 month after a stroke or transient ischaemic attack (TIA) and that the DVLA and the insurance company should be informed.

* *Influenza*. Arrange for annual immunization, as well as pneumococcal immunization in those aged 65 and over.

* Check that the patient knows about the relevant statutory and voluntary organizations.

* Arrange relief admissions and other support for the carers (e.g. attendance allowance) in consultation with the stroke team.

PRIMARY PREVENTION OF STROKE

Prevention should be targeted towards patients with one or more of these factors.

* *Hypertension.* Control blood pressure to < 140/85 mmHg (see page 135). A meta-analysis of 17 trials, in which the mean reduction in diastolic BP was 5–6 mmHg, gave an NNT of 20 to prevent one major vascular event in 5 years among older patients and an NNT of 60 for younger patients (MacMahon, Neal and Rodgers 1995).

* *Atrial fibrillation.* Advise the patient about anticoagulation or antiplatelet treatment according to risk (see page 158). The risk of stroke is reduced by anticoagulants by two thirds (OR 0.39 (95%CI 0.26 to 0.59)). At a baseline annual risk of 4% that gives an NNT of 40 (Benavente, Hart, Koudstaal, *et al.* 2004). Patients at lower risk may choose aspirin or no treatment.

* *Aspirin.* Recommend aspirin in primary prevention only in high-risk patients (see page 165) (Hart, Halperin, McBride, *et al.* 2000).

* *Cholesterol.* Assess the patient's risk from all occlusive arterial disease. The Heart Protection study (Heart Protection Study Collaborative Group 2004) shows that treatment with simvastatin 40 mg daily prevents stroke in patients at high risk. In this case high risk was defined as having occlusive cardiovascular disease other than stroke, or diabetes, or hypertension in men aged at least 65. Stroke risk was reduced by 25% (95%CI 15 to 34%) giving an NNT of 84 over 5 years. This benefit was independent of age, gender, blood pressure or baseline cholesterol level. A greater benefit came from the 22% reduction in all major vascular events (NNT 19 over 5 years).

* *ACE inhibition.* In the HOPE study ramipril decreased the risk of stroke by 32% despite lowering the BP by only 4/3 mm Hg (Bosch, Yusuk, Pogue *et al.* 2002). Some specialists recommend it in patients at high risk: age 55 or over, with CVD or diabetes plus one additional risk factor (Schrader and Luders 2002).

* *Alcohol.* Advise the patient to keep to the national guidelines for alcohol consumption of < 21 units per week for a male and < 14 units per week for a female. Regular light to moderate consumption of alcohol seems to decrease the risk of ischaemic stroke by reducing atherothrombotic events. Heavy drinking or binge drinking can increase the risk of stroke with an odds ratio of 1.64 (95%CI 1.39 to 1.93) (Reynolds, Lewis, Nolen, *et al.* 2003).

* *Smoking.* Encourage smokers to stop (see page 498) or reduce. Studies have found a dose–response relationship between the amount of cigarettes smoked per day and the relative risk of stroke (Higa and Davanipour 1991).

* Encourage *lifestyle and behaviour modifications* (including moderate exercise for 30 minutes on 5 days a week) that are effective in the prevention of cardiovascular disease and stroke (Batty and Lee 2002). Weight (a BMI > 28) and a large girth (waist circumference > 99 cm) are independent risk factors for stroke, at least in older men (Dey, Rothenberg, Sundh, *et al.* 2002).

TRANSIENT ISCHAEMIC ATTACK (TIA)

> **GUIDELINE**
>
> National Collaborating Centre for Chronic Conditions. 2008. *Stroke: National Clinical Guideline for Diagnosis and Initial Management of Acute Stroke and Transient Ischaemic Attack (TIA).* NICE guideline. Royal College of Physicians, London

* A TIA is a sudden focal neurological disturbance lasting less than 24 hours. The risk of a subsequent stroke is 8–12% in the first week and 11–15% in the first month, despite preventative measures (Coull, Lovett and Rothwell 2004). A meta-analysis has shown that, where a stroke is preceded by a TIA, almost half of them were in the 7 days before the stroke (Rothwell and Warlow 2005).

* The likelihood of a subsequent stroke must be assessed so that urgent investigation can be provided for those most at risk.

* Check that the symptoms are due to a TIA. Differentiate TIA from:

(a) transient cerebral symptoms caused by hypoperfusion due to cardiac disease;

(b) cerebral tumour. Patients with sensory TIAs, jerking TIAs, loss of consciousness or speech arrest should be assumed to have a tumour until proved otherwise;

(c) epilepsy. A careful history of the attacks from an observer is important;

(d) migraine;

(e) traumatic brain injury;

(f) subdural haematoma;

(g) subarachnoid haemorrhage.

* Note that a patient with a TIA that seems to be in the vertebro-basilar distribution, as manifested, for instance, by vertigo, bilateral visual loss or diplopia, should be managed in the same way as one with a TIA in the carotid distribution, except that the ABCD^2 score is likely to be lower.

ASSESS THE URGENCY OF REFERRAL USING ABCD^2

ABCD^2

Score the patient's risk of stroke in the next 30 days as follows:

- Age $\geq$ 60: 1 point.
- Blood pressure $\geq$ 140/90: 1 point if either systolic or diastolic reaches those levels.
- Clinical features: 2 points if weakness; if not, 1 point if speech affected.
- Duration: 2 points if event lasted $\geq$ 60 minutes; 1 point if 10–59 minutes.
- Diabetes: 1 point.

Significance of the score (Tsivgoulis, Spengos, Manta, et al. 2006)

A study of patients admitted to the Oxford Neurology Department found, using the 6 point ABCD score (omitting diabetes), an overall stroke risk at 30 days of 9.7%. None of the strokes occurred in those with a score of 2 or less. Above this the stroke risks were as follows:

- a score of 3: stroke risk 3.5%;
- a score of 4: stroke risk 7.6%;
- a score of 5: stroke risk 21.3%;
- a score of 6: stroke risk 31.3%.

Referral

* Score of 4 or more: refer to the rapid access TIA clinic (or equivalent local facility) to be seen within 24 hours of the onset of symptoms.

* Score < 4 but other worrying features, e.g. crescendo TIAs, with two or more TIAs occurring in one week: refer to the rapid access TIA clinic (or equivalent local facility) to be seen within 24 hours of the onset of symptoms.

* Score < 4, or the TIA occurred over a week before presentation, refer to the rapid access TIA clinic (or equivalent local facility) to be seen within 7 days.

OTHER MEASURES

* *Aspirin:* give 300 mg to be taken immediately unless contraindicated. One possible contraindication is a patient with a minor stroke who has not had a haemorrhage excluded by CT scan. In these patients, wait 2 weeks from the event before starting aspirin. If aspirin is not tolerated use clopidogrel or modified release dipyridamole 200 mg b.d. If the TIA/stroke occurs in a patient already taking aspirin 75 mg, increase to 300 mg daily, then to a dipyridamole/aspirin combination/ then to clopidogrel.

* *Prevention:* Treat as for stroke.

* *Driving:* Advise as for stroke.

RECURRENT TIAS

* If the TIA occurred in a patient already taking aspirin 75 mg daily, change to 300 mg daily, then to an aspirin/dipyridamole combination, then to clopidogrel.

* Check that a treatable cardiac or carotid cause has been excluded.

* Tighten control of other risk factors for stroke (BP, cholesterol, glucose, etc.).

* Admit if the TIAs assume a crescendo pattern.

* Refer if recurrent attacks continue despite the above measures.

PATIENT ORGANIZATION

The Stroke Association, Stroke House, 240 City Road, London EC1V 2PR. Helpline 0845 30 33 100 www.

stroke.org.uk. It offers posters and leaflets explaining the FAST (Face Arm Speech Test)

Local Stroke Clubs can be accessed through the community rehabilitation team

MOTOR NEURONE DISEASE

GUIDELINES

Motor Neurone Disease Association. Evidence-based Clinical Guidelines in MND: *Making and Communicating the Diagnosis; Respiratory Management; Nutritional Management.* Available: www.mndassociation.org. Choose 'For professionals' then 'Sharing good practice' then 'Clinical guidelines'

* Refer every patient for confirmation of the diagnosis.
* Explain what little is known about the disease. Offer referral to the Motor Neurone Disease (MND) association regional care development adviser.
* Support the patient and family as you would in any terminal illness. The median survival is only 3–4 years, with older patients having the worst prognosis. Always make a further appointment, rather than waiting for the patient or family to contact you with a problem.
* *Ventilation.* Discuss at an early stage with the patient and the family the fact that ventilation may become necessary. Non-invasive ventilation (i.e. via facemask), at night only, in those with good bulbar function prolongs life by a median of 7 months with improvement in the quality of life (McDermott and Shaw 2008). If bulbar function fails, tracheostomy or ventilation may become necessary. Discuss this well before it becomes necessary; there is often no time to discuss it with them during a crisis (Shneerson 1996).
* *Nutrition.* In the early stages of dysphagia, refer to a speech therapist and a dietician. Offer referral for consideration of insertion of a gastrostomy tube, or a nasogastric tube, *before* the patient becomes weak through malnutrition. Standard criteria for tube feeding are when > 10% of premorbid weight has been lost, or when the patient finds

eating an ordeal because of choking or because it takes too long (McDermott and Shaw 2008).
* Refer for physiotherapy, occupational therapy, speech therapy for help with speech as well as eating, district nursing, health visitor and social work assistance as appropriate. In each case do this pro-actively, not when a serious problem has developed.
* *Hospice care.* Introduce this idea well before it is needed. Short-term admission as respite care will establish a link with the hospice and help the patient to make a decision about what he or she wants to happen in the terminal stages.
* *Drug treatment.* If riluzole is initiated by the responsible neurologist, share the patient's care with the specialist according to an agreed shared care protocol (NICE 2001). Riluzole prolongs life in amyotrophic lateral sclerosis by an average of 3–4 months (McDermott and Shaw 2008).

END OF LIFE CARE IN MND

* *Musculoskeletal pain.* Consider physiotherapy to relieve the stiffness associated with prolonged immobility. Treat with NSAIDs and opioids. Use opioids early rather than late in patients with pain, as well as to ease the distress of terminal respiratory failure (Norris 1992). Treat muscle spasms with baclofen, dantrolene or diazepam, although evidence for their use in MND is lacking. Refer for endurance-type exercises of moderate intensity, if the local physiotherapy service can offer it. It offers significant improvement in spasticity (Ashworth, Satkunam and Deforge 2004).
* *Dribbling.* Treat dribbling with anticholinergics, e.g. sublingual hyoscine 0.3 mg t.d.s. or hyoscine hydrobromide transdermal patches.
* *Dry mouth.* Try pineapple chunks or apple or lemon juice to stimulate saliva.
* Consider referral for tracheostomy for sputum retention or stridor, or for recurrent aspiration of food or drink.
* *Choking spasms.* Give sublingual lorazepam and leave a supply with the patient for future occasions. They relieve the laryngeal spasm associated with inhalation of food, drink or saliva.

* *Respiratory failure*. Consider referral for ventilatory support if the quality of life is otherwise sufficiently good. Be prepared to ease the distress of dying from respiratory failure with oral morphine while the patient is able to swallow and s.c. or i.v. diazepam or morphine in the terminal stage (Jennings, Davies, Higgins and Broadley 2004).

PATIENT ORGANIZATION

Motor Neurone Disease Association, PO Box 246, Northampton NN1 2PR; 08457 626262; www.mndassociation.orgs

MULTIPLE SCLEROSIS

GUIDELINE

National Institute for Health and Clinical Excellence. 2003. *Multiple Sclerosis. Management of Multiple Sclerosis in Primary and Secondary Care.* Clinical Guideline No. 8. Online. Available: www.nice.org.uk

The NICE guidance, above, sets out the following principles:

(a) the diagnosis should be made rapidly by a specialist neurologist, and every patient, once diagnosed, should have access to neurological and specialist neurological rehabilitation services as the need arises;

(b) the patient should be actively involved in all decisions. To do this the patient needs clear verbal and written information;

(c) the patient and any family or other carers need emotional as well as practical support from the medical services;

(d) whenever the patient is assessed, attention should be paid to any 'hidden' factors (e.g. emotional state, fatigue, bladder and bowel problems) as well as to the presenting symptom. The NICE guidance includes a useful checklist of issues to consider (see Appendix 17)

(e) the GP should be pro-active in the prevention of avoidable morbidity e.g. contractures, inhalation, pressure sores, or renal infections.

The MS Society booklet for GPs stresses the role of the GP as patient's advocate. The GP may not know how to manage every problem raised by this complex illness but he or she should know someone who does and should make the referral. Even if the patient is already authorized to self refer direct, the GP may be needed to expedite the appointment if the first offer of an appointment is not sufficiently prompt (Multiple Sclerosis Society 2006).

A BETTER PROGNOSIS IS ASSOCIATED WITH

(a) Young age at onset.
(b) Female gender.
(c) A relapsing and remitting course.
(d) Initial symptoms: sensory or optic neuritis.
(e) First manifestations affecting only one CNS region.
(f) High degree of recovery from initial bout.
(g) Longer interval between first relapses.
(h) Low number of relapses in the first 2 years.
(i) Less disability at 5 years after onset.

* *Prognosis*. Explain what is known about the disease and how good the prognosis is; 76% of MS patients are alive 25 years after the onset, which is 85% of that seen in age- and sex-matched controls. Point out the positive prognostic features (see box above) if they apply.

* *Relapses*. At the start of an acute disabling relapse give methylprednisolone 500 mg orally daily for 3–5 days, after discussion with the patient of the risks and benefits. Giving the same dose intravenously is not feasible in primary care because the high-dose intravenous preparation should be given over 30 minutes. Steroids can hasten recovery, but there is no evidence that the long-term course is altered (Filippini, Brusaferri, Sibley, *et al.* 2001). No more than three courses should be given in one year. Also consider what help the patient needs, in the way of care and equipment, because of the relapse and whether referral to the specialist neurological rehabilitation service is needed.

* *Beta-interferon* in patients with relapsing remitting MS reduces the occurrence of exacerbations by 20% (RR 0.8, 95% CI0.73 to 0.88) and progression of the disease by 31% (RR 0.69, 95% CI0.55 to 0.87) 2 years after randomization (Rice, Incorvaia, Munari, *et al.* 2001). However, the non-inclusion of dropouts in the studies puts even this modest benefit in doubt; and evidence of benefit after 2 years is currently lacking.

Evidence for glatiramer is less compelling (DTB 2001). Both drugs must be given by injection. NICE determined in 2002 that the drugs should not be prescribed at NHS expense in the UK (NICE 2002). However, the UK Department of Health currently allows prescription under very limited circumstances (see below); they have funded a web site which explains to the patient what they are likely to be offered and helps them decide whether to accept it.

CANDIDATES FOR BETA-INTERFERON OR GLATIRAMER

In the UK, under the 'risk-sharing scheme' set out in Health Service Circular 2002/004 (DoH 2002), the following patients are entitled to disease modifying treatment (beta-interferon or glatiramer) at NHS expense as part of a cost-effectiveness study:

(a) those with relapse-remitting MS; and

(b) those with secondary progressive MS in which relapses are the dominant feature,

provided they meet the eligibility criteria of the Association of British Neurologists. These are set out in NICE guideline No. 8 (see box above). Go to www.nice. org.uk, search on 'Multiple sclerosis', open the guideline and search on 'Table 3'.

Treatment is to be initiated at a specialist MS treatment centre. Those already on treatment may continue until they and their consultant agree it is time to stop. Clinicians may also prescribe the drugs at NHS expense if they deem it clinically necessary.

* *Mitoxantrone* and other immunomodulatory drugs show some evidence of benefit but there are few trials of each drug, side-effects are frequent and no cost-effectiveness studies have been conducted (Bryant, Clegg and Milne 2001). NICE considers that they should not be used except by an expert in MS, preferably as part of a trial. However, a more recent Cochrane review found evidence that azathioprine can reduce the number of relapses and slow progression on a par with beta-interferon (Casetta, Iuliano and Filippini 2007).

REGULAR REVIEW

Check that there is a key worker to whom the patient has immediate access and who is co-ordinating all members of the multidisciplinary team. If there is no such person then, by default, the role falls to the GP.

At every review check the following even if the patient does not volunteer that there is a problem:

* *Fatigue*, which is common and not the same as sleepiness. The fatigue may be physical or mental, so that the patient can concentrate for only a short period of time. Check for an underlying cause: e.g. depression, chronic pain, disturbed sleep. The most useful manoeuvre is to explain that the fatigue is real and that it is a part of the syndrome.

* *Spasticity*. The evidence of benefit from therapy is poor (Shakespeare, Boggild and Young 2001). Treat any precipitating cause, such as infection or pain. Otherwise management should be supervised by the specialist rehabilitation service. The components of a treatment programme are:

    (a) stretching exercises by physiotherapist, patient or family.

    (b) a skeletal muscle relaxant, e.g. baclofen or gabapentin, or, if they fail, diazepam or dantrolene. Start low and increase the dose slowly. Up to 100 mg/day of baclofen may be required. If stopping, reduce the dose over several weeks. Abrupt withdrawal of baclofen may result in hallucinations or seizures;

    (c) consider an evening dose of diazepam if spasms or clonus interfere with sleep;

    (d) refer, if spasticity is still uncontrolled, for consideration of intrathecal baclofen.

* *Weakness*. Refer to the specialist rehabilitation service for training in exercises and techniques to maximize strength. Check that a risk assessment for pressure ulcers has been performed on any patient who uses a wheelchair.

* *Contractures*. These may develop around any joint whose muscles are weak or spastic. Contractures lead to further reductions in mobility and difficulties in handling. Prevent them by instructing the patient or carer in passive stretching of the joint. Refer to the specialist team if a contracture does develop.

* *Pressure sores*. Check that all wheelchair users have been assessed for pressure sore risk and appropriate preventive measures are in place.

* *Depression and anxiety.* A major depressive episode occurs in > 50% at some stage. Search for it and treat it as actively as in a patient without MS.
* *Emotionalism.* Consider a trial of an antidepressant (a TCA or SSRI).
* *Dysphagia.* If the patient has bulbar signs (dysarthria, ataxia, or abnormal eye movements), or if there has been a chest infection, assess swallowing formally.
* *Dysarthria.* If communication is affected refer to a speech and language therapist.
* *Pain* may be neuropathic or musculoskeletal. The former needs a trial of carbamazepine, gabapentin, or amitriptyline, see page 677; the latter needs physiotherapy and analgesics.
* *Visual problems* that are not corrected with glasses need assessment by an ophthalmologist. Optic neuritis is the commonest cause of visual loss.
* *Cognitive impairment*, if suspected, should be formally assessed and the results used to inform the management of every aspect of the patient's care.
* *Bladder problems*: see below.
* *Constipation.* Can usually be managed with adequate fluid, bulk laxatives and stool softeners. More severe constipation may require osmotic agents, bowel stimulants, anal stimulation, suppositories, or enemas. Bedridden patients may develop faecal impaction unresponsive to these measures and require manual disimpaction. Faecal incontinence may be minimized by adherence to a schedule for bowel movements and by early detection of impaction.
* *Sexual problems.* The precise nature of the sexual dysfunction will determine the treatment. Physical difficulty from spasticity may be alleviated by premedication with baclofen, and a fast-acting anticholinergic such as oxybutynin may calm urinary urgency. Sexual dysfunction should not be automatically attributed to MS. It may be necessary to investigate hormonal levels and to obtain urological or gynaecological consultation. Manual lubrication with gel is a ready solution to vaginal dryness. Erectile dysfunction may be treated by sildenafil at NHS expense in the UK. If it fails, older treatments may succeed (vacuum devices, intracavernous injections or a penile implant; see page 373).
* *The health and state of mind of any carers*, see page 626.

THE BLADDER

* *Urgency.* See whether access to the toilet can be made easier and give an anticholinergic, e.g. oxybutynin or tolterodine.
* *Minor incontinence.* Consider desmopressin 100–400 mcg nocte orally or 10–40 mcg intranasally, for night-time incontinence. It works by reducing the volume of urine produced. The same dose once in any 24 hour period may be useful to tide a patient over a time when there is no toilet within reach, e.g. on a journey. Padding may help a patient of either sex.
* *More severe incontinence*, occurring more than once a week: refer to a continence service. The patient needs ultrasound assessment for a residual urine and consideration of intermittent or even long-term catheterization. Meanwhile, supply pads for a woman and a penile drainage device for a man.
* *Urinary infection.* Once treated, order an ultrasound scan for residual urine, if not already performed. Residuals in excess of 15 ml are abnormal. If the residual is above 50 ml, or if there have been > 3 confirmed infections in a year, refer to a continence service. If catheterization is needed, intermittent self-catheterization is better than an indwelling catheter if the patient can manage it.

OTHER ISSUES

■ *Pregnancy* does not appear to influence the course of the disease overall. There may be fewer relapses during the pregnancy with a slight increase in the risk of relapse after delivery.
■ *Immunizations.* A patient should have all routine immunizations as well as an annual influenza vaccination. There is no evidence that they precipitate relapse.
■ *Employment.* Check that the patient knows about the assistance that is available from disability employment advisors and the Access to Work scheme.

END OF LIFE CARE

While MS is not often fatal in itself, life is shortened by an average of 6–11 years and it may complicate a death from another condition. See Motor neurone disease for a discussion of end of life care (page 311).

PATIENTS' ORGANIZATION

The Multiple Sclerosis (MS) Society, 372 Edgware Road, London NW2 6ND. National helpline: 0808 800 8000; www.mssociety.org.uk

HUNTINGTON'S DISEASE

GUIDELINE

Rosenblatt A, Danen NG, Nance MA, Paulsen JS. 2002. *A Physician's Guide to the Management of Huntington's Disease*, 2nd edition. Huntington's Disease Association

- The diagnosis should always be made by a specialist.
- Genetic testing may be requested by people who are at risk because of their family history. The arguments in favour and against are complex and the discussion is best handled by experienced staff at a genetics centre.
- Management should be in the hands of a specialist team; but the GP may be the first person to detect a new problem and needs to understand the principles of management.

MANAGEMENT

- Involuntary movements may be helped by three groups of drugs: neuroleptics, benzodiazepines and dopamine depleting agents. They have the problems respectively of parkinsonism and tardive dyskinesia; of drowsiness and ataxia; and of depression and hypotension. Some patients can be managed by ensuring an environment free from stress, with padding of chair and bed and weights on wrists and ankles to reduce movements.
- The impairment of voluntary movements does not respond to medication but useful

improvement can be achieved by behavioural methods. Dysphagia can improve with a change of food type, usually to a slightly more liquid food, and by developing a habit of eating slowly. A speech therapist can help with speech and with dysphagia. An occupational therapist can make the home safer for a patient at risk of falling.

- The problems posed by cognitive impairment can be reduced by training the family to communicate with the patient in a simple way. Explain that a patient who seems to be unaware of his or her disability may have a neurological basis for the unawareness and is not 'just being difficult'.
- The specific psychiatric disorders that are associated with Huntington's disease (HD), namely depression, mania, obsessive-compulsive disorder, may respond to the same treatment as would be appropriate for a patient without HD.

COPING WITH THE COGNITIVE IMPAIRMENT

- Explain to the family, and to the patient if the impairment is not too advanced, the principles of coping with cognitive impairment (see pages 305 and 603).
- Explain that HD has certain specific problems and suggest solutions to them:
  (a) Difficulty with initiating and organizing tasks: use lists and prompt the patient to do things.
  (b) Perseveration of thoughts or actions: gently ease the patient on to something else.
  (c) Impulsivity and irritability: reduce stress with a regular schedule, respond with calmness and try to find out what has prompted it.
  (d) Difficulty with attention: do one thing at a time.
  (e) Lack of insight: it is a feature of the disease – not a sign that the patient is being difficult.

Other points that may have escaped the attention of the specialist team:

- Advise the patient, if a driver, of the need to notify the DVLA and insurance company of the condition once it is diagnosed (though not when a genetic diagnosis has been made in a well patient).

* Raise the question of an advance directive (see page 22). It can be a great help if the patient decides certain key issues, and records the decision, when still competent to do so. Some key issues are: preferred place of terminal care when the need arises, whether to be given a gastrostomy tube when no longer able to swallow, whether to be resuscitated when in a terminal state.

* Check what the family has been told about who else is at risk of developing the disease and what decision has been made about genetic testing. Record this in those patients' records.

PATIENT GROUPS

Huntington's Disease Association, Neurosupport Centre, Liverpool L3 8LR. Tel. 0151 298 3298; www. hda.org.uk

Scottish Huntington's Association. Suite 135, St James Business Centre, Linwood Road, Paisley PA3 3AT, Scotland. Tel. 0141 848 0308. www.hdscotland.org

Huntington's Disease Association, Northern Ireland, C/O Dept of Medical Genetics, Belfast City Hospital Trust, Lisburn Road, Belfast BT9 7AB, Northern Ireland. www.hdani.org.uk

---

PARAPLEGIA

Every patient with paraplegia will be under the care of a consultant. The GP, however, is likely to be the doctor to whom certain problems present. A proactive approach can make a difference to the patient's quality of life.

SPASTICITY

Use established drugs (baclofen, dantrolene sodium, diazepam, clonidine) singly or in combination on a trial basis. The place of newer drugs (tizanidine, cannabinoids) is not yet clear. Attempts to control troublesome spasticity should not be abandoned without referral for consideration of intrathecal baclofen (Taricco, Adone, Pagliacci, *et al.* 2001).

URINARY TRACT INFECTION

* Always confirm suspected urinary tract infections with an MSU.

* Do not give antibiotics if the patient is catheterized unless there are systemic symptoms or *Proteus* is grown (see page 413).

AUTONOMIC DYSREFLEXIA

This is reflex sympathetic overactivity, giving rise to vasoconstriction resulting in hypertension, severe headache, visual disturbance, anxiety and pallor. The parasympathetic system slows the heart and causes flushing and sweating above the lesion. It only occurs in patients with lesions above T6.

(a) Sit the patient up.

(b) Remove the cause (e.g. distended bladder, UTI, loaded colon or anal fissure). If catheterizing or disimpacting, allow the lidocaine jelly at least 2 minutes to act. Both activities can exacerbate autonomic dysreflexia. If flushing a catheter through, use fluid at body temperature.

(c) If the systolic pressure is > 150 mmHg, give nifedipine 5–10 mg. Get the patient to bite the capsule and swallow the liquid. Alternatively, use glyceryl trinitrate (GTN) 300 mg sublingually. Patients with a high level paraplegia usually have a systolic pressure of 90–110 (Paralyzed Veterans of America/ Consortium for Spinal Cord Medicine 2001).

(d) Monitor the BP at least every 5 minutes. It may fluctuate rapidly. If hypotension occurs, lie the patient down and raise the legs.

(e) Admit urgently to hospital if not settling.

(f) If it does settle, warn the patient that it may recur as the medication wears off, and that they should call for help at the first sign of recurrence.

PRESSURE ULCERS

Prevention

* Avoid prolonged immobilization in the same position, i.e. for over 2 hours.

* Identify pressure areas and protect them.

* Ensure that someone inspects at risk areas daily: ischii, sacrum, trocanters, and heels.

* Refer for an exercise programme to retain posture, muscle strength.

* Refer to a dietician to ensure adequate nutrition.

❋ Warn patients to make contact if a red patch does not improve within 24 hours after relieving the pressure on the area (Paralyzed Veterans of America 2000).

Treatment

❋ Treat sores or ulcers intensively, and admit early if not resolving e.g. within 2–4 weeks.

PSYCHOLOGICAL ASPECTS

❋ Be aware of the fact that the patient may be suffering:
  (a) a severe grief response to the loss of function and independence;
  (b) a feeling of fear and vulnerability;
  (c) difficulties with their changing relationships with those around them.
❋ Be prepared to raise the issue of sexuality. Avoid the temptation to think of the individual as asexual. Sexual function and fertility are possible with appropriate support. Recommend publications from the Spinal Injuries Association (see box below).

ADVICE FOR PATIENTS AND PROFESSIONALS

Spinal Injuries Association, SIA House, 2 Trueman Place, Oldbrook, Milton Keynes MK6 2HH
  Helpline: 0800 980 0501; www.spinal.co.uk
  Apparelyzed is a web site dedicated to the support of those with spinal injuries. www.apparelyzed.com

ESSENTIAL TREMOR

For details of the diagnosis of tremor see *Evidence-based Diagnosis in Primary Care* by A. F. Polmear (editor), published by Butterworth-Heinemann, 2008.

SYSTEMATIC REVIEW

Ferreira J, Sampaio C. 2008. What are the effects of drug treatments in people with essential tremor of the hand? *Clinical Evidence*. Online. Available: www.clinicalevidence.org

❋ Ask what effect the tremor is having. A quarter of those who consult about tremor retire early or change jobs because of it.
❋ *Mild cases:* patients may choose not to take any medication. Check that they are not exacerbating the tremor with, for instance, caffeine. They may have noticed the improvement given by alcohol that is seen in 50–70% of patients.
❋ *Cases where the patient is more bothered:* use propranolol 30 mg/day up to 160–320 mg/day (Cleeves and Findley 1988). If the tremor improves but the patient cannot tolerate propranolol, try another beta-blocker, e.g. atenolol or metoprolol.
❋ *Cases not responding to propranolol or in whom it is contraindicated:* consider
  (a) phenobarbital or primidone, but depression and cognitive impairment are common;
  (b) topiramate, but it is associated with nausea, weight loss and paraesthesiae.
Anecdotal evidence exists for other drugs including benzodiazepines, gabapentin and calcium channel blockers. Of these benzodiazepines are most likely to be effective but with the danger of dependence developing. One way of reducing this risk is for the patient whose tremor is worsened by stress only to take the drug in a stressful situation.
❋ *Severe cases uncontrolled by medication:* consider referral for neurosurgery, either electrode implantation or thalamotomy (Schuurman, Bosch, Bossuyt, *et al.* 2000), or for local botulinum toxin injection.

References

Aben, I., Denollet, J., Lousberg, R., et al., 2002. Personality and vulnerability to depression in stroke patients. Stroke 33, 2391–2395.

Alldredge, B., Gelb, A., Isaacs, S., et al., 2001. A comparison of lorazepam, diazepam, and placebo for the treatment of out-of-hospital status epilepticus. N. Eng. J. Med. 345, 631–637.

Anderson, C., Mhurchu, C., Rubenach, S., et al., 2000. Home or hospital for stroke rehabilitation? Results of a randomized controlled trial. Stroke 31, 1024–1031.

Anon., 1990. Changing view of prognosis of epilepsy. BMJ 301, 1112–1114.

Anon., 2000. Sodium valproate for migraine prevention. Bandolier Nov. Available on www.jr2.ox.ac.uk/bandolier/booth/migraine/valpr.html.

Anon., 2001. More evidence on chronic headache: antidepressants for chronic headache. Bandolier Nov, 93–96.

Ashworth, N., Satkunam, L., Deforge, D., 2004. Treatment for spasticity in amyotrophic lateral sclerosis/motor neurone disease (Cochrane Review). In: The Cochrane Library, Issue 3. John Wiley, Chichester, UK.

Bates, D., Ashford, E., Dawson, R., et al., 1994. Subcutaneous sumatriptan during the migrainous aura. Neurology 44, 1587–1592.

Batty, G., Lee, I.-M., 2002. Physical activity for preventing strokes. BMJ 325, 350–351.

Bell, G., Gaitatzis, A., Bell, C., et al., 2008. Drowning in people with epilepsy. Neurology 71, 578–582.

Benavente, O., Hart, R., Koudstaal, P., et al., 2004. Oral anticoagulants for preventing stroke in patients with non-valvular atrial fibrillation and no previous history of stroke or transient ischemic attacks (Cochrane Review). In: The Cochrane Library, Isssue 1. John Wiley, Chichester, UK.

Bosch, J., Yusuk, S., Pogue, J., et al., 2002. Use of ramipril in preventing stroke: double blind randomised trial. BMJ 324, 699–702.

Breen, D., Davenport, R., 2006. Teratogenicity of antiepileptic drugs. BMJ 333, 615–616.

British Association for the Study of Headache, 2004. Guidelines for all doctors in the diagnosis and management of migraine and tension-type headache. Available: www.eguidelines.co.uk.

Brown, K., Sloan, R., Pentland, B., 1998. Fluoxetine as a treatment for post-stroke emotionalism. Acta Psychiatr. Scand. 98, 455–458.

Browne, T., Holmes, G., 2001. Primary care: epilepsy. N. Engl. J. Med. 344, 1145–1151.

Bryant, J., Clegg, A., Milne, R., 2001. Systematic review of immunomodulatory drugs for the treatment of people with multiple sclerosis: is there good quality evidence on effectiveness and cost? J. Neurol. Neurosurg. Psychiatry 70, 574–579.

Casetta, I., Iuliano, G., Filippini, G., 2007. Azathioprine for multiple sclerosis. Cochrane Database Syst. Rev. 17 (4),CD003982.

Chadwick, D., 1987. Overuse of monitoring of blood concentrations of antiepileptic drugs. BMJ 294, 723–724.

Chadwick, D., Taylor, J., Johnson, T., 1996. Outcomes after seizure recurrence in people with well-controlled epilepsy and the factors that influence it. Epilepsia 37, 1043–1050.

Choudhury, K., Clough, C., 1998. Subcutaneous apomorphine in Parkinson's disease. BMJ 316, 641.

Chronicle, E., Mulleners, W., 2004. Anticonvulsant drugs for migraine prophylaxis (Cochrane Review). In: The Cochrane Library, Isssue 3. John Wiley, Chichester, UK.

Cleeves, L., Findley, L., 1988. Propranolol and propranolol-LA in essential tremor: a double blind comparative study. J. Neurol. Neurosurg. Psychiatry 51, 379–384.

Clough, C., 1989. Non-migrainous headaches. BMJ 299, 70–72.

Codispoti, J., Prior, M., Fu, M., et al., 2001. Efficacy of nonprescription doses of ibuprofen for treating migraine headache: a randomized controlled trial. Headache 41, 665–679.

Colman, I., Brown, M., Innes, G., et al., 2004. Parenteral metoclopramide for acute migraine: meta-analysis of randomised controlled trials. BMJ 329, 1369–1373.

Coull, A., Lovett, J., Rothwell, P., 2004. Population based study of early risk of stroke after transient ischaemic attack or minor stroke: implications for public education and organisation of services. BMJ 328, 326–328.

Crawford, P., Hall, W.W., Chappell, B., et al., 1996. Generic prescribing for epilepsy: is it safe? Seizure 5, 1–5.

Crosby, N., Deane, K., Clarke, C., 2004. Amantadine in Parkinson's disease (Cochrane Review). In: The Cochrane Library, Isssue 3. John Wiley, Chichester, UK.

de Goede, C., Keus, S., Kwakkel, G., et al., 2001. The effects of physical therapy in Parkinson's disease: a research synthesis. Arch. Phys. Med. Rehab. 82, 509–515.

Deane, K., Ellis-Hill, C., Playford, E., et al., 2001. Occupational therapy for patients with Parkinson's disease (Cochrane Review). In: The Cochrane Library, Isssue 3. Update Software, Oxford.

Deane, K., Jones, D., Playford, E., et al., 2001. Physiotherapy for patients with Parkinson's disease (Cochrane Review). In: The Cochrane Library, Isssue 3. Update Software, Oxford.

Deane, K., Whurr, R., Clarke, C., et al., 2004. Non-pharmacological therapies for dysphagia in Parkinson's disease (Cochrane Review). In: The Cochrane Library, Isssue 3. John Wiley, Chichester, UK.

Deane, K., Whurr, R., Playford, E., et al., 2004. Speech and language therapy versus placebo or no intervention for dysarthria in Parkinson's disease (Cochrane Review). In: The Cochrane Library, Isssue 3. John Wiley, Chichester, UK.

Dey, D., Rothenberg, E., Sundh, V., et al., 2002. Waist circumference, body mass index, and risk of stroke in older people. J. Am. Geriatr. Soc. 50, 1510–1518.

Dobson, R., 2004. Half of UK patients taking drugs for epilepsy continue to have seizures. BMJ News Roundup 328, 68.

DoH, 2002. Health Service Circular 2002/004. Department of Health, London. Available: www.dh. gov.uk.

Donaghy, M., Chang, C., Poulter, N., 2002. Duration, frequency, recency, and type of migraine and the risk of ischaemic stroke in women of childbearing age. J. Neurol. Neurosurg. Psychiatry 73, 747–750.

DTB, 1994. Drug treatment of epilepsy. Drug. Ther. Bull. 32, 45–48.

DTB, 2001. Glatiramer acetate for multiple sclerosis. Drug. Ther. Bull. 39, 41–43.

Edmeads, J., Lainez, J., Brandes, J., et al., 2001. Potential of the Migraine Disability Assessment (MIDAS) Questionnaire as a public health initiative and in clinical practice. Neurology 56 (Suppl. 1), S29–S34.

Filippini, G., Brusaferri, F., Sibley, W., et al., 2001. Corticosteroids or ACTH for acute exacerbations in multiple sclerosis (Cochrane Review). In: The Cochrane Library, Isssue 4. Update Software, Oxford.

Gandelman, M., 1994. Review of carbamazepine-induced hyponatraemia. Prog. Neuro-Psychopharm. Biol. Psych. 18, 211–233.

Granella, F., Sances, G., Pucci, E., et al., 2000. Migraine with aura and reproductive life events: a case control study. Cephalalgia 20, 701–707.

Hankey, G., 2004. Informal care giving for disabled stroke survivors. BMJ 328, 1085–1086.

Hanna, N., Black, M., Sander, J., et al., 2002. The national sentinel clinical audit of epilepsy-related deaths: report 2002: epilepsy - death in the shadows. The Stationery Office, Norwich.

Harari, D., Coshall, C., Rudd, A., et al., 2003. New-onset fecal incontinence after stroke. Stroke 34, 144–150.

Harbison, J., Hossain, O., Jenkinson, D., et al., 2003. Diagnostic accuracy of stroke referrals from primary care, emergency room physicians, and ambulance staff using the Face Arm Speech Test. Stroke 34, 71–76.

Hart, R., Halperin, J., McBride, R., et al., 2000. Aspirin for the primary prevention of stroke and other major vascular events. Arch. Neurol. 57, 326–332.

He, J., Whelton, P., Vu, B., et al., 1998. Aspirin and risk of hemorrhagic stroke: a meta-analysis of randomized controlled trials. JAMA 280, 1930–1935.

Heart Protection Study Collaborative Group, 2004. Effects of cholesterol-lowering with simvastatin on stroke and other major vascular events in 20 536 people with cerebrovascular disease or other high risk conditions. Lancet 363, 757–767.

Higa, M., Davanipour, Z., 1991. Smoking and stroke. Neuroepidemiology 10, 211–212.

Holroyd, K., O'Donnell, F., Stensland, M., et al., 2001. Management of chronic tension-type headache with tricyclic antidepressant medication, stress management therapy and their combination. JAMA 285, 2208–2215.

Intercollegiate Working Party on Stroke, 2002. National Clinical Guidelines for Stroke: Update 2002. Royal College of Physicians, London.

Intercollegiate Working Party for Stroke, 2004. National Clinical Guidelines for Stroke, second ed. Royal College of Physicians, London.

Jacoby, A., Johnson, A., Chadwick, D., for The Medical Research Council Antiepileptic Drug Withdrawal Study Group, 1992. Psychosocial outcomes of anti-epileptic drug discontinuation. Epilepsia 33, 1123–1131.

Jennings, A., Davies, A., Higgins, J., Broadley, K., 2004. Opioids for the palliation of breathlessness in terminal illness (Cochrane Review). In: The Cochrane Library, Isssue 3. John Wiley, Chichester, UK.

Katzenschlager, R., Sampaio, C., Costa, J., Lees, A., 2004. Anticholinergics for symptomatic management of Parkinson's disease (Cochrane Review). In: The Cochrane Library, Isssue 3. John Wiley, Chichester, UK.

Kotila, M., Numminen, H., Waltimo, O., et al., 1998. Depression after stroke: results of the FINNSTROKE Study. Stroke 29, 368–372.

Koudstaal, P., 2004. Anticoagulants versus antiplatelet therapy for preventing stroke in patients with nonrheumatic atrial fibrillation and a history of stroke or transient ischemic attacks (Cochrane Review). In: The Cochrane Library, Isssue 1. John Wiley, Chichester, UK.

Krymchantowski, A., 2004. Acute treatment of migraine. Breaking the paradigm of monotherapy. BMC Neurol. 4, 4. Available on BioMed Central at www. biomedcentral.com/1471-2377/4/4.

Kurth, T., Schurks, M., Logroscino, G., et al., 2008. Migraine, vascular risk, and cardiovascular events in women: prospective cohort study. BMJ 337, 383–387.

Lees, K., Bath, P., Naylor, A., 2000. Secondary prevention of transient ischaemic attack and stroke. BMJ 320, 991–994.

Lees, A., Katzenschlager, R., Head, J., et al., 2001. Ten-year follow-up of three different initial treatments in de-novo PD. Neurology 57, 1687–1694.

Leonardi-Bee, J., Bath, P., Bousser, M.-G., et al., 2005. Dipyridamole for preventing recurrent ischemic stroke and other vascular events: a meta-analysis of individual patient data from randomized controlled trials. Stroke 36, 162–168.

Linn, F.H.H., Wijdicks, E.F.M., van der Graaf, Y., et al., 1994. Prospective study of sentinel headache in aneurysmal subarachnoid haemorrhage. Lancet 344, 590–593.

Lipton, R., Stewart, W., Stone, A., et al., 2000. Stratified care vs step care strategies for migraine: the Disabilities in Strategies of Care (DISC) Study: a randomized trial. JAMA 284, 2599–2605.

McDermott, C., Shaw, P., 2008. Diagnosis and management of motor neurone disease. BMJ 336, 658–662.

MacGregor, E., Chia, H., Vohrah, R., Wilkinson, M., 1990. Migraine and menstruation: a pilot study. Cepalalgia 10, 305–310.

MacMahon, S., Neal, B., Rodgers, A., 1995. Blood pressure lowering for the primary and secondary prevention of coronary and cerebrovascular disease. Schweizerische Medizinische Wochenschrift. Journal Suisse de Medecine 125, 2479–2486.

Marras, C., Rochon, P., Lang, A., 2002. Predicting motor decline and disability in Parkinson Disease. Arch. Neurol. 59, 1724–1728.

Marson, A., Al-Kharusi, A., Alwaidh, M., et al., 2007a. The SANAD study of effectiveness of valproate, lamotrigine, or topiramate for generalised and unclassifiable epilepsy: an unblinded randomised controlled trial. Lancet 369, 1016–1026.

Marson, A., Al-Kharusi, A., Alwaidh, M., et al., 2007b. The SANAD study of effectiveness of carbamazepine, gabapentin, lamotrigine, oxcarbazepine, or topiramate for treatment of partial epilepsy: an unblinded randomised controlled trial. Lancet 369, 1000–1015.

Marson, A.G, Kadir, Z.A, Chadwick, D.W, et al., 1996. New anti-epileptic drugs: a systematic review of their efficacy and tolerability. BMJ 313, 1169–1174.

Mayo, N., Wood-Dauphinee, S., Cote, R., et al., 2000. There's no place like home: an evaluation of early supported discharge for stroke. Stroke 31, 1016–1023.

Medical Research Council Antiepileptic Drug Withdrawal Study Group, 1993. Prognostic index for recurrence of seizures after remission of epilepsy. BMJ 306, 1374–1378.

Meenan, R., Saha, S., Chou, R., et al., 2002. Effectiveness and Cost-Effectiveness of Echocardiography and Carotid Imaging in the Management of Stroke. Evidence Report/Technology Assessment No. 49. Agency for Healthcare Research and Quality, Rockville, MD.

Melchart, D., Linde, K., Berman, B., et al., 2001. Acupuncture for idiopathic headache. Cochrane Database of Syst. Rev. (1), CD001218. DOI: 10.1002/14651858.CD001218.

Multiple Sclerosis Society, 2006. A Guide to MS for GPs and Primary Care Teams. Available: www.mssociety.org.uk.

National Collaborating Centre for Chronic Conditions, 2008. Stroke: National Clinical Guideline for Diagnosis and Initial Management of Acute Stroke and Transient Ischaemic Attack (TIA), NICE guideline. Royal College of Physicians, London.

Nelson-Piercy, C., De Swiet, M., 1996. Low-dose aspirin may be used in prophylaxis (letter). BMJ 313, 691.

NICE, 2001. Guidance on the Use of Riluzole for the treatment of Motor Neurone Disease: National Institute for Clinical Evidence Care Guideline. Available: www.nice.org.uk.

NICE, 2002. Beta Interferon and Glatiramer Acetate for the Treatment of Multiple Sclerosis. National Institute for Clinical Excellence, London. Technology Appraisal Guidance No. 32. Available: www.nice.org.uk.

NICE, 2004. Newer Drugs for Epilepsy in Adults: NICE Technology Appraisal 76. Available: www.nice.org.uk.

Norris, F., 1992. Motor neurone disease. BMJ 304, 459–460.

O'Brien, M., Gilmour-White, S., 1993. Epilepsy and pregnancy. BMJ 307, 492–495.

Oldman, A., Smith, L., McQuay, H., Moore, A., 2002. Pharmacological treatments for acute migraine: quantitative systematic review. Pain 97, 247–257.

Olesen, J., 1995. Analgesic headache. BMJ 310, 479–480.

Outpatient Service Trialists, 2003. Therapy-based rehabilitation services for stroke patients at home (Cochrane Review). In: The Cochrane Library, Isssue 1. Update Software, Oxford.

Paralyzed Veterans of America, 2000. Pressure Ulcer Prevention and Treatment Following Spinal Cord Injury: A Clinical Practice Guideline for Health Care Professionals. PVA, Washington (DC).

Paralyzed Veterans of America/ Consortium for Spinal Cord Medicine, 2001. Acute management of autonomic dysreflexia: individuals with spinal cord injury presenting to health-care facilities. PVA, Washington (DC).

Pittler, M., Ernst, E., 2004. Feverfew for preventing migraine (Cochrane Review). In:

The Cochrane Library, Isssue 3. John Wiley, Chichester, UK.

PROGRESS Collaborative Group, 2001. Randomised trial of a perindopril-based blood-pressure-lowering regimen among 6105 individuals with previous stroke or transient ischaemic attack. Lancet 358, 1033–1041.

Rascol, O., Goetz, C., Koller, W., et al., 2002. Treatment interventions for Parkinson's disease: an evidence based assessment. Lancet 359, 1589–1598.

Reynolds, K., Lewis, B., Nolen, J., et al., 2003. Alcohol consumption and risk of stroke: a meta-analysis. JAMA 289, 579–588.

Rice, G., Incorvaia, B., Munari, L., et al., 2001. Interferon in relapsing-remitting multiple sclerosis (Cochrane Review). In: The Cochrane Library, Isssue 4. Update Software, Oxford.

Rothwell, P., Eliasziw, M., Gutnikov, S., et al., 2004. Endarterectomy for symptomatic carotid stenosis in relation to clinical subgroups and timing of surgery. Lancet 363, 915–924.

Rothwell, P., Gutnikov, S., Warlow, C., et al., 2003. Reanalysis of the final results of the European Carotid Surgery Trial. Stroke 34, 514–523.

Rothwell, P., Warlow, C., 2005. Timing of TIAs preceding stroke: time window for prevention is very short. Neurology 64, 817–820.

Ryan, R., Elkind, A., Baker, C.C., et al., 1997. Sumatriptan nasal spray for the acute treatment of migraine. Neurology 49, 1225–1230.

Schrader, J., Luders, S., 2002. Preventing stroke. BMJ 324, 687–688.

Schrag, A., Ben-Shlomo, Y., Quinn, N., 2002. How valid is the clinical diagnosis of Parkinson's disease in the community? J. Neurol. Neurosurg. Psychiatry 73, 529–534.

Schuurman, P., Bosch, D., Bossuyt, P., et al., 2000. A comparison of continuous thalamic stimulation and thalamotomy for suppression of severe tremor. N. Engl. J. Med. 342, 461–468.

Scottish Intercollegiate Guidelines Network, 2003. Diagnosis and Management of Epilepsy in Adults. SIGN Guideline No. 70. Available: www.sign.ac.uk.

Scottish Intercollegiate Guidelines Network, 2008. The Diagnosis and Management of Headache in Adults. SIGN Guideline No. 107. Edinburgh. Available: www.sign.ac.uk.

Shakespeare, D., Boggild, M., Young, C., 2001. Anti-spasticity agents for multiple sclerosis (Cochrane Review). In: The Cochrane Library, Isssue 4. Update Software, Oxford.

Shneerson, J., 1996. Motor neurone disease. BMJ 313, 244–245.

Shorvon, S., 1991. Medical assessment and treatment of chronic epilepsy. BMJ 302, 363–366.

Silberstein, S., 2001. Headache and female hormones. Curr. Opin. Neurol. 14, 323–333.

Sirven, J., Sperling, M., Wingerchuk, D., et al., 2001. Early versus late antiepileptic drug withdrawal for people with epilepsy in remission (Cochrane Review). In: The Cochrane Library, Isssue 3. Update Software, Oxford.

Stroke Unit Trialists' Collaboration, 2004. Organised inpatient (stroke unit) care for stroke (Cochrane Review). In: The Cochrane Library, Isssue 1. John Wiley, Chichester UK.

Sumatriptan Cluster Headache Study Group, 1991. Treatment of acute cluster headache with sumatriptan. N. Engl. J. Med. 325, 322–326.

Taricco, M., Adone, R., Pagliacci, S., et al., 2001. Pharmacological interventions for spasticity following spinal cord injury (Cochrane Review). In: The Cochrane Library, Isssue 4. Update Software, Oxford.

Taylor, S., Tudur Smith, C., Williamson, P., et al., 2001. Phenobarbitone versus phenytoin monotherapy for partial onset seizures and generalised onset tonic-clonic seizures (Cochrane Review). In: The Cochrane Library, Isssue 4. Update Software, Oxford.

Tronvik, E., Stovner, L., Helde, G., et al., 2003. Prophylactic treatment of migraine with an angiotensin II receptor blocker. JAMA 289, 65–69.

Tsivgoulis, G., Spengos, K., Manta, P., et al., 2006. Validation of the ABCD score in identifying individuals at high early risk of stroke after a transient ischaemic attack: a hospital-based case series study. Stroke 37, 2892–2897.

van Vliet, J., Bahra, A., Martin, V., et al., 2003. Intranasal sumatriptan in cluster headache. Neurology 60, 630–633.

Vickers, A., Rees, R., Zollman, C., et al., 2004. Acupuncture for chronic headache in primary care: large, pragmatic, randomised trial. BMJ 328, 744–747.

Ward, A., Begg, A., Kent, R., et al., 2004. Community management and referral of spasticity following stroke. Available: www.eguidelines.co.uk.

Wardlaw, J., del Zoppo, G., Yamaguchi, T., Berge, E., 2004. Thrombolysis for acute ischaemic stroke (Cochrane Review). In: The Cochrane Library, Isssue 1. John Wiley, Chichester, UK.

Welch, K., 1994. Migraine and pregnancy. Adv. Neurol. 64, 77–81.

Wiart, L., Petit, H., Joseph, P., et al., 2000. Fluoxetine in early post-stroke depression: a double-blind placebo-controlled study. Stroke 31, 1829–1832.

Williams, B., Poulter, N., Brown, M., et al., 2004. British Hypertension Society guidelines for hypertension management 2004 (BHS-IV): summary. BMJ 328, 634–640.

Willoughby, B., Thomson, R., Chopra, R., 2004. Validation of a method to establish practice-based stroke and TIA registers. Br. J. Gen. Pract. 54, 127–129.

Wonderling, D., Vickers, A., Grieve, R., McCarney, R., 2004. Cost effectiveness analysis of a randomised trial of acupuncture for chronic headache in primary care. BMJ 328, 747–749.

Chapter 11

Gynaecological problems

CHAPTER CONTENTS

DYSMENORRHOEA

REVIEW

Proctor M, Farquhar C. 2007. Dysmenorrhoea. *Clinical Evidence*. London: BMJ Publishing Group. Available: www.clinicalevidence.com

Guideline

Royal College of Obstetricians and Gynaecologists. *The Initial Management of Chronic Pelvic Pain*. Available: www.rcog.org.uk (search on 'Dysmenorrhoea')

PRIMARY DYSMENORRHOEA

- Dysmenorrhoea is common. In about 20% of women it is severe enough to interfere with daily activities.
- Dysmenorrhoea is more common in women with an early age of menarche, longer duration of menstruation and in those who smoke.
- * Reassure the patient that this is not a sign of disease. An examination of the abdomen is worthwhile as part of that reassurance as well as to exclude gross pelvic pathology. The need for a vaginal examination will depend on the individual circumstances. It should be performed if the patient is sexually active.
- * Give an *NSAID*, alone or in addition to an analgesic. If taken from just before or at the onset of menstruation until pain subsides, they are effective in about 80%. Examples are

DOI: 10.1016/B978-0-7020-3053-6.00011-8

ibuprofen 1200 mg daily, mefenamic acid 750–1500 mg daily or naproxen, although adverse effects may be more common with the latter (Marjoribanks, Proctor and Farquhar 2006).

* Give aspirin, paracetamol or compound analgesics (Zhang and Po 1998).

* Consider a trial of the combined oral contraceptive (COC). It is commonly used despite the lack of evidence either way about its benefit.

* Consider also:
  (a) *Thiamine* 100 mg daily. In one study it was more effective than placebo (Gokhale 1996).
  (b) *Vitamin E.* Two RCTs have shown significant improvement in pain relief if vitamin E is taken prior to the onset of menses and until the third or fourth day. The doses ranged from 500 units to around 2000 units a day. However, there is now evidence of harm from taking regular vitamin E doses above 400 IU a day (Miller, Pastor-Barriuso, Dalal, *et al.* 2005).
  (c) *Toki-shakuyaku-san*, a herbal remedy, which may reduce pain after 6 months.
  (d) Acupressure which may be as effective as ibuprofen and high frequency TENS.

* *Women who are still in pain.* Consider referral for all those not responding.

SECONDARY DYSMENORRHOEA

* Examine vaginally. Take an HVS and swabs for *Chlamydia*. Refer for laparoscopy women in whom there is suspicion of pelvic pathology.

* *Chronic pelvic pain.* This affects about one in six women. It is a symptom with a number of contributory factors including gynaecological factors and non-gynaecological factors (e.g. irritable bowel syndrome, nerve entrapment) as well as psychological and social factors. Allow enough time for the woman to tell her story. Recommend a pain diary and review. Refer women who also have dyspareunia and low-grade pain throughout the cycle; they may have subclinical endometriosis, adenomyosis or low-grade pelvic inflammatory disease despite a normal pelvic examination.

* Otherwise, treat symptomatically as for primary dysmenorrhoea, although symptom control is less likely to be successful. Refer all women, if the pain persists, to a gynaecologist.

* *IUD.* Consider removing an intrauterine contraceptive device, if present.

ENDOMETRIOSIS

Farquhar C. Endometriosis. *Clinical Evidence*, London: BMJ Publishing Group, 2007. Available: www.clinicalevidence.com

Royal College of Obstetricians and Gynaecologists. *The Investigation and Management of Endometriosis.* 'Green top' clinical guideline 24. London: Available: www.rcog.org.uk (search on 'endometriosis')

* Refer for laparoscopy patients in whom you suspect the diagnosis. The interpretation of the finding of endometriosis can, however, be difficult. It is found in about half of women presenting with dysmenorrhoea. In some of these it may be co-incidental, in that it is present in 2–22% of women who have no symptoms. In addition to dysmenorrhoea, consider the diagnosis particularly in those with deep dyspareunia, chronic pelvic pain, ovulation pain and those with cyclical symptoms without excessive bleeding.

* *Where endometriosis has been diagnosed.* Treat as follows. The effectiveness of the different medical treatments are similar although their adverse effects differ (Farquhar and Sutton 1998).

  ■ Patients not wishing to become pregnant: consider:
    (a) *A low-dose oral contraceptive.* Give three packets of a combined oral contraceptive back to back, followed by a 1 week break. Continue for 9 months in the first instance (Moore, Kennedy and Prentice 2001).
    (b) *Progestogens* continuously for 6 months, e.g. norethisterone 10–20 mg daily. Dydrogesterone appears to be no better than placebo (Farquhar 2001; Vercellini, Cortesi and Crosignani 1997).

(c) *Danazol* 400 mg daily for 2 months decreasing to 200 mg daily, then 100 mg daily, at 2-monthly intervals. Maintain the patient on the lowest effective dose for 6 months. Occasionally patients need 600–800 mg daily. Warn the patient about the possible side-effects of acne, weight gain, muscle cramps, oedema and irreversible voice changes (DTB 1999; Pattie, Murdoch, Theodoros, *et al.* 1998). Non-hormonal contraception is essential if the patient is sexually active

(d) *Gonadorelin analogues.* Refer for complete ovarian suppression for up to 6 months. Non-hormonal contraception is essential if the patient is sexually active (DTB 1999).

(e) *Levonorgestrel-releasing intrauterine system (LNG-IUS).* The evidence suggests that the LNG-IUS reduces pain and that this is maintained for at least 3 years

■ Patients wishing to become pregnant:

(a) consider using NSAIDs, as in primary dysmenorrhoea: or

(b) refer for consideration of surgical ablation or excision of endometriosis. This is an effective alternative to medical management (Sutton, Ewen, Whiltelaw, *et al.* 1994).

PATIENT ADVICE

National Endometriosis Society, 50 Westminster Palace Gardens, Artillery Row, London SW1P 1RL, tel. 020 7222 2781; helpline 0808 808 2227; www.endo.org.uk
  RCOG. *Endometriosis: What You Need to Know*, 2007, available by following the link to *The Investigation and Management of Endometriosis.* 'Green top' clinical guideline as above

MENORRHAGIA

Duckitt K, McCully K. Menorrhagia. *Clinical Evidence*, London: BMJ Publishing Group, 2008. Online. Available: http://clinicalevidence.bmj.com

Guideline

National Institute for Health and Clinical Excellence. *Heavy Menstrual Bleeding.* Clinical Guideline 44, 2007. Available: www.nice.org.uk

● Menorrhagia is defined as regular bleeding with a loss of more than 80 ml of blood per month.

● Menorrhagia is suggested by a history of bleeding that cannot be controlled with tampons alone, and by having to get up during the night to change.

● Two thirds of women who have a blood loss of more than 80 ml per month have to limit normal activities and have anaemia.

● NICE prefers to define menorrhagia as excessive blood loss that interferes with a woman's quality of life.

● NICE also stresses that the presence of other menstrual symptoms will influence a woman's assessment of the severity of her blood loss.

● 50% of women referred for menorrhagia have depression or anxiety as their primary problem (DTB 1994a).

● One in 20 women aged 30–55 years consults her GP each year with menorrhagia (RCOG 1999).

CLINICAL ASSESSMENT

✳ Check that there is no intermenstrual or post-coital bleeding.

✳ Check that there are no other menstrual symptoms, such as pain or pelvic pressure, which might suggest an underlying pathology. For details of the diagnosis of menorrhagia see *Evidence-based Diagnosis in Primary Care* by A. F. Polmear (editor) published by Butterworth-Heinemann, 2008.

✳ Check that the patient has had a recent smear as offered by the current recall system.

✳ Ascertain the impact the bleeding is having on the patient's life.

✳ Do not perform a pelvic and abdominal examination unless the history suggests an underlying pathology.

✳ Check Hb; two thirds will be anaemic.

✳ Exclude hypothyroidism only if there are signs or symptoms.

* Consider haematological abnormalities, e.g. von Willebrand's disease or thrombocytopenia, especially in women who have a family history of easy bleeding or who have bled heavily since the menarche.
* Refer to a gynaecologist for assessment if:
  (a) the patient is over 45; or
  (b) there is suspicion of an organic cause (fibroids, pelvic pain, dyspareunia); or
  (c) there is any postcoital, intermenstrual, or irregular bleeding, or any sudden change in blood loss; or
  (d) medical treatment is unsuccessful.

TREATMENT

* *Levonorgestrel-releasing intrauterine system (LNG-IUS)(Mirena)).* This appears to be the most effective non-surgical treatment (National Institute for Health and Clinical Excellence 2007), and is licensed for the treatment of menorrhagia. The patient should be warned that irregular bleeding may occur in the first 6 months and that progestogen-type adverse effects are possible: breast tenderness, acne and headaches. A pelvic examination is needed before insertion.
* *Tranexamic acid.* Start on the first day of each cycle and continue until heavy bleeding has ceased. Tranexamic acid 1 g q.d.s decreases bleeding by up to 70% (National Institute for Health and Clinical Excellence 2007).
* *NSAIDs.* Give mefenamic acid 500 mg t.d.s or naproxen 500 mg b.d.. Taken shortly before or at the start of menstruation and continued during heavy loss, they can decrease bleeding by 20–50%. They are especially useful if there is dysmenorrhoea.
* *The combined oral contraceptive (COC)* is commonly used but there is insufficient evidence at present to adequately assess its effectiveness (National Institute for Health and Clinical Excellence 2007). It is especially useful if there is also dysmenorrhoea and if contraception is required.
* *Progestogens.* Give them in tablet form for 21 days of each cycle. Giving them for the second half of each cycle only is no better than placebo (Lethaby, Irvine and Cameron 2001). Alternatively they can be given by injection in the same way as for contraception.
* *IUD.* If an IUD is in situ either give an NSAID or an antifibrinolytic or change to a progestogen-releasing IUD.

* *Women not responding.* Consider referral for:
  (a) ultrasound to exclude endometrial polyps and other pathology such as fibroids. Also consider endometrial sampling in the patient over 40 years of age;
  (b) endometrial ablation or hysterectomy. Endometrial ablation has a shorter hospital stay, and less time off work but a proportion of women will have further bleeding and will require further surgery (Gannon, Holt, Fairbank, *et al.* 1991).

FLOODING

* Give norethisterone:
  (a) 15 mg b.d. for 2 days, then 10 mg b.d. for 2 days, then 15 mg once daily for 2 days, followed by 10 mg once daily for 14 days. The patient should expect a bleed 2–3 days after stopping the norethisterone; or
  (b) 20 mg b.d. for 5 days.

DELAYING A PERIOD

* Give norethisterone 5 mg b.d. or t.d.s 3 days prior to the expected period. If that fails, double the dose on the next occasion. Continue it until it is convenient to have the period. The next period can be expected 2–3 days after stopping norethisterone.

IRREGULAR PERIODS

TEENAGERS

* *Reassure* the patient that irregular periods are common after the menarche and that a regular cycle will probably establish itself without treatment.
* *If the patient is sufficiently bothered.* Give a progestogen cyclically, from day 10 to day 25 or day 1 to day 21, for 3 months. There is, however, no reason to think that this will speed up the establishment of normal periods.
* *COC* can be considered especially if contraception is required or they have dysmenorrhoea.
* *Very infrequent periods.* These girls need assessment (see page 328).

WOMEN IN THEIR REPRODUCTIVE YEARS

* Exclude pregnancy.
* Check whether irregular periods or amenorrhoea have always been a feature. They may have PCOS (see page 328).
* Check whether the irregularity is due to the progestogen-only pill (POP) (see page 356).
* Look for weight loss, excessive exercise (see page 514), recent stress, hirsutism, galactorrhoea or infertility (see page 369).
* Take blood for TFTs, prolactin, free androgen index, LH and FSH on day 2 of the cycle.
* If results are normal and the patient wishes to become pregnant consider referral for clomiphene.
* If the results are normal and pregnancy is not desired, COC or cyclical progestogens can be considered.
* If the results are abnormal, refer to an endocrinologist or gynaecologist as appropriate.

OLDER WOMEN

* Distinguish the irregularity due to ovarian failure from the pathological pattern of intermenstrual bleeding, which should be referred.
* Consider cyclical progestogens if the patient is sufficiently bothered.
* The COC will regulate bleeding and provide contraception. The known risks of thrombosis and breast carcinoma should be discussed with the patient and documented.
* HRT can be considered if there are other symptoms of the menopause and the bleeding is not pathological.

POSTMENOPAUSAL WOMEN

> **GUIDELINE**
>
> Scottish Intercollegiate Guidelines Network (SIGN). *Investigation of Postmenopausal Bleeding.* Available: www.sign.ac.uk

Postmenopausal bleeding is generally accepted as an episode of bleeding 12 months or more after the last period.

* Refer (to be seen within 2 weeks) if:
  (a) There has been more than one episode of bleeding or a single heavy episode;
  (b) Women on tamoxifen, especially if they have been on it for more than 5 years. There is a four-fold increase in incidence in endometrial cancer.
* Refer (to be seen within 4–6 weeks) any other women with postmenopausal bleeding. Ideally, perform a pelvic examination before referral as this may influence the referral.

For the management of bleeding in women taking HRT see page 336.

INTERMENSTRUAL BLEEDING (IMB)

* Examine:
  (a) for anaemia;
  (b) the pelvis for abnormalities with a bimanual examination;
  (c) the cervix for abnormalities, and take a smear and swabs;
  (d) the vulva and vagina.
* Take a pregnancy test if appropriate.
* Refer any patient with gynaecological pathology or with persistent IMB.
* *Premenstrual spotting.* Reassure the patient if the loss is light and premenstrual. It is probably due to failure of the corpus luteum, and should settle within a few cycles. Give cyclical progestogens, day 12–26 (i.e. in the luteal phase), to women sufficiently troubled by the symptoms.
* *Women on the COC:* check compliance. If the examination is normal and bleeding persists, consider changing the pill (see page 350).
* *Women with an IUD:*
  (a) Take endocervical swabs and a high vaginal swab (HVS).
  (b) If there is no infection, remove the IUD but remember to discuss alternative contraception.
  (c) Reassess in 3 months.

AMENORRHOEA

> **REVIEW**
>
> Clinical Knowledge Summaries. 2009. *Amenorrhoea.* Available: www.cks.nhs.uk/amenorrhoea

PRIMARY AMENORRHOEA

Girls aged 14–16 years

* Refer any girl aged 14 who has no breast development.
* Refer any girl whose breast development began more than 2 years ago and who has not yet menstruated.

Girls aged 16 and over

* Examine her for evidence of endocrine disorders and weight disturbance.
* Look at the external genitalia and secondary sexual characteristics, and check for an imperforate hymen (associated with cyclical pain).
* Refer to a gynaecologist.

SECONDARY AMENORRHOEA

Secondary amenorrhoea exists when a woman has not menstruated for 6 months, having had a previously established cycle.

* In the history, note particularly:
  (a) any weight loss (if the patient's weight is less than 45 kg and she is of average height she is unlikely to menstruate);
  (b) contraception. Amenorrhoea may occur with use of the levonorgestrel-releasing intrauterine system, with depot medroxyprogesterone, or following use of the COC;
  (c) excessive exercise (see page 514);
  (d) recent stress;
  (e) the character of the cycles prior to the amenorrhoea.
* Exclude pregnancy.
* Take blood for LH and FSH, free testosterone, prolactin, oestradiol and TFTs.
* Refer to a gynaecologist if:
  (a) the FSH is high (≥ 30 IU/l) and the patient is under the age of 45. This indicates premature ovarian failure; or
  (b) the free testosterone is raised or the LH level is > 10. This suggests polycystic ovary syndrome (see below); or

(c) the prolactin is over 800 mIU/l. This suggests a pituitary adenoma. Repeat the test if the level is between 400 and 800 mIU/l. Check for drugs that can cause hyperprolactinaemia, e.g. SSRIs; or
(d) the oestradiol is low.

POLYCYSTIC OVARY SYNDROME (PCOS)

GUIDELINES

RCOG. 2007. *Long-term Consequences of Polycystic Ovary Syndrome. Evidence-based Clinical Guideline.* RCOG, London. Available: www.rcog.org.uk (search on 'PCOS')

Rotterdam ESHRE/ASRM-sponsored PCOS Consensus Workshop Group. 2004. Revised 2003 consensus on diagnostic criteria and long-term health risks related to polycystic ovary syndrome. Fertil Steril 81, 19–25. Available: http://humrep.oxfordjournals.org/cgi/content/abstract/19/1/41

Anon. 2001. Tackling polycystic ovary syndrome. Drug Ther Bull 39, 1–5

* Polycystic ovary syndrome is a common problem affecting, according to ultrasound diagnosis, about 20% of women of reproductive age, only approximately half of whom have clinical or biochemical signs of anovulation or androgen excess.
* The characteristic features include:
  (a) truncal obesity;
  (b) oligomenorrhoea/amenorrhoea;
  (c) hirsutism;
  (d) acne;
  (e) raised serum free testosterone or free testosterone index;
  (f) raised luteinizing hormone.
* Patients with PCOS are twice as likely to develop diabetes (Wild, Pierpoint, Mckeigue, *et al.* 2000). By the age of 40, up to 40% will have type 2 diabetes (Lord, Flight and Norman 2003). They have a higher prevalence of features associated with metabolic syndrome; hypertension, dyslipidaemia, visceral obesity, insulin resistance and hyperinsulinaemia.

DIAGNOSIS

Consider the diagnosis if two of the following three criteria are met:

(a) Polycystic ovaries on USS (either 12 or more follicles in at least one ovary or increased ovarian volume ($> 10 \, \text{cm}^3$).

(b) Oligo- or anovulation: as suggested by menstrual cycles longer than 35 days or < 10 periods a year.

(c) Clinical and/or biochemical signs of hyperandrogenism. Clinical signs include acne, hirsutism and androgenic alopecia. The biochemical confirmation required is a raised free testosterone. A raised LH/FSH ratio is no longer considered useful in the diagnosis because of its inconsistency.

* Exclude adrenal hyperplasia, hyperprolactinaemia, androgen secreting tumours and Cushing's syndrome. If the latter is suspected on clinical grounds refer to an endocrinologist.
* Check TFTs, serum prolactin and free testosterone. If there is clinical evidence of hyperandrogenism and the total testosterone is greater than 5 nmol/l check the level of 17-hydroxyprogesterone.
* If one of the criteria above is met but not the other, order a pelvic USS for ovarian cysts.

MANAGEMENT

* Explain what little is known about the syndrome: that the ovaries produce excess female hormone (LH) which stimulates the ovary to produce excess testosterone which, in turn, causes acne and hirsutism. Associated with this is a tendency to insulin resistance, manifested by overweight and the development of diabetes.
* *CVD risk.* Check the serum lipids and the fasting sugar, or the fasting and 2 hour sugars if obese (BMI $> 30 \, \text{kg/m}^2$ or $> 25 \, \text{kg/m}^2$ in South Asian women, in whom insulin resistance is more common). Cardiovascular risk calculators have not been validated in PCOS. Hypertension should be treated but lipid lowering agents should only be introduced by a specialist.
* *Diabetes.* Screen all women with PCOS on an annual basis for diabetes. If the fasting glucose is borderline ($> 5.5 \, \text{mmol/l}$) and the body mass is greater than 30 arrange a glucose tolerance test.
* *Snoring.* Ask about snoring and sleep apnoea. PCOS appears to be a risk factor independently of BMI in sleep apnoea.
* *Weight.* Advise about weight loss through diet (especially low GI see page 507) and exercise. Loss of weight has been reported to result in resumption of ovulation, improvement in fertility, increased SHBG and reduced levels of insulin.

Management of symptoms

* *Acne*; see page 567.
* *Hirsutism* see page 244. First-line treatment is with a combination of cyproterone acetate and ethinylestradiol (as Dianette) although a desogestrel-containing COC may be as effective. Second-line treatments are spironolactone or finasteride. Contraception is required as they carry the theoretical risk of feminizing a male fetus (Farquhar, Lee, Toomath, *et al.* 2000). Warn that benefit is unlikely before about 6 months of any of these treatments.
* *Lack of regular periods.* This may predispose to endometrial hyperplasia and later carcinoma. The Royal College of Gynaecologists (UK) recommends that a withdrawal bleed should be induced every 3–4 months with progestogens (for at least 12 days) or the COC. Women who do not have withdrawal bleeds should be referred to a gynaecologist.
* *Lack of ovulation.* Refer to a gynaecologist. Metformin 500 mg t.d.s., although unlicensed for this use, can induce ovulation, as well as reducing fasting insulin concentrations, blood pressure and LDL-cholesterol. However, the Royal College of Gynaecologists (UK) states that 'long term use of insulin sensitising agents cannot as yet be recommended'. Patients are increasingly aware and ask for metformin treatment but this is ahead of the evidence and outside the product licence (Harborne, Fleming, Lyall, *et al.* 2003).
* *Infertility.* Refer. A combination of metformin and clomifene is more effective than either alone. Both laparoscopic electrocautery and ovarian drilling have been shown to have long-term benefits in ovulation and normalization of serum androgens.

VAGINAL DISCHARGE

For details of the diagnosis of vaginal discharge see *Evidence-based Diagnosis in Primary Care* by A. F. Polmear (editor), published by Butterworth-Heinemann, 2008.

REVIEW

Spence D, Melville C. 2007. Vaginal discharge. BMJ 335, 1147–1151

Guideline

FFPRHC and BASHH Guidance. 2006. The management of women of reproductive age attending non-genitourinary medicine settings complaining of vaginal discharge. J Fam Plann Reprod Health Care 32, 33–42

* Ask about the type of discharge, the timing, whether it smells, whether it itches and whether there is pelvic pain.
* Ask the woman what she thinks it is and, when asking whether it seems related to sexual activity, ask tactfully about the number of sexual partners.
* Examine the vulva and test the vaginal pH using narrow range pH paper. There are no grounds for a *routine* bimanual or speculum examination nor for a swab. However, bimanual examination is needed if the history raises the possibility of pelvic infection; swabs are needed in those at high risk of sexually transmitted infections, and in those in whom the clinical picture does not suggest bacterial vaginosis or candida.

Interpretation of findings:

■ Smelly white discharge with pH > 4.5: **bacterial vaginosis.**
■ White curdy discharge, usually with vulval soreness and itch, erythema, and possibly fissuring and satellite lesions; pH > 4.5: **candidiasis.**
■ Smelly yellow or green frothy discharge with pH < 4.5, perhaps with dysuria: **trichomonas.**

When the clinical picture is not typical of bacterial vaginosis nor of candidiasis, or the patient is under age 25 or has had a new sexual partner in the last year, take 'triple swabs':

■ HVS for *Trichomonas*, the clue cells of bacterial vaginosis, and *Candida*.
■ Endocervical swab in transport medium for gonorrhoea.
■ Endocervical swab for a chlamydial DNA amplification test.

Patients with sexually transmitted infections are best managed in the GUM clinic (see page 71).

MANAGEMENT: CANDIDA

GUIDELINE

Clinical Effectiveness Group (Association for Genitourinary Medicine and Medical Society for the study of Venereal Disease). 2007. *Management of Vulvovaginal Candidiasis.* Available: www.bashh.org (choose 'Guidelines').

* Give general advice to avoid local irritants, and avoid tight fitting synthetic clothing (Bingham 1999).
* Treat only if symptomatic.
* Prescribe a topical imidazole. Cure rates are 80–95%. Give it either as a single dose or as a short course at night, usually for 3 nights. Oral imidazoles are no more effective (Watson, Grimshaw, Bond, *et al.* 2002) but they have more side-effects. In addition, they are contraindicated in pregnancy.
* *Male partners.* There is no evidence to support the treatment of asymptomatic male sexual partners (Bisschop, Merkus, Scheyground, *et al.* 1986).
* *COC.* Do not stop the COC. Its use is not associated with candidiasis.
* *Pregnancy.* Asymptomatic colonization is more common in pregnancy (30–40%). Treat symptomatic patients with topical azoles, but a longer course may be necessary.

RECURRENT CANDIDIASIS (≥ 4 SYMPTOMATIC EPISODES PER YEAR)

* Check the urine for glucose approximately 2 hours after a meal or glucose load. Note that this would be inadequate as a screening test for diabetes in any other situation.

* Exclude other risk factors; iron deficiency anaemia, thyroid disease, frequent antibiotic use, corticosteroid use, immunodeficiency.
* Screen for other vaginal infections.
* Give either:
  (a) an imidazole pessary daily for 2 weeks then weekly for 6 months; or use a pessary only when an infection is most likely, e.g. after intercourse or when taking a broad-spectrum antibiotic. These treatment regimens are empirical and are not based on randomized controlled trials; or
  (b) fluconazole 150 mg orally every 3 days for three doses then weekly for 6 months. Approximately 90% of women remain disease free at 1 year. If there is relapse between doses consider giving twice weekly fluconazole 150 mg.
* Consider giving certirizine 10 mg daily for 6 months or zafirlucast 20 mg b.d. for 6 months. Allergy may be an important component especially in women with atopy.
* *Candida of the gut.* There is no evidence to suggest that eradication of candida from the gut is helpful.
* *Probiotics/Lactobacillus.* Evidence does not support the use of oral or topical *Lactobacillus* in prevention of vulvovaginal candidiasis.
* *Alteration of vaginal pH.* Suggest a trial of a pH lowering agent, e.g. AciGel.

MANAGEMENT: BACTERIAL VAGINOSIS

GUIDELINE

Clinical Effectiveness Group of the Association for Genitourinary Medicine and the Medical Society for the Study of Venereal Diseases. 2001. *National Guideline for the Management of Bacterial Vaginosis.* Available: www.bashh.org.uk. (choose 'Guidelines').

Systematic review

Joesoef M, Schmid G. 2004. Bacterial vaginosis. *Clinical Evidence* BMJ Publishing Group, London. Available: www.clinicalevidence.com
    Association of Medical Microbiologists. *Management of Abnormal Vaginal Discharge in Women - Quick Reference Guide.* http://www.hpa.org.uk (search for 'Vaginal discharge')

* Bacterial vaginosis is characterized by a reduction in lactobacilli and an overgrowth of predominantly anaerobic organisms (*Gardnerella vaginalis, Mycoplasma hominis, Prevotella* species, *Mobiluncus* species).
* Approximately 50% of women with the condition are asymptomatic.
* It is not regarded as sexually transmitted. It can arise and remit spontaneously in women regardless of sexual activity. However, it is more common in women liable to sexually transmitted infections.
* *Partners.* No evidence has been found supporting the treatment of partners of women affected by bacterial vaginosis (Potter 1999).
* Treatment is indicated for:
  (a) symptomatic women;
  (b) pregnant women with a history of recurrent miscarriage;
  (c) women undergoing termination of pregnancy. They are at greater risk of pelvic inflammatory disease if the bacterial vaginosis is untreated.
* Give metronidazole 400–500 mg b.d. for 5–7 days; or intravaginal metronidazole gel (0.75%) once daily for 5 days; or metronidazole 2 g as a single oral dose: or intravaginal clindamycin cream (2%) once daily for 7 days. The cure rate is 70–80%.
* *Pregnancy and lactation.* Symptomatic women in pregnancy should be treated with metronidazole. Lactating women should be treated with intravaginal metronidazole.

PELVIC INFLAMMATORY DISEASE (PID)

GUIDELINE

RCOG. *Management of Acute Pelvic Inflammatory Disease. Evidence-based Clinical Guideline.* London: RCOG, 2009. www.rcog.org.uk (search on 'Acute pelvic inflammatory disease').

Systematic review

Ross J. 2005. Pelvic inflammatory disease. *Clinical Evidence.* BMJ Publishing Group, London. Available: www.clinicalevidence.com

- PID is usually the result of ascending infection from the endocervix. *Neisseria gonorrhoeae* and *Chlamydia trachomatis* have been identified as causative agents, whilst *Mycoplasma genitalium*, anaerobes and other organisms commonly found in the vagina may also be implicated.
- PID has a high morbidity; about 20% of affected women become infertile, 20% develop chronic pelvic pain, and 10% of those who conceive have an ectopic pregnancy (Metters, Catchpole, Smith, *et al.* 1998).
- Repeated episodes of PID are associated with a four- to six-fold increase in the risk of permanent tubal damage (Hills, Owens, Marchbanks, *et al.* 1997).
- PID may be asymptomatic.
- 10–20% of women with PID will develop perihepatitis.
- A delay of only a few days in receiving treatment markedly increases the risk of long-term sequelae (Hills, Joesoef, Marchbanks, *et al.* 1993). Because of this, and the lack of definitive diagnostic criteria, a low threshold for the empirical treatment of PID is recommended.

DIAGNOSIS

- Symptoms can include fever, lower abdominal pain, deep dyspareunia, abnormal bleeding, abnormal vaginal or cervical discharge. On examination there may be cervical excitation and adnexial tenderness.
- Clinical diagnosis is correct in only 65–90% of cases compared to laparoscopy. Even laparoscopy can miss mild cases but it remains the most reliable investigation. In the UK it is not recommended in all cases but should be performed when there is diagnostic doubt.
- * If not referring, perform the following:
  - (a) endocervical swabs for gonococcus and chlamydia. Negative microbiological tests do not exclude a diagnosis of PID; in at least 50% of cases no specific organism is identified. Screen for the same diseases in any sexual partners;
  - (b) urinalysis, pregnancy test, and MSU specimen to look for other causes of lower abdominal pain;

- (c) blood for ESR or C-reactive protein. A raised level would support the diagnosis (Miettinen, Heinonen, Laippala, *et al.* 1993).
- * Recommend rest and provide adequate analgesia.
- * Recommend that unprotected intercourse be avoided until the woman and her partner(s) have completed treatment and follow up. If it is not possible to screen for gonorrhoea and chlamydia in the sexual partner(s) give empirical treatment for both gonorrhoea and chlamydia (Haddon, Heason, Fay, *et al.* 1998; Groom, Stewart, Kruger, *et al.* 2001).
- * If an IUD is in situ, and this is the preferred method of contraception, leave it in place. Remove it only if the condition fails to respond to treatment and other causes of pain have been excluded (Teisala 1989; Larsson and Wennergren 1981; Soderberg and Lingren 1981).
- * Drug treatment.
  - (a) ofloxacin 400 mg b.d plus metronidazole 400 mg b.d. for 14 days; or
  - (b) in women at high risk of gonococcal infection: ceftriaxone 250 mg i.m. as a single dose then 14 days of oral doxycycline 100 mg b.d. and metronidazole 400 mg b.d.
- * Review daily in case admission becomes necessary.

ADMISSION

Admit patients if:
- (a) the illness is severe;
- (b) not responding after 3 days of oral therapy;
- (c) unable to tolerate oral drugs;
- (d) a pelvic mass is present;
- (e) the patient is pregnant;
- (f) there is diagnostic uncertainty;
- (g) the patient suffers from immunodeficiency;
- (h) the patient is above the usual age for PID. An alternative diagnosis, e.g. ovarian carcinoma, is more likely.

FOLLOW-UP FOR ALL PATIENTS

- * Review within 72 hours. Refer if there is little improvement.
- * Review again in 4 weeks to ensure:
  - (a) there is adequate clinical response;
  - (b) there was compliance with the antibiotics;

(c) to trace, investigate and treat the woman's partner(s) if an STD is diagnosed (Robinson and Kell 1995). One study of women with acute salpingitis found that 30 out of 34 male contacts had urethritis (Kinghorn, Duerden and Hafiz 1986). Another study found that 60% of contacts had relevant infections, and that in most of these it was asymptomatic (Kamwendo, Johansson, Moi, *et al.* 1993). Consider referral to a GUM clinic for contact tracing;

(d) to stress the significance of the disease and the sequelae.

* Discuss with the patient her need for safer sex.
* Advise the patient to ask for antibiotic cover (e.g. doxycycline 200 mg stat or metronidazole 2 g stat) if she ever needs a termination of pregnancy (TOP) or a dilatation and curettage (D&C).
* Advise the patient to seek advice promptly if the symptoms return.

PATIENT INFORMATION

Download the RCOG leaflet 'Acute pelvic inflammatory disease' available on the RCOG web site, www.rcog. org.uk (search on 'Acute pelvic inflammatory disease')

PREMENSTRUAL SYNDROME

SYSTEMATIC REVIEW

Kwan I, Onwude JL. 2006. Premenstrual syndrome. *Clinical Evidence*. BMJ Publishing Group, London. www.clinicalevidence.com

---

* 95% of women have symptoms related to their menstrual cycle; in 5% they are disabling. More than 150 symptoms have been reported.
* Diagnosis depends not on the type of symptom, but on the timing of the symptoms and their cyclicity. Symptoms present 1–14 days prior to menstruation and disappear at the onset or by the day of the heaviest flow. If behavioural symptoms persist throughout the cycle then consider a psychological/psychiatric disorder.
* Ask the patient to keep a menstrual and symptom diary for at least 2 months. She can score symptoms according to their severity.

* Listen sympathetically. It is a real entity. This alone can be therapeutic.
* Give simple advice:

   (a) *Dietary advice.* Explain that some women seem more sensitive to blood sugar changes at this time of the cycle, and this may be the cause of food cravings, panic reactions, irritability and aggression. Advise patients to reduce their refined sugar intake as well as their caffeine intake. Small frequent carbohydrate snacks seem effective in about 30% of women.

   (b) *Stress management.* Explain that although it is not the cause of the syndrome, stress is harder to cope with during the premenstrual period. Relaxation methods, yoga, meditation and exercise can be of benefit.

THERAPEUTIC OPTIONS

* *SSRI.* Consider using an SSRI. There is good evidence of their efficacy (Wyatt, Dimmock and O'Brien 2002) and they may be effective if used in the luteal phase alone. Side-effects may limit their acceptability.
* *Breast tenderness, bloating and irritability* may be improved by taking spironolactone 100 mg daily from day 12 until the onset of menstruation.
* *NSAIDs* given for 7 days prior to menses and 4 days after the onset, have been shown to improve a number of symptoms but not breast tenderness.
* *Aerobic exercise.* 45 minutes of low and moderate exercise (50–70% of maximum) three times a week has been shown to reduce symptoms.
* *Oestrogens* may improve or in some cases worsen the situation. The COC can prove helpful, especially in those women requiring contraception. Women who experience symptoms during their pill-free week can take three consecutive packets back-to-back. A lower dose of oestrogen, as HRT, may help some women but cyclical progestogens must also be used in women with an intact uterus.
* *Danazol* has been shown to be effective. Adverse effects are common (masculinization and weight gain) with continuous use but may not occur with luteal phase use alone.
* *Vitamin B$_6$ (pyridoxine)* 50–100 mg daily. This recommendation is based on limited

information from poor quality trials, but the evidence suggests that B_6 may be of benefit.

* *Breast tenderness.* Consider bromocriptine 1.25 mg b.d. but adverse effects are common.

Note: Progestogens have been found unhelpful in the treatment of PMS.

Note: Evening primrose oil. There is no evidence that it is helpful in PMS.

PATIENTS NOT RESPONDING

* Refer to a gynaecologist for the consideration of suppression of ovarian function. Treatment options include high-dose danazol, high-dose oestrogen, gonadotrophin-releasing hormone analogues with add-back HRT.

PATIENT SUPPORT

National Association for Premenstrual Syndrome (NAPS), www.pms.org.uk
Premenstrual Society, PO Box 429, Addlestone, Surrey KT15 1DZ, helpline 01932 872560 (11 am–6 pm, weekdays only)

OVARIAN CANCER SCREENING

* The analysis of the first stage of the UK Collaborative Trial of Ovarian Cancer Screening (UKCTOCS) trial showed an 89% detection rate using CA125 levels and a 75% detection rate using transvaginal ultrasound. With the latter there was high number of false positives. The value of a National Screening programme will not be known until 2015.

* Many women will request screening for ovarian cancer on the basis of their family history. Some useful figures can be used to reassure many women (see Table 11.1).

Table 11.1   Ovarian cancer risk

NUMBER OF FIRST DEGREE RELATIVES WITH OVARIAN CANCER	LIFETIME RISK OF DEVELOPING OVARIAN CANCER
0	1%
1	5%
2	15%
> 2	? 50%

* Women at 'higher risk' may be eligible for screening and genetic testing and if they fall into one of the following groups, may be referred to the UK Familial Ovarian Cancer Screening Study (UKFOCSS) or for genetic testing by the local genetics service. Women at 'higher risk' are those with:

(a) two or more first degree relatives with ovarian cancer; or

(b) one first degree relative with ovarian cancer and one first degree relative with breast cancer diagnosed under 50 years of age; or

(c) one ovarian cancer and two breast cancers diagnosed under 60 years in first degree relatives;

(d) known BRCA-1 or BRCA-2 mutations in the family; or

(e) three colorectal cancers, at least one diagnosed under 50 years of age, and one ovarian cancer, all first degree relatives of each other.

(f) affected relatives with any of the above combinations, who are related by second degree through an unaffected male and there is an affected sister (i.e. paternal transmission is occurring).

Note: A first degree relative is a parent, sibling or child. A second degree relative is a grand-parent, aunt or uncle or cousin.

Weak family history. Women with one close relative with epithelial ovarian cancer diagnosed before the age of 50 may also wish to be referred for advice but may not be offered regular screening.

PATIENT INFORMATION

'Ovarian cancer screening'. www.cancerhelp.org.uk

GESTATIONAL TROPHOBLASTIC DISEASE: HYDATIDIFORM MOLE AND CHORIOCARCINOMA

RCOG. 2004. *The Management of Gestational Trophoblastic Neoplasia.* Guideline No. 38. Royal College of Obstetricians and Gynaecologists, London. Available from www.rcog.org.uk (search on 'gestational trophoblastic neoplasia')

- Gestational trophoblastic disease is uncommon in the UK, with a calculated incidence of 1/714 live births. The incidence is highest in women from Asia (incidence 1/387) compared to non-Asian women (incidence 1/752).
- In the UK there is an effective registration and treatment programme with high cure rates.
- Once the diagnosis of hydatidiform mole has been made, follow-up will be needed for between 6 months and 2 years. The aim is to detect the occurrence of choriocarcinoma.
- Once treated, serum estimations of levels of human chorionic gonadotrophin (HCG) levels should be performed according to protocols from the regional expert units (London, Sheffield and Dundee).
- The combined oral contraceptive pill and hormone replacement are safe to use once HCG levels have reverted to normal.
- Women should be advised not to conceive until the HCG level has been normal for 6 months or follow-up has been completed (whichever is the sooner). The risk of further recurrence is 1 in 55. After any further pregnancy, urine and blood samples should be taken to exclude disease recurrence.
- Women who undergo chemotherapy should not attempt to conceive until a year after completion of treatment.

* Refer all women with persistent bleeding:
  (a) after the evacuation of retained products of conception;
  (b) after normal pregnancy;
  (c) after miscarriage.
* Send for histology any products of conception passed at home.
* If no products of conception are available, check HCG 4 weeks after the loss of the pregnancy.

PATIENT INFORMATION

The Hydatidiform Mole and Choriocarcinoma UK information service, www.hmole-chorio.org.uk

SCREENING CENTRES

Trophoblastic Tumour Screening and Treatment Centre. Department of Oncology, Charing Cross Hospital, Fulham Palace Road, London W6 8RF. Tel. 020 8846 1409, fax 020 8748 5665

Trophoblastic Tumour Screening and Treatment Centre. Weston Park Hospital, Whitham Road, Sheffield S10 2SJ. Tel. 0114 226 5202. Fax. 0114 226 5511

Hydatiform Mole Follow-up (Scotland) Department of Obstetrics and Gynaecology, Ninewells Hospital, Dundee DD1 9SY. Tel. 01382 632748. Fax. 01382 632096

THE MENOPAUSE

ESTABLISHING THE DIAGNOSIS

No investigations are routinely indicated. FSH levels fluctuate markedly during the perimenopause and so are of limited value in symptomatic women, in whom a clinical history can form the basis of diagnosis. There is little place for LH, oestradiol and progesterone estimation in clinical practice (Hope, Rees and Brockie 1999).

* Consider taking serial FSH measurements in the following circumstances:
  (a) Women with symptoms under the age of 40 because of the implications of premature ovarian failure.
  (b) Women with symptoms who have had a hysterectomy with ovarian conservation. They are at risk of an early menopause.
* Take FSH levels:
  (a) 4–8 weeks apart when the woman is not on HRT or hormonal contraception. FSH levels of greater than 30 IU/l are generally considered to be in the postmenopausal range.
  (b) On day 2 or 3 of menses in women with menstrual bleeding; a FSH level of 10–12 IU/l, is considered to be raised (American Association of Clinical Endocrinologists 1999).
* *Abnormal bleeding.* Refer women, without starting HRT, if they give a history of abnormal bleeding, e.g. sudden change in menstrual pattern, intermenstrual bleeding, postcoital bleeding or a postmenopausal bleed (Hope, Rees and Brockie 1999; Korhonen, Symons, Hyde, *et al.* 1997).

INITIAL MANAGEMENT

* Counsel women about the menopause. Ideally, all perimenopausal women should be given the opportunity to discuss the menopause, with particular reference to the symptomatology,

common misconceptions and treatment options.

* Take the opportunity to discuss lifestyle issues (smoking cessation, diet and exercise). Hormone replacement therapy (HRT) is no longer recommended as a general prophylactic measure because, above all, of the increased risk of breast cancer, but individual women may judge that, for them, the benefit outweighs the risks (see below).

* *Osteoporosis.* Identify those patients at high risk of osteoporosis and investigate and treat, if appropriate (see page 278). HRT is no longer indicated for the prevention of osteoporosis, except in those with an early menopause.

* *Vasomotor symptoms.*

   (a) *HRT* is extremely effective in controlling these symptoms (MacLennan, Lester and Moore 2001). Because of the possible harms, use the lowest effective dose for the shortest time possible, see below.

   (b) *Progestogens.* A trial of megestrol 20 mg b.d. for 4 weeks found that 74% of patients given megestrol had a decrease of 50% or more in the frequency of hot flashes, compared to 20% on placebo (Loprinzi, Michalak, Quella, *et al.* 2003). A withdrawal bleed is likely on cessation of treatment.

   (c) *SSRIs and related drugs.* A meta-analysis has found some evidence of benefit, with paroxetine performing best. However, even paroxetine reduced flushes by only one or two a day compared to placebo (Nelson, Vesco, Haney, *et al.* 2006).

   (d) *Gabapentin.* A trial of 12 weeks of 900 mg/day reduced the hot flash composite score by 54% against 31% with placebo (Guttuso, Kurlan, McDermott, *et al.* 2003).

   (e) *Diet.* Discuss the limited evidence that suggests that phytoestrogens may be helpful in relieving vasomotor symptoms (Scambia, Mango, Signorile, *et al.* 2000; Anon. 1998). They are plant substances, found in soya beans, chickpeas, red clover and cereals, that stimulate the oestrogen receptors.

   (f) *Consider clonidine* for those unable to take HRT or an SSRI (Edington and Chagnon 1980; Nagamani, Kelver and Smith 1987).

   (g) *Black cohosh*, with or without other natural remedies has been shown to be ineffective (Newton, Reed, LaCroix, *et al.* 2006).

* *Vaginal dryness.* Treatment options include:

   (a) HRT (see below).

   (b) local oestrogens. These can be given per vaginum daily until symptoms have ceased, then twice weekly for 3–6 months. There is some systemic absorption of the oestrogen and therefore if used long-term oral progestogen should be taken for 10 days of each month (Loprinzi, Michalak, Quella, *et al.* 2003).

   (c) vaginal lubricants. These include KY jelly, Replens (a non-hormonal aqueous moisturizer) and Senselle (a water-based lubricant), although the latter two are not available on the NHS.

* *Urinary symptoms.*

   (a) Symptoms related to urogenital atrophy will respond to oestrogen by any route. Maximum benefit will not be seen for at least the first month, and may take up to a year (Cardozo, Bachmann, McClish, *et al.* 1998).

   (b) Stress incontinence is unlikely to respond to oestrogen replacement therapy alone. Refer patients who are sufficiently troubled to a gynaecologist.

* *Psychological symptoms.* Psychological symptoms may relate to a woman's hormonal status but, equally, the menopause may become a 'scapegoat' for patients with underlying emotional problems (Hunter 1996). Counselling may be helpful, but many will improve when their physical symptoms improve (Gath and Iles 1990). Depression may need treatment in its own right.

HORMONE REPLACEMENT THERAPY (HRT)

REVIEW AND RECOMMENDATIONS

Medicines and Healthcare Products Regulatory Agency/Commission on Human Medicines (MHRA/CHM). 2007. Drug Safety Update 1 (2), 2–6 available: www.mhra.gov.uk

HRT may be indicated in the following:

- Women with an early menopause (before age 45) mainly for the prevention of osteoporosis. It may also give some protection in this young age group against cardiovascular disease. It is usually given until age 50.
- Women under the age of 65 with severe vasomotor and other symptoms of the menopause who understand the risks and are prepared to take HRT for a limited period. Analysis of the Women's Health Initiative results has shown no increase in breast cancer, myocardial infarction or stroke in women < 60 years old who use HRT for 5 years or less (Rossouw, Prentice, Manson, et al. 2007).
- * Record that the risks of HRT have been explained and an informed decision taken by the patient.
- * Review the decision at least annually.

BENEFITS AND RISKS
Benefits

- *Symptom relief.* Improvement in vasomotor symptoms occurs in a few weeks, and in vaginal symptoms in 3 months. Improvement in mental function is less certain. The mental health of women with vasomotor symptoms seems to improve on HRT but those without vasomotor symptoms worsen, with poorer physical functioning and lower energy levels compared to those on placebo (Hlatky, Boothroyd, Vittinghoff, et al. 2002). Overall, HRT does not improve the quality of life (Hays, Ockene, Brunner, et al. 2003).
- *Osteoporosis.* Combined HRT protects against hip fracture in unselected postmenopausal women [RR 0.66 (95%CI 0.45 to 0.98)] and reduces the risk of all fractures [RR 0.76 (95%CI 0.69 to 0.85)]. This represents five fewer hip fractures per 10,000 person years, an NNT of 2000 for 1 year (Rossouw, Anderson, Prentice, et al. 2002). In women at high risk of fracture the absolute benefit will be greater. The benefit is dose related (see Table 11.2). However, the benefit on fracture risk is lost within 3 years of stopping HRT (Heiss, Wallace, Anderson, et al. 2008).

Table 11.2   Minimum doses of oestrogen needed for bone conservation

DRUG	DOSAGE	FREQUENCY
Oestradiol	1–2 mg	Daily*
Oral conjugated equine oestrogens	0.625 mg	Daily
Transdermal oestradiol patch	50 mg	Daily
Oestradiol gel	1.5 g (two measures)	Daily
Oestradiol implants	50 mg	6 monthly

*Although 1 mg or 2 mg oral oestradiol can be used for prevention of osteoporosis, the bone protective effect is dose related. Some products are licensed for osteoporosis prevention at 2 mg only, while others are licensed at 1 mg and 2 mg.

- *Prevention of carcinoma of the colon.* HRT appears to reduce the risk of developing colonic carcinoma by 20% (RR 0.80 95%CI 0.74 to 0.86) (Nelson, Humphrey, Nygren, et al. 2002).

Harms

- *Cardiovascular disease.* The use of combined HRT in healthy postmenopausal women is associated with an increase in coronary heart disease [RR 1.29 (95%CI 1.02 to 1.63)] and in stroke [RR 1.41 (95%CI 1.07 to 1.85)] (Rossouw, Anderson, Prentice, et al. 2002). The risk is greater in women on combined HRT more than 10 years after the menopause.
- *Breast cancer.* The use of combined HRT in healthy postmenopausal women is associated with an increase in breast cancer risk [RR 1.24 (95%CI 1.01 to 1.54)] (Rossouw, Anderson, Prentice, et al. 2002). If women who did not take the medication were excluded, the relative risk rose to 1.49. For more detail see the box below.
- *Endometrial cancer.* Unopposed oestrogen is associated with an extra five cases per 1000 women over 5 years. The use of combined preparations reduces, but does not eliminate, this risk with an estimated risk of two extra cases per 1000 women over 10 years.
- *Ovarian cancer.* Long-term combined or oestrogen-only HRT is associated with a small increased risk of ovarian cancer. This excess risk disappears within a few years of stopping HRT.
- *Venous thromboembolism (VTE).* The incidence of VTE in postmenopausal women is about double

TYPE OF HRT	AGE	BASELINE RISK PER 1000 WOMEN OVER 5 YEARS	ADDITIONAL CASES PER 1000 WOMEN USING HRT FOR 5 YEARS	ADDITIONAL CASES PER 1000 WOMEN USING HRT FOR 10 YEARS
Oestrogen–only (post hysterectomy)	< 60	42	5	12
	60–69	82	6	17
Combined HRT	< 60	37	14	40
	60–69	70	22	64

Table 11.3   Major risks and benefits of HRT

Risks are from cancers of breast, endometrium and ovary, from venous thromboembolism, heart disease and stroke. Benefits are the reduction in fracture of the femur and colorectal cancer. The benefits are subtracted from the risks to give the figures above. Adapted from: MHRA. UK Public Assessment Report. Hormone-replacement therapy: safety update. September 2007.

that of premenopausal women and the risk increases with age. In women on HRT this risk is further increased with a hazard ratio of 2.1 (95%CI 1.39 to 3.25) (Rossouw, Anderson, Prentice, *et al.* 2002). The highest risk occurs in the first 6 months to a year of use. This means that, in women aged 50–60 HRT will cause an extra four cases for every 1000 women using HRT for 5 years. The risk may be less in women using a patch than in those on oral HRT (RCOG 2004).

- *Dementia.* Combined HRT appears to double the risk of dementia, although it has no effect on the number of women developing mild cognitive impairment (Shumaker, Legault, Rapp, *et al.* 2003).

- From the Women's Health Initiative it is possible to calculate that, overall, HRT is associated with 19 excess serious adverse events per 10,000 women years of use. This risk is greater the longer the period of use and the greater the age of the user (see Table 11.3).

FACTS ABOUT HRT AND BREAST CANCER

HRT increases the risk of breast cancer, starting from the end of the third year (Rossouw, Anderson, Prentice, *et al.* 2002). The risk reverts to normal 1 year after stopping HRT (Beral, Million Women Study Collaborators 2003).

The exact risk depends on the type of HRT. With combined HRT (oestrogen and progestogen) it is double [HR 2.0 (95%CI 1.88 to 2.12)] while with unopposed oestrogen it is increased by a third (HR 1.30 (1.21 to 1.40)) and with tibolone it is increased by almost a half (HR 1.45 (1.25 to 1.68)) (Rossouw, Anderson, Prentice, *et al.* 2002).

Overall, this gives a number needed to harm of 167 over 5.6 years, which is a rate of six additional breast cancers per 1000 women over that period (Rossouw, Anderson, Prentice, *et al.* 2002).

Risk increases with duration of use, so that, after 10 years, combined HRT is associated with 19 extra breast cancers per 1000 women (Beral, Million Women Study Collaborators 2003). With unopposed oestrogen the risk is five extra, and with tibolone six extra cancers per 1000 women over 10 years use.

Contrary to previous information from observational studies, breast cancers in women on HRT are larger and at a more advanced stage than those in women on placebo (Rossouw, Anderson, Prentice, *et al.* 2002).

OTHER ISSUES TO DISCUSS

Explain that taking HRT means that cyclical bleeding will return if the woman has an intact uterus and a cyclical preparation is used. Irregular bleeding is common with continuous preparations.

Explain that evidence from randomized trials suggests that HRT does not cause extra weight gain in addition to that normally gained at the time of the menopause (Norman, Flight and Rees 2001).

Contraindications

Oestrogen replacement therapy is absolutely contraindicated in very few patients. Even in women in whom treatment appears contraindicated, oestrogen therapy may be prescribed under supervision of a specialist menopause clinic if the woman's symptoms are particularly severe (Rees and Purdie 1999).

Absolute contraindications include:

(a) acute-phase myocardial infarction, pulmonary embolism or deep vein thrombosis (DVT);

(b) active endometrial or breast cancer;

(c) pregnancy;

(d) undiagnosed breast mass;

(e) uninvestigated abnormal vaginal bleeding;

(f) severe active liver disease.

Note: Many contraindications given in prescribing data sheets are derived from high-dose combined oral contraceptives, and are, in the view of most experts, not applicable to HRT (Rees and Purdie 1999).

HRT use in women with comorbidity (relative contraindications)

(a) *History of thromboembolic disease.* Women with a personal or family history of thromboembolism should be offered screening for thrombophilia before starting (see page 640). Those with a personal history of VTE should not take HRT unless the woman decides that, for her, the benefits outweigh the risks (RCOG 2004). She may choose prophylactic anticoagulation, though that has its own risks. A transdermal route may reduce the risk of VTE. A specialist opinion would be wise in those with thrombophilia.

(b) *Past history of endometrial cancer.* Refer women who want to consider HRT to the appropriate specialist. Although conventional advice is that oestrogens are contraindicated, small studies of endometrial cancer survivors have not shown an adverse effect on survival.

(c) *Diabetes and gall bladder disease.* Use a transdermal preparation.

(d) *Liver disease.* Refer to a specialist clinic.

(e) *Endometriosis.* Refer to a specialist clinic.

(f) *Fibroids.* HRT may enlarge fibroids, causing heavy or painful withdrawal bleeds. Warn patients to report pain or pressure effects on the bladder or bowel.

(g) *Migraine* is not a contraindication to HRT. There is no evidence that the risk of stroke is increased by the use of HRT in women with migraine (Bousser, Conard, Kittner, *et al.* 2000).

(h) *Hypertension.* There is no evidence that HRT raises blood pressure (Rees and Purdie 1999).

INITIAL ASSESSMENT

* Take a history and assess the woman's menopausal status.

* Check for contraindications to HRT therapy: especially risk factors for cardiovascular disease and a history of breast cancer or venous thromboembolism.

* Check BP, BMI and serum lipids.

* Advise the woman about breast awareness. Check that mammography screening is in place if over 50 years. Mammography is not needed before commencing HRT unless the woman is at high risk of breast cancer (Hope, Rees and Brockie 1999).

* Check that regular cervical screening is taking place.

* Give lifestyle advice, as above.

TREATMENT

General principles

Oestrogens

* Start at the lowest possible dose of oestrogen (especially in the older women who tend to get more oestrogenic side-effects) and increase at 3-monthly intervals if necessary to achieve optimum symptom control.

* Give oestrogens continuously, and only give them without progestogens if the woman has had a hysterectomy.

Progestogens

These must be added for endometrial protection in women with a uterus. Most products contain either C-19 derivatives (norethisterone/levonorgestrel) which are more androgenic, or C-21 derivatives (medroxyprogesterone acetate/dydrogesterone) which are less androgenic.

* Change to a less androgenic preparation if the patient is troubled by progestogenic side-effects.

Perimenopausal women with an intact uterus

* Use a cyclical regimen (monthly or 3-monthly). The majority of women will have a bleed towards the end of the progestogen phase.

Postmenopausal women with an intact uterus:

* Use:
  (a) a cyclical regimen; or
  (b) a continuous combined regimen. Continuous regimens induce an atrophic endometrium

and so do not produce a withdrawal bleed, although irregular bleeding can occur in the first 4–6 months. Bleeding should be investigated if it persists for longer than 6 months, becomes heavier rather than less, or if it occurs after amenorrhoea; or

(c) tibolone. This combines oestrogenic and progestogenic activities, and weak androgenic activity. It is indicated for the treatment of vasomotor symptoms and osteoporosis prophylaxis. It must only be started at least 1 year after the menopause. There is evidence that it improves libido (Kokcu, Cetinkaya, Yanik, *et al.* 2000).

Alternative modes of delivery

■ *Oestrogen implants*. Repeat every 4–8 months. Occasionally vasomotor symptoms can return despite supraphysiological plasma concentrations of oestradiol (tachyphylaxis). Check plasma oestradiol levels have returned to normal (less than 1000 pmol/l) before inserting a new implant.

■ *Transdermal patches and gels*. These avoid the first-pass metabolism in the liver and deliver a more constant level of hormone. Patches come as either reservoir or matrix patches. Skin reactions are less common with the matrix patches.

■ *Intrauterine system*. The levonorgestrel releasing system (LNG-IUS) is now licensed for 4 years' usage for the delivery of progestogen to protect the endometrium. A 5-year follow-up concludes that the LNG-IUS effectively protects against endometrial hyperplasia (Varila, Wahlstrom and Rauramo 2001). It provides contraception, and it is the only way a non-bleed regimen may be achieved in the perimenopause.

MANAGING THE SIDE–EFFECTS OF HRT

Bleeding

Patients on HRT should only be referred urgently (in the UK under the 2 week rule) if the bleeding continues after the HRT has been stopped for 4 weeks.

Bleeding on cyclical combined therapy

∗ Check when the bleeding occurs. These regimens should produce regular predictable bleeds starting towards or soon after the end of the progestogenic phase.

∗ Consider poor compliance, drug interactions or gastrointestinal upset.

∗ Try stopping HRT to see if it is the cause of the bleeding.

∗ If bleeding problems are due to HRT, alter the progestogen:

(a) heavy or prolonged bleeding: increase the dose or duration of progestogen, or change the type of progestogen to a more androgenic type (see page 339);

(b) bleeding early in the progestogenic phase: increase the dose or change the type of progestogen;

(c) painful bleeding: change the type of progestogen;

(d) irregular bleeding: change the regimen or increase the dose of progestogen.

∗ *No bleeding* whilst taking a cyclical regime reflects an atrophic endometrium and occurs in 5% of women, but pregnancy needs to be excluded in perimenopausal women.

∗ Refer if there is:

(a) a change in the pattern of withdrawal bleeds and breakthrough bleeding that persists for more than 3 months;

(b) unexpected or prolonged bleeding that persists for more than 4 weeks after stopping HRT: refer urgently.

Bleeding on continuous combined therapy or tibolone

∗ Explain to patients that the risk of bleeding is 40% in the first 4–6 months.

∗ Make sure the patient was at least 1 year postmenopausal before she started the regimen.

∗ Bleeding beyond 6 months requires further investigation.

∗ Bleeding that occurs after a period of amenorrhoea requires further investigation.

Oestrogen–related side–effects

● Oestrogenic side-effects include fluid retention, bloating, breast tenderness and enlargement, nausea, headache, leg cramps and dyspepsia.

∗ Encourage the patient to persist with therapy for 12 weeks, as most side-effects resolve with time.

∗ For persistent side-effects consider:

(a) reducing the dose; or

(b) changing the oestrogen type (swap between the two main forms of oestrogen: oestradiol and conjugated equine oestrogens); or

(c) changing the route of delivery.

* *Nausea and gastric upset.* Change the timing of the oestrogen dose, e.g. try taking it with food or at bedtime.

Progestogen–related side–effects

Progestogen-related side-effects tend to occur in a cyclical pattern during the progestogenic phase of cyclical HRT. Continuous combined products contain lower doses of progestogens and side-effects are less likely. Side-effects include fluid retention, breast tenderness, headaches, mood swings, depression, acne, lower abdominal pain and backache.

* Encourage the patient to persist with therapy for about 12 weeks, as some side-effects will resolve.
* Various changes in the progestogens may be helpful, but remember not to reduce the dose or duration below that which protects the endometrium. Options:

(a) reduce the duration but not below 10 days per cycle;

(b) reduce the dose of progestogen; or

(c) change the progestogen type (either C-19 or C-21 derivatives; see page 339); or

(d) change the route of progestogen (oral, transdermal, vaginal or intrauterine); or

(e) reduce the frequency of how often the progestogen is taken by switching to a long-cycling regime, in which progestogens are administered for 14 days every 3 months. This is only suitable for women with scant periods or who are postmenopausal; or

(f) change to a continuous combined therapy which often reduces progestogenic side-effects with established use, but it is only suitable for postmenopausal women.

FOLLOW–UP OF WOMEN ON HRT

* See after 3 months, then 6 monthly.
* Check for compliance, bleeding patterns and side-effects.
* Check that the patient is up to date with her cervical smears and mammograms.

Note: There is no need to check the BP except as good practice in any well-person screening.

HOW LONG TO CONTINUE?

* *Symptomatic relief.* Guidelines recommend that HRT be given 'for the shortest possible time' but there is no way of predicting how long this is. Most authorities recommend that HRT given for symptom relief be stopped within 5 years. In the WHI trial HRT was stopped after 5.7 years. Half the women with vasomotor symptoms at the start of the trial reported moderate or severe symptoms after stopping (Ockene, Barad, Cochrane, *et al.* 2005). If troublesome symptoms recur on withdrawal HRT can be restarted for 6–12 months at a time.

* *Osteoporosis prevention when no more appropriate alternative exist.* Five years treatment is the minimum period for which benefit has been shown, yet after this the risks, especially of breast cancer, rise. The fact that the benefit rapidly drops off after stopping HRT must be set against the risks associated with longer-term use.

STOPPING TREATMENT

HRT may be stopped abruptly or gradually. There is no evidence that either approach is better in terms of preventing the return of symptoms.

* For gradual reduction reduce the strength of oestrogen every 1–2 months, then take it on alternate days for 1–2 months then stop. At this stage:

  ■ if using a calendar pack, take alternate tablets from the pack so that the regimen includes progestogen for the second half of the cycle;

  ■ if using a patch, cut the patch in half once the lowest dose has been reached. If using the half-patch cyclically, use the progestogen-containing half-patch for the second half of the cycle.

* Review after a few months. If troublesome symptoms have recurred consider restarting therapy at the lowest possible dose and titrating up as necessary. If only local symptoms persist, use a vaginal preparation.

● *Stopping HRT prior to surgery.* The RCOG does not consider that this is necessary but recommends prophylactic measures instead: antithromboembolic stockings and low molecular weight heparin (RCOG 2004).

HRT AND CONTRACEPTION

- Perimenopausal women cannot be assumed to be infertile.
- Routine HRT preparations do not suppress ovulation and are not contraceptive.
- * Contraception should be continued for 1 year after the last menstrual period (LMP) for women over 50 years, or for 2 years after the LMP for women under the age of 50 years.
- * Perimenopausal women may use:
  - (a) barrier methods, IUD or LND-IUS, as well as HRT; or
  - (b) the low dose COC instead of HRT; or
  - (c) the progestogen-only pill (POP), possibly combined with HRT, although there are theoretical concerns that the oestrogen component of HRT may interfere with the action of the POP on the cervical mucus (Pitkin 2000).

WHEN HAS THE MENOPAUSE OCCURRED WHEN MASKED BY HRT OR COC?

It is important to know this so that a realistic idea of how long the woman needs to remain on contraception can be calculated (see above); 80% of women are postmenopausal by the age of 54 years (DTB 1994b).

- * Discontinue HRT or COC for 6–8 weeks then check FSH and repeat after a further 4–8 weeks (Gebbie 1998). If both FSH levels are above 30 IU/l, stop contraception after a further year. If a spontaneous period occurs, or FSH is less than 30 IU/l, continue contraception and repeat the test in 1 year.
- * *Women on the POP.* Check the FSH without stopping the POP.

PATIENT ORGANIZATIONS

British Menopause Society. 4-6 Eton Place, Marlow, Bucks SL7 2QA, tel. 01628 890199; www.the-bms.org
The Menopause Amarant Trust. 80 Lambeth Road, London SE1 7PW, helpline 01293 413000. www. amarantmenopausetrust.org.uk
Women's Health Information Service. 52 Featherstone Street, London EC1Y 8RT, tel. 020 7251 6333; helpline 0845 125 5254; www. womenshealthlondon.org.uk

CERVICAL SCREENING

A summary of updated national guidelines within the cervical screening programme. Available: www. cancerscreening.nhs.uk/ (choose 'Cervical')

- The NHS screening programme requires that all women between the age of 25 and 64 are offered a smear:
  - Aged 25: first invitation
  - 25–49: 3 yearly
  - 50–64: 5 yearly
  - 65+: only screen those who have not been screened since the age of 50 or have had a recent abnormal test.

The advisory committee on cervical screening reviewed the policy on screening (June 2009) and concluded that there should be no change in policy on age of starting screening and that the harms of screening under this age outweigh the benefits.

- Evidence for the programme:
  - (a) In 2000 there were 2424 new registrations for invasive cervical cancer in England (National Statistics, Cancer registrations in England, 2000).
  - (b) Cervical cancer incidence fell by 42% between 1988 and 1997 (England and Wales). This fall was directly related to the cervical screening programme (National Statistics 2000).
  - (c) In 1995 there were 10.4/100,000 newly diagnosed cases, by 1999 this had fallen to 9.3/100,000 (National Statistics 1999).
  - (d) Cervical cancer screening saves approximately 4500 lives in England and prevents 3900 cases per year in the UK (Peto, Gilham, Fletcher, *et al.* 2004; Sasieni, Cuzick, Lynch-Farmery *et al.* 1996).
- The major risk groups are:
  - (a) women with many sexual partners or whose partners have had many partners;
  - (b) smoking. It doubles a woman's risk.
- Liquid based cytology (LBC) has reduced the number of inadequate samples from over 9% to 2.9% in 2008. Results are received faster and there is less pressure on the workforce. The changeover to LBC was completed in October 2008.

ACTION ACCORDING TO THE SMEAR RESULT

An inadequate smear

- Smears cannot be interpreted (inadequate) if the specimen is obscured by inflammatory cells/blood, does not contain the right type of cells or is incorrectly labelled.

* Repeat an inadequate smear after between 6 weeks and 3 months. Repeating the smear within 6 weeks does not allow adequate tissue re-growth. Refer if there are two further inadequate smears, repeated at 3-monthly intervals (preferably mid-cycle).

Borderline or mild dyskaryosis ± human papilloma virus

In the absence of signs or symptoms:

1. treat vulval warts if present (see page 72);
2. repeat the smear in 6 months.

- If still borderline, repeat in a further 6 months and if still unchanged, refer for colposcopy.
- If negative, repeat in a further 6 months. If still negative the woman can revert to 3-yearly smears.

Note: Opinion is divided over whether this represents best practice. The most recent guideline falls between the two camps by describing referral after two mildly dyskaryotic smears as the 'minimum standard' and referral after 1 smear as 'best practice' (Luesley and Leeson 2004) (see next column). The possibility that a woman is likely to default from follow-up would sway the balance in favour of immediate referral.

Moderate or severe dyskaryosis

* Refer for early colposcopy. Stress that this is part of the screening process and does not mean that the patient has cancer.

* Advise the woman to continue her contraception, including the COC; pregnancy makes management more difficult.

FOLLOW-UP AFTER COLPOSCOPY AND TREATMENT

* Follow-up at 6 months (by gynaecologist).
* Then smear yearly for 10 years (GP or gynaecologist).
* If normal, then revert to 3-yearly smears.

FOLLOW UP AFTER HYSTERECTOMY

* Routine smears for 10 years prior to hysterectomy and negative for CIN at hysterectomy, vault cytology not required.
* Less than 10 years routine smears prior to hysterectomy and negative for CIN at hysterectomy, single vault smear required then no further follow-up required.
* CIN present at hysterectomy but fully excised, vault smears at 6 and 18 months then no further follow-up if negative.
* CIN present at hysterectomy with incomplete or uncertain excision, follow up as if cervix still in situ.

EVIDENCE FOR AND AGAINST REFERRAL AFTER A SINGLE SMEAR SHOWING MILD DYSKARYOSIS (CIN 1) (ALTS GROUP 2003)

In a recent trial patients were randomized to having a repeat smear, with colposcopy if positive, or to immediate colposcopy.

Against immediate referral

- Of patients in the 'repeat smears' group, only 19% needed a colposcopy.
- Progression to CIN 3 was similar in both groups at 15%.

In favour of immediate referral

- Where CIN 3 did develop it was detected later in the 'repeat smears' group.
- 3% of cases of CIN 3 were missed in the 'repeat smears' group (but detected at colonoscopy at the end of the trial).

Conclusion

- Repeating a mildly dyskaryotic smear saves resources at a small risk of missing a case.

Table 11.4   Terminology used during cervical screening

Cytological terms	Histological equivalent*
Mild dyskaryosis	CIN 1 (mild dysplasia) outer 1/3 of epithelium
Moderate dyskaryosis	CIN 2 (moderate dysplasia) 1/3 to 2/3 of epithelium
Severe dyskaryosis	CIN 3 (severe dysplasia or carcinoma in situ) full thickness of the epithelium with breakdown of structure between basement membrane and epithelium

CIN = cervical intraepithelial neoplasia.
*The correlation between status on smear and on histology is not close.

References

ALTS Group, 2003. A randomized trial on the management of low-grade sqamous intraepithelial lesion cytology interpretations. Am. J. Obstet. Gynaecol. 188, 1393–1400.

American Association of Clinical Endocrinologists, 1999. AACE medical Guidelines for Clinical Practice for Management of Menopause. American Association of Clinical Endocrinologists. www.aace.com.

Anon. 1998. Alternatives for the menopause. Bandolier, Oct. 56–59.

Austoker, J., 1994. Screening for cervical cancer. BMJ 309, 241–248.

Beral, V., Million Women Study Collaborators, 2003. Breast cancer and hormone-replacement therapy in the Million Women Study. Lancet 362, 419–427.

Bingham, J.S., 1999. What to do with patients with recurrent vulvovaginal candidiasis. Sex. Transm. Infect. 75, 225–227.

Bisschop, M.P., Merkus, J.M., Scheyground, H., et al., 1986. Co-treatment of the male partner in vaginal candidosis: a double blind randomised controlled study. Br. J. Obstet. Gynaecol. 93, 79–81.

Bousser, M.G., Conard, J., Kittner, S., et al., 2000. Recommendations on the risk of ischaemic stroke associated with use of combined oral contraceptives and hormone replacement therapy in women with migraine. The International Headache Society Task Force on Combined Oral Contraceptives & Hormone Replacement Therapy. Cephalalgia 20, 155–156.

Cardozo, L., Bachmann, G., McClish, D., et al., 1998. Meta-analysis of estrogen therapy in the management of urogenital atrophy in postmenopausal women: second report of the Hormones and Urogenital Therapy Committee. Obstet. Gynecol. 92, 722–727.

DTB, 1994a. Surgical management of menorrhagia. Drug. Ther. Bull. 32, 70–72.

DTB, 1994b. Hormone replacement therapy. Drug. Ther. Bull. 34, 81–84.

DTB, 1999. Managing endometriosis. Drug. Ther. Bull. 37, 25–29.

Edington, R.F., Chagnon, J.P., 1980. Clonidine for menopausal flushing. Can. Med. Assoc. J. 123, 23–26.

Farquhar, C., 2001. Endometriosis. Clinical Evidence, Issue 5. BMJ Publishing Group, London Available: www.clinicalevidence.org.

Farquhar, C., Lee, O., Toomath, R., et al., 2000. Spironolactone versus placebo or in combination with steroids for hirsutism and/or acne (Cochrane Review). In: The Cochrane Library, Issue 4. Update Software, Oxford.

Farquhar, C., Sutton, C., 1998. The evidence for the management of endometriosis. Curr. Opin. Obst. Gynecol. 10 (4), 321–332.

Gannon, M.J., Holt, E.M., Fairbank, J., et al., 1991. A randomised trial comparing endometrial resection and abdominal hysterectomy for the treatment of Menorrhagia. BMJ 303, 1362–1364.

Gath, D., Iles, S., 1990. Depression and the menopause. BMJ 300, 1287–1288.

Gebbie, A.E., 1998. Contraception for women over 40. In: Studd, J. (ed.), The management of the Menopause, Annual Review. Parthenon Publishing, London, pp. 67–80.

Gokhale, L.B., 1996. Curative treatment of primary (spasmodic) dysmenorrhoea. Indian J. Med. Res. 103, 227–231.

Groom, T.M., Stewart, P., Kruger, H., et al., 2001. The value of a screen and treat policy for Chlamydia trachomatis in women attending for termination of pregnancy. J. Fam. Plann. Reprod. Health Care 27, 69–72.

Guttuso, T., Kurlan, R., McDermott, M.P., et al., 2003. Gabapentin's effects on hot flashes in postmenopausal women: a randomized controlled trial. Am. Coll. Obstet. Gynaecologists 101, 337–345.

Haddon, L., Heason, J., Fay, T., et al., 1998. Managing STIs identified after testing outside genitourinary medicine departments: one model of care. Sex. Transm. Infect. 74, 256–257.

Harborne, L., Fleming, R., Lyall, H., et al., 2003. Descriptive review of the evidence for the use of metformin in polycystic ovary syndrome. Lancet 361, 1894–1901.

Hays, J., Ockene, J.K., Brunner, R.L., et al., 2003. Women's Health Initiative Investigators. Effects of estrogen plus progestin on health-related quality of life. N. Engl. J. Med. 348, 1839–1854.

Heiss, G., Wallace, R., Anderson, G. L., et al., 2008. Health risks and benefits 3 years after stopping randomized treatment with estrogen and progestin. JAMA 299, 1036–1045.

Hills, S.D., Joesoef, R., Marchbanks, P.A., et al., 1993. Delayed care of pelvic inflammatory disease as a risk factor for impaired fertility. Am. J. Obstet. Gynecol. 168, 1503–1509.

Hills, S.D., Owens, L.M., Marchbanks, P.A., et al., 1997. Recurrent chlamydial infections increase the risks of hospitalisation for ectopic pregnancy and pelvic inflammatory disease. Am. J. Obstet. Gynecol. 176, 103 107.

Hlatky, M.A., Boothroyd, D., Vittinghoff, E., et al., 2002. Quality-of-life and depressive symptoms in postmenopausal women after receiving hormone therapy: results from the Heart and Estrogen/Progestin Replacement Study (HERS) trial. JAMA 287, 591–597.

Hope, S., Rees, M., Brockie, J., 1999. Hormone Replacement Therapy – a Guide for Primary Care. Oxford University Press, Oxford.

Hunter, M.S., 1996. Depression and the menopause. BMJ 313, 350–351.

Kamwendo, F., Johansson, E., Moi, H., et al., 1993. Gonorrhoea, genital chlamydia infection and non-specific urethritis in male partners of hospitalized women treated for acute pelvic inflammatory disease. Sex. Transm. Dis. 20, 143–146.

Kinghorn, G.R., Duerden, B.I., Hafiz, S., 1986. Clinical and microbiological investigation of women with acute salpingitis and their consorts. Br. J. Obstet. Gynaecol. 93, 869–880.

Kokcu, A., Cetinkaya, M.B., Yanik, F., et al., 2000. The comparison of effects of tibolone and conjugated estrogen-medroxyprogesterone acetate therapy on sexual performance in postmenopausal women. Maturitas 36, 75–80.

Korhonen, M.O., Symons, J.P., Hyde, B.M., et al., 1997. Histological classification and pathological findings for endometrial biopsy specimens obtained from 2964 perimenopausal and postmenopausal women undergoing screening for continuous hormone replacement therapy. Am. J. Obstet. Gynaecol. 176, 377–380.

Larsson, B., Wennergren, M., 1981. Investigation of Cu-IUD for possible effect on frequency and healing of PID. Contraception 24, 137–149.

Lethaby, A., Irvine, G., Cameron, I., 2001. Cyclical progestogens for heavy menstrual bleeding (Cochrane Review). In: The Cochrane Library, Issue 3. Update Software, Oxford.

Loprinzi, C.L., Michalak, J.C., Quella, S.K., et al., 2003. Megestrol acetate for the prevention of hot flashes. N. Engl. J. Med. 331, 347–352.

Lord, J.M., Flight, I.H.K., Norman, R.J., 2003. Metformin in polycystic ovary syndrome: systematic review and meta-analysis. BMJ 327, 951–955.

Luesley, D., Leeson, S. (eds.), 2004. Colposcopy and Programme Management: Guidelines for the NHS Cervical Screening Programme. NHS Cancer Screening Programmes (NHSCSP publication No. 20).

MacLennan, A., Lester, S., Moore, V., 2001. Oral oestrogen replacement therapy versus placebo for hot flushes (Cochrane Review). In: The Cochrane Library, Issue 3. Update Software, Oxford.

Marjoribanks, J., Proctor, M.L., Farquhar, C., 2006. Nonsteroidal anti-inflammatory drugs for primary dysmenorrhoea. Cochrane Database Syst. Rev. www.library.nhs.uk (choose 'Cochrane library').

Metters, J.S., Catchpole, M., Smith, C., et al., 1998. Chlamydia trachomatis: Summary and Conclusions of CMO's Expert Advisory Group. Department of Health, London.

Miettinen, A.K., Heinonen, P.K., Laippala, P., et al., 1993. Test performance of ESR & C-reactive protein in assessing the severity of acute PID. Am. J. Obstet. Gynecol. 169, 1143–1149.

Miller, E.R., Pastor-Barriuso, R., Dalal, D., et al., 2005. Meta-analysis: high-dosage vitamin E supplementation may increase all-cause mortality. Ann. Intern. Med. 142, 37–47.

Moore, J., Kennedy, S., Prentice, A., 2001. Modern combined oral contraceptives for pain associated with endometriosis (Cochrane Review). In: The Cochrane Library, Issue 3. Update Software, Oxford.

Nagamani, M., Kelver, M.E., Smith, E. R., 1987. Treatment of menopausal flashes with transdermal administration of clonidine. Am. J. Obstet. Gynecol. 156, 561–565.

National Institute for Health and Clinical Excellence, 2007. Heavy Menstrual Bleeding. Clinical Guideline 44. Available: www.nice.org.uk.

National Statistics, 1999. MB1 No 28 Cancer Statistics Registrations 1995–1997; National Statistics MB1 No 30 Registrations of cancer diagnosed in 1999.

National Statistics, 2000. Health Quarterly Statistics 07, Autumn 2000.

Nelson, H.D., Humphrey, L.L., Nygren, P., et al., 2002. Postmenopausal hormone replacement therapy: scientific review. JAMA 288, 872–881.

Nelson, H.D., Vesco, K.K., Haney, E., et al., 2006. Nonhormonal therapies for menopausal hot flashes. JAMA 295, 2057–2071.

Newton, K.M., Reed, S.D., LaCroix, A.Z., et al., 2006. Treatment of vasomotor symptoms of menopause with black cohosh, multibotanicals, soy, hormone therapy or placebo. Ann. Intern. Med. 145, 869–879.

Norman, R.J., Flight, I.H.K., Rees, M. C.P., 2001. Oestrogen and progestogen hormone replacement therapy for peri-menopausal and post-menopausal women: weight and body fat distribution (Cochrane Review). In: The Cochrane Library, Issue 3. Update Software, Oxford.

Ockene, J.K., Barad, D.H., Cochrane, B.B., et al., 2005. Symptom experience after discontinuing use of estrogen plus progestin. JAMA 294, 183–191.

Pattie, M.A., Murdoch, B.E., Theodoros, D., et al., 1998. Voice changes in women treated for endometriosis and related conditions: the need for comprehensive vocal assessment. J. Voice 12, 366–371.

Peto, J., Gilham, C., Fletcher, O., et al., 2004. The cervical cancer epidemic that screening has prevented in the UK. Lancet 364, 249–256.

Pitkin, J., 2000. Contraception and the menopause. Maturitas 1, S29–S36.

Potter, J., 1999. Should sexual partners of women with bacterial vaginosis receive treatment? Br. J. Gen. Pract. 49, 913–918.

RCOG, 1999. The Initial Management of Menorrhagia. Evidence-based clinical guidelines, No. 1. Royal College of Obstetricians and Gynaecologists, London.

RCOG, 2004. Hormone Replacement Therapy and Venous Thromboembolism. Royal College of Obstetricians and Gynaecologists Guideline No.19. Available: www.rcog.org.uk.

Rees, M., Purdie, D.W., 1999. Management of the Menopause. BMS Publications. The Handbook of the BMS, London.

Robinson, A.J., Kell, P., 1995. Male partners of women with pelvic infection should be traced (letter). BMJ 311, 630.

Rossouw, J.E., Anderson, G.L., Prentice, R.L., et al., 2002. Writing Group for the Women's Health Initiative Investigators. Risks and benefits of estrogen plus progestin in healthy postmenopausal women: principal results from the Women's Health Initiative randomized controlled trial. JAMA 288, 321–333.

Rossouw, J.E., Prentice, R.L., Manson, J.E., et al., 2007. Postmenopausal hormone therapy and risk of cardiovascular disease by age and years since menopause. JAMA 297, 1465–1477.

Sasieni, P.D., Cuzick, J., Lynch-Farmery, E., et al., 1996. Estimating the efficacy of screening by auditing smear histories of women with and without cervical cancer. Br. J. Cancer 73, 1001–1005.

Scambia, G., Mango, D., Signorile, P. G., et al., 2000. Clinical effects of a standardised soy extract in postmenopausal women: a pilot study. Menopause 7, 105–111.

Shumaker, S.A., Legault, C., Rapp, S. R., et al., 2003. WHIMS Investigators. Estrogen plus progestin and the incidence of dementia and mild cognitive impairment in postmenopausal women: the Women's Health Initiative Memory Study: a randomized controlled trial. JAMA 289, 2651–2662.

Soderberg, G., Lingren, S., 1981. Influence of an IUD on the course of acute salpingitis. Contraception 24, 137–143.

Sutton, C.J., Ewen, S.P., Whiltelaw, N., et al., 1994. Prospective, randomized, double-blind, controlled trial of laser laparoscopy in the treatment of pelvic pain associated with minimal, mild, and moderate endometriosis. Fertil. Steril. 62, 696.

Teisala, K., 1989. Removal of an IUD and the treatment of acute PID. Ann. Med. 21, 63–65.

Varila, E., Wahlstrom, T., Rauramo, I., 2001. A 5-year study of the use of a levonorgestrol intra-uterine system in women receiving hormone replacement therapy. Fertil. Steril. 76, 969–973.

Vercellini, P., Cortesi, I., Crosignani, P.G., 1997. Progestogens for symptomatic endometriosis – a critical analysis of the evidence. Fertil. Steril. 68 (3), 393–401.

Watson, M.C., Grimshaw, J.M., Bond, C.M., et al., 2002. Oral versus intra-vaginal imidazole and triazole anti-fungal treatment of uncomplicated vulvovaginal candidiasis (thrush) (Cochrane Review). In: The Cochrane Library, Issue 1. Update Software, Oxford.

Wild, S., Pierpoint, T., Mckeigue, P., et al., 2000. Cardiovascular disease in women with PCOS at long term follow up: a retrospective cohort study. Clin. Endocrinol. 52, 595–600.

Wyatt, K.M., Dimmock, P.W., O'Brien, P.M.S., 2002. Selective serotonin reuptake inhibitors for premenstrual syndrome. Cochrane Database Syst. Rev.

Zhang, W.Y., Po, A.L., 1998. Efficacy of minor analgesics in primary dysmenorrhoea: a systematic review. Br. J. Obstet. Gynaecol. 105 (7), 780–789.

Chapter 12

Contraception and sexual problems

CHAPTER CONTENTS

INFORMATION FOR PROFESSIONALS

Glasier A, Gebbie A. 2008. Handbook of Family Planning and Reproductive Healthcare, Churchill Livingstone, London
   Faculty of Sexual & Reproductive Healthcare. www.fsrh.org

Information for patients

FPA, 50 Featherstone Street, London EC1Y 8QU, Helpline 0845 122 8690; Available: www.fpa.org.uk

When giving contraceptive advice it is good practice if this is backed up with appropriate and accessible written information. The Family Planning Association (FPA) provides a range of leaflets covering all methods, which is regularly revised and is available through the local Health Promotion Unit or from the website (above). These leaflets should be used when a patient is deciding on a method, initiating a method and from time to time as a refresher. However, leaflets are not a substitute for discussion (Jones 2008).

Patients wanting to go to a family planning clinic or who are being referred from general practice can get details of a convenient clinic from the FPA. Their website allows a search on a map with details right down to street level.

© 2011 Elsevier Ltd.
DOI: 10.1016/B978-0-7020-3053-6.00012-X

HORMONAL CONTRACEPTION

COMBINED ORAL CONTRACEPTIVE (COC) PILL

Effectiveness

With perfect use of the COC failure rates are as low as 0.3% in the first year (Trussell 2007). However, with typical use this rises to 8%.

Assessment of the patient (Clinical Effectiveness Unit 2006a)

The following are the essential components of the assessment before initiating the COC:

(a) menstrual and obstetric history;

(b) history of migraine – presence of aura;

(c) past or current illnesses which might represent contraindications;

(d) family history of venous thromboembolism (VTE), MI, cerebrovascular accident (CVA), hypertension and breast cancer;

(e) current drug therapy (prescribed and OTC);

(f) allergies;

(g) blood pressure (BP) measurement (defer starting the COC until 8 weeks after delivery in women who have had pre-eclampsia, even if the BP is normal);

(h) baseline height/weight: BMI (important, as it is a risk factor for VTE).

(i) No blood tests are necessary before first prescription of a COC without specific clinical indication.

(j) In asymptomatic women breast and pelvic examinations are not recommended before first prescription of a COC (Stewart, Harper, Ellertson, et al. 2001).

Contraindications

UK Medical Eligibility Criteria give four categories of condition in which use of the COC is (or is not) contraindicated (Clinical Effectiveness Unit 2009):

■ UKMEC1 is a condition for which there is no restriction on use of the method.

■ UKMEC2 is when the advantages of the method generally outweigh the theoretical or proven risks.

■ UKMEC3 is when the theoretical or proven risks usually outweigh the advantages. Provision of a method requires expert clinical judgement and/or a referral to a specialist contraceptive provider.

■ UKMEC4 is a condition which represents an unacceptable health risk and the method should not be used.

UNACCEPTABLE HEALTH RISK (UKMEC4) (CLINICAL EFFECTIVENESS UNIT 2006A; 2009A)

(a) *Breast feeding* – < 6 weeks postpartum (Clinical Effectiveness Unit 2009b).

(b) *Smoking* – aged > 35 years and smoking > 15 cigarettes/day.

(c) *Cardiovascular disease* – multiple risk factors for arterial cardiovascular disease such as older age, smoking, diabetes and hypertension.

(d) *Hypertension* – BP ≥ 160 systolic or ≥ 95 diastolic.

(e) *Vascular disease* – peripheral vascular disease, hypertensive retinopathy and TIAs.

(f) *Venous thromboembolism* – current or past history.

(g) *Major surgery with prolonged immobilization.*

(h) *Known thrombogenic mutations* – such as Factor V Leiden, prothrombin variant G20210A, protein S, protein C and antithrombin III deficiencies.

(i) *Ischaemic heart disease* – current or past history.

(j) *Stroke* – history of CVA.

(k) *Valvular heart disease* – complicated by pulmonary hypertension, atrial fibrillation, history of infective endocarditis.

(l) *Migraine*, with aura (MacGregor 2007). The following suggest transient ischaemia and preclude use of the COC: loss of a part of the visual field; unilateral weakness/paraesthesiae; disturbance of speech; first ever migraine attack after starting COC; status migrainosus. Migraine without aura is relatively safe (this includes blurred vision, photophobia, phonophobia and flashing lights affecting the whole visual field) for those who did not first develop it while on the COC.

(m) *Breast cancer* – current.

(n) *Diabetes* – nephropathy, retinopathy, neuropathy or other vascular disease.

(o) *Viral hepatitis* – acute or flare.

(p) *Cirrhosis* – severe (decompensated).

(q) *Liver tumours* – benign (hepatocellular adenoma) or malignant (hepatoma).

(r) *SLE* – with positive or unknown antiphospholipid antibodies.

RISKS USUALLY OUTWEIGH BENEFITS (UKMEC3) (CLINICAL EFFECTIVENESS UNIT 2006A; 2009A)

(a) *Breastfeeding* – between 6 weeks and 6 months postpartum and primarily breast feeding (Clinical Effectiveness Unit 2004a).

(b) *Postpartum* (in non-breast feeding women) (Brechin and Penney 2004) – < 21 days.

(c) *Smoking* – aged ≥ 35 years and smoking < 15 cigarettes/day; aged ≥ 35 years and stopped smoking < 1 year ago.

(d) *BMI* – ≥ 35.

(e) *Multiple risk factors for arterial cardiovascular disease.*

(f) *Hypertension* – on treatment with BP adequately controlled; elevated BP 140–159 systolic or 90–94 diastolic.

(g) *FH of VTE* – in a first degree relative aged < 45 years.

(h) *Immobility* – wheelchair use, debilitating illness.

(i) *Hyperlipidaemia* – e.g. familial hypercholesterolaemia.

(j) *Migraine* – past history of migraine with aura ≥ 5 years ago, at any age.

(k) *Breast cancer* – past history of and no evidence of recurrence for 5 years; carriers of known mutations associated with breast cancer, e.g. BRCA1.

(l) *Gallbladder disease* – symptomatic medically treated or current.

(m) *History of cholestasis* – past COC-related.

(n) *Potent enzyme-inducing drugs* – rifampicin, rifabutin and certain antiepileptic drugs (see page 350).

Arterial and venous thrombosis

The risk factors for VTE and arterial disease should be assessed separately. Age is a risk factor common to both conditions. Many of the risk factors can be viewed as being on a sliding scale, for instance there is not suddenly a problem with age on the 35th birthday. Smoking status, weight and immobility are the only factors that may be changed in the future and the suitability for the COC reviewed.

CHOOSING A COMBINED PILL

- Pill formulations contain one of eight progestogens.
- The initial dose of oestrogen should normally be in the range 20–35 mcg combined with a low or standard dose of progestogen.
- A monophasic COC containing 30 mcg ethinylestradiol with norethisterone or levonorgestrel is a suitable first pill.
- As from June 1999, desogestrel- and gestodene-containing pills were recommended again as first-line COCs, following the pill scare of October 1995 (Anon. 1999). However, in view of the apparent increased risk of VTE with these preparations [relative risk (RR) 1.7 compared to levonorgestrel or norethisterone pills (Kemmeren, Algra and Grobbee 2001)] the slightly increased risk of VTE should be explained to the patient (see Table 12.1) and these pills should not be used in those with a risk factor for VTE. Norgestimate containing pills have similar rates of VTE to levonorgestrel pills (Jick, Kaye, Russmann and Jick 2006).
- For all COCs the risk of VTE is greatest in the first year of use. For COCs containing levonorgestrel, for instance, the RR for VTE in the first year is 6.6 compared to women not taking the pill, falling to 1.3 after 5 years use (Brechin and Penney 2004).
- Desogestrel- and gestodene-containing pills are probably best avoided for young first-time users.

Table 12.1 Risks of venous thromboembolism	
Background rate of VTE in healthy non pregnant women not taking a COC	5/100,000/year
Healthy women taking levonorgestrel or norethisterone COCs	15/100,000/year
Healthy women taking gestodene or desogestrel COCs	25/100,000/year
Pregnancy	60/100,000/year

VTE = venous thromboembolism.
COC = combined oral contraceptive.

Their risk of VTE is 3.1 times the risk they would run with a levonorgestrel or norethisterone preparation (Kemmeren, Algra and Grobbee 2001). These brands may be useful, however, for those who have side-effects, for acne sufferers or those with cycle control problems.

■ Co-cyprindiol (ethinylestradiol with cyproterone acetate) is licensed as an acne treatment but is an effective contraceptive too. It should be used only in those with significant acne. There is a higher risk of VTE than with levonorgestrel pills: RR 3.9 (Vasilakis-Scaramozza and Jick 2001).

■ Women react individually to the pill; if side-effects are experienced, it is well worth trying at least one other brand before abandoning the method.

RECOMMENDATIONS

> Recommend the information leaflet from the FPA on www.fpa.org.uk

Higher doses of oestrogen

Formulations containing 50 mcg of ethinylestradiol should not be used unless specific individual circumstances warrant a higher dose:

(a) long-term use of an enzyme-inducing drug. NICE recommends that women taking enzyme-inducing anti-epileptic drugs are started on 50 mcg; if breakthrough bleeding (BTB) occurs, the dose may be increased to 75 mcg or 100 mcg daily (Stokes, Shaw, Juarez-Garcia, *et al.* 2004);

(b) persistent BTB on a standard strength COC, provided no other cause is found;

(c) past true COC method failure, suggesting unusually rapid metabolism or malabsorption (an alternative is tricycling and shortening the pill-free interval (PFI) to 4 days – see below).

Special cases

* Recommend an alternative method when there has been a previous failure of COC or

where pill efficacy may be reduced because the patient:

(a) is on long-term hepatic enzyme-inducing drugs, e.g. for fungal infection, TB, epilepsy, daytime sleepiness or HIV, or taking OTC drugs e.g. St John's wort (consult BNF) (Clinical Effectiveness Unit 2005a); or

(b) has severe malabsorption.

* If an alternative method is unacceptable, consider:

(a) starting a high-dose pill, or two low-dose pills, to give at least 50 mcg of ethinylestradiol; or

(b) running three packs of pills together (the 'tricycle' regimen) plus reducing the 3-monthly PFI to 4 days;

* If breakthrough bleeding still occurs, try 75 mcg or 100 mcg per day (Stokes, Shaw, Juarez-Garcia *et al.* 2004).

Phased preparations

(a) Give a better bleeding pattern for a lower monthly dose (has been shown for levonorgestrel preparations) (Rosenberg and Long 1992);

(b) are more expensive than fixed-dose preparations, not least because these products attract two dispensing fees (biphasics) or three dispensing fees (triphasics) in the UK;

(c) have a reduced margin for error, especially early in the packet;

(d) may cause premenstrual tension-like symptoms towards the end of the packet;

(e) are less flexible when a patient wants to postpone a period.

TAKING THE PILL: PROCEDURE AND ADVICE

Starting the pill (Clinical Effectiveness Unit 2006a)

(a) *Days 1–5 of the cycle.* If started on or before day 5, then no other precautions are necessary.

(b) *After day 5*, other precautions should be used for the first 7 days.

(c) *Changing from a hormonal method.* COC can be started immediately if the previous method has been used consistently and correctly, or if it is

Table 12.2	How a clinician can be reasonably certain a woman is not pregnant (Clinical Effectiveness Unit 2006a; Anon 2005)

- There should be no symptoms or signs of pregnancy and any ONE of the following criteria should be met:
- no sex since the start of the last normal menstrual period; or
- she has been correctly and consistently using a reliable* method of contraception; or
- she is within the first 7 days of her cycle; or
- she is within the first 7 days after an abortion or miscarriage; or
- she is fully breastfeeding, amenorrhoeic and < 6 months postpartum; or
- she is not breast feeding and is < 3 weeks postpartum or has had no unprotected sex since delivery.
- A pregnancy test adds weight to the diagnosis, but only if 3 weeks have elapsed since the date of last sex.

*The author does not regard condoms, *coitus interruptus* or fertility awareness as reliable enough to exclude the possibility of pregnancy.

reasonably certain she is not pregnant (Table 12.2). There is no need to wait for the next period.

(d) *After childbirth*. If starting at the end of the third week postpartum, no other precautions are needed. A later start necessitates extra precautions for 7 days. Note that the earliest recorded ovulation after delivery is day 30 (Guillebaud 1989), so waiting until a postnatal examination is not an option unless a woman is exclusively breastfeeding.

(e) *After miscarriage or TOP*. Start within 7 days. If starting later, extra precautions are needed for 7 days. The earliest recorded ovulation after TOP is day 16 (Guillebaud 1989).

Changing the pill

(a) Same or higher strength oestrogen but the same progestogen. Start it after the 7-day break. No extra precautions are necessary.

(b) Lower strength oestrogen or a different progestogen. Omit the 7-day break. If the break is not omitted, extra precautions are needed for 7 days.

Postponing a bleed

This is possible (see below).

STOPPING THE COC

Alternative methods of contraception are needed from the day of stopping the COC, not the end of the PFI.

ADVICE
Mode of action

The main action of the pill is to suppress the normal cycle so that ovulation does not occur; the 'periods' while on the pill are withdrawal bleeds. Within 7 days of use the ovaries are fully suppressed. Conversely, during the PFI there is no significant follicular development, unless the PFI is lengthened beyond 7 days.

Risks

(a) Venous thromboembolism. The risk of VTE while using any COC is increased but is less than the risk of VTE during pregnancy (see Table 12.1) (Brechin and Penney 2004).

(b) Myocardial infarction. The risk of MI on a COC is confined to smokers (RR 9.5 compared to non-smokers not on COC) (Khader, Rice, John and Abueita 2003) and those with arterial risk factors. Women who do not smoke, who have their BP checked and who do not have hypertension or diabetes are at no increased risk of MI on a COC, regardless of their age.

(c) Ischaemic stroke. The risk of ischaemic stroke in COC users is increased (RR 2.7) (Chan, Ray, Wai, *et al.* 2004). Among women with no history of migraine, who do not smoke, have their BP checked and who do not have hypertension, the risk is less.

(d) Gallstones. COCs may accelerate the presentation of cholelithiasis in those who are predisposed. Their use should be avoided in those with known gallbladder disease. They can be used after cholecystectomy (UKMEC2) but usually not after medical treatment for gallstones (UKMEC3).

(e) Hypertension. COCs can induce hypertension, particularly in the early months of use (Poulter 1996). About 1% of COC users become clinically hypertensive with modern formulations. Pill-induced hypertension should not be treated with antihypertensive drugs, but the pill should be stopped and observation continued.

(f) Cancer. Overall, the balance of risks and benefits of the COC on cancer is beneficial. There is an increased risk of cancer of the cervix; this is mitigated by a large reduction in risk of cancer of the ovary (RR 0.73) (Collaborative Group on Epidemiological Studies of Ovarian Cancer 2008) and the endometrium (Weiderpass, Adami, Baron, *et al.* 1999) and by a reduction in the risk of cancer of the colon (RR 0.82) (Fernandez, La Vecchia, Balducci, *et al.* 2001). The COC probably accelerates development of cancer of the cervix caused by chronic infection with oncogenic HPV; with 5 years or more of use the RR is 1.90 (International Collaboration of Epidemiological Studies of Cervical Cancer 2007). The literature on the COC and breast cancer is conflicting but some good quality studies show no increased risk (Clinical Effectiveness Unit 2010b). Both UK cohort studies show no increased risk: RRs of 1.0 (Vessey and Painter 2006) and 0.90 (Hannaford, Iversen, Macfarlane, *et al.* 2010) respectively. By the age of 40–44, however, COC use is associated with 30 extra cancers per 100,000 women.

(g) Inflammatory bowel disease. IBD may be associated with VTE, hepatobiliary disease and osteoporosis, all of which would need to be taken into consideration when considering suitability for the COC (Clinical Effectiveness Unit 2009c). Also, the efficacy of the COC may be reduced in women with Crohn's disease who have small bowel disease and malabsorption.

Side–effects

There are side-effects, but most wear off after the first few cycles, especially bloating, nausea and breast tenderness. Nausea may be reduced by taking the pill at night.

Non–contraceptive benefits

The following have all been shown to be beneficial effects of the COC: lighter, shorter bleeding (less anaemia), less dysmenorrhoea, less PMS, less PID, fewer ectopic pregnancies, less benign breast disease, a bone sparing effect, fewer functional ovarian cysts, less hospitalization for fibroids and less symptomatic endometriosis. The COC tends to improve acne. There is little to choose between COC formulations. COCs need to be taken for at least 6 months for their full effect on the skin to become apparent. Evidence for the use of co-cyprindiol, if a COC fails to improve acne, is of poor quality (Arowojolu 2009).

Bleeding

Withdrawal bleeds are usually lighter than periods. BTB may occur during the first two or three cycles. BTB is not a reason for stopping the pill in mid-packet.

Missed pills (Clinical Effectiveness Unit 2006a)

The most risky time for pills to be forgotten is on either side of the pill-free week. Forgetting in the middle of a packet is less likely to give rise to breakthrough ovulation or pregnancy.

If more than 24 hours late, this is classed as 'missed pills' and the agreed rules are as in Figure 12.1.

Diarrhoea or vomiting

This requires extra precautions for the period of illness and for 7 days afterwards, as above. If this would run into the pfi, the pfi should be omitted. However, it is known that diarrhoea has to be of dysenteric proportions to reduce pill absorption.

Drugs for infections (Clinical Effectiveness Unit 2005a and 2010c)

Certain antibiotics may reduce the effectiveness of the COC. Ampicillin, amoxicillin, co-amoxiclav, broad-spectrum cephalosporins and tetracyclines may possibly alter the reabsorption of oestrogen (this does not occur with narrow-spectrum antibiotics, nor with trimethoprim or erythromycin). Rifampicin, rifabutin, griseofulvin and some antiretroviral drugs (notably ritonavir-boosted protease inhibitors) induce liver enzymes. Oral antifungal agents have also been associated with anecdotal reports of COC failure.

＊ Extra precautions should be taken during the treatment and for 7 days thereafter. If this runs into the PFI the next packet should be started without a break. Rifampicin and rifabutin are such powerful enzyme-inducers that extra precautions should be taken for 4 weeks even

Figure 12.1 Action to be taken if pills are missed. *Faculty of Family Planning and Reproductive Health Care Clinical Effectiveness Unit. 2005. WHO selected practice recommendations for contraceptive use update. 'Missed pills: new recommendations. J Fam Plann Reprod Health Care 31, 153–155. Reproduced with permission.*

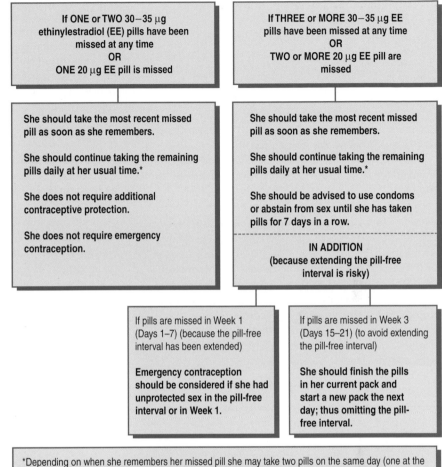

If ONE or TWO 30–35 µg ethinylestradiol (EE) pills have been missed at any time
OR
ONE 20 µg EE pill is missed

She should take the most recent missed pill as soon as she remembers.

She should continue taking the remaining pills daily at her usual time.*

She does not require additional contraceptive protection.

She does not require emergency contraception.

If THREE or MORE 30–35 µg EE pills have been missed at any time
OR
TWO or MORE 20 µg EE pill are missed

She should take the most recent missed pill as soon as she remembers.

She should continue taking the remaining pills daily at her usual time.*

She should be advised to use condoms or abstain from sex until she has taken pills for 7 days in a row.

IN ADDITION
(because extending the pill-free interval is risky)

If pills are missed in Week 1 (Days 1–7) (because the pill-free interval has been extended)

Emergency contraception should be considered if she had unprotected sex in the pill-free interval or in Week 1.

If pills are missed in Week 3 (Days 15–21) (to avoid extending the pill-free interval)

She should finish the pills in her current pack and start a new pack the next day; thus omitting the pill-free interval.

*Depending on when she remembers her missed pill she may take two pills on the same day (one at the moment of remembering and the other at the regular time) or even at the same time.

after a 2-day course and elimination of PFIs during this time (Clinical Effectiveness Unit 2006a).

* *Long-term antibiotics:* If starting the patient on long-term treatment, extra precautions need to be taken for the first 3 weeks. Thereafter, if the bleeding pattern is normal, adequate contraception can be presumed.

Surgery

The COC should be stopped from 4 weeks before until 2 weeks after any major surgery, varicose vein surgery or sclerotherapy, or any operation likely to be followed by immobilization (e.g. leg surgery) (Clinical Effectiveness Unit 2009). It is otherwise not necessary to stop the COC.

POSTPONING OR AVOIDING BLEEDS

Monophasic pills

Patients on a fixed-dose combined pill can postpone the next withdrawal bleed by starting the next packet immediately, omitting the PFI.

Phased preparations

* If on Synphase, another packet can be taken immediately following the first.
* If taking other phased preparations there would be an abrupt drop in progestogen levels if the above regimen were followed, leading to a risk of bleeding. Advise:
  (a) tablets from the last phase of a spare packet can be taken, to give 7 (TriNovum) or 10

(Logynon, Triadene) or 14 (Binovum) days' postponement; or

(b) a packet can be started of the next higher dose monophasic pill, omitting the PFI. With Qlaira, the 17 highest dose tablets should be used.

If postponement by a few days is needed, e.g. to avoid a bleed at weekends, the necessary number of pills from a fresh pack should be taken, and the rest of that pack thrown away. If on phased preparations, they should follow the principles above.

Note: ED preparations. In all the above advice, the seven inactive pills in ED preparations should be discarded.

Extended use of the COC has become widespread; running several or all packets together reduces bleeding days and menstrual cycle related symptoms (Archer 2006). When used continuously for 1 year, 18% of women achieve amenorrhoea by 3 months of use and 88% by 10 months (Miller and Hughes 2003). Extended use can be at the personal preference of the woman according to how often she wishes to bleed; or recommended on medical grounds, e.g. for low bone density, endometriosis, PMS or withdrawal headaches.

FOLLOW-UP

* The patient should be seen again at 3 months, or earlier if side-effects occur. Do not give repeat prescriptions without someone seeing the patient and at least checking the blood pressure.
* Once established on the pill, see the patient 6-monthly and:
    (a) assess whether there are any new risk factors, including migraine;
    (b) check whether the patient is smoking;
    (c) ask about side-effects;
    (d) check BP (discontinue if BP increases to and remains at 160/95 mmHg). If the BP is satisfactory 2 years after commencement of the COC, BP checks can be extended to annually in women without risk factors or relevant diseases.

CHANGING THE PILL BECAUSE OF SIDE-EFFECTS

When changing a pill because of side-effects, the choice lies between changing oestrogen/progestogen dominance and changing to a pill with a different progestogen (see below).

Breakthrough bleeding (BTB)

BTB occurs in up to 30% of users in the first few cycles, but tends to settle by the third cycle. Unless prior warning of this is given, discontinuation rates will be high, especially in the young.

* *If BTB occurs in the first 3 months*, ask whether pills have been missed; encourage the patient to persevere.
* *If BTB continues beyond 3 months*, exclude lesions of the cervix and problems with taking the pill, e.g. vomiting. Also encourage smokers to quit, as they are more likely to have BTB (Rosenberg, Waugh and Stevens 1996). Give a pill with a higher progestogen dose, change to a progestogen with better cycle control, e.g. gestodene, or change to a triphasic formulation of the same progestogen. If this fails consider increasing the oestrogen content as well.
* *If BTB occurs when previous control had been good*, exclude lesions of the cervix, chlamydia infection, interacting drugs, gastrointestinal disorder and a change to a vegetarian diet.

Absent withdrawal bleeds (WB)

* Explain that this is not unsafe and does not signify overdosage.
* Missing one WB does not need any action. If two are missed, exclude pregnancy.
* If the patient is concerned despite reassurance, consider a switch to a triphasic pill.

Oestrogen withdrawal headache during pill-free interval

* Consider advising the patient to use three packets consecutively without a break, followed by a 7-day break (tricycle regimen).

COMBINED TRANSDERMAL PATCH

Recommend the information leaflet from the FPA on www.fpa.org.uk

● At present there is only one product, Evra (Clinical Effectiveness Unit 2004b). This patch releases norelgestromin 150 mcg/day and ethinylestradiol 20 mcg/day into the circulation. The patch is applied weekly for 21 days and the fourth week is patch-free. Suitable sites are the upper outer arm, upper torso (excluding breast), buttock or lower abdomen.

- Effectiveness is similar to the COC. The same contraindications apply as for the COC. Also the same drug interactions as for the COC must be presumed. Breakthrough bleeding and spotting and breast tenderness are more common than with the COC in the first two cycles.

If a patch is partly detached for less than 24 hours, it should be reapplied to the same site or replaced with a new patch immediately. No additional contraception is needed and the next patch should be applied on the usual change day.

If a patch remains detached for more than 24 hours or if the user is not aware when the patch became detached she should stop the current contraceptive cycle and start a new cycle by applying a new patch, giving a new 'day 1' – additional precautions must be used concurrently for the first 7 days of the new cycle.

If application of a new patch at the start of a new cycle is delayed, contraceptive protection is lost. A new patch should be applied as soon as remembered giving a new 'day 1' – additional non-hormonal methods of contraception should be used for the first 7 days of the new cycle. If intercourse has occurred during this extended patch-free interval, a possibility of fertilization should be considered.

If applications of a patch in the middle of the cycle is delayed (i.e. the patch is not changed on day 8 or day 15):

(a) for up to 48 hours, apply a new patch immediately; next patch change day remains the same and no additional precautions are required

(b) for more than 48 hours, contraceptive protection may have been lost. Stop the current cycle and start a new 4-week cycle immediately by applying a new patch giving a new 'day 1'. Additional precautions should be used for the first 7 days of the new cycle.

If the patch is not removed at the end of the cycle (day 22), remove it as soon as possible and start the next cycle on the usual change day, after day 28. No extra precautions are required.

COMBINED VAGINAL RING (CLINICAL EFFECTIVENESS UNIT 2009D)

NuvaRing was launched in 2009. It releases 120 mcg etonogestrel and 15 mcg ethinylestradiol/day from an ethylene vinyl acetate copolymer ring with an outer diameter of 54 mm. The same contraindications and drug interactions apply as for the COC. Tampon use has no effect on the systemic absorption of the hormones released from NuvaRing. A ring can be removed, e.g. for sex, for up to 3 hours. Prior to dispensing, NuvaRing is stored at 2–8°c. Once dispensed, storage is at room temperature and the shelf life is 4 months.

- Women use a ring for 3 weeks followed by a ring-free week during which time they have a withdrawal bleed. A new ring is needed for each 4-week cycle.
- NuvaRing has high effectiveness no different from the combined pill, especially when adherence is good (Oddsson, Leifels-Fischer, de Melo, *et al.* 2005; Ahrendt, Nisand, Bastianelli, *et al.* 2006).
- Cycle control is better than with the combined pill (Bjarnadóttir, Tuppurainen and Killick 2002; Oddson, Leifels-Fischer, Wiel-Masson, *et al.* 2005; Roumen, op ten Berg and Hoomans 2006; Merki-Feld and Hund 2007).
- The ring can, however, cause leucorrhoea, vaginal discomfort, vaginitis and ring-related events comprising foreign body sensation, coital problems and expulsion (Oddsson, Leifels-Fischer, de Melo, *et al.* 2005; Ahrendt, Nisand, Bastianelli, *et al.* 2006).

If the ring-free interval is extended beyond 7 days, the woman should insert a new ring as soon as she remembers. Extra precautions should be used for the next 7 days. If unprotected sex took place during the ring-free interval, the use of emergency contraception can be considered or a pregnancy test done after 3 weeks.

If the ring was temporarily outside the vagina, it should be rinsed in lukewarm water and reinserted. If the ring was outside the vagina for less than 3 hours, no further action is necessary. If the ring was outside the vagina for more than 3 hours, extra precautions should be used for the next 7 days. If the loss in continuity of use of the ring for more than 3 hours occurs in the third week of use, a new ring should be inserted without the ring-free interval.

If the ring is left in place for more than 3 weeks, this is acceptable up to a total of 4 weeks, even if there is then a ring-free week. If the ring has been left in the vagina for longer than 4 weeks, pregnancy should be excluded before another ring is inserted.

PROGESTOGEN-ONLY PILL (POP) (CLINICAL EFFECTIVENESS UNIT 2008A)

There are four traditional POPs available. A POP containing desogestrel (Cerazette) was launched in 2002 (Clinical Effectiveness Unit 2003b). This is much more likely than traditional POPs to inhibit ovulation, but comparative data on efficacy is lacking. Available data show that effectiveness is similar to the COC (Trussell 2007) but traditional POPs are probably less effective than COCs.

PATIENTS FOR WHOM THE POP IS PARTICULARLY INDICATED

(a) *Older women:* those over 45 years old without risk factors, and those over 35 years old who smoke.
(b) *Those with medical contraindications to oestrogen*, including a personal history of VTE.
(c) *Those with risk factors for arterial disease*, including hypertension, diabetes mellitus, migraine with aura and smokers aged > 35.
(d) *Lactating mothers*; progestogen in the breast milk has no adverse effect on the baby (Clinical Effectiveness Unit 2009b).
(e) *Those who choose it*, especially those aged over 25 or 30 years, and who accept that it may be less reliable than the COC.

UNACCEPTABLE HEALTH RISK (UKMEC4) (CLINICAL EFFECTIVENESS UNIT 2009A)

(a) Breast cancer – current.

RISKS USUALLY OUTWEIGH BENEFITS (UKMEC3) (CLINICAL EFFECTIVENESS UNIT 2009A)

(a) *Ischaemic heart disease* – current or past history, if occurred when on POP.
(b) *Stroke* – history of CVA, if occurred when on POP.

(c) *Breast cancer* – past and no evidence of current disease for 5 years.
(d) *Cirrhosis* – severe (decompensated).
(e) *Liver tumours* – benign (hepatocellular adenoma) and malignant (hepatoma).
(f) *SLE* – with positive or unknown antiphospholipid antibodies.
(g) *Enzyme-inducing drugs* – see page 350.

TAKING THE POP: PROCEDURE AND ADVICE

Recommend the information leaflet from the FPA on www.fpa.org.uk

Starting the POP:

(a) *Days 1–5 of the cycle*. If started on or before day 5 then no other precautions need be taken.
(b) *After day 5*. Extra precautions should be taken for the first 2 days.
(c) *Switch from COC*. If changing from a COC, go straight on to the POP without a 7-day break. Extra precautions are not necessary but it may be necessary to take the pill at a different time of day.
(d) *Postpartum*. Start at 3 weeks postpartum. Extra precautions are only needed for the next 7 days if starting later than that.

Note: Time of day. Traditional POPs must be taken regularly at the same time each day (ideally at least 4 hours before the most frequent time of intercourse to ensure maximal mucus-thickening effect).

Advice

(a) *Efficacy*. Efficacy is lowest in women with no alteration in cycle activity and is greatest in those with complete suppression of cycles and consequent amenorrhoea. Roughly 40% of women continue to ovulate, in 40% there is variable interference with the follicular and luteal phase, and in 20% ovulation is inhibited completely.
(b) *Bleeding pattern*. From (a) it follows that 40% have similar cycles to their normal pattern, 40% have shorter cycles (which may gradually lengthen towards normal over time) with episodes of spotting or breakthrough bleeding and 20% have long cycles or amenorrhoea.

(c) *Safety.* There is no evidence of increased cardiovascular risk (Heinemann, Assmann, DoMinh and Garbe 1999). However, there is limited evidence of an increased risk of breast cancer for use in the previous 5 years (RR 1.17), but no increase 10 or more years after stopping (Collaborative Group on Hormonal Factors in Breast Cancer 1996).

(d) *Antibiotics.* The POP is not affected by antibiotics, except rifampicin, rifabutin and griseofulvin (see (h) below).

(e) *Missed pills.* If one or more pills are missed or delayed for more than 3 hours then: take one pill as soon as remembered; take the next pill at the usual time (this may mean taking two pills in one day); continue taking pills, one daily; extra precautions need to be taken for 2 days. For Cerazette the instructions are the same, except the window is 12 hours instead of 3 hours. Emergency contraception can be considered, if unprotected sex occurs during this 2-day period.

(f) *Diarrhoea or vomiting.* If vomiting or diarrhoea occur, continue to take the pill regularly but take extra precautions during the attack and for the next 2 days.

(g) *Obesity.* There is no evidence that the efficacy of POPs is reduced in women weighing over 70 kg; the licensed use of one pill per day is recommended.

(h) *Enzyme-inducing drugs.* Those on enzyme-inducing drugs are best advised not to rely on POPs (Clinical Effectiveness Unit 2005a and 2008a).

SIDE-EFFECTS
Non-menstrual

These are the usual progestogenic ones such as headaches, tender breasts, acne, depression, weight gain and loss of sexual drive. But because the dose of progestogen is so low, these side-effects are not that common and often not severe.

Irregular bleeding

* Examine to exclude a pathological cause.
* Do not change to another POP. There is no suggestion that with traditional POPs changing

brand will improve menstrual or non-menstrual side-effects.
* Suggest a change to another method.

Abdominal pain of gynaecological origin

* Consider ectopic pregnancy. If it can be excluded, then refer for ultrasound. It may be due to a functional ovarian cyst. Such a cyst usually resolves without treatment.

Amenorrhoea when cycles have been present

* Exclude pregnancy before assuming that it is due to the POP.
* Encourage the woman to persevere with the POP. She is in the group least likely to become pregnant with it.

INJECTABLE PROGESTOGENS (CLINICAL EFFECTIVENESS UNIT 2008B)

Recommend the information leaflet from the FPA on www.fpa.org.uk

PREPARATIONS

* Depot medroxyprogesterone acetate (DMPA) – Depo-Provera: 150 mg in 1 ml. Mix the preloaded syringe thoroughly before administration.
* Norethisterone enantate (NE) – Noristerat: 200 mg in 1 ml. Warm the vial close to body temperature before administration.

Note: NE is not licensed for long-term use. When used for longer than 16 weeks, this use outside the licence must be discussed with the patient.

INDICATIONS

The indications are similar to those for the POP. Patients for whom injectable progestogens are especially indicated are women:

(a) *likely to forget* (or to worry about forgetting) to take daily pills;
(b) *for whom higher dose long-term progestogens are beneficial,* e.g. those with fibroids or endometriosis;

(c) *with sickle-cell disease:* DMPA improves the blood picture and reduces the number of crises (Westhoff 2003).

UNACCEPTABLE HEALTH RISK (UKMEC4) (CLINICAL EFFECTIVENESS UNIT 2009A)

(a) *Breast cancer* — current.

RISKS OUTWEIGH BENEFITS (WHO3) (CLINICAL EFFECTIVENESS UNIT 2009A)

(a) *Vascular disease* - ischaemic heart disease, peripheral vascular disease, hypertensive retinopathy or TIAs. Injectables have hypo-oestrogenic effects and reduce HDL levels.
(b) *Stroke* – history of CVA.
(c) *Unexplained vaginal bleeding* – before evaluation.
(d) *Breast cancer* – past and no evidence of current disease for 5 years.
(e) *Diabetes* – with nephropathy, retinopathy, neuropathy, other vascular disease.
(f) *Cirrhosis* – severe (decompensated).
(g) *Liver tumours* – benign (hepatocellular adenoma) or malignant (hepatoma).
(h) *SLE* – with positive or unknown antiphospholipid antibodies.

BEFORE STARTING

Discuss with the patient the following:

Advantages

Injectables are effective and independent of coitus, with no oestrogenic side-effects. They are 'invisible', which may be important to some women, e.g. those in controlling or abusive relationships. They decrease the risk of endometrial cancer, pelvic inflammatory disease, ectopic pregnancy, fibroids and iron deficiency anaemia (Westhoff 2003). They may enhance lactation and relieve premenstrual and menstrual symptoms. Seizure control has been reported to be improved in some epileptics.

Effectiveness

Injectables are a very effective means of contraception: perfect use failure rates are $< 0.7\%$ for DMPA in the first year and $< 1.0\%$ for NE. Typical use failure rates are 3%. Blood levels of DMPA are not affected by drugs including enzyme-inducers; there is no justification for increasing the dose or reducing injection intervals for this reason (Clinical Effectiveness Unit 2005a). With NE, care is needed with concurrent antiretroviral therapy, certain anti-epileptics and rifampicin/rifabutin (UKMEC2).

Side–effects

■ *Erratic bleeding.* This will occur in most women initially. Prolonged episodes of bleeding may occur, but are rarely heavy and decrease over time (WHO 1987).
  * Examine (especially the cervix).
  * Give either:
    (a) the next injection early (but not earlier than 4 weeks after the last one); or
    (b) a short course of oestrogen, e.g. the COC, if no contraindication; or
    (c) a course of mefenamic acid.
  * Refer if the above do not control the bleeding.
  * Alternatively the patient may prefer to discontinue the method.
■ *Amenorrhoea.* This is likely, more so the longer the method is used. The amenorrhoea rate with DMPA is around 70% at 12 months (Canto De Cetina, Canto and Ordoñez Luna 2001). With NE, episodes of bleeding are the more usual pattern and the amenorrhoea rate at 12 months is 25%. Explain that these methods make the lining of the womb so thin that there is no monthly shedding. Many women find the amenorrhoea a very acceptable side-effect.
  * Exclude pregnancy (beware of weight gain at successive visits with nausea or breast symptoms).
  * Discuss other concerns. There is concern that injectables can lower ovarian oestradiol production; see 'bone mineral density' below. There is a lack of consensus on any action to be taken with continuous amenorrhoea for over 5 years. Some authorities have recommended checking serum oestradiol but this is not a useful proxy indicator for bone mineral density. Bone densitometry is the test of choice but is expensive and not always freely available.
■ *Weight gain.* This is possible, through appetite stimulation, although some studies show no effect on weight (Westhoff 2003). The weight gain is not generally the result of fluid retention. Modification of diet and behaviour will tend to

counteract the weight gain. Any weight gain is less likely with NE.

■ *Return of fertility.* This may be delayed, with a mean time to ovulation of 18 weeks from the expiry of the last dose of DMPA (maximum 49 weeks). Return of fertility is much faster with NE: mean of 4 weeks and maximum of 26 weeks (Fotherby and Howard 1986).

Risks

■ *Reduced bone mineral density.* DMPA reduces BMD in many women who use it. However, so far, no studies have shown an increased risk of osteoporosis or fractures. When a reduction in BMD occurs, it takes place over the first 2–3 years and then tends to level off. The reduction is generally less than 1 SD, i.e. not into the osteopenic range (Curtis and Martins 2006). After discontinuation of DMPA, BMD consistently returns towards or to baseline values in women of all ages (Kaunitz, Arias and McClung 2008). Patterns of BMD recovery are similar to those seen after cessation of lactation. Available evidence does not justify the requirement of a limit to the duration of DMPA use, even in adolescents. Care is needed in high-risk groups: smokers, BMI < 19, thyroid disease, long-term antiepileptic therapy and those with a family history of osteoporosis. Avoid in those on oral steroids.

■ *Cancer.* There is limited evidence of an increased risk of breast cancer for use in the previous 5 years (RR 1.17), but no increase 10 or more years after stopping (Collaborative Group on Hormonal Factors in Breast Cancer 1996). DMPA has a strong protective effect against endometrial cancer (RR 0.21) (WHO 1991).

INITIATING TREATMENT AND FOLLOW-UP

Schedule for the injections

✳ Give the first injection within 5 days of the onset of menstruation, within 3 weeks of delivery, or 1–5 days after miscarriage or termination. The patient should use additional precautions for 7 days after the first injection unless it was given as above.

✳ Use the upper outer quadrant of the buttock or the lateral thigh. The deltoid is used when the patient is obese, as it is important the drug reaches muscle. Warn the patient not to massage the site as this may speed up drug release.

✳ Give subsequent injections: Depo-Provera 150 mg 12-weekly; Noristerat 200 mg 8-weekly.

If the patient returns late for the next injection of DMPA or NE, proceed as in Table 12.3.

ETONOGESTREL-RELEASING IMPLANT: IMPLANON (CLINICAL EFFECTIVENESS UNIT 2008c)

Recommend the information leaflet from the fpa on www.fpa.org.uk

● Implanon releases a mean etonogestrel dose of 40 mcg/day.

● Subdermal implants should only be inserted and removed if specific practical training has been obtained and a minimum number of implants are inserted and removed to keep up the necessary skills.

● Implanon has the advantage that it lasts for 3 years but is reversible should the need arise. It has a high effectiveness, 0.05% in the first year, higher even than vasectomy (Trussell 2007). Pregnancies in women using Implanon are generally due to non-insertion and drug interactions (Harrison-Woolrych and Hill 2005). The return of fertility after removal of Implanon is immediate; ovulation occurs mostly within 3 weeks of removal. Implanon has a beneficial effect on dysmenorrhoea. Implanon is more cost-effective than the COC (National Collaborating Centre for Women's and Children's Health 2005).

● Disadvantages are the discomfort of insertion and removal.

● *Practicalities.* If it is implanted other than on days 1–5 of the menstrual cycle, extra precautions are needed for the first 7 days, if there is no previous method providing cover. For postpartum women, including those who are breastfeeding, insert at up to 3 weeks postpartum. Following abortion or miscarriage, insert at up to 5 days. The patient should use additional precautions for 7 days after insertion unless timed as above.

Table 12.3   Management of late injections of injectable progestogens (Clinical Effectiveness Unit 2008)

TIMING OF INJECTION	HAS UNPROTECTED SEX OCCURRED?	CAN THE INJECTION BE GIVEN?	IS EMERGENCY CONTRACEPTION INDICATED?[a]	IS ADDITIONAL CONTRACEPTION OR ABSTINENCE ADVISED?	SHOULD A PREGNANCY TEST BE PERFORMED?
Up to 14 weeks since last DMPA injection or up to 10 weeks since last NET-EN injection	Not applicable, as long as next injection is given 14 weeks since last DMPA injection or 10 weeks since last NET-EN injection or before	Yes	No	No	No
When an injection is overdue: 14 weeks + 1 day or more since last DMPA injection; or 10 weeks + 1 day or more since last NET-EN injection	No (abstained or used barrier methods)	Yes	No	Yes, for the next 7 days	No, if abstained Yes, if used barrier methods, but at least 21 days later
	Yes, but only in the last 3 days[b]	Yes	Yes, should offer Levonelle 1500 or a copper IUD	Yes, for the next 7 days	Yes, at least 21 days later
	Yes, but only in the last 4–5 days[b]	Yes	Yes, should offer a copper IUD	No, if opts for copper IUD	Yes, at least 21 days later
	Yes, more than 5 days ago[b]	No	No	Yes, for 21 days until a pregnancy test is confirmed negative and for a further 7 days after giving injection	Yes, at the initial presentation and at least 21 days later

(a) If EC is declined, decisions about ongoing use of DMPA/NET-EN should be tailored to the individual woman. Alternative methods if required should then be considered.
(b) Not applicable if unprotected sex occurred within 14 weeks of last DMPA injection or 10 weeks of last NET-EN injection.
Reproduced with permission of the Faculty of Sexual & Reproductive Healthcare.

UNACCEPTABLE HEALTH RISK (UKMEC4) (CLINICAL EFFECTIVENESS UNIT 2009A)

(a) *Breast cancer* – current.

RISKS OUTWEIGH BENEFITS (UKMEC3) (CLINICAL EFFECTIVENESS UNIT 2009A)

(a) *Ischaemic heart disease* – current or past history.
(b) *Stroke* – history of CVA, if occurred when using implant.
(c) *Unexplained vaginal bleeding* – before evaluation.
(d) *Breast cancer* – past history and no evidence of current disease for 5 years.
(e) *Cirrhosis* – severe (decompensated).
(f) *Liver tumours* benign (hepatocellular adenoma) or malignant (hepatoma).
(g) *SLE* – with positive or unknown antiphospholipid antibodies.

MONITORING

● There is no reason to check weight and blood pressure.
● There is no reason to do any routine follow up.

PROBLEMS WITH THE IMPLANT

Menstrual

Bleeding patterns are variable even in an individual over time. Frequent irregular bleeding, spotting and prolonged bleeding are all possible – heavy bleeding is rare. Amenorrhoea occurs in 22% of users and infrequent bleeding in 34% (Mansour, Korver, Marintcheva-Petrova and Fraser 2008). Those who discontinue tend to be from the groups with less favourable patterns: prolonged bleeding (18%) and frequent bleeding (7%).

Problematic bleeding can be treated as per injectables (see page 358). Some clinicians add a progestogen such as Cerazette or norethisterone; there are no data to support this.

Non-menstrual

Acne, mastalgia, headache, weight gain, abdominal pain, emotional lability and depression.

NON-HORMONAL METHODS OF CONTRACEPTION

INTRAUTERINE DEVICES (IUD) (CLINICAL EFFECTIVENESS UNIT 2007A)

Recommend the information leaflet from the FPA on www.fpa.org.uk

- Typical use failure rates for copper IUDs are 0.8% in the first year (Trussell 2007).
- IUDs should only be fitted if specific practical training has been obtained and a minimum number of devices are fitted to keep up the necessary skills.
- All IUDs with frames have copper on the stem and/or on the arms. GyneFix is a frameless device with six copper cylinders on a thread. Modern copper-containing IUDs are clinically effective and safe for at least 5 years. The TT380 Slimline and TCu380A QuickLoad are effective for 10 years.
- The risk of perforation associated with insertion of IUDs is 1 in 1000.
- IUDs do not offer any protection against sexually transmitted infections (STIs) but previous studies that purported to show an increased risk of pelvic inflammatory disease (PID) have now been shown to be flawed (Grimes 2000). There is no evidence that prophylactic use of antibiotics for IUD insertion is of significant benefit in healthy women (Grimes, Schulz and Stanwood 2004).
- Currently available high-load IUDs protect against ectopic pregnancy when compared to using no contraception.
- Cumulative expulsion rates at 5 years for copper IUDs are around 5%. Expulsion may occur at any time after insertion, but is most likely in the early cycles, especially during menstruation. Patients who are older and of higher parity are less likely to expel their device.

UNACCEPTABLE HEALTH RISK (UKMEC4) (CLINICAL EFFECTIVENESS UNIT 2009A)

(a) Pregnancy.
(b) Puerperal sepsis.
(c) Immediately after septic abortion.
(d) Insertion before evaluation of unexplained vaginal bleeding.
(e) Gestational trophoblastic disease – with persistently elevated β-hCG levels or malignant disease.
(f) Cervical or endometrial cancer – current.
(g) STI (current purulent cervicitis, chlamydial infection or gonorrhoea) or PID – current.
(h) Pelvic TB.

RISKS USUALLY OUTWEIGH BENEFITS (UKMEC3) (CLINICAL EFFECTIVENESS UNIT 2009A)

(a) Postpartum insertion between 48 hours and 4 weeks postpartum – in women who are breast feeding, not breast feeding or post-Caesarean section.
(b) Distortion of the uterine cavity – e.g. congenital malformation, submucous fibroids.
(c) Ovarian cancer.

ADVERSE EFFECTS

Heavier periods, intermenstrual bleeding, dysmenorrhoea

* Warn the patient that these are common in the first few cycles after insertion.
* Examine for infection or malposition of the device.
* Prescribe NSAIDs, which may reduce pain and bleeding (see page 323).
* Remove the IUD if it appears to be associated with a change in bleeding pattern. If the pattern does not return to normal, refer for gynaecological assessment.

Pelvic infection

* Symptoms of infection require examination and endocervical swabs for STIs.
* Treat with antibiotics (see page 331).

* If the symptoms settle, the IUD can be left in place.
* *Actinomyces-like organisms (ALOs)* may be found on a cervical smear.
  (a) If the patient is asymptomatic, leave the IUD in place;
  (b) If the patient has symptoms, i.e. pain or discharge, remove the IUD and investigate the patient for pelvic pain/STIs, treat with antibiotics as appropriate and consider referral to GUM or gynaecology.

Pregnancy

* If symptoms suggest an ectopic pregnancy, admit to hospital; 6% of pregnancies that occur with an IUD in place are ectopic.
* If a scan indicates that the pregnancy is intrauterine, gently remove the IUD if the threads are visible and the pregnancy is less than 12 weeks. This will halve the miscarriage rate. If the pregnancy is > 12 weeks or no threads are seen, refer early for antenatal assessment.

Lost threads

* Teach the patient to feel for the threads after each period, or on the first of the month if there is amenorrhoea with the IUS (see page 363).
* If the threads are not palpable, warn the patient temporarily to use other precautions, and arrange for USS.
* If USS confirms that the device is in situ, leave in place until it is due to be changed. Repeat vaginal examination yearly, and only repeat USS if there is reason to suspect expulsion.

TIMING OF INSERTION

* Insertion can be at any time during the menstrual cycle if it is reasonably certain a woman is not pregnant (Table 12.2).
* Do not insert before 4 weeks postpartum.
* An IUD can be safely fitted immediately after a first trimester abortion (spontaneous or therapeutic), although this carries an increased risk of expulsion (Grimes, Schulz and Stanwood 2004).

REMOVAL OR REFIT

* *Women aged 40 and over:* an IUD fitted after the age of 40 can be left as the only means of contraception until the menopause. When there has been 6 months of amenorrhoea it should be removed; later removal may be difficult because of cervical stenosis. If a woman presents more than 6 months after the menopause with a device in situ, attempt to remove it. If difficulty is encountered try again after a short course of treatment with topical oestrogen.

TIMING OF REMOVAL

* *If pregnancy is desired*, the IUD may be removed at any time.
* *If pregnancy is not desired*, remove the IUD when the patient is established on a hormonal method or when barrier methods have been used carefully since the last period.
* *Emergency contraception* may be necessary if intercourse has occurred within the last 5 days and removal of the IUD is urgent (see page 365).

PROPHYLACTIC ANTIBIOTICS FOR CARDIAC DISEASE

For women with previous endocarditis or with a prosthetic heart valve it is no longer recommended to give antibiotic prophylaxis during IUD insertion or removal (NICE 2008).

FOLLOW-UP

* Review after 6 weeks. Thereafter followup is not necessary.
* Ask about menstrual blood loss, pelvic pain, vaginal discharge and discomfort to the partner.
* Do a pelvic examination and check the presence of the threads.

INTRAUTERINE SYSTEM (MIRENA) (CLINICAL EFFECTIVENESS UNIT 2007A)

Recommend the information leaflet from the FPA on www.fpa.org.uk

The steroid reservoir contains 52 mg levonorgestrel. It is licensed for contraception and menorrhagia (for 5 years) and for endometrial protection (4 years). It is more cost-effective than the COC (National Collaborating Centre for Women's and Children's Health 2005).

● *Protection after insertion.* The IUS takes 7 days to provide effective contraceptive protection. Unless the IUS is inserted within the first 7 days of the cycle, extra precautions are advised for the next 7 days. If there has been a risk of conception it would be inappropriate to insert an IUS that cycle.

● *The IUS in older women.* Women who have the IUS inserted at the age of 45 or over for contraception can retain the device until the menopause is confirmed or until contraception is no longer required.

Advantages of the IUS over IUDs

(a) It reduces blood loss instead of increasing it and is a form of therapy for menorrhagia, even in the presence of fibroids.

(b) It can reduce dysmenorrhoea.

(c) It is more reliable as a contraceptive, with a failure rate of 0.2% in the first year compared to 0.8% for copper IUDs. The IUS approximates in effectiveness to female sterilization.

(d) It has a very low rate of ectopic pregnancy.

Disadvantages of the IUS

(a) The initial cost is much more than IUDs.

(b) It is slightly more difficult to insert than a copper IUD because of a wider insertion diameter.

(c) The patient may have irregular slight bleeding in the first 3 months of use.

(d) Progestogenic side-effects (headache, breast tenderness, nausea, mood changes, acne) are possible, especially to begin with, as there is some systemic absorption; the rate of occurrence is no different from IUDs after 5 years.

Patients for whom the IUS is particularly indicated

∗ As an alternative to sterilization when the family is complete.

∗ Those with menorrhagia.

∗ Those in whom the COC is contraindicated.

∗ Those with learning disabilities or physical disabilities needing long-term contraception.

Unacceptable health risk (UKMEC4) (Clinical Effectiveness Unit 2009a)

In addition to the conditions listed for the IUD:

(a) breast cancer – current.

Risks usually outweigh benefits (UKMEC3) (Clinical Effectiveness Unit 2009a)

In addition to conditions listed for the IUD:

(a) *ischaemic heart disease* – current or past history, if developed while IUS in situ;

(b) *cirrhosis* – severe (decompensated);

(c) *liver tumours* – benign (hepatocellular adenoma) and malignant (hepatoma);

(d) *SLE* – with positive or unknown antiphospholipid antibodies.

BARRIER METHODS (CLINICAL EFFECTIVENESS UNIT 2007B, C)

Recommend the information leaflet from the FPA on www.fpa.org.uk

These have the advantage of protecting against STIs and HPV, as well as pregnancy. However, efficacy is utterly dependent on consistent use before/during sex; there is considerable potential for user failure, especially among young people.

Condoms and diaphragms made of latex rubber can be damaged by oil-based products such as:

(a) baby oil/bath oil/body oil/Vaseline;

(b) suntan oil/massage oil;

(c) cream/ice cream/salad cream;

(d) lipstick/hair conditioner;

(e) many antithrush preparations;

(f) progesterone pessaries.

MALE CONDOMS

Male condoms give a pregnancy rate of 2–15% in the first year. Non-latex condoms are now available (Gallo, Grimes, Lopez and Schulz 2006) in addition to latex rubber products; they cannot be damaged by oil-based products.

* Ensure the couple knows to use condoms bearing the CE mark and preferably also the British Standards Institution Kitemark.
* Advise the couple about use of emergency contraception in the event of a mishap.

FEMALE CONDOM

Femidom is a loose-fitting polyurethane sheath with two flexible rings which is inserted into the vagina. It is pre-lubricated with dimeticone, an odourless, non-spermicidal lubricant. It lines the vagina and covers some of the vulva. It is disposable and comes in one size. Its failure rate is 5–21% in the first year.

DIAPHRAGMS

Diaphragms are more effective than the condom, and have the advantage that they do not need to be inserted and removed at the time of intercourse. They are not, however, as effective a protector as condoms against STIs. They have a failure rate of 6–16 % in the first year. They come in sizes rising in steps of 5 mm and in the form of coiled spring, arcing spring or flat spring. Coil spring and arcing diaphragms are also available in silicone. Correct size and type is determined on vaginal examination.

(a) The diaphragm should be inserted before sex and left in place for at least 6 hours after the last act of sex.
(b) A strip of spermicide about 5 cm long should be placed on the upper side of the diaphragm before insertion. If sex takes place more than 3 hours later, more spermicide should be inserted, either as a pessary or as cream with an applicator.
(c) The diaphragm must be washed in warm soapy water, dried after use and stored in a cool place in its container to maintain its shape.
  * Check the fit and comfort after 1 week and discuss again the routine for its use.
  * See after 3 months and then annually, but more frequently if there are difficulties or if there is a weight change of more than 3 kg. Prescribe a new diaphragm annually.

CERVICAL CAPS

These had rather gone out of fashion, but a revival is under way with the FemCap (Clinical Effectiveness Unit 2004c) made of silicone. Failure rates are 10–18% in the first year. Before starting, sizing is needed by a doctor or nurse. FemCap comes in three sizes and is reusable.

* Diaphragms and caps should not be used if the woman has a history of toxic shock syndrome (UKMEC3).
* Condoms, diaphragms and caps should not be used in people with latex allergy (UKMEC3).

FERTILITY AWARENESS

Fertility awareness or natural family planning relies on avoidance of intercourse around the time of ovulation. Failure rates can be as low as 2.6% in the first year when multiple indicators are used to define the beginning and the end of the fertile period (European Natural Family Planning Study Groups 1993) – but this high efficacy is only achieved by highly motivated and well-trained couples. Expert training is essential; advise the patient to contact Fertility UK (see box) for information about local classes. Computerized thermometers and saliva testing kits are on sale but they are unevaluated and cannot be recommended.

> **PATIENT INFORMATION**
>
> Fertility UK, Bury Knowle Health Centre, 207 London Road, Headington, Oxford, OX3 9JA; Available: www.fertilityuk.org

Recognized indicators are:

(a) waking (basal) body temperature changes;
(b) changes in cervical secretions;
(c) cervical changes;
(d) calculation based on cycle length;
(e) minor changes, e.g. Mittelschmerz (mid-cycle pain).

Combining indicators is best; the combination of temperature and cervical secretions (sympto-thermal) is commonly used.

Persona is a fertility monitor that measures estrone-3-glucuronide and LH in the urine and predicts fertile days for an individual by storing information on the woman's biochemistry and cycle length. It requires eight urine tests per cycle. A red light indicates fertile days and a green light non-fertile days. A yellow light indicates that a urine test is required. It must be realized that when this device is used by the non-NFP fraternity without combining indicators, failure rates will be higher. Nevertheless, a failure rate of 6.2% in the first year is predicted in such a population (Bonnar, Flynn, Freundl, *et al.* 1999).

EMERGENCY CONTRACEPTION (CLINICAL EFFECTIVENESS UNIT 2006B)

HORMONAL PREPARATIONS

- *The progestogen-only method* is available as levonorgestrel 1500 mcg: Levonelle 1500 on prescription and as Levonelle One Step as a pharmacy item.
- Ulipristal acetate 30 mg (ellaOne), a progesterone receptor modulator on prescription only.

IUD INSERTION

- *Insertion of a copper-IUD* can be considered if:
  (a) the patient presents within 5 days of unprotected intercourse; or
  (b) within 5 days of the calculated time of ovulation if intercourse took place more than 5 days before presentation, whether or not further intercourse has taken place in the last 5 days.
- Patients who have failed to take oral contraception correctly:
  (a) *COC.* Either method can be considered for a patient who misses three or more pills (see Figure 12.1);
  (b) *POP.* Either method can be considered for a patient who has unprotected sex during the 48-hour window after regular pill taking has been re-established after missed pills.

REGIMEN FOR HORMONAL EMERGENCY CONTRACEPTION

- One tablet of Levonelle 1500 taken within 72 hours of (the first episode of) unprotected intercourse.

- One tablet of ulipristal taken within 120 hours of (the first episode of) unprotected intercourse.

CONTRAINDICATIONS

(a) Suspected pregnancy.

(b) *IUD.* Contraindications to the insertion of an IUD apply except that, in an emergency, an IUD can be inserted with antibiotic cover in a patient at risk of PID. Contraindications to the long-term use of an IUD do not apply because the IUD can be removed after the next period.

(c) Ulipristal should not be used in those needing oral steroids such as asthma or in those on drugs which increase gastric pH e.g. antacids, H2-receptor antagonists or proton pump inhibitors.

SPECIAL SITUATIONS

(a) *Enzyme-inducing drugs.* These may be prescribed or bought OTC. Patients taking enzyme-inducing drugs should take two Levonelle 1500 pills instead of one. Ulipristal should not be used in those taking enzyme-inducers.

(b) *Previous ectopic pregnancy.* Patients should understand that neither method will protect against a further ectopic pregnancy.

(c) The woman who wants the most reliable method or in whom there has been multiple exposure; use an IUD.

(d) Use of hormonal contraception is possible immediately following administration of Levonelle, with use of condoms or abstinence for 7 days (2 days for POP). When ulipristal is used, there is a possibility that it may reduce the efficacy of hormonal methods for up to a week, so advise condoms or abstinence for 2 weeks after administration.

MANAGEMENT

The treatment of choice is usually Levonelle, even in low-risk situations, in view of patient anxiety and the safety of the method. Ulipristal can be offered for those presenting between 72 and 120 hours after unprotected intercourse. But patients should be informed about the copper IUD method and its greater effectiveness.

∗ Establish from the consultation:
  (a) date of LMP;

(b) whether the LMP was normal;

(c) the normal menstrual cycle length and probable date of ovulation;

(d) *all* the occasions of unprotected sexual intercourse (UPSI) in the last cycle;

(e) number of hours since first episode of UPSI;

(f) the method of contraception normally used.

* Warn the woman that the maximum risk of pregnancy after midcycle UPSI is about 9% (Wilcox, Dunson, Weinberg, *et al.* 2001), but depends on the inherent fertility of the couple.

* Explain to the patient that:

(a) the method is not guaranteed. The average risk of pregnancy from a single episode of coitus is 3% (Wilcox, Dunson, Weinberg, *et al.* 2001). The progestogen-only method and ulipristal reduce this risk by around 85%. The IUD is more effective, reducing the risk by 99% (Liying and Bilian 2001);

(b) if the hormonal method is given, barrier methods must be used until the next period, which may be a little earlier or later than expected. The COC may then be started;

(c) she should re-attend if the next period does not come, or she has any other worries;

(d) if vomiting occurs within 2 hours of taking the dose she should re-attend urgently.

FOLLOW-UP

* If a normal period has not occurred, exclude pregnancy and bear in mind the possibility of ectopic pregnancy.

* Discuss the long-term need for contraception. Use the opportunity to counsel the young and inexperienced. Consider whether a supply of Levonelle 1500 in advance might be appropriate for a woman who does not wish planned contraception but who anticipates the need for occasional emergency contraception after unplanned sex. In a US study it increased the use of emergency contraception without reducing the use of routine contraception (Jackson, Bimla Schwarz, Freedman and Darney 2003).

CONTRACEPTION IN SPECIAL CASES

CONTRACEPTION AND YOUNG PEOPLE (CLINICAL EFFECTIVENESS UNIT 2010A)

INFORMATION AND ADVICE

Brook Helpline. Free confidential counselling service for young people. Tel. 0800 0185023; Available: www.brook.org.uk

Sexwise for under 18-year-olds with problems with sex, relationships and contraception. Helpline 0800 282930; Available: www.maketherightdecision.co.uk

In England and Wales, provision of contraceptive advice and treatment by health professionals to those aged under 16 is governed by a health circular issued on 29 July 2004 (Anon. 2004a). Advice and treatment may be given, according to the Fraser guidelines, without parental knowledge when the young person:

(a) has sufficient maturity to understand the moral, social and emotional implications of the treatment;

(b) cannot be persuaded to inform the parents or allow them to be informed;

(c) is very likely to begin, or to continue, sexual intercourse with or without contraception;

(d) would be likely to suffer in terms of physical or mental health if no contraceptive advice or treatment were given;

(e) has their best interests served by being given contraceptive advice or treatment without parental consent.

Young people continue to have concerns about the possibility of breaches of confidentiality. Improving young people's trust in the confidentiality of their practice should help remove one of the main obstacles that deter some teenagers from seeking early sexual health advice (Donovan, Hadley, Jones, *et al.* 2000). Every practice should develop its own confidentiality policy.

* *Legal aspects*. Inform the patient (and, if she gives her consent, her parents) of the legal situation – it is an offence for a person to have sexual contact with a girl under the age of 16, even if the girl consents (Sexual Offences Act 2003).

* *Smoking*. Discuss the importance of not smoking, especially if the COC is to be used.

* Discuss the risks of contracting STIs, especially chlamydia, and how condoms protect against transmission.
* Raise the advantages, both psychological and physical, of not having sex at a young age.

COMBINED ORAL CONTRACEPTIVE

* Warn the patient that BTB can occur in the first few packets, is not harmful, and to come in and discuss the problem rather than stop the pill.
* Stress the value of using the condom as well to reduce the risk of STIs including HIV (dual protection). Young people should be shown how to use condoms.

CONTRACEPTION AND OLDER WOMEN (CLINICAL EFFECTIVENESS UNIT 2010B)

* Women over 40 are more likely to have irregular cycles, but ovulation still occurs in around 35% of these cycles and there is still need for contraception.
* Current advice is for contraception to be continued in women aged 40–50 until there has been 2 years' amenorrhoea, and in women over 50 until there has been 1 year's amenorrhoea.

Women on the COC

* *Age.* Healthy non-smokers without risk factors may continue until the age of 50.
* Advise women who have stopped the COC at 50 to use the POP, barrier methods or spermicide until they have had 1 year's amenorrhoea. If menstruating on the POP, follow the advice below.

Women on the POP (Clinical Effectiveness Unit 2010b)

* When amenorrhoea occurs in those who have been having periods, stop the POP but use other precautions for 1 year if aged over 50, for 2 years if aged 50 or less.
* Alternatively, check the FSH.
* Those women who have always had amenorrhoea on the POP can have their FSH checked after age 50.

Hormone replacement therapy (HRT)

HRT is not contraceptive as the natural oestrogens do not necessarily inhibit ovulation.

* *Women started on HRT before the menopause* should continue contraception (barrier or IUD, possibly the POP) until there is reason to think that they have reached the menopause, e.g. at age 50. It is impossible to assess the timing of the natural menopause in women using HRT. If a woman is unwilling to discontinue HRT for 3–4 months to allow accurate assessment of FSH levels, then barrier contraception, an IUD or the POP can be used until the age of 55, at which time loss of natural fertility can be assumed.
* *Women on the COC* do not need HRT until the COC is stopped.

CONTRACEPTION AND LEARNING DISABILITY (COOPER 2000)

Contraception is most likely to be considered in women with learning disability who:

(a) are entering a sexual relationship. There is a 40% chance of learning disability in children born to a couple where both parents have learning disability;
(b) are in danger of being exploited.

* *Consent.* Consult a consultant psychiatrist if there is doubt about the ability to give consent. The majority of patients with moderate and mild learning disability are able to give consent.
* *Sex education.* Refer to the local community learning disability team, social services department, education department or voluntary organization.
* *Epilepsy.* If patients are on enzyme-inducing antiepileptics, the dose of the COC needs to be higher (see page 350). Those on the POP should change method.

STERILIZATION (ANON 2004B; BRECHIN 2006)

When counselling for sterilization the following should be borne in mind:

(a) Both partners should ideally be seen together.

(b) Patients should be made aware of the high efficacy of alternative long-acting reversible contraceptive methods (National Collaborating Centre for Women's and Children's Health 2005).

(c) The possibility of death of partner or child should be covered.

(d) The possibility of relationship breakdown should be discussed.

(e) The pros and cons of male versus female sterilization should be explained.

WHICH PARTNER SHOULD BE STERILIZED?

Sometimes it is not the partner who presents her-/himself who is subsequently sterilized. Points to be raised here are:

(a) Vasectomy is more effective than tubal occlusion: 1 in 2000 lifetime pregnancy risk (when postoperative semen analysis is adhered to) compared with 1 in 200 for tubal occlusion (all varieties of technique). Effectiveness of the Filshie clip is a little more favourable, but the data are less robust.

(b) Vasectomy is a more minor operation.

(c) Vasectomy is safer as it is usually performed under local anaesthesia.

(d) A man has a longer reproductive span to lose.

(e) A man is more likely to feel threatened (fear of loss of sexual drive and sexual prowess).

REVERSAL

If a patient wants a reversal of sterilization, patency rates of around 90% can be achieved with microsurgical techniques but fertility is lower: 31–92% in females and 9–82% in males (rates tend to be at the low end of this range when the vasectomy was performed more than 10 years previously).

When counselling a patient, be aware that risk factors for subsequent regret about sterilization include:

(a) age < 30;

(b) no children;

(c) not in a relationship;

(d) association in time with pregnancy (full term or abortion);

(e) crisis in relationship or not in mutually faithful relationship;

(f) coercion by partner or health professional;

(g) psychological or psychosocial issues.

TERMINATION OF PREGNANCY (ANON. 2004C)

The Abortion Act 1967, as amended by the Human Fertilisation and Embryology Act 1990, allows termination of pregnancy (TOP) if two doctors agree that:

(a) The continuance of the pregnancy would involve risk to the life of the pregnant woman greater than if the pregnancy were terminated; or

(b) The termination is necessary to prevent grave permanent injury to the physical or mental health of the pregnant woman; or

(c) The pregnancy has not exceeded its 24th week and the continuance of the pregnancy would involve risk, greater than if the pregnancy were terminated, of injury to the physical or mental health of the pregnant woman; or

(d) The pregnancy has not exceeded its 24th week and the continuance of the pregnancy would involve risk, greater than if the pregnancy were terminated, of injury to the physical or mental health of any existing child(ren) of the family of the pregnant woman; or

(e) There is a substantial risk that if the child were born it would suffer from such physical or mental abnormalities as to be seriously handicapped.

Note: There is no time limit for grounds (a), (b) and (e).

- Mortality for a TOP is 0.2 per 100,000 compared to 6 per 100,000 for death in childbirth.

- The risk of serious complications and death increases with advancing gestation, so do not be responsible for delays in referral.

- TOP is not associated with an increase in breast cancer risk.

- There are no proven associations between TOP and subsequent ectopic pregnancy, placenta praevia or infertility.

- TOP may be associated with a small increase in the risk of subsequent miscarriage or pre-term delivery.

- Higher quality studies show no higher risk of mental health sequelae in those who have TOPs compared to women with unintended pregnancies who continue (Charles, Polis, Sridhara and Blum 2008).

* Counsel the woman to help her come to her own informed decision about TOP that she will not regret and to lessen the risk of emotional disturbance whatever decision is reached.

* Ensure that she is aware of the alternative of continuing the pregnancy and keeping the baby or giving it up for adoption.

* Check she is not under pressure from partner or parent.

* Discuss the need for and if possible plan future contraception, including information about emergency contraception if not already known about.

* Arrange a follow-up appointment 2 weeks after the termination to check for medical and psychological sequelae.

* Early medical TOP with mifepristone and misoprostol up to 9 weeks' gestation (Fiala and Gemzell-Danielsson 2006) is now widely available. Check that she does not have any contraindications e.g. severe asthma not controlled by therapy, chronic adrenal failure.

THE PATIENT UNDER 16 YEARS OLD (ANON. 2004A)

Involve the parents or guardians, with the patient's consent. They will be needed to sign the consent form as well as to support the patient before and after the termination.

If the patient refuses to inform a parent or guardian, she has the right, under the Family Law Reform Act 1969, to consent to treatment herself, provided she understands the nature of the procedure including its risks and complications. If a competent child consents to treatment, a parent cannot override that consent.

INFERTILITY

For details of the diagnosis of fertility problems see *Evidence-based Diagnosis in Primary Care* by A. F. Polmear (editor), published by Butterworth-Heinemann, 2008.

NICE

Fertility: Assessment and Treatment for People with Fertility Problems. National Institute for Health and Clinical Excellence, February 2004. **www.rcog.org.uk**

Review

Taylor A, Braude P. 2004. *ABC of subfertility.* BMJ Books, London

* Reassure the couple that 75% of couples achieve conception within 6 months, and 84% by 12 months. If the woman is aged 35 the success rate is 94% over 3 years. If the woman is aged 38 the success rate is 77% over 3 years.

* Start investigations as soon as the couple voices anxiety about conceiving. Explain that in 30% of cases the problem lies with the male alone, in 30% with the female alone, and that in the remainder it is mixed or unexplained.

* Aim to consider referral after 1 year, or sooner if there is good reason to predict difficulties, e.g. oligo- or amenorrhoea, abnormal sperm count, a history of PID or maternal age over 35. Refer the couple direct to a tertiary centre holding the contract for the treatment of subfertility, not to a general gynaecology clinic.

INVESTIGATIONS

Assessment of the woman

(a) History should include details of menstrual cycle, previous pregnancies, pelvic infections or operations. Regular periods are a reliable guide to the fact that the woman is ovulating. Check that they are having intercourse at the woman's most fertile time (as well as throughout the cycle). Do not bother with temperature charts.

(b) Check that the woman is rubella immune and taking folic acid.

(c) Screen for *Chlamydia*.

(d) Examine for evidence of pelvic pathology.

(e) *Progesterone level*. Take blood 7 days before menstruation is due. A level of > 16 nmol/l suggests ovulation, and a level of > 30 nmol/l confirms it. Borderline levels may be due to a deficient luteal phase, or to mistimed sampling. Levels < 16 nmol/l confirm that the cycle was anovulatory.

(f) *Measure FSH and LH* in a woman with irregular cycles in whom it is impossible to predict when to check the blood progesterone.

Note: There is no value in measuring TFTs or prolactin in women with regular menses in the absence of galactorrhoea or symptoms of thyroid disease.

Assessment of the man

(a) Medical history should include operations on or infections of the testes and operations on the prostate.

(b) Drug history – sulfasalazine, tetracyclines, allopurinol, anabolic steroids, cannabis and cocaine have all been shown to interfere with male reproductive function.

(c) Examine him, including genitals and secondary sexual characteristics.

(d) Screen for *Chlamydia.*

(e) Arrange for semen analysis. Semen should be produced by masturbation 3 days after the last ejaculation, and examined within an hour.

(f) If the count is low, repeat after 3 months and refer to a specialist fertility clinic if still low. However, if the count is severely low, refer after a single count.

(g) Warn the patient that even a 'normal' sperm count does not mean that there is not some sperm dysfunction which can only be detected on more sophisticated tests.

NORMAL VALUES FOR SEMEN (WHO)

(a) Volume: ≥ 2 ml.

(b) pH 7.2 or higher.

(c) Concentration: ≥ 20 million per ml.

(d) Total sperm number ≥ 40 million per ejaculate.

(e) Motility: $\geq 50\%$ with $\geq 25\%$ showing progressive motility;

(f) vitality: $> 75\%$ live.

(g) morphology (strict criteria): $> 15\%$ normal forms;

(h) white blood cells: < 1 million per ml.

ADVICE

Advice to the couple should routinely be:

(a) Both should stop smoking.

(b) The woman should drink no more than one or two units of alcohol once or twice weekly while trying to conceive.

(c) Men who drink heavily should cut their drinking to no more than 3–4 units in any day.

(d) Women and men with a BMI > 30 should lose weight whether or not ovulation is a problem.

(e) Men should avoid soaking in hot baths, wearing tight underwear and remaining seated for many hours at a time.

(f) Couples should be advised to have regular sex throughout the cycle, every 2–3 days; there is no evidence that use of temperature charts and LH detection tests to time sex improves pregnancy rates.

Use of clomifene in general cannot be justified in general practice in view of the increased risk of multiple pregnancy and ovarian cancer. An exception to this is if a woman, who previously conceived using it, presents again with anovulatory cycles.

The role of the GP after referral

∗ Administer the drugs for assisted conception according to a protocol agreed with the specialist clinic.

∗ Support the couple throughout the drawn-out process of investigation and treatment.

Infertility Network UK is a self-help organization which supplies literature and runs support networks. Tel. 0800 008 7464; Available: www.infertilitynetworkuk.com
    The Human Fertilization and Embryology Authority, 21 Bloomsbury Street, London WC1B 3HF, Tel. 020 7291 8200 www.hfea.gov.uk has books and videos about assisted conception

ADOPTION

PATIENT CONTACT

The Director, British Association for Adoption and Fostering, Saffron House, 6–10 Kirby Street, London EC1N 8LS, tel. 020 7421 2600; www.baaf.org.uk

SEXUAL PROBLEMS

REVIEW

Tomlinson J (ed). 2005. ABC of Sexual Health. Malden: Blackwell.

- Sexual problems may have a physical or psychological origin, but often they are mixed.
- All patients with sexual problems develop 'performance anxiety', where they are not relaxed and spontaneous in love making, are alert to further failure and become a spectator of their own sexual performance.
- In about 30% of patients, the partner also has a problem.
- ∗ In any consultation about sexual problems it is important to ascertain:
  - (a) what is the real complaint?
  - (b) why is the problem being presented now?
  - (c) is the desire for change real?
  - (d) who is really complaining, the patient or the partner?
  - (e) what are the expectations of the patient?
- ∗ Consider the following psychological aspects in any patient presenting with a problem:
  - (a) *Ignorance and misunderstanding.* This includes faulty sex education and technique, inability to communicate sexual needs, and unrealistic expectations due to stereotyped views of expected behaviour and performance.
  - (b) *Anger and resentment.* This often remains unresolved, with the couple unable to communicate their feelings to each other clearly. It often arises where the partners are unable to express their feelings as children because of excessive unresolved anger in their parents. It may occur in response to relationship difficulties, financial difficulties, children, in-laws or stress at work.
  - (c) *Shame, embarrassment and guilt.* This may be due to a negative sexual attitude laid down in childhood, where the parents looked upon sexuality as 'bad'. Traumatic sexual experiences may add to these fears.
  - (d) *Anxiety/fear about sex.* Fear of closeness, vulnerability, letting go and failure may lead to a self-perpetuating cycle of anxiety.
  - (e) *Poor self-image* may contribute to lack of interest in sex and sexual response. Changes in women may occur after operations, especially mastectomy or hysterectomy, postmenopausally and after childbirth. Both sexes commonly suffer after redundancy and when depressed.

INFORMATION FOR PATIENTS

Litvinoff S. 2001. *The Relate Guide to Sex in Loving Relationships.* London: Vermilion.
   Self-help material on the internet: the 'Sex and relationships' section at www.netdoctor.co.uk

Patient contact

Sexual Advice Association, Suite 301, Emblem House, London Bridge Hospital, 27 Tooley Street, London SE1 2PR, Tel. 020 7486 7262; www.sda.uk.net

ERECTILE DYSFUNCTION (HACKETT, DEAN, KELL, *ET AL.* 2007)

For details of the diagnosis of erectile dysfunction see *Evidence-based Diagnosis in Primary Care* by A. F. Polmear (editor), published by Butterworth-Heinemann, 2008.

Erectile dysfunction (ED) occurs in 10–15% of men but varies with age, with some degree of dysfunction being experienced by 40% of men at age 40 and by 70% at age 70. ED in an otherwise asymptomatic man may be a marker for underlying cardiovascular disease. Although at least 50% of the patients referred to specialist clinics have an organic component, anxiety about the situation will make things worse.

- ∗ From the history, assess particularly whether:
  - (a) the ED has arisen suddenly, with a precipitating cause, and is variable, with erections occurring in the early morning but not during intercourse. These patients are likely to have a psychological cause for the problem; or
  - (b) the onset was gradual, is constant, with partial or poorly sustained erections and no full early morning erections. These patients are likely to have a physical cause, although a psychological component is frequently superimposed.
- ∗ Consider the psychological aspects discussed above (under sexual problems).

* Be alert to psychiatric problems including generalized anxiety states (excessive adrenergic constrictor tone), depression, psychosis, body dysmorphic disorder, gender identity problems and alcoholism.

* Check for the cause being an adverse drug reaction to beta-blockers, thiazides, spironolactone, cimetidine, antidepressants, phenothiazine antipsychotics and, especially, alcohol.

* Examine:
  (a) blood pressure, heart rate, waist circumference and weight;
  (b) genitalia (includes testicular size, fibrosis in the shaft of the penis and retractibility of the foreskin).

Further examination may sometimes be indicated by age or findings in the history especially cardiovascular, neurological, endocrine and urinary systems.

WORK-UP

(a) Fasting blood glucose and lipids.

(b) Testosterone (if history or examination suggest possible hypogonadism or if required to reassure patient). Take blood at 9 am and not within 3 months of serious illness, which can depress the testosterone level.

ED as a risk factor for cardiovascular disease

● Observational studies show that factors associated with ED are similar to those associated with CVD (sedentary lifestyle, obesity, smoking, hypercholesterolaemia and the metabolic syndrome).

● ED seems to carry an independent risk for CVD of 1.46, making it as powerful a predictor of CVD as smoking.

When a man presents with ED which appears to be vascular in origin, assess his risk of CVD. Manage that risk according to the guidance on page 164.

TREATMENT IN GENERAL PRACTICE

* *Exercise and weight loss*. In the Massachusetts Male Aging Study (MMAS) men who started exercise in midlife had a 70% reduced risk for ED later in life. There is some evidence that exercise and weight loss, in those with established ED, leads to a significant reduction in ED.

Phosphodiesterase type-5 inhibitor

These are facilitators rather than initiators of erections and require sexual stimulation in order to facilitate an erection; they have a slower onset of action than injected or transurethral alprostadil (see below). Sildenafil and vardenafil are relatively short-acting PDE5 inhibitors, having a half life of about 4 hours (suitable for occasional use), whereas tadalafil has a longer half life of 17.5 hours (suitable for longer periods, e.g. over a weekend).

* In the UK, prescribe a PDE5 inhibitor at NHS expense to men with any of the conditions approved by the Department of Health (see the BNF), marking the prescription SLS, and giving enough (usually) for one treatment a week. A private prescription can be issued to any patient who does not come within the DoH guidelines (Health Services Circular HSC 1999/148).

● Studies have shown that patients often take PDE5 inhibitors incorrectly and that almost half of previous non-responders respond if the drugs are taken correctly.

* Instruct the patient to:
  (a) take sildenafil or vardenafil 30–60 minutes before intercourse and tadalafil several hours before intercourse;
  (b) avoid excessive food or alcohol although absorption is less of a problem with tadalafil.

* Beware the drug interaction with nitrates and nicorandil in those with cardiovascular comorbidity.

Non-responders

Patients should use the drug eight times at maximal dosage before being classified as a non-responder.

* Recheck testosterone and prolactin levels in non-responders. PDE5 inhibitors are less effective in those with low or low-normal testosterone levels and there is some evidence of improved response with testosterone replacement.

Counselling may be successful in psychogenic impotence, and is appropriate for couples who do not wish to be referred:

* See the couple together.

* Recommend a manual, e.g. *The Relate Guide to Sex in Loving Relationships* (see box above).

* Instruct the couple on the sensate focus programme. Instructions can be downloaded from the web, e.g. at www.personalmd.com/healthtopics/crs/touch.htm.
* Set 'homework' assignments for the couple; these can be tailored to meet specific needs.

Referral

* Refer those not responding for sex therapy via the local family planning clinic or Relate. The outcome is successful in 50–80% of cases.
* Refer for relationship counselling those whom you sense have larger relationship or personality problems.
* Refer to a urologist those with physical causes, those who have not responded to PDE5 inhibitors or who have contraindications to it, and those with psychological causes that are proving intractable. Possible treatments are:
  (a) hormone replacement therapy in those with hypogonadism;
  (b) alprostadil – as injections into the corpus cavernosum or transurethrally;
  (c) vacuum devices;
  (d) penile prostheses.

DETAILS OF THERAPISTS ARE AVAILABLE FROM

British Association for Sexual and Relationship Therapy, tel. 020 8543 2707; www.basrt.org.uk
    Institute of Psychosexual Medicine, 12 Chandos Street, London W1G 9DR, tel. 020 7580 0631; www.ipm.org.uk

---

LACK OF SEXUAL DESIRE (BASSON 2006)

This is the commonest presenting female sexual dysfunction. A low level of sexual desire is usually accompanied by low levels of arousal and sexual excitement and infrequent orgasms and is frequently associated with sexual dissatisfaction. Underlying psychological difficulties are frequent. These may relate specifically to sex, e.g. previous sexual abuse, or they may relate to a more widespread psychological disorder.

Physical illness and drugs/ substances are also possible causes.
    Women specifically lose sexual desire:

(a) postpartum;
(b) because of pain;
(c) where their partner's performance repeatedly leads to frustration, as in premature ejaculation or ED.

In general, psychological interventions and sex therapy are of greater benefit than drugs.

* Check for the presence of depression and anxiety (see pages 452 and 463)
* Reassure the patient that sexual desire varies at different times of life and that loss of desire is not necessarily abnormal.
* Enquire whether she wants to improve her sexual desire or whether it is her partner's wish.
* Consider factors that may be contributing (see above).
* Recommend the website of (the British Association for Sexual and Relationship Therapy www.basrt.org.uk) which discusses the problem of lack of desire.
* Offer counselling along the lines described under erectile dysfunction.

DYSPAREUNIA (WEIJMAR SCHULTZ, BASSON, BINIK ET AL. 2005)

This may be primary, or secondary to a physical cause, and considerable skill may be needed to unravel the problem.

* Distinguish from the history and examination between:
  (a) lack of lubrication due to lack of interest;
  (b) vaginismus, which usually becomes apparent at vaginal examination (see below);
  (c) vulval or vaginal causes: infections, vulvar vestibulitis syndrome, lichen sclerosus, lichen planus, urethral caruncle, postmenopausal vaginitis, postepisiotomy syndrome. Those for whom there is no specific treatment may benefit from 5% lidocaine ointment applied 20 minutes before sexual intercourse; they can also be referred to specialist physiotherapists.

(d) pelvic causes with tenderness on rocking the cervix or palpating the fornices, e.g. endometriosis, pelvic infection, ovarian pathology;

(e) psychogenic causes, where vulval burning or pain is due to somatization of other difficulties.

Where a physical cause is not found, CBT and SSRIs have been found to be beneficial.

INFORMATION FOR PATIENTS AND THEIR PARTNERS

Vulval Pain Society, PO Box 7804, Nottingham NG3 5ZQ; www.vulvalpainsociety.org

---

VAGINISMUS

This consists of a phobia of penetration and involuntary spasm of the pubococcygeal and associated muscles surrounding the lower third of the vagina. Such women may avoid having cervical smears and sometimes present with infertility.

* Explore the root cause. It may be:

(a) fear of the unknown or the patient's ignorance of her own anatomy;

(b) a past history of unpleasant experiences such as rape, sexual abuse or severe emotional trauma; or previous dyspareunia;

(c) a defence mechanism against growing up and becoming a woman. (A common pattern is for the patient to live close to her parents, remaining the daughter and marrying an unassertive man.)

* Desensitize simple cases by encouraging the woman to examine herself, and also encourage her partner to be confident enough to insert a finger into the vagina. Some women may prefer to use vaginal trainers.

* Refer to a sex therapist if this simple approach fails. Hypnotherapy may be helpful (McGuire and Hawton 2003).

PATIENT CONTACT

The Vaginismus Support Group. Resolve, PO Box 820, London N10 3AW. The group has no website or email address

---

DISORDERS OF ORGASM

Anxiety tends to delay a woman's orgasm, but accelerates a man's.

PREMATURE EJACULATION (WALDINGER 2007)

This is present when ejaculation occurs sooner than either partner would wish, usually before penetration or soon after. Interest in sex may be reduced in both partners.

* Advise the patient that, with practice, he can learn to delay ejaculation. The stop/start technique can be taught by therapists or learnt from the book cited above. In essence, when, during caressing or during intercourse, a man feels he is close to climax he should stop being stimulated and relax for 30 seconds. Stimulation can then recommence until he is close to climax again, when the relaxation is repeated. If this fails, the woman should squeeze the penis at the base of the glans between finger and thumb during relaxation phases.

* Clomipramine 25 mg daily or paroxetine 20 mg each evening are effective in delaying ejaculation.

RETARDED EJACULATION

This is usually a sign of long-standing sexual inhibition. Often the patient can ejaculate by masturbation, but not intravaginally.

* Explore any feelings of anxiety and guilt.

* Start a sensate focus programme (see above).

* If 'home therapy' fails, refer for psychosexual counselling.

ORGASMIC PROBLEMS IN WOMEN (MESTON, HULL, LEVIN AND SIPSKI 2004)

* A woman who has never achieved an orgasm may have deep-seated psychological reasons for being afraid to let go. She may need 'permission' to investigate her body's own responses further, either by masturbation or vibrator. When she has learnt how to relax, she should be encouraged to tell her partner and incorporate caressing into their usual lovemaking.

* Women who have lost the ability to achieve orgasm may need counselling, especially about their current relationship or a recent loss of self-image.

* Check that she is not taking drugs that inhibit orgasm, e.g. clonidine, and that her failure to achieve orgasm is not due to neurological disease or pelvic surgery. Total hysterectomy does not impair ability to achieve orgasm (Farrell and Kieser 2000).

References

Ahrendt, H.J., Nisand, I., Bastianelli, C., et al., 2006. Efficacy, acceptability and tolerability of the combined contraceptive ring, NuvaRing, compared with an oral contraceptive containing 30 μg ethinyl estradiol and 3 mg of drospirenone. Contraception 74, 451–457.

Anon., 1999. Combined oral contraceptives containing desogestrel or gestodene and the risk of venous thromboembolism. Curr. Prob. Pharmacovigilance 25, 12.

Anon., 2004a. Best Practice Guidance for Doctors and Other Health Professionals on the Provision of Advice and Treatment to Young People Under 16 on Contraception, Sexual and Reproductive Health. Department of Health, London.

Anon., 2004b. Male and Female Sterilisation. Evidence-based guideline no. 4, 2nd ed. Royal College of Obstetricians & Gynaecologists, London.

Anon., 2004c. The Care of Women Requesting Induced Abortion. Evidence-based guideline No. 7, 2nd ed. Royal College of Obstetricians & Gynaecologists, London.

Anon., 2005. Selected Practice Recommendations for Contraceptive Use, 2nd ed. World Health Organization, Geneva.

Archer, D.F., 2006. Menstrual-cycle-related symptoms: a review of the rationale for continuous use of oral contraceptives. Contraception 74, 359–366.

Arowojolu, A.O., Gallo, M.F., Grimes, D.A., Garner, S.E., 2009. Combined oral contraceptive pills for treatment of acne. Cochrane Database of Systematic Reviews. Issue 3, Art No. CD004425.

Basson, R., 2006. Sexual desire and arousal disorders in women. NEJM 354, 1497–1506.

Bjarnadóttir, R.I., Tuppurainen, M., Killick, S.R., 2002. Comparison of cycle control with a combined contraceptive vaginal ring and oral levonorgestrel/ethinyl estradiol. Am. J. Obstet. Gynecol. 186, 389–395.

Bonnar, J., Flynn, A., Freundl, G., et al., 1999. Personal hormone monitoring for contraception. Br. J. Fam. Plann. 24, 128–134.

Brechin, S., Bigrigg, A., 2006. Male and female sterilisation. Curr. Obs. Gynaecol. 16, 39–46.

Brechin, S., Penney, G.C., 2004. Venous Thromboembolism and Hormonal Contraception. Guideline no. 40. 1-13., Royal College of Obstetricians & Gynaecologists, London.

Canto De Cetina, T.E., Canto, P., Ordoñez Luna, M., 2001. Effect of counselling to improve compliance in Mexican women receiving depot-medroxyprogesterone acetate. Contraception 63, 143–146.

Chan, W.S., Ray, J., Wai, E.K., et al., 2004. Risk of stroke in women exposed to low-dose oral contraceptives: a critical evaluation of the evidence. Arch. Intern. Med. 164, 741–747.

Charles, V.E., Polis, C.B., Sridhara, S.K., Blum, R.W., 2008. Abortion and long-term mental health outcomes: a systematic review of the evidence. Contraception 78, 436–450.

Clinical Effectiveness Unit, 2003b. Desogestrel-only pill (Cerazette). J. Fam. Plann. Reprod. Health Care 29, 162–164.

Clinical Effectiveness Unit, 2004b. Norelgestromin/ethinyloestradiol transdermal contraceptive system (Evra®). J. Fam. Plann. Reprod. Health Care 30, 43–45.

Clinical Effectiveness Unit, 2004c. FemCap. Faculty of Family Planning & Reproductive Healthcare, London.

Clinical Effectiveness Unit, 2005a. Drug interactions with hormonal contraception. J. Fam. Plann. Reprod. Health Care 31, 139–150.

Clinical Effectiveness Unit, 2006a. First Prescription of Combined Oral Contraception. Faculty of Family Planning and Reproductive Healthcare, London.

Clinical Effectiveness Unit, 2006b. Emergency contraception. J. Fam. Plann. Reprod. Health Care 32, 121–128.

Clinical Effectiveness Unit, 2007a. Intrauterine contraception, 2nd ed. Faculty of Sexual & Reproductive Healthcare, London. http://www.fsrh.org.

Clinical Effectiveness Unit, 2007b. Male and female condoms. Faculty of Family Planning & Reproductive Healthcare, London.

Clinical Effectiveness Unit, 2007c. Female Barrier Methods. Faculty of Family Planning & Reproductive Healthcare, London.

Clinical Effectiveness Unit, 2008a. Progestogen-only Pills. Faculty of

Sexual & Reproductive Healthcare, London.

Clinical Effectiveness Unit, 2008b. Progestogen-only Injectable Contraception. Faculty of Sexual & Reproductive Healthcare, London.

Clinical Effectiveness Unit, 2008c. Progestogen-only Implants. Faculty of Sexual & Reproductive Healthcare, London.

Clinical Effectiveness Unit, 2009a. UK medical eligibility criteria. Faculty of Sexual and Reproductive Healthcare, London.

Clinical Effectiveness Unit, 2009b. Postnatal sexual and reproductive health. Faculty of Sexual and Reproductive Healthcare, London.

Clinical Effectiveness Unit, 2009c. Sexual and reproductive health for individuals with inflammatory bowel disease. Faculty of Sexual and Reproductive Healthcare, London.

Clinical Effectiveness Unit, 2009d. Combined vaginal ring (NuvaRing). Faculty of Sexual and Reproductive Healthcare, London.

Clinical Effectiveness Unit, 2010a. Contraceptive choices for young people. Faculty of Sexual and Reproductive Healthcare, London.

Clinical Effectiveness Unit, 2010b. Contraceptive choices for women aged over 40 years. Faculty of Sexual and Reproductive Healthcare, London.

Clinical Effectiveness Unit, 2010c. Antiepileptic drugs and contraception. Faculty of Sexual and Reproductive Healthcare, London.

Collaborative Group on Epidemiological Studies of Ovarian Cancer, 2008. Ovarian cancer and oral contraceptives: collaborative reanalysis of data from 45 epidemiological studies including 23 257 women with ovarian cancer and 87 303 controls. Lancet 371, 303–314.

Collaborative Group on Hormonal Factors in Breast Cancer, 1996. Breast cancer and hormonal contraceptives: collaborative reanalysis of individual data on 53 297 women with breast cancer and 100 239 women without breast cancer from 54 epidemiological studies. Lancet 347, 1713–1727.

Cooper, E., 2000. Couples with learning disabilities. In: Killick, S. (ed.), Contraception in Practice. Martin Dunitz, London, pp. 229–240.

Curtis, K.M., Martins, S.L., 2006. Progestogen-only contraception and bone mineral density: a systematic review. Contraception 73, 470–487.

Donovan, C., Hadley, A., Jones, M., et al., 2000. Confidentiality and Young People. Royal College of General Practitioners and Brook, London.

European Natural Family Planning Study Groups, 1993. Prospective European multi-center study of natural family planning (1989–1992): interim results. Adv. Contracep. 9, 269–283.

Farrell, S.A., Kieser, K., 2000. Sexuality after hysterectomy. Obstet. Gynecol. 95, 1045–1051.

Fernandez, E., La Vecchia, C., Balducci, A., et al., 2001. Oral contraceptives and colorectal cancer risk: a meta-analysis. Br. J. Cancer 84, 722–727.

Fiala, C., Gemzell-Danielsson, K., 2006. Review of medical abortion using mifepristone in combination with a prostaglandin analogue. Contraception 74, 66–86.

Fotherby, K., Howard, G., 1986. Return of fertility in women discontinuing injectable contraceptives. J. Obstet. Gynaecol. 6, S110–S115.

Gallo, M.F., Grimes, D.A., Lopez, L.M., Schulz, K.F., 2006. Non-latex versus latex male condoms for contraception. Cochrane Database Syst. Rev. (1), CD003550.

Grimes, D., 2000. Intrauterine device and upper-genital-tract infection. Lancet 356, 1013–1019.

Grimes, D.A., Lopez, L.M., Schulz, K.F., Stanwood, N.L., 2004. Immediate Post-abortal Insertion of Intrauterine Device. Cochrane Database of Systematic Reviews. Issue 4, Art No. CD001777.

Grimes, D.A., Schulz, K.F., 1999. Antibiotic prophylaxis for intrauterine contraceptive device insertion. Cochrane Database of Systematic Reviews. Issue 3, Art No. CD001327.

Guillebaud, J., 1989. Contraception and sterilization. In: Turnbull, A., Chamberlain, G. (eds), Obstetrics. Churchill Livingstone, Edinburgh, pp. 1135–1152.

Hackett, G., Dean, J., Kell, P., et al., 2007. Guidelines on the Management of Erectile Dysfunction. British Society for Sexual Medicine, Lichfield. http://www.bssm.org.uk/downloads/BSSM_ED_Management_Guidelines_2007.pdf.

Hannaford, P.C., Iversen, L., Macfarlane, T.V., Elliott, A.M., Angus, V., Lee, A.J., 2010. Mortality among contraceptive pill users: cohort evidence from Royal College of General Practitioners' Oral Contraception Study. BMJ 340, c927.

Harrison-Woolrych, M., Hill, R., 2005. Unintended pregnancies with the etonogestrel implant (Implanon): a case series from postmarketing experience in Australia. Contraception 71, 306–308.

Heinemann, L.A.J., Assmann, A., DoMinh, T., Garbe, E., 1999. Oral progestogen-only contraceptives and cardiovascular risk: results from the Transnational Study on Oral Contraceptives and the Health of Young Women. Eur. J. Contracept. Reprod. Health Care 4, 67–73.

International Collaboration of Epidemiological Studies of Cervical Cancer, 2007. Cervical cancer and hormonal contraceptives: collaborative reanalysis of individual data for

16 573 women with cervical cancer and 35 509 women without cervical cancer from 24 epidemiological studies. Lancet 370, 1609–1621.

Jackson, R.A., Bimla Schwarz, E., Freedman, L., Darney, P., 2003. Advance supply of emergency contraception: effect on use and usual contraception - a randomized trial. Obstet. Gynecol. 102, 8–16.

Jick, S.S., Kaye, J.A., Russmann, S., Jick, H., 2006. Risk of nonfatal venous thromboembolism with oral contraceptives containing norgestimate or desogestrel compared with oral contraceptives containing levonorgestrel. Contraception 73, 566–570.

Jones, S., 2008. Legal aspects of family planning. In: Glasier, A., Gebbie, A, (eds), Handbook of Family Planning and Reproductive Healthcare, 5th ed. Churchill Livingstone, Edinburgh, pp 249–267.

Kaunitz, A.M., Arias, R., McClung, M., 2008. Bone density recovery after depot medroxyprogesterone acetate injectable contraception use. Contraception 77, 67–76.

Kemmeren, J.M., Algra, A., Grobbee, D.E., 2001. Third generation oral contraceptives and risk of venous thrombosis: meta-analysis. BMJ 323, 131–134.

Khader, Y.S., Rice, J., John, L., Abueita, O., 2003. Oral contraceptive use and risk of myocardial infarction: a meta-analysis. Contraception 68, 11–17.

Liying, Z., Bilian, X., 2001. Emergency contraception with Multiload Cu-375SL IUD: a multicentre clinical trial. Contraception 64, 107–112.

MacGregor, E.A., 2007. Migraine and use of combined hormonal contraceptives: a clinical review. J. Fam. Plann. Reprod. Health Care 33, 159–169.

McGuire, H., Hawton, K., 2003. Interventions for vaginismus. Cochrane Database Syst. Rev. CD001760.

Mansour, D., Korver, T., Marintcheva-Petrova, M., Fraser, I.S., 2008. The effects of Implanon® on menstrual bleeding patterns. Eur. J. Contracept. Reprod. Health Care 13 (Suppl. 1), 13–28.

Marchbanks, P.A., McDonald, J.A., Wilson, H.G., et al., 2002. Oral contraceptives and the risk of breast cancer. NEJM 346, 2025–2032.

Merki-Feld, G.S., Hund, M., 2007. Clinical experience with NuvaRing in daily practice in Switzerland: cycle control and acceptability among women of all reproductive ages. Eur. J. Contracept. Reprod. Health Care 12, 240–247.

Meston, C.M., Hull, E., Levin, R.J., Sipski, M., 2004. Disorders of orgasm in women. J. Sex. Med. 1, 66–68.

Miller, L., Hughes, J.P., 2003. Continuous combination oral contraceptive pills to eliminate withdrawal bleeding: a randomized trial. Obstet. Gynecol. 101, 653–661.

National Collaborating Centre for Women's and Children's Health, 2005. Long-acting reversible contraception (NICE guideline). RCOG, London. http://www.nice.org.uk.

NICE, 2008. Prophylaxis against infective endocarditis. NICE clinical guideline 64, National Institute for Health and Clinical Excellence, London.

Oddson, K., Leifels-Fischer, B., Wiel-Masson, D., et al., 2005. Superior cycle control with a contraceptive vaginal ring compared with an oral contraceptive containing 30mcg ethinylestradiol and 150mcg levonorgestrel: a randomized trial. Hum. Reprod. 20, 557–562.

Oddsson, K., Leifels-Fischer, B., de Melo, N.R., et al., 2005. Efficacy and safety of a contraceptive vaginal ring (NuvaRing) compared with a combined oral contraceptive: a 1-year randomized trial. Contraception 71, 176–182.

Poulter, N.R., 1996. Oral contraceptives and blood pressure. In: Hannaford, P.C., Webb, A.M.C, (eds), Evidence-guided Prescribing of the Pill. Parthenon, Carnforth, pp. 77–88.

Rosenberg, M.J., Long, S.C., 1992. Oral contraceptives and cycle control: a critical review of the literature. Adv. Contracept. 8 (Suppl. 1), 35–45.

Rosenberg, M.J., Waugh, M.S., Stevens, C.M., 1996. Smoking and cycle control among oral contraceptive users. Am. J. Obstet. Gynecol. 174, 628–632.

Roumen, F.J.M.E., op ten Berg, M.M.T., Hoomans, E.H.M., 2006. The combined contraceptive ring (NuvaRing): first experience in daily clinical practice in the Netherlands. Eur. J. Contracept. Reprod. Health Care 11, 14–22.

Stewart, F.H., Harper, C.C., Ellertson, C.E., et al., 2001. Clinical breast and pelvic examination requirements for hormonal contraception. JAMA 285, 2232–2239.

Stokes, T., Shaw, E.J., Juarez-Garcia, A., et al., 2004. Clinical guidelines and evidence review for the epilepsies: diagnosis and management in adults and children in primary and secondary care. Royal College of General Practitioners, London.

Trussell, J., 2007. Contraceptive efficacy. In: Hatcher, R.A., Trussell, J., Nelson, A.L., Cates, W., Stewart, F.H., Kowal, D., (eds), Contraceptive technology, 19th ed. Ardent Media, New York, pp. 747–826.

Vasilakis-Scaramozza, C., Jick, H., 2001. Risk of venous thromboembolism with cyproterone or levonorgestrel contraceptives. Lancet 358, 1427–1429.

Vessey, M., Painter, R., 2006. Oral contraceptive use and cancer. Findings in a large cohort study, 1968–2004. Br. J. Cancer 95, 385–389.

von Hertzen, H., Piaggio, G., Ding, J., et al., 2002. Low dose mifepristone and two regimens of levonorgestrel for emergency contraception: a WHO multicentre randomised trial. Lancet 360, 1803–1810.

Waldinger, M.D., 2007. Premature ejaculation: state of the art. Urol. Clin. North Am. 34, 591–599.

Weiderpass, E., Adami, H., Baron, J.A., et al., 1999. Use of oral contraceptives and endometrial cancer risk. Cancer Causes Control 10, 277–284.

Weijmar Schultz, W., Basson, R., Binik, Y., et al., 2005. Women's sexual pain and its management. J. Sex. Med. 2, 301–316.

Westhoff, C., 2003. Depot-medroxyprogesterone acetate injection (Depo-Provera®): a highly effective contraceptive option with proven long-term safety. Contraception 68, 75–87.

Wilcox, A.J., Dunson, D.B., Weinberg, C.R., et al., 2001. Likelihood of conception with a single act of intercourse: providing benchmark rates for assessment of post-coital contraceptives. Contraception 63, 211–215.

Wingo, P.A., Austin, H., Marchbanks, P.A., et al., 2007. Oral contraceptives and the risk of death from breast cancer. Obstet. Gynecol. 110, 793–800.

World Health Organization, 1987. A multicentred phase III comparative trial of depot-medroxyprogesterone acetate given three-monthly at doses of 100mg or 150mg: II. The comparison of bleeding patterns. Contraception 35, 591–610.

World Health Organization, 1991. Collaborative study of neoplasia and steroid contraceptives. Depot medroxyprogesterone acetate (DMPA) and risk of endometrial cancer. Int. J. Cancer 49, 186–190.

Chapter 13

Obstetric problems

CHAPTER CONTENTS

© 2011 Elsevier Ltd.
DOI: 10.1016/B978-0-7020-3053-6.00013-1

PREPREGNANCY CARE

- Whilst prepregnancy counselling offers an opportunity to reinforce good health habits and identify potential problems for pregnancy early, there is no evidence from randomized controlled trials that women who attend such visits have better health or pregnancy outcomes. In one large cohort study only a small proportion of women planning pregnancy followed recommendations for nutrition and lifestyle (Inskip, Crozier, Godfrey, et al. 2009).
- GPs may have the opportunity to identify risk factors before conception. This can be done either at a specific consultation or when the opportunity arises, e.g. as part of contraceptive care, or when seeing patients with diabetes or hypertension.

If a woman does present for a prepregnancy visit this can be used as a time to encourage her to:

(a) stop smoking;
(b) take 400 mcg of folic acid a day (explain that folic acid supplements have been shown to reduce the risk of neural tube defects by 50–70% (Rush 1994);
(c) avoid alcohol or at most take two units a week;
(d) take a healthy diet; particularly avoiding soft cheeses and liver.

At the same time the doctor can:

(a) consider the risk of inherited disorders;
(b) assess medical conditions (e.g. hypertension, diabetes, epilepsy, hyperthyroidism);
(c) assess whether the woman has an eating disorder or is overweight;
(d) check that the patient is immune to rubella and has an up-to-date cervical smear;
(e) warn the patient to avoid contact with chickenpox or exposed shingles. In the US and Australia varicella vaccination is offered to non-immune women.

GENETIC DISORDERS

All couples should be referred for genetic counselling if they request it, or there are risk factors that need further investigation. The list of identifiable conditions is increasing, and studies suggest that clinicians across specialties are poor at appreciating which conditions have identifiable genetic components (Harris, Lane, Harris, et al. 1999). If there is any doubt, contact the nearest department of clinical genetics for advice. Children or adults with a major abnormality or disease, even if not at present thought to be genetic in origin, should have blood stored at a regional genetics laboratory for later analysis.

Those at higher risk are:

(a) couples with a personal or family history of an abnormality that is presumed to be genetic in origin. They should be referred for genetic counselling or have blood taken by the GP on the advice of the geneticist. Important examples are:
  - cystic fibrosis;
  - Huntington's chorea;
  - Duchenne and other muscular dystrophies;
  - polycystic kidneys;
  - intellectual disability, which may be due to fragile-X syndrome.
(b) Couples belonging to a high risk ethnic group (see below).
(c) *Older women.* The risk of having a baby with Down's syndrome is 1:400 at age 35, rising to 1:100 at age 40 and 1:30 at age 45. Around the age of 37 the risk of chromosomal abnormality is greater than the risk of miscarriage after amniocentesis. Recommend the leaflet *Testing for Down's Syndrome in Pregnancy*, available from www.screening.nhs.uk/annbpublications.
(d) *Consanguineous couples.* First degree cousins have a slight but significant increase in congenital malformations. This is likely to be higher if there is a family history of congenital disease. Caucasian first degree cousins should be offered screening for cystic fibrosis, even where there is no family history.

DISEASES IN HIGH–RISK ETHNIC GROUPS
Sickle cell and thalassaemia

- Women from areas where malaria has been common are at increased risk of carrying the sickle cell or thalassaemia traits: Africa, the Caribbean, the Middle East, the Indian subcontinent, South America, South and South-East Asia and the Mediterranean (see page 638).

- In the UK all pregnant women are offered screening for thalassaemia using the MCH measurement as part of the routine blood count.
- Women, or potential fathers, from an ethnic group at risk are also offered a test for sickle cell and related haemoglobin variants.
- At a prenatal consultation a couple may choose to undergo screening because of the ethnic group to which they belong or because of a positive family history. When assessing ethnic origin try to go back at least two generations. Discuss the appropriate test with the laboratory and send the completed Family Origin Questionnaire with the blood samples. This is available from the sickle cell and thalassaemia screening programme (http://sct.screening.nhs. uk then search for 'Family origin questionnaire').

* Refer to the obstetrician all couples who are both heterozygous for sickle cell or thalassaemia, or where the mother is and the father is unknown.

PATIENT INFORMATION

Sickle Cell Society, 54 Station Road, London NW10 4UA. Tel: 020 8961 7795. Helpline 0800 001 5660. www.sicklecellsociety.org
   NHS Sickle Cell and Thalassaemia Screening Programme. www.screening.nhs.uk/annbpublications
   UK Thalassaemia Society, 19 The Broadway, Southgate Circus, London N14 6PH. Tel: 020 8882 0011. Free Adviceline: 0800 731 109. www.ukts.org
      www.thalassemia.ca (Canadian)
      www.thalassaemia.cdc.net.my/links.html (Sarawak but with excellent international links)

Jewish population: Tay–Sachs

Tay–Sachs disease is an incurable neurodegenerative disorder that begins around 6 months of age. Babies born with it live for only a few years. People of Ashkenazi (Eastern European) Jewish descent are most at risk.

* Consider referral of both prospective parents for testing for *Tay–Sachs* trait. One in 25 of Jewish descent is positive. In London refer to the Genetics Centre at Guy's and St Thomas' Hospital, London: www.guysandstthomas.nhs. uk (search on Tay–Sachs). Tel 020 7188 1364. Outside London send a sample to the Regional Genetics Centre.

PATIENT INFORMATION

For information about the disease: http://www.ygyh. org/tay/whatisit.htm
   The National Tay-Sachs and Allied Diseases Association (USA), www.ntsad.org

---

PREVIOUS OBSTETRIC HISTORY

(a) *Down's syndrome.* Make certain that all women who have had a previous pregnancy affected by Down's syndrome have received genetic counselling, regardless of the age at which they conceived.

(b) *Previous miscarriages* (see below). Inform all patients, if asked, that the overall incidence of miscarriage is around 15%. However, women whose last pregnancy was normal have a risk of miscarriage of only 5%, whereas women whose last pregnancy ended in miscarriage have a 20–25% chance of a miscarriage (Regan, Braude, Trembath, *et al.* 1989). Women with three consecutive miscarriages have a 40% chance of the next pregnancy ending in miscarriage.

(c) *Recurrent miscarriages.* Refer to a gynaecologist for assessment all women who have had three consecutive miscarriages. Reassure them, however, that they still have a 60% chance of a normal pregnancy and that it is common for no cause to be identified. Consider earlier referral if:

- the woman requests it;
- there is a family history of miscarriage or of congenital disease;
- there is a relevant medical problem; or
- there is an urgency to achieve a live birth, as in the older woman.

INVESTIGATIONS TO CONSIDER UNDERTAKING PRIOR TO REFERRAL FOR RECURRENT MISCARRIAGE

(a) Pelvic ultrasound.
(b) LH on day 7.
(c) Blood group and antibodies.
(d) Anticardiolipin antibodies (IgM and IgG).
(e) Lupus anticoagulant.
(f) Protein C, protein S, factor V Leiden.
(g) Karyotyping of both partners (and of fetal products if available).

(d) Family history or previous infant with neural tube defects:

All women in this category should receive folic acid prior to conception. Give 5 mg daily, starting 1 month prior to stopping contraception, and continue throughout the first trimester.

Women should also receive advice about antenatal diagnosis (see below).

(e) Size, gestation and maturity of previous infants:

- *Previous baby less than 2500 g:* stress the importance of not smoking and drinking alcohol and explain that she is at increased risk of intrauterine growth retardation. Careful symphysis-fundal measurements should be performed at each visit, ideally, by the same experienced practitioner. The woman should be referred early in pregnancy for assessment by a specialist obstetrician.
- *Large previous baby:* check that a modified glucose tolerance test has been performed.

MEDICAL HISTORY

HYPERTENSION (see page 394)

* This should be assessed before a woman gets pregnant, as it may be masked by the fall in blood pressure in the first half of pregnancy.

* Discuss the most appropriate drug with the relevant specialist before conception.

DIABETES (see page 396)

* Explain that diabetes is associated with an increase in congenital abnormalities (about double), but that this can be decreased significantly by good control of the blood sugar prior to and during pregnancy (Steel, Johnstone, Hepburn, *et al.* 1990; Nachum, Ben-Shlomo, Weiner *et al.* 1999).

EPILEPSY

Women with epilepsy are more likely to have unplanned pregnancies due to contraceptive failure and twice as likely to have a fetal malformation. Not all malformations may be attributable to antiepileptic drugs (Fairgrieve, Jackson, Jonas, *et al.* 2000). Sodium valproate increases the risk of neural tube defects 50 times, to about 1.5%. With carbamazepine the rate is 1%. There are few data on the safety of newer drugs. There is no convincing evidence that any one drug is safer than another (DTB 1994a).

* Discuss with the neurologist:

- whether to stop anticonvulsants in any woman who has been free of convulsions for 2 years; but counsel the patient about the risks of untreated epilepsy in pregnancy. Convulsions may lead to stillbirth; or
- whether to change anticonvulsants or reduce their dose in those in whom they cannot be stopped.

* Make it clear that even on anticonvulsants there is a 90% chance of a normal outcome, that prenatal diagnosis is effective in picking up neural tube defects (see page 386) and that many defects can be corrected after birth.

* Ensure that all women with epilepsy are offered:

- *folic acid.* Those continuing antiepileptic medication should take folic acid 5 mg daily from 3 months before conception until the end of the 12th week. Those stopping their drugs need only take 400 mcg daily from 1 month before conception;
- an anomaly ultrasound examination at 18/19 weeks; and
- *vitamin K.* Give vitamin K 10 mg orally daily for the last 4 weeks of pregnancy to women on enzyme-inducing antiepileptic treatment.

* Educate a woman's partner about what to do should she have a seizure, as epilepsy may be less predictable.

ASTHMA

- Asthma is one of the commonest chronic medical conditions and around 5% of pregnant women will require asthma medication during pregnancy (Olesen, Steffensen, Nielsen, *et al.* 1999).
- Asthma increases the risk of IUGR by 24% overall, and by 47% in those with severe asthma (Bracken, Triche, Belanger, *et al.* 2003).
- Women with asthma should continue on their asthma medication, including preventers, as the risk of uncontrolled asthma poses a greater risk to the fetus than continuing preventive medication (Martel, Rey, Beauchesne, *et al.* 2005).

OTHER MEDICATION

A decision should be taken about the need to stop other drugs which are associated with fetal abnormalities, e.g. warfarin and lithium. The NICE guideline *Antenatal and postnatal mental health: clinical management and service guidance*, available on www.nice.org.uk, discusses the risks associated with psychotropic medication.

PSYCHIATRIC HISTORY

Mental illness is a common 'indirect' cause of maternal mortality. Seeking a history early in pregnancy and ensuring effective follow-up in late pregnancy and the early post-natal period is essential.

INFECTION

(a) *Rubella*. All women should have rubella antibodies tested before each pregnancy; immunity can be lost between one pregnancy and the next.

(b) *Hepatitis B*. All women should be offered screening for hepatitis B early in pregnancy as selective screening has been shown to miss cases of HBV due to the time pressures of routine clinical practice.

(c) *Listeria*. Advise women to avoid soft cheeses, chilled ready-to-eat foods (unless thoroughly re-heated) and patés, prior to and during pregnancy. They should avoid contact with sheep at lambing time, and with silage. Advise women to reheat food to steaming hot and thaw frozen foods in a microwave or refrigerator. Listeriosis is rare but can occur in outbreaks.

(d) *Toxoplasmosis*. Women contemplating pregnancy should be warned about the risks of handling soil, cat faeces or raw meat, and of eating undercooked meat and unwashed vegetables and fruit. 80% of British women are not immune at the time of pregnancy. Routine screening is not recommended.

(e) *HIV*. All women should be offered screening for HIV early in pregnancy by midwives or doctors trained in pre- and post-test counselling (Brocklehurst 2000).

(f) *Genital herpes and warts* (see page 72). Management is only an issue in the last weeks of pregnancy.

PATIENT INFORMATION (ON HEPATITIS B, HIV, SYPHILIS AND RUBELLA)

www.screening.nhs.uk/annbpublications and choose 'Infectious diseases in pregnancy'

PRENATAL AND ANTENATAL ADVICE

LIFESTYLE

* *Alcohol*. Counsel the woman to reduce her alcohol consumption to a minimum (at the most one or two units once or twice a week). Complete abstinence is now recommended by the Department of Health, the BMA, the RCOG and the WHO. However, the evidence relating to the possibility of fetal damage from very low levels of alcohol intake does not provide a clear answer about the risk. A more powerful argument in favour of total abstinence is that women who drink a little in pregnancy may easily overstep the limits without realizing it (Head to Head 2007).

* *Smoking*. Rather than asking: *'Do you smoke?'* women should be asked *'What best describes your smoking? Daily, Every once in a while, or I don't currently smoke?'* All women who smoke should be offered a smoking cessation intervention. Advise about the risks. Provide information. Assess willingness to quit. Assist to quit using a cognitive behavioural intervention. Arrange for additional support if unsuccessful (see page 498).

* *Coffee*. Heavy coffee drinking (eight or more cups a day) is associated with a tripling of the risk of stillbirth (OR = 3.0; 95%CI 1.5 to 5.9) (Wisborg, Kesmodel, Bech, *et al.* 2003). A recent study found that caffeine intake as low as 200 mg (two cups of coffee or five cups of tea or five cans of caffeinated fizzy drinks) was associated with a doubling of the rate of miscarriage and that lower intakes were not without risk (Weng, Odouli and Li 2008). However, a Danish randomized trial failed to show any effect on birth weight or length of gestation from reducing caffeine intake, suggesting that the association of caffeine with poor outcomes may be due to one or more confounding factors (Bech, Obel, Henriksen, *et al.* 2007).

* *Other drugs.* All women should be asked about their use of prescription and non-prescription drugs. Women using non-prescription drugs should be referred to the appropriate drug service for assistance in quitting.

NUTRITION

Recommend a balanced diet – low in fat with adequate iron, fresh fruit and vegetables. Avoid soft cheeses (see Listeria above). Recommend the article in Bandolier Extra: *A Healthy Pregnancy*, available on www.medicine.ox.ac.uk/bandolier/ Extraforbando/healpreg.pdf.

Anaemia

* Check Hb in all women with a previous history or at high risk of anaemia, e.g. vegans, multiple pregnancies, and those with a short interval between pregnancies.
* Check the serum ferritin in those women who have a history of iron-deficiency anaemia, even if the haemoglobin is normal.

Vitamin D

* All women should be counselled about the importance of adequate vitamin D intake during pregnancy and whilst breast feeding. There is no evidence to recommend routine supplementation.
* Women who are high risk should take 10 mcg of vitamin D per day (Health Start Vitamins for women). These are:
  (a) women of South Asian, African, Caribbean or Middle Eastern family origin;
  (b) women who have limited exposure to sunlight, such as women who are predominantly housebound, or usually remain covered when outdoors;
  (c) women who eat a diet particularly low in vitamin D, such as women who consume no oily fish, eggs, meat, vitamin D-fortified margarine or breakfast cereal;
  (d) women with a prepregnancy body mass index above 30 kg/m^2.

Folic acid

* Recommend that all women take 400 mcg of folic acid a day from before conception until the end of the 12th week. This will prevent 95% of neural tube defects (DTB 1994b).

Vitamin A

* Advise all women to limit intake of vitamin A to 700 mcg/day and not to eat liver or liver products, e.g. sausage or paté, because of their high vitamin A content. High levels of vitamin A may be teratogenic.

EXERCISE

* Advise women that beginning or continuing a moderate course of exercise during pregnancy is not associated with adverse outcomes.
* Inform women about sports that have a danger: contact sports, high-impact sports and vigorous racquet sports that may involve the risk of abdominal trauma, falls or excessive joint stress, and scuba diving, which may result in fetal birth defects and fetal decompression disease.

SEXUAL INTERCOURSE IN PREGNANCY

* Advise women that sexual intercourse in pregnancy is not known to be associated with any adverse outcomes.

CAR TRAVEL

Seatbelts are used less frequently in the back seat than the front.

* Advise about the correct use of seatbelts in pregnancy:
  (a) Above and below the bump, not over it.
  (b) Use three-point seatbelts with the lap strap placed as low as possible beneath the 'bump', lying across the thighs with the diagonal shoulder strap above the bump lying between the breasts.
  (c) Adjust the fit to be as snug as comfortably possible.

TRAVEL OVERSEAS

See Chapter 2 for information about overseas travel. For advice about immunization in pregnancy see Appendix 19.

Malaria. Pregnant women are advised to avoid travel to malarious areas. However, advice is available for those whose travel is essential, see the

Health Protection Agency document *Guidelines for Malaria Prevention in Travellers from the UK* available from www.hpa.org.uk (choose 'Topics A–Z', then 'M' for malaria).

ROUTINE ANTENATAL CARE

GUIDELINE

Antenatal Care: Routine Care for the Healthy Pregnant Woman. 2008. National Collaborating Centre for Women's and Children's Health. Commissioned by the National Institute for Health and Clinical Excellence. NICE Clinical Guideline 62. http://www.nice.org.uk

- The woman should be the focus of maternity care.
- Midwifery and GP-led models of maternity care are safe for low-risk women.
- Women with the following conditions may require specialist care:
  - (a) a current medical problem (e.g. diabetes, epilepsy, hypertension);
  - (b) a psychiatric disorder (on medication);
  - (c) drug use such as heroin, cocaine (including crack cocaine) and ecstasy;
  - (d) HIV or hepatitis B virus (HBV) infected;
  - (e) an autoimmune disorder;
  - (f) obesity (BMI 35 or more at first contact) or underweight (BMI less than 18 at first contact);
  - (g) women who are particularly vulnerable (e.g. teenagers) or who lack social support;
  - (h) multiple pregnancy.
- Women who have experienced any of the following in previous pregnancies also need specialist care:
  - (a) recurrent miscarriage (three or more consecutive pregnancy losses) or a mid-trimester loss;
  - (b) severe pre-eclampsia, HELLP syndrome or eclampsia;
  - (c) rhesus isoimmunization or other significant blood group antibodies;
  - (d) uterine surgery including Caesarean section, myomectomy or cone biopsy;
  - (e) antenatal or postpartum haemorrhage on two occasions;
  - (f) retained placenta on two occasions;
  - (g) puerperal psychosis;
  - (h) grand multiparity (more than six pregnancies);
  - (i) a stillbirth or neonatal death;
  - (j) a small-for-gestational-age infant (less than 5th centile);
  - (k) a large-for-gestational-age infant (greater than 95th centile);
  - (l) a baby weighing less than 2500 g or more than 4500 g;
  - (m) a baby with a congenital anomaly (structural or chromosomal).
- Women at risk of gestational diabetes should be offered an oral glucose tolerance test (OGTT) at 16–18 weeks and at 28 weeks. Those at high risk are women with a high BMI, previous gestational diabetes, a previous macrosomic baby, a family history of diabetes and an ethnic origin with a high prevalence of diabetes.
- Risk factors for postnatal depression (see page 403) should be noted at this stage, in order to facilitate earlier detection should it occur. There is little evidence that it can be prevented by intervention in the antenatal period (NICE 2007).
- Care providers should:
  - (a) make sure that pregnancy care is woman-centred and that they use effective communication skills to ensure that women make informed choices about their care;
  - (b) be aware that there is a huge amount of information presented to women during pregnancy and they should provide written information and resources in plain language;
  - (c) ensure women are given an opportunity to discuss information at antenatal visits.

Because of the increase in information to be processed by pregnant women, early antenatal appointments should be scheduled to allow discussion time.

BOOKING – PRIOR TO 12 WEEKS

- (a) Take a full medical and obstetric history if the patient is new to the practice.
- (b) Recommend folic acid 400 mcg daily until week 12 if the patient is not already taking it.
- (c) Assess risk and discuss the model of maternity care appropriate for the woman.

(d) Estimate EDD. Offer early ultrasound (10–13 weeks) to determine gestation. Offer 18–20 week ultrasound for structural anomalies.

(e) Provide information on diet and lifestyle. Routine iron supplementation is not recommended. Advise about reducing the risk of listeriosis, toxoplasmosis, and salmonellosis.

(f) Offer a smoking cessation programme, if a smoker.

(g) Check blood group and rhesus D (RhD) status.

(h) Offer screening for anaemia, red-cell autoantibodies, hepatitis B virus, HIV, rubella, asymptomatic bacteriuria, syphilis. Tests for sickle cell trait and thalassaemia if at risk.

(i) Offer screening for Down's syndrome.

(j) Measure BMI and blood pressure (BP) and test urine for proteinuria.

(k) Assess psychosocial well-being. Ask about feelings and fears. Ask about relationships and supports. Consider asking about intimate partner violence. Ask the two screening questions for depression (see page 452) and, if the answers are positive, ask if this is something the patient would like help with (NICE 2007).

FOLLOW–UP APPOINTMENTS

Reducing the number of visits is not associated with worse outcomes, except that women may be less satisfied (Villar, Carroli, Khan-Neelofur, *et al.* 2001; Sikorski, Wilson, Clement, *et al.* 1996). Ten visits can provide essential care (booking, and weeks 16, 18–20, 25, 28, 31, 34, 36, 38, 40). Visits should be long enough to allow women to have concerns voiced and addressed. Some women will require more visits. Multiparous women may need as few as six (booking and 28, 34, 36, 38, 41 weeks).

Current evidence does NOT support the following *as routine*:

(a) repeated maternal weighing;

(b) breast examination;

(c) pelvic examination;

(d) antenatal screening to predict post-natal depression using EPDS;

(e) iron supplementation;

(f) vitamin D supplementation;

(g) screening for cytomegalovirus, hepatitis C virus, group B streptococcus, toxoplasmosis, bacterial vaginosis, gestational diabetes mellitus;

(h) formal fetal movement counting;

(i) antenatal electronic cardiotocography;

(j) ultrasound scanning after 24 weeks;

(k) umbilical artery Doppler USS;

(l) uterine artery Doppler USS to predict pre-eclampsia.

AT EACH APPOINTMENT CHECK

(a) The patient's general health and psychosocial well-being.

(b) BP.

(c) Symphysis–fundal height, plotted in cm on a chart.

(d) Fetal movements or fetal heart sounds.

(e) Presentation (after 34 weeks).

PRENATAL DIAGNOSIS AND SCREENING

SCREENING TESTS

Pregnant women should be offered screening for structural anomalies and chromosomal abnormalities by appropriately trained staff. If there is a family history of another genetic disorder the woman should be referred to a specialist service for genetic counselling.

STRUCTURAL ABNORMALITIES

Ultrasonography should be offered between 18 and 20 weeks.

Routine ultrasonography can detect the more obvious forms of congenital abnormality, e.g. cranial and neural tube defects, severe skeletal dysplasia and abnormalities of the heart, chest and abdominal organs. Hydrocephalus may be detected later. As technology and training improve the range of anomalies detectable before birth continues to increase.

Fetoscopy

Visualization of the fetus is necessary for the assessment of some external malformations. It is also used for laser treatment of twin-to-twin transfusion syndrome.

CHROMOSOMAL ABNORMALITIES

Women need:

(a) to understand that screening is a risk assessment and not a diagnostic test;

(b) to be informed that diagnostic tests are invasive and have a risk of miscarriage;

(c) information about the performance of a screening test based on *their* age, as maternal age is a key component of all screening tests: younger women (< 25) having screening tests will have a low screen positive rate (1%) and a 30% detection rate whilst older women (> 40) will have a high screen positive rate (50%) and a 90% detection rate (Three Centres Consensus Guidelines on Antenatal Care Project 2001);

(d) to be informed that most women having a screen positive result will **not** have a Down's syndrome affected pregnancy.

Types of screening tests for chromosomal abnormalities

A number of screening tests exist yet availability varies between countries and centres. Check with your local maternity unit to confirm availability.

Tests with detection rates greater than 75% and false positive rates less than 3% are:

(a) **combined first trimester screening** – (Nuchal Translucency @ 11.5–14 weeks, hCG and PAPP-A @ 8–12 weeks);

(b) **second trimester maternal serum screening** – **the quadruple test** (hCG, AFP, uE3, inhibin A) performed between 14 and 20 weeks;

(c) **the integrated test** (Nuchal Translucency, PAPP-A + hCG, AFP, uE3, inhibin A);

(d) **the serum integrated test** (PAPP-A + hCG, AFP, uE3, inhibin A) can be performed between 11 and 20 weeks.

Methods (a), (c) and (d) involve tests at different stages of pregnancy. A result is only reported when all tests have been performed.

Diagnostic tests for chromosomal abnormalities

Chorionic villus biopsy (CVB)

This is usually performed after 11 weeks and allows women to consider termination of pregnancy in the first trimester, but has a miscarriage rate of 1.2%. There is also a further 1–2% chance of needing an amniocentesis to establish the diagnosis. CVB performed before 10 weeks may rarely cause limb abnormalities (Lilford 1991).

Amniocentesis

This is usually performed at 15–16 weeks, which will allow women to consider termination by 20 weeks. It is associated with a miscarriage rate of 1%. Polymerase chain reaction technology allows results for Down's and Edward's syndrome in 48 hours, usually backed by culture results for other chromosomal anomalies available 2 weeks later.

PROBLEMS IN PREGNANCY

NAUSEA AND VOMITING

Around 80% of pregnant women experience nausea during the first trimester and around 50% experience vomiting. These problems can vary from being minor to severe and disabling.

* Reassure the woman that most cases of nausea and vomiting settle by 20 weeks and that it does not harm the fetus.

* Consider over-the-counter or prescribed treatment if the vomiting has severe consequences on the quality of life (on day-to-day activities, including interfering with household activities, restricting interaction with children, greater use of healthcare resources and time lost off work). Ensure that women remain adequately hydrated, avoid exhaustion and consider the following (Jewell and Young 2003):

(a) acupressure at P6 (seabands) and ginger may be of benefit;

(b) antihistamines (promethazine, prochlorperazine) reduce nausea and vomiting but can cause drowsiness. There is no evidence that they are teratogenic;

(c) vitamin B_6 may be of benefit alone, but the evidence is not strong. There are concerns about the toxicity of B_6 at high dose. Limit the maximum daily dose to 10 mg.

* If associated with reflux, advise:

(a) a biscuit before getting up;

(b) small frequent meals;

(c) a low sodium, low sugar antacid for heartburn;

(d) stop iron if it is making symptoms worse.

* Prescribe an H_2 receptor antagonist, e.g. ranitidine 150 mg b.d., to patients with reflux not controlled on the above measures. A lesser dose is no better than placebo (Larson, Patatanian, Miner Jr, *et al.* 1997). A PPI is likely to be more effective but toxicity has occurred in animal studies.

* In late pregnancy exclude: UTI, pre-eclampsia and surgical causes of vomiting.

* *Hyperemesis gravidarum.* Admit if the weight loss is more than 5% with ketosis. If this diagnosis is suspected give thiamine 100 mg i.v. once per week.

HEARTBURN

Heartburn is common in pregnancy and becomes more common as the pregnancy progresses.

* Suggest lifestyle modifications (see page 204).
* Alginate antacids, e.g. Gaviscon.
* Ranitidine and omeprazole are effective but the manufacturers advise against their use unless essential. No association between use of these drugs and fetal malformations has been found (Nikfar, Abdollahi, Moretti, *et al.* 2002).

PELVIC PAIN

Symphysis pubis dysfunction is a collection of signs and symptoms of discomfort and pain in the pelvic area, including pelvic pain radiating to the upper thighs and perineum. It can be debilitating. There is no evidence that any treatment helps but referral to a physiotherapist and pelvic support may be of value.

VAGINAL BLEEDING AND MISCARRIAGE

For details of the diagnosis of bleeding in pregnancy see *Evidence-based Diagnosis in Primary Care* by A. F. Polmear (editor), published by Butterworth-Heinemann, 2008.

> **GUIDELINE**
>
> Stillbirth and Neonatal Death Society. 1995. *Pregnancy Loss and the Death of a Baby: Guidelines for Professionals. SANDS.* Available from SANDS (see below)

Rhesus status. If a rhesus-negative patient bleeds, anti-D immunization is recommended (see page 396). The dose depends upon the preparation used. Give it within 72 hours of the bleeding starting, although, if a longer period has elapsed, it may still give some protection.

ECTOPIC PREGNANCY

Ectopic pregnancy is usually associated with mild vaginal bleeding as well as pain. A negative pregnancy test (i.e. an HCG level below 50 IU/l) virtually excludes it. Intrauterine pregnancies should be visible on transvaginal ultrasound when serum HCG exceeds 1000 IU/l.

* Admit any patient in whom the possibility of an ectopic is anything more than remote. It is the commonest cause of death in the first trimester and remains in the top five causes of death in pregnancy (Department of Health 1991).

SUSPECTED MISCARRIAGE UP TO 14 WEEKS PREGNANCY

> **GUIDANCE**
>
> Ankum WM, Wieringa-de Waard M, Bindels PJE. 2001. Management of spontaneous miscarriage in the first trimester: an example of putting informed shared decision making into practice. BMJ 322, 1343–1346
>
> Cahill DJ. 2001. Managing spontaneous first trimester miscarriage. BMJ 322, 1315–1316

● Women referred to specialist care tend to undergo surgical evacuation, sometimes unnecessarily.

● If provided with appropriate counselling, most women who miscarry in the first trimester will choose expectant management. About 81% of these complete their miscarriage without intervention (Luise, Jermy, May, *et al.* 2002).

* Perform a vaginal examination to assess the cervix.

* Do not use a pregnancy test to see whether the pregnancy is viable; too many false positives and false negatives occur.

Threatened miscarriage

* If there is modest loss, minor pain and the os is closed, manage at home. Rest will reduce the amount of loss, although it will not affect the outcome.

* Arrange for an ultrasound detection of fetal heart movements. They are reliably detectable from the 6th week, and may be detectable earlier. If they are present, the pregnancy has a 95% chance of continuing (Everett and Preece 1996). Clinical judgment without ultrasound is unreliable (Wieringa-de Waard, Bonsel, Ankum, *et al.* 2002).

* Prepare the patient for what may happen. 50% will progress to a complete miscarriage in the next 8 days although slight blood loss may continue for up to 50 days. Increased bleeding is a sign that the miscarriage is about to complete spontaneously and so should not *necessarily* lead to admission. However 12% of those managed expectantly will need admission for evacuation (Wieringa-de Waard, Ankum, Bonsel, *et al.* 2003).

If bleeding and pain settle:

(a) Advise the patient that, if the pregnancy continues, the risk of abnormality is no greater than in patients who have not bled. (There is a higher risk of antepartum haemorrhage and early neonatal death, but it is difficult to justify telling the patient this unless asked.)

(b) Arrange an ultrasound scan to confirm that the pregnancy is viable.

(c) If a vaginal examination has not been performed, do so to look for local causes of bleeding, e.g. erosion, polyp or carcinoma.

Inevitable miscarriage

* If there is considerable loss, pain and the os is open, refer to hospital.

* Products of conception may be present on vaginal examination. Removal should only be attempted if you have intravenous access and can maintain fluid balance and resuscitate in the event of shock.

* If bleeding is heavy, give Syntometrine 1 ml i.m. while waiting for the ambulance.

The decision as to whether to perform an evacuation of retained products of conception (ERPC) will be made by the gynaecologist. Not performing ERPC is as effective in four out of five women, but requires greater follow-up (Nielsen and Hahlin 1995). The complications of infection or bleeding are similar with either approach. In addition, surgical intervention carries a 1:50 risk of perforation (Trinder, Brocklehurst, Porter, *et al.* 2006).

Complete miscarriage

* If products have been lost, pain and bleeding have stopped and the os is closed:

(a) inform the patient that the miscarriage is probably complete;

(b) tell the patient to contact you if more bleeding occurs;

(c) discuss with the parents whether to send the products of conception for histology. Some may wish to have some tissue returned to them so that a burial service can be held. This can provide a focus for their grief. Even if no tissue is available, it is possible for a memorial service to be held;

(d) arrange for an ultrasound to confirm that the miscarriage is complete.

Follow-up after miscarriage

* Arrange to meet all patients who have miscarried about 4 weeks afterwards. Be aware that the patient has suffered a bereavement, and may need counselling. 50% are still likely to feel depressed (Friedman 1989).

* Attend to any physical issues and the possible need for contraception. The traditional advice to have two normal periods before trying to conceive again may be more important to allow time for the grieving process than for any physical reason.

* Be aware that women are distressed by the fact that no reason for the miscarriage can usually be given. Many feel unreasonable guilt and feel 'brushed off' by being reassured that miscarriage is common (Wong, Crawford, Gask, *et al.* 2003). Explain that early miscarriage is due either to an abnormality of fetal development, or to a failure of implantation.

* Explain that one miscarriage is followed by a slight or even no increase in risk of subsequent miscarriages (Everett 1997). Investigations are

unlikely to be fruitful unless three or more pregnancies have miscarried (see page 381). Having three consecutive miscarriages gives a patient a subsequent risk of 40%. Referral for investigation is then traditional, but earlier referral may be justified as discussed above.

PATIENT INFORMATION AND SUPPORT

The Miscarriage Association, c/o Clayton Hospital, Northgate, Wakefield, West Yorkshire, WF1 3JS, helpline 01924 200799, administration 01924 200795 for leaflets about all aspects of miscarriage, ectopic pregnancy and molar pregnancy. www.miscarriageassociation.org.uk
  Other sites include: http://www.miscarriagesupport.org.nz/ (New Zealand) http://www.connectedscotland.org.uk/scimnet/index.asp (Scotland); http://www.fertilityplus.org/faq/miscarriage/resources.html (international)

SUSPECTED MISCARRIAGE AFTER 14 WEEKS' PREGNANCY

The more advanced the pregnancy, the more advisable it is to admit the patient to hospital at the onset of bleeding, whether or not there has been pain. After 14 weeks, painless bleeding is due to placenta praevia until proved otherwise. Bleeding with severe pain is likely to be due to abruptio placentae.

∗ Do not do a vaginal examination in these patients.

PATIENT INFORMATION AND SUPPORT

For parents whose baby is stillborn or dies soon after birth, SANDS (the Stillbirth and Neonatal Death Society), 28 Portland Place, London W1B 1LY. Helpline 020 7436 5881. Administration 020 7436 7940
  Websites: www.uk-sands.org; www.sandsvic.org.au; www.nationalshareoffice.com/default.asp (United States)

ABDOMINAL PAIN

Abdominal pain may be due to a variety of causes, some of which are serious and which may present in an atypical way. Any cause which could occur outside pregnancy (e.g. renal calculus) must be considered.

In the first 20 weeks, consider:

(a) miscarriage;
(b) ectopic pregnancy;
(c) urinary infection;
(d) appendicitis;
(e) impaction of a retroverted uterus;
(f) red degeneration of a fibroid (the maximum incidence is 12–18 weeks, but it may occur at any time);
(g) torsion of an ovary or tube;
(h) haematoma of the round ligament;
(i) accident to an ovarian cyst.

After 20 weeks, consider, in addition:

(a) labour;
(b) abruptio placentae;
(c) haematoma of the rectus abdominis;
(d) red degeneration of a fibroid;
(e) uterine rupture;
(f) dehiscence of the pubic symphysis.

INFECTION OR CONTACT WITH INFECTIOUS DISEASE

RUBELLA CONTACT

● If a pregnant woman is infected with rubella, the risk to the fetus is greatest up to 11 weeks but 30% of fetuses between 11 and 16 weeks are affected.
● Women experiencing infection before 16 weeks should be offered counselling regarding termination of pregnancy.
● If a pregnant woman is affected between 16 and 19 weeks, the risk of fetal damage is less than 2%. Deafness is the most likely problem.
● After 19 weeks the risk appears very low (Jones 1990).
● Accidental immunization in pregnancy has not been associated with embryopathy.

Rubella contact before 16 weeks

If the pregnancy is less than 16 weeks; regardless of whether the woman has had rubella or the vaccination or antibodies were previously detected (Best, Banatuala, Morgan-Capner, et al. 1989):

∗ Take blood for rubella antibodies.

(a) If IgG is present and the blood was taken within 12 days of contact, inform the woman that she is immune and that there is little need to worry.

(b) If IgG is present but the blood was taken more than 12 days after contact, request IgM levels. If IgM shows recent infection, discuss the risks of fetal abnormality and the question of termination of pregnancy.

(c) If IgG is absent, repeat IgM 2 weeks later. If she has seroconverted, discuss the question of termination of pregnancy as above. The value of immunoglobulin in protecting the fetus is doubtful.

(d) Any IgG-negative woman should be immunized in the puerperium.

Note: If a woman contracts rubella and decides to continue the pregnancy, fetal blood sampling (from the umbilical vein) from 20 weeks onwards can indicate whether the baby has contracted it by assessing fetal IgM.

Note: IgM can persist for up to a year after rubella. Only act on an IgM result if it is consistent with the clinical picture or with a reliable history of exposure (Best, O'Shea, Tipples, *et al.* 2002).

VARICELLA (CHICKENPOX)

> **GUIDELINE**
>
> RCOG. *Chickenpox in Pregnancy.* Available: http://www.rcog.org.uk/resources/Public/Chickenpox_No13.pdf

- A congenital varicella syndrome, including limb deformities and scarring, may occur in 1–2% of pregnancies where the mother contracts chickenpox (though not shingles) up to, but not after, 20 weeks gestation (Royal College of Obstetricians and Gynaecologists 2001).

- Exposure to chickenpox after 20 weeks and before 36 weeks does not appear to be associated with fetal abnormalities.

* *A woman who is not known to be immune* and who is in contact with chickenpox in the first trimester: check her varicella antibodies urgently, and give VZIG if not immune (see page 52).

* *Give aciclovir* to a pregnant woman who develops chickenpox at a gestation of > 20 weeks, starting within 24 hours of the appearance of the rash. Monitor any pregnant woman with chickenpox carefully. 10% develop pneumonia.

* Offer an ultrasound anomaly scan to women contracting chickenpox before 20 weeks gestation.

* If a mother contracts chickenpox in the 5 days prior to giving birth or within 2 days of giving birth the baby should be given VZIG.

CYTOMEGALOVIRUS

CMV infection is now the commonest congenital infection worldwide. The birth incidence is between 0.2 and 2.5%, and 10% of these infections will produce an affected neonate. Consequences of infection can include deafness and developmental disability; this is commoner with primary infection and occurs in up to 20% of cases. Two thirds of congenital infections are thought to result from primary maternal infection and one third from recurrent infection in the mother. Ganciclovir is effective in the neonate but has not been proven to be of benefit if given to the mother during pregnancy. Advice to a woman who seroconverts to CMV during pregnancy is difficult and such cases should be referred for tertiary centre advice.

TOXOPLASMOSIS

Toxoplasmosis causes fetal infection in about 15% of cases in the first trimester, rising to 70% in the third. The risk of serious fetal damage if the fetus is infected is, however, greater in early pregnancy. Overall, up to 90% of infected babies escape long-term damage. Most maternal cases are asymptomatic. The incidence of children born with definite or probable toxoplasmosis is very low.

Where there is concern, check serology as soon as possible after conception and monthly thereafter. IgM may stay positive for months; timing infection in relation to pregnancy stage requires IgG avidity testing at the National Reference Laboratory. In the case of infection, the woman may be offered USS and amniocentesis to detect fetal abnormality, and fetal blood sampling between 20 and 24 weeks. Even if FBS demonstrates fetal infection, it cannot indicate whether the fetus has been damaged (Robinson 1991). Treatment with spiramycin in pregnancy is safe but of unproven benefit.

LISTERIA

Maternal infection may be asymptomatic or associated with fever. The infection carries a risk of miscarriage, stillbirth or the birth of an infected baby. Symptoms in the mother are so non-specific that the diagnosis is rarely made during the acute illness, especially since the only useful diagnostic test is blood culture. Women with fever for 48 hours who are pregnant and who have no obvious other source of infection should have a blood culture specifying listeria. Treatment is with i.v. ampicillin.

GROUP B STREPTOCOCCAL (GBS) INFECTION (ROYAL COLLEGE OF OBSTETRICIANS AND GYNAECOLOGISTS 2003A)

GBS is the commonest severe infection in infants in the first 7 days of life.

Situations in which neonatal GBS infection is more likely are:

- neonatal GBS infection in a previous baby;
- vaginal, urinary or intestinal GBS present in the woman in this pregnancy;
- preterm (before 37 weeks) labour;
- prolonged (> 18 hours) rupture of membranes;
- fever during labour (> 38°C).
- * Consider women at risk, as above, for intravenous antibiotics during labour, or the newborn baby for antibiotics until blood cultures show that there is no BGS present.
- * Recommend to the woman the excellent leaflet available from Group B Strep Support on www.gbss.org.uk.

HEPATITIS A

Reassure the mother that the infant will not be harmed although it may be infected if occurring shortly before term.

HEPATITIS B

Hepatitis B is not influenced by pregnancy, but if the mother is infected there is a risk of acute infection of the fetus or neonate.

For the management of babies born to HbSAg positive mothers, see page 39.

HERPES SIMPLEX

Genital herpes (Royal College of Obstetricians and Gynaecologists 2003b)

Primary infection at delivery gives a 20–50% risk of neonatal herpes, which is frequently fatal. Recurrent herpes at delivery gives a risk of 1–2%. LSCS is therefore only recommended if the patient is suffering her first attack during labour. Viral shedding is less in subsequent attacks and maternal IgG crosses the placenta to provide some fetal protection. There is little value in taking viral swabs in the last month of pregnancy in those with a history of infection but without active lesions. Aciclovir in the last month of pregnancy reduces viral shedding and vertical transmission (Braig, Luton, Sibony, et al. 2001).

Labial herpes

The mother, and indeed any family or friends with labial herpes, should refrain from direct contact with the baby (i.e. kissing) once born.

Genital warts (see page 72)

Respiratory papillomatosis in the child is strongly related to maternal genital warts during pregnancy. However the risk is small (6.9 cases per 1000 live births, against a risk of 0.03 per 1000 live births with no such maternal history) and is not reduced by Caesarean section (Silverberg, Thorsen, Lindeberg, et al. 2003).

HIV

- A mother who is HIV positive has a risk of fetal infection of 15–25%, but this can be substantially reduced by delivery by Caesarean section and/or antiretroviral therapy. Screening should be offered to all women. Some babies will be HIV antibody positive at birth due to maternal antibody, but will become negative as maternal antibody is cleared.
- Breastfeeding doubles the chance of vertical transmission and is not recommended. If a woman must breastfeed then exclusive breastfeeding rather than mixed feeding should be recommended as neonatal seroconversion may be greatest with the bowel inflammation secondary to artificial feeds.

- Zidovudine can reduce the chance of vertical transmission if given to the mother antenatally and during labour, and to the baby postpartum (Connor, Sperling, Gelber, et al. 1994).
- Pregnancy does not appear to hasten the onset of AIDS in women who are HIV positive.

PARVOVIRUS B 19 INFECTION (FIFTH DISEASE/ SLAPPED CHEEK SYNDROME) (MORGAN–CAPNER AND CROWCROFT 2002)

- This is common in schools and nurseries especially in April and May. If a woman is exposed in the first 20 weeks of pregnancy there is an increased risk of intrauterine death (excess risk 9%) and if infection occurs between 9–20 weeks, fetal anaemia leading to hydrops fetalis (3%, of whom half die – included in the excess 9%). The consequences usually occur with 3–5 weeks of maternal infection.
- Maternal asymptomatic infection is as likely to damage the fetus as symptomatic infection.
* Check antibodies in all women exposed as soon as possible, informing the lab of the clinical details.
  (a) If specific IgG is detected and specific IgM not detected the woman can be reassured that she has had past infection.
  (b) If specific IgM is detected but specific IgG is not a further sample should be tested immediately. Refer all women who are positive to an obstetrician.
  (c) If specific IgG and IgM are not detected a further sample should be tested after 1 month.

PRURITIS

* Pruritis, without jaundice, is the commonest manifestation of obstetric cholestasis, which, in turn, is associated with premature birth in 60%, fetal distress in up to 33% and intrauterine death in up to 2% (Milkiewicz, Elias, Williamson, et al. 2002). Although most women with pruritis in pregnancy do not have obstetric cholestasis, it should be considered in every case because of its serious implications.

* Check LFTs. Transaminases are raised in 60% of cases of obstetric cholestasis, though only 25% have a raised bilirubin.
* Refer all affected patients. Most obstetricians will deliver the baby at 37 weeks.

EXCESSIVE WEIGHT GAIN

- A woman's BMI should be calculated at the first booking appointment.
- The average weight gain in pregnancy is 10–12.5 kg (0.65 kg first quarter, 4 kg by mid-pregnancy, 8.5 kg by the third quarter, 12.5 kg by term). Over a quarter of the total gain is due to fat deposition in the middle two quarters of pregnancy.
- The ideal weight gain depends on the prepregnancy BMI. A woman with a BMI that is low or normal has fewest obstetric and neonatal adverse outcomes if her weight gain is < 10 kg. A woman with a BMI 25–30 does best if her weight gain is < 9 kg and an obese woman does best with a weight gain < 6 kg (Cedergren 2007). Excessive weight gain may be associated with an increased incidence of pre-eclampsia. Check BP, urine and the presence of oedema.
- Despite the above, there is no evidence that the regular weighing of patients is of benefit and it is not recommended.
- *Obesity.* Obesity is associated with an increase in congenital malformations and first trimester abortions, gestational diabetes, hypertension, macrosomia, stillbirth, prolonged labour and Caesarean birth. All women with obesity should be seen by an obstetrician and monitored closely for weight gain, blood pressure and diabetes (Stotland 2009).
- *Eating disorders* are common in pregnancy; the disorder may worsen or improve as the pregnancy progresses (Ward 2008). Women with a recognized eating disorder should be referred to an obstetrician and the eating disorder service, early in pregnancy. Suggested screening questions at each antenatal visit are:
  (a) What is your current eating pattern? Are you restricting your dietary intake? Do you binge? Do you vomit or take laxatives after eating?
  (b) How do you feel about your shape and weight?

(c) What is your weight? Are you gaining weight appropriately?

(d) What is your mood like? Do you feel low or anxious?

(e) What exercise are you taking? Are you exercising too much?

FUNDAL HEIGHT

- At 22 weeks the fundus should have reached the umbilicus, and at 32 weeks the lower rib border.
- The symphysis-to-fundus height in centimetres should be within two of the number of weeks gestation between 20 and 36 weeks; after 36 weeks it should be within ±3 cm.
- * If the fundus is over 3 cm less than dates, refer for exclusion of fetal IUGR, or oligohydramnios.
- * If the fundus is 3 cm more than dates, refer for assessment for possible multiple pregnancy or hydramnios.

HYPERTENSION

- Blood pressure falls early in the first trimester as the fall in peripheral resistance exceeds the rise in cardiac output. Blood pressure reaches its nadir by 16 weeks, plateaus until 22 weeks and then increases towards term.
- *Pregnancy induced hypertension(PIH):* blood pressure which rises to exceed 90 mmHg diastolic on more than one occasion, in the second half of pregnancy, resolves after delivery and is *not* complicated by proteinuria. The International Society for the Study of Hypertension in Pregnancy has chosen this definition, rather than one based on a relative rise in diastolic pressure, because of the fact that any rise in pressure varies according to when the baseline was taken; and because a relative rise seems to correlate less well with outcomes than the use of an absolute cut-off point.
- *Pre-eclampsia:* this is defined in the same way as above, but is associated with proteinuria of > 300 mg/24 hours, raised creatinine, abnormal liver function tests, neurological symptoms, low platelet count, and IUGR. The terms PIH and pre-eclampsia should not be used interchangeably as the former is not associated

with poor maternal or fetal outcome, whilst pre-eclampsia is a leading cause of maternal and fetal morbidity.

- *Antihypertensives* do not lessen the risk of developing pregnancy-induced hypertension or alter its progression, but protect against stroke and possibly placental abruption.
- *Aspirin* prophylaxis (75 mg daily) may prevent the development of pre-eclampsia and moderate the condition once it has started (Askie, Duley, Henderson-Smart, *et al.* 2007).
- *Measuring the blood pressure.* Use phase 4 diastolic pressure and not phase 5, which may be misleadingly low in pregnancy (MacGillivray and Thomas 1991).
- * **Chronic hypertension:** predates pregnancy or appears prior to 20 weeks gestation. A blood pressure of ≥ 140/90 before 20 weeks suggests pre-existing hypertension and needs specialist assessment.

PRE-ECLAMPSIA

GUIDELINE

Milne F, Redman C, Walker J, *et al.* 2005. The pre-eclampsia community guideline (PRECOG). BMJ 330, 576–580

Women with any of the following should be referred for specialist assessment before 20 weeks of gestation:

- previous pre-eclampsia;
- multiple pregnancy;
- underlying medical conditions:

    (a) pre-existing hypertension or booking diastolic blood pressure ≥ 90 mmHg;

    (b) pre-existing renal disease or booking proteinuria (≥ + on more than one occasion or ≥ 300 mg/24 hours);

    (c) pre-existing diabetes;

    (d) presence of antiphospholipid antibodies.

Women with any two or more of the following should be referred for specialist assessment before 20 weeks of gestation:

- first pregnancy;
- more than 10 years since last baby;
- age more than 40 years;
- body mass index ≥ 35;

- family history of pre-eclampsia (mother or sister);
- booking diastolic blood pressure ≥ 80 mmHg.

Any woman with suspected pre-eclampsia should be managed in conjunction with specialist advice. This will usually be undertaken in a special day assessment centre.

Action to be taken if new hypertension is discovered after 20 weeks:

- diastolic 90–99: refer to specialist clinic to be seen within 48 hours;
- diastolic 90–99 plus a symptom associated with pre-eclampsia: refer for same day assessment;
- diastolic 90–99 plus proteinuria: refer for same day assessment;
- BP 160/100 to 169/109: refer for same day assessment;
- BP 160/90 or above, plus proteinuria plus a symptom associated with eclampsia: admit immediately;
- BP 170/110 or above: admit immediately.

Note: Symptoms associated with pre-eclampsia: headache, visual disturbance, nausea, vomiting and epigastric pain.

Long-term follow-up (Magee 2007)

Women who have had pre-eclampsia are at higher long-term risk of cardiovascular disease and also higher risk that the disease may occur earlier.

- Inform them that their risk of CVD when young is still low but that they should concentrate on prevention.
- Counsel all women who have had pre-eclampsia about a healthy lifestyle (see page 166).
- Screen for the emergence of other risk factors for CVD at an earlier stage than usual.

ECLAMPSIA

- This is a medical emergency with a high maternal mortality. The patient must be resuscitated, and transferred to hospital as fast as possible. There is now good evidence that the anticonvulsant of choice to prevent further fits is magnesium sulphate.
- *Recurrence and follow up*: Many women will have post-traumatic stress disorder when their

normal physiological pregnancy has been taken from them. It is important to explain what happened and the relatively low chance of recurrence in future pregnancies (20%). Many units offer uterine artery Doppler as a screening test in subsequent pregnancies, with the possibility that aspirin, or vitamins C and E (antioxidants; Chappell, Seed, Briley, *et al.* 1999), can reduce this rate further.

PROTEINURIA

A trace of protein is acceptable. It may be due to contamination with vaginal secretions or to a delay since the urine was passed.

Proteinuria in the absence of raised blood pressure (Milne, Redman, Walker, *et al.* 2005)

* *One plus (+).* Arrange for a midstream urine for culture and microscopy and check the urinary spot protein:creatinine ratio. Review in 1 week. If culture and microscopy are negative but the protein:creatinine ratio is positive, check the serum creatinine, the 24-hour urinary protein and refer. Continue to look for pre-eclampsia. 10% of patients who develop eclampsia have proteinuria without a raised blood pressure (Douglas and Redman 1994).
* More than +: arrange to be seen in a specialist clinic within 48 hours.
* At least + with a symptom associated with pre-eclampsia: refer for same day assessment.

Using the different tests for proteinuria (Chappell and Shennan 2008)

- *The protein dipstick* is prone to both false negatives and false positives. Although recommended by NICE for the routine assessment of urinary protein in antenatal care, it is the least useful of the available tests.
- *The urinary spot protein:creatinine ratio* has few false negatives but rather more false positives. It is therefore a good screening test (if it is negative the patient almost certainly does not have significant proteinuria) but a more accurate test is required to confirm a positive finding. A positive result is considered to be ≥ 30 mg/mmol.

- *24 hour-urinary protein* remains the most accurate test available, with a cut-off of 300 mg/24 hours. False negatives occur when women forget to collect every sample; and different laboratories use different assays and so get different results.

BACTERIURIA

2–10% of pregnant women have asymptomatic bacteriuria. If untreated, 30% will develop a urinary infection. Antibiotics are very effective in preventing pyelonephritis (Smaill 2001).

* Treat with ampicillin, amoxicillin, cephalosporin or nitrofurantoin according to sensitivities.
* Repeat the MSU 2 weeks after treatment.

GLYCOSURIA

This occurs in 70% of pregnant women. If glycosuria is detected:

* Repeat the urine test on a second morning specimen (i.e. the second urine sample passed in the morning while the patient is still fasting).
* If still positive arrange for a modified glucose tolerance test (see page 228). If the sugar level is raised (fasting sugar ≥ 7 mmol/l or the 2-hour sugar ≥ 7.8 mmol/l), refer the patient urgently.

Gestational diabetes

GUIDELINE

NICE. 2008. *Diabetes in Pregnancy: Management of Diabetes and its Complications from Preconception to the Postnatal Period.* Clinical Guideline 63, available: www.nice.org.uk

- A patient should be managed intensively (see page 397) if her 2-hour sugar is over 9 mmol/l or her fasting glucose is over 6 mmol/l. For most patients, however, diet will be sufficient to control blood sugars. Active management with diet, blood glucose monitoring and, if necessary, metformin or insulin has been shown to reduce the risk of serious perinatal complications (Crowther, Hiller, Moss, *et al.* 2005). Recheck the modified GTT 6 weeks postpartum to be sure that it has returned to normal.

- Warn the patient of her 20–30% chance of developing diabetes in the next 5 years. This risk can be decreased by maintenance of a 'diabetic diet' after pregnancy.

ANAEMIA

- As the plasma volume increases in pregnancy, the haemoglobin falls. Only a haemoglobin < 11 g/dl (WHO) in the first trimester, or < 10.5 g/dl at 28 weeks, is considered to be anaemia.
- Routine iron supplementation is not recommended.
- A low serum ferritin is not a reliable guide to iron deficiency in pregnancy. It may reflect a shift of iron stores to the increased red cell mass rather than a low total body iron. However, there is no better, non-invasive, test.

ANAEMIA DEVELOPING IN PREGNANCY

* Check full blood count, film and serum ferritin. Check B_{12} and red cell folate if there is macrocytosis.
* Start iron in treatment doses if the haemoglobin is below 10 g/dl or MCV below 82 fl, e.g. give ferrous sulphate 200 mg t.d.s. and folic acid 5 mg daily. The addition of folate can almost double the rise in haemoglobin regardless of the patient's folate status (Juarez-Vazquez, Bonizzoni and Scotti 2002).
* Repeat Hb in 2 weeks. It should rise by about 0.8 g/dl per week.
* If there has been no response:
  (a) exclude occult infection, especially urinary; and either
  (b) consider arranging for parenteral iron; or
  (c) if the serum ferritin is normal, check the serum B_{12} and red cell folate (if not already checked) and continue combined iron and folate.
* If the Hb remains low, seek expert advice. Consider an Hb electrophoresis regardless of the apparent ethnic origin.

RHESUS–NEGATIVE WOMEN

* Check antibodies at booking and in primagravida at 28 and 36 weeks; in multigravida, monthly from 24 weeks. If the

maternal anti-D levels are 0.5–10.0 IU, antibody levels are needed every 2 weeks. A level above 10 means that fetal blood sampling is needed and referral to a fetal medicine unit is indicated. If gestation allows, delivery, rather than intra-uterine transfusion, may be the preferred option. It is important to realize (and explain) that subsequent pregnancies may behave similarly.

* Offer routine anti-D immunization to all Rhesus-negative women at 28 and at 34 weeks if non-sensitized, except where the patient:
  (a) is certain she will not have another child after the present pregnancy; or
  (b) is in a stable relationship with the father of the child and the father is known to be RhD negative (NICE 2002).

A leaflet for patients is available from NICE (www.nice.org.uk/pdf/Anti_d_patient_leaflet.pdf).

* In addition to routine antenatal anti-D immunization, offer it postnatally and if a sensitizing event occurs antenatally, namely:
  (a) abdominal trauma including external cephalic version;
  (b) chorionic villus biopsy and amniocentesis;
  (c) antepartum haemorrhage;
  (d) ectopic pregnancy;
  (e) termination of pregnancy or ERPC;
  (f) threatened or complete miscarriage after 12 weeks;
  (g) interuterine death.
* Use 250 IU up to 20 weeks of pregnancy. Give 500 IU thereafter, followed by a Kleihauer test for fetal haemoglobin. If the feto-maternal haemorrhage exceeds 4 ml red cells, a further dose will be needed.

ABNORMAL LIE

* Check the lie from 32–34 weeks onwards. If a transverse lie is found at 32 weeks or later, then either:
  (a) refer; or
  (b) arrange a scan and reassess at 36 weeks. Refer if still transverse.

Note: A breech presentation should be seen at the hospital by 37–38 weeks.

HIGH HEAD

A 'high head' is one that lies completely out of the pelvis. Make sure that the bladder and rectum are empty before accepting that the head is high.

* *Primipara:* refer by 36 weeks.
* *Multipara:* refer if still high at 38 weeks.

PREMATURE RUPTURE OF MEMBRANES

All women suspected of rupturing membranes should be referred for specialist assessment. After 35 weeks gestation the specialist is likely to recommend induction of labour. Before 35 weeks a short inpatient stay with antibiotic cover is more likely.

POST-MATURITY

If the expected date of delivery was established by USS in early pregnancy, routine induction of labour at 41 weeks reduces perinatal mortality (Crowley 2002). Routine induction does not cause a rise in the rate of LSCS, nor in lower maternal satisfaction.

Women who have not given birth by 41 weeks should be offered a pelvic examination and membrane sweep and discussion and information about induction of labour.

SPECIFIC MEDICAL CONDITIONS AND PREGNANCY

ASTHMA

Deterioration occurring during pregnancy is usually due to a reduction in therapy because of a fear that it will harm the fetus.

* Explain that poorly controlled asthma has been linked to IUGR.
* Explain that beta-sympathomimetics, inhaled steroids and ipratropium are safe while oral steroids and theophylline have been linked to preterm delivery.

DIABETES (TYPE 1 AND 2)

Optimum control of blood sugars should be achieved by the time of conception to reduce the risk of congenital malformation. Because of the higher risk of neural tube defects women with diabetes should take 5 mg (instead of 400 mcg) of folate daily before conception until the end of the 12th week. The GP should emphasize the importance of good control throughout pregnancy, even if the majority of the management will be done by the hospital.

* Patients should be referred to the diabetes clinic and seen 2-weekly before 28 weeks and then weekly.
* Insulin dose may need to be doubled or tripled, and will need to be reduced immediately after delivery to the prepregnant dose.
* Patients on oral hypoglycaemic drugs should be changed to insulin.
* Blood sugar profiles should show the majority of readings (pre-meals) below 6 mmol/l.
* Aim to keep the HbA_{1c} at 6 or below.
* Discontinue ACEI and ACEII inhibitors before conception or as soon as pregnancy is confirmed. Substitute with a more suitable drug.
* Discontinue statins before pregnancy or as soon as pregnancy is confirmed.
* Women should have serial ultrasound scans to exclude macrosomia and placental insufficiency. They should have examination of the fetal heart at 18–20 weeks.

THYROID DISORDERS

Pre-existing thyroid disease

● *Hypothyroidism.* Thyroid requirements change little during pregnancy, and the fetus is not affected by maternal thyroxine (Girling and de Swiet 1992). Thyroid function should be checked at booking and at 36 weeks.
● *Hyperthyroidism.* Refer all pregnant women with hyperthyroidism to an endocrinologist as soon as they present. It is important that they remain euthyroid throughout the pregnancy. Propylthiouracil is the preferred drug during pregnancy, given at the lowest effective dose to reduce the risk of fetal hypothyroidism and goitre (Marx, Amin and Lazarus 2008).

Postnatal thyroiditis

● Up to 10% of women develop transient autoimmune thyroiditis after delivery. This is usually between 1 and 3 months and may present with features of hyperthyroidism, but more commonly with those of hypothyroidism, i.e. fatigue and lethargy, at a time when she is understandably tired anyway. Thyroxine is necessary for 6 months, followed by repeat TFTs. Antithyroid drugs are not usually needed for the hyperthyroid state, but beta-blockers may be given to control symptoms.

* Follow the patient with yearly TFTs. Up to 20% develop hypothyroidism in the subsequent 4 years (DTB 1995).

EPILEPSY

● The association between epilepsy and treatment with congenital malformations has been discussed (page 382). 20% of patients have an increase of fits during pregnancy due either to poor compliance or to a fall in serum levels because of the physiological changes of pregnancy. Fits are more common when tired.

* Do not stop anticonvulsants or reduce their dose if a woman presents already pregnant. Any teratogenic effect will have already occurred. Liaise with her neurologist to plan the rest of the pregnancy. In general it is not necessary to monitor serum levels of anticonvulsant in pregnancy, but to be guided by the clinical condition, and only to increase the dose of a drug if the frequency of fits increases. A patient who drives or for whom a single fit would be a disaster may prefer drug level monitoring (O'Brien and Gilmour-White 1993).
* Encourage the patient to take her treatment correctly. Poor compliance is the main reason for fits in pregnancy.
* Ensure that an anomaly ultrasound is performed at 18–19 weeks.
* Recommend folic acid 5 mg daily to all epileptic women until the end of the 12th week (see page 382). This is particularly important in patients taking sodium valproate or carbamazepine or who have a history of a previous baby with a neural tube defect (DTB 1994b).
* Prescribe Vitamin K 10 mg daily for the last 4 weeks of pregnancy to reduce the risks of maternal and fetal bleeding, in those taking

enzyme-inducing drugs, i.e. phenytoin, barbiturates and carbamazepine.
* Reassure women that the majority have a normal delivery and that epilepsy is not an indication for elective Caesarean section.

INFLAMMATORY BOWEL DISEASE (FERGUSSON, MAHSU–DORNAN AND PATTERSON 2008)

* Inflammatory bowel disease is not worsened by pregnancy and may improve. If the disease is quiescent at the time of conception it remains so in two thirds of patients. If the disease is active two thirds of patients will have ongoing active disease.
* Women with inactive disease have no increased risk of an adverse outcome. Women with active disease have up to a 35% miscarriage rate. Crohn's disease has an increased risk of low birth weight, preterm delivery, and adverse perinatal outcome.
* Assessment of IBD in pregnancy is based on clinical factors, e.g. abdominal pain, stool frequency and bleeding. Pregnancy affects haemoglobin concentration, ESR and serum albumin. C-reactive protein is not altered by pregnancy.
* Reassure the woman that it is most important to achieve the best control of the disease possible and that this seems to give the best outcome. All women should be seen urgently by the gastroenterology and obstetric team.
* For the safety of commonly used drugs for inflammatory bowel disease see Caprilli R, Gassull MA, Escher JC, *et al*. 2006. *European evidence based consensus on the diagnosis and management of Crohn's disease: special situations.* Gut 55(Supplement 1), i36–i58.

DEPRESSION

REVIEW AND GUIDELINE

O'Keane V, Marsh MS. 2007. Depression during pregnancy. BMJ 334, 1003–1005
    NICE. *Antenatal and Postnatal Mental Health: Clinical Management and Service Guidance.* Clinical Guideline 45; 2007. Available: www.nice.org.uk

* Rates of depression are higher during pregnancy than at any other point in a woman's life.
* About half of postnatal depression starts during pregnancy.
* Two thirds of women with recurrent depression will relapse during pregnancy if they stop their antidepressants after conception.
* Depression during pregnancy is associated with poorer outcomes, especially preterm delivery.
* Women depressed during pregnancy are more likely to drink alcohol and smoke and less likely to attend antenatal appointments.
* If major depression is present and drug treatment is being considered, the following are relevant and should be shared with the patient:
  (a) TCAs (amitriptyline, imipramine and nortriptyline) are safer for the fetus than other antidepressants;
  (b) TCAs are more dangerous in overdosage than SSRIs;
  (c) fluoxetine is the SSRI of choice during pregnancy, but not when breastfeeding, because it is present in breast milk in high concentrations;
  (d) SSRIs, taken after 20 weeks gestation, may be associated with a risk of persistent pulmonary hypertension in the neonate;
  (e) paroxetine in the first trimester is associated with an increased risk of congenital abnormalities (especially cardiac) and pulmonary hypertension;
  (f) venlafaxine may cause high blood pressure and greater difficulty in withdrawal in the neonate;
  (g) all antidepressants may cause withdrawal symptoms in the neonate, although these are usually mild. The possible symptoms are hypotonia, excessive crying, sleeping difficulties and mild respiratory distress.

DRUG MISUSE

* *Amphetamines and cocaine*: stop the drugs immediately.
* *Benzodiazepines:* withdraw over 4 weeks (see page 489).
* *Barbiturates*: arrange admission. If there is any delay maintain the patient on phenobarbital.

✳ *Opiates*: arrange an urgent outpatient appointment. Maintain the patient on oral methadone meanwhile.

INTRAPARTUM CARE

POLICY STATEMENT

Royal College of GPs and the BMA. 1997. *General Practitioners and Intrapartum Care: Interim Guidance.* Available from BMA House, Tavistock Square, London WC1H 9JP

This section does not cover the clinical aspects of delivery.

● The guidance above defines three levels of GP involvement in intrapartum care:
  (a) the GP provides general medical care only, with the responsibility to refer a patient to another professional to provide intrapartum care if the patient wishes to deliver at home;
  (b) the GP attends a patient in labour as non-specialist back-up for the midwife, with the midwife taking responsibility for the delivery;
  (c) the GP provides intrapartum care and has the competence, over and above that of the average GP, to do so. The GPC of the BMA advises GPs that, in order to assume this role, they must be skilled in the identification of abnormalities of labour, in perineal suturing, in the resuscitation of mother and baby and the insertion of an i.v. line (GPC 1999).

● It is the policy of the two relevant Royal Colleges that women who wish to have a home birth should be able to do so.

● There is growing evidence that the risks of planned home delivery have been overemphasized in the UK, with a perinatal hazard associated with planned home births of < 1% (Northern Region Perinatal Mortality Survey Co-ordinating Group 1996).

● Home delivery is valued by those who choose it, even in those who are transferred to hospital during labour (Davies, Hey, Reed, *et al.* 1996).

WHEN A WOMAN REQUESTS A HOME DELIVERY

✳ Check that there are no medical or obstetric contraindications. Some contraindications, e.g. previous retained placenta, can be dealt with by 'domino', where most of labour takes place at home with the briefest possible admission for the delivery.

✳ Refer to the community midwife, who has a statutory duty to provide a service at home, whether or not a GP is willing to provide maternity services.

POSTNATAL CARE

✳ See the mother and baby within 24 hours of discharge, and then again as often as needed.

MOTHER

✳ *Examine* fundal height, perineum, lochia and breasts.

✳ *Feeding*. If necessary, reinforce the midwife's advice on breastfeeding (see below).

✳ *Contraception*. Hormonal methods should not be started before 4 weeks or before bleeding has stopped.

✳ *Rest*. Stress the need for rest in the first week, but also that the mother should be ambulant from day 2 to prevent deep vein thrombosis.

✳ *Pelvic exercises*. Urge the patient to perform pelvic exercises from the first day.

✳ Warn the patient that she will inevitably receive conflicting advice from professionals, family and friends. Parents need to develop their own solutions.

✳ *Depression*. Ensure there is time to talk about her emotional well-being.

BABY

✳ Examine the baby, unless this has already been done in hospital.

✳ Vitamin K. If it has not already been given i.m., give it orally according to local guidelines (see page 83). If the baby is breastfed, it will need to be repeated at 1 and at 4 weeks.

* Registration. Encourage early registration of the baby with the registrar; the start of Child Allowance is dependent on this. Register the baby with the practice.

AT 6 WEEKS

Review the patient's experiences.

* Does she have any outstanding questions about what happened during labour or birth?
* Is she getting enough sleep? Who is sharing in the work of caring for the baby? How is she feeling in herself? Is she feeling depressed? How is she getting along with her partner (if she has one)? Is she getting any time away from the baby?
* Ask about pain in her breasts, back, perineum.
* Ask about urinary and faecal incontinence, haemorrhoids, constipation.
* Ask about sex. Around 90% of women will report having sex by 10 weeks postpartum, while 2% report not attempting sex by 1 year (Glazener 1997). An explanation that libido is often low in the first year may relieve a couple who are finding that this is the case.
* Perform a vaginal examination only if symptoms dictate or if a smear is due (Noble 1993).
* Offer contraceptive advice.
* *Prevention of sudden infant death syndrome.* Reinforce the importance of:
  (a) the sleeping position (see page 82);
  (b) not smoking;
  (c) not giving the baby a duvet.

BREASTFEEDING

Advantages of breastfeeding

● *Advantages for the baby:* less infection, less chance of atopy or diabetes, better bonding.
● *Advantages for the mother:* a lower risk of breast and ovarian cancer, weight loss, and less postpartum bleeding. It is also cheaper.

Problems with breastfeeding

The majority of problems centre round the infant's attempts to remove milk. The baby needs to be in a comfortable position in order to allow jaw and tongue to drain the milk ducts under the areola.

* Check that mother and baby are managing the following:
  (a) the baby's chest against the mother's chest, with the baby's chin to the breast;
  (b) the mouth wide open;
  (c) both lips curled back;
  (d) the lower lip at the junction of the areola and breast;
  (e) rhythmical movements of jaw muscles.

PATIENT INFORMATION

Successful Breast Feeding, published by the Royal College of Midwives, 15 Mansfield Street, London W1M OBE

The following documents give advice for women about breast-feeding:

http://www.addenbrookes.org.uk/docs/cp/wo/cpwo001_breastfeed_wellterm.pdf

http://www.dh.gov.uk/assetRoot/04/08/44/52/04084452.pdf

Failing lactation

* Suckling is the strongest stimulus. Ensure that the baby is suckling well (see above).
* Advise the mother to go to bed for 2 days with the baby, to feed on demand (mother and baby).
* In general drugs should not be used, but a short course of domperidone may restore prolactin secretion.

Sore nipples

GUIDANCE

The Breastfeeding Network. *Differential Diagnosis of Nipple Pain.* 2009. Available: www.breastfeedingnetwork.org.uk

These are usually due to the baby's tongue rubbing the nipple rather than the areola.

* Check that the nipple is positioned in an upwards direction towards the roof of the baby's mouth.

* Allow breast milk to dry on the nipple when not feeding, or, if the skin is broken, use white soft paraffin.

Skin infection

This may be due to candida infection and may present as localized soreness, as pain around the areola and nipple, or as pain in the breast after a feed.

* Treat the mother with miconazole cream and the baby with miconazole oral gel, whether the baby has signs of infection or not. It is unnecessary for the mother to remove the cream before feeding.

* Consider using oral fluconazole if local treatment alone is not working. This use is not licensed but WHO recognizes fluconazole as compatible with breastfeeding. Download the above leaflet for guidance on dosing. The unlicensed use must be discussed with the mother and documented.

Blocked duct

This presents as a hard lump anywhere in the breast.

* Get the mother to massage the breast while feeding the baby from that breast.

* The baby's position should be altered so that the lower lip is nearer the blocked duct.

Breast engorgement

The pain of engorgement is one of the commonest reasons for stopping breastfeeding in the first 2 weeks. Treatment is disappointing with cabbage leaves, ultrasound and cold packs being no better than placebo (Snowden, Renfrew and Woolridge 2001).

* Give simple analgesia and support.

* Attempt to prevent engorgement by removing any obstacles to easy breastfeeding.

Mastitis

Early mastitis is inflammatory, not infectious, and may respond to effective emptying of the breast plus an NSAID (Thomsen, Espersen, Maigaards, *et al.* 1984).

* Reassess the feeding position of the baby to ensure that milk is removed completely.

* Prescribe an NSAID.

* Treat with flucloxacillin for 10–14 days if the patient is unwell, febrile or there is any suspicion of abscess formation. Use erythromycin if the patient is allergic to penicillin. Warn mothers that the milk will change in taste and feeding may be harder initially, or that the baby may develop diarrhoea and need to feed more frequently.

* *Breast abscess.* If an abscess forms which is large enough to need draining, admit the patient for incision and drainage.

Suppression of lactation

This usually takes 4–5 days after stopping breastfeeding. It may be very painful and require analgesia and a supportive bra. It is usually not necessary to use drugs. However, after stillbirth, or if there is another good reason to stop lactation, use bromocriptine 2.5 mg at night for 2 nights then 2.5 mg b.d. for 3 weeks. If used for a shorter period, a number of patients relapse.

VAGINAL BLEEDING AFTER 24 HOURS

● The traditional management of excessive bleeding more than 24 hours after delivery (secondary PPH) is surgical. However, ERPC yields placental tissue in less than 30% of these cases, and so the majority of patients do not benefit.

* *Mild bleeding.* Give:

(a) ergometrine 0.5 mg i.m. then 0.5 mg t.d.s. orally for 4 days; and

(b) antibiotics, e.g. amoxicillin/erythromycin ± metronidazole for 5 days.

* *Severe bleeding*, or if the os still admits one finger after 7 days: admit. Admit more readily if there is no one at home to look after the patient, if she is already anaemic, febrile or otherwise unwell (DTB 1992).

FEVER

✴ *Endometritis.* Patients with fever, pain and foul-smelling lochia are likely to need admission, but early cases could be treated at home with amoxicillin/erythromycin and metronidazole (see page 402).

✴ Be aware that DVT and UTI can cause fever without localized symptoms.

DEPRESSION

For details of the diagnosis of postnatal depression see *Evidence-based Diagnosis in Primary Care* by A. F. Polmear (editor), published by Butterworth-Heinemann, 2008.

● Depression after birth is experienced by one in seven women in the year after childbirth. It is distinct from the transient 'blues' of the first 10 days, and from a puerperal psychosis, which is likely to need admission.

● The issue of antenatal screening for postnatal depression remains controversial. At present the evidence does not support routine screening and no screening tool can be recommended for use during routine antenatal care (Austin and Lumley 2003).

● There is a lack of robust evidence to support unequivocally the use of routine postnatal screening for depression and the recommendations of guideline groups differ. SIGN notes that, while evidence is lacking, many screening programmes have been implemented to screen for depression at 6 weeks and 3 months postpartum (SIGN 2002). The Edinburgh Postnatal Depression Scale (EPDS) (Cox, Holden and Sagovsky 1987) may be administered by a trained professional (see Appendix 20) as part of that screening process, but with the understanding that it is a screening, not a diagnostic, tool. Clinical assessment is needed to establish the diagnosis. Between 30% and 70% of women who screen positive with the EPDS are not depressed (Oates 2003). The UK National Screening Committee puts the point more strongly, recommending it as a checklist, not a screening tool, which may be used as part of the assessment of a woman's mood (National Screening Committee UK 2004).

Factors associated with developing depression in the year after childbirth are:

(a) perceived lack of social, emotional and practical support, particularly from a partner (Astbury, Brown, Lumley and Small 1994; Paykel, Emms, Fletcher, *et al.* 1980; Kumar and Robson 1984;

(b) physical health problems (Brown and Lumley 1998);

(c) exhaustion (Small, Brown, Lumley and Astbury 1994);

(d) infant factors: unsettled/ 'difficult' babies (Miller, Barr and Eaton 1993; Murray, Stanley, Hooper, *et al.* 1996);

(e) negative life events (Paykel, Emms, Fletcher, *et al.* 1980; Small, Brown, Lumley, Astbury 1994; O'Hara 1986);

(f) a previous psychiatric history, although this will only account for a small number of the women who experience depression (Watson, Elliot, Rugg and Brough 1984).

There is little or no evidence of any direct association between depression after birth and hormonal factors (Kendell 1985; Adler, Cook, Davidson, *et al.* 1986; O'Hara, Schlechte, Lewis, *et al.* 1991). There have been inconclusive findings about the link between type of delivery and socioeconomic status and the development of depression (Astbury, Brown, Lumley and Small 1994; Paykel, Emms, Fletcher, *et al.* 1980; Watson, Elliot, Rugg and Brough 1984).

✴ During the postnatal visit every woman should have the opportunity to speak about how she is feeling and how she is coping with the transition to motherhood. Some simple questions that may assist women to talk about how they are really feeling are (Gunn, Southern, Chondros, *et al.* 2003):

(a) How are you feeling?

(b) How are you sleeping?

(c) How is your relationship going?

(d) Who is sharing in the work of caring for the baby?

(e) How much time do you get to yourself?

(f) How do you find being a mother?

Management of postnatal depression

● Antenatal and postnatal interventions offered routinely to all women in an effort to prevent postnatal depression have been ineffective (Lumley, Austin and Mitchell 2004) apart from the IMPACT programme consisting of a re-designed community midwifery model of care (MacArthur, Winter, Bick, *et al.* 2002).

- Antenatal and postnatal interventions offered only to those women perceived to be at a higher risk of developing depression have been ineffective (Lumley, Austin and Mitchell 2004).
- Interventions offered to women identified as experiencing depression have been effective and there is strong evidence that postnatal counselling (from active listening to cognitive behavioural therapy) will reduce depression with a number needed to treat of two to three (Lumley, Austin and Mitchell 2004). Simple nondirective counselling by health visitors, weekly for 8 weeks, doubles the recovery rate (Holden, Sagovsky, Cox, *et al.* 1989).

* Check for physical health problems – women experiencing the common postnatal physical problems are more likely to be depressed. Ask about:
  - tiredness. Consider checking Hb and ferritin, and TFTs (see page 396);
  - backache;
  - sexual problems;
  - perineal pain;
  - mastitis and feeding problems;
  - urinary and faecal incontinence;
  - constipation and haemorrhoids.

* *Offer counselling/psychotherapy.* Cognitive behavioural therapy is as effective as fluoxetine in reducing postnatal depression. The choice of treatment can be made by the woman herself (Appleby, Warner, Whitton and Faragher 1997).

* *Offer an antidepressant* to the 3–5% of women whose depression is moderate or severe (Oates 2003) and for whom an effective form of counselling/psychotherapy is not immediately available, or who chooses an antidepressant. An SSRI is recommended. If she is breastfeeding the choice is between an SSRI which is present in breast milk at low levels, e.g. sertraline but not fluoxetine or citalopram, or a TCA, which, with the exception of doxepin, appear safe in lactation (Spigset and Martensson 1999). Prescribing antidepressants for a lactating woman is a case-specific, risk-benefit decision (Wisner, Perel and Findling 1996).

* Consider referral if a multidisciplinary mental health team is able to offer more than the primary health care team. Ideally, if the woman requires admission, this should be to a mother and baby facility.

* Refer urgently, to be seen within 24 hours, any woman with ideas of suicide or of harming the baby.

EXHAUSTION

Around 70% of women will experience extreme tiredness and exhaustion in the 6 months after giving birth (Watson, Elliot, Rugg and Brough 1984). Tiredness is common, even among women who are not depressed. It is uncommon to find a specific cause – but anaemia, iron deficiency and thyroid problems should be considered. Lack of sleep is one of the commonest causes. Taking note of the baby's sleep patterns, excluding depression, offering time to talk, encouraging time-out from childcare and encouraging sharing the work of looking after the baby are all simple support strategies.

COMMON PHYSICAL PROBLEMS

Physical problems are common: around 44% of women will experience backache, 26% sexual problems (see page 401), 21% haemorrhoids, 21% perineal pain, 17% mastitis (see page 402), 13% bowel problems 11% urinary incontinence 6%; faecal incontinence (Brown and Lumley 1998; MacArthur, Bick and Keighley 1997).

Unfortunately, there is little evidence to guide our management of postpartum incontinence or perineal pain. Three quarters of women with urinary incontinence at 3 months postpartum still had the problem 6 years later, despite conservative nurse-led pelvic floor and bladder training management of urinary and faecal incontinence (Glazener, Herbison, MacArthur, *et al.* 2005).

NEONATAL JAUNDICE

* *Jaundice within 24 hours of birth:* admit.
* *Deep jaundice developing after 24 hours:*

(a) admit if the baby is unwell or is at risk because of prematurity, small for dates or birth asphyxia;

(b) otherwise, arrange for a serum bilirubin. If the level is 290 mol/l or above, discuss with the paediatric team.

* *Jaundice still present at 2 weeks:* test the urine for bilirubin and the serum for conjugated bilirubin. If either is positive, admit. The baby may have biliary atresia. The earlier surgery is performed, the more successful it is likely to be (Mackinlay 1993).

* *Admit if jaundice is associated with any of the following:*

(a) pale fatty stools;

(b) dark yellow urine;

(c) failure to thrive;

(d) poor feeding;

(e) a tendency to bleed or bruise;

(f) an enlarged liver or spleen, or ascites.

References

Adler, E., Cook, M., Davidson, D., et al., 1986. Hormones, mood and sexuality in lactating women. Br. J. Psych. 148, 74–79.

Appleby, L., Warner, R., Whitton, A., Faragher, B., 1997. A controlled study of fluoxetine and cognitive-behavioural counselling in the treatment of postnatal depression. Br. Med. J. 314, 932–936.

Askie, L.M., Duley, L., Henderson-Smart, D.J., et al., 2007. Antiplatelet agents for prevention of pre-eclampsia: a meta-analysis of individual patient data. Lancet 369, 1791–1798.

Astbury, J., Brown, S., Lumley, J., Small, R., 1994. Birth events, birth experiences and social differences in postnatal depression. Aust. J. Public Health 18 (2), 176–184.

Austin, M.P., Lumley, J., 2003. Antenatal screening for postnatal depression: a systematic review. Acta Psychiatr. Scand. 107, 10–17.

Bech, B.H., Obel, C., Henriksen, T.B., et al., 2007. Effect of reducing caffeine intake on birth weight and length of gestation: randomised controlled trial. BMJ 334, 409–412.

Best, J.B., O'Shea, S., Tipples, G., et al., 2002. Interpretation of rubella serology in pregnancy – pitfalls and problems. BMJ 325, 147–148.

Best, J.M., Banatuala, J.E., Morgan-Capner, P., et al., 1989. Fetal infection after maternal reinfection with rubella: criteria for defining reinfection. BMJ 299, 773–775.

Bracken, M.B., Triche, E.W., Belanger, K., et al., 2003. Asthma symptoms, severity, and drug therapy: a prospective study of effects on 2205 pregnancies. Obstet. Gynecol. 102, 739–752.

Braig, S., Luton, D., Sibony, O., et al., 2001. Acyclovir prophylaxis in late pregnancy prevents recurrence of genital herpes and viral shedding. Eur. J. Obstet. Gynecol. Reprod. Biol. 96, 55–58.

Brocklehurst, P., 2000. Interventions aimed at decreasing the risk of mother-to-child transmission of HIV infection. Cochrane. Database. Syst. Rev. Available: www.nelh.nhs.uk/cochrane.asp.

Brown, S., Lumley, J., 1998. Maternal health after childbirth: results of an Australian population based survey. Br. J. Obstet. Gynaecol. 105, 156–161.

Cedergren, M.I., 2007. Optimal gestational weight gain for body mass index categories. Obstet. Gynecol. 110, 759–776.

Chappell, L.C., Seed, P.T., Briley, A.L., et al., 1999. Effect of anti-oxidants on the occurrence of pre-eclampsia in women at increased risk: a randomised trial. Lancet 354, 810–816.

Chappell, L.C., Shennan, A.H., 2008. Assessment of proteinuria in pregnancy. BMJ 336, 968–969.

Connor, E.M., Sperling, R.S., Gelber, R., et al., 1994. Reduction of maternal–infant transmission of human immunodeficiency virus type 1 with zidovudine treatment. N. Engl. J. Med. 331, 1173–1180.

Cox, J.L., Holden, J.M., Sagovsky, R., 1987. Detection of postnatal depression. Br. J. Psychiatry. 150, 782–786.

Crowley, P., 2002. Interventions for preventing or improving the outcome of delivery at or beyond term (Cochrane Review). In: The Cochrane Library. Update Software, Oxford Issue 1. Available: www.nelh.nhs.uk/cochrane.asp.

Crowther, C.A., Hiller, J.E., Moss, J.R., et al., 2005. Effect of treatment of gestational diabetes mellitus on pregnancy outcomes. N. Engl. J. Med. 352, 2477–2486.

Davies, J., Hey, E., Reed, W., et al., 1996. Prospective regional study of planned home births. BMJ 313, 1302–1306.

Department of Health, 1991. Report on Confidential Enquiries into Maternal Deaths in the UK 1988–90. HMSO.

Douglas, K.A., Redman, C.W.G., 1994. Eclampsia in the United Kingdom. BMJ 309, 1395–1400.

DTB, 1992. The management of postpartum haemorrhage. Drug Ther. Bull. 30, 89–92.

DTB, 1994a. Epilepsy and pregnancy. Drug Ther. Bull. 32, 49–51.

DTB, 1994b. Folic acid to prevent neural tube defects. Drug Ther. Bull. 32, 31–32.

DTB, 1995. The practical management of thyroid disease in pregnancy. Drug Ther. Bull. 33, 75–77.

Everett, C., 1997. Incidence and outcome of bleeding before the 20th week of pregnancy: prospective study from general practice. BMJ 315, 32–34.

Everett, C.B., Preece, E., 1996. Women with bleeding in the first 20 weeks of pregnancy: value of general practice ultrasound in detecting fetal heart movement. Br. J. Gen. Pract. 46, 7–9.

Fairgrieve, S., Jackson, M., Jonas, P., et al., 2000. Population based, prospective study of the care of women with epilepsy in pregnancy. BMJ 321, 674–675.

Fergusson, C.B., Mahsu-Dornan, S., Patterson, R.N., 2008. Inflammatory disease in pregnancy. BMJ 337, 170–173.

Friedman, T., 1989. Women's experiences of general practitioners' management of miscarriage. J. R. Coll. Gen. Pract. 39, 456–458.

Girling, J.C., de Swiet, M., 1992. Thyroxine doses during pregnancy in women with primary hypothyroidism. Br. J. Obstet. Gynaecol. 99, 368–370.

Glazener, C., Herbison, P., MacArthur, C., et al., 2005. Randomised controlled trial of conservative management of postnatal urinary and faecal incontinence: six year follow up. BMJ doi:10.1136/bmj.38320.613461.82.

Glazener, C., 1997. Sexual function after childbirth: woman's experiences, persistent morbidity and lack of professional recognition. Br. J. Obstet. Gynaecol. 104, 330–335.

GPC, 1999. The role of the GP involved in intrapartum care. BMA. Available: www.bma.org.uk; choose 'Committees' then 'GPC Guidance' then 'General Practitioners and maternity medical services'.

Gunn, J., Southern, D., Chondros, P., et al., 2003. Guidelines for assessing postnatal problems: introducing evidence based guidelines in Australian general practice. Fam. Pract. 20, 382–389.

Harris, R., Lane, B., Harris, H., et al., 1999. National confidential enquiry into counselling for genetic disorders by non-geneticists: general recommendations and specific standards for improving care. Br. J. Obstet. Gynaecol. 106, 658–663.

Head to Head, 2007. Is it all right for women to drink small amounts of alcohol in pregnancy? BMJ 335, 856–857.

Holden, J.M., Sagovsky, R., Cox, J.L., 1989. Counselling in a general practice setting: controlled study of health visitor intervention in treatment of postnatal depression. BMJ 298, 223–226.

Inskip, H.M., Crozier, S.R., Godfrey, K.M., et al., 2009. The Southampton Women's Survey Study Group. Women's compliance with nutrition and lifestyle recommendations before pregnancy: general population cohort study. BMJ 338, b481.

Jewell, D., Young, G., 2003. Interventions for nausea and vomiting in early pregnancy. Cochrane Database Syst. Rev. Issue 4, CD000145. DOI: 10.1002/14651858.CD000145.

Jones, G., 1990. Congenital rubella in Great Britain. Health Trends 22, 73–76.

Juarez-Vazquez, J., Bonizzoni, E., Scotti, A., 2002. Iron plus folate is more effective than iron alone in the treatment of iron deficiency anaemia in pregnancy: a randomised, double blind clinical trial. BJOG 109, 1009–1014.

Kendell, R., 1985. Emotional and physical factors in the genesis of puerperal mental disorders. J. Psychosom. Res. 29, 3–11.

Kumar, R., Robson, K., 1984. A prospective study of emotional disorders in childbearing women. Br. J. Psych. 144, 35–47.

Larson, J.D., Patatanian, E., Miner Jr., P.B., et al., 1997. Double-blind, placebo-controlled study of ranitidine for gastroesophageal reflux symptoms during pregnancy. Obstet. Gynecol. 90, 83–87.

Lilford, R.J., 1991. The rise and fall of chorionic villus sampling. BMJ 303, 936–937.

Luise, C., Jermy, K., May, C., et al., 2002. Outcome of expectant management of spontaneous first trimester miscarriage: observational study. BMJ 324, 873–875.

Lumley, J., Austin, M.P., Mitchell, C., 2004. Intervening to reduce depression after birth: a systematic review of the randomized trials. Int. J. Tech. Assess. Health Care 20, 128–144.

MacArthur, C., Bick, D., Keighley, M.R., 1997. Faecal incontinence after childbirth. Br. J. Obstet. Gynaecol. 104, 46–50.

MacArthur, C., Winter, H., Bick, D., et al., 2002. Effects of redesigned community postnatal care on women's health 4 months after birth: a cluster randomised trial. Lancet 359, 378–385.

MacGillivray, I., Thomas, P., 1991. Recording diastolic blood pressure in pregnancy (letter). BMJ 302, 179.

Mackinlay, G.A., 1993. Jaundice persisting beyond 14 days after birth. BMJ 306, 1426–1427.

Magee, L.A., 2007. Pre-eclampsia and increased cardiovascular risk. BMJ 335, 945–946.

Martel, M.J., Rey, E., Beauchesne, M.F., et al., 2005. Use of inhaled corticosteroids during pregnancy and risk of pregnancy induced hypertension: nested case-control study. BMJ 330, 230.

Marx, H., Amin, P., Lazarus, J.H., 2008. Hyperthyroidism and pregnancy. BMJ 336, 663–667.

Milkiewicz, P., Elias, E., Williamson, C., et al., 2002. Obstetric cholestasis. BMJ 324, 123–124.

Miller, A., Barr, R., Eaton, W.O., 1993. Crying and motor behaviour of six-week-old infants and postpartum maternal mood. Paediatrics 92 (4), 551–558.

Milne, F., Redman, C., Walker, J., et al., 2005. Pre-eclampsia community guideline (PRECOG): how to screen for and detect onset of pre eclampsia in the community. BMJ 330, 576–580.

Morgan-Capner, P., Crowcroft, N.S., 2002. On behalf of the PHLS Joint Working Party of the Advisory Committees of Virology and Vaccines and Immunisation Guidelines on the management of, and exposure to, rash illness in pregnancy (including consideration of relevant antibody screening programmes in pregnancy). Available: www.hpa.org.uk.

Murray, L., Stanley, C., Hooper, R., et al., 1996. The role of infant factors in postnatal depression and mother-infant interactions. Dev. Med. Child Neurol. 38, 109–119.

Nachum, Z., Ben-Shlomo, I., Weiner, E., et al., 1999. Twice daily versus four times daily insulin dose regimens for diabetes in pregnancy: randomised controlled trial. BMJ 319, 1223–1227.

National Screening Committee UK, 2004. Postnatal depression. Available: www.nsc.nhs.uk choose 'National electronic Library for Screening' then search on 'Postnatal'.

NICE, 2002. Guidance on the use of routine antenatal anti-D prophylaxis for RhD-negative women. NICE May. Available: www.nice.org.uk.

NICE, 2007. Antenatal and postnatal mental health: clinical management and service guidance. Clinical Guideline 45. Available: www.nice.org.uk.

Nielsen, S., Hahlin, M., 1995. Expectant management of first-trimester spontaneous abortion. Lancet 345, 84–86.

Nikfar, S., Abdollahi, M., Moretti, M.E., et al., 2002. Use of proton pump inhibitors during pregnancy and rates of major malformations: a meta-analysis. Dig. Dis. Sci. 47, 1526–1529.

Noble, T., 1993. The routine 6-week vaginal examination. BMJ 307, 698.

Northern Region Perinatal Mortality Survey Co-ordinating Group, 1996. Collaborative survey of perinatal loss in planned and unplanned home births. BMJ 313, 1306–1309.

O'Brien, M.D., Gilmour-White, S., 1993. Epilepsy and pregnancy. BMJ 307, 492–495.

Oates, M., 2003. Postnatal depression and screening: too broad a sweep? Br. J. Gen. Pract. 53, 596–597.

O'Hara, M., 1986. Social support, life events, and depression during pregnancy and the puerperium. Arch. Gen. Psychiatry 43, 569–573.

O'Hara, M., Schlechte, W., Lewis, D.A., et al., 1991. Prospective study of postpartum blues: biologic and psychosocial factors. Arch. Gen. Psychiatry 48, 801–806.

Olesen, C., Steffensen, F.H., Nielsen, G.L., et al., 1999. Drug use in first pregnancy and lactation: a population-based survey among Danish women. The EUROMAP group. Eur. J. Clin. Pharmacol. 55, 139–144.

Paykel, E.S., Emms, E.M., Fletcher, J., et al., 1980. Life events and social support in puerperal depression. Br. J. Psychiatry 136, 339–346.

Regan, L., Braude, P.R., Trembath, P.L., et al., 1989. Influence of past reproductive performance on risk of spontaneous abortion. BMJ 299, 541–545.

Robinson, R., 1991. Surveying rare diseases of childhood. BMJ 303, 1091.

Royal College of Obstetricians and Gynaecologists, 2001. Chickenpox in Pregnancy. Clinical Green Top Guideline No. 13. Online. Available: www.rcog.org.uk (choose 'Good practice' then 'Clinical green top guidelines').

Royal College of Obstetricians and Gynaecologists, 2003a. Prevention of early onset neonatal Group B streptococcal disease. Clinical Green Top Guideline No. 36. Available: www.rcog.org.uk (choose 'good practice' then 'clinical green top guidelines').

Royal College of Obstetricians and Gynaecologists, 2003b. Management of genital herpes in pregnancy. Clinical Green Top Guideline No. 30. Available: www.rcog.org.uk (choose 'Good practice' then 'Clinical green top guidelines').

Rush, D., 1994. Periconceptional folate and neural tube defect. Am. J. Clin. Nutr. 59 (Suppl. 2), 511S–515S.

SIGN, 2002. Postnatal depression and puerperal psychosis. Scottish Intercollegiate Guidelines Network. Available: www.sign.ac.uk.

Sikorski, J., Wilson, J., Clement, S., et al., 1996. A randomised controlled trial comparing two schedules of antenatal visits: the antenatal care project. BMJ 312, 546–553.

Silverberg, M.J., Thorsen, P., Lindeberg, H., et al., 2003. Condyloma in pregnancy is strongly predictive of juvenile-onset recurrent respiratory papillomatosis. Obstet. Gynaecol. 101, 645–652.

Smaill, F., 2001. Antibiotics for asymptomatic bacteriuria in pregnancy (Cochrane Review). In: The Cochrane Library. Update Software, Oxford Issue 4 Available: www.nelh.nhs.uk/cochrane.asp.

Small, R., Brown, S., Lumley, J., Astbury, J., 1994. Missing voices:

what women say and do about depression after childbirth. J. Reprod. Infant. Psychol. 12, 89–103.

Snowden, H.M., Renfrew, M.J., Woolridge, M.W., 2001. Treatments for breast engorgement during lactation (Cochrane Review). In: The Cochrane Library. Update Software, Oxford Issue 4. Available: www.nelh.nhs.uk/cochrane.asp.

Spigset, O., Martensson, B., 1999. Fortnightly review: drug treatment of depression. BMJ 318, 1188–1191.

Steel, J.M., Johnstone, F.D., Hepburn, D.A., et al., 1990. Can pre-pregnancy care of diabetic women reduce the risk of abnormal babies? BMJ 301, 1070–1074.

Stotland, N.E., 2009. Obesity and pregnancy. BMJ 338, 107–110.

Thomsen, A.C., Espersen, T., Maigaards, S., et al., 1984. Course and treatment of milk stasis, noninfectious inflammation of the breast, and infectious mastitis in nursing women. Am. J. Obstet. Gynecol. 149, 492–495.

Three Centres Consensus Guidelines on Antenatal Care Project, 2001. Melbourne: Mercy Hospital for Women, Southern Health. Women's and Children's Health, Melbourne, Australia.

Trinder, J., Brocklehurst, P., Porter, R., et al., 2006. Management of miscarriage: expectant, medical or surgical? Results of randomised control trial. BMJ 332, 1235–1238.

Villar, J., Carroli, G., Khan-Neelofur, D., et al., 2001. Patterns of antenatal care for low-risk pregnancy (Cochrane Review). In: The Cochrane Library. Update Software, Oxford Issue 4. Available: www.nelh.nhs.uk/cochrane.asp.

Ward, V.B., 2008. Eating disorders in pregnancy. BMJ 336, 96.

Watson, J., Elliot, S., Rugg, A.J., Brough, D., 1984. Psychiatric disorder in pregnancy and the first postnatal year. Br. J. Psychiatry 144, 453–462.

Weng, X., Odouli, R., Li, D.K., 2008. Maternal caffeine consumption during pregnancy and the risk of miscarriage: a prospective cohort study. Am. J. Obstet. Gynecol. 279, e1–e8.

Wieringa-de Waard, M., Ankum, W.M., Bonsel, G.J., et al., 2003. The natural course of spontaneous miscarriage: analysis of signs and symptoms in 188 expectantly managed women. Br. J. Gen. Pract. 53, 704–708.

Wieringa-de Waard, M., Bonsel, G.J., Ankum, W.M., et al., 2002. Threatened miscarriage in general practice: diagnostic value of history taking and physical examination. Br. J. Gen. Pract. 52, 825–829.

Wisborg, K., Kesmodel, U., Bech, B.H., et al., 2003. Maternal consumption of coffee during pregnancy and stillbirth and infant death in first year of life: prospective study. BMJ 326, 420–422.

Wisner, K., Perel, J., Findling, R.L., 1996. Antidepressant treatment during breast-feeding. Am. J. Psychiatry 153, 1132–1137.

Wong, M.K.Y., Crawford, T.J., Gask, L., et al., 2003. A qualitative investigation into women's experiences after a miscarriage: implications for a primary healthcare team. Br. J. Gen. Pract. 53, 697–702.

Chapter 14

Urinary problems

CHAPTER CONTENTS

© 2011 Elsevier Ltd.
DOI: 10.1016/B978-0-7020-3053-6.00014-3

URINARY TRACT INFECTIONS

UNCOMPLICATED LOWER URINARY TRACT INFECTION IN NON-PREGNANT WOMEN OF CHILD-BEARING AGE

For details of the diagnosis of dysuria in women
see *Evidence-based Diagnosis in Primary Care* by
A. F. Polmear (editor), published by Butterworth-
Heinemann, 2008.

REVIEWS

Hummer-Pradier E, Kochen MM. 2002. Urinary tract
infections in adult general practice patients. Br J Gen
Pract 52, 752–761
   Bowler I. 2003. Diagnosis and treatment of urinary
tract infections in general practice. Trends Urol,
Gynaecol Sexual Health April, 33–35

Guidelines
*Diagnosis of Urinary Tract Infection- Quick Reference
Guide.* Health Protection Agency. http://www.hpa.org.
uk/infections/topics_az/primary_care_guidance/
uti_guide_290404.rtf

SIGN. 2006. Clinical Guideline 88: *Management of Suspected Bacterial Urinary Tract Infection in Adults.* http://www.sign.ac.uk/guidelines/fulltext/88/index.html

CYSTITIS / UNCOMPLICATED LOWER URINARY TRACT INFECTION

- Half of women who present with frequency and dysuria do not have bacterial infection (Hamilton-Miller 1994). Half of those with bacterial infections resolve within 3 days without antibiotics (Brumfitt and Hamilton-Miller 1994). The key to management is in distinguishing an uncomplicated from a complicated UTI (acute pyelonephritis, unusual organism, structural predisposition, refractory, recurrent, or systemic symptoms) and in avoiding unnecessary antibiotics in those without infection or in the elderly with asymptomatic bacteriuria.

- The management of uncomplicated lower UTI in women can be as effective *over the telephone* as if the patients are seen in person (Barry, Hickner, Ebell, *et al.* 2001), although this must be done with caution, given GMC advice on prescribing antibiotics in this manner. A strong history of typical cystitis symptoms is sufficient to diagnose a UTI, but where there is doubt or if the symptoms are refractory or relapse then it is better to do a urine dipstick test and consider the need for an MSU.

  - If *positive for nitrites and/or leucocytes*, assume that this is infection and treat with antibiotics without sending an MSU. Where positive for leucocytes but not nitrites, remember that the symptoms may represent 'urethral syndrome' (see below).

  - If *positive for protein and/or blood only*, then consider the diagnosis and differentials further.

  - If *negative for all four tests*, send an MSU for microscopy and culture without starting antibiotics. 95% will have a negative MSU and do not require antibiotics at this stage (MeReC Bulletin 1995). 'Urethral syndrome' is still possible with these results.

- ✳ *If treating, give antibiotics for 3 days.* This is as effective as a 7-day course (Brumfitt and Hamilton-Miller 1994; Christiaens, De Meyere, Verschraegen, *et al.* 2002). Seven days are,

however, appropriate when treating the elderly, men, children, and catheterized patients, and 10 days for pregnant women. A single dose is less effective than a three day course but may be justified when compliance is likely to be a problem. For the 3-day course use trimethoprim 200 mg BD, although resistance can be above 25% in some areas. Most infections respond even if reported as resistant *in vitro*, as the urine concentration of the drug exceeds that of the sensitivity disk (MeReC Bulletin 1995). Alternatives are nitrofurantoin 50 mg q.d.s. where renal function is normal, and cefalexin 250 mg q.d.s.–500 mg t.d.s. (Christiaens, De Meyere, Verschraegen, *et al.* 2002). Co-amoxiclav should only be used when there are grounds to suspect resistant organisms (Committee for Safety of Medicines 1997). Reserve quinolones for complicated infections such as acute pyelonephritis (Baerheim 2001).

- ✳ Patients with resistant organisms may need a change of antibiotics. Women who are infected with unusual organisms (e.g. *Proteus* or *Pseudomonas*) need a repeat MSU and further investigation if still present.

- ✳ Explain to the patient that symptoms should clear within 7 days (i.e. may persist after the 3 days of antibiotics). Advise the patient to return if symptoms are still severe after 3 days or persist after 7 days.

- ✳ *Prevention*. In women with recurrent infection offer self-help advice, below. Cranberry juice has variable evidence available (Stothers 2002; Kontiokari, Sundqvist, Nuutinen, *et al.* 2001; Jepson, Mihaljevic and Craig 2004).

WHICH MSU RESULTS ARE ABNORMAL?

Bacterial counts of 10^5/ml are 'significant' and reported on MSU results, but lower counts may be found with organisms that are difficult to culture (e.g. *Staphylococcus saprophyticus*, *Chlamydia*, *Gardnerella*). Counts of 10^3 and 10^4/ml should be repeated if the symptoms suggest infection. Organisms without cells can be ignored, except in pregnant women and young children. Cells without organisms need further investigation, unless the MSU was taken after antibiotics had been started. Repeat the MSU and refer if cells are still present. Females aged > 40 years old with a refractory UTI with haematuria or recurrent UTIs with haematuria need a referral to a urologist.

Recurrence of symptoms

* Repeat the MSU, or do one for the first time, and assess whether the patient is suffering from:
  (a) relapse – the organism is the same;
  (b) re-infection – a different organism is present; or
  (c) the urethral syndrome, see below.

Relapse

* Treat, with an antibiotic to which the original organism was sensitive, for 7 days.
* Look for a reason for the failure to clear the original infection. Consider stones and chronic retention. Repeat the dipstick test for protein and haematuria.

Re-infection(s)

* Consider using a different antibiotic; the new organisms are likely to be resistant to the one originally used.

Frequent re-infection

* *Investigations.* After more than three infections in a short period of time, consider an ultrasound scan, an abdominal X-ray of the urinary tract, and urea, electrolytes and creatinine, to rule out underlying abnormalities. If normal, there is no need for specialist referral, but consider prophylaxis.
* *Prophylaxis.* Consider low-dose prophylaxis in those with at least four attacks per year. Use nitrofurantoin 100 mg at night or trimethoprim 100 mg at night for 6 months in the first instance. They will more than halve the number of attacks (NNT 1.85 to prevent one recurrence) (Albert, Huertas, Pereiro, *et al.* 2004). If an infection occurs while on prophylaxis, use a different drug as treatment. The use of cranberry juice has gained some evidence since an inconclusive 2004 Cochrane Review, but only for reducing the risk of recurrent UTIs (Stothers 2002; Kontiokari T, Sundqvist K, Nuutinen M, *et al.* 2001) in those women using tablets twice daily or drinking juice thrice daily for 12 months, and not for treating an acute UTI (Jepson, Mihaljevic and Craig 2004). The NNT to reduce the risk of a further symptomatic UTI in those 12 months was 5–8 (Stothers 2002; Kontiokari T, Sundqvist K, Nuutinen M, *et al.* 2001).

Infections occurring after intercourse

* Advise emptying the bladder after intercourse.

* Give a single dose of antibiotics to be taken within 2 hours of intercourse, e.g. trimethoprim 200 mg or nitrofurantoin 50 mg, or, as third line, a quinolone (Albert, Huertas, Pereiro, *et al.* 2004).

Asymptomatic bacteriuria

* Asymptomatic bacteriuria in the elderly requires no treatment (SIGN clinical guideline 88 (2006) referenced above), but does in pregnancy.

SELF-HELP

Recommend that patients:
(a) increase fluids;
(b) increase the frequency of micturition (practise double voiding, i.e. attempting to pass urine a second time immediately after the first);
(c) empty the bladder before sleep and after sexual intercourse;
(d) wear loose-fitting cotton underwear and avoid tights;
(e) avoid external sanitary towels;
(f) make sure a diaphragm, if worn, fits comfortably (or change contraceptive method);
(g) use a lubricant, e.g. K-Y jelly, if vaginal dryness makes intercourse painful;
(h) wipe from front to back (should be routine) and wash the vulva with soapy water;
(i) consider drinking cranberry juice or taking cranberry juice tablets daily in evidence-based quantity (Stothers 2002; Kontiokari T, Sundqvist K, Nuutinen M, *et al.* 2001).

URETHRAL SYNDROME

The diagnosis will have been made on the basis of repeated attacks of frequency and dysuria with repeatedly sterile MSUs.

* Examine to exclude:
  (a) vaginal infection, especially candida, chlamydia, trichomonas, gardnerella or gonorrhoea;
  (b) urethral herpes or warts;
  (c) significant anterior prolapse;
  (d) atrophic vaginitis.
* Arrange 3-monthly MSUs to exclude intermittent infection. Ask for counts as low as 10^2 to be reported.

* Ask the patient to keep a diary of input, output and symptoms for 1 week, and consider managing as for detrusor instability (see Urge incontinence, below).
* *Self-help*. Patients should:
  (a) alkalinize the urine, e.g. with potassium citrate mixture;
  (b) avoid coloured toilet paper, scented soaps, bubble baths, douches, antiseptics, talcum powder, vaginal deodorants and deodorised tampons;
  (c) ensure that sexual intercourse is not traumatic because, for instance, of lack of lubrication.
* Do not treat with antibiotics, as overgrowth with lactobaccilli and candida may be encouraged (Anon. 1991).
* *If symptoms are disabling*, refer to a urologist.

LOWER URINARY TRACT INFECTION IN MEN

For details of the diagnosis of dysuria in men see *Evidence-based Diagnosis in Primary Care* by A. F. Polmear (editor), published by Butterworth-Heinemann, 2008.

Initial assessment and management

* Consider possible causes: prostate problems, congenital urinary tract problems, phimosis, previous urinary tract surgery, immunodeficiency, or anal intercourse.
* Examine: the abdomen (for a palpable bladder); the testes and epididymis to assess the extent of infection; the prostate; and the urethral meatus for discharge.
* Exclude diabetes with a fasting glucose.
* Arrange for an MSU before, and 7–14 days after finishing, antibiotics.
* Treat with antibiotics for 7 days in the first instance (trimethoprim, nitrofurantoin or cefalexin) and review the MSU results.
* If ill, admit.

Further management

* Investigate all men with a USS and an abdominal X-ray of the urinary tract. This has been shown to detect all pathology that would

have been detected on IVP as well as some that would have been missed (Andrews, Brooks and Hanbury 2002). If negative, referral is not necessary.
* If infection recurs, refer and consider low-dose prophylaxis until seen by a urologist.

Note: Most episodes of dysuria in young men will be due to urethritis. Consider referral to a GUM clinic.

ACUTE PROSTATITIS

* Send an MSU, plus urethral swabs if there is any suggestion of a sexually transmitted infection (see page 70).
* Start antibiotics, e.g. trimethoprim 200 mg b.d., ciprofloxacin 500 mg b.d., or erythromycin 500 mg q.d.s., all of which penetrate prostatic fluid well. Continue for 2 weeks in those that resolve promptly but 4–6 weeks in those that respond more slowly.
* Give analgesics, e.g. an NSAID for symptomatic relief.
* Admit patients who are ill or in whom rectal examination suggests a prostatic abscess.

CHRONIC PROSTATITIS

REVIEW

McNaughton Collins M, MacDonald R, Wilt T. 1999. Interventions for chronic abacterial prostatitis. Cochrane Database of Systematic Reviews, Issue 4. Accessed 2009. Available: www.nelh.nhs.uk/cochrane.asp

Guideline

Clinical Knowledge Summaries. *Prostatitis – chronic.* http://www.cks.nhs.uk/prostatitis_chronic#-367474

Only 5–10% of patients with this symptom complex (perineal pain, lower urinary tract symptoms, variable dipstick and MSU results) have bacterial infection.

* Establish the diagnosis: order microscopy and culture on the *first part of the stream of the first urine passed in the morning*. Threads of white cells suggest prostatitis. If negative, repeat it after prostatic massage, with the patient's consent.

* *If culture positive*: treat with doxycycline 200 mg o.d. or ciprofloxacin 500 mg b.d. for up to 12 weeks or until symptoms have completely settled, whichever is the longer, and only then if an MSU is clear. Repeat the MSU at 4 weeks and advise an early review if symptoms return. If a sexual infection was implicated, check that the partner been adequately assessed and treated.

* *If culture negative*: no treatment has been clearly shown to aid resolution (McNaughton Collins, MacDonald and Wilt 1999). Offer a trial of NSAIDs for symptomatic relief and referral to a urologist if symptoms are not resolving. The value of referral is to confirm the diagnosis and assist in explaining it to the patient.

LOWER URINARY TRACT INFECTION IN OTHER SITUATIONS

CHILDREN

See page 118.

PREGNANCY

All women are screened for bacteriuria at the first antenatal visit.

* Treat bacteriuria, whether or not symptoms are present, with cefalexin 500 mg t.d.s., or nitrofurantoin 50 mg q.d.s., both for 10 days.
* Repeat an MSU 7 days after completion of treatment, and then monthly until delivery.
* *Acute pyelonephritis:* admit.
* *Second UTI during pregnancy:* refer to an obstetrician.

POSTMENOPAUSAL WOMEN

> **REVIEW**
>
> Cardozo L. 1996. Post-menopausal cystitis. BMJ 313, 129.

Recurrent UTIs are common after the menopause, affecting more than 10% of women. This is in addition to symptoms due to urogenital atrophy. Treatment in the elderly with antibiotics should be for 7 days.

* *Oestrogen therapy.* Prescribe low-dose oestrogen therapy in those with no contraindications.

It has been shown to change the colonization of the vagina and decrease infections. Topical treatment may be sufficient.

* *Culture-negative 'cystitis'.* Organize a further culture if symptoms persist, asking specifically for *Ureaplasma urealyticum* and *Mycoplasma hominis*. Consider treating with tetracycline or erythromycin for 3 months, if present.
* Refer for urodynamic investigation women not responding to the above measures or unsuitable for oestrogen.
* *Interstitial cystitis.* Treatment is palliative and should be decided by the urologist. The options are:
  (a) oral therapy with, e.g., a tricyclic antidepressant; or
  (b) intravesicular with, e.g., dimethyl sulfoxide.

> **PATIENT SUPPORT**
>
> The Cystitis and Overactive Bladder Foundation, 76 High Street, Stony Stratford, Bucks MK11 1AH, tel. 01908 569169; www.cobfoundation.org

CATHETERIZED PATIENTS

● 90% of patients with an indwelling catheter have bacteriuria after 17 days (DTB 1998). Dipsticks are of little value when catheterized, and asymptomatic bacteriuria does not usually need treatment.

● Infection cannot be prevented by topical antimicrobials applied to the meatus, nor by irrigation with antimicrobials or antiseptics. The best defence against infection is to open the closed drainage system as infrequently as possible.

* *Give antibiotics* for 7 days only if the patient is clearly symptomatic, if the infection is systemic (i.e. the patient is febrile), or if the causative organism is *Proteus*. *Proteus* may give rise to triple-phosphate stones and is worth eradicating with antibiotics.
* *If giving antibiotics,* remove the catheter if the patient can manage without it for a few days. Insert a new one once the urine is sterile.
* Consider whether intermittent catheterization by the patient, or a suprapubic catheter, might be a better option.
* Wash the meatus daily with soap and water.

* Only give antibiotics prophylactically if they are needed to prevent endocarditis or if patients do badly with UTIs, e.g. many patients catheterized with multiple sclerosis.

ACUTE PYELONEPHRITIS

* Admit if too ill to take oral fluids, or if pregnant. Otherwise:
* Arrange an MSU.
* Prescribe a 7-day course of antibiotics, choosing one to give the widest antibacterial cover, e.g. ciprofloxacin 500 mg b.d., or co-amoxiclav 625 mg t.d.s. Give it for 2 weeks if there is an underlying structural abnormality.
* Consider the need for analgesics.
* Review the patient and the MSU result and confirm that the antibiotic was appropriate.
* Repeat the MSU 7 days after the antibiotics are finished.
* *Follow-up:* consider a USS and an abdominal X-ray of the urinary tract, see page 411.

URINARY INCONTINENCE

GUIDELINE

Scottish Intercollegiate Guidelines Network. 2004. *Management of Urinary Incontinence in Primary Care.* SIGN Guideline No. 79 December. http://www.sign.ac.uk/pdf/sign79.pdf

Reviews

Holroyd-Leduc JM, Straus SE. 2004. Management of urinary incontinence in women: scientific review. JAMA 291, 986–995. Comment in Evidence-Based Medicine 2004 9, 173 (analysis by Harper D).
   The National Prescribing Centre. 2000. Drug treatment of urinary incontinence in adults. MeReC Bulletin 11(3)

● Up to 20% of women and 10% of men living at home aged 65 suffer from incontinence, as do up to 7% of women aged 45 (MeReC 1997).
● Only a quarter of women with incontinence consult a doctor about it spontaneously (Burgio, Matthews and Engel 1991).

● It is possible to help 70% of patients with incontinence. A practice must decide either to offer a full assessment and management programme itself, or to refer patients to a continence adviser (Duckett 1996). The use of a nurse with only 3 weeks training can lead to improvement or cure in 68% of patients against 5% in controls (O'Brian and Long 1995). Referral times for continence advisers and physiotherapists can be long. District nurses, practice nurses and health visitors may also have (or can get) appropriate training.

The history

* Be ready to ask anyone about incontinence if they have a condition which puts them at risk. A question like 'do you ever have trouble holding your water?' is less threatening than the word 'incontinence'.
* Check, from the history, for other urinary symptoms. Incontinence is usually part of a larger problem. Consider benign prostatic hypertrophy (BPH) in older men and perform an IPS score if indicated (see Appendix 24).
* Identify the type of incontinence from the history: stress, urge, overflow or continuous, or a mixture. Many sufferers have at least two types.
* Ask about precipitating events: excess fluids or alcohol, behavioural or cognitive problems, and poor mobility or access to a toilet.
* Check for other underlying conditions. Constipation and UTIs are leading causes of incontinence in the elderly. Neurogenic incontinence may present with a mixture of symptoms. Cauda equina syndrome is a surgical emergency: results are poor when surgery is undertaken > 48 hours after first presentation (Markham 2004).

The examination

* Examine the abdomen, the genitals and prostate in men, with a pelvic examination in women, and a rectal examination in both sexes for constipation and for the integrity of the anal reflex.
* Proceed to the BPH guidance for further evaluation (below) in men where this is the suspected cause of the incontinence, as well as performing the investigations below.

The investigations

* Dip the urine for sugar and evidence of infection. Consider an MSU.
* Frequency/volume diary.
* Consider the use of a validated questionnaire for incontinence severity and quality of life (see Annex 1 of the SIGN guideline above).
* Consider a urinary ultrasound scan to assess residual volume, especially if there is a possibility that overflow incontinence is present or if the patient does not respond promptly to the measures below. A residual volume of 200 ml or more is abnormal. In men a residual volume > 100 ml is associated with other problems relating to BPH.
* Consider referral for urodynamic studies if the type of incontinence is not clear or if a trial of treatment fails.
* *Refer to a urologist or gynaecologist*, as appropriate, at this stage if there is:
  (a) a severe vaginal or uterine prolapse;
  (b) a pelvic mass (to be seen within 2 weeks in the UK);
  (c) a vesical fistula;
  (d) persistent or recurrent infection;
  (e) evidence of bladder outflow obstruction;
  (f) evidence of a large residual urine.
* Refer to a neurologist if there appears to be a neurological cause. The possibility of cauda equina syndrome or myelopathy needs urgent discussion with the neurosurgeons (or orthopaedic surgeons).

MANAGEMENT OF PRIMARILY STRESS INCONTINENCE (MEN AND WOMEN)

* *Reduce intra-abdominal pressure* by weight loss, the avoidance of constipation and reducing cough by stopping smoking.
* Increase external sphincter tone (87% cured or improved) (US Department of Health and Human Services 1992):
  (a) by pelvic floor exercises for men and women. Give the patient a copy of the DTB handout (see 'Patient information' below). Teach the patient to practice stopping the flow of urine momentarily midstream and then continue tensing those same muscles for 4 seconds at a time with 4 seconds rest, for a total of 1 hour

a day in 'ten tightening' bursts. Short, repeated bouts of exercises are the most useful. Continue for 3 months before deciding that exercises have not helped;
  (b) use of intravaginal weighted cones for women (available through urologists or local chemists). The patient inserts the lowest weight cone, with the pointed end downwards, and learns to retain the cone. The weight of the cones is steadily increased to 100 g (see the DTB handout below);
  (c) by referral to an appropriate physiotherapist for electrical stimulation therapy.
* *Postmenopausal women with an atrophic vagina.* The Women's Health Initiative has shown that oral oestrogen, with or without progestogen, significantly *worsened* continence, both in those troubled by incontinence at the start of the trial and in those who had no incontinence at the start of the trial (Hendrix, Cochrane, Nygaard, et al. 2005). No clear-cut evidence exists for local oestrogen.
* *Referral.* Refer those with troublesome symptoms that do not respond to the measures above. Surgery cures or improves 85% of those operated on. Operations include the older open abdominal retropubic suspension procedures as well as the newer and less invasive suburethral sling procedures (including those using trans-vaginal tape).
* *Consider prescribing duloxetine in addition to pelvic floor exercises.* It has an NNT for reduction of stress incontinence by > 50% of 5.7 (95%CI 4.5 to 7.8). However, most women report adverse effects, with nausea the most common, and one in five women in trials stop the drug (Anon. 2004).

MANAGEMENT OF PRIMARILY URGE INCONTINENCE (MEN AND WOMEN)

* Reduce excessive fluid intake and try avoiding caffeine.
* *Bladder retraining* (87% cured or improved) (US Department of Health and Human Services 1992).

Instruct the patient to:

(a) keep a frequency/volume chart for a week;
(b) return for discussion of the pattern the diary reveals. In addition, check that the total

volume of urine passed does not suggest that the patient is drinking too much;

(c) practise holding the urine when the urge to pass it is there; and

(d) slowly increase the interval between voiding up to 2–3 hours.

* *Anticholinergic drugs* are helpful in up to 83% (Malone-Lee, Walsh, Maugourd, *et al.* 2001), but are limited by side-effects. Undertake a trial for 6 weeks and, if working, review again after 6 months. Use oxybutynin, tolterodine, trospium or propiverine; the last three are more expensive than oxybutynin but may have fewer adverse effects (Anon. 2001). 60% show marked improvement or cure in the presence of detrusor instability. Flavoxate and imipramine are no longer used because of lack of efficacy and adverse effects respectively (Haeusler, Leitich, van Trotsenburg, *et al.* 2002).

* *Desmopressin nasal spray* in a single evening dose may help night-time symptoms in those aged 5–65 years old, including those with multiple sclerosis.

* *Oestrogen* given orally does not help incontinence in postmenopausal women (see above), in contrast to the conclusions of a Cochrane Review based on smaller earlier studies (Moehrer, Hextall and Jackson 2003). The case for local oestrogen is unclear.

* *Referral.* Refer to a urologist for consideration of augmentation cystoplasty those still sufficiently troubled by symptoms despite treatment and who might be candidates for surgery.

PATIENT SUPPORT

The Cystitis and Overactive Bladder Foundation, 76 High Street, Stony Stratford, Bucks MK11 1AH, tel. 01908 569169; www.cobfoundation.org

---

MANAGEMENT OF PRIMARILY OVERFLOW INCONTINENCE

* Refer for assessment by a urologist, neurologist or other specialist, according to the cause.

MANAGEMENT OF INCONTINENCE IN THE FRAIL ELDERLY OR COGNITIVELY IMPAIRED

* Assess:
  (a) *is it due to infection?* Older people often do not experience the typical symptoms of urinary infection. Send an MSU where possible;
  (b) *is it a symptom of another physical illness or of dementia?*
  (c) *are drugs causing or exacerbating the situation?* e.g. diuretics, sedatives;
  (d) *are there issues of practicality and mobility?* How easy is it to get to the toilet? Can mobility be improved? Can clothing be made easier to unfasten?

* Encourage the patient to pass urine regularly to try to pre-empt the incontinence.

COPING WITH INCONTINENCE: CONSERVATIVE 'CONTAINMENT' ADVICE FOR ALL

* Where the situation does not respond to any of the above measures, a continence adviser will be able to advise the patient on appliances, some of which are prescribable. Others may be available through the social services (including bath and laundry allowance) (see also page 8).

Bedding protection

* *Plastic mattress covers and one-way sheets* can be bought if not available from the community nursing service. They not only increase comfort but also reduce bedsores.

Pads and appliances

* *Inco pads* may be available from the community nursing service.
* *Cellulose wadding* can be prescribed.
* *Body-worn pads and waterproof pants* usually have to be bought, e.g. Urocare, Kanga and Kanga pouch.
* *Collecting devices* such as commodes, pans and urinals can be bought from pharmacists or hired from the Red Cross.
* *Penile sheaths* are available on prescription. Conveen provide a free sizing kit (catalogue

no. 6902) and sheaths from 17 mm to 35 mm. Downs Medical offer a free advice service and small, medium and large sheaths.

Urinary drainage bags

* Assess the patient's requirements: the length of tubing (short for wearing on the thigh or long on the calf); the type of tap (selection should depend on the patient's dexterity); the capacity needed (350, 500, 750 ml).
* Night bags hold 2 litres and should only be used for bed-bound patients or overnight.

URINARY CATHETERS AND PROBLEM-SOLVING

> **GUIDELINE**
>
> National Institute for Clinical Excellence. 2003. *Infection Control: Prevention of Healthcare-associated Infection in Primary and Community Care.* NICE Clinical Guideline No. 2. Available: www.nice.org.uk

Infection makes catheterization an unattractive solution but one that is likely to be necessary in those with retention or neurogenic bladder dysfunction, with severe pressure ulcers, who are terminally ill, or who cannot cope with less invasive appliances.

* Choose intermittent catheterization over an indwelling catheter if it is feasible.
* *Catheters* for long-term use should always be silicone with a 10 ml balloon. If a catheter is unlikely to be needed for more than 3 weeks, use a cheaper latex catheter.
* *Catheter insertion* should be performed using a no-touch technique and clean, but not necessarily sterile, gloves.
* *Catheter changes* should only be done when there is malfunction or contamination.
* *Urine samples* should be taken from a sampling port, not by disconnecting the bag, nor from the bag drainage outlet.
* *Debris* may be reduced by acidification of the urine with ascorbic acid. Encrustation ends up affecting half of all long-term catheters and is associated with infection by *Proteus*. When a patient starts to develop encrustation, plan a regular catheter change before the encrustation becomes troublesome.

Infection

* See page 413. Inflammation around the urethral meatus may be related to encrustation of the catheter and/or infection.

Bypass

* This is caused by obstruction of the catheter or by detrusor instability, not by the catheter being too small.
* Check that the bag is lower than the bladder; change the catheter and see if the old one was blocked; use a small bulb size, e.g. 5 ml; exclude and, if necessary, treat bladder stones and infection; and if there is no improvement use anticholinergic drugs, e.g. oxybutynin (Foster, Upsdell and O'Reilly 1990).

Catheterizing a patient in chronic retention

* *Haematuria* is inevitable if the bladder has been distended for some time. Clamping to release the urine in stages does not prevent this.
* *Diuresis* may occur after the obstruction is relieved. Diuretic doses may need to be reduced. Admit patients whose diuresis is severe.

> **PATIENT INFORMATION**
>
> Treatment notes: 'Incontinence due to having a baby', 'Have you got a prostate problem?' and 'Help for your overactive bladder'. Drug and Therapeutics Bulletin (DTB): Treatment Notes. Available on CD-Rom or free to NHS clinicians via www.nelh.nhs.uk (choose 'Drug and Therapeutics Bulletin' – Athens password needed from your local postgraduate medical library)
>
> The Bladder and Bowel Foundation provides a continence nurse helpline for medical advice: 0845 345 0165. http://www.bladderandbowelfoundation.org
>
> Incontinence Advisory Service, Disabled Living Foundation, 380–384 Harrow Road London W9 2HU, tel. 020 7289 6111; helpline 0845 130 9177; http://www.dlf.org.uk

ERIC (Enuresis Resource and Information Centre for children and young adults). 34 Old School House, Britannia Road, Kingswood, Bristol BS15 8DB, tel. 0117 960 3060; http://www.eric.org.uk

DIFFICULTY VOIDING

BLADDER OUTFLOW PROBLEMS IN MEN AND BENIGN PROSTATIC HYPERTROPHY (BPH)

For details of the diagnosis of lower urinary tract symptoms in men see *Evidence-based Diagnosis in Primary Care* by A. F. Polmear (editor), published by Butterworth-Heinemann, 2008.

GUIDELINES

Speakman MJ, Kirby RS, Joyce A, *et al.* 2004. British Association of Urological Surgeons. Guideline for the primary care management of male lower urinary tract symptoms. BJU Int 93, 985–990

Kirby R. 2004. New guideline will aid management of BPH in primary care. Guidelines in Practice **7** (June), 17–27. Available: www.eguidelines.co.uk (choose 'Guidelines in practice' then 'June 2004')

NICE. 2001. *Referral Advice.* http://www.nice.org.uk/page.aspx?o=201960

Reviews

Webber R. 2003. Benign prostatic hyperplasia. Clinical Evidence BMJ: search date July 2003. http://www.clinicalevidence.com/ceweb/conditions/index.jsp

Wilt TJ, N'Dow J. 2008. Benign prostatic hyperplasia. Part 1–Diagnosis. BMJ 336, 146–149. Part 2–Management. BMJ 336, 206–210

BPH is the commonest cause of bladder outflow problems in men and occurs with increasing age and with variable symptoms. Once symptoms are present, the 'rule of thirds' applies with 1/3 deteriorating, 1/3 remaining stable, and 1/3 improving over time (Ball, Feneley and Abrams 1981).

The history

* Take a history for relevant symptoms and score them (see Appendix 24). BPH is very common, with 41% of men > 50 years old reporting moderate or severe symptoms.
* Consider differential diagnoses: UTI, diabetes, prostatitis, medications, or lifestyle factors such as fluid and alcohol intake.
* Identify whether the patient has:
  (a) voiding/obstructive symptoms (poor flow, hesitancy, terminal dribbling and incomplete emptying);
  (b) filling/overactive bladder symptoms (frequency, urgency, urge incontinence, small volume urinating and nocturia).
These terms have replaced the older ones of bladder outflow obstruction and detrusor instability because of the poor correlation between the symptoms and objective findings of obstruction and instability (Abrams 1995).

* Is there nocturia out of proportion to other lower urinary tract symptoms (LUTS)? Nocturia three or more times a night raises the possibility of nocturnal polyuria, which can be defined as a nocturnal urine volume > 35% of the total 24-hour urine volume (Marinkovic, Gillen and Stanton 2004). This suggests a disturbance of the normal diurnal excretory rhythm. It can occur in chronic renal disease, diabetes mellitus, diabetes insipidus, right-sided heart failure, or can be an adverse effect of phenytoin, digoxin, lithium, diuretics and excess vitamin D. Any of these would need treatment followed by reassessment of the LUTS. In the absence of a treatable cause it may respond to restriction of fluid at night, diuretics in the morning, compression stockings for those with oedema, or desmopressin at night.
* Are there 'filling symptoms' with no evidence of obstruction? Manage as for urge incontinence (see page 415).

The examination

* Examine the abdomen for signs of chronic retention and pelvic or renal masses.
* Consider performing a digital rectal examination to examine for prostate size, to exclude sinister features, and as an aid to management decisions.

However, note that men with lower urinary tract symptoms are no more likely than others to have prostate cancer and there is an argument that a digital rectal examination (and PSA testing) are not routinely indicated with lower urinary tract symptoms (see the Wilt and N'Dow 2008 BMJ reviews above).

The investigations

* Perform a dipstick urinalysis.
* Test the blood for urea, creatinine and electrolytes, fasting glucose and consider (with informed consent) a PSA, though men with BPH are no more likely than others to have prostate cancer.
* Consider ordering an ultrasound scan (with post-void residual volume) where there is a suspicion of chronic retention or an obstructive uropathy (e.g. palpable bladder, raised creatinine, overflow incontinence); uroflowmetry may also be available locally. Refer if the post-voiding residual volume is > 100 ml.

The immediate management

* Admit those with acute urinary retention or acute renal failure.
* Refer to be seen urgently (in the UK within 2 weeks) (National Institute for Clinical Excellence 2001) those with macroscopic haematuria, a nodular or firm or irregular prostate, a raised PSA for the patient's age (see page 421), culture-negative dysuria (provided it is not due to a sexually transmitted disease), chronic urinary retention with overflow incontinence, or abnormal urinary cytology, where done.
* Refer to be seen 'soon' (in 4–8 weeks) those with recurrent UTIs or microscopic haematuria.
* Refer, at a timescale appropriate to the individual, those with chronic kidney disease or with refractory symptoms affecting the quality of life.

The management of those not needing/ wanting referral after viewing investigation results

Offer the patient a choice from the following options according to how bothered he is by his symptoms and whether he is at increased risk of progression of the obstruction. Explain that surgery is by no means inevitable. In one study only 7% required surgery over the next 3 years (Wasson, Reda, Bruskewitz, et al. 1995).

(a) *Lifestyle advice and consider 'watchful waiting'.* This is a key first line approach to management. Advice includes advising a fluid intake reduced to 2 l/day and avoiding caffeine. Recommend bladder training to those with 'filling symptoms'. Briefly, this means gradually lengthening the time between passing urine. Explain that avoiding excess fluid or alcohol intake, and avoiding constipation, will help to reduce the risk of acute retention. Review medications that might predispose to retention (especially anticholinergics).

(b) *Drugs*

* *Use an alpha blocker* in those with mild symptoms without risk factors for progression and where a quick symptomatic response is required. They are generally the first line drugs for BPH. If there is benefit, it is felt within 4–6 weeks and lasts for at least 3 years. A trial in the individual patient is therefore feasible, using the IPS Score to follow a trend (see Appendix 24). All alpha-blockers share this effect; a considerable saving can be made by choosing the least expensive. A reduction in BP from the less selective alpha -blockers such as doxazosin might be beneficial in hypertensive patients.

* *Use a 5-α reductase inhibitor* (finasteride, dutasteride) in those at higher risk of progression (see box). Given to men with a large prostate or raised PSA, it will reduce the risk of acute retention and the likelihood of prostatectomy by 50–60%. Use the other risk factors to sway the decision in cases of doubt (Lepor, Williford, Barry, et al. 1996). No symptomatic benefit may be seen for 3–6 months. If there is benefit, it is sustained while the drug is continued. Libido and erection problems occur in 9%, and there are risks of gynaecomastia, reduced ejaculate volume and presence of the drug in semen (such that condoms are advised). PSA rates are, on average, halved, to be remembered when performing future PSAs.

* *Use a combination of the two* in those more troubled by their symptoms. A study of 3047 men with at least moderately symptomatic

BPH found that clinical progression of symptoms over 4 years occurred in 17% on placebo, in 10% on either finasteride or doxazosin, and in only 5% on both drugs (McConnell, Roehrborn, Bautista, *et al.* 2003).

* *Antimuscarinics:* where BPH has caused a predominantly overactive bladder presentation consider these drugs in addition to bladder training. There is little evidence to suggest that they can precipitate acute urinary retention even in the presence of severe BPH.

* *Saw Palmetto* has only weak and conflicting evidence for efficacy in treating BPH symptoms, summarized in the CKS section on BPH by searching at http://www.cks.nhs.uk/clinical_topics.

RISK FACTORS FOR PROGRESSION OF BLADDER OUTFLOW PROBLEMS IN MEN

- A large prostate (> 30 cc).
- A PSA > 1.4 ng/ml regardless of age.
- Age > 70 years.
- IPSScore > 7 (at least 'moderate' severity).
- A low flow rate (< 12 ml/sec).
- A post-voiding residual volume > 100 ml on ultrasound.

(c) *Surgery* (usually transurethral resection of prostate, TURP) is much more effective than drugs in improving symptoms and flow rates, but only in two thirds of those who undergo it. It is most likely to be successful in those most bothered by their symptoms (Wasson, Reda, Bruskewitz, *et al.* 1995). It does, however, carry not only the short-term risks of any operation but also, in the case of TURP (Brookes, Donovan, Peters, *et al.* 2002), the risk of incontinence in one third although only 6% are bothered by it. After TURP, 9% need reoperation within 5 years. The rates for sexual dysfunction vary according to the type of surgery but the main techniques all worsen ejaculatory dysfunction (Emberton, Neal, Black, *et al.* 1996).

Review patients at 6–12 weeks if on an alpha-blocker; otherwise at 3–6 months

* Consider whether medications are working and tolerated, whether further medications need to

be used in combination, whether lifestyle advice should be repeated, and whether a referral to a urologist is now indicated.

* Check creatinine and PSA annually.

CARCINOMA OF THE PROSTATE

GUIDELINES

NICE. 2005. Clinical Guideline 27. *Referral for Suspected Cancer.* http://www.nice.org.uk/nicemedia/pdf/cg027niceguideline.pdf
    NICE. 2008. Clinical Guideline 58. *Prostate Cancer.* http://www.nice.org.uk/nicemedia/pdf/CG58NICEGuideline.pdf

Prostate cancer raises difficult issues relating to screening and the question of the value of treatment in the asymptomatic man in whom carcinoma is discovered incidentally. Symptomatic patients will benefit from referral. Nearly 10,000 die annually in the UK from prostate cancer. For details of the diagnosis of carcinoma of the prostate see *Evidence-based Diagnosis in Primary Care* by A. F. Polmear (editor), published by Butterworth-Heinemann, 2008.

PSA COUNSELLING AND INTERPRETATION

THE PATIENT EXPERIENCE

Chapple A, Ziebland S, Shepperd S, *et al.* 2002. Why men with prostate cancer want wider access to prostate specific antigen testing: qualitative study. BMJ 325, 737–781
    Thornton H, Dixon-Woods M. 2002. Prostate specific antigen testing for prostate cancer. BMJ 325, 725–726

Population screening for cancer of the prostate is not recommended in the UK (Muir Gray 2004), but should be available for a man who requests it and is able to give informed consent.

Risk factors for cancer of the prostate

(a) *Age.* Half of men aged > 80 have prostate cancer but most are asymptomatic and will die of other causes. Guidance suggests that PSA screening should not be offered to an asymptomatic man over 75 years old with < 10 years life expectancy.

(b) *Family history.* A family history of cancers of the prostate, breast, ovary, bladder and kidney increase the risk.

(c) *Race.* African Americans have a rate that is double that of whites. Asian and Oriental men have the lowest rates.

Counselling for the patient who requests PSA screening (NHS Centre For Reviews and Dissemination 1997; Chan and Sulmasy 1998)

Explain the following points:

(a) a rectal examination is considered as well as the blood test;

(b) if screening is positive, a biopsy may be needed. The biopsy itself is uncomfortable, risks infection and is followed by haematuria or haematospermia for up to three weeks in 1/3. The mortality is 1:10,000;

(c) only about one in three who have a positive PSA turn out to have cancer. Conversely, even biopsy will miss 20% of cancers;

(d) it is not clear that early treatment saves lives or improves other outcomes; and the treatments that may be offered can have potentially severe adverse effects including effects on sexual functioning, and continence. Studies are conflicting on the benefits of screening, and the CMO of England has advised to continue to screen asymptomatic men if they ask for it and are appropriately informed. Where the patient has symptoms or signs suggestive of prostate cancer (see NICE guidance on referring suspected cancer, above), PSA testing is more likely to be useful. Consider performing a digital rectal examination (DRE) and a PSA where there is unexplained haematuria, lower urinary tract symptoms, erectile dysfunction, bone pain, low back pain or weight loss. Refer urgently patients with an abnormal DRE or where the PSA is rising or above the age-specific thresholds (see below). Repeat the PSA after 1–3 months if borderline and refer urgently if rising;

(e) the stress and anxiety of knowing that you have or might have cancer is considerable and will affect life insurance applications.

PSA INTERPRETATION

1. The upper limit of normal rises with age and was revised in the BAUS BPH 2004 guideline (above):
   - Age < 50: 2.5ng/ml.
   - Age 50–59: 3.0.
   - Age 60–69: 4.0.
   - Age 70+: 5.0.

2. Probability of cancer at different levels of PSA:
   - PSA 4–10: 25%.
   - PSA > 11 or more: 66%.
   - PSA > 60: usually indicates metastatic prostate cancer.

3. Repeat a borderline level in 2 weeks; the result can alter by up to 30%.

4. Double the result if the patient has been taking finasteride or dutasteride for 6 months or more. Conversely, an enlarged prostate due to BPH can double the PSA level without indicating cancer.

5. Rectal examination does not raise the PSA but more invasive manoeuvres (even catheterization) can, as can UTI, prostatitis and benign prostatic hypertrophy.

Treatment options

This remains controversial. NICE guidance has been issued (see above NICE CG58) and there are various options:

(a) 'Active surveillance'. Especially appropriate for men whose life expectancy is < 10 years and those reluctant to face radical treatment.

(b) Radical (potentially curative) therapy. Surgery carries a risk of incontinence that is mild in 4–21% and total in up to 7%. Erectile dysfunction varies between 20% and 80%.

(c) Hormone therapy or orchidectomy (androgen deprivation), is indicated for non-curable disease that is not organ-confined. Early treatment in the form of androgen deprivation prolongs survival in advanced local and in metastatic disease (MRC Prostate Cancer Working Party Investigators Group 1997). 'Hormone escape' disease refers to a rising PSA despite hormonal measures. The life expectancy is about 6 months. Drug options are:

   - LHRH analogues, e.g. goserelin and leuprorelin, can improve quality of life but not life expectancy. They may also cause hot flushes, reduced libido, erectile dysfunction, gynaecomastia and an initial tumour flare;

■ non-steroidal anti-androgens, e.g. flutamide and bicalutamide, can be used as adjunctive therapy for total androgen blockade.

URINARY STONES

REVIEWS

Dawson C, Whitfield H. 1996. Urinary stone disease. BMJ 312, 1219–1221

Holdgate A, Pollock T. 2004. Nonsteroidal anti-inflammatory drugs (NSAIDs) versus opioids for acute renal colic (Cochrane Review). In: the Cochrane Library, Issue 4

* *Consider:* a family history of urinary stones, dehydration, urinary infection (especially by *Proteus*), hypercalcaemia, hyperuricaemia, and a chronic obstructive uropathy.
* *Analgesia.* Use an NSAID parenterally, e.g. diclofenac 75 mg i.m. Opioids may be necessary if that fails; use morphine not pethidine.
* Check for microscopic haematuria with a dipstick. If negative, reconsider the diagnosis (Dawson and Whitfield 1996). Check MSU and serum urea, electrolytes and creatinine.
* Arrange an urgent KUB (X-ray film), and an IVU (IVP) or ultrasound scan according to local guidelines:
  (a) to establish the diagnosis;
  (b) to assess the size, position and number of stones;
  (c) to look for obstruction.
* *Admit* for:
  (a) uncontrolled pain;
  (b) unable to drink adequate liquids;
  (c) infection;
  (d) complete uni- or bilateral obstruction on IVU;
  (e) known renal insufficiency;
  (f) known to have a single kidney.
* *Refer to outpatients* all those not requiring admission.
* Instruct the patient to save any stone passed by passing urine through a filter, e.g. a woman's stocking. Send it for analysis.

Once the patient is discharged from follow-up

* If conservative management has been chosen, support the patient with the information that 90% of small stones (< 5 mm) pass spontaneously and that 50% of stones that are 5–10 mm in diameter also pass (Clinical Knowledge Summaries, www.cks.nhs.uk – search on 'Renal colic-acute'). Although dehydration is a risk factor for developing stones, there is no evidence to support the practice of recommending an increased water intake as part of treatment (Qiang and Ke 2004).
* Check that an attempt has been made to find a cause, i.e. serum calcium and uric acid and a 24-hour urinary calcium. If there is a family history or the patient has recurrent stones, the following should also be checked:
  (a) 24-hour urine for pH, oxalate, phosphate and uric acid;
  (b) random urine for cystine.
* If an abnormality is found:
  (a) Treat *hypercalciuria* and calcium phosphate calculi with a low calcium diet and consider the use of bendroflumethiazide or potassium citrate.
  (b) Treat *hyperuricaemia* and urate calculi with allopurinol.
  (c) Explain the importance of avoiding dehydration.
  (d) Give dietary advice for oxalate stones (avoid chocolate, tea, rhubarb, spinach) and calcium stones (reduce amount of dairy products).

ASYMPTOMATIC PROTEINURIA IN MEN AND NON-PREGNANT WOMEN

GUIDELINE

Renal Unit, Royal Infirmary of Edinburgh (EdREN). 2009. *How to Manage Asymptomatic Proteinuria.* http://renux.dmed.ed.ac.uk/EdREN/Unitbits/ProtGuide. html

Protein+ or more on dipstick is likely to be significant, but false positives (40%) and negatives (< 20%) for urinary tract disease occur. False positives can result from a sample being highly concentrated or alkaline, or taken after exercise, during a fever, during menstruation, or in the presence of vaginal or urethral discharge. False negatives occur in dilute or acidic urine or in non-albuminuric proteinuria.

INTERPRETATION

- Proteinuria which is absent on waking suggests orthostatic proteinuria (but beware of diagnosing this in patients over 30 years old).
- Proteinuria that disappears on repeat testing may have been idiopathic transient proteinuria, which is found particularly below the age of 20 years, or may have been associated with another medical condition, e.g. UTI or heart failure. Repeat after a further 6 months.
- Proteinuria that is intermittent but not showing one of the patterns above: investigate as for persistent proteinuria and, if no grounds for referral are found, repeat the dipstick test, blood pressure and serum creatinine 6–12 monthly.
- Persistent proteinuria: investigation is needed.

INVESTIGATIVE STRATEGY IF A DIPSTICK SHOWS PERSISTENT PROTEINURIA+ OR ++

- ✷ History, including urinary tract symptoms, family history of renal disease and medications.
- ✷ Examination, including abdomen and loins, blood pressure, weight and oedema.
- ✷ Investigations:
  - (a) MSU and check the dipstick for haematuria (1+ is significant).
  - (b) Urine for albumin/creatinine ratio (ACR) to quantify the degree of proteinuria (see Appendix 26).
  - (c) Serum urea, creatinine and electrolytes. The GFR can be calculated (see page 425).
  - (d) Fasting blood sugar.
  - (e) Serum protein electrophoresis and urinary Bence Jones protein if other features (anaemia, bone pain) suggest myeloma or the patient is over 50 years old.

MANAGEMENT

- ✷ *Protein+++ or more: refer promptly that day* (by telephone discussion with the nephrologists). The protein loss is likely to be heavy enough

to lead to nephrotic syndrome (proteinuria > 3.5 g/day or urinary albumin/creatinine ratio > 300 mg/mmol).

- ✷ *Protein+ or ++:* Take an MSU and confirm that there is *persisting* proteinuria with a second and a third sample a week apart, at least one taken on waking.
- ✷ Refer less urgently to nephrology outpatients those:
  - (a) with a protein excretion of more than 1 g/day (consider sending a request-for-advice letter if proteinuria is between 150 mg and 1 g/day), or a albumin/creatinine ratio of > 120 mg/mmol, even if they have a primary condition which is likely to be the cause (e.g. diabetes);
  - (b) with a protein excretion of 250 mg/l or an albumin/creatinine ratio of > 30 mg/mmol if they *also* have a raised creatinine or hypertension. Refer with more urgency if the creatinine is clearly rising over weeks;
  - (c) with a decreased creatinine clearance (see page 425);
  - (d) with any proteinuria and a family history of renal disease.
- ✷ If proteinuria is present but does not meet the above criteria for referral, repeat the investigations 6-monthly until it resolves or does meet those criteria. Continue to check the BP, serum creatinine and a dipstick for haematuria.

ASYMPTOMATIC HAEMATURIA

For details of the diagnosis of haematuria see *Evidence-based Diagnosis in Primary Care* by A. F. Polmear (editor), published by Butterworth-Heinemann, 2008.

MACROSCOPIC HAEMATURIA

- ✷ Check that it is not due to menstruation or other bleeding.
- ✷ Check the urine with a dipstick, send MSU for culture and blood for urea, creatinine and electrolytes.
- ✷ Where the MSU is negative for red blood cells consider 'beetrooturia', obstructive jaundice and (rarely) porphyria. However, if

these are not present and repeat dipstick is still positive, believe the dipstick. Red cells may have lyzed on the journey to the laboratory.

* Refer any patient with painless macroscopic haematuria urgently to a urologist. The exception is haematuria during a proven UTI, which does not need further investigation provided a test for haematuria 7 days after completing antibiotics is clear. However, women aged over 40 with recurrent haematuria with UTIs, or refractory haematuria despite treating a UTI successfully, need an urgent urology referral, and men with a first UTI may also need referring even if the haematuria resolves (National Collaborating Centre for Primary Care 2004).

MICROSCOPIC HAEMATURIA

GUIDELINE

Joint Consensus Statement on the Initial Assessment of Haematuria. Renal Association and British Association of Urological Surgeons. 2008. http://www.renal.org and search on 'haematuria'

Review

Bakker M, Boon D. 2009. 10-minute consultation: haematuria. BMJ 338, b1324

- Screening is not routinely recommended (poor specificity).
- Aspirin, warfarin, etc., are not an 'excuse' for haematuria.
- The patient should collect an early morning urine sample in a plain white bottle for dipstick analysis. False positives occur after exercise, during menstruation or a UTI. An MSU is usually not necessary in primary care to confirm the microscopic haematuria.
- A finding of 1+ or more is significant when persistent in two out of three early morning urines over 4–6 weeks. Almost half of these patients will have glomerular disease, the proportion rising in the younger patient (Topham, Harper, Furness, *et al.* 1994).

- Common causes are:
  (a) *urological*: BPH, prostatitis, urological cancers (especially > 40 years old) or calculi;
  (b) *renal*: glomerular disease is relatively more common in those < 40 years old, especially IgA nephropathy; polycystic kidney disease.

INVESTIGATIVE STRATEGY IF PERSISTENT UNEXPLAINED MICROSCOPIC HAEMATURIA

Adapted from the British Association of Urological Surgeons and the Renal Association (see above reference).

(a) Always consider the history and examination. Is the patient ill or do they have 'red flags' for urological cancer? Urological symptoms + haematuria makes a urology referral to exclude underlying pathology appropriate.

(b) Consider age, BP and the presence of significant proteinuria. A renal cause is more likely if the patient is < 40 years old, is unwell, or there is proteinuria, a raised BP, or ankle oedema. Quantify the proteinuria. An albumin:creatinine ratio (ACR) > 30 mg/mmol or a protein:creatinine ratio (PCR) > 50 mg/mmol is significant.

(c) Assess renal function by measuring serum urea, electrolytes, creatinine and an estimated glomerular filtration rate (eGFR).

(d) Referral
  ■ *If the patient is ≥ 40 years old* consider urgent urology/haematuria clinic referral to exclude cancer and, where excluded, consider nephrology referral if the eGFR is persistently < 60, or the ACR is ≥ 30 mg/mmol, or the PCR is ≥ 50 mg/mmol, or the BP ≥ 140/90 mmHg.
  ■ If the patient is < 40 years old, consider nephrology referral with appropriate urgency if necessary if any of the factors listed are present.

(e) Where no cause is found after referral, monitor annually with BP, creatinine, eGFR and an ACR or PCR urine test. Consider urology (re-)referral if haematuria becomes symptomatic or macroscopic. Consider nephrology (re-)referral if the ACR or PCR deteriorate as above, or if the eGFR falls persistently to < 30 or falls by > 5 per year or > 10 per 5 years (NICE CKD clinical guideline, referenced below).

CHRONIC KIDNEY DISEASE (CKD)

GUIDELINES

National Kidney Foundation–K/DOQI. 2002. Clinical practice guidelines for chronic kidney disease: evaluation, classification and stratification. Am J Kidney Dis 39 (suppl 1), S1–S266

Renal Association. 2007. *Consensus Conference on Early Chronic Kidney Disease.* http://www.renal.org/ CKDguide/consensus.html

NICE. 2008. Clinical Guideline 73: *Chronic Kidney Disease.* http://www.nice.org.uk/nicemedia/pdf/ CG073FullGuideline.pdf

SIGN 2008. Clinical Guideline 103: *Diagnosis and Management of Chronic Kidney Disease.* http://www. sign.ac.uk/guidelines/fulltext/103/index.html

Department of Health. 2005. The National Service Framework for Renal Services. Part Two: *Chronic Renal Disease, Acute Renal Failure and End of Life Care.* February 2005. Available: www.dh.gov.uk (search on 'Chronic kidney disease')

- The incidence of CKD is rising due to an ageing population and increases in the incidence of the main causes, e.g. diabetes. There is an accompanying growing incidence of the need for renal replacement therapy (RRT) for end-stage CKD.
- Most patients with CKD are asymptomatic. Nearly half of all patients with CKD are in the stage 3A/B area, with much smaller numbers for stages 4 and 5.
- The principal causes of CKD in the UK are (from common to uncommon): diabetes mellitus, hypertension (these two cause three quarters of all CKD), vasculitis and glomerulonephritis, pyelonephritis, renovascular disease and obstructive uropathies. Adult polycystic kidney disease (APKD), medications and amyloidosis are less common. CKD, diabetes and proteinuria are interlinked and are strong, independent risk factors for cardiovascular disease and increased mortality. This, plus the rising incidence of CKD, plus the relatively new system for classification and management have led to CKD becoming a quality and outcomes framework (QOF) criterion in England.

- Management should be based on an estimated glomerular filtration rate (eGFR). The serum creatinine alone is an insensitive measurement of renal function, only becoming abnormal after considerable renal function decline. A study in primary care showed that using the eGFR increased the detection of CKD from 22% to 85% (Akbari, Swedko, Clark, *et al.* 2004). NICE and SIGN guidance aims to increase the detection of CKD in at-risk groups and thus assist in reducing the rates of associated cardiovascular disease and mortality, and in identifying and referring those at risk of progression to end-stage CKD requiring RRT.
- Calculating eGFRs $(ml/min/1.73m^2)$:

Use the modification of diet in renal disease (MDRD) formula based on values for creatinine, urea and albumin, and the patient's age, race and gender. UK labs are now routinely providing eGFRs. If not, it can be requested.

Age is never an 'excuse' for a low eGFR. Consider the whole picture, trend and comorbidity when considering further assessment and management.

ASSESSMENT AND MANAGEMENT OF CKD

Patients at risk of developing CKD

* Screen those with predisposing factors for CKD, e.g. hypertension, diabetes, cardiovascular disease, persistent haematuria or proteinuria, nephrotoxic drugs, structural renal problems or calculi, BPH, a family history of CKD stage 5, or multisystem disease, e.g. SLE.
* Perform annual serum creatinine, eGFR and a urinary protein:creatinine ratio (PCR) or albumin:creatinine ratio (ACR). NICE supports the ACR over PCR in diabetes and for detection, but the PCR is increasingly used for monitoring in non-diabetics.

Action to be taken on finding an eGFR < 60 or a normal eGFR with other signs of kidney damage

* Consider if the patient is ill, raising the suspicion of glomerulonephritis. If so, act according to the clinical picture, not just the laboratory results.
* Consider a repeat creatinine and eGFR with the patient fasted and well-hydrated, off oral

NSAIDs. Consider past creatinine levels to assess the stability of the result. Note that the eGFR may fall by 25% as a result of taking an ACE-inhibitor. If giving an ACE-inhibitor, monitor closely, stop if > 25% deterioration in eGFR or > 30% rise in creatinine. Such deterioration raises the possibility of renal artery stenosis.

* Beware of misinterpreting the eGFR because of the fact that serum creatinine is dependent on muscle mass. In those with high muscle mass the eGFR will be underestimated whilst in those with low muscle mass (including amputees and paraplegics) it will be overestimated. Equally, significant oedema and pregnancy cause problems with using the eGFR.

* Beware of over-interpreting eGFR changes where values are > 60. Look instead for a > 20% rise in the creatinine.

* Repeat a new finding of eGFR < 60 in 2 weeks and ensure three eGFRs are assessed over 3 months. At least two < 60 suggests a true reduced eGFR and CKD. Consider the rate of progression and whether this is likely to be a problem, based on the patient's age and comorbidity. Significant progression is more likely if there is also significant proteinuria.

* Consider renal ultrasound if there is a family history of APKD, or there are obstructive urinary symptoms, persistent haematuria, significant progression of eGFR decline, or possibly in CKD stages 4/5.

* Monitor blood and urine tests according to the CKD stage identified. Plan future monitoring to identify progression early. Most complications occur at eGFRs < 60. Check urea, creatinine, electrolytes, eGFR, BP and ACR or PCR at least annually. Check the calcium and phosphate in CKD stages 4/5; check the Hb in CKD stages 3B/4/5;

Further management

* *Consider referral*: CKD stages 4/5 (for consideration of RRT), ACR > 70 mg/mmol or PCR > 100 mg/mmol (heavy proteinuria suggests progression and/or underlying disease), ACR > 30 mg/mmol or PCR > 50 mg/mmol with persistent haematuria (1+ on dipstick), significant eGFR deterioration (> 5/year, > 10/5 years), suspected renal artery stenosis or genetic kidney disease, or uncontrolled hypertension despite four antihypertensives.

* *Medications review:* consider drugs that may be causing a reduced eGFR, and those whose dosage is affected by reduced renal function.

* Consider the need for smoking cessation and healthy lifestyle advice.

* Control hypertension to 120–139/< 90 mmHg (120–129/< 80 mmHg with diabetes or ACR > 70 mg/mmol). Use an ACE-inhibitor first-line.

* Give an ACE-inhibitor (or angiotensin-2 receptor antagonist) to maximal dosage if the patient has diabetes and significant microalbuminuria; or ACR > 70 mg/mmol; or CKD and Hypertension and ACR > 30 mg/mmol.

* Optimize the management of risk factors for CKD progression: CVD, significant proteinuria, hypertension, diabetes, smoking, chronic use of oral NSAIDs, and urinary outflow obstruction. Asian and black ethnicity are also risk factors for progression.

* Anaemia (Hb < 11 g/dl), acidosis, and metabolic bone disease are all complications increasingly prevalent from CKD stage 3B downwards and may require referral or primary care-initiated assessment, dependent upon local guidance. In CKD stages 3/4/5 iron deficiency anaemia is likely at ferritin levels < 100 mcg/l. NICE has published guidance on anaemia in CKD, and after excluding other causes iron can be given to get the ferritin to > 200 mcg/l. If this fails refer for consideration of erythropoietin therapy aiming in adults for a Hb of 10.5–12.5g/dl.

* Monitoring should depend on the stage of CKD (see CKD classification Table 14.1 for frequency). Check urea, creatinine and eGFR, BP, ACR or PCR and FBC at CKD stage 3A and worse. Also check calcium and phosphate at CKD stage 3B and worse.

* If monitoring shows an ACR > 70 mg/mmol or PCR > 100 mg/mmol no repeat is needed; this is heavy proteinuria requiring referral. However, an ACR 30–70 mg/mmol needs to be repeated on the first morning sample to confirm the proteinuria. Haematuria is also grounds for referral when persistent. In diabetes an ACR > 2.5 mg/mmol in men and > 3.5 mg/mmol in women is significant and needs repeat confirmation on an early morning ACR.

The above plan assumes that the patient is not suffering from another condition that makes an active approach inappropriate.

Table 14.1 Classification and key actions for CKD (adapted from NICE guidance, see above)

STAGE OF KIDNEY DISEASE	GRF (ML/MINUTE/ 1.73M^2)	ACTION
Stage 1. Evidence of kidney damage* but normal GFR	≥90	Address CVD risk factors, treat comorbidity. Monitor annually
Stage 2. Evidence of kidney damage* and mildly reduced GFR	60–89	As above. Monitor annually
Stage 3A. Moderately reduced GFR	45–59	Closer monitoring 6-monthly
Stage 3B. Moderately reduced GFR	30–44	Check for complications; treat / refer. 6-monthly monitoring
Stage 4. Severely reduced GFR	15–29	Refer to a nephrologist to consider RRT. 3-monthly monitoring
Stage 5. Established kidney failure	<15	RRT possibly indicated (haemodialysis, peritoneal dialysis, transplantation). 6-weekly monitoring

Key: GFR = the glomerular filtration rate; cardiac risk can be calculated over 10 years (see page 165); RRT = Renal Replacement Therapy. CKD Stage 3 was split into 3A and 3B following the Consensus conference and ensuing statement on early CKD (see above reference).
*Kidney damage: persistent proteinuria, haematuria, anatomical abnormalities, e.g. polycystic or scarred, shrunken kidneys, biopsy-proven glomerulonephritis.
Based on the National Kidney Foundation classification (National Kidney Foundation-K/DOQI 2002) and a revision splitting CKD stage 3 (the most prevalent stage) to be of increased utility, reflected in the 2008 NICE guidance.

References

Abrams, P., 1995. Managing lower urinary tract symptoms in older men. BMJ 310, 1113–1117.

Akbari, A., Swedko, P.J., Clark, H.D., et al., 2004. Detection of chronic kidney disease with laboratory reporting of estimated glomerular filtration rate and an educational program. Arch. Int. Med. 164, 1788–1792.

Albert, X., Huertas, I., Pereiro, I., et al., 2004. Antibiotics for preventing recurrent urinary tract infection in non-pregnant women (Cochrane Review). In: The Cochrane Library. Issue 4.

Andrews, S., Brooks, P.T., Hanbury, D.C., 2002. Ultrasonography and abdominal radiography versus intravenous urography in investigation of urinary tract infection in men: prospective incident cohort study. BMJ 324, 454–456.

Anon. 1991. The mysterious 'urethral syndrome' (letter). BMJ 303, 361–362.

Anon. 2001. Managing incontinence due to detrusor instability. DTB 39, 59–64.

Anon. 2004. Duloxetine for female stress urinary incontinence. Bandolier 129, 4–5. www.jr2.ox.ac.uk/bandolier.

Baerheim, A., 2001. Empirical treatment of uncomplicated cystitis. BMJ 323, 1197–1198.

Ball, A.J., Feneley, R.C., Abrams, P.H., 1981. The natural history of untreated 'prostatism'. Br. J. Urol. 53, 613–616.

Barry, H.C., Hickner, J., Ebell, M.H., et al., 2001. A randomized controlled trial of telephone management of suspected urinary tract infections in women. J. Fam. Pract. 50, 589–594.

Brookes, S.T., Donovan, J.L., Peters, T.J., et al., 2002. Sexual dysfunction in men after treatment for lower urinary tract symptoms: evidence from randomised controlled trial. BMJ 324, 1059–1061.

Brumfitt, W., Hamilton-Miller, J.M.T., 1994. Consensus viewpoint on management of urinary infections. J. Antimicrob. Chemother. 33 (Suppl. A), 147–153.

Burgio, K.L., Matthews, K.A., Engel, B.T., 1991. Prevalence, incidence and correlates of urinary incontinence in healthy middle-aged women. J. Urol. 146, 1255–1259.

Chan, E.C.Y., Sulmasy, D.P., 1998. What should men know about prostate-specific antigen screening before giving informed consent? Am. J. Med. 105, 266–274.

Christiaens, T.C., De Meyere, M., Verschraegen, G., et al., 2002. Randomised controlled trial of nitrofurantoin versus placebo in the treatment of uncomplicated urinary tract infection in adult women. Br. J. Gen. Pract. 52, 729–734.

Committee for Safety of Medicines, 1997. Revised indications for co-amoxiclav. Curr. Prob. Pharmacovigil. 23, 8. Available: www.mca.gov.uk/.

Dawson, C., Whitfield, H., 1996. Urological emergencies in general practice. BMJ 312, 838–840.

DTB, 1998. Managing urinary tract infection in women. Drug Ther. Bull. 36, 30–32.

Duckett, J.R.A., 1996. Women with urinary incontinence should be referred to a specialist. BMJ 313, 754.

Emberton, M., Neal, D.E., Black, N., et al., 1996. The effect of prostatectomy on symptom severity and quality of life. Br. J. Urol. 77, 233–247.

Foster, M.C., Upsdell, S.M., O'Reilly, P.H., 1990. Urological myths. BMJ 301, 1421–1423.

Haeusler, G., Leitich, H., van Trotsenburg, M., et al., 2002. Drug therapy of urinary urge incontinence: a systematic review. Obstet. Gynaecol. 100, 1003–1016.

Hamilton-Miller, J.M., 1994. The urethral syndrome and its management. J. Antimicrobial. Chemother. 33 (Suppl. A), 63–73.

Hendrix, S.L., Cochrane, B.B., Nygaard, I.E., et al., 2005. Effects of estrogen with and without progestin on urinary incontinence. JAMA 293, 998–1001.

Jepson, R.G., Mihaljevic, L., Craig, J.C., 2004. Cranberries for treating urinary tract infections (Cochrane Review). In: The Cochrane Library. Issue 4.

Kontiokari, T., Sundqvist, K., Nuutinen, M., et al., 2001. Randomised trial of cranberrylingonberry juice and Lactobacillus GG drink for the prevention of urinary tract infections in women. BMJ 322, 1571–1573.

Lepor, H., Williford, W.O., Barry, M.J., et al., 1996. Veterans Affairs Cooperative Studies Benign Prostatic Hyperplasia Study Group. The efficacy of terazocin, finasteride, or both in benign prostatic hyperplasia. N. Engl. J. Med. 335, 533–539.

McConnell, J.D., Roehrborn, C.G., Bautista, O.M., et al., 2003. The long-term effects of doxazosin, finasteride, and combination therapy on clinical progression of benign prostatic hypertrophy. N. Engl. J. Med. 349, 2387–2398.

McNaughton Collins, M., MacDonald, R., Wilt, T., 1999. Interventions for chronic abacterial prostatitis. Cochrane Database Syst. Rev Issue 4. www.wiley.com/cochrane.

Malone-Lee, J.G., Walsh, J.B., Maugourd, M.F., et al., 2001. Tolterodine: a safe and effective treatment for older patients with overactive bladder. J. Am. Geriatr. Soc. 49, 700–705.

Marinkovic, S.P., Gillen, L.M., Stanton, S.L., 2004. Managing nocturia. BMJ 328, 1063–1066.

Markham, D.E., 2004. Cauda equina syndrome: diagnosis, delay and litigation risk. MDU 20 (1), 12–15.

MeReC, 1995. Urinary tract infection. MeReC. Bull. 6, (8), 29–32. (See also the Health Protection Agency guideline referenced at the top of the UTI section).

MeReC, 1997. Urinary incontinence in adults. MeReC Bulletin 8 (part 1), 33–36 (part 2) 41–44.

Moehrer, B., Hextall, A., Jackson, S., 2003. Oestrogens for urinary incontinence in women. Cochrane Database Syst. Rev Issue 2.

MRC Prostate Cancer Working Party Investigators Group, 1997. Immediate versus deferred treatment for advanced prostatic cancer: initial results of the Medical Research Council trial. Br. J. Urol. 79, 235–246.

Muir Gray, J.A., 2004. New concepts in screening. Br. J. Gen. Pract. 54, 292–298.

National Collaborating Centre for Primary Care, 2004. Referral guidelines for suspected cancer; draft for second consultation. September. Available:http://www.nice.org.uk/pdf/RSC_2ndcons_Full_version.pdf.

National Institute for Clinical Excellence, 2001. Referral advice: a guide to appropriate referral from general to specialist services. Available: www.nice.org.uk.

National Kidney Foundation-K/DOQI., 2002. Clinical practice guidelines for chronic kidney disease: evaluation, classification and stratification. Am. J. Kidney Dis. 39 (Suppl. 1), S1–S266.

NHS Centre for Reviews and Dissemination, 1997. Screening for prostate cancer. Effectiveness Matters 2 (2).

O'Brian, J., Long, H., 1995. Urinary incontinence: long-term effectiveness of nursing intervention in primary care. BMJ 311, 1208.

Qiang, W., Ke, Z., 2004. Water for preventing urinary calculi. In: The Cochrane Library, Issue 4.

Stothers, L., 2002. A randomized trial to evaluate effectiveness and cost effectiveness of naturopathic cranberry products as prophylaxis against urinary tract infection in women. Can. J. Urol. 9, 1558–1562.

Topham, P.S., Harper, S.J., Furness, P.N., et al., 1994. Glomerular disease as a cause of isolated microscopic haematuria. Q. J. Med. 87, 329–335.

US Department of Health and Human Services, 1992. Urinary incontinence in adults. Agency for Health Care and Policy Research (AHCPR), Rockville MD.

Wasson, J.H., Reda, D.J., Bruskewitz, R.C., et al., 1995. A comparison of transurethral surgery with watchful waiting for moderate symptoms of benign prostatic hyperplasia. The Veterans Affairs Cooperative Study Group on Transurethral Resection of the Prostate. N. Engl. J. Med. 332, 75–79.

Chapter 15

Surgical problems

CHAPTER CONTENTS

© 2011 Elsevier Ltd.
DOI: 10.1016/B978-0-7020-3053-6.00015-5

ORTHOPAEDIC PROBLEMS IN PRIMARY CARE

HEAD AND NECK INJURY

Indications for referral to the accident and emergency department (NICE 2007)

(a) History of unconsciousness; or an altered conscious state at the time of the examination (Glasgow Coma Score (GCS) < 15).

(b) Any amnesia for events before or after the trauma.

(c) History of trauma involving a dangerous mechanism (see below).

(d) Suspected foreign body or penetrating injury; or clinical signs of skull fracture e.g. crepitus, skull depression, 'bogginess', serious scalp laceration or haematoma, blood or CSF in the nose or ear, or CSF in the wound, new deafness, bruising behind one or both ears, or a black eye without associated damage around the eye.

(e) Convulsion.

(f) Persistent headache.

(g) Any vomiting since the injury.

(h) Focal neurological signs at the time of examination, including ill defined signs such as loss of balance.

(i) Complicating medical factors (e.g. anticoagulant use, a bleeding disorder, or alcohol or drug misuse).

(j) Difficulty in assessing the patient, due e.g. to intoxication.

(k) Age 65 or over.

(l) Previous cranial neurosurgery.

(m) Suspicion of non-accidental injury.

(n) Any other cause for concern.

NICE recommends that the GP use discretion in the following situations:

(a) irritability or altered behaviour, especially in infants and young children;

(b) adverse social factors; usually the patient should not be unsupervised at home for the next 48 hours;

(c) visible trauma to the head that does not meet the criteria above but which still causes the GP concern;

(d) concern by the patient or carer about the situation.

Phone ahead to alert the Department if the GCS has been 8 or below (see Table 15.1), asking for the appropriate professionals to be standing by.

Criteria for imaging in adults

The investigation of choice is a CT scan; but note that the criteria for a scan are stricter than those for referral for assessment at A&E:

(a) GCS < 13 at any time;

(b) GCS < 15 at 2 hours after the trauma;

(c) suspicion of open or depressed skull fracture;

(d) evidence of basal skull fracture;

(e) post-traumatic seizure;

(f) focal neurological deficit;

(g) more than one episode of vomiting;

(h) pre-traumatic amnesia > 30 minutes;

(i) any amnesia or loss of consciousness with one of the following: age ≥ 65, a bleeding disorder, or a dangerous mechanism of injury (see box).

Note: If a patient with a minor head injury, with or without a normal skull X-ray (SXR) but no CT scan, is not improving, do not hesitate to refer back for a scan (Voss, Knottenbelt and Peden 1995). One in seven who are sent back despite a normal SXR will have an abnormal scan.

WHAT CONSTITUTES A DANGEROUS MECHANISM IN RELATION TO HEAD AND NECK INJURY?

- A pedestrian or cyclist hit by a motor vehicle.
- A person thrown from a motor vehicle.
- A high speed motor vehicle collision.
- A diving accident.
- A fall of > 1 metre, e.g. down at least five stairs, or of > 3 metres in a child.
- Being hit on the head by a high-speed projectile.
- Any other high-energy mechanism.

Table 15.1	Glasgow Coma Scale (Jennett and Teasdale 1974)		
PARAMETER	RESPONSE	SCORE	ALTERNATIVE IN PRE–VERBAL CHILDREN OR INTUBATED PATIENTS
Best eye response	Spontaneous	4	
	To speech	3	
	To pain	2	
	None	1	
Best verbal (or grimace) response	Orientated	5	Normal spontaneous facial activity
	Confused	4	Less than normal facial activity
	Inappropriate	3	Vigorous grimace
	Incomprehensible sounds	2	Mild grimace
	None	1	None
Best motor response to painful stimulus	Obeys commands	6	
	Localizes pain	5	
	Withdrawal from pain	4	
	Abnormal flexion to pain	3	
	Extension to pain	2	
	None	1	
	TOTAL	3–15	

Notes on reporting the patient's score:
1. report the three parameters (eyes, verbal and motor) separately e.g. E3, V3, M4.
2. if reporting a combined score report it out of 15, e.g. 10/15.
3. report the time when the assessment was made.

Care of the cervical spine in the context of head injury

While waiting for the ambulance to collect a patient with a head injury, immobilize the cervical spine in any patient:

(a) whose GCS has been < 15; or

(b) with neck pain or tenderness; or

(c) with focal neurological signs or paraesthesiae in the limbs; or

(d) with any other suspicion of cervical spine injury.

See below for more details of the management of neck injury.

If the patient is not admitted, warn the patient's attendant, verbally and in writing, to report:

(a) unusual drowsiness;

(b) severe headache;

(c) vomiting;

(d) visual disturbance or deafness;

(e) strange behaviour;

(f) anything else worrying.

* Record the warning in the patient's notes.

* Give paracetamol or codeine for headache, but nothing stronger.

NECK INJURY

Any patient who has suffered blunt trauma to the head or neck may have suffered a cervical fracture or dislocation. The more obvious head injury may mask this.

The Canadian C-spine rule is highly sensitive (99.4%) though not very specific (45.1%) (Stiell, Clement, McKnight, *et al.* 2003). In other words, a negative assessment means that the patient almost certainly does not have traumatic cervical spine injury, but a positive assessment increases the risk of cervical spine injury only slightly. For a more detailed discussion of this issue see *Evidence-based Diagnosis in Primary Care* by A. F. Polmear (editor), published by Butterworth-Heinemann, 2008.

Using the rule, a cervical spine X-ray is needed if:

1. there is a high-risk factor that mandates radiography (age 65 or over, a dangerous type of trauma, or paraesthesiae in the extremities, in a patient with neck pain or midline cervical tenderness); or

2. there is a contraindication to assessment of neck movement (see below); or

3. neck movements are assessed and the patient cannot rotate the neck actively 45° to left and right.

Assessment of neck movements is considered safe if one of the following is present:

■ the accident was a simple rear-end motor vehicle collision;

■ the patient is sitting up when seen or has been walking about at any time since the accident;

■ the onset of neck pain was delayed; or

■ there is no midline tenderness.

HEAD INJURY IN YOUNG CHILDREN

In infants and children the same criteria for CT scanning apply but with the following alterations:

a) witnessed loss of consciousness > 5 minutes;

b) GCS < 14 when assessed;

c) any amnesia for > 5 minutes (antegrade or retrograde);

d) vomiting three or more times;

e) suspicion of non-accidental injury.

And for infants only:

a) GCS < 15 when assessed;

b) Bruise, swelling or laceration > 5 cm across on the head.

General points about young children

● Small children can be difficult to assess. Refer if in doubt.

● The inability to rouse a child is a worrying sign. Refer. Sleepiness alone is not worrying.

● Persistent crying may indicate that the child has a headache; small children will not usually complain of headache.

● If the child does not cry immediately after head trauma, suspect moderate to severe head injury and refer.

● NICE recommends that any child who qualifies for imaging should be assessed by a clinician experienced in detecting non-accidental injury.

Skull fractures in children (Haslam 1996)

● Radiological evidence of a skull fracture is found in almost one third of children with a history of head injury. These children are normally neurologically intact at the time of examination and remain so.

● Nearly 50% of children who die of an acute brain injury have no evidence of a skull fracture.

● Subdural haematoma is twice as likely in the absence of a skull fracture after head injury in children compared with adult head injury without skull fracture.

● Epidural haematoma occurs in 50% children with skull fracture.

● Location and type of skull fracture are rarely correlated with symptoms and physical findings in children who have suffered head trauma.

● Depressed skull fractures require surgical decompression if the depression is more than 3–5 mm.

TREATMENT AFTER HEAD INJURY

* NICE recommends that a patient discharged from hospital who was judged to be sufficiently severely injured to warrant imaging or admission should see the GP within 1 week. The GP should have the possibility of referral to a professional trained in the assessment and management of brain injury sequelae (NICE 2007).

* Explain that headache, dizziness, tinnitus, poor concentration and balance and fatigue are common. They usually subside over 2 weeks in minor injury but may take 6 months (Greenwood, McMillan, Brooks, *et al.* 1994). Sadly, almost half are still disabled at 1 year. A study from Glasgow (Thornhill, Teasdale, Murray, *et al.* 2000) found that 47% of patients with mild head injury (GCS 13–15) had moderate or severe disability 1 year later, a rate not significantly better than those with moderate or severe head injury.

* *Depression or anxiety.* Consider treatment with antidepressants on the usual criteria (see pages 451 and 464) (NNT 5 (95% CI 4 to 7)) (Gill and Hatcher 2001).

* *Agitation and aggression.* Evidence to guide management is sparse but beta-blockers seem to benefit patients (Fleminger, Greenwood and Oliver 2003).

* Post-traumatic stress disorder (see page 461). Check specifically for this if the trauma was violent. It is amenable to cognitive behavioural therapy (Bryant, Moulds, Guthrie and Nixon 2003).

Note: Prophylactic antiepileptic drugs reduce early seizures after moderate to severe head injury when given within hours and continued for several weeks (RRR 66% (95% CI = 46 to 79%); NNT 16 (95% CI = 11 to 35)) but do not reduce late seizures, neurological disability, or death (RRR 15% (95% CI = −11 to 51)) (Schierhout and Roberts 1998).

REHABILITATION AFTER A HEAD INJURY

● Residual problems, which are common after severe head injury, can be reduced by rehabilitation.

● Neuropsychiatric problems are common after minor head injury.

* Attempt to keep the patient in a rehabilitation programme and consider re-referring patients still troubled by cognitive, behavioural and emotional disturbances.

PATIENT ORGANIZATION

HEADWAY: the brain injury association. Tel. 0115 924 0800. Helpline 0808 800 2244. www.headway.org.uk

WHIPLASH INJURY

ACUTE

● Whiplash injury is self-limiting in the absence of bone or nerve injury (Cassidy, Carroll, Cote, *et al.* 2000).

● The traditional therapy of rest, a soft collar and gradual self-mobilization leads to more long-term disability than an active approach (Rosenfield, Seferiadis, Carlsson, *et al.* 2003).

● Impending compensation delays recovery (Cassidy, Carroll, Cote, *et al.* 2000).

● Careful examination is important as imaging studies are rarely helpful. The act of examination helps to relieve anxiety and encourages self-management (Livingstone 2000).

* Check for weakness, with or without pain in one or both arms. It would suggest nerve root involvement. This is an unusual complication of whiplash but requires urgent specialist evaluation.

* Reassure that 90% make some recovery within 6 months, although up to 40% of these patients have some neck pain after 15 years (Binder 2001).

* Give paracetamol with or without codeine and/or an NSAID and recommend that they be taken regularly.

* Encourage normal activities rather than rest. It speeds resolution (Borchgrevink, Kaasa, McDonagh, *et al.* 1998).

* Consider referring to a physiotherapist for training in active mobilization of the neck.

* Resist over-treatment; instead, try to reward the patient for getting better. Discourage symptom diaries (Livingstone 2000).

CHRONIC WHIPLASH INJURY

- This is arbitrarily defined as symptoms from a whiplash injury still present after 6 months. Studies show that between 14% and 42% of patients with whiplash still have symptoms at 6 months (Poorbaugh, Brismee, Phelps, *et al.* 2008).
- Symptoms that form part of the syndrome of whiplash-related disorders, apart from neck pain and stiffness, are headache, dizziness, paraesthesiae in the upper limbs and psychological distress.
- The general practitioner is torn between, on the one hand, helping the patient focus on the recovery that will eventually come, and, on the other, referring those likely to fare badly, as early as possible.
- * In patients whose initial pain was mild to moderate and who are not significantly disabled by their symptoms, continue the approach outlined above: mild analgesia, avoidance of further investigations, encouragement to remain active, while remaining alert to the possibility of anxiety and depression. When the patient is focusing on the possibility of compensation rather than on recovery, explore ways of bringing litigation to an end as quickly as possible.
- * Refer to a pain clinic a patient who has risk factors for a poor prognosis. These are: severe initial pain, more symptoms, and greater initial disability (Carroll, Holm, Hogg-Johnson, *et al.* 2008). Of referred patients, 46% (95% CI 22 to 79%) will improve with treatment (Binder 2001).

BREAST PROBLEMS

For details of the diagnosis of breast problems see *Evidence-based Diagnosis in Primary Care* by A. F. Polmear (editor), published by Butterworth-Heinemann, 2008.

REFERRAL CRITERIA FOR BREAST PROBLEMS (NHS CANCER SCREENING PROGRAMMES AND CANCER RESEARCH UK 2003)

Refer urgently if there is:

- a new discrete lump in a woman age > 45; or
- other signs of cancer: ulceration, a skin nodule or skin distortion.

Lump: refer, but not necessarily urgently, if there is:

(a) a new discrete lump in a younger woman; or

(b) a new lump in pre-existing nodularity; or

(c) asymmetrical nodularity in a woman with a strong family history of cancer or who is age 35 or over. In a younger woman only refer if the asymmetry persists after the next period; or

(d) an abscess; or

(e) recurrence of a previously drained cyst.

- Young women with tender, lumpy breasts and older women with symmetrical nodularity, provided there is no localized abnormality, do not need referral to specialist.
- For women with recurrent multiple cysts, aspiration is acceptable by a GP with the necessary skills.

Discharge: refer if there is discharge from the nipple without a lump and the patient is:

(a) 50 years old or over; or

(b) under 50 with discharge that is:

- bilateral and heavy enough to stain clothing; or
- bloodstained; or
- persistent from a single duct.

Women aged under 50 who have nipple discharge that is from more than one duct or is intermittent and is neither bloodstained nor troublesome do not require referral to a breast specialist.

Other problems: refer if there is:

(a) nipple abnormality: eczema or a retracted or distorted nipple; or

(b) a change in breast contour (best seen with arms raised while patient sitting upright); or

(c) a dimple or change in skin texture of the breast; or

(d) localized, non-cyclical breast pain; or

(e) intractable cyclical breast pain which fails to respond to medical treatment; or

(f) a strong family history of breast cancer (see page 436).

BREAST PAIN WITHOUT A LUMP – MASTALGIA (BUNDRED 2004)

- The pain of cyclical mastalgia is almost always derived from the breast itself; non-cyclical breast pain may be derived from the breast or, especially if unilateral, the chest wall.
- Nearly 70% women have breast pain at some time in their life, most commonly aged 30–50 years.

- Cyclical pain resolves within 3 months in 20–30% of women. Non-cyclical pain is more difficult to treat but eventually resolves in nearly 50%.
- Women with minor and moderate degrees of breast pain who do not have a discrete palpable lesion can be managed in general practice. Refer women with intractable pain or postmenopausal women with persistent unilateral pain. They may have cancer despite the absence of a lump.
- There is no evidence of effectiveness for many potential remedies: evening primrose oil, vitamin E, LHRH analogues, progestogen orally or topically, pyridoxine, antibiotics or diuretics. Gestrinone may be effective but adverse effects are likely to outweigh any benefit.

* Discuss the need to stop oral contraceptives or HRT, if taken. If a patient taking HRT in the form of a conventional oestrogen/progestogen combination wishes to continue, consider changing to tibolone (Colacurci, Mele, De Franciscis, *et al*. 1998).
* Recommend analgesics, a supportive bra and a low-fat, high-carbohydrate, diet, which can reduce breast pain and tenderness (Boyd, McGuire, Shannon, *et al*. 1988).
* If pain is more severe, use danazol for 3–6 months (200 mg daily reducing to 100 mg daily once pain is controlled). Danazol can be confined to the 2 weeks before menstruation in order to reduce adverse effects further. Pain relief continues for at least 6 months after stopping the drug (NNT = 3, 95%CI 2 to 5) (Kontostolis, Stefanidis, Navrozoglou, *et al*. 1997). If pain recurs, give further 6-month courses as necessary.
* Consider bromocriptine, as an alternative to danazol, starting at 1.25 mg nocte and increasing to a maximum of 2.5 mg b.d. However, its side-effects may outweigh any benefit (Mansell and Dogliotti 1990). If the response is good, treat for 6 months. If the pain recurs, further 6-month courses may be given.
* An alternative, for which the evidence of only one small RCT exists, is a topical NSAID. Topical diclofenac, 50 mg applied to the breast three times daily for 6 months, led to complete resolution of pain in half of women compared to placebo (NNT 2.1 (1.6 to 2.9)) (Bandolier 2004).

In patients with severe pain not helped by the above:

* Consider tamoxifen, although it is unlicensed for this use. 10 mg daily during those days in which the pain is felt is as effective as 20 mg with fewer adverse effects. However, hot flushes and vaginal dryness are still possible. Contraception is essential. Specialist advice and review after 6 months is recommended.
* Consider lisuride, although the only evidence of benefit is from one, possibly biased, trial. 200 mcg daily for 2 months gave an NNT of 2 (95%CI 2 to 3) to achieve > 50% reduction of pain scores (Kaleli, Aydin, Erel, *et al*. 2001). Fibrotic reactions have been described in patients taking lisuride for Parkinson's disease and the CSM recommends baseline CXR, ESR and creatinine.

BREAST CANCER SCREENING AND BREAST CANCER

General practitioners have a role in supporting the breast screening programme but should know its limitations.

- A GP with 2000 patients will see nearly two new cases of breast cancer annually (incidence = 118 per 100,000) while she/he will be looking after five women with breast cancer (prevalence = 0.5%). That is equivalent to a lifetime risk for each woman of 1 in 11.
- 5% of screening mammograms are abnormal and need further assessment. Only 5% of these turn out to show cancer.
- At an initial screen up to 20% of the breast cancers found will be in situ, 20–25% will be invasive lesions under 1 cm in diameter, and 25% will be invasive lesions between 1 and 2 cm in diameter (Miller, To, Baines and Wall 2000).
- Mammography misses 10% of cancers.
- Over 90% of breast cancers are found by women themselves.

Information the GP needs to support the breast cancer screening programme

(a) *Women under 50*. A large Canadian RCT showed no benefit from mammography in women aged 40–49 (Miller, To, Baines, *et al*. 2002).
(b) *Women aged 50–70*. There is a large body of evidence for regular screening mammography (Kerlikowske, Grady, Rubin, *et al*. 1995; Tabár,

Vitak, Chen, *et al.* 2001). Five-year survival in those in whom cancer is found is almost 75% and 10-year mortality is reduced by 25–30% (Blanks, Moss, McGahan, *et al.* 2000).

(c) *Women over 70* are still entitled to be screened but they need to initiate the appointment; they will not be recalled by the screening service. There is no reason to think that screening is less valuable over the age of 70 and the GP should encourage women to contact the service.

(d) *Women with symptoms between routine mammography.* Women should continue to be aware of minimal symptoms and to report these without delay to their GP even if they have been recently screened. A woman with symptoms should be referred for investigation to a surgeon with a special interest in breast disease working in a hospital that can provide a multidisciplinary approach to breast disease.

(e) *Women with breast cancer.* Women who have undergone surgery for breast cancer should have mammography yearly for the first 5 years and then 2-yearly.

(f) *Women receiving hormone replacement therapy.* Women aged 50–64 on HRT do not need more frequent screening. Women do not need a baseline mammogram before receiving HRT. However, HRT does increase the risk of breast cancer. The hazard ratio (HR) for breast cancer for women on HRT containing oestrogen and progestin is 1.24 (95%CI 1.01 to 1.54) compared to placebo. If women who do not take the medication are excluded it rose to 1.49. In other words, a woman who actually takes HRT increases her risk of breast cancer by 50% and that increase in risk starts after the end of the 3rd year (Chlebowski, Hendrix, Langer, *et al.* 2003).

Put another, less alarming, way, 2.28% of women on placebo developed breast cancer against 2.88% on HRT; an increase of 0.6%. This gives a number needed to harm of 167 over 5.6 years, which is a rate of six additional breast cancers per 1000 women over that period.

Combined HRT (oestrogen and progestogen) carried the greatest risk [HR 2.0 (95%CI 1.88 to 2.12)] while that for unopposed oestrogen was 1.30 (1.21 to 1.40) and for tibolone 1.45 (1.25 to 1.68).

Risk increased with duration of use, so that, after 10 years, combined HRT was associated with 19 extra breast cancers per 1000 women.

The risk declines once HRT is stopped so that it is back to baseline after 5 years (Million Women Study Collaborators 2003).

Women with a family history of breast cancer (NICE 2004)

* Assess the patient's risk (see below). Refer any patient with a risk that is at least moderate to a specialist breast unit. Refer women with a family history of a known genetic mutation direct to tertiary care.

* Reassure women with a family history that does not meet these criteria, with an explanation of the fact that breast cancer is so common that it will occur in many families where the risk in other members is not sufficiently raised for special surveillance to be needed. However, certain women with a relative with breast cancer who do not meet the criteria but who have other risk factors should be discussed with a breast specialist. Those factors are: a Jewish origin; or a history of breast cancer on the paternal side; or a history of tumours that may be associated with an increased risk of breast cancer (see note below).

* Women with at least moderate risk are likely to be offered annual mammography from age 40–49 and 3-yearly from age 50. Exceptionally, mammography may be offered from age 30–39.

* *Lifestyle.* Explain how lifestyle can affect breast cancer risk. Breast feeding and exercise can reduce risk while overweight, and possibly alcohol, may increase it.

* *HRT.* Explain that HRT increases the risk of breast cancer (see above). Advise a woman who decides to take it to use the lowest possible dose for the shortest possible time and to aim to stop by the age of 50. If possible, use an oestrogen-only product.

* *Combined oral contraception (COC).* Explain that it is associated with an increased risk of breast cancer and that, over the age of 35, the combination of increasing age, genetic risk and oral contraception make it hazardous. Under the age of 35 the risk of breast cancer is so low that any increase because of the COC is minimal. A patient with a *BRCA1* mutation

may decide to take oral contraception as protection against ovarian cancer. Specialist advice would be wise.

GENETIC RISK FOR WOMEN WITH A FAMILY HISTORY OF BREAST CANCER (NICE 2006)

Women at high risk (lifetime risk 30% or over)

- Two first degree female relatives diagnosed before an average age of 50.
- One first degree female relative and one second degree female relative, diagnosed before an average age of 50.
- Three or more first or second degree relatives diagnosed at any age.
- One first degree male relative diagnosed at any age.
- One first degree relative with bilateral breast cancer where the first cancer was diagnosed before age 50.
- One first or second degree relative with bilateral cancer, and one second degree relative with at least unilateral cancer, at any age.
- One relative with ovarian cancer and one with breast cancer, both diagnosed at any age, where one of them is a first degree relative and the other at least a second degree relative.

Moderate risk (lifetime risk 17–30%)

- One first-degree female relative with breast cancer diagnosed under the age of 40.
- One first-degree female relative and one first or second degree female relative diagnosed over an average age of 50.
- Those with at least one first or second degree relative with breast cancer diagnosed above the age of 40, but not falling into any of the above categories: only refer to secondary care if at least one other risk factor is present:
  - (a) Jewish ancestry;
  - (b) paternal family history (two or more relatives with breast cancer on father's side); or
  - (c) unusual cancers (e.g. bilateral or male).

Note 1: A first degree relative is a parent, or sibling, or child. A second degree relative is a grandparent, or grandchild, or aunt or uncle, or niece or nephew. A third degree relative is a great grandparent, or great grandchild, or great aunt or uncle, or first cousin, or grand niece or nephew.

All must be blood relatives of the patient and on the same side of the family.

Note 2: A woman with Jewish ancestry has a 5–10 times increased risk of carrying the BRCA1 or BRCA2 mutations.

Note 3: Non-breast cancers in the family which increase the risk of breast cancer: ovarian cancer; sarcoma at age < 45; glioma or childhood adrenal cortical carcinoma; multiple cancers at young ages.

Note 4: Consider referring more readily women from small families (e.g. with no sisters or aunts) who have therefore had less chance that a positive family history would show itself.

Note 5: Consider referring a woman with a third degree relative with breast cancer if that relative was male, or the cancer was bilateral.

Self-examination

Self-examination using a set technique has not been shown to reduce the mortality rate from breast cancer, while it does increase the rate of referral and of biopsy (Kosters and Gotzsche 2003). As a result women are encouraged to be 'breast aware' rather than to examine themselves regularly in a certain way. This means that a woman should be familiar with:

- the shape of her breasts, both with her arms raised and lowered;
- the skin and where it puckers or dimples;
- any pain or discomfort she feels at different times in her cycle;
- any lumps or thickenings in the breast and armpit which have always been there;
- the shape of the nipples and the degree to which they discharge.

If she then notices something which she fears is abnormal she will be in a position to judge whether it represents a change.

INFORMATION FOR PATIENTS

CancerBACUP: Helpline 0808 800 1234. www.cancerbacup.org.uk

CancerHelp (the information service of Cancer Research UK): 0207 061 8355 www.cancerhelp.org.uk

Be Breast Aware. A leaflet from the NHS Breast Screening Programme and Cancer Research UK, available for the Department of Health Publications orderline website: www.orderline.dh.gov.uk or by phoning 0300 123 1002

PERIPHERAL VASCULAR DISEASE

For details of the diagnosis of intermittent claudication see *Evidence-based Diagnosis in Primary Care* by A. F. Polmear (editor), published by Butterworth-Heinemann, 2008.

INTERMITTENT CLAUDICATION

- The prevalence in the population is 1.7% to 2.2% rising to 5% in those aged 55–74 (McDermott and McCarthy 1995).
- Once the finding of peripheral vascular disease (PVD) has been confirmed, the patient needs all appropriate measures to reduce the risk of coronary heart disease and stroke as well as reducing the risk of progression of the peripheral lesion (see page 168).

PROGNOSIS FOR PVD

- 75% remain stable or improve over 5 years. 20% develop worsening claudication and 1% require amputation. Mortality is two to three times that of others of the same age and sex without claudication. These results are hugely better than those expected before the use of aspirin and statins when 30% died within 5 years (DTB 2002).

EVALUATION WHEN PVD IS SUSPECTED

- ✳ Check the history for CHD risk factors. Ask about erectile dysfunction.
- ✳ Examine for femoral, popliteal and foot pulses; bruits, including iliac bruits; limb temperature; and venous filling time to determine whether arterial disease is present and, if so, where the obstruction is (McGee and Boyko 1998).
- ✳ Check the abdomen for a palpable aortic aneurysm.
- ✳ Check the ankle-brachial index (ABI; Table 15.2) (Hiatt 2001).
- ✳ Check blood tests: Hb, creatinine and electrolytes, lipid profile. Check the fasting blood sugar; 20% of claudicants are diabetic. Check LFTs; a statin is likely to be needed.
- ✳ Perform other investigations: urinary protein, ECG.

Table 15.2   The ankle–brachial index (ABI)

ABI	INTERPRETATION
> 1.3	Non-compressible, i.e. the artery is calcified at the ankle – test invalid
0.91 to 1.3	Normal
0.5 to 0.9	Mild to moderate peripheral arterial disease
0.00 to 0.49	Severe peripheral arterial disease

An ABI > 1.4 carries a risk of cardiovascular mortality that is equivalent to a ratio < 0.9 (Resnick, Lindsay, McDermott, *et al.* 2004).

TO MEASURE ABI

- ✳ Measure systolic pressure in both arms. Use the higher.
- ✳ Measure systolic pressure in the dorsalis pedis and the posterior tibial arteries of each leg with the cuff placed just above the malleoli. Use the higher on each side. A portable Doppler ultrasound is the most reliable way to measure the pressure.
- ✳ Calculate the ABI for each leg as the ankle systolic over the brachial systolic pressure.

MANAGEMENT AND SECONDARY PREVENTION (TIERNEY, FENNESSY, BOUCHIER AND HAYES 2000)

Treat those who are asymptomatic but have an ABI that is clearly abnormally low (e.g. < 0.7) as though they had claudication. Their risk of other cardiovascular events is the same as those with symptoms (DTB 2002). Only about a quarter of those with peripheral arterial disease have claudication (Makin, Silverman and Lip 2002).

- ✳ *Stop smoking.* Doing so reduces stroke risk, preventing one stroke for every 67 hypertensive men, smoking at least 20 cigarettes/day, who stop for 5 years (Wannamethee, Shaper, Whincup, *et al.* 1995). It also slows the progression of the limb ischaemia (Hiatt 2001).
- ✳ *Exercise* despite pain. This can increase the distance that can be walked by 150% and improve rest pain (Leng, Fowler and Ernst 2004). Walking should be for at least 30 minutes at least three times a week for at least 6 months before benefit is likely (Gardner and Poehlman 1995). Be specific and ask to see the patient frequently at first to report progress. Only about

half of patients actually walk as recommended, citing lack of supervision and lack of specific instruction as reasons for this poor performance (Bartelink, Stoffers, Biesheuvel, *et al.* 2004). Warn the patient who is not used to walking to avoid trauma to the feet (e.g. blisters) which could be hazardous in ischaemic legs.

* *Check the patient's footwear.* Tight socks and garters can compromise the circulation.
* *Antiplatelet therapy* is indicated in all cases. Low-dose aspirin given to 100 patients with peripheral vascular disease will protect nine from acute arterial occlusion over 19 months (Antiplatelet Trialists' Collaboration 1994). Antiplatelet drugs reduce all cardiovascular events in patients with claudication by 23% (Scottish Intercollegiate Guidelines Network 2006). Use clopidogrel if aspirin is contraindicated or not tolerated.
* *Lower cholesterol.* Aim for a total cholesterol < 4.0 mmol/l and an LDL-cholesterol < 2.0 mmol/l (see page 168). As well as reducing the risk of cardiovascular events, this will improve walking distance and the ABI as early as 6 months after starting treatment (Mondillo, Ballo, Barbati, *et al.* 2003).
* *Treat hypertension* in those with a sustained BP of 140/90 or above, even though lowering the blood pressure may initially worsen symptoms. Use the same sequence of drugs you would use in a patient without PVD. Fears have been raised about two classes of drugs in PVD:
  1. that beta-blockers would worsen claudication. This has not been borne out by trials, although their use in critical leg ischaemia would possibly be unwise (DTB 2002).
  2. that ACE inhibitors may precipitate renal failure. One study found that 59% of patients referred for peripheral angiography had stenosis of one or both renal arteries (Choudhri, Cleland, Rowlands, *et al.* 1990). However, they reduce mortality in those at risk of cardiovascular disease without renal artery stenosis and so are indicated if an ultrasound scan of the renal arteries has excluded stenosis, or if serum creatinine is measured before and after starting the ACE inhibitor and there is no rise (see page 139).

     A small study from Australia found that ramipril markedly improved the distance walked (Ahimastos, Lawler, Reid, *et al.* 2006) quite apart from the benefits of its action in relation to cardiovascular disease.

* *Treat diabetes*, if present, meticulously. The combination of diabetes and PVD puts the feet even more at risk.
* *Treat obesity*, even though no studies have specifically noted the effect of doing so in PAD.

REFERRAL

* Refer if walking distance is 50% less than normal or < 100 yards.
* Refer if there is rest pain.
* *Patients under 50.* Refer all young patients presenting with intermittent claudication. They are more likely to have a non-atheromatous cause for their claudication.
* *Refer urgently* if the limb is at risk. Patients with a short history of rest pain and critical ischaemia on examination need urgent admission for heparin and assessment for arterial surgery.
* *Admit immediately* if there is acute limb ischaemia, as shown by a pale, pulseless, painful and cold limb.

Revascularization is indicated if the limb is at risk because of critical ischaemia but rarely for claudication alone.

* Angioplasty is the treatment of choice if the lesion is amenable.
* Mortality after aorto-iliac (A-I) reconstruction is 3% and after femoro-popliteal (F-P) reconstruction is 1%.
* 80–90% of large grafts (e.g. A-I) remain patent for 5–10 years but smaller grafts especially those with poor run-off, do less well (Makin, Silverman and Lip 2002).

DRUG TREATMENT

Pentoxifylline, naftidrofuryl, cilostazol, cinnarizine, and inositol nicotinate may all improve walking distance slightly, but no more than exercise. Unlike exercise, there is no evidence that they improve the prognosis. They may be indicated in patients with severe symptoms despite 3–6 months of medical treatment. The best evidence is for cilostazol (Burns, Gough and Bradbury 2003) and naftidrofuryl (De Backer, Vander Stichele, Lehert, *et al.* 2009).

BUERGER'S DISEASE

* Refer to exclude embolic disease, especially if a cardiac murmur or arrhythmia is present; the differential diagnosis includes multiple emboli. If Buerger's disease is confirmed:
* Explain the importance of stopping smoking; the disease is almost entirely smoking related.
* Refer if digital gangrene develops.

RAYNAUD'S PHENOMENON (ISENBERG AND BLACK 1995)

Evaluation when Raynaud's phenomenon is suspected

* *Young patients* with a typical history of episodes in which the extremities turn white then blue or red, before recovering completely need no investigations.
* *Patients in whom the onset is aged 30 or over,* or who have evidence of other disorders, need investigations: Hb, ESR, antinuclear antibodies, other autoantibodies (especially cold agglutinins), U&Es, LFTs, TFTs.

TREATMENT

Mild symptoms

* Check that the patient is not taking medication which may exacerbate it: beta-blockers, ergotamine, oral contraceptives.
* Encourage the patient to keep the hands warm and not to smoke.

Moderate symptoms

* Calcium-channel blockade (e.g. long-acting nifedipine 20–30 mg daily).
* Sildenafil or another phosphodiesterase inhibitor. Although not licensed for this, early work suggests that they can relieve pain and promote ulcer healing in secondary Raynaud's phenomenon and possibly in primary Raynaud's (Levien 2006).

A 2-week trial of each drug will establish whether it is of any benefit.

Severe symptoms

* Refer, especially if there is ulceration or gangrene. They may benefit from i.v. prostacyclin.

PATIENT ORGANIZATION

The Raynaud's and Scleroderma Association, 112 Crewe Road, Alsager, Cheshire ST7 2JA. Tel. 01270 872776. www.raynauds.org.uk

ABDOMINAL AORTIC ANEURYSM (AAA)

* Screening for aortic aneurysm can almost halve the number of AAA-related deaths in men aged 65–79, although it does not seem to reduce all-cause mortality (Greenhalgh and Powell 2007). In the UK men are offered a screen at the age of 65.
* All cause mortality for patients with small aneurysms 6 years after diagnosis is 30% regardless of whether 'watchful waiting' or operation is chosen (UK Small Aneurysm Trial Participants 1998).
* The 30-day mortality after repair of asymptomatic aneurysms is < 5%. For ruptured aneurysms it is over 80% (BHF 2003).
* Elective surgical repair is recommended to patients when:
  (a) the aneurysm diameter is > 5.5 cm; or
  (b) the growth rate is > 1 cm/year; or
  (c) the aneurysm becomes tender; or
  (d) iliac or thoracic repair is needed.
* Order an abdominal USS for men aged 60 with a family history of a first degree relative with AAA. Their risk is increased four to ten-fold (BHF 2003). Subsequent scans are usually performed every 3–5 years or as agreed by the local vascular team and radiology department.
* Refer all clinically detectable aneurysms unless the quality of life precludes surgery.
* Order an USS if the aorta appears prominent but it is not clear clinically whether it is aneurysmal.
* Admit any aneurysm that is tender. Rupture may be imminent.

* Organize a CHD secondary prevention programme for all patients after detection of AAA (see page 168).

ANAL PROBLEMS

FISSURE

The healing rate of fissure when treated with placebo is 35% over the course of most published studies. Topical preparations hardly improve on this (Nelson 2003). Sphincterotomy is successful in 90% but at the risk of incontinence in 10%.

* Check that the fissure is not secondary to another disease: sexually transmitted infection, inflammatory bowel disease, or rectal or anal carcinoma.
* Recommend fibre to keep the stool soft. If there is constipation treat that vigorously.
* Recommend a lubricant, e.g. KY jelly, while waiting for spontaneous healing. Lidocaine gel is no more effective and carries the risk of sensitization.
* Institute a trial of a topical preparation, e.g. glyceryl trinitrate 0.4% rectal ointment. Headaches are common. A result superior to placebo is more likely in chronic than in acute fissures (Scholefield, Bock, Marla, *et al.* 2003). Topical calcium-channel blockers may be equally effective with less headache but they are not available in the UK.
* Refer patients who are not improving to a surgeon with a view to sphincterotomy, if the patient wishes to take the risk of subsequent incontinence. Anal stretch is no longer recommended, being less effective with a risk of incontinence that is greater than sphincterotomy.

HAEMORRHOIDS

* Check for pointers towards underlying disease: altered bowel habit, tenesmus, weight loss, tiredness, or abdominal pain. Refer any patient with a 'red flag' for colorectal carcinoma (see page 217), including rectal bleeding over the age of 45 that is not obviously due to haemorrhoids.
* Examine the abdomen and the rectum digitally and with a proctoscope.
* Treat constipation with a change to a high-fibre diet which should continue for life.

* Explain that any itching is due to a failure to clean the anus after defecation. Recommend wet wipes or soap and water. If there is leakage recommend petroleum jelly as a barrier after cleaning.
* Discuss the question of referral. First and second degree haemorrhoids are likely to be treated with injections of sclerosant, rubber banding, infrared coagulation or cryotherapy. Third or fourth degree haemorrhoids are more likely to need haemorrhoidectomy.
* Be prepared to prescribe powerful analgesia to patients after surgical haemorrhoidectomy. The operation is often performed as a day case and the post-operative course can be very painful (Acheson and Scholefield 2008).

PRURITUS ANI

* Examine the anus and rectum, looking for secondary causes: haemorrhoids, extensive skin tags, infection, infestation, malignancy, and other dermatological conditions. Threadworm infestation is the commonest cause of secondary pruritus ani, and is suggested by itching that is worse at night and where others in the family are itching.
* If the problem is primary, explain that the anus is being irritated, probably by faecal material and possibly by soap or other irritants. The treatment is to keep the anus clean and dry. This means:
  (a) washing the anus after each bowel movement with soap and water (washing the soap off well) or by using a 'wet wipe';
  (b) drying the anus with a towel or hairdryer. The obese and others who report that the area is always moist should insert a soft cotton tissue between the buttocks and wear cotton underwear;
  (c) repeating the cleansing during the day if prone to seepage through the anus.
* Other practical measures are to avoid scratching (keeping the fingernails trimmed), and to note whether certain foods worsen the problem.
* Those whose sleep is disturbed might benefit from a 1-week course of sedative antihistamine at night and/or a 1-week course of a mild steroid ointment, such as Anusol-HC.

GALLSTONES (CHOLELITHIASIS)

✳ *Do not refer patients with asymptomatic gallstones* unless they fall into one of the categories below. They are often discovered during evaluation of other problems and are best left alone unless symptoms appear. Only 20% will develop pain over the next 20 years. On a population basis, people with stones are no more likely to have pain than those without. If, however, the gallbladder is removed, the prevalence of pain is greater than if it is left in situ. Even doctors think that up to 30% of cholecystectomies are inappropriate (Johnson 1993).

✳ *Refer patients with symptomatic gallstones.* Cholecystectomy is indicated as half will develop severe symptoms or complications over the next 20 years.

✳ Also refer:

(a) patients who are jaundiced;

(b) children with pigment stones;

(c) where the risk from complications is high: e.g. where a patient has diabetes (diabetics have a 20% chance of developing emphysematous cholecystitis), or is on long-term parenteral nutrition or is immunosuppressed;

(d) where there is a risk of cancer (Tait and Little 1995):

■ the gallbladder is non-functioning, or there is scarring, calcification or thickening; or

■ the gallbladder epithelium shows adenomyosis or papillomatosis; or

■ the history is chronic.

✳ Treat severe pain with diclofenac IM. It seems to reduce the progression to acute cholecystitis (Indar and Beckingham 2002). Treat less severe pain with an NSAID orally.

OUTCOMES OF CHOLECYSTECTOMY

● 90% patients will be symptom free after cholecystectomy.

● 5–10% patients will continue to be troubled by pain. Some of these people will have retained bile duct stones; others will have biliary dyskinesia (see below).

Post–cholecystectomy syndrome

● This is caused by *biliary dyskinesia* which is a structural or functional disorder of the ampulla of Vater. Patients experience periodic colicky pain with variable associated findings of transient elevation of bilirubin or liver enzymes, suggesting cholestasis, or elevation of serum amylase and lipase levels.

● The biliary tree, and less often the pancreatic duct, may be dilated on direct cholangiography and pancreatography.

● Sphincter pressures may be elevated when measured during endoscopic ductal manometry. Small residual calculi are discovered in some patients.

● Endoscopic sphincterotomy may be curative in patients with objective findings but is controversial in patients with pain alone.

● Episodic pain caused by papillary disorders may have been responsible for the symptoms that prompted cholecystectomy and may be the cause of continued pain after surgery.

CHOLECYSTITIS

Admit patients with acute cholecystitis, especially if the hospital has a policy of early surgery. Surgery during the attack reduces the number of days in hospital with no increase in adverse effects (Papi, Catarci and D'Ambrosio 2004). If admission is not possible, patients with acute cholecystitis can be managed successfully at home if the diagnosis is clear and the condition relatively mild. However, it carries risks: without a scan the diagnosis may be wrong; and 20% of patients need emergency surgery because of overwhelming infection or perforation of the gallbladder (Indar and Beckingham 2002). Overall the mortality rate from acute cholecystitis is 10%.

TREATMENT OF ACUTE CHOLECYSTITIS IN PRIMARY CARE

✳ Encourage fluids and a bland fat-free diet.

✳ Give adequate analgesia.

✳ Give oral antibiotics covering aerobic and anaerobic bacteria (co-amoxiclav; or a cephalosporin plus metronidazole).

* Request FBC, LFTs and U&Es – many hospitals can provide results within 24 hours if notified.
* Request an abdominal USS as an outpatient to confirm the diagnosis – refer to the surgeons for cholecystectomy if gallstones are confirmed.
* Refer immediately if jaundiced (cholangitis is a medical emergency) or there is no improvement within 48–72 hours or if the patient is too ill to take oral fluids and antibiotics.

INGUINAL HERNIA

* A recent US study found that patients managed by 'watchful waiting' for minimally symptomatic hernia had no more pain or discomfort after 2 years than those offered surgery (Fitzgibbons, Hurder-Giobbie, Gibbs, *et al.* 2006).
* The danger of incarceration or obstruction from an uncomplicated inguinal hernia is low: in the above study only two out of 364 men allocated to 'watchful waiting' rather than surgery had developed these complications over 4 years: a rate (0.5%) that was lower than that of surgical complications following prophylactic repair (22%).
* 31% of patients offered 'watchful waiting' requested surgery in the subsequent 4 years, mainly because of an increase in pain. The success rate of their operations was the same as for those operated on at the start of the trial.
* Offer surgery to those in sufficient pain or discomfort to want it, but warn that there is a 10% chance that they will experience chronic pain following surgery, sufficient to interfere with everyday activities (Cunningham, Temple, Mitchell, *et al.* 1996).
* Reassure those whose symptoms do not warrant surgery at this stage that delaying surgery is very unlikely to be harmful and may mean that they never need it.

VARICOSE VEINS

* Ascertain the reason for the patient's concern. If it is swelling, heaviness, aching or itching, check that the symptoms are due to the varicose veins (i.e. that they are worse after prolonged standing, and relieved by a support stocking or by elevation). If it is cosmetic,

warn that varicose veins may recur after surgery. If it is a fear of haemorrhage or deep vein thrombosis, explain that haemorrhage is rare and that deep vein thrombosis is unrelated to varicosities.
* Refer in the following situations (NICE 2001):
  ■ ulcer, whether healed or not;
  ■ progressive skin changes;
  ■ recurrent superficial thrombophlebitis;
  ■ symptoms, as above, which appear to be related to the veins, and which are adversely affecting the patient's quality of life. However, warn that surgery may well have no effect on the symptoms (Bradbury, Evans, Allan, *et al.* 1999).
* Refer more urgently if an ulcer is progressing or is painful despite treatment.
* Refer urgently if a varicose vein has bled and is at risk of rebleeding.
* Admit if a varicose vein is currently bleeding (meanwhile tell the patient to lie down with the leg elevated while waiting for the ambulance).

Evidence of peripheral arterial disease (ABI < 0.8) argues in favour of referral (see page 437). These patients should not use compression bandaging or support stockings.

SUPERFICIAL WOUNDS

The expertise of general practitioners in relation to wounds varies hugely. The general principle should be: only deal with wounds that you are competent to manage; refer if in doubt.

BURNS

WHO CAN BE MANAGED WITHOUT REFERRAL? (HUDSPITH AND RAYATT 2004)

Patients with:

(a) a burn affecting < 5% of the body area (see Table 15.3); and
(b) a superficial partial-thickness burn only; and
(c) the ability to care for themselves.
* Superficial partial-thickness burns are pink, blister, blanche on pressure, and sensation to pinprick is intact. Deep partial-thickness burns are red but do not blanch on pressure and pinprick is not felt as being sharp. Full thickness

Table 15.3	Guide to the extent of a burn in an adult
AREA BURNT	**PERCENTAGE OF TOTAL BODY SURFACE AFFECTED**
One side of one hand	1.5%
Whole face or whole of the back of the head	3.5%
Whole of the back or front of one hand and arm	5%
Whole of the back or front of one foot, leg and thigh	9%
Whole of front or back of torso	13%

Do not include mere erythema in the calculation of the area affected.

Values in children are different. The smaller the child, the more the head represents a greater percentage of the whole than in adults.

burns are white or charred, and are also insensate. Full-thickness burns need early surgery.

● A simpler guide than Table 15.3 to estimating burnt surface area is to count the patient's own handprint as 1%. See how many handprints can be fitted into the burnt area.

FIRST AID

1. Remove any clothing unless it is stuck to the burn.
2. Cool the burn for 20 minutes with tepid tap water. This is worthwhile up to 20 minutes after the injury. Avoid very cold water; vasoconstriction can worsen the damage.
3. Give appropriate analgesia. Opioids may be needed.
4. Remove any dead tissue. Leave small blisters intact; the rate of infection is lower than if the blister is aspirated or de-roofed (Swain, Berge, Wakeley, *et al.* 1987). However, it is customary to de-roof large ones with sterile scissors (Benson, Dickson and Boyce 2006).
5. Cover the burn with Clingfilm or put a clean plastic bag over a burnt hand. If they are not available, cover the burn with a clean cotton sheet. Leave it on until the patient is either seen in hospital or a dressing can be applied in general practice.
6. Leave burns on the face and perineum exposed.

DRESSINGS IN GENERAL PRACTICE

(a) Tulle dressings, impregnated with paraffin. Cover the dressing with cotton gauze and a crepe bandage. Change the dressing after 2 days, then every 3–5 days.
(b) Calcium alginate dressings, e.g. Sorbsan or Kaltostat, for exuding burns.
(c) Occlusive dressings, e.g. Opsite, Tegaderm, Spyroflex, Granuflex or Tegasorb. These are less bulky than the above and permit the patient to wash without the wound getting wet. They should only be changed weekly. They should not be used if infection is present, or there has been a delay in presentation or the wound is dirty.

Flamazine (silver sulfadiazine) cream on gauze is no longer favoured after trials showing it to be inferior to other dressings (Apostoli and Caula 2004).

TETANUS PROPHYLAXIS

Burn wounds are easily contaminated. Provide a booster if necessary (see page 50).

Refer the above patients:

(a) if healing is incomplete after 2 weeks;
(b) if there is invasive sepsis needing i.v. antibiotics.

DOG AND CAT BITES

About 250,000 people attend minor injury units or emergency departments in the UK each year because of a dog bite (Morgan and Palmer 2007). Many more victims regard their injury as too trivial to seek medical help. Because a small number go on to develop severe infection, or unsightly scarring, the injury can only be regarded as trivial in retrospect.

The following advice is based on consensus; there is little evidence on the management of this problem.

First aid (National Health Service 2009; DTB 2004)

Irrigate the wound thoroughly with warm tap water. If it is bleeding, allow it to continue to do so.

* Do not suture in primary care.
* Give analgesia if necessary.
* Elevate the arm or leg if that is where the patient has been bitten.

* Decide on the need to refer to the emergency department. This is advised in:
  (a) penetrating wounds, in which nerves, tendons or other tissues could be injured. This includes the skull in infants with bites to the head;
  (b) bites to the face or to poorly vascularized areas (cartilage of the ear or nose);
  (c) wounds that need debridement, suturing or reconstructive surgery;
  (d) wounds that have already developed infection that is severe, or not responding to treatment or where the patient is systemically unwell;
  (e) patients vulnerable to infection, because of diabetes, cirrhosis or low immunocompetence.
* Decide on the need for antibiotics, if not sending to the emergency department. Give them for:
  (a) all cat (or human) bites that have broken the skin;
  (b) all bites to the head, genitals, hands or feet;
  (c) puncture wounds, crush wounds and wounds with devitalized tissue;
  (d) patients vulnerable to infection (see above);
  (e) patients with prosthetic valves or joints.

Use co-amoxiclav for 7 days; or metronidazole plus doxycycline in those intolerant of co-amoxiclav. However, antibiotics are unnecessary if the bite occurred over 48 hours before and there is no evidence of infection.

* *Tetanus.* Check the patient's tetanus status and give a booster if necessary.
* *Rabies.* Consider the risk of rabies if the bite occurred abroad (see page 59).
* Warn patients who are not referred to look for signs of infection and report them.
* Review all, except the most trivial, within 48 hours.

SNAKE BITES (WARRELL 2005)

In the UK this means a bite from the only native venomous snake, the adder (*Vipera berus*).

* Keep the patient quiet and still. If the bite is on a limb, immobilize it to reduce blood flow.
* Do not apply a tourniquet or a compression bandage or interfere with the wound in any way.
* Transfer to hospital immediately. The danger is of an anaphylactoid reaction to the venom

which may appear within minutes of the bite, or hours later.

* If a systemic reaction occurs while the patient is still in your care, give an oral antihistamine, a parenteral antihistamine or intramuscular adrenaline accordingly to the severity of the reaction. Shock, or closure of the upper airway or severe bronchospasm would warrant the latter. Make sure a written note of what you have given accompanies the patient to hospital.

WEEVER FISH STINGS

These are common in people who swim or paddle in the Mediterranean or North Atlantic. It feels at first like a scratch but rapidly worsens to a **severe** pain after 2–3 minutes. Swelling and redness will be visible. The pain eases within a few hours if left untreated.

* Immerse the affected area in hot water (as hot as can be tolerated). This denatures the protein-based venom. Pain is reduced within 10–20 minutes but keep the affected part in very hot water for 30–90 minutes. The longer the delay before heat is applied the longer it needs to be continued.
* Remove any spines from the wound with tweezers.
* Prescribe or advise analgesia.
* Warn the patient to return if signs of infection develop.

LACERATIONS (CLINICAL KNOWLEDGE SUMMARIES 2009A)

* Control bleeding – 10 minutes of pressure usually suffices, unless a vein or an artery is damaged.
* Clean the wound with sterile normal saline solution or tap water.
* Check for:
  ■ damage to peripheral nerves (altered sensation beyond the wound or weakness of muscles supplied by nerves in the vicinity of the wound) and tendons.
  ■ damage involving the blood supply to structures beyond the wound. *This advice is particularly important for lacerations of face and limbs.*

- evidence of *any* infection in a hand wound.
- evidence of serious cellulitis in a wound over a joint.
- foreign bodies. If shattered glass was involved, X-ray for further fragments is needed.
- devitalized tissue which will need extensive debridement.

If a problem is detected, refer to the local emergency department or plastic surgery team.

* Decide if you are competent to close the laceration – if not, refer to the local emergency department. Facial lacerations where a good cosmetic result is needed are usually better sutured in secondary care. Before referring check for intraoral penetration – 'through and through' wounds require specialist attention.

  - Only use adhesive strips, rather than sutures, if the wound is ≤ 5 cm, there are no risk factors for infection, the wound margins come together easily without leaving a dead space beneath the skin, *and* the wound will not be subject to excessive flexing, tension or wetting.
  - After suturing apply a clear vapour-permeable dressing, or an absorbent dressing (e.g. Melolin) for wounds with more exudation.
  - Give the patient written instructions on wound care, including the need to keep it dry and to return if the wound becomes infected.

* Check *tetanus status* – provide a booster if necessary.

* *Removal of sutures.* Healing times vary with the site of the laceration and the age of the patient. When in doubt it is better to remove sutures earlier than later; the cosmetic result is better. Slight gaping of wound can be treated with *Steristrips*. Remove sutures as follows:

  - face: after 3–5 days;
  - upper limb, scalp, trunk: after 5–7 days;
  - lower limb, back: after 7–10 days;
  - over a joint: 10–14 days.

Always remove sutures if the suture line is moist and red – this signals local wound infection. If there is no improvement, or pus develops, commence oral antibiotics (flucloxacillin or erythromycin).

* *People with diabetes, vascular disease or suppressed immunity.* Give prophylactic antibiotics for all but the smallest of wounds.

WOUNDS AT HIGH RISK OF INFECTION (CLINICAL KNOWLEDGE SUMMARIES 2009B)

If the risk of infection is high, e.g. because of contamination with soil, faeces, saliva or pus, or the patient is at high risk of infection, e.g. because of diabetes or immunosuppression:

* Do not close the laceration. Keep the wound open with a non-adherent dressing.
* Give co-amoxiclav if the wound is contaminated, otherwise use flucloxacillin. If the patient is intolerant of penicillins use erythromycin.
* Refer to the emergency department for human tetanus immunoglobulin, regardless of the patient's immunization status, if the wound is contaminated with manure or soil AND is at high risk for tetanus (puncture wound, devitalized tissue or foreign body present, OR untreated for > 6 hours).
* Warn the patient to keep the wound dry and to report any sign of infection.
* Review in 3–5 days and close the wound if there is no infection.

COMMON POSTOPERATIVE COMPLICATIONS

- With reduced hospital stays for surgical patients and an upsurge in day case surgery family doctors are facing a rising incidence of postoperative problems. In general, early referral back to the patient's surgeon is encouraged for all but the most trivial of complications.
- Major surgery triggers a catabolic response that is followed by anabolic activity. Patients can experience dramatic loss of weight and suffer fatigue during the weeks and months after major surgery. Nutritional deficiency may occur during recovery if the diet does not meet the needs of the healing process.
- Low mood after operations is common. This can be a bereavement reaction, especially if patients have had a major amputation or suffered the removal of vital structures. Disfigurement and deformity after surgery can cause a great deal of distress. Standard

care for depressive illness can be deployed with success for such cases.

● Pain: postoperative pain syndromes are protean. Often there is no clear explanation for the pain. The symptoms are very real for the patient and require a sympathetic approach to achieve control (see page 676). Referral to the local pain clinic is advised if there is no identifiable reason for the pain and simple measures for controlling the pain have not succeeded.

ABDOMINAL WOUNDS

* *Cellulitis*. Use an antibiotic which covers streptococci and staphylococci, e.g. erythromycin or co-amoxiclav.
* *Abscess*. Incise or refer immediately.
* *Serous ooze*. Refer for an early outpatient appointment.
* *Dehiscence*. Cover with clean tissues or a towel and admit immediately. Treat shock with i.v. morphine.

LOWER LIMB IMMOBILIZATION

Continue the measures for the prevention of venous thromboembolism (VTE) started in hospital:

■ Low molecular weight heparin, given daily for the duration of the immobilization, significantly reduces the risk of VTE. Some surgeons give it to all with lower limb immobilization; others reserve it for those at higher risk, e.g. those > 40 years old and those with a lower limb fracture (Testroote, Stigter, de Visser, *et al.* 2008). NICE, in the first draft of its advice (March 2009) (NICE 2009), recommends specific durations of treatment: 28–35 days for elective hip replacement or following hip fracture; 10–14 days following knee replacement.

■ Graduated compression stockings should be worn after all inpatient surgery, until the patient has returned to full activity. Exceptions to this are those with peripheral artery disease, peripheral neuropathy and other conditions of the legs which put the circulation or health of the skin at risk. NICE recommends that in certain higher risk situations the stockings be thigh length, while a group of Australian

authors points out that below knee stockings are more practical with no evidence that they are less effective (Phillips, Gallagher and Buchan 2008).

GASTROINTESTINAL SURGERY

* Be aware of the possibility of:
  (a) B_{12} deficiency after terminal ileum resection or gastric surgery;
  (b) malabsorption after small bowel resection;
  (c) blind loop syndrome after colonic surgery.

ANAL SURGERY

* Salt baths three times a day, and especially after stool.
* Dab the anus dry with a paper towel.
* Keep stool soft but not bulky. Use a laxative (but not fibre) and glycerol suppositories.
* Prevent impaction with lidocaine gel administered into the anal canal via a nozzle.
* If impaction occurs, use a stool-softening enema, e.g. Micolette or Fletcher's Enemette.
* Treat diarrhoea promptly; it will excoriate the perianal wound.

ARTERIAL SURGERY

* Refer immediately if:
  (a) a graft blocks that was previously patent; or
  (b) emboli occur distal to a graft.
* Refer urgently to outpatients if a pulsatile swelling appears at the site of a graft. It is probably an anastomotic aneurysm.
* Suspect graft infection if a patient with a graft develops a fever without obvious cause.

EYE SURGERY

* Refer immediately if any of the following occur:
  (a) hyphaema;
  (b) intraocular infection;
  (c) iris prolapse;
  (d) acute glaucoma;
  (e) retinal detachment (1–2% of all cataract extractions);

(f) iritis which was not present on discharge;

(g) postoperative conjunctivitis not settling after 10 days of antibiotic/steroid topically.

GYNAECOLOGICAL SURGERY

* *Termination*: re-admit if bleeding is more than a normal period. There may be retained products of conception.

* *Fever* is frequently due to urinary infection after catheterization. Otherwise, after hysterectomy, consider vault haematoma, which will need re-referral.

* *Laparoscopy* may cause diaphragmatic irritation with shoulder-tip pain. It will settle.

TONSILLECTOMY

* *Throat pain and otalgia.* Give antibiotics.

* *Tonsillar bed infection.* Give antibiotics.

* *Haemorrhage.* Admit if the loss is more than one cupful or continues for more than 24 hours. Even milder haemorrhage may require admission if there is not adequate supervision at home (Kuo, Hegarty, Johnson, *et al.* 1995).

UROSURGERY

* *Cystoscopy:* haematuria more than 24 hours after cystoscopy may signify infection. Patients need an MSU, antibiotics, and rest. If severe, take blood for Hb, give tranexamic acid 1 g t.d.s. and consider admission.

* *TURP:* haematuria, urgency, dysuria, frequency and incontinence may take 2–3 weeks to resolve. Worsening symptoms from the second week suggest infection.

ENDOCRINE SURGERY

* Be aware of the possibility of:

  (a) hypocalcaemia after thyroid surgery;

  (b) Addison's disease after pituitary/adrenal gland surgery;

  (c) diabetes mellitus after pancreatic surgery;

  (d) diabetes insipidus after pituitary/brain surgery;

  (e) premature ovarian failure after gynaecological procedures.

RETURNING TO WORK AFTER OPERATIONS

The following guidance is for open surgery. Timings can often be halved if the operation was performed by laparoscopy. The timings assume that recovery was uncomplicated.

(a) *Time off is not usually needed after:* vasectomy; varicose vein injections; anal dilatation; pilonidal sinus, provided the patient can be released for regular dressings.

(b) *2 weeks for sedentary workers, 4 weeks for heavy workers:* unilateral inguinal or femoral hernia; appendicectomy.

(c) *4 weeks for sedentary workers, 6 weeks for heavy workers:* bilateral inguinal hernias; small umbilical or incisional hernias.

(d) *4 weeks for sedentary workers, 12 weeks for heavy workers:* gastric and duodenal surgery; femoro-popliteal grafts.

(e) *6 weeks for sedentary workers, 12 weeks for heavy workers:* cholecystectomy; abdominal or vaginal hysterectomy; large incisional or umbilical hernias; repair of a previous inguinal hernia repair; colectomy; aorto-iliac and aortic grafts; coronary artery bypass and heart valve surgery; nephrectomy; an abdominal wound weakened by postoperative infection or haematoma.

SPECIAL CASES

(a) *Simple mastectomy:* as soon as the wound has healed.

(b) *Varicose vein ligation, anal fistula:* 2 weeks.

(c) *Haemorrhoidectomy, deep vein thrombosis, TURP:* 4 weeks.

(d) *Retinal detachment:* if surgery is successful, the heaviest manual work should be avoided permanently.

Individual differences in personality, wound size, wound healing, the presence of other illnesses and the type of work performed will all lead to variation in the advice given. For further details, see:

■ Palmer KT, Cox RAF, Brown I. *Fitness for Work: The Medical Aspects*; 4th edition: Oxford Medical Publications 2007;

■ The Working Fit website: www.workingfit.com;

■ The recommendations of the Royal College of Surgeons of England: www.rcseng.ac.uk/patient_information/return-to-work.

References

Acheson, A., Scholefield, J., 2008. Management of haemorrhoids. BMJ 336, 380–383.

Ahimastos, A., Lawler, A., Reid, C., et al., 2006. Brief communication: ramipril markedly improves walking ability in patients with peripheral arterial disease. Ann. Int. Med. 144, 660–664.

Antiplatelet Trialists' Collaboration, 1994. Collaborative overview of randomised trials of antiplatelet therapy - II: maintenance of vascular graft or arterial patency by antiplatelet therapy. BMJ 308, 159–168.

Apostoli, A., Caula, C., 2004. Treatment of burns is controversial. BMJ 329, 292.

Bandolier, 2004. Topical NSAID for mastalgia. Bandolier July.

Bartelink, M.L., Stoffers, H., Biesheuvel, C., et al., 2004. Walking exercise in patients with intermittent claudication. experience in routine clinical practice. Br. J. Gen. Pract. 54, 196–200.

Benson, A., Dickson, W., Boyce, D., 2006. ABC of wound healing: burns. BMJ 332, 649–652.

BHF, 2003. Abdominal Aortic Aneurysms. British Heart Foundation Factfile, London. Available: www.bhf.org.uk/factfiles.

Binder, A., 2001. Neck Pain. BMJ Publishing Group.

Blanks, R., Moss, S., McGahan, C., et al., 2000. Effect of NHS breast screening programme on mortality from breast cancer in England and Wales, 1990–8: comparison of observed with predicted mortality. BMJ 321, 665–669.

Borchgrevink, G., Kaasa, A., McDonagh, D., et al., 1998. Acute treatment of whiplash neck injuries. Spine 23, 25–31.

Boyd, N., McGuire, V., Shannon, P., et al., 1988. Effect of a low-fat high-carbohydrate diet on symptoms of cyclical mastopathy. Lancet 2, 128–132.

Bradbury, A., Evans, C., Allan, P., et al., 1999. What are the symptoms of varicose veins? Edinburgh vein study cross sectional population survey. BMJ 318, 353–356.

Bryant, R., Moulds, M., Guthrie, R., Nixon, R., 2003. Treating acute stress disorder following mild traumatic brain injury. Am. J. Psychiatry 160, 585–587.

Bundred, N., 2004. Breast pain. Clin. Evid. 12, 1–2.

Burns, P., Gough, S., Bradbury, A., 2003. Management of peripheral arterial disease in primary care. BMJ 326, 584–588.

Carroll, L., Holm, L., Hogg-Johnson, et al., 2008. Course and prognostic factors for neck pain in whiplash-related disorders (WAD): results of the Bone and Joint Decade 2000-2010 Task Force on Neck Pain and its Associated Disorders. Spine 33 (Suppl. 4), S83–S92.

Cassidy, J., Carroll, L., Cote, P., et al., 2000. Effect of eliminating compensation for pain and suffering on the outcome of insurance claims for whiplash injury. N. Engl. J. Med. 342, 1179–1186.

Chlebowski, R., Hendrix, S., Langer, R., et al., 2003. Influence of estrogen plus progestin on breast cancer and mammography in healthy postmenopausal women. JAMA 289, 3243–3253.

Choudhri, A., Cleland, J., Rowlands, P., et al., 1990. Unsuspected renal artery stenosis in peripheral vascular disease. BMJ 301, 1197–1198.

Clinical Knowledge Summaries, 2009a. Laceration – low risk of infection. National Library for Health. Available: www.cks.library.uk (search on Laceration).

Clinical Knowledge Summaries, 2009b. Laceration - high risk of infection. National Library for Health. Available: www.cks.library.uk (search on Laceration).

Colacurci, N., Mele, D., De Franciscis, P., et al., 1998. Effects of tibolone on the breast. Eur. J. Obstet. Gynecol. Reprod. Biol. 80, 235–238.

Cunningham, J., Temple, W., Mitchell, P., et al., 1996. Pain in the post-repair patient. Ann. Surg. 224, 598–602.

De Backer, T., Vander Stichele, R., Lehert, P., et al., 2009. Naftidrofuryl for intermittant claudication: meta-analysis based on individual patient data. BMJ 338, 703.

DTB, 2002. Managing peripheral arterial disease in primary care. Drug. Ther. Bull. 40, 5–8.

DTB, 2004. Managing bites from humans and other mammals. Drug Ther. Bull. 42 (9), 67–70.

Fitzgibbons, J.J., Hurder-Giobbie, A., Gibbs, J., et al., 2006. Watchful waiting vs. repair of inguinal hernia in minimally symptomatic men: a randomized clinical trial. JAMA 295, 285–292.

Fleminger, S., Greenwood, R., Oliver, D., 2003. Pharmacological management for agitation and aggression in people with acquired brain injury. The Cochrane Database Syst. Rev. Issue 1.

Gardner, A., Poehlman, E., 1995. Exercise rehabilitation programs for the treatment of claudication pain: a meta-analysis. JAMA 274, 975–980.

Gill, D., Hatcher, S., 2001. A systematic review of the treatment of depression with antidepressant drugs in patients who also have a physical illness (Cochrane Review). In: The Cochrane Library, Issue 4. Update Software, Oxford.

Greenhalgh, R., Powell, J., 2007. Screening for aortic aneurysm. BMJ 335, 732–733.

Greenwood, R., McMillan, T., Brooks, D., et al., 1994. Effects of case management after severe head injury. BMJ 308, 1199–1205.

Haslam, R., 1996. Head injuries. Nelson Textbook of Pediatrics, 15th ed. Saunders WB, Philadelphia.

Hiatt, W., 2001. Medical treatment of peripheral arterial disease and claudication. N. Engl. J. Med. 344, 1608–1621.

Hudspith, J., Rayatt, S., 2004. First aid and treatment of minor burns. BMJ 328, 1487–1489.

Indar, A., Beckingham, I., 2002. Acute cholecystitis. BMJ 325, 639–643.

Isenberg, D., Black, C., 1995. ABC of rheumatology: Raynaud's phenomenon, scleroderma, and overlap syndromes. BMJ 310, 795–798.

Jennett, B., Teasdale, G., 1974. Assessment of coma and impaired consciousness. A practical scale. Lancet 2, 81–84.

Johnson, A., 1993. Gall stones: the real issues. BMJ 306, 1114–1115.

Kaleli, S., Aydin, Y., Erel, C., et al., 2001. Symptomatic treatment of premenstrual mastalgia in premenopausal women with lisuride maleate: a double-blind placebo-controlled randomized study. Fertil. Steril. 75, 718–723.

Kerlikowske, K., Grady, D., Rubin, S., et al., 1995. Efficacy of screening mammography: a meta-analysis. JAMA 273, 149–154.

Kontostolis, E., Stefanidis, K., Navrozoglou, I., et al., 1997. Comparison of tamoxifen with danazol for treatment of cyclical mastalgia. Gynecol. Endocrinol. 11, 393–397.

Kosters, J., Gotzsche, P., 2003. Regular self-examination or clinical examination for early detection of breast cancer. Cochrane Database Syst. Rev. Issue 2, CD003373.

Kuo, M., Hegarty, D., Johnson, A., et al., 1995. Early post-tonsillectomy morbidity following hospital discharge: do patients and GPs know what to expect? Health Trends 27, 98–100.

Leng, G., Fowler, B., Ernst, E., 2004. Exercise for intermittent claudication. The Cochrane Database Syst. Rev. Issue 4. The Cochrane Collaboration. John Wiley & Sons, Ltd.

Levien, T., 2006. Phosphodiesterase inhibitors in Raynaud's phenomenon. Ann. Pharmacother. 40, 1388–1393.

Livingstone, M., 2000. Whiplash injury: why are we achieving so little? J. R. Soc. Med. 93, 526–529.

Makin, A., Silverman, S., Lip, G., 2002. Antithrombotic therapy in peripheral vascular disease. BMJ 325, 1101–1104.

Mansell, R., Dogliotti, L., 1990. European multicentre trial of bromocriptine in cyclical mastalgia. Lancet 335, 190–193.

McDermott, M., McCarthy, W., 1995. Intermittent claudication: the natural history. Surg. Clin. N. Am. 75, 581–606.

McGee, S., Boyko, E., 1998. Physical examination and chronic lower-extremity ischemia: a critical review. Arch. Intern. Med. 158, 1357–1364.

Miller, A., To, T., Baines, C., et al., 2002. The Canadian National Breast Screening Study-1: breast cancer mortality after 11 to 16 years of follow-up: a randomized screening trial of mammography in women age 40 to 49 years. Ann. Int. Med. 137, 305–312.

Miller, A., To, T., Baines, C., Wall, C., 2000. Canadian National Breast Screening Study-2: 13 year results of a randomised trial in women aged 50–59 years. J. Natl. Cancer. Inst. 92, 1490–1498.

Million Women Study Collaborators, 2003. Breast cancer and hormone-replacement therapy in the Million Women Study. Lancet 362, 419–427.

Mondillo, S., Ballo, P., Barbati, R., et al., 2003. Effects of simvastatin on walking performance and symptoms of intermittant claudication in hypercholesterolemic patients with peripheral vascular disease. Am. J. Med. 114, 359–364.

Morgan, M., Palmer, J., 2007. Dog bites. BMJ 334, 413–417.

National Health Service, 2009. Bites – human and animal – management. Clinical Knowledge Summaries.http://cks.library.nhs.uk/home.

Nelson, R., 2003. Non surgical therapy for anal fissure (Cochrane Review). In: The Cochrane Library, Issue 4. John Wiley & Sons, Ltd, Chichester.

NHS Cancer Screening Programmes and Cancer Research UK, 2003. Guidelines for referral of patients with breast problems, 2nd ed. (with amendments). HMSO, London. Available: www.cancerscreening.nhs.uk.

NICE, 2001. Referral advice: varicose veins. National Institute for Health and Clinical Excellence, London. Available: www.nice.org.uk.

NICE, 2004. Familial Breast Cancer. The classification and care of women at risk of familial breast cancer in primary, secondary and tertiary care. NICE. Available: www.nice.org.uk.

NICE, 2006. Familial Breast Cancer. The classification and care of women at risk of familial breast cancer in primary, secondary and tertiary care. NICE. Available: www.nice.org.uk.

NICE, 2007. Head Injury – Triage, Assessment, Investigation and Early Management of Head Injury in Infants, Children and Adults. Clinical Guideline 56. National Institute for Health and Clinical

Excellence, London. Available onwww.nice.org.uk.

NICE, 2009. Venous thromboembolism: reducing the risk of venous thromboembolism in patients admitted to hospital. NICE Clinical Guideline. 1st draft March 2009. Available: www.nice.org.uk.

Papi, C., Catarci, M., D'Ambrosio, L., 2004. Timing of cholecystectomy for acute calculous cholecystitis. Am. J. Gastroenterol. 99, 147–155.

Phillips, S., Gallagher, M., Buchan, H., 2008. Use graduated compression stockings postoperatively to prevent deep vein thrombosis. BMJ 336, 943–944.

Poorbaugh, K., Brismee, J., Phelps, V., et al., 2008. Late whiplash syndrome: a clinical science approach to evidence-based diagnosis and management. Pain Pract. 8, 65–87.

Resnick, H., Lindsay, R., McDermott, M., et al., 2004. Relationship of high and low ankle brachial index to all-cause and cardiovascular disease mortality. Circulation 109, 733–739.

Rosenfield, M., Seferiadis, A., Carlsson, J., et al., 2003. Active intervention in patients with whiplash-associated disorders improves long-term prognosis. Spine 28, 2491–2498.

Schierhout, G., Roberts, I., 1998. Prophylactic antiepileptic agents after head injury: a systematic review. J. Neurol. Neurosurg. Psychiatry 64, 108–112.

Scholefield, J., Bock, J., Marla, B., et al., 2003. A dose finding study with 0.1%, 0.2%, and 0.4% glyceryl trinitrate ointment in patients with chronic anal fissures. Gut 52, 264–269.

Scottish Intercollegiate Guidelines Network, 2006. Diagnosis and Management of Peripheral Arterial Disease: SIGN. Clinical Guideline No. 89 Available: www.sign.ac.uk.

Stiell, I., Clement, C., McKnight, R., et al., 2003. The Canadian C-spine rule versus the NEXUS low-risk criteria in patients with trauma. N. Engl. J. Med. 349, 2510–2518.

Swain, A., Berge, S., Wakeley, C., et al., 1987. Management of blisters in minor burns. BMJ 295, 181.

Tabár, L., Vitak, B., Chen, H.H., et al., 2001. Beyond randomized controlled trials: organized mammographic screening substantially reduces breast carcinoma mortality. Cancer 91, 1724–1731.

Tait, N., Little, J., 1995. The treatment of gallstones. BMJ 311, 99–102.

Testroote, M., Stigter, W., de Visser, C., et al., 2008. Low molecular weight heparin for prevention of venous thromboembolism in patients with lower-leg immobilization. Cochrane Database Syst. Rev. Issue 4, CD006681.

Thornhill, S., Teasdale, G., Murray, G., et al., 2000. Disability in young people and adults one year after head injury: prospective cohort study. BMJ 320, 1631–1635.

Tierney, S., Fennessy, F., Bouchier Hayes, D., 2000. ABC of arterial and vascular disease: secondary prevention of peripheral vascular disease. BMJ 320, 1262–1265.

UK Small Aneurysm Trial Participants, 1998. Mortality results for randomised controlled trial of early elective surgery or ultrasonographic surveillance for small abdominal aortic aneurysms. Lancet 352, 1649–1655.

Voss, M., Knottenbelt, J., Peden, M., 1995. Patients who re-attend after head injury: a high risk group. BMJ 311, 1395–1398.

Wannamethee, S., Shaper, A., Whincup, P., et al., 1995. Smoking cessation and the risk of stroke in middle-aged men. JAMA 274, 155–160.

Warrell, D., 2005. Treatment of bites by adders and exotic venomous snakes. BMJ 331, 1244–1247.

Chapter 16

Psychiatric problems

CHAPTER CONTENTS

DEPRESSION

- 25% to 40% of GP consultations have a significant psychological component (Goldberg and Lecrubier 1995). Of these only about 5% are referred to specialist services.
- Recent research has shown how specific questions help to elicit crucial information about the patient's mental state.
- Qualitative research has shown the importance of the patient's relationship with the GP in such situations. Patients value an empathetic, interested doctor with whom they have a continuing relationship (Buszewicz, Pistrang, Barker, *et al.* 2006).

For details of the diagnosis of depressive illness see *Evidence-based Diagnosis in Primary Care* by A. F. Polmear (editor), published by Butterworth-Heinemann, 2008.

GUIDELINES

NICE. 2004. *Depression: Management of Depression in Primary and Secondary Care*. National Institute for Health and Clinical Excellence; Clinical Guideline 23. www.nice.org.uk
   Anderson IM, Ferrier IN, Baldwin RC, *et al.* 2008. Evidence-based guidelines for treating depressive disorders with antidepressants: a revision of the 2000 British Association for Psychopharmacology guidelines. J Psychopharmacol 22, 343–396

- GPs fail to diagnose up to half of their patients with a major depressive illness, and often fail to

© 2011 Elsevier Ltd.
DOI: 10.1016/B978-0-7020-3053-6.00016-7

treat adequately those whom they do recognize (Freeling, Rao, Paykel, *et al.* 1985; Anderson, Nutt and Deakin 2000).

- Depression in people from the African–Caribbean, Asian, refugee and asylum-seeking communities is often overlooked, although the prevalence is 60% higher than in the white population (Department of Health 1999). People from black and minority ethnic communities are much less likely to be referred to psychological therapies (Department of Health 1999).

- Those patients whose depression is most likely to be missed are those with somatic complaints or with physical illness, those with long-standing depression, those who do not look depressed and those who do not realize they are depressed (Freeling, Rao, Paykel, *et al.* 1985; Gill and Hatcher 2002).

- Depression is often accompanied and masked by anxiety (Goldberg and Bridges 1987), yet treatment of the anxiety alone is insufficient and may appear to worsen the depression.

PRESENTING COMPLAINTS

* Screen for depression in patients with low mood or with a past history or who are at risk because of physical illness or other mental illnesses such as anxiety or dementia. Ask two specific questions: during the past month have you felt:
  (a) low, depressed or hopeless?
  (b) little interest or pleasure in doing things?
     (Whooley, Avins, Miranda, *et al.* 1997).

* If the answer to either question is yes, confirm the diagnosis of depression using the DSM-IV criteria as follows. Used by GPs this is highly specific (Van Weel-Baumgarten, Van Den Bosch, Van Den Hoogen, *et al.* 2000). However, if the score conflicts with clinical judgement, treat it as a checklist only, and act on your clinical judgment.

A *major depressive illness* exists if the patient has low mood or diminished interest or pleasure for at least 2 weeks, occurring most of the day or nearly every day, and a positive score on at least five of the following:

(a) depressed mood;
(b) loss of interest or pleasure;
(c) change in weight or altered appetite almost every day;

(d) disturbed sleep;
(e) agitation or slowing of movement or speech;
(f) fatigue or loss of self-energy;
(g) guilt or low esteem;
(h) poor concentration;
(i) recurrent suicidal thoughts or acts.

Minor depression is characterized by three or four of the above. The evidence that it responds to antidepressant drugs is poor, unless it lasts for at least 2 years, when it may be called *dysthymia*, which may respond to drugs (Barrett, Williams, Oxman, *et al.* 2001).

Cautions

- The scoring system cannot be used in patients reacting appropriately to a life crisis or who are schizophrenic.

- To score as positive, the symptoms should indicate significant distress or impairment in functioning.

- No scoring system can be totally accurate. Modify the result in the light of the patient's circumstances. A past or family history of major depression, for instance, would increase the chance of major depression in a patient whose score does not reach that threshold.

- The distinction between major and minor depression on the DSM-IV criteria should not be confused with mild, moderate and severe depression on the ICD-10 criteria (WHO 2003), where the scoring is out of 10, not 9, and includes an assessment of functioning, rather than a more rigid count of symptoms. This leads to the imperfect correlation between the two scores shown in Table 16.1.

DIFFERENTIAL DIAGNOSIS

* *Schizophrenia.* Look for evidence of schizophrenia, which may present with depression. If delusions or hallucinations are also present, depression should not be the initial diagnosis.

* *Bipolar affective disorder.* Ask about a past history of a manic episode or hypomania. The management of bipolar affective disorder is different (see page 478). A study in US primary care looked at the prevalence of a current diagnosis of depression plus a positive screen

Table 16.1   Depression: definitions and scoring

ICD-10 DEFINITION	ICD-10 SCORES	EQUIVALENT DSM-IV DEFINITION
Mild depression	2–3. The patient is distressed but able to continue functioning	Minor depression
Moderate depression	4 or more. The patient is likely to have great difficulty in continuing with normal activities	Minor or major depression
Severe depression	Several symptoms are marked and distressing, typically loss of self-esteem and ideas of worthlessness and guilt. Suicidal thoughts are common and a number of somatic symptoms are usually present. Hallucinations or delusions also mean that the episode is severe, regardless of other symptoms	Major depression

for bipolar affective disorder. In the adult primary care population, 4% had both but the GPs who were managing the depression did not detect concurrent bipolar affective disorder in any of these patients (Das, Olfson, Gameroff, *et al.* 2005).

* *Iatrogenic cause.* Check for drugs that can cause depression, e.g. antihypertensives, H_2-blockers, steroids and beta-blockers.
* *Life events.* Ask about recent life events such as recent childbirth, bereavement, termination of pregnancy, loss of job, work stress, family illness or divorce. They may have triggered the depression.

MANAGEMENT OF DEPRESSION

The GP will manage 90% of depressed patients without referral to a specialized mental health service. The following steps are common to almost all severities of depression.

* *Life events.* Identify relevant life events which may have precipitated the illness and focus on small steps that might be taken to reduce their impact.
* Explore the impact of the depression on behaviour and relationships at home and work.
* Explain the nature of the illness, its treatment and good prognosis.
* Discuss the link between physical symptoms and mood.
* Encourage the patient not to make major or irreversible decisions about work or family until their mental state improves.
* *Exercise.* Recommend exercise, to the same extent as for cardiovascular fitness, for at least 10 weeks, even (or especially) on days when the

patient feels like staying in bed (Dunn, Trivedi, Kampert, *et al.* 2005). 'High dose' exercise 3 days a week is likely to lead to remission in one in five depressed patients compared to controls. The depressed patient will have little motivation and will need supervision. Refer to an exercise referral scheme if one is available.

* *Light therapy.* Recommend it for seasonal affective disorder. However, if using artificial lights, exposure to a bank of lights is needed for 1 hour a day, preferably in the morning. Similar benefit is seen with exposure to natural light, even if the sky is cloudy (Jorm, Christensen, Griffiths and Rodgers 2002). Exposure to daylight could usefully be combined with exercise.
* *Discuss drug therapy and counselling* (see below).
* *Follow up.* Explain the need for and frequency of follow-up.
* *Patient information.* Provide one of the leaflets listed in the box on page 453 and give the patient details of sources of information and support.

REFERRAL

Refer to a specialist mental health service if:

(a) psychotic features are present; or the depression is severe;
(b) the history suggests a bipolar illness;
(c) there is a significant risk of suicide or severe neglect;
(d) other forms of treatment are needed, e.g. cognitive behavioural therapy, if they are not available in primary care;
(e) the patient is a child or adolescent with major depressive illness;

(f) there has been a poor response to an appropriate antidepressant in maximum dosage, with good compliance, taken for an adequate period of time;

(g) there is social isolation, little family support, or poor compliance.

SPECIFIC TREATMENT OF MINOR DEPRESSION (OR MILD DEPRESSION ON THE ICD-10 CRITERIA)

* Explain the possible options:

(a) 'watchful waiting'. The patient may choose to return in, say, 2 weeks without treatment other than the general measures described above;

(b) guided self-help. The patient works through a written or computer programme which is usually designed along cognitive behavioural lines (see 'information for patients' below). A simple guide is available on www. whoguidemhpcuk.org; choose 'Patient Resources' then 'Depression' then 'Dealing with Depressive Thinking'. NICE has approved a computerized CBT programme, 'Beating the Blues', for mild to moderate depression, suitable for those with no computer experience. If the GP is unable to offer access to it using NHS funding, the patient can access it, for a considerable fee, on www.beatingtheblues.co.uk/connect;

(c) counselling or psychotherapy. There is evidence that brief cognitive behavioural therapy, problem-solving therapy and other forms of counselling, are beneficial.

* Explain that antidepressants are usually ineffective in minor depression unless it has lasted for 2 years (i.e. dysthymia). Any possible benefit is likely to be outweighed by the adverse effects. However, a patient with a past history of major depression who presents with minor depression may choose to take an antidepressant at this stage.

* Discuss complementary therapies with a patient interested in that approach. The best evidence lies with St John's wort. At a dose of hypericum extract of 350 mg t.d.s. it is superior to placebo and as good as imipramine 100 mg daily in mild–moderate depression (Philipp, Kohnen and Hiller 1999; Woelk 2000), and as good as paroxetine in moderate to severe depression in

one study using 900–1800 mg St John's wort daily (Szegedi, Kohnen, Dienel, *et al.* 2005). It has mild monoamine oxidase inhibitor (MAOI) properties so should not be combined with other antidepressants and caution may be needed with diet (Breckenbridge 2000). It is an inducer of drug-metabolizing enzymes and so can reduce the effectiveness of the following: oral contraceptives, warfarin, digoxin, theophylline, ciclosporin, indinavir. It may also reduce the effectiveness of other HIV protease inhibitors, non-nucleoside reverse transcriptase inhibitors, and anticonvulsants (phenytoin, carbamazepine and phenobarbital) (Mills, Montori, Wu, *et al.* 2004). Because of these problems, and lack of information about effective doses and preparations, NICE advises practitioners not to recommend it nor to prescribe it (NICE 2004a).

SPECIFIC TREATMENT OF MAJOR DEPRESSION (OR MODERATE–SEVERE DEPRESSION ON THE ICD-10 CRITERIA)

* *Offer an antidepressant.* The NICE guideline recommends an SSRI because they are as effective as tricyclics but with a 10% less chance of being discontinued because of adverse effects. Cost-effectiveness studies, in which doctors' time is costed as well as drug expenditure, favour SSRIs, or are at least neutral (Stewart 1998; Simon, Heiligenstein, Revicki, *et al.* 1999). However, both types of drug have considerable, but different, adverse effects. Attempt to make a choice that is the best for that patient (see below).

* Explain to the patient that:

(a) even if their depression is a reaction to life-events, they are as likely to benefit from an antidepressant as if it was endogenous;

(b) they will not notice any improvement for the first 10 days to 3 weeks but that adverse effects are most likely to occur in this period and then lessen;

(c) that antidepressants are not addictive. They will not develop craving or tolerance, but there is the possibility of a discontinuation reaction especially if stopped abruptly;

(d) stopping the drug early increases the risk of relapse. All patients should take the drug for

6 months after recovery. Anyone with a recent previous episode of major depression should take it for 2 years, as should other people at high risk of relapse, e.g. the elderly (see below).

* *Prescribe a generic preparation.* There is some evidence that venlafaxine is more effective than other antidepressants (Smith, Dempster, Glanville, *et al.* 2002) but adverse effects may also be greater (Cipriani, Geddes and Barbui 2007). A recent study suggests that the risk-benefit profile from 117 RCTs favours sertraline (Cipriani, Furukawa, Salanti, *et al.* 2009).

* Drug dosage
  (a) If choosing a tricyclic, start at the equivalent of amitriptyline 75 mg daily and expect to increase to 150 mg daily. A much criticized meta-analysis (Furukawa, McGuire and Barbui 2002) has suggested that the lower doses may be adequate. Such studies, and their critics, inevitably examine the mean response of a large number of patients. In clinical practice what matters is the response of that individual. Assess the effect of the lower dose and increase the dose monthly if the response is inadequate.
  (b) If choosing an SSRI start at the standard dose. Evidence that subsequent dose increases are beneficial is poor (although higher doses are effective in other conditions).

* *Follow-up.* See the patient 1 week after starting a drug in order to discuss any adverse effects (e.g. agitation or akathisia on an SSRI) and to check on compliance. A quarter of patients either never cash in their prescription or only do so once (Boardman and Walters 2009). If an SSRI is causing agitation, a 2-week course of a benzodiazepine is an alternative to stopping the drug. Slowly increase the time between consultations as the patient responds.

* *Response.* Do not be disappointed by a partial response. Studies of published and unpublished studies combined show that the effect size of all antidepressants is 'small' (NNT = 6) (Boardman and Walters 2009) and certainly less than the claims of manufacturers, based on published studies alone (Turner and Rosenthal 2008).

* *Maintenance.* Continue the drug for at least 6 months after remission. This reduces the relapse rate from 50% to 20%. A reduction in

dose should only be made if side-effects are a problem. Consider treatment for 1–2 years if there has been a previous episode in the recent past or the patient is at high risk because of age, family history, or other features (see below).

FACTORS WHICH WILL INFLUENCE THE CHOICE OF AN ANTIDEPRESSANT

(a) *The elderly:* avoid highly anticholinergic drugs (e.g. amitriptyline, clomipramine, doxepin, imipramine and maprotiline).

(b) *Young people:* the CSM has concluded that the majority of SSRIs are contraindicated in children and adolescents up to the age of 18 because of poor efficacy and a possible increase in the risk of self-harm and suicide. Fluoxetine seems to be an exception to this. The CSM also cautions that very young adults may be at similar risk, even though such a risk has not been detected in trials (CSM Expert Working Group 2004).

(c) *Pregnancy:* avoid SSRIs; a Danish cohort study suggests an increased risk of congenital malformations (Wogelius, Norgaard, Grislum, *et al.* 2006). Use tricyclics with caution; neonatal irritability has been reported with imipramine.

(d) *Prostatism or glaucoma:* avoid all anticholinergic drugs.

(e) *Cardiac disease:* avoid tricyclics and venlafaxine; the best evidence for use in ischaemic heart disease is for sertraline.

(f) *Suicide risk:* there is no evidence that one class of drugs poses a greater risk of suicide (Cipriani, Barbui and Geddes 2005) but intuitively doctors will avoid the more toxic tricyclics.

(g) *Lethargy:* avoid sedative drugs, e.g. amitriptyline, clomipramine, dosulepin, doxepin, maprotilene, mianserin, trazodone and trimipramine.

(h) *Anxiety or insomnia:* use a sedative drug.

(i) *Obesity:* use an SSRI.

(j) *Epilepsy:* avoid SSRIs.

(k) *Other drugs:* all classes of antidepressants show considerable interaction with other drugs, but any one interaction rarely applies to all classes and may not be seen with all members of one class. Choose an antidepressant tailored to the patient's other medication.

MANAGEMENT OF A POOR RESPONSE TO DRUG THERAPY

* Check that the patient was taking the drug correctly. An apparent relapse could be due to a discontinuation reaction in a patient who has omitted one or more doses.

* Where there is evidence that an increased dose may be associated with an improved response, and there are no adverse effects, consider increasing the dose gradually, waiting for 4 weeks each time before deciding that the response is inadequate.

* If dosage increase is not a possibility, assess whether referral is needed or whether the patient's condition allows the trial of another drug. Make a choice, according to any adverse effects experienced with the first drug, between another SSRI, a tricyclic (but not dosulepin), or a member of a different class, e.g. moclobemide, mirtazapine or reboxetine. Because it is a RIMA, moclobemide cannot be started until the previous antidepressant has washed out of the system. For a tricyclic this is 1 week but for fluoxetine it is 5 weeks. The STAR*D study found that putting non-responders through four steps of antidepressant treatment (either increased dosage or a change of drug) increased the rate of remission from 37% with step 1 to 67% by step 4, in those who adhered to treatment (Rush, Trivedi, Wisniewski, et al. 2006). Against these impressive-sounding results is the fact that drop-out rates were high and the percentage remitting fell with each step.

* Consider combining psychotherapy with drug treatment. Response is greater than with either alone, even if this is just because patients who also receive psychotherapy are more likely to take their drugs (Pampallona, Bollini and Tibaldi 2004).

STOPPING MAINTENANCE THERAPY AND MANAGING DISCONTINUATION REACTIONS

* Tail off, over 4 weeks, any antidepressant that has been given for 8 weeks or more, to reduce the risk of a discontinuation reaction (Haddad, Lejoyeux and Young 1998). A long-acting drug (e.g. fluoxetine or sertraline) may be given at the same dose but every other day, then every third day. A short-acting drug (e.g. paroxetine or citalopram) should be given daily at decreasing dosage. Tablets may be cut in half or a liquid form prescribed.

* Warn the patient that a discontinuation reaction is possible on stopping an antidepressant. The incidence is unclear. Estimates based on reports of adverse drug reactions suggest that it is uncommon (5% with paroxetine, < 1% with other SSRIs; Price, Waller, Wood, et al. 1996) but such reports rely on the reporting doctor making the diagnosis. A retrospective analysis of patients discontinuing antidepressants found that a reaction occurred in 31% who had taken clomipramine, in 17% who had taken a short-acting SSRI (paroxetine or fluvoxamine), and in only 1.5% who had taken a long-acting SSRI (fluoxetine or sertraline) (Coupland, Bell and Potokar 1996). Even if half of these are due to a placebo effect (Haddad, Lejoyeux and Young 1998), the study suggests that the reaction is common with the shorter acting drugs.

* Explain that a discontinuation reaction is unlikely to feel like a recurrence of depression. Dizziness, paraesthesia, tremor, anxiety, nausea and palpitations are the commonest symptoms. They occur within days of stopping the drug and last for 10 days on average.

* If a discontinuation reaction occurs:
  - A mild reaction: explain what is happening and continue the planned reduction, if the patient agrees.
  - A more severe reaction: either:
    (a) increase the dose to the last dose that gave no reaction; or
    (b) change the patient to a longer acting drug of the same class; and
    (c) prepare to tail off over a longer period, e.g. 3–6 months.

* Review patients 4 weeks after finally stopping the drug to ensure they remain well. Advise them to return at the earliest sign of a recurrence.

HOW TO DISTINGUISH AN ANTIDEPRESSANT DISCONTINUATION REACTION FROM A RETURN OF THE UNDERLYING DISORDER

(a) Its onset is within days (against weeks for a recurrence of depression).

(b) It resolves with 24 hours of restarting the antidepressant.

(c) Although the patient may report mood disturbance (low mood, irritability, anxiety) there are likely to be somatic symptoms as well (numbness, paraesthesiae, dizziness, headache, myalgia, fatigue, insomnia with vivid dreams).

COGNITIVE BEHAVIOURAL THERAPY/ COUNSELLING/OTHER PSYCHOTHERAPIES

- In patients at the mild–moderate end of the spectrum of major depression, cognitive and interpersonal therapies can be as effective as antidepressants and may prevent relapse (Gloaguen, Cottraux, Cucherat, *et al.* 1998). In a meta-analysis, antidepressants and psychotherapy both resulted in remission at a mean of 16 weeks in 46% of patients against 24% of controls (Casacalenda, Perry and Looper 2002).

- More patients would choose counselling than drugs if given the choice (Chilvers, Dewey, Fielding, *et al.* 2001).

- In major depression, a combination of antidepressants and cognitive behavioural therapy can be more effective than either alone (Timonen and Liukkonen 2008). Other psychotherapies have not shown a benefit from being combined with drugs.

- Most of the evidence for the benefit of psychological therapies in depression lies with certain techniques only, mainly cognitive behavioural, interpersonal, and problem-solving ones (Mynors-Wallis, Gath, Day, *et al.* 2000), and cannot be assumed to exist for all forms of counselling (DoH 2001).

- A 6-year follow-up study suggests that a course of cognitive behavioural therapy, in addition to drug therapy, leads to fewer subsequent relapses than drug therapy alone (40% versus 90% in a study of 40 patients) (Fava, Ruini and Rafanelli 2004).

PREVENTION OF RECURRENCE

- The continuing nature of the condition and the benefit to be gained from early intervention argue strongly for depression to be managed as a chronic disease, with a systematic approach to follow-up by a dedicated team following agreed protocols (Scott 2006).

- 75% of patients with a first episode of major depression have a recurrence within the next 10 years (Angst 1997). A second episode during the next 4 years requires full initial treatment, followed by psychiatric referral to consider prophylaxis with long-term antidepressant medication. In the first 3 years this will reduce the rate of recurrence from 41% to 18%. Only slightly more patients withdraw from treatment on an antidepressant than on placebo (OR 1.3) (95%CI 1.07 to 1.59) (Geddes, Carney, Davies, *et al.* 2003).

- Long-term prophylaxis after a single episode may be appropriate in the following because their risk of recurrence is even higher:
  (a) the elderly;
  (b) those with a first-degree relative with bipolar disorder or recurrent major depression.

* As a minimum, consider a 3-monthly telephone review by a doctor or nurse over the 2 years after treatment is stopped. In a US study it increased remission over 2 years by 33% (95% CI 7 to 46%) (Rost, Nutting, Smith, *et al.* 2002).

INFORMATION FOR PATIENTS

The Samaritans. Tel. 0845 7909090. Email: jo@samaritans.org. Website: www.samaritans.org
   The Mental Health Foundation has fact sheets for patients as well as other resources on www.mentalhealth.org.uk
   The WHO Guide to Mental and Neurological Health in Primary Care has information for patients available on www.whoguidemhpcuk.org choose 'patient resources'.
   Royal College of Psychiatry leaflet 'Help is at Hand: Depression', available: www.rcpsych.ac.uk/info/index.htm

Books
Butler G, Hope A. 2007. *Manage your Mind: The Mental Fitness Guide*. OUP, Oxford
   Rowe D. 2003. *Depression: The Way Out of Your Prison*. Brunner-Routledge, London
   Lewinsohn PM *et al.* 1992. *Control your Depression*. Simon and Schuster
   Burns DD. 1999. *Feeling Good: The New Mood Therapy*. Avon Books

POSTNATAL DEPRESSION

GUIDELINE

SIGN. *Postnatal Depression and Puerperal Psychosis.*
Scottish Intercollegiate Guidelines Network 2002.
Available: www.sign.ac.uk

- Postnatal depression occurs in 10–15% of women in the first year after delivery, usually in the first 6 months. The symptoms are almost always present at 6 weeks. It is distinct from the transient 'blues' of the first 10 days, and from a puerperal psychosis which is likely to need admission.
- Those most at risk are those:
  - (a) with previous psychological disturbance in pregnancy;
  - (b) with poor social support;
  - (c) with a poor marital relationship;
  - (d) with recent stressful events;
  - (e) with an episode of the 'baby blues'.
- The strongest risk factors for puerperal psychosis are a personal or family history of an affective psychosis. A woman who has one episode of puerperal psychosis has a 25–57% risk of a recurrence in a subsequent pregnancy. The risk of non-puerperal affective psychosis at some stage is even greater.
- Every practice should be aware of the need to identify 'at risk' patients during the antenatal period and should ensure that they receive more intensive help after birth. Risk factors should be identified during pregnancy and the primary care team need to decide:
  - (a) what extra care this group should receive; and
  - (b) who is responsible for identifying this condition as early as possible.
- Patients often do not realize that they are depressed, and doctors recognize it even less frequently. Women often present with a feeling of not coping rather than with classic symptoms of depression.

The SIGN guideline recommends that every woman should be screened for depression at 6 weeks and 3 months postpartum. The Edinburgh Postnatal Depression Scale (EPDS) (Cox, Holden and Sagovsky 1987) may be administered by a trained professional (see Appendix 20) as part of that screening process, but with the understanding that it is a screening, not a diagnostic, tool. Clinical assessment is needed to establish the diagnosis. The UK National Screening Committee puts the point more strongly, recommending it as a check-list, not a screening tool, which may be used as part of the assessment of a woman's mood (National Screening Committee UK 2004).

If the EPDS is not available, ask four simple questions:

(a) How are you feeling?
(b) How are you sleeping?
(c) How are you eating?
(d) Are you enjoying the baby?

IF DEPRESSION IS FOUND

- Check TFTs in those complaining mainly of tiredness (see page 240).
- *Counsel*. Simple, non-directive counselling by health visitors, weekly for 8 weeks, doubles the recovery rate (Holden, Sagovsky and Cox 1989).
- Explain to the patient that she is ill: it is not her fault and does not mean that she is a poor mother.
- *Literature*. Recommend one of the sources of information below, or print it off for the patient.
- *Antidepressants*. Offer drug treatment on the same basis that you would offer it to a non-puerperal patient, i.e. if major depressive illness is present. SIGN recommends that tricyclics (other than doxepin) or SSRIs (fluoxetine, paroxetine and sertraline) may be used and the patient may continue to breastfeed. This goes beyond the manufacturers' advice and indeed a mother should be told that the SSRIs, especially, will be excreted in the breast milk but that there is no evidence that this is harmful to the baby. However, the baby may experience a discontinuation reaction (see page 456). Use a long-acting drug and tail off breastfeeding (or the drug if still breastfeeding) slowly.
- Consider referral if a multidisciplinary mental health team is able to offer more than the primary healthcare team.
- Refer immediately for urgent psychiatric assessment any woman with ideas of suicide or of harming the baby or with symptoms of puerperal psychosis.

SUICIDE AND SUICIDAL RISK

- Two thirds of successful suicides are mentally ill (Owens, Lloyd and Campbell 2004), mostly with undiagnosed depression. In the elderly the prevalence of mental illness in suicides rises to up to 95% (O'Connell, Chin, Cunningham and Lawlor 2004).
- The risk of completed suicide in the first 9 days of drug treatment is 38 times that of the risk in a patient who has been on treatment for at least 3 months (Jick, Kaye and Jick 2004). This is independent of the type of antidepressant used.
- There is no evidence that SSRIs increase the risk of suicide in adults, though they appear to do so in children and adolescents. On the contrary, it seems likely that effective treatment of depression offers the most hope of reducing the risk of suicide. Even in adolescents the risk of suicide is greater in the month before starting antidepressants than in the first month on therapy (Brent 2007).
- Suicide is uncommon even in major depressive illness. One study found that only 4% of patients admitted because of depression killed themselves (Bostwick and Pankratz 2000). Furthermore, that 4% is hard to detect, though an attempt should be made.
- In all patients with depression, assess the risk. For instance, ask a series of questions, only stopping when the answer is no:
  1. Have you thought how nice it would be if you did not wake up one morning?
  2. Have you thought of killing yourself?
  3. Have you decided how to do it?
  4. Have you decided when to do it?

- Judge the risk according to the following risk factors:
  (a) a history of previous attempts, especially if determined or violent methods were used, or if a suicide note was left;
  (b) intense feelings of hopelessness and worthlessness;
  (c) major mental illness including depression;
  (d) suicidal ideation or evidence of planning, e.g. if the patient has decided when to do it, and if a sudden and infallible method has been chosen (Boardman and Walters 2009);
  (e) chronic physical illness or in much pain;
  (f) recent bereavement or other significant loss including job;
  (g) males. The male: female ratio for suicide is 4:1;
  (h) old age. The risk age > 75 is three times that of age 15–24;
  (i) alcohol or other substance misuse;
  (j) previous inpatient psychiatric treatment;
  (k) family history of mental illness, suicide or alcoholism;
  (l) AIDS or HIV-positive patients;
  (m) unmarried, separated or divorced, especially if living alone.

MANAGEMENT OF SUICIDAL PATIENTS

Low risk

- Manage at home patients who have thoughts of suicide but who have:
  (a) no clear suicidal plans or past history of a serious suicidal attempt;
  (b) good rapport with their GP or local psychiatric services;
  (c) 24-hour home support;
  (d) a stable personality;
  (e) no psychotic illness, chronic physical illness, or drug or alcohol misuse
- *Drugs.* If prescribing, give small quantities of medication, initially.

High risk

- Refer urgently to the mental health team. Check that the patient meets the previously agreed local criteria for same-day referral.

A domiciliary visit by a psychiatrist may be indicated (even if a patient refuses all offers of help).

* If the GP and psychiatrist cannot visit together, make sure that the GP is notified immediately of the outcome of the visit.
* Ensure that the carers can provide observation for 24 hours a day, until the risk diminishes. The family may need help to provide this level of care. If drug treatment is started, a relative or carer ought to be asked to supervise the medication.

Follow-up after attempted suicide

Often the first time a GP hears about a suicidal patient is when a hospital discharge report is received. When this occurs the doctor should:

(a) review the records to see if the patient has recently attended;
(b) discuss the management with the mental health care team, if the patient has a severe longstanding mental illness;
(c) identify anything that might indicate the patient was a suicide risk;
(d) enter suicide attempt on summary card and on computer;
(d) ask the patient to make an appointment to see the GP for review;
(e) follow-up to:
- identify depression or other precipitating life events;
- assess the need for treatment including counselling;
- make a care plan to review outcome and prevent recurrence;
(f) start treatment as below if indicated.

SUPPORT ORGANIZATIONS

The Samaritans. Tel. 0845 7909090. Email: jo@samaritans.org. Website: www.samaritans.org
PAPYRUS (prevention of young suicide). Helpline 08000 684141. www.papyrus-uk.org

HELPING THOSE BEREAVED BY SUICIDE

Grief after suicide seems to be particularly intense and often associated with shame and guilt. On average 6 people have intense grief for every suicide (Hawton 2003). Identify the people most likely to be affected and give them a chance to talk about their feelings.

* If their grief is intense, refer for counselling, or recommend self-help literature or self-help groups, according to its severity.

SUPPORT ORGANIZATIONS

Survivors of Bereavement by Suicide (SOBS). National helpline 0844 5616855. www.uk-sobs.org.uk
Winston's Wish is specifically for children bereaved by suicide. Helpline 08452 030405. www.winstonswish.org.uk
CRUSE offers support to all those who are bereaved. Day by Day helpline 0844 4779400. Young Person's helpline 0808 808 1677. www.crusebereavementcare.org.uk
The Compassionate Friends helps parents and siblings who have lost a child, including from suicide. Helpline 08451 232304. www.tcf.org.uk

STRESS REACTIONS

● Stress reactions may be:
(a) acute and brief;
(b) an adjustment reaction which may last a few months; or
(c) post-traumatic stress disorder (PTSD), with a delay between the stress and the onset of symptoms.
● Stress may be a reaction to loss or trauma. Symptoms may be those of anxiety, depression, abnormal behaviour or inability to cope with normal events. Symptoms may have been present for a long time before help is sought.
● Stressful events include:
(a) crime or accidents involving psychological and/or physical trauma;
(b) bereavement, including siblings in a family where a child has died;
(c) termination of pregnancy, miscarriage;
(d) redundancy, loss of job, occupational stress;
(e) divorce, separation, relationship difficulties;
(f) housing or financial problems;
(g) surviving a disaster;
(h) having to perform in front of an audience, or have work appraisal;
(i) seeking asylum;
(j) drug or alcohol withdrawal.

MANAGEMENT

* Identify underlying precipitating events and the steps taken by the patient to modify or cope with the situation.
* Exclude a physical or drug cause for the symptoms (drug or alcohol withdrawal, sudden stopping of a beta-blocker, hyperthyroidism).
* Identify others who might help, e.g. Relate, Citizens' Advice Bureau, Victim Support, union representative, local police domestic violence unit.
* Review what support can be obtained from family, friends, work colleagues and sources of community support.
* Discuss coping strategies.
* Assess the need for counselling.
* Decide if short-term time off work might be helpful.
* Consider prescribing a beta-blocker if somatic symptoms (shaking and tachycardia) are prominent. Avoid anxiolytic drugs but if the symptoms are very severe give them for a maximum of 2 weeks.

POST-TRAUMATIC STRESS DISORDER (PTSD)

The risk of developing PTSD varies according to the nature of the trauma and the susceptibility of the patient, ranging from 10% following a road traffic accident, 32% following a myocardial infarct (Jones, Chung, Berger, *et al.* 2007), to 57% following rape (Hull 2004). A study from the Netherlands suggests that non-traumatic life events (e.g. divorce or unemployment) may be more frequently the cause of PTSD than trauma (Mol, Arntz, Metsemakers, *et al.* 2005). Presentation may be delayed for several months after the event. In the US the lifetime prevalence is 8% (American Psychiatric Association 2000a). An Israeli study found that only 2.4% of patients with PTSD had been detected by their GPs (Munro, Freeman and Law 2004).

* Look for PTSD specifically in patients who have had a extremely traumatic incident in their lives. The cues to the diagnosis are where, at least 1 month after the event, the patient's life is disturbed by:

* intrusive symptoms; memories, flashbacks and nightmares; and
* avoidance of thoughts, activities, situations associated with the event; emotional numbing; and
* symptoms of autonomic arousal, e.g. hypervigilance, insomnia, irritability, excessive anger, and impaired concentration and/or memory.
* Check whether the patient has taken refuge in drug or alcohol misuse.
* In severe cases assess the risk of suicide.

MANAGEMENT

* *Debriefing.* Do not routinely offer debriefing after a traumatic event. It appears to be useless and may be harmful (Bisson 2004). A follow-up appointment 1–2 months after the event is more likely to be useful. Even then, beware of overdiagnosing it in a patient who is recovering spontaneously from a traumatic event.
* Provide information for patient and family (see box).
* Encourage discussion of the precipitatory event once PTSD has developed.
* Encourage the patient to discuss his or her feelings and fears.
* Explain how avoiding things that remind the patient of the trauma prolongs the syndrome.
* Draw up a gradual plan to face avoided activities and situations.
* *Alcohol.* Warn about the need to avoid excess use of alcohol. If the patient is already misusing alcohol or other drugs, treatment of the misuse must come before treatment of the PTSD.
* *Psychological therapy.* Refer for trauma-focused CBT if symptoms are present 3 months after the event. Refer at 1 month if symptoms are severe (NICE 2005a).
* *Antidepressants.* SSRIs reduce all symptoms of PTSD as well as treating any associated anxiety and depression. Sertraline has been shown to increase the response rate from one-third (with placebo) to a half, although the reduction in symptoms was small (Jick, Kaye and Jick 2004). It may take 8 weeks before effects are seen and high doses may be needed. If effective, continue for at least 6 months in total, or at least

12 months if the PTSD has lasted more than 3 months, to avoid relapse. There is an impression that patients do better if the drugs are started early in the course of the condition. NICE recommends paroxetine and mirtazapine for general use and other antidepressants for use by mental health specialists (NICE 2005b).

* *Other drugs.* Consider a beta-blocker for a patient disabled by startle and hyperarousal symptoms. The evidence for benzodiazepines is poor. However, consider a night-time short-acting benzodiazepine for a patient exhausted by poor sleep. Explain the disadvantages (dependence and tolerance) and obtain the patient's agreement that it will only be used, at the most, twice a week, while waiting for the SSRI to take effect.

* Inform the patient about the resources listed below.

PATIENT ORGANIZATIONS

Victim Support: emotional and practical support for victims of crime. Supportline: 0845 3030900. Email: support@victimsupport.org.uk. Website: www.victimsupport.org

Refugee Support Centre: counselling for refugees and asylum seekers in London. Tel. 020 7820 3606

Information Centre about Asylum and Refugees (ICAR). www.icar.org.uk

Medical Foundation for Care of Victims of Torture. www.torturecare.org.uk. The Foundation requests that written referrals are made. See the website for details of the four regional offices

Combat Stress (Ex-Services Mental Welfare Society) supports ex-service people with PTSD. Email: contactus@combatstress.org.uk. Website: www.combatstress.org.uk

Information: MIND has an excellent booklet. Call the Mindinfoline 0845 766 0163 or download it from www.mind.org.uk (choose 'Information' then 'Booklets – understanding' then 'Understanding post-traumatic stress disorder')

INSOMNIA

For details of the diagnosis of insomnia see *Evidence-based Diagnosis in Primary Care* by A.F. Polmear (editor), published by Butterworth-Heinemann, 2008.

* Insomnia may be primary, or secondary to another mental or physical disorder or to medication. Common causes of insomnia are depression, anxiety, menopausal symptoms, restless legs syndrome, pain and drugs. Half of patients with insomnia have a specific mental disorder and an overlapping half have a physical disorder (NICE 2004b).

* Patients with secondary insomnia need treatment both of the underlying condition and of the insomnia. A study of patients with rheumatoid arthritis found that treating insomnia with a short-acting benzodiazepine improved morning stiffness as well as improving sleep (Walsh, Muehlbach, Lauter, *et al.* 1996).

* Sedatives do significantly increase sleep duration and quality but at the risk of adverse effects, especially cognitive impairment next day and daytime sleepiness (Glass, Lanctot, Herrmann, *et al.* 2005). They also have addictive potential.

* Check that the insomnia is not due to an underlying disorder which needs treatment in its own right. Drugs which can cause insomnia include SSRIs and venlafaxine, and high dose steroids.

* Explain that failing to sleep is a natural part of a reaction to stress and not harmful; and that worrying about not sleeping makes sleep harder to achieve.

* Check that the patient is not using alcohol to sleep. In non-dependent drinkers it does improve sleep in the first part of the night but at the expense of early morning rebound awakening. Dependent drinkers lose even this early benefit.

* Explain that simple rules will help (see below) and offer an leaflet, e.g. www.mentalneurologicalprimarycare.org (choose 'Patient resources' then 'Sleep problems'). Behavioural techniques can be more effective than drug treatment, with longer-lasting benefit, but they take longer to administer (Sivertsen, Omvik, Pallesen, *et al.* 2006).

* Offer medication only if the patient's functioning is affected by the lack of sleep and the reason for the insomnia is temporary (e.g. jet lag or changing shifts). Obtain the patient's agreement that the course will not extend beyond 14 days because of the dangers of

dependence, tolerance and difficulties on withdrawal. Use a short-acting benzodiazepine. The National Institute for Clinical Excellence has assessed the 'Z drugs' (zaleplon, zolpidem and zopiclone), and found insufficient evidence to recommend them over the cheaper benzodiazepines (NICE 2004b).

* Be aware that some specialists in sleep disorders think that the approach set out in the BNF and repeated above is too draconian; and that the evidence of tolerance and dependence, when short-acting benzodiazepines are used for true primary insomnia, is poor (Wilson and Nutt 2003). A compromise position is to prescribe a short-acting benzodiazepine for, say 14 nights, to be repeated every 2 months, allowing the patient to use them when the need is greatest.

* Consider a tricyclic antidepressant in those for whom all other approaches have failed or are inappropriate. Dependence is not a problem but daytime drowsiness, and other adverse effects, are. Consider it an option of last resort. An early resort to drugs will distract the patient from the changes in lifestyle, and in their mental attitude to insomnia, that are necessary.

* Do not prescribe melatonin for most types of insomnia. A meta-analysis has shown that it is ineffective both in secondary insomnia and in jet lag (Buscemi, Vandermeer, Hooton, *et al.* 2006). It may be useful in people with delayed sleep phase syndrome (in which the patient's circadian rhythm is off kilter) (Buscemi, Vandermeer, Hooton, *et al.* 2004).

* Consider referral for cognitive behavioural therapy if the patient is sufficiently troubled by the problem. Even long-term users of hypnotics can benefit, with improved sleep, improved quality of life and reduction in use of hypnotics (Morgan, Dixon, Mathers, *et al.* 2003).

SIMPLE RULES TO REDUCE INSOMNIA

(a) Go to bed and get up at the same time, even at weekends. It helps set your 'internal clock'.

(b) Prepare for sleep by doing something restful in the half hour before bed. Avoid exercise in the 3 hours before bed. Refuse to discuss exciting or worrying things in bed; keep the bed for sleep and sex.

(c) Make sure the room is dark and quiet. Use earplugs if you have to.

(d) Avoid caffeine from about 4 pm. This may include chocolate and tea as well as coffee and cola.

(e) If you find yourself worrying, write down what the problem is, and when you are going to think about it properly. Worrying about something at night magnifies a problem that may seem perfectly soluble in the day.

(f) Distract yourself with thoughts of something pleasant: gardening, sex, an imaginary dinner party in which you light a candle in front of each of your friends and visualize their faces in detail. You need something more interesting than counting sheep.

(g) If you still can't sleep, don't lie there fretting. Get up, sit somewhere warm, do something restful, and go back to bed when you feel sleepy.

(h) However tired you feel in the day, don't nap. It will mean you sleep even less well at night.

(i) If you've slept badly, accept it and lead a full day. Most people can function on less sleep than they think they need.

INFORMATION FOR PATIENTS

The Royal College of Psychiatrists has leaflets and audio tapes on www.rcpsych.ac.uk (Choose 'Publications' then 'Factsheets and leaflets' then 'Sleep problems')

The *WHO Guide to Mental and Neurological Health in Primary Care* has a leaflet on insomnia on www.mentalneurologicalprimarycare.org (choose 'Patient resources' then 'Sleep problems')

ANXIETY DISORDERS

For details of the diagnosis of anxiety disorders see *Evidence-based Diagnosis in Primary Care* by A.F. Polmear (editor), published by Butterworth-Heinemann, 2008.

● Anxiety disorders are more common than depression, rarely present as pure anxiety, are even less frequently diagnosed, yet the majority of patients will respond to treatment: usually an SSRI or cognitive behavioural therapy.

● Detection of an anxiety disorder is improved if the GP uses a few screening questions (Katon and Roy-Byrne 2007).

- In few conditions is a positive, persistent and supportive stance by the doctor more important. The patient's instincts will be to avoid facing up to situations that provoke anxiety while treatment relies on facing up to them.
- Almost all anxiety disorders can be managed in primary care, especially if a member of the team is trained in cognitive behavioural therapy. However, any patient sufficiently distressed by an anxiety disorder who has not responded to primary care management should be offered referral to a specialist mental health service.
- Individual SSRIs and related drugs are licensed in the UK for one or more types of anxiety but not for all types. There is every reason to think that this is a quirk of licensing and that the benefits are common to all drugs of that class.
- Do not lead the patient to expect a cure; they are likely to be disappointed. Most, however, can expect significant improvement with treatment.
- Anxiety disorders rarely start in mid life or later. Such a presentation suggests another underlying disorder, especially depression or alcohol misuse.

Table 16.2	Prevalences of the anxiety disorders in the general population (Ballenger and Tylee 2003; American Psychiatric Association 2000b)

CONDITION	LIFETIME PREVALENCE
Generalized anxiety disorder	5%
Panic disorder (PD)	2–3%
Panic attacks without reaching the criteria for PD	10%
Agoraphobia	6%
Social anxiety	13%
Specific phobias	7–11%
Obsessive compulsive disorder (OCD)	2–3%
Obsessive or compulsive symptoms without reaching the criteria for OCD	8%

Note that most patients suffer from more than one condition. Note that the prevalence in a primary care population will be higher, since patients with anxiety present more frequently, usually with somatic complaints.

GENERALIZED ANXIETY

NICE. 2004. *Management of Anxiety (Panic Disorder, with or without Agoraphobia, and Generalized Anxiety Disorder) in Adults in Primary, Secondary and Community Care.* National Institute for Health and Clinical Excellence, Clinical Guideline 22. Available: www.nice.org.uk

* Check whether the patient also suffers from other mental conditions which need treatment in their own right: e.g. panic disorder, obsessive-compulsive disorder, phobia, depression, post-traumatic stress disorder, or the misuse of alcohol or drugs.
* Check that there is no physical condition which is mimicking the symptoms of anxiety: e.g. thyrotoxicosis or asthma.

MANAGEMENT OF A CRISIS

It may take a crisis to bring the patient to seek help. Immediate treatment is needed to tide the patient over and gain the confidence of patient and family.

* Give a brief but clear explanation of what is happening and that effective help is available.
* Consider prescribing anxiolytics for 2–4 weeks with the clear understanding that this is crisis management only. Use a benzodiazepine, although, in a patient who has misused a benzodiazepine in the past, a sedating antihistamine or an antipsychotic may be preferred. Warn of the risks of dependence, sedation, industrial accidents and road traffic accidents (Gale and Oakley-Browne 2004a). Outside the UK a longer term role for benzodiazepines is accepted, with the view that dependence and tolerance is rare when prescribed for anxiety (Ballenger and Tylee 2003).
* Arrange an early appointment to begin definitive treatment for the condition.

LONG-TERM TREATMENT

* Explain how anxiety causes physical symptoms and how they in turn increase anxiety. Offer a leaflet (see below).

* Assess the patient's disability. How does it affect family relationships, sex, work, and physical and mental state? Is a job at risk? Is alcohol or caffeine intake excessive?

* Explain the options:

  (a) *Cognitive behavioural therapy (CBT)*. CBT has the strongest evidence of benefit (Gale and Oakley-Browne 2004b). A 1–2 hour weekly session will be needed for a total of 8–20 hours with a trained professional. Briefly, it involves training the patient to act and think differently from their usual manner until a new response to life becomes natural to them. However, do not 'oversell' it to the patient. Even in randomized controlled trials only half have recovered at 6-month follow-up (Fisher and Durham 1999). Those who do show some response continue to improve for at least 2 years after treatment has ended (Dugas, Ladouceur and Leger 2003). Anxiety management, without cognitive restructuring, can achieve similar benefit (Gale and Davidson 2007).

  (b) *An SSRI*. Almost half of patients show significant improvement with follow-up periods of up to 6 months. However, this yields an NNT of only 5 (because a number improve on placebo) (Kapczinski, Lima and Souza 2003). Although this seems an easier option than CBT there are disadvantages: benefit may not be seen for some weeks and maximum benefit not for 6 months; anxiety may worsen in the first few weeks; at least 6 months treatment will be needed; and, while not addictive, there is the possibility that the patient will notice a discontinuation reaction, especially if the drug is stopped suddenly. In patients who cannot take an SSRI use a tricyclic antidepressant.

  (c) *Self-help*, using a written approach with supportive visits to the doctor or nurse. This is also CBT but without a personal therapist; the patient needs to find the motivation to succeed and be comfortable with reading and with acting on the written word.

* *Recommend a self-help group*, whichever treatment the patient chooses. Some can assist the patient in a CBT approach but all will provide support and help the patient realize that he or she is not the only one with this problem.

* *Follow-up*. Unless the patient will be seeing a therapist within 2 weeks, arrange for follow-up along the following lines: at 2, 4 and 6, weeks then at 3 and 6 months. This applies whether the patient decides on an SSRI or self-help, or is waiting to see a CBT therapist.

PRACTICAL DETAILS WHEN PRESCRIBING AN SSRI FOR ANXIETY

1. Start with a low dose to minimize the increase in anxiety seen with standard doses. For instance, start with paroxetine 5 mg daily for 2 weeks and double the dose every fortnight until reaching 20 mg daily. This means cutting up tablets or prescribing the liquid.

2. If the response at 8 weeks is inadequate, increase slowly to the maximum recommended dose.

3. Treat for a minimum of 6 months after a response is achieved. Patients who show some response at 2 months may continue to improve over the subsequent 6 months.

4. Decide, with the patient, how long to continue to prevent relapse. Treatment for 1 to 2 years is likely to be needed if the condition is longstanding.

5. With prolonged use, sexual dysfunction becomes the most significant adverse effect. For men with erectile dysfunction, sildenafil and related drugs can be used (although not on the NHS in the UK).

6. When stopping the drug, tail it off in fortnightly steps over 1 to 2 months according to what dose was used. If a discontinuation reaction occurs, go back a step and tail off more slowly.

SPECIAL SITUATIONS

* *The patient who fails to respond to an SSRI* or in whom it is contraindicated or not tolerated: consider a tricyclic antidepressant in the same doses as for depression. An alternative is pregabalin, originally used in partial seizure epilepsy. Give it twice daily (Pohl, Feltner, Fieve, *et al.* 2005) with a maximum dose of 200 mg/day; further dosage increases are of no benefit.

* *The patient whose anxiety returns when the SSRI is stopped.* It can be hard to distinguish a discontinuation reaction from the return of anxiety. The symptoms (dizziness, numbness, tingling, nausea, headache, sweating, insomnia

and feeling anxious) are common to both. Sometime the patient is clear that the symptoms feel different from the original anxiety. If in doubt, restart the SSRI and taper the dose more slowly.

* *The patient whose physical symptoms of anxiety are crippling:* consider a beta-blocker, although there is a dearth of evidence (Gale and Oakley-Browne 2004c). A long-acting preparation will be needed.

INFORMATION FOR PATIENTS

Self-help group

No Panic is a charity that provides information, written treatment programmes and telephone support for those with anxiety, phobias and obsessive compulsive disorders. Helpline 0808 808 0545. www.nopanic.org.uk

Leaflets

WHO Guide to Mental and Neurological Health in Primary Care, Available on www.whoguidemhpcuk.org
   Royal College of Psychiatrists' leaflet 'Help is at hand: anxiety and phobias'. Available: on www.rcpsych.ac.uk/info/index.htm

Books

Butler G, Hope T. 2007. *Manage Your Mind: The Mental Fitness Guide*. OUP, Oxford

---

PANIC DISORDER

* Follow the management outlined under Generalized Anxiety, but without the offer of a benzodiazepine. It is even more important to explain the link between the feeling of panic and the physical symptoms it produces, since patients often see it as a physical illness.

* Offer the same triad of behavioural therapy or CBT, an SSRI, or self-help. In addition, NICE has approved the use of computer-assisted CBT (NICE 2006). *Fearfighter* is an 8–12 week course of treatment accessed by the patient via a computer with internet access. The patient needs a password to access the programme, for which PCT approval is needed.

* If there has been no response after 12 weeks of an SSRI, consider a tricyclic antidepressant.

* The details in the box 'Information for patients' are the same as for generalized anxiety.

* Give the patient a copy of *'First Aid for a Panic Attack'* (see below).

* Do not offer a benzodiazepine or another anxiolytic. They are less effective than SSRIs, and they are inappropriate in a disorder that usually lasts over 4 weeks and where dependence can occur. They do not treat the depression that is often co-existent, or which may emerge as the panic disorder is treated.

* Consider a long-acting beta-blocker. It will abolish some of the somatic symptoms of panic and may help the subjective terror as well (Mol, Arntz, Metsemakers, *et al.* 2005). However, it will not lead to a lasting cure and may distract the patient from the need to enter more definitive therapy (i.e. CBT).

* Monitor progress with two questions:
  - how many panic attacks have you had since I last saw you?
  - how severe were they, on a scale of 1 to 5, where 1 is very mild and 5 is extremely severe?

* Prepare yourself, if not the patient, for a relatively poor response to treatment. A Cochrane review (Furukawa, Watanabe and Churchill 2007) found that, 2 years after the start of treatment, 60% of patients had not achieved a sustained response. Combining psychotherapy with an antidepressant was more likely to achieve a response in the short-term than either alone, with a NNT of 10. In other words, if 10 patients are treated with both treatments one more will respond than if treated with one *or* the other. However, follow-up of 1 or 2 years found that the combination of psychotherapy and antidepressant was better than antidepressant alone (NNT 6) but no better than psychotherapy alone.

'FIRST AID' FOR A PANIC ATTACK – INSTRUCTIONS FOR THE PATIENT

■ Panic always subsides, even if it can take an hour.
■ If some situation has triggered the attack, try to stay in the situation. Leaving can make it harder to go back later.
■ Breathe slowly but not deeply. Deep breathing can mean you hyperventilate and develop more symptoms.

- Check your watch. What seems like an hour may only be 5 minutes.
- Distract yourself, e.g. read every detail of the label on something on the supermarket shelf.
- Have something you say to yourself during the attack, e.g. 'It's only a panic attack. I'm not going to faint or vomit (or whatever you most fear) – and so what if I do?'
- Don't use alcohol. Attacks are more likely as the alcohol wears off.
- Check whether caffeine has played a part in triggering the attack.

SOCIAL ANXIETY/SOCIAL PHOBIA

Patients with social anxiety often think they are excessively shy, rather than suffering from a treatable mental disorder.

* Take even more care than usual to explain the nature of the condition. The concept of 'an overactive circuit deep in the brain' may be acceptable to a patient who already understands the concept of, for instance, an overactive thyroid.

* Follow the management outlined under *Generalized anxiety*, but without the offer of a benzodiazepine. An SSRI, exposure therapy and a combination of the two are all effective during treatment. A large study suggests that those treated with exposure therapy alone continue to improve in the 6 months after treatment whereas those treated with sertraline, with or without exposure, show some loss of benefit (Haug, Blomhoff, Hellstrom, *et al.* 2003). If the SSRI is continued long-term, the benefit is sustained and a treatment course of a minimum of 6 months, following remission, is needed (Schneier 2003).

* Offer a beta-blocker to a patient with a circumscribed social anxiety which is disabling and where the somatic symptoms (tremor, palpitations) are preventing the patient from functioning. Performing musicians are the prime example. Warn the patient that they will find it hard not to become psychologically reliant on the drug. However, they may prefer this to the loss of their chosen career.

PHOBIAS

- Phobias require energetic management if they present early in order to prevent them from becoming fixed. Even those presenting late are amenable to treatment if the patient is willing to undergo therapy. All patients with phobias need treatment.
- Many patients who are phobic do not present with the phobia but with a consequence of it: alcohol or drug misuse, truancy, failure to attend appointments at the surgery, anxiety or depression. Failure to discover the underlying phobia will result in a failure of treatment.

* Offer referral for CBT, an SSRI, or a self-help programme along CBT lines (see *Generalized anxiety*).

* In those patients who choose to be treated without referral, use the following programme, with or without treatment with an SSRI:

  (a) Urge the patient not to avoid the phobic situation. Avoidance increases the strength of the phobia.

  (b) Teach the patient the rules of 'first aid' during an attack of panic (see page 466).

  (c) Plan a programme of gently increasing exposure to the phobia. Do this with imaginary exposure if real exposure is not possible. Exposure must be daily, and the patient must stay in the phobic situation until the panic has subsided. Ask the patient to keep a diary to discuss at each appointment.

  (d) Ask what would be 'the worst possible scenario'. Often it turns out to be unpleasant but acceptable. Usually it is that other people will see that the patient is being phobic. Being prepared to 'own up' to a phobia is often a great step forward.

* Recommend *Manage your Mind: the Mental Fitness Guide* by Gillian Butler and Tony Hope for details of strategies that patients can use for themselves.

* *Drug treatment at the time of the phobic event:* avoid giving benzodiazepines for a phobia that poses a problem more than occasionally. The patient is likely to become even less able to face the situation without drugs than before treatment began. Consider a beta-blocker, e.g. propranolol 40 mg 1–2 hours before exposure to the phobic situation in those who cannot tolerate the physical symptoms of panic.

SPECIFIC PHOBIAS

- *Fear of flying.* Exposure therapy, either using a computer stimulation, or just sitting in an aircraft and imagining that it is flying, show marked short-term benefits, with over half of patients who previously refused to fly, managing to fly. However, the effect does not last and is almost completely lost after 6 months (Maltby, Kirsch, Mayers, *et al.* 2002). It is therefore most suitable for someone who has to make a one-off flight. Several organizations offer exposure therapy. For instance, Aviatours (tel: 01252 793250. www.aviatours.co.uk) offers training courses in association with British Airways. Virgin Atlantic offers 'Flying Without Fear' courses (tel: 01423 714900. www.flyingwithoutfear.info/).

- *Fear of medical or dental procedures.* Cognitive behavioural therapy is the most effective treatment, but most patients present too late, when the need for help is urgent. Diazepam 10 mg 1–2 hours before the event has been shown to reduce anxiety significantly more than placebo, although the placebo effect is also marked (Wilner, Anziano, Johnson, *et al.* 2002).

- *Patients with agoraphobia* are likely to find themselves unable to attend a primary care clinic and even more likely to have difficulty attending a specialist centre. Treatment in primary care, using an SSRI and a simple CBT approach (above) will be successful in some and allow others to improve enough to participate in more definitive therapy.

INFORMATION FOR PATIENTS

Self-help group

Triumph over Phobia has details of local groups. Tel. 0845 600 9601. Email: info@topuk.org Website: www.triumphoverphobia.com

Leaflets

WHO Guide to Mental and Neurological Health in Primary Care, available on www.whoguidemhpcuk.org
 Royal College of Psychiatrists' leaflet 'Help is at hand: anxiety and phobias', available: www.rcpsych.ac.uk/info/index.htm

---

Books

Butler G. 1999. *Overcoming Social Anxiety and Shyness: A Self-help Guide Using Cognitive Behavioural Techniques*, Robinson.
 Butler G, Hope T. 2007. *Manage Your Mind: The Mental Fitness Guide.* OUP, Oxford

OBSESSIVE COMPULSIVE DISORDER (OCD)

- Be on the alert for the diagnosis: patients are often reluctant to admit to the disorder. In patients whose symptoms raise the possibility of OCD ask specific questions: 'do you find yourself doing things repeatedly in a way you can't control?' and 'do you find yourself bothered by certain thoughts that you can't get out of your mind?'. Conditions which raise the possibility of OCD include depression, anxiety, eating disorders, fear of illness, fear of causing others harm, skin disorders that suggest repeated hand washing.

- Once OCD is diagnosed, check for depression. One third with OCD are currently depressed and two thirds will become depressed at some stage (Ballenger and Tylee 2003).

- Assess the risk of self-harm and suicide.

- The NICE guideline (NICE 2005b) suggests a stepped-care approach, with the starting point being the recognition of the disorder and the offer of information about the condition and the support groups that are available (see box). Later steps involve the provision of self-help material, referral for cognitive behavioural therapy (CBT), and the offer of an SSRI (see below).

- Involve the family or carers in the process of finding out about the disease and its treatment.

- When functional impairment is at least moderate, offer an SSRI as described under *Generalized anxiety*. Expect the response to take even longer (up to 12 weeks) than with other forms of anxiety. Expect to continue it for at least 1 year.

- If the patient cannot take an SSRI, consider clomipramine (Ballenger and Tylee 2003). NICE advises against other tricyclic antidepressants.

- Offer CBT if it is available. It involves gradual exposure of the patient to situations which provoke anxiety while not allowing the patient the relief of using a ritual to relieve that anxiety. At the same time the therapist retrains the patient in different patterns of thought. Patients who refuse CBT at first because it sounds too threatening may accept it after partial remission with drug treatment. CBT appears to offer most hope for lasting remission.

* If the patient responds then relapses after discharge, refer back urgently, before the pattern of behaviour becomes firmly established.

PATIENT INFORMATION

Pedrick C, Hyman B. 2005. *The OCD Workbook: Your Guide to Breaking Free from Obsessive-compulsive Disorder.* 2nd edition. A Harbinger Self-help Workbook.
    NICE. 2005. Treating obsessive-compulsive disorder (OCD) and body dysmorphic disorder in adults, children and young people. Understanding NICE guidance – information for people with OCD or BBD, their families and carers, and the public. CG31. www.nice.org.uk

Patient support

OCD Action on www.ocdaction.org.uk or via the helpline: 0845 3906232. The website includes aids to self-diagnosis, blogs by people with the condition, and information about support groups

---

UNEXPLAINED SOMATIC COMPLAINTS

REVIEW

Goldberg R, Dennis H, Novack M, Gask L. 1992. The recognition and management of somatization: what is needed in primary care training. Psychosomatics 33, 55–61

There is a group of patients characterized by:

■ voluminous records;
■ frequent attendances for physical symptoms intensively investigated by many hospital referrals with no cause found;
■ repeated reassurance, which does not alter the belief that physical illness is the underlying cause;
■ repeated demands for further investigations and referrals.

Management is directed at preventing the above pattern by firm intervention once diagnosed. Further referrals and investigations should be restricted to a minimum, while the GP maintains a relationship with the patient in the hope that the underlying psychopathology will emerge so that it can be treated. As a minimum, such a firm stance will limit damage to the patient, and the health service.

MANAGEMENT

* Acknowledge that the symptoms are real and explain the relationship between somatic and psychological symptoms.
* When a new symptom is presented, investigate the possibility of physical and mental causes in parallel; and be explicit about what you are doing.
* Look for underlying mental disorders: alcohol or drug misuse, depression or anxiety. If the condition begins in a patient over the age of 30, an underlying mental disorder is likely.
* Resist the temptation to 'try' drugs for symptomatic relief if the real problem is the patient's concern about an undiagnosed physical problem. Stop, one by one, any medication that is not necessary.
* Ascertain whether the patient is becoming an invalid, in the hope of avoiding more symptoms. Encourage regular exercise.
* Try to see the patient in regular scheduled appointments. It may, in the long-term, reduce the number of requests for home visits or for emergency appointments.
* Offer a second opinion from another partner, but if the second doctor confirms your opinion, resist attempts to 'shop around' for further opinions.
* Consider a single referral to a specialist, with a statement of your diagnosis of somatization disorder. If your diagnosis is confirmed refuse requests for further referrals. Far from providing reassurance, they will continue to focus the patient's attention on the pursuit of yet more tests which will finally discover the diagnosis.
* Refer to a liaison psychiatrist or cognitive behavioural therapist if the patient will accept it. CBT has been shown to produce significant lasting improvement in somatization disorder (Allen, Woolfolk, Escobar, *et al.* 2006).

* If the patient still resists the diagnosis of somatization, consider a compromise position: that, even if the symptoms are physical in origin, a serious cause for them has been excluded. Offer a low dose tricyclic antidepressant for its analgesic effect.

DELIBERATE SELF-HARM

National Institute for Health and Clinical Excellence. 2004. *Self-harm: The Short-term Physical and Psychological Management and Secondary Prevention of Self-harm in Primary and Secondary Care:* NICE Guideline No. 16. Online. Available: www.nice.org.uk

- In the UK one in 10 teenagers deliberately self-harms. Of them, over 24,000 are admitted to hospitals each year, usually because of overdoses or cutting (NHS Direct 2004). Seven out of eight are female.
- It is the strongest single predictor of successful suicide, being found in 40–60% of suicides (Hawton, Zahl and Weatherall 2003). However, that does not make it a useful predictor of suicide. Of self-harmers in the UK, only 0.7% kill themselves within a year and 3% in 15 years.
- Two out of three self-harmers consult their GP in the subsequent 3 months (Bennewith, Stocks, Gunnell, *et al.* 2002). One in six will harm themselves again within a year. However, attempting to assess the risk of repeated self-harm is unlikely to be successful (Kapur, Cooper, Rodway, *et al.* 2005).
- A large study of an intervention in which patients were sent an invitation to consult following an episode of self-harm failed to show any benefit in terms of reducing repeated episodes (Bennewith, Stocks, Gunnell, *et al.* 2002). Indeed, systematic review has failed to identify benefit from any treatment (Soomro 2004).
  * Ask what the patient did, what precipitated it and whether the problem is still present. Assume it is evidence of serious emotional distress.
  * Assess the current mental state and the suicidal risk.
  * Look for other problems – medical illness, social problems, past or present physical or sexual abuse.
  * Manage according to what is found. The underlying problem may be trivial (an impulsive act, immediately regretted) or grave (a psychotic illness). Among those who are not mentally ill, being unclear about the reason for the self-harm is a bad prognostic sign, as is male sex and being an older rather than a younger adolescent (Royal College of Psychiatrists 1998). Self-harm in people over 65 years of age is especially associated with depression and suicide (NICE 2004c).
  * Teach the patient ways of reducing the risk of serious harm, while the underlying problem is being attended to (Mental Health Foundation 2004):
    - *harm minimization:* e.g. make a small cut rather than a large one, or take aspirin rather than paracetamol and never more than four at once;
    - *distraction:* have a plan of something to do once the urge to self-harm starts to build up, e.g. go for a run or play music very loudly;
    - *identify someone* you can talk to when you feel in danger.

ACUTE PSYCHOTIC DISORDERS

The possibility of acute psychosis is raised by the following:

- hallucinations;
- delusions;

- disorganized or strange speech;
- agitation or bizarre behaviour;
- extreme and labile emotional states;
- family concern about recent changes in personality, behaviour or function.

INITIAL ASSESSMENT

* Obtain a careful history from family or friends of recent events and changes in the patient's behaviour.
* Ask about drug or alcohol misuse.
* Assess the mental state including the risk of suicide and of harm to others.
* Make a differential diagnosis if this is a first episode. Consider the possibilities of acute confusional state, drug-induced psychosis and epilepsy. An episode that is related to cannabis use probably signifies an underlying psychosis triggered by the cannabis.
* If this is a relapse, review past management and outcomes.
* Decide if admission or referral is necessary.
* Explain to the family what you think is wrong and what action is needed. If feasible, give the patient the same information and obtain consent.

When there is a risk of violence

First, try to calm the patient. The NICE guideline for handling violence in the in-patient setting (NICE 2005) applies in the community too:

* Appoint one member of staff to relate to the patient. Others should move away.
* Encourage the patient to move to a safe place.
* If there is a weapon, ask the patient to put it in a neutral place, not to hand it over.
* Explain to the patient throughout, in a calm manner, what you are doing.
* Ask the patient open questions, e.g. tell me what's going on.

DRUG TREATMENT

* If the situation is not urgent, leave a decision about medication to the admitting psychiatrist, or specialist mental health team, if the patient is not admitted.

* If medication is needed urgently, and the patient agrees to it, give an oral atypical antipsychotic (e.g. amisulpride, olanzapine, quetiapine, risperidone or zotepine but not clozapine) (NICE 2002). Use a dose at the lower end of the range if this is a first attack; otherwise use a dose that proved effective last time. However, if the patient was previously well controlled on a conventional antipsychotic, restart that.
* If a patient initially refuses medication that is urgently needed, spending time, in a calm manner, can often win the patient's confidence. Do not deny the patient's delusions or hallucinations but say something like: 'I can see you are pretty upset about all this and I can help with that'.
* Rarely, an agitated or aggressive patient needs rapid tranquillization. Tranquillization makes subsequent assessment difficult, it is traumatic for the patient, and sedated patients need observation, which may not be possible. If there is no alternative to forcible tranquillization do it only when sufficient police, or mental health staff, have arrived. For a strong patient, four male officers are likely to be needed.

Alternatives:

(a) lorazepam 2–4 mg orally or, preferably, sublingually; or
(b) haloperidol 5–10 mg orally; or, if refused,
(c) lorazepam 1–2 mg i.m; have flumazenil available for use if oversedated; or haloperidol 5–10 mg i.m. Give procyclidine 10 mg i.m. at the same time to counter any exrapyramidal adverse effects.

If two drugs are needed combine lorazepam and haloperidol.

* After rapid tranquillization, check pulse, blood pressure and respiratory rate while waiting for the ambulance to arrive. Ask the crew to continue monitoring with pulse oximetry in the ambulance.

PRECAUTIONS WHEN VISITING A DISTURBED PATIENT AT HOME

* Ensure there is no past history of violence or delusions focused on the GP.
* If necessary, organize support and do not go alone.

* Try to ensure that a relative or friend is present.
* Tell someone in the practice whom you are visiting and when.
* Arrange for the practice staff to phone you after a specified time.
* Have an action plan if you do not respond to the phone call.

REFERRAL AND ADMISSION

Refer all patients suffering from acute psychosis to the psychiatrist or specialist mental health team. The specialist services will usually decide whether the patient needs admission or can be managed at home.

Admission is usually required in acute psychosis especially if:

(a) it is the first episode; or
(b) there is a significant risk of suicide, violence or neglect; or
(c) the patient is non-compliant or has serious side-effects; or
(d) there is coexisting alcohol or drug misuse.

Consider managing at home a patient who is suffering from a relapse of a known mental illness with a previous good response to treatment, where the patient agrees to restart, is at low risk, where home care is safe, and community support available.

Driving. A patient suffering from an acute psychosis or relapse of bipolar affective disorder should not drive and the DVLA must be informed.

COMPULSORY ADMISSION

MENTAL HEALTH ACTS

The WHO Guide to Mental and Neurological Health in Primary Care. Available: www.whoguidemhpcuk.org (choose 'Legal issues')
   England and Wales: www.dh.gov.uk (search on 'Mental Health Act')

INDICATIONS FOR USE OF THE MENTAL HEALTH ACT (ENGLAND AND WALES) 1983

This account includes amendments made to the Mental Health Act up to 2008. It focuses on sections of the Act most relevant to general practice.

The Mental Health Act can only be used if the following conditions are met:

(a) the patient is suffering from a mental disorder of a nature or degree which warrants detention in a hospital for assessment (or assessment followed by medical treatment) for at least a limited period; and
(b) he or she ought to be detained in the interests of his or her own health or safety, or with a view to the protection of others; and
(c) there is no alternative management other than compulsory admission to hospital.

● 'Mental disorders' are mental illness, psychopathic disorder, mental impairment and severe mental impairment. The latter two disorders refer to patients with learning difficulties associated with abnormally aggressive or seriously irresponsible conduct.
● Although often called by relatives or neighbours, the doctor's role is to safeguard the patient's welfare and not that of the relatives or neighbours, unless they are in danger.
● A patient can be admitted compulsorily even when he or she poses no danger, provided that he or she is sufficiently ill (e.g. acutely psychotic) to need compulsory admission because treatment is urgently needed for the sake of the patient's health.
● An approved mental health professional (AMHP) is responsible for making the application for compulsory admission, for co-ordinating the medical assessment of the patient, providing the forms and arranging for the transport of the patient to hospital.
● Every practice, and PCT, should have agreed on a procedure for the management of psychiatric crises. Appendix 21 is an example.

THE ASSESSMENT UNDER THE ACT

* Obtain all available information, from the patient's records and from available friends and family. Try to find out who is the next of kin: they have the right to be informed, to object to detention, and to insist that a detained patient be discharged, unless that patient poses a danger.
* Telephone the AMHP and agree a plan. This should include whether to involve a second doctor or the police at this stage.

✱ If admission looks likely, contact the duty psychiatrist to discuss the availability of a bed and the need for his or her attendance.

✱ If the decision is made not to admit the patient, work out a care plan. Essential features are that family members know whom to call in an emergency, and that intensive follow-up arrangements are put in place.

WHICH SECTION OF THE ACT SHOULD BE USED?

How desperate is the situation?

■ *The patient is about to injury him or herself or others.* The doctor may restrain the patient or give emergency treatment knowing that under common law such action is defensible if done in good faith. Such action would normally be followed by an admission under the Act using Section 2 (28 days) although if the emergency continues Section 4 (72 hours) might be needed.

■ *Admission is needed and is so urgent that*:

(a) the doctor cannot leave the patient; and

(b) waiting for an approved clinician (usually an approved psychiatrist) would cause 'undesirable delay'.

Use Section 4 (detention for 72 hours). This requires assessment by a doctor and an AMHP. Admission must take place within 24 hours of the assessment or the application whichever is earlier. The fact that attendance by the approved clinician is inconvenient is not grounds for the use of this section.

■ *Admission is needed but there is time to wait for an approved clinician.* Use Section 2 (28 days). This is the preferred section and will be used in almost all cases. It requires assessment by a mental health professional approved under Section 12 of the Act (the 'first' doctor) and by a doctor with previous knowledge of the patient (the 'second' doctor) and an AMHP. Admission must take place within 5 days or the application is void. Arrange to see the patient together if possible, although the Act allows the two doctors to examine the patient up to 5 days apart.

FURTHER CLARIFICATIONS

● The 'second' doctor should be one with previous knowledge of the patient. However, if no such doctor is available, any doctor may sign provided he or she does not work in the same hospital as the 'first' doctor.

● In theory the application for compulsory admission may be made by the next of kin. In practice this is rarely wise: an AMHP is needed to ensure that the formalities are observed, that a full assessment is made, and to avoid later recriminations within the family if the next of kin made such a decision.

● It is occasionally possible to commit a patient to hospital under the Act even if he or she agrees to informal admission. A psychiatrist may recommend this course of action if, from previous knowledge of the patient, a judgment is made that an apparent agreement to informal admission is not likely to be sustained. If taking this line of action, the reasons for doing so must be stated on the form.

● Once an application has been signed, decide how to escort the patient into an ambulance. Given time and patience it is usually possible to achieve it without force. If force is needed it is the role of the police rather than the ambulance crew (see page 471).

● Drug or alcohol dependency is not, in itself, grounds for compulsory admission. This is only possible if the person also suffers from a mental disorder as defined in the Act. If a patient is under the influence of drugs or alcohol so that a proper assessment cannot be made, it should be postponed until such assessment is possible.

● Learning difficulty is not grounds for compulsory admission under Sections 3 or 4 unless associated with 'abnormally aggressive or seriously irresponsible conduct'. However, the other relevant sections, including section 2, can be used.

● Psychopathic disorder is defined as 'a persistent disorder or disability of mind (whether or not including significant impairment of intelligence) that results in abnormally aggressive or seriously irresponsible conduct on the part of the person concerned'. It is grounds for compulsory admission, regardless of whether it is treatable, provided that the other criteria are met. Only in using Section 3 is it necessary that the pyschopathy should be 'treatable', i.e. that treatment should be necessary to alleviate or prevent deterioration in the patient's condition.

OTHER SECTIONS OF VALUE

Section 3 allows for detention for 6 months. It is occasionally used in the community instead of Section 4 if the patient is already known to the psychiatric services. In practice it is almost always used once the patient is in hospital and before a section 2 or 4 has expired.

Section 7 allows the appointment of a guardian for up to 6 months. The guardian has the power to insist that the patient live at a specified place, attend for work, training, or medical appointments.

Section 136 allows the police to remove a person from a public place to a hospital or police station, for a maximum period of 72 hours, if they are:

(a) suffering from a mental disorder; and
(b) in immediate need of care and control.

Section 135 allows a magistrate to authorize a police officer (with a doctor and AMHP) to enter any premises to which access has been denied, and remove the patient to a place of safety if there is reasonable cause to suspect that the person is:

(a) suffering from a mental disorder; and
(b) is being ill-treated or neglected or not kept under proper control; or
(c) is unable to care for themselves and lives alone.

The GP can usually gain entry legally without using Section 135, for instance by asking the neighbours to open the door, or by using his or her relationship with the patient to get the door open.

A Community Treatment Order (CTO) ensures that assessment and treatment are carried out in the community with the responsible clinician having the power to recall the patient to hospital if necessary.

REGULATIONS FOR SCOTLAND AND NORTHERN IRELAND

These follow similar principles to those for England and Wales but the brief details of the Acts are as follows (Table 16.3 and Table 16.4):

For emergency detention the following must apply:

(a) the person has a mental disorder which causes his or her decision-making to be 'significantly impaired';
(b) it is necessary as a matter of urgency to detain the person for assessment;
(c) the person's health, safety or welfare, or the safety of another person, would be at significant risk if he or she was not detained;

Table 16.3	Mental Health (Care and Treatment) (Scotland) Act 2003 (see www.nes.scot.nhs.uk/mha/)		
TYPE OF COMPULSION	**PROFESSIONALS**	**DURATION**
Emergency detention	GP, and MHO if practicable	72 hours
Short-term detention	GP and MHO	28 days
Compulsory treatment order	MHO, AMP and patient's GP or another AMP	6 months
Power of entry	MHO obtains from sheriff or JP	Single event

GP, general practitioner; MHO, mental health officer; AMP, approved medical practitioner.

(d) making arrangements for the possible granting of a short-term detention certificate (see below) would involve 'undesirable delay'.

For short-term detention the same four criteria must apply except that it need not be a matter of urgency, and detention is for assessment or treatment.

For a compulsory treatment order the following must apply:

(a) the patient has a mental disorder;
(b) medical treatment is available which would be likely to prevent the disorder worsening, or would be likely to alleviate the symptoms or effects of the disorder;
(c) there would be a significant risk to the patient or to any other person if the patient was not provided with such treatment;
(d) the patient's ability to make decisions about the provision of medical treatment is significantly impaired because of his or her mental disorder;
(e) the making of the compulsory treatment order is necessary.

A compulsory treatment order may authorize detention in hospital or impose certain requirements on the patient in the community (a community-based compulsory treatment order).

The Act also allows for the removal to a place of safety of a person who is exposed to ill-treatment or neglect, or who is unable to look after him or herself or property/financial affairs. It further allows for a person to be removed from a public place to a place of safety where it is in the interests of that person, or where it is necessary to protect other people (NHS Education for Scotland 2004).

Table 16.4		Mental Health (Northern Ireland) Order 1986	
SITUATION	SECTION	PROFESSIONALS	DURATION
Emergency	4	GP and ASW or relative	7 days
Power of entry	129	ASW obtains from JP. GP and police enter.	Single event

ASW, approved social worker; GP, general practitioner; JP, justice of the peace; MHO, mental health officer; AMP, approved medical practitioner.
For more details, see: www.psychiatry.ox.ac.uk/cebmh/whoguidemhpcuk/mha.html

ADVICE FOR PATIENTS AND PROFESSIONALS

MIND provides a leaflet on the Act available on www.mind.org.uk (search on 'Mental Health Act')
  The WHO Guide to Mental and Neurological Health in Primary Care. Available: www.whoguidemhpcuk.org (Choose 'Legal issues'). It contains information for patients and professionals

CHRONIC SCHIZOPHRENIA

GUIDELINE

National Collaborating Centre for Mental Health. 2002. *Schizophrenia.* Full national clinical guideline on core interventions in primary and secondary care. Commissioned by the National Institute for Health and Clinical Excellence. Available: www.nice.org.uk

- About 1% of a practice population will suffer from schizophrenia at some time in their life, more in cities and in immigrant communities. Between 25 and 40% will lose contact with secondary services while still chronically ill (DTB 1994).
- Structured care offers a chance of improving the management of such patients.
- In 2002 an average UK GP looked after 12 patients with schizophrenia, half of them without current involvement of the specialist mental health services (Picchioni and Murray 2007).

STRUCTURED CARE

This entails:
(a) Establishing a register of patients with severe and enduring mental illness. This can be done from existing clinical codes, from repeat prescriptions for psychotropic drugs, from addresses of hostels and homes catering for the mentally ill, and opportunistically;
(b) Using the register to ensure that patients are seen at least 6-monthly. Seek out patients who default from follow-up;
(c) Working with local mental health teams to identify agreed policies and guidelines for treatment, referral, and the management of relapse;
(d) Adapting existing computer templates to record long-term follow-up and undertaking practice audit of the above goals.

REFERRAL

* Arrange for urgent assessment of the following:
  - those presenting for the first time;
  - those posing a risk to themselves or to others;
  - those relapsing, or showing the prodrome of a relapse;
  - those at risk of relapse because of:
    (a) a deterioration in their home circumstances; or
    (b) poor compliance; or
    (c) abuse of drugs or alcohol;
  - those suffering from side-effects of medication or who are not taking it.
Such an assessment is better done at home than in the outpatient department if possible.
  Patients will also need to be referred, although not necessarily urgently, if:
- they are becoming increasingly disabled by their illness; or
- a care plan needs to be drawn up, as when a patient moves to a new area; or
- the patient or family request referral or the therapeutic relationship has broken down.

GENERAL MANAGEMENT

* *Education.* The patient and the family need to know:
  (a) that 85–90% recover from the first episode in the following 2 years (WHO 1979). In the

5 years following the first episode, half do not relapse, or relapse but recover completely between episodes. 20% will never have another episode (Picchioni and Murray 2007);

(b) how to identify early signs of relapse. Looking for early warning signs can prevent relapse or reduce its severity (Falloon, Laporta, Fadden and Graham-Hole 1993). The Early Warning Signs Form (see Appendix 22) can be used to help with this;

(c) how to obtain early treatment;

(d) that avoiding extremes of expressed emotion by family members, whether hostility or overprotectiveness, can reduce the risk of relapse.

* *Advance directives.* Discuss the use of advance directives with patient and family. These indicate what the patient wants to happen if a relapse occurs. If one is drawn up, the patient, and primary and secondary care, all need copies.

* Check that the patient has been offered the benefits of case management. In the UK this takes the form of the care programme approach, in which a specialist team assists the patient with daily living, in the understanding of the condition and in its management.

* If fit for sheltered work, liaise with the mental health team or the disablement resettlement officer (see page 4).

* Assess the patient's housing needs.

* Help the patient to claim the disability living allowance if eligible (see page 6).

DRUG TREATMENT

● Early drug treatment seems to lead to better medium- and long-term outcomes (Loebel, Lieberman, Alvir, *et al.* 1992).

● Without drugs, 60% of patients relapse in the 9 months after an acute attack. Maintenance with antipsychotics reduces this by over a half.

● Atypical antipsychotics are now first line drugs in the UK, although, if a patient is successfully treated with a conventional antipsychotic, it should not be changed (NICE 2002). Atypical antipsychotics are chosen because of the lower incidence of extrapyramidal adverse effects and possibly greater effect on cognition and on negative symptoms. However, they are no more effective than typical antipsychotics and overall they have as many, but different, adverse effects (Picchioni and Murray 2007). The exceptions to this are clozapine and olanzapine, which may be more effective than other drugs (Citrone and Stroup 2006).

● The choice of long-term medication should be made by the psychiatrist and patient together. It will be needed for at least 1–2 years after a relapse and monitoring will be needed for 2 years after that.

● All antipsychotics are associated with an increased risk of sudden cardiac death as well as of stroke. An expert working group of the CSM recommends a baseline ECG in those at increased risk of cardiovascular events: e.g. the elderly, and those with a personal or family history of heart disease (MHRA 2006). The MHRA recommends that all patients taking an antipsychotic should have regular monitoring of serum potassium, especially during an illness that can lead to potassium loss, e.g. diarrhoea.

RELAPSE

Ascertain whether the relapse is due to the patient discontinuing medication. If it is:

* assess the reason for stopping treatment, e.g. the presence of side-effects, failure to obtain a prescription, etc.;

* decide if restarting previous medication is appropriate and acceptable;

* review the need for urgent psychiatric assessment;

* if assessment is needed but will be delayed, and there is concern about medication, phone for advice from the psychiatrist.

MEDICATION REVIEW

Patients need a medication review at least once every 6 months (Primary Care Schizophrenia Consensus Group 2005). The repeat prescription slip should indicate when a medication review is due. Someone in the practice needs to be responsible for ensuring such patients have attended for this review, and to know what action to take if the patient defaults. The medication review will include:

■ assessment of mental state and compliance;

■ presence of adverse effects or drug interactions. Adverse effects with conventional antipsychotics are likely to be extrapyramidal; with atypical antipsychotics they are likely to be weight gain and hyperprolactinaemia;

- existence of drug or alcohol problems;
- whether the patient has been admitted in the past 6 months;
- patients on clozapine need monitoring for agranulocytosis, weekly for 6 months then monthly in the UK. Organizing this is the responsibility of the prescriber. If delegated to primary care a written protocol is needed.

SIDE-EFFECTS OF MEDICATION

Conventional antipsychotics

- Extra-pyramidal adverse effects. If they occur, discuss management with the specialist. The main options are:
  (a) reduce the dose of the antipsychotic;
  (b) add an anticholinergic drug, e.g. orphenadrine 50 mg t.d.s. Avoid procyclidine, which is a stimulant and can be abused. Try to withdraw an anticholinergic after 3 months without symptoms. Tetrabenazine may help in tardive dyskinesia;
  (c) change to an atypical antipsychotic. Clozapine is the treatment of choice.
- Neuroleptic malignant syndrome occurs in 0.5%.

Atypical antipsychotics

- Weight gain;
- Dizziness and postural hypotension in the early stages;
- Diabetes;
- Extra-pyramidal adverse effects, but they are uncommon and usually respond to dose reduction.

All anti-psychotics

- Palpitations. Repeat the ECG. If the QT interval is prolonged but is ≤ 500 ms, reduce the dose. If it is > 500 ms, stop the drug (MHRA 2006).

PSYCHOTHERAPY

Good evidence exists for both cognitive behavioural therapy and family therapy (NICE 2002). A minimum course of 6 months of either is needed. If they are available they should be offered as well as medication.

ANNUAL REVIEW

The annual review is likely to be more comprehensive if a checklist or computer template is used. Topics to cover are:

(a) current mental state including the presence of depression, delusional thoughts, anxiety, hallucinations, signs of self-neglect. Half of patients with schizophrenia develop depression at some stage. It carries a higher risk of suicide than depression in other patients (Jones and Buckley 2003);
(b) problems, crises or admissions since last seen;
(c) daily activities, employment, training, income and disability benefits;
(d) substance misuse, which is likely in half of patients;
(e) accommodation needs;
(f) carers, relationships, dependants (children), home support;
(g) assessment of physical health including weight, blood pressure, cervical screening, smoking status, family planning needs, fasting sugar, assessment of CVD risk. In the US an annual ECG is recommended in those on an antipsychotic which can prolong the QT interval;
(h) medication review and blood tests if necessary;
(i) whether care is GP only or shared with psychiatrist, CPN, or social worker;
(j) assessment of carer's needs.

CARERS' NEEDS (see page 626)

People who care for someone with severe and enduring mental illness should have:

(a) a needs assessment at regular intervals;
(b) a care plan which is reviewed annually;
(c) links with local carer support groups.

Carers need to be identified and this information should be put on their summary card or computer problem list. The practice should have a carers' register and a practice policy on whom to assess, when and by whom. Social services should record each carer's needs, and draw up an agreed care plan which includes:

(a) information about the mental health needs of the patient;
(b) how to identify a relapse and what action to take;
(c) advice on benefits, housing and employment;

(d) arrangements for short-term breaks;

(e) social support including access to carers' support groups;

(f) information about appeals or complaints procedures.

The plan should be confirmed in writing and communicated to the primary care team. The GP is the professional most likely to identify signs of stress or deteriorating health of a carer. The plan will indicate who should review the carer's needs at such times and the GP can initiate this.

PATIENT ORGANIZATIONS

Rethink Severe Mental Illness, 89 Albert Embankment, London SE1 7TP. General enquiries tel. 0845 456 0455; national advice line 020 7840 3188; www.rethink.org

MIND, Mindinfoline 0845 766 0163; www.mind.org.uk

SANE, Saneline tel. 0845 767 8000; email support via the website www.sane.org.uk

Patient information

The WHO Guide to Mental and Neurological Health in Primary Care provides information for patients. It is available online: www.whoguidemhpcuk.org (Choose 'Patient resources' then 'Psychoses')

The Royal College of Psychiatrists. Available: www.rcpsych.ac.uk (Choose 'Mental health info' then 'Schizophrenia')

Carer information

Wilkinson G, Kendrick T, Moore B. 1999. *A Carer's Guide to Schizophrenia*. RSM Press, London

---

BIPOLAR AFFECTIVE DISORDER

GENERAL MANAGEMENT

* Check that the patient has had a recent assessment by a specialist and that everyone is clear who the key worker is, in case of difficulties.
* Explain the nature of the condition to the patient and family.
* Agree on what the warning signs of relapse are for that individual (see Appendix 22).
* Draw up a plan of action for when relapse occurs. This will depend on the form the relapse

takes; in hypomania it may mean removing cheques, debit and credit cards from the patient; in depression it may mean intensifying social support. In mania it may involve supplying medication (an anti-psychotic or a benzodiazepine) to be taken at the first sign of relapse.

* Explore whether stressors seem to trigger a relapse: irregular hours, lack of sleep, use of alcohol or drugs.
* Enter the patient on the practice register of patients with severe mental illness.
* Ensure recall for annual reviews (see page 475).
* Offer information about the local and national support that is available (see box).

DURING EPISODES OF DEPRESSION

* Manage as for depression (see page 454) but with an antimanic agent as well (e.g. lithium, an antipsychotic, valproic acid (rather than sodium valproate) or carbamazepine) or with lamotrigine, after discussion with the patient's specialist (Goodwin 2003). It is likely that the specialist will recommend that the antidepressant be used short-term only. Long-term use is associated with inducing mania, with rapid cycling (more frequent episodes) and mixed states in which mania and depression co-exist (Berk, Dodd, Berk, *et al.* 2005). This adverse effect may only be associated with tricyclic antidepressants (Scottish Intercollegiate Guidelines Network 2005).

DURING EPISODES OF MANIA OR HYPOMANIA

* Avoid unnecessary confrontation.
* Check if there was a trigger for the relapse and whether it can be rectified.
* Assess the risk of impulsive behaviour, e.g. financial or business recklessness.
* Assess the need for admission, including compulsory admission, or for referral to the community mental health team.
* Tell the family who to contact if the patient becomes very agitated or severely disruptive.
* Identify the carer's needs. In chronic illness consider respite care.

MEDICATION

* Discuss the options with the patient's specialist. They are likely to involve:

  (a) an oral antipsychotic or valproic acid or carbamazepine. Olanzapine is probably more effective than the other options but at the expense of greater sedation and weight gain (Macritchie, Geddes, Scott, *et al.* 2003);

  (b) increasing lithium while keeping the blood level within the therapeutic range;

  (c) short-term use of a benzodiazepine for night sedation;

  (d) tailing off an antidepressant if one is being taken.

* Do not expect dramatic improvement. Even in the ideal setting of clinical trials only about half the patients have a 50% improvement of symptoms over 3–4 weeks (Keck 2003).

* Prepare to taper off the antipsychotic over at least 2 weeks once in full remission. Continued use can precipitate depression.

PREVENTION OF RELAPSE

Lithium is the first line drug. Alternatives are carbamazepine or, especially if depression is the major problem, lamotrigine.

Lithium

The GP needs to:

(a) Ensure clear agreement on who is responsible for monitoring lithium treatment.

(b) Have an agreed protocol for monitoring blood levels, identifying side-effects and taking appropriate action. Put the patient on the recall register for monitoring blood levels.

(c) Provide the patient with a written description of drug side-effects and what to do if these develop e.g. lithium toxicity in *The WHO Guide to Mental and Neurological Health in Primary Care* (see below).

(d) Check the patient knows to maintain adequate fluid intake and avoid dehydration and NSAIDs.

(e) Check that the patient understands that the lithium should not be stopped, unless toxicity occurs, as relapse may occur.

(f) *Lithium levels.* Check lithium levels every 3 months. Take blood 12 hours after the last dose. Levels of 0.4–0.8 mmol/l are adequate for maintenance but in acute mania a level of 0.8–1 mmol/l is necessary.

(g) *Change in dose.* If the dose is changed, check levels weekly for 4 weeks, then monthly for 3 months and then 3-monthly.

(h) Check thyroid and renal function annually.

(i) Warn women of reproductive age that lithium is an enzyme inducer which reduces the efficacy of the combined oral contraceptive, and that it carries a risk of teratogenicity as well.

Management of suspected lithium toxicity

Symptoms of toxicity include muscle weakness, shaking, trembling, fasciculation, nausea, vomiting or diarrhoea, ataxia, confusion, slurred speech, toxic psychosis, convulsions, coma and cardiac arrhythmias.

* Check the lithium level and U&Es.

* Stop lithium. Levels usually fall to safety within 24 hours. If the lithium level is more than 1.5 mmol/l, or there is diarrhoea and vomiting, stop lithium immediately and seek urgent specialist advice.

* Identify the cause of the toxicity before restarting lithium.

* If no cause is found, restart at a lower dose.

* Monitor levels monthly for 3 months after toxicity for which there was no obvious reason.

SUPPORT AND ADVICE FOR PATIENTS AND FAMILIES

Manic Depression Fellowship. Tel. 08456 340 540; www.mdf.org.uk

The Mental Health Foundation. They do not offer advice or support and there is no helpline, but the website has useful information: www.mentalhealth.org.uk

WHO Guide to Mental and Neurological Health in Primary Care. www.whoguidemhpcuk.org (choose 'Patient resources' then 'Bipolar disorder')

DEALING WITH VIOLENCE

GUIDANCE

Braithwaite R. 1992. *Violence: Understanding, Intervention and Prevention.* Oxford: Radcliffe Professional Press

Every practice needs a policy for dealing with violent patients. Many of these patients have a past history of violent or threatening behaviour. A typical policy would include:

(a) a notice in the waiting room stating that physical or verbal abuse, racism, threats or violence to staff will result in removal from the practice;

(b) panic buttons in consulting rooms and a clear procedure to follow if one is set off;

(c) clear guidelines on who should deal with an aggressive, abusive or violent patient in the waiting room;

(d) how risks will be assessed and what action will be taken (Shaw 2000);

(e) a protocol for the management of a patient whose delusions are focused on a specific doctor or nurse;

(f) written indications on when to call the police and who should do so;

(g) guidance on how to deal with home visit requests to a potentially violent patient;

(h) sympathetic support for staff exposed to violent situations;

(i) a policy of informing local GPs that a violent patient who has been removed from the practice list may want to register with them;

(j) a record kept of all such incidents;

(k) a way to report these incidents as 'significant events' so that lessons can be learnt by others.

References

Allen, L., Woolfolk, R., Escobar, J., et al., 2006. Cognitive-behavioral therapy for somatization disorder: a randomized controlled trial. Arch. Int. Med. 166, 1512–1518.

American Psychiatric Association, 2000a. Posttraumatic stress disorder. Diagnostic and Statistical Manual of Mental Disorders, 4th ed. text revision. American Psychiatric Association, Washington DC.

American Psychiatric Association, 2000b. Diagnostic and Statistical Manual of Mental Disorders, 4th ed. text revision. American Psychiatric Association, Washington DC.

Anderson, I., Nutt, D., Deakin, J., 2000. Evidence-based guidelines for treating depressive disorders with antidepressants: a revision of the 1993 British Association for Psychopharmacology guidelines. J. Psychopharmacol. 14, 3–20.

Angst, J., 1997. A regular review of the long-term follow-up of depression. BMJ 315, 1143–1146.

Ballenger, J., Tylee, A., 2003. Anxiety. Mosby.

Barrett, J., Williams, J., Oxman, T., et al., 2001. Treatment of dysthymia and minor depression in primary care. J. Fam. Pract. 50, 405–412.

Bennewith, O., Stocks, N., Gunnell, D., et al., 2002. General practice based intervention to prevent repeat episodes of deliberate self harm; cluster randomised controlled trial. BMJ 324, 1254–1257.

Berk, M., Dodd, S., Berk, J., et al., 2005. Diagnosis and management of patients with bipolar disorder in primary care. Br. J. Gen. Pract. 55, 662–664.

Bisson, J., 2004. Post-traumatic stress disorder: what are the effects of preventive psychological interventions? Clin. Evid. Available: www.clinicalevidence.com.

Boardman, J., Walters, P., 2009. Managing depression in primary care: it's not only what you do it's

the way that you do it. Br. J. Gen. Pract. 59, 76–78.

Bostwick, J., Pankratz, V., 2000. Affective disorders and suicide risk: a reexamination. Am. J. Psychiatry 157, 1925–1932.

Breckenbridge, A., 2000. Important interactions between St John's wort (*Hypericum perforata*) preparations and prescribed medicines. Committee on Safety of Medicines, 29 Feb.

Brent, D., 2007. Antidepressants and suicidal behavior: cause or cure? Am. J. Psychiatry 164, 989–991.

Buscemi, N., Vandermeer, B., Hooton, N., et al., 2004. Melatonin for treatment of sleep disorders. Agency for Healthcare Research and Quality, Rockville, MD. Evidence report/technology assessment No. 108.

Buscemi, N., Vandermeer, B., Hooton, N., et al., 2006. Efficacy and safety of exogenous melatonin for secondary sleep disorders and sleep disorders accompanying sleep restriction: meta-analysis. BMJ 332, 385–388.

Buszewicz, M., Pistrang, N., Barker, C., et al., 2006. Patients experiences of GP consultations for psychological problems: a qualitative study. Br. J. Gen. Pract. 56, 496–503.

Casacalenda, N., Perry, J., Looper, K., 2002. Remission in major depressive disorder: a comparison of pharmacotherapy, psychotherapy, and control conditions. Am. J. Psychiatry 159, 1354–1360.

Chilvers, C., Dewey, M., Fielding, K., et al., 2001. Antidepressant drugs and generic counselling for treatment of major depression in primary care: randomised trial with patient preference arms. BMJ 322, 772–775.

Cipriani, A., Barbui, C., Geddes, J., 2005. Suicide, depression, and antidepressants. BMJ 330, 373–374.

Cipriani, A., Furukawa, T., Salanti, G., et al., 2009. Comparative efficacy and acceptability of 12 new-generation antidepressants: a multiple-treatments meta-analysis. Lancet 373, 746–758.

Cipriani, A., Geddes, J., Barbui, C., 2007. Venlafaxine for major depression. BMJ 334, 215–216.

Citrone, L., Stroup, T., 2006. Schizophrenia, clinical antipsychotic trials of intervention effectiveness (CATIE) and number needed to treat: how can CATIE inform clinicians? Int. J. Clin. Pract. 60, 933–940.

Coupland, N., Bell, C., Potokar, J., 1996. Serotonin reuptake inhibitor withdrawal. J. Clin. Psychopharmacol. 16, 356–362.

Cox, J.L., Holden, J.M., Sagovsky, R., 1987. Detection of postnatal depression. Br. J. Psychiatry 150, 782–786.

CSM Expert Working Group, 2004. Safety of selective serotonin reuptake inhibitor antidepressants. Committee on Safety of Medicines, London. Available: http://www.mca.gov.uk/aboutagency/regframework/csm/csmhome.htm.

Das, A., Olfson, M., Gameroff, M., et al., 2005. Screening for bipolar disorder in a primary care practice. JAMA 293, 956–963.

Department of Health, 1999. National Service Framework for Mental Health. The Stationery Office, London. Available: www.dh.gov.uk.

DoH, 2001. Treatment choice in psychological therapies and counselling: evidence based clinical practice guideline. Department of Health, London. Available: www.dh.gov.uk.

DTB, 1994. Long-term management of people with psychotic disorders in the community. Drug Ther. Bull. 32, 73–77.

Dugas, M., Ladouceur, R., Leger, E., 2003. Group cognitive-behavioral therapy for generalized anxiety disorder: treatment outcome and long-term follow-up. J. Consult. Clin. Psychol. 71, 821–825.

Dunn, A., Trivedi, M., Kampert, J., et al., 2005. Exercise treatment for depression: efficacy and dose response. Am. J. Prev. Med. 28, 1–8.

Falloon, I., Laporta, M., Fadden, G., Graham-Hole, V., 1993. Managing Stress in Families: Cognitive and Behavioural Strategies for Enhancing Coping Skills. Routledge, London.

Fava, G., Ruini, C., Rafanelli, C., 2004. Six-year outcome of cognitive behavior therapy for prevention of recurrent depression. Am. J. Psychiatry 161, 1872–1876.

Fisher, P., Durham, R., 1999. Recovery rates in generalized anxiety disorder following psychological therapy: an analysis of clinically significant change in the STAI-T across outcome studies since 1990. Psychol. Med. 29, 1425–1434.

Freeling, P., Rao, B., Paykel, E., et al., 1985. Unrecognised depression in general practice. BMJ 290, 1880–1883.

Furukawa, T., McGuire, H., Barbui, C., 2002. Meta-analysis of effects and side effects of low dosage tricyclic antidepressants in depression: systematic review. BMJ 325, 991–995.

Furukawa, T., Watanabe, N., Churchill, R., 2007. Combined psychotherapy plus antidepressants for panic disorder with or without agoraphobia. Cochrane Database Syst. Rev. (1) CD004364.

Gale, C., Davidson, O., 2007. Generalised anxiety disorder. BMJ 334, 579–581.

Gale, C., Oakley-Browne, M., 2004a. Generalised anxiety disorder: what are the effects of drug treatments? Benzodiazepines. Clin. Evid. Available: www.clinicalevidence.com.

Gale, C., Oakley-Browne, M., 2004b. Generalised anxiety disorder: what are the effects of cognitive therapy? Clin. Evid. Available: www.clinicalevidence.com.

Gale, C., Oakley-Browne, M., 2004c. Generalised anxiety disorder: what are the effects of drug treatments? Beta-blockers. Clin. Evid. Online. Available: www.clinicalevidence.com.

Geddes, J., Carney, S., Davies, C., et al., 2003. Relapse prevention with antidepressant drug treatment in depressive disorders: a systematic review. Lancet 361, 653–661.

Gill, D., Hatcher, S., 2002. Antidepressants for depression in medical illness (Cochrane Review). In: The Cochrane Library. Issue 1. Update Software, Oxford.

Glass, J., Lanctot, K., Herrmann, N., et al., 2005. Sedative hypnotics in older people with insomnia: meta-analysis of risks and benefits. BMJ 331, 1169–1173.

Gloaguen, V., Cottraux, J., Cucherat, M., et al., 1998. A meta-analysis of the effects of cognitive therapy in depressed patients. J. Affect. Disord. 49, 59–72.

Goldberg, D., Bridges, K., 1987. Screening for psychiatric illness in general practice: the general practitioner versus the screening questionnaire. J. R. Coll. Gen. Pract. 37, 15–18.

Goldberg, D., Lecrubier, Y., 1995. Form and frequency of mental disorders across centres. In: Ustun, B., Sartorius, N. (eds.), Mental illness in general health care: an international study. WHO, John Wiley, Chichester, pp. 323–334.

Goodwin, G., 2003. Evidence-based guidelines for treating bipolar disorder: recommendations from the British Association for Psychopharmacology. J. Psychopharmacol. 17, 149–173.

Haddad, P., Lejoyeux, M., Young, A., 1998. Antidepressant discontinuation reactions. BMJ 316, 1105–1106.

Haug, T., Blomhoff, S., Hellstrom, K., et al., 2003. Exposure therapy and sertraline in social phobia: 1 year follow-up of a randomised controlled trial. Br. J. Psychiatry 182, 312–318.

Hawton, K., Zahl, D., Weatherall, R., 2003. Suicide following deliberate self-harm: long-term follow-up of patients who presented to a general hospital. Br. J. Psychiatry 182, 537–542.

Hawton, K., 2003. Helping people bereaved by suicide. BMJ 327, 177–178.

Holden, J., Sagovsky, R., Cox, J., 1989. Counselling in a general practice setting: controlled study of health visitor intervention in treatment of postnatal depression. BMJ 298, 223–226.

Hull, A., 2004. Primary care management of post-traumatic stress disorder. Prescriber April 1940–48.

Jick, H., Kaye, J., Jick, S., 2004. Antidepressants and the risk of suicidal behaviors. JAMA 292, 338–343.

Jones, P., Buckley, P., 2003. Schizophrenia. Mosby.

Jones, R., Chung, M., Berger, Z., et al., 2007. Prevalence of post-traumatic stress disorder in patients with previous myocardial infarction consulting in general practice. Br. J. Gen. Pract. 57, 808–810.

Jorm, A., Christensen, H., Griffiths, K., Rodgers, B., 2002. Effectiveness of complementary and self-help treatments for depression. MJA 176, S84–S96.

Kapczinski, F., Lima, M., Souza, J., 2003. Antidepressants for generalized anxiety disorder. Cochrane Database Syst. Rev. (2).

Kapur, N., Cooper, J., Rodway, C., et al., 2005. Predicting the risk of repetition of self harm: cohort study. BMJ 330, 394–395.

Katon, W., Roy-Byrne, P., 2007. Anxiety disorders: efficient screening is the first step in improving outcomes. Ann. Int. Med. 146, 390–392.

Keck, P., 2003. The management of acute mania. BMJ 327, 1002–1003.

Loebel, A., Lieberman, J., Alvir, J., et al., 1992. Duration of psychosis and outcome in first-episode schizophrenia. Am. J. Psychiatry 149, 1183–1188.

Macritchie, K., Geddes, J., Scott, J., et al., 2003. Valproate for acute mood episodes in bipolar disorder (Cochrane Review). In: The Cochrane Library. Issue 1. Update Software, Oxford.

Maltby, N., Kirsch, I., Mayers, M., et al., 2002. Virtual reality exposure therapy for the treatment of fear of flying: a controlled investigation. Journal of Consulting and Clinical Psychiatry 70, 1112–1118.

Mental Health Foundation, 2004. Self harm. Mental Health Foundation. Available: www.mentalhealth.org.uk.

MHRA, 2006. Cardiac arrhythmias associated with antipsychotic drugs. Curr. Prob. Pharmacovigilance 31, 9.

Mills, E., Montori, V., Wu, P., et al., 2004. Interaction of St John's wort with conventional drugs: systematic review of clinical trials. BMJ 329, 27–30.

Mol, S., Arntz, A., Metsemakers, J., et al., 2005. Symptoms of post-traumatic stress disorder after non-traumatic events: evidence from an open population study. Br. J. Psychiatry 186, 494–499.

Morgan, K., Dixon, S., Mathers, N., et al., 2003. Psychological treatment for insomnia in the management of long-term hypnotic drug use: a pragmatic randomised controlled trial. Br. J. Gen. Pract. 53, 923–928.

Munro, C., Freeman, C., Law, R., 2004. General practitioners' knowledge of post-traumatic stress disorder: a controlled study. Br. J. Gen. Pract. 54, 843–847.

Mynors-Wallis, L., Gath, D., Day, A., et al., 2000. Controlled trial of problem solving treatment, antidepressant medication, and combined treatment for major depression in primary care. BMJ 320, 26–30.

NHS Direct, 2004. Self harm: NHS Direct. www.nhsdirect.nhs.uk.

NHS Education for Scotland, 2004. Education for Frontline Staff. Mental Health (Care and Treatment) (Scotland) Act: Available: www.nes.scot.nhs.uk/mha.

NICE, 2002. Schizophrenia: core interventions in the treatment and management of schizophrenia in primary and secondary care. National Institute for Clinical Excellence. Available: www.nice.org.uk.

NICE UK, 2004. Postnatal depression. Available: www.nsc.nhs.uk. Choose 'National electronic Library for Screening' then search on 'Postnatal'.

NICE, 2004a. Depression: management of depression in primary and secondary care. NICE Clinical Guideline 23 Available: www.nice.org.uk.

NICE, 2004b. Zaleplon, zolpidem and zopiclone for the short-term management of insomnia. National Institute for Clinical Excellence. Technology Appraisal Guidance 77. Available www.nice. org.uk.

NICE, 2004c. Self-harm: the short-term physical and psychological management and secondary prevention of self-harm in primary and secondary care. National Institute for Clinical Excellence. Guideline No. 16. Available: www.nice.org.uk.

NICE, 2005. Violence: the short-term management of disturbed/violent behaviour in psychiatric inpatient settings and emergency departments. NICE clinical guideline 34. Available: www. nice.org.uk.

NICE, 2005a. Post-traumatic stress disorder: the management of PTSD in adults and children in primary and secondary care. NICE Clinical Guideline 26. Available: www.nice.org.uk.

NICE, 2005b. Obsessive-compulsive disorder: core interventions in the treatment of obsessive-compulsive disorder and body dysmorphic disorder. NICE Clinical Guideline 31. Available: www.nice.org.uk.

NICE, 2006. TA97. Depression and anxiety - computerised cognitive behavioural therapy (CCBT). Available: www.nice.org.uk.

O'Connell, H., Chin, A.V., Cunningham, C., Lawlor, B., 2004. Recent developments: suicide in older people. BMJ 329, 895–899.

Owens, C., Lloyd, K., Campbell, J., 2004. Access to health care prior to suicide: findings from a psychological autopsy study. Br. J. Gen. Pract. 54, 279–281.

Pampallona, S., Bollini, P., Tibaldi, G., 2004. Combined pharmacotherapy and psychological treatment for depression: a systematic review. Arch. Gen. Psychiatry 61, 714–719.

Philipp, M., Kohnen, R., Hiller, K., 1999. Hypericum extract versus imipramine or placebo in patients with moderate depression: randomised multicentre study of treatment for eight weeks. BMJ 319, 1534–1539.

Picchioni, M., Murray, R., 2007. Schizophrenia. BMJ 335, 91–95.

Pohl, R., Feltner, D., Fieve, R., et al., 2005. Efficacy of pregabalin in the treatment of generalized anxiety disorder: double-blind, placebo-controlled comparison of BD versus TID dosing. J. Clin. Psychopharmacol. 25, 151–158.

Price, J., Waller, P., Wood, S., et al., 1996. A comparison of the post-marketing safety of four selective serotonin re-uptake inhibitors including the investigation of symptoms occurring on withdrawal. Br. J. Clin. Pharmacol. 42, 757–763.

Primary Care Schizophrenia Consensus Group, 2005. Guidelines for the Care of Schizophrenia in General Practice. Available: www.eguidelines.co.uk.

Rost, K., Nutting, P., Smith, J., et al., 2002. Managing depression as a chronic disease: a randomised trial of ongoing treatment in primary care. BMJ 325, 934–937.

Royal College of Psychiatrists, 1998. Managing Deliberate Self-harm in Young People. Council Report CR64. Royal College of Psychiatrists, London.

Rush, A., Trivedi, M., Wisniewski, S., et al., 2006. Acute and longer-term outcomes in depressed outpatients requiring one or several treatment steps: a STAR✳D report. Am. J. Psychiatry 163, 1905–1917.

Schneier, F., 2003. Social anxiety disorder. BMJ 327, 515–516.

Scott, J., 2006. Depression should be managed like a chronic disease. BMJ 332, 985–986.

Scottish Intercollegiate Guidelines Network, 2005. Bipolar affective disorder. SIGN Guideline No. 82, Edinburgh. Available: www.sign. ac.uk.

Shaw, J., 2000. Assessing the risk of violence in patients. BMJ 320, 1088–1089.

Simon, G., Heiligenstein, J., Revicki, D., et al., 1999. Long-term outcomes of initial antidepressant drug choice in a 'real world' randomized trial. Arch. Fam. Med. 8, 319–325.

Sivertsen, B., Omvik, S., Pallesen, S., et al., 2006. Cognitive behavioral therapy vs zopiclone for treatment of chronic primary insomnia in older adults: a randomized controlled trial. JAMA 295, 2851–2858.

Smith, D., Dempster, C., Glanville, J., et al., 2002. Efficacy and tolerability of venlafaxine compared with selective serotonin reuptake inhibitors and other antidepressants: a meta-analysis. Br. J. Psychiatry 180, 396–404.

Soomro, G., 2004. Deliberate self-harm. In: Clinical Evidence. BMJ Publishing Group, London.

Stewart, A., 1998. Choosing an anti-depressant: effectiveness based pharmacoeconomics. J. Affect. Disord. 48, 125–133.

Szegedi, A., Kohnen, R., Dienel, A., et al., 2005. Acute treatment of moderate to severe depression with hypericum extract WS 5570 (St John's wort): randomised controlled double blind non-inferiority trial versus parowetine. BMJ 330, 503–506.

Timonen, M., Liukkonen, T., 2008. Management of depression in adults. BMJ 336, 435–439.

Turner, E., Rosenthal, R., 2008. Efficacy of antidepressants. BMJ 336, 516–517.

Van Weel-Baumgarten, E., Van Den Bosch, W., Van Den Hoogen, H., et al., 2000. The validity of the diagnosis of depression in general practice: is using criteria for diagnosis as a routine the answer? Br. J. Gen. Pract. 50, 284–287.

Walsh, J., Muehlbach, M., Lauter, S., et al., 1996. Effects of triazolam on sleep, daytime sleepiness, and morning stiffness in patients with rheumatoid arthritis. J. Rheumatol. 23, 245–252.

WHO, 1979. Schizophrenia: An International Follow-up Study. John Wiley & Sons, Chichester.

WHO, 2003. International Statistical Classification of Diseases and Related Health Problems. 10th revision. Available: www.who.int.en (search on 'ICD 10').

Whooley, M.A., Avins, A.L., Miranda, J., et al., 1997. Case-finding instruments for depression: two questions are as good as many. J. Gen. Int. Med. 12, 439–445.

Wilner, K., Anziano, R., Johnson, A., et al., 2002. The anxiolytic effect of the novel antipsychotic ziprasidone compared with diazepam in subjects anxious before dental surgery. J. Clin. Psychopharmacol. 22, 206–210.

Wilson, S., Nutt, D., 2003. Insomnia: recommended practice management. Prescriber October 5, 45–57.

Woelk, H., for the Remotiv/Imipramine Study Group, 2000. Comparison of St John's wort and imipramine for treating depression: randomised controlled trial. BMJ 321, 536–539.

Wogelius, P., Norgaard, M., Grislum, M., et al., 2006. Maternal use of selective serotonin reuptake inhibitors and risk of congenital malformations. Epidemiology 17, 701–704.

Chapter 17

Substance abuse

CHAPTER CONTENTS

ALCOHOL PROBLEMS

GUIDELINES

Lingford-Hughes AR, Welch S, Nutt DJ. 2004. Evidence-based guidelines for the pharmacological management of substance misuse, addiction and comorbidity: recommendations from the British Association for Psychopharmacology. J Psychopharm 18, 293–335

Scottish Intercollegiate Guidelines Network. 2003. *The Management of Harmful Drinking and Alcohol Dependence in Primary Care.* A national clinical guideline. Edinburgh, SIGN. Available: www.sign.ac.uk and look under 'Guidelines' and 'Mental Health'

National Health and Medical Research Council (NHMRC). 2009. *Australian Guidelines to Reduce Health Risks from Drinking Alcohol.* Available: www. nhmrc.gov.au and search on 'Alcohol'

- In England in 2007, 33% of men and 16% of women were classified as hazardous drinkers. Among adults age 16–74, 9% of men and 4% of women showed some signs of alcohol dependence (NHS Information Centre Lifestyles Statistics 2009).
- There were 863,300 alcohol-related admissions to hospital in 2007/8. This is an increase of 69% since 2002/3. In 2007, there were 6541 deaths directly due to alcohol and it is estimated that alcohol related harm cost the NHS £2.7 billion (NHS Information Centre Lifestyles Statistics 2009).

© 2011 Elsevier Ltd.
DOI: 10.1016/B978-0-7020-3053-6.00017-9

- In 2009, the Department of Health (England and Wales) advised:
  - (a) limits of up to 3-4 units per day for men and 2-3 for women;
  - (b) a daily tally rather than a weekly one;
  - (c) that these maximum sensible limits should not be drunk every day (Department of Health, Home Office, Department for Education and Skills, Department for Culture Media and Sport 2007).
- UK guidelines recognize the dangers of binge drinking and define it as drinking more than 8 units for men and more than six for women on one occasion. Exceeding these limits more than doubles the mortality over non-drinkers (Department of Health, Home Office, Department for Education and Skills, Department for Culture Media and Sport 2007; National Health Committee (New Zealand) 1999; National Health and Medical Research Council 2009).
- Alcohol dependent patients consult their GPs about twice as frequently as other patients in a practice (Buchan, Buckley, Deacon, et al. 1981; Anderson 1985).

SCREENING AND DETECTION

The Alcohol Harm Reduction Strategy for England recommends targeted screening for people that present with symptoms or conditions that could be linked to problem drinking (Prime Minister's Strategy Unit 2004).

Two well-validated brief screening questionnaires are:

- (a) Alcohol Use Disorders Identification Test (AUDIT) (Babor, Higgins-Biddle, Saunders, et al. 2001);
- (b) the Fast Alcohol Screening Test (FAST) (Hodgson, Alwyn, John, et al. 2002).
- AUDIT is the gold standard screening tool and will take around 2 minutes to complete. FAST can be completed in an average time of 20 seconds (Hodgson, Alwyn, John, et al. 2002).
- AUDIT has been validated in a wide variety of settings. It is 92% sensitive and 94% specific in the detection of harmful and hazardous drinking when patients score 8 or more. There is an abbreviated AUDIT-C which asks the first three questions only (Bradley, DeBenedetti, Volk, et al. 2007). See Appendix 23.
- * Consider alcohol as a cause of 'black-outs', accidents, obesity, pancreatitis, dyspepsia,

impotence, anxiety or panic, depression, insomnia, a poor employment record, or a criminal record.

- * When new patients register with a GP they should be asked about weekly and maximum daily alcohol consumption, or an appropriate screening tool should be used (Scottish Intercollegiate Guidelines Network 2003).

FAST

For the first three questions score 0 for never, 1 for less than monthly, 2 for monthly, 3 for weekly and 4 for daily or almost daily
Ask:

1. Men: how often do you have eight or more drinks on one occasion? Women: how often do you have six or more drinks on one occasion?
   - If 0 is scored then there is no need to continue – the patient is not misusing alcohol.
   - If 3 or 4 is scored then there is no need to continue – the patient is a hazardous, harmful or dependent drinker.
2. How often during the last year have you been unable to remember what happened the night before because you had been drinking?
3. How often during the last year have you failed to do what was normally expected of you because of drink?
4. In the last year has a relative or friend, or a doctor or other health workers been concerned about your drinking or suggested you cut down?
   - Score 0 for no, 2 for yes, on one occasion and 4 for yes, on more than one occasion

The minimum score is 0 and the maximum score is 16. The score for hazardous drinking is 3 or more. A positive score does not make a diagnosis of alcohol misuse but indicates that more detailed investigation is necessary.

ASSESSING AND MANAGING PATIENTS WHO DRINK EXCESSIVELY

- * Ask the patient to keep a drink diary for the next week to confirm the amount drunk.
- * Assess whether drinking is at dependent levels that will require detoxification (see page 487).
- * Examine for signs of chronic liver disease and be alert for the wide variety of physical problems alcohol can cause.
- * Take blood for:
  - (a) *a full blood count* (for macrocytosis);

(b) *liver function tests*, including gamma-glutamyl transferase (GGT). Note that the GGT is raised in only one third of those with an alcohol problem, and that a raised level is not specific for alcohol abuse (Bernadt, Mumford, Taylor, *et al.* 1982). However, a raised MCV and a raised GGT detects 75% of problem drinkers (Ashworth and Gerada 1997).

* Check that the drinking is not secondary to some other disorder, e.g. anxiety, phobia, depression or insomnia.
* Be aware of social factors such as employment in the licensing trade, a family history of alcohol problems and a lack of social support.
* *Driving.* Assess in a patient who drives whether the drinking is putting other people at risk (see page 12) (DVLA 2009).
* *Occupation.* Assess whether the patient's job means that other people are being put at risk.
* *Follow up* after 1 month, then 3-monthly for as long as the patient seems to be at risk.

Brief interventions in alcohol use

● There is good evidence that brief interventions are effective in primary care at lowering alcohol consumption (Anderson 1993; Kaner, Dickinson, Beyer, *et al.* 2007).
● Around 8 patients will need to be given a brief intervention in order to achieve a reduction of drinking to non-hazardous levels in one patient (Ockene, Adams, Hurley, *et al.* 1999; WHO Brief Intervention Study Group 1996; Fleming, Mundt, French, *et al.* 2002).
● Brief interventions are variable: they can consist of a short chat or could involve structured sessions of motivational interviewing. The essential elements of brief interventions are included in the FRAMES model (Miller and Sanchez 1991).

MANAGEMENT OF ALCOHOL-DEPENDENT DRINKERS

● Alcohol-dependent drinkers can be identified by the severity of the withdrawal from alcohol. The dangers of fits are real. Untreated, delirium tremens has a mortality of 10–20% (Chick 1989). Alcohol withdrawal is characterized by:
(a) Tremulous state and perceptual disturbance from 6–24 hours. There will be autonomic

overactivity with tremor, sweating, retching, anxiety, illusions and transient hallucinations.
(b) The peak time for seizures is 36 hours and the peak time for delirium is 72 hours (Raistrick 2000).

● The risk of delirium tremens is significant in a patient who has been drinking 12 units a day or more. However, 'DTs' may occur with consumption as low as 8 units a day and as late as 72 hours after stopping drinking (Chick 1989).
● Wernicke-Korsakoff syndrome (WKS) is a disorder with a spectrum of presentations from acute to chronic. Only 20% present with the classic acute triad of eyes signs, global confusion and ataxia of gait (Feeney and Connor 2008).

* Prescribe oral thiamine but if there is concern about acute Wernicke's encephalopathy then high dose parenteral thiamine should be given where there are facilities for resuscitation (small risk of anaphylaxis) (Scottish Intercollegiate Guidelines Network 2003).

Community detoxification

* A benzodiazepine, such as chlordiazepoxide or diazepam, is the drug of choice (Lingford-Hughes, Welch and Nutt 2004; Mayo-Smith 1997).
* Clomethiazole (former name chlormethiazole) should not be used in alcohol detoxification in primary care.
* Refer to the community alcohol team patients with dependent drinking and the following characteristics:
(a) no support at home;
(b) multiple drug problems, including benzodiazepine dependence;
(c) other psychiatric problems, especially depression with suicidal ideas;
(d) physical illness, e.g. jaundice or pancreatitis; known WKS; history of cardiovascular disease;
(e) a previous history of fits or delirium tremens;
(f) severe dependence; or
(g) previous failed attempts at abstinence.
* Consider referring to the community alcohol team patients who do not come into the above categories but who would benefit from the

specialist care or individual or group counselling that they can provide.

* Involve family, friends and organizations to provide support. Family members who enrol in Al-Anon facilitation therapy can succeed in getting previously unmotivated drinkers into treatment (Miller, Meyers and Tonigan 1999).

* Evidence from randomized controlled trials (RCTs) supports the use of the 12-Step Facilitation Programme of AA (Longabaugh, Wirtz, Zweben, *et al.* 1998).

* Ensure that you, as physician, have experience in the management of alcohol withdrawal or discuss the plan with a colleague who has.

* Enlist the support of any community-based staff, e.g. community alcohol nurse.

* Advise the patient to take 1 week off work and stay at home.

* Obtain the patient's agreement not to take alcohol while on sedative drugs.

* Enlist another person to give the patient the drugs; or arrange for the pharmacist to dispense daily.

* Tailor the benzodiazepine dose to the patient. The Severity of Alcohol Dependence Questionnaire (SADQ) (Stockwell, Murphy and Hodgson 1983) can be used to anticipate appropriate regimens but is no substitute for daily clinical assessment. A typical regimen for covering uncomplicated withdrawal might be 10 mg diazepam q.d.s. on day 1 reducing to 0 over 7 days.

* See daily at first to assess the physical condition and ensure compliance. Examine to check for tremor, sweating, raised pulse and BP suggesting inadequate dosing. Reduce the dose if the patient is over-sedated.

* Treatment may be required for 7–10 days but refuse requests for further supplies of benzodiazepines after the detoxification.

* Admit under the physicians any patient who convulses or becomes confused, agitated, paranoid or hallucinates or who develops other new neurological signs.

LONG-TERM MANAGEMENT

* There is good evidence to support the use of some medications in improving drinking behaviour as an adjunct to psychosocial

interventions. There is no good evidence about who might respond to this approach.

* Follow up regularly.

* Agree on a contract with a clear goal; this should be abstinence for patients who have needed help with withdrawal.

* Look again for any underlying psychiatric disorder. Do not attempt this assessment until at least 2 weeks after the patient has stopped drinking as depression may resolve with abstinence.

* Attend again to the patient's social situation. Homeless patients do better in hostels catering specially for those with alcohol problems and, indeed, can be successfully detoxified there (Haigh and Hibbert 1990).

* Consider (especially in the period immediately after detoxification but only as an adjunct to psychosocial interventions):

  (a) *acamprosate and naltrexone*. Can be used to help with maintaining abstinence. Acamprosate reduces craving and can aid in achieving abstinence with a NNT of around 12 to prevent one relapse (Carmen 2004; Slattery, Chick, Cochrane, *et al.* 2003). Naltrexone also reduces craving and can decrease relapses when used for short-term treatment (Srisurapanont and Jarusuraisin 2004).

  (b) *disulfiram*. Used for negative reinforcement it will cause a severe aversive reaction to any alcohol with symptoms including flushing, vomiting, palpitations and hypotension. Evidence of benefit is limited to situations where it is supervized and there is a partner or friend who can give it to the patient every day (Slattery, Chick, Cochrane, *et al.* 2003; Chick, Gough, Falkowski, *et al.* 1992; Hughes and Cook 1997; Garbutt, West and Carey 1999). Patients must be clear that it is dangerous to drink from 12 hours before the first dose until 1 week after the last dose.

SELF-HELP GROUPS

Alcoholics Anonymous; see telephone directory or www.alcoholics-anonymous.org.uk

Al-Anon Family Groups UK and Eire 24-hour Helpline 020 7403 0888

Drinkline (National Alcohol 24-hour Helpline) 0800 917 8282

BENZODIAZEPINE WITHDRAWAL

GUIDELINES

Lingford-Hughes AR, Welch S, Nutt DJ. 2004. Evidence-based guidelines for the pharmacological management of substance misuse, addiction and comorbidity: recommendations from the British Association for Psychopharmacology. J Psychopharm 18, 293–335

Department of Health (England) and the devolved administrations (2007). *Drug Misuse and Dependence: UK Guidelines on Clinical Management.* London: Department of Health (England), the Scottish Government, Welsh Assembly Government and Northern Ireland Executive. Available: www.dh.gov.uk (search on 'Drug misuse and dependence')

Lader M, Russell J. 1993. Guidelines for the prevention and treatment of benzodiazepine dependence: summary of a report from the Mental Health Foundation. Addiction 88, 1707–1708

Ford C, Roberts K, Barjolin J. 2005. *Guidance on Prescribing Benzodiazepines to Drug Users in Primary Care.* SMMGP. Available: www.smmgp.org.uk (under 'Resource library' and 'Guidance documents')

ADVICE OF THE UK COMMITTEE ON THE SAFETY OF MEDICINES

1. Benzodiazepines are indicated for the short-term relief (2–4 weeks only) of anxiety that is severe, disabling or subjecting the individual to unacceptable distress, occurring alone or in association with insomnia or short-term psychosomatic, organic or psychotic illness.
2. The use of benzodiazepines to treat short-term 'mild' anxiety is inappropriate and unsuitable.
3. Benzodiazepines should be used to treat insomnia only when it is severe, disabling, or subjecting the individual to extreme distress.

The following guidelines apply to two distinct populations of patients – those who have taken benzodiazepines long-term for a disorder such as insomnia or anxiety but do not abuse their prescription, and those who abuse their prescription or buy their benzodiazepines, often as part of polydrug use. Dependence can affect individuals in both groups. Every practice needs a policy to avoid initiating dependence in patients given benzodiazepines. For example:

(a) Benzodiazepines will only be used for the short-term relief of severe anxiety or insomnia, or for specific medical emergencies such as alcohol detoxification or the management of convulsions.
(b) Short-acting compounds (such as lorazepam) will not be given for daytime use.
(c) No repeat prescriptions will be given except to those already established as long-term users.
(d) Patients not already on benzodiazepines will be prescribed short-term courses of no more than 4 weeks.
(e) Current benzodiazepine users will be identified and invited to attend to discuss withdrawal. The invitation will be repeated annually until the drug is withdrawn. An exception to this might be the older patient maintained long-term symptom-free on the same dose.
(f) An annual audit of the number of benzodiazepine users will be conducted to monitor success and to learn from failures.

MANAGEMENT OF WITHDRAWAL

- Withdrawal symptoms can be distinguished from a return of anxiety and include:
  (a) disordered perceptions: feelings of unreality, increased sensory perception, or a sensation of movement;
  (b) serious psychiatric and neurological adverse effects: convulsions or acute psychosis.
- Symptoms typically emerge in the first week after stopping or reducing the dose. Occasionally they occur in patients on a stable dose, and are temporarily abolished by an increase in the dose. They usually last for up to 3 months but may last for over a year.
- Withdrawal symptoms may be seen in patients who have been on benzodiazepines for as little as 3 weeks and they occur in up to almost half of patients who have taken them for over 3 months (Kan, Breteler and Zitman 1997).
- Two thirds will be able to stop with some disturbance of sleep but without the true withdrawal syndrome. They may, however, need help in finding a different solution to the problem for which they were taking the benzodiazepine.

* Offer withdrawal with explanation to all patients on long-term benzodiazepines who have become dependent inadvertently following therapeutic use. Record the discussion in the notes.

* Refer patients who are misusing other drugs or alcohol, as well as benzodiazepines, to the specialist services. Concurrent withdrawal of more than one drug is not recommended.

* Refer patients requiring very high doses or who are injecting the drugs. A number of withdrawal regimens have been used. There is a spectrum of possibilities with the two proposed below at opposite ends of the spectrum. The two principles behind all regimens are to use a long-acting benzodiazepine and to reduce slowly, or very slowly.

Rapid withdrawal

For patients who give no indication that a withdrawal syndrome is likely.

* Reduce the benzodiazepine dose by a quarter of the original dose every 2 weeks and see the patient each time. If true withdrawal symptoms develop then change to a slow withdrawal.

Slow withdrawal

For patients in whom a withdrawal syndrome is likely (because of evidence of tolerance or previous symptoms of withdrawal).

* Change patients on short-acting to long-acting benzodiazepines, e.g. diazepam. For equivalent doses see box. If the changeover proves difficult, do it in stages, e.g. in a patient using lorazepam 2 mg daily, change 500 mcg lorazepam to 5 mg diazepam at a time.

EQUIVALENT (ROUGHLY) DOSES TO DIAZEPAM 5 MG
Chlordiazepoxide 15 mg.
Loprazolam 0.5–1 mg.
Lorazepam 500 mcg.
Lormetazepam 0.5–1 mg.
Nitrazepam 5 mg.
Oxazepam 15 mg.
Temazepam 10 mg.

* Prescribe 2 mg diazepam tablets for daily collection if there is concern about abuse or diversion.

* Avoid starting on doses greater than 30 mg diazepam daily. Consider referral for those with high-dose dependency.

* Start with a plan agreed with the patient, e.g. reducing the daily dose by 1/8 per fortnight, with smaller reductions in the final stages. Expect to take several months or even a year. If the patient has been obtaining the drug illegally, start with a dose considerably below the amount claimed.

* Be prepared to renegotiate the plan if the patient develops severe withdrawal effects. Keep patients on each dose long enough for them to settle before the next reduction.

* If the patient requests a slower rate of reduction because of psychological rather than physical dependence, it is better to keep to the agreed plan and intensify support.

* Be prepared for the emergence of anxiety, depression or insomnia, and manage accordingly. Patients on long-term benzodiazepines often have inappropriate reactions to difficulties in their lives. Withdrawal of the drug must be accompanied by re-education by the GP or referral, for instance, to a benzodiazepine-withdrawal support group.

* *Symptom control.* For patients struggling to tolerate the symptoms of withdrawal, consider using other drugs temporarily:
  (a) promethazine 25 mg at night for insomnia;
  (b) propranolol 10–40 mg t.d.s. for somatic symptoms;
  (c) tricyclic antidepressants, e.g. amitriptyline 25–75 mg daily, for depression and anxiety (but not isolated insomnia).

* Avoid using buspirone or major tranquillizers. They may make withdrawal worse. Do not use zopiclone or clomethiazole; they have cross-dependency with benzodiazepines.

PATIENT INFORMATION
UK National Drugs helpline. Talk to Frank. Tel. 0800 776600. Available: www.talktofrank.com. This resource is good on the illicit use of benzodiazepines rather than the problem of unintentional addiction

OPIATE MISUSE

GUIDELINES

Department of Health (England) and the devolved administrations. 2007. *Drug Misuse and Dependence: UK Guidelines on Clinical Management*. London: Department of Health (England), the Scottish Government, Welsh Assembly Government and Northern Ireland Executive. Available: www.dh.gov.uk and search on 'Drug misuse and dependence'

Ford C, Morton S, Lintzeris N, *et al.* 2004. *Guidance for the use of Buprenorphine for the Treatment of Opioid Dependence in Primary Care*. Royal College of General Practitioners. Available: www.rcgp.org.uk and search on 'buprenorphine'.

Ford C, Barnard J, Bury J, *et al.* 2005. *Guidance for the use of Methadone for the Treatment of Opioid Dependence in Primary Care*. Royal College of General Practitioners. Online: www.rcgp.org.uk and search on 'Methadone'

- The UK Department of Health guidelines stress that drug misusers have the same right as other patients to medical services. The UK General Medical Council has ruled that it is unethical for a doctor to withhold treatment on the basis of a judgment that the patient's activities or lifestyle might have contributed to their condition (Department of Health (England) and the devolved administrations 2007).
- The guidelines stress the importance of:
  (a) shared care, primarily shared between primary and secondary care; and
  (b) a multidisciplinary approach.
- *Notification.* In the UK doctors are expected to report drug misusers, on the standard reporting forms, to the regional or national drug misuse database or centre (see BNF) when they start treatment for their misuse. Data are anonymized. The doctor is not obliged to notify the patient of this procedure. Reporting is required not only for opioids and cocaine but also for any other drug that is being misused and for which treatment is given.
- Long-term follow-up of heroin users show that their mortality rates are nearly 12 times greater than the general population. Those that inject opiates are 22 times more likely to die than

non-injectors (Department of Health (England) and the devolved administrations 2007).
- UK research has shown that around 40% of heroin users that enter treatment will achieve long-term abstinence (Gossop, Marsden, Stewart, *et al.* 2003).

Seeing a patient where violence is a possibility

* Try not to see the patient alone.
* Ask staff to check on you at regular intervals during the consultation.
* If visiting, consider having a mobile phone 'open' to the surgery so that the consultation can be monitored.

HARM MINIMIZATION FOR ALL USERS

* *Needle exchange.* Ensure that the user knows about the local needle exchange scheme and the risk of HIV and hepatitis B and C. Explain that infection can be acquired from sharing spoons or the same water supply as well as from sharing needles and syringes. Give a copy of *Harm Minimization: Advice about Safer Drug Use* available on www.whoguidemhpcuk.org (choose 'patient resources' then 'Drug misuse').
* *Injecting risks.* Explain that cleaning equipment is not as good as using sterile needles and syringes. Cleaning reduces HIV risk but may not protect against hepatitis C. If they do clean then be sure that the user knows to:
  (a) draw up thin, undiluted household bleach and squirt it down the sink, twice;
  (b) draw up clean cold water and squirt it down the sink, three times.
* Discuss safe injecting techniques:
  (a) never inject alone;
  (b) inject *with* the blood flow;
  (c) rotate sites and avoid infected areas and swollen limbs;
  (d) avoid the neck, groin, breast, feet and hands;
  (e) mix powders with sterile water and filter the solution before injecting;
  (f) dispose of equipment safely. Sharps bins are available at needle exchanges.
* Offer immunization against hepatitis B (see page 39).
* Offer hep C and HIV antibody testing with counselling (see page 75).

* *Safe sex.* Check that the user is using condoms. Drug users are a high-risk group for HIV and may acquire it sexually.
* *Specialist help.* Encourage the patient to attend the local substance misuse clinic.
* *Admission.* Arrange urgent admission for the few patients in whom it is important, i.e. the woman in late pregnancy and those physically ill (e.g. those with multiple abscesses or septicaemia).

PATIENTS SEEKING HELP – ASSESSMENT PROCESS

● Care should be shared between primary and secondary care. The level of intervention in primary care will depend on the experience available in the primary health-care team and the ease of access to a specialist unit.
● Treatment is normally facilitated through a keyworker. This can be the GP but is commonly a nurse or voluntary sector drugs worker. The keyworker has several roles including: developing and agreeing the care plan, information and advice on drug misuse, interventions to prevent relapse, harm reduction work and motivational interventions, helping to address social needs and monitoring the family situation including child protection risk.
* Refer to the specialist services patients:
  (a) with other serious mental or physical health problems; or
  (b) misusing more than one drug; or
  (c) with a serious forensic history; or
  (d) needing specialist psychological interventions or help with housing or employment; or
  (e) needing a residential rehabilitation programme; or
  (f) not responding to an oral substitute regimen.

The following guidelines are appropriate where a GP delivers the bulk of the medical care.

First appointment

* Discover what has prompted the patient to present at this time and what he or she expects from the consultation. Assess their motivation to change.

* *Substance use history.* Assess the past and current drug situation. Check which other drugs are being used, including alcohol.
* Assess the patient's psychological and physical state; check injection sites for needle marks. If female, establish whether she is pregnant. Refer patients with severe mental health problems to the mental health team.
* Assess the social situation, including contacts with other drug users. Establish whether there is a child-care issue, whether a court case is pending and whether the patient is working and housed.
* *Infections.* Assess the need for HIV and hepatitis B and C screening.
* *Previous treatment.* Ask about previous episodes of care. If the patient is new to the practice, contact the previous GP.
* *Drug screen.* Send urine to the laboratory for a full drug screen or take an oral swab. Immediate testing kits for urine are reliable and will also confirm urine temperature to ensure sample belongs to the patient. Almost all drugs of misuse are detectable 24 hours after ingestion. Heroin is detectable for 48 hours after use and methadone for 7–9 days.
* *Confirming opiate use.* Aim to get at least two samples on separate occasions before prescribing.
* *Take blood,* with informed consent, for creatinine, LFTs, hepatitis B and C serology and HIV antibodies.
* Do not prescribe any psychoactive drugs at this stage, other than one of the drugs listed below for symptomatic relief.
* *Driving.* Advise the patient that if they hold a driving license it is their responsibility to notify the DVLA.
* Keep full records of the discussion.

If the assessment and drug screen confirms opiate use

* If necessary, discuss any planned pharmacological treatment with a specialist or a specialized generalist before the appointment.
* Agree a treatment plan with the patient: either withdrawal, or maintenance on methadone or buprenorphine. A written contract between doctor and patient can be helpful.

* Whichever option is chosen, draw up a contract specifying what you will prescribe and that the patient agrees to keep appointments, not to consult other doctors and not to take other drugs.
* Discuss the necessary changes in lifestyle: the patient may need to give up all friends who are themselves users. It may be possible to arrange residential rehabilitation for when the patient is drug free.
* Recommend Narcotics Anonymous or Release and any other source of support.
* Agree who will provide support from the statutory services. This might be the community drug team, community psychiatric nurse, probation officer, social worker or street agency.

METHADONE MAINTENANCE

* Methadone maintenance has been shown to be more effective than withdrawal in keeping patients in treatment (Ball and Ross 1991) and it results in lower heroin use rates (Sees, Delucchi, Masson, *et al.* 2000; Tober and Strang 2003; Mattick, Breen, Kimber, *et al.* 2003; Faggiano, Vigna-Tagliant, Versino, *et al.* 2003).
* Higher doses (60–120 mg/day) are associated with better outcomes than lower doses (Farrell, Ward and Mattick 1994).
* Methadone maintenance has the potential to reduce crime and reduce HIV transmission, as well as to reduce illicit opiate use; but it should be given as part of a structured programme (Farrell, Ward and Mattick 1994; Marsch 1998).
* Methadone can be used during pregnancy.
* There is considerable evidence that the first 2 weeks of methadone treatment is a time of increased risk of death due to methadone toxicity.
* Risk factors for overdose during induction are: low opioid tolerance; use of CNS depressant drugs, including alcohol; too high an initial dose; increases in dose that are too rapid; slow methadone clearance.
* Converting other opioids to methadone or buprenorphine equivalents is difficult to accurately predict. Street drugs are notoriously variable in purity. Careful induction is required.
* The MHRA recommended in 2006 that 'patients with the following risk factors for QT interval prolongation are carefully monitored whilst taking methadone: heart or liver disease, electrolyte abnormalities, concomitant treatment with the potential to cause QT interval prolongation. In addition, any patient requiring more than 100 mg of methadone per day should be closely monitored' (MHRA 2006).

Methadone induction

* Start with doses of 10–30 mg daily. Start at the lower doses if there are risk factors for overdose present (see above).
* Specify the pharmacy to be used and speak personally to the pharmacist about every prescription.
* Ask the pharmacist to supervise the patient taking the methadone. There is indirect evidence that supervised consumption may reduce drug-related death (Department of Health (England) and the devolved administrations 2007). After 3 months without difficulties, dispensing may move to unsupervised with less frequent pick-ups (if stable and no high risk behaviour).
* Increase in 5–10 mg increments every 3–4 days. Patients should be seen daily by a trained pharmacist but review personally during induction (daily if necessary) if there are any concerns regarding supervision.
* Do not prescribe tablets; there is a risk they can be crushed and injected.
* Prescribe methadone liquid 1 mg in 1 ml oral solution. Some users will prefer the sugar-free preparation. Specify this on the prescription.
* Write the prescription in ink on a FP10 (MDA) in England, GP10 in Scotland. State the form and strength of the preparation, with the dose and the total dose in words and figures with the amount in each instalment and the frequency of instalments. Up to 14 days treatment may be prescribed, to be dispensed daily with two doses on Saturday if the chemist is shut on Sunday. Order three doses for public holiday weekends.
* Provide information on the risk of overdose, get full consent, and document this in the notes.

Ongoing care

* Increase the dose incrementally to a level (usually 60–120 mg) where the patient reports feeling comfortable and is no longer using illicit

heroin. It can take several weeks to reach the desired dose.

* Review 2–4 weekly once stable.
* Continue to address physical, emotional, social and legal issues once the patient is stable.
* Random urine or oral fluid tests may be helpful, at least every 3–4 months.
* If the patient omits 2 or more days of methadone then they should be assessed for intoxication and withdrawal. Tolerance to methadone may have been lost and it may be necessary to reduce the dose or start a new induction.
* If the patient claims that a prescription has been lost or stolen do NOT provide a duplicate prescription for methadone. (This issue should be covered in the initial contract.)

BUPRENORPHINE MAINTENANCE

● Buprenorphine is a mixed opioid agonist-antagonist and is an effective intervention for use in the maintenance treatment of opioid dependent patients.
● It can be offered as an alternative to methadone maintenance treatment, though it may not be as effective as high dose methadone maintenance treatment (Mattick, Kimber, Breen, *et al.* 2003; Lintzeris, Bell, Bammer, *et al.* 2002).
● Higher doses of buprenorphine (more than 8 mg) are more effective in maintenance treatment than lower doses (Lintzeris 2002; Lintzeris, Bammer and Rushworth 2003).
● Starting buprenorphine with opiates in the system can result in a sudden unpleasant precipitated withdrawal as the buprenorphine has a higher affinity for opiate receptors than heroin.
● Unlike methadone, buprenorphine can be increased rapidly to the appropriate level but similar precautions should be taken to assess those at most risk during the induction.
* Buprenorphine should also be supervised by a pharmacist for the first 3 months. Supervision can be more challenging because it is a sublingual tablet that is slow to dissolve. It may be necessary to crush the tablets and this should be discussed with the pharmacist before prescribing.
* First dose should be delayed until patient has features of opiate withdrawal (or at least 6–12 hours after last heroin use).

* A typical initial dose would be 4–8 mg, increasing to 8–16 mg on day 2 if required.
* Effective maintenance doses are usually achieved at 12–24 mg per day.
* Review every 2–4 days until stabilization.
* Review 2–4 weekly once stable.

For both methadone and buprenorphine it is recommended that patients be encouraged to remain in treatment for at least 12 months to achieve enduring lifestyle changes.

WITHDRAWAL AND DETOXIFICATION

Detoxification is the process of supporting safe and effective discontinuation of opiates in dependent users while minimizing withdrawal symptoms. It should be available to anybody who has expressed an informed choice to become abstinent from opiates.

* Advise on the physical and psychological effects of withdrawal; and how these can be managed.
* Advise on the loss of tolerance after detoxification and the subsequent increased risk of overdose and death from illicit drug use if there is a relapse.
* Stress the importance of continued support to maintain abstinence.

There is a substantial evidence base for three main types of pharmacotherapy: methadone, buprenorphine and α-2 adrenergic agonists (Lingford-Hughes, Welch and Nutt 2004; Amato, Davioli, Ferri, *et al.* 2003; Gowing, Ali and White 2003; Gowing, Farrell, Ali, *et al.* 2003). All are effective in reducing withdrawal symptoms.

The options are:

(a) symptom control alone if only mild to moderate symptoms are predicted; or
(b) detoxification on lofexidine if more severe symptoms are predicted but the patient is stable on a low or moderate dose of illicit opiate; or
(c) a methadone or buprenorphine reduction programme.

Note: There is no place for dihydrocodeine, which has to be taken four times a day and so cannot be supervised.

Symptom control

● While there is no evidence to suggest they improves outcome, withdrawing from opiates can be an unpleasant experience and symptomatic relief should be offered.

* If severe symptoms are likely, offer a 4-day course of:
  (a) loperamide hydrochloride or co-phenotrope to prevent and treat diarrhoea; and
  (b) mebeverine to treat stomach cramps; and
  (c) metoclopramide or prochlorperazine for nausea and vomiting; and
  (d) NSAIDs or paracetamol for muscle pains and headaches; and
  (e) low doses of diazepam (e.g. 4–6 mg t.d.s.); can be used to treat agitation and anxiety but care should be taken if there is a history of benzodiazepine abuse.

Detoxification with lofexidine

● The α-2 agonist lofexidine is effective in opiate withdrawal (Gowing, Farrell, Ali, *et al.* 2003). Clonidine is not recommended in routine practice.

● Lofexidine will reduce the symptoms of opiate withdrawal but will not abolish the craving for the drug. It suppresses noradrenergic neuronal hyperactivity during opiate withdrawal (Washton, Resnick and Geyer 1983).

* Give 200 mcg twice a day, and increase by 200 mcg twice a day until symptoms are controlled, up to a maximum of 2.4 mg/day. Continue for 7–10 days, then tail off over a further 2–4 days.

* Check the blood pressure at baseline and again daily for the first 3 days. Stop lofexidine if there is significant hypotension.

Detoxification with methadone or buprenorphine

● Stabilize on methadone and buprenorphine as described above.

● There is no clear evidence over whether methadone or buprenorphine is more effective for detoxification.

● It is recommended that usually detoxification is carried out using the medicine on which the patient has been stabilized.

  * Reduce methadone by around 5 mg every 1–2 weeks. The dose can be reduced to 0 in around 12 weeks.

  * Reduce buprenorphine initially by 2 mg every 2 weeks. Final reductions of 400 mcg can be made.

PATIENT INFORMATION

UK National Drugs helpline. Talk to Frank. Tel. 0800 776600. www.talktofrank.com
  Narcotics Anonymous, helpline 0845 373 3366. www.ukna.org
  Release, helpline 0845 4500 215. www.release.org.uk
  Drugs in School, helpline tel. 0808 8000 800

Information and help for relatives

ADFAM National, which offers counselling for family and friends of drug users. www.adfam.org.uk
  Families Anonymous, which runs self-help groups for parents of drug users. Helpline 0845 1200 660. www.famanon.org.uk

---

OTHER SUBSTANCES

CANNABIS

GUIDELINE

National Health Committee (New Zealand). Guidelines for recognising, assessing and treating alcohol and cannabis abuse in primary care. July 1999. Online: www.nzgg.org.nz and search on 'Cannabis'

● The most common symptoms of cannabis dependence are difficulties controlling use and withdrawal (Swift, Hall and Teeson 2001a, b).

● Only 17% of long-term users who try to quit are abstinent 1 year after treatment (Stephens, Roffman and Simpson 1994).

● The evidence suggests a causal link between cannabis and psychosis. Estimates suggest that cannabis may account for 10% of cases of psychosis but most users will not have any problems (Fergusson, Poulton, Smith, *et al.* 2006).

* Ask about cannabis use in younger patients who are also using alcohol and tobacco.

* Explain the dangers: subtle specific cognitive defects (memory loss, poor concentration), chronic bronchitis and carcinoma of the lung and oropharynx, precipitation of latent psychosis (Hall and Degenhardt 2001) and possible infertility, as well as deterioration in relationships and performance at work.

* Explain that withdrawal symptoms are likely to be mild and short-lived: insomnia, sweating, anxiety, restlessness, lethargy, anorexia, nausea, tremor and paranoia.
* Agree a goal along the line of the approach taken with problem drinkers and arrange to see the patient again. Brief interventions of this sort can be as effective as extensive ones (Stephens, Roffman and Simpson 1994; Copeland, Swift, Roffman, *et al.* 2001).

PATIENT INFORMATION FOR TEENAGERS

www.talktofrank.com is also available on UK freephone 0800 77 66 00 and by email frank@talktofrank.com

PSYCHOSTIMULANTS: AMPHETAMINES, COCAINE AND ECSTASY

GUIDELINES

Department of Health (England) and the devolved administrations. 2007. *Drug Misuse and Dependence: UK Guidelines on Clinical Management*. London: Department of Health (England), the Scottish Government, Welsh Assembly Government and Northern Ireland Executive. Online: www.dh.gov.uk and search on 'Drug misuse and dependence'

Linsford-Hughes AR, Welch S, Nutt DJ. 2004. Evidence-based guidelines for the pharmacological management of substance misuse, addiction and comorbidity: recommendations from the British Association for Psychopharmacology. J Psychopharm 18, 293–335

Jenner L, Baker A, Whyte I, *et al.* 2007. *Management of Patients with Psychostimulant use Problems – Guidelines for General Practitioners*. Canberra, Australian Government Department of Health and Ageing. Online: www.nationaldrugstrategy.gov.au and search on 'psychostimulants'

Ford C. 2004. *Guidance for Working with Cocaine and Crack Users in Primary Care*. Royal College of General Practitioners. Online: http://www.rcgp.org.uk and search on 'Cocaine'

* Psychostimulant use has been increasing steadily in UK, Australia and New Zealand over the past decade.

* There is a lack of evidence supporting pharmacological treatment for stimulant abuse and dependence and psychosocial interventions such as cognitive management are the mainstay of treatment (Lingford-Hughes, Welch and Nutt 2004; Department of Health (England) and the devolved administrations 2007).
* Craving for stimulants is real. Withdrawal symptoms mainly take the form of psychiatric reactions, including depression, anxiety, agitation and acute psychosis.
* Do not give substitute drugs.
* Refer high risk patients (dependent alcohol/benzodiazepine use) for specialist supervision during detoxification.
* Warn patients about the possible lengthy withdrawal process as mood fluctuations, irritability and sleep disorders may persist for several months.
* Monitor dependent patients after cessation for at least 2–4 weeks but defer diagnosing depression in this period as mood symptoms will often abate with continued cessation.
* The use of SSRIs with simultaneous stimulant use has been associated with serotonin toxicity (Jenner, Baker, Whyte, *et al.* 2004).
* Arrange for counselling and social support.

AMPHETAMINES

* Highly dependent individuals show poorer performance on tests of cognitive functioning, especially with memory and concentration (McKetin and Mattick 1998).
* There is substantial evidence that amphetamines can produce a distinctive psychotic episode with a good short-term prognosis in people with no pre-existing mental health problems (Bell 1973).
* Acute psychostimulant-induced psychotic episodes may be indistinguishable from paranoid schizophrenia. In most cases of drug related psychoses there is a significant improvement in symptoms after 2–4 days with only a minority of patients experiencing persistent symptoms beyond 1 month.
* Use of amphetamines may act as a stressor or trigger for a psychotic disorder that does not resolve naturally after cessation (Jenner, Kavanagh, Greenaway, *et al.* 1998).

- Psychological therapies such as cognitive behavioural therapy, motivational approaches and relapse prevention strategies may assist with continued cessation (Jenner, Baker, Whyte, et al. 2004; Baker, Kay-Lamkin, Lee, et al. 2003).
- There has previously thought to be a limited place for the use of dexamphetamine and some prescribing still occurs in the UK. However, the evidence of benefit is unconvincing and it should not ordinarily be prescribed (Department of Health (England) and the devolved administrations 2007).
- * Refer patients presenting with behavioural disturbance related to amphetamine use for a psychiatric assessment.

COCAINE

- Excessive doses can cause severe medical problems, and even death, from pulmonary oedema, heart failure, myocardial infarction, cerebral haemorrhage, stroke and hyperthermia.
- There is a dangerous interaction between alcohol and cocaine which may result in death.
- The after-effects of crack use may include fatigue, depression, paranoid ideation and depersonalization as people 'come down' from the high.
- Psychosocial interventions such as cognitive behavioural therapy, motivational interviewing, the Minnesota (12-step) method and relapse prevention are the mainstay of treatment (Ford 2004).
- * Provide as multi-faceted and intensive a programme as possible, as more intensive psychosocial programmes are associated with better outcomes (Crits-Cristoph, Siqueland, Blaine, et al. 1999; Higgins, Sigmon, Wong, et al. 2003).
- * Refer cocaine users to Cocaine Anonymous (tel. 0800 612 0225; www.cauk.org.uk).

ECSTASY

- Ecstasy is the street name usually applied to 3,4-methylenedioxymethamphetamine or MDMA.
- The most significant adverse effects of ecstasy use are hyperthermia and hyponatraemia or 'water intoxication', both of which can be fatal.

- Psychosocial interventions such as cue exposure/response prevention, contingency management, multifaceted behavioural therapy and relapse prevention are the mainstay of treatment.
- There have been several reports of serotonin toxicity associated with the use of psychostimulants in the recent past, particularly MDMA (ecstasy).
- Serotonin toxicity may be a mild, self-limiting condition or potentially fatal with symptoms such as muscle rigidity, coma, seizures, hypertension or hypotension. When toxicity is severe, rhabdomyolysis with hyperkalaemia, acidosis and frank renal failure may result (Jenner L, Baker A, Whyte I, et al. 2004; Dean and Whyte 2004).
- * Suspect serotonin toxicity if there is recent use of a serotonergic agent. (Peak rise time for cocaine is 20–40 minutes after administration and for an amphetamine is 2–3 hours) and three of the following are present: altered mental status, agitation, tremor, shivering, diarrhoea, hyperreflexia, myoclonus (may be severe enough to mimic seizures), ataxia, fever; and/or diaphoresis.
- * Educate patients about early warning signs (muscle rigidity, increasing body temperature, increasing agitation, severe headaches, etc.).
- * Treat with mechanical cooling (cold packs, fans and fluids) and immediate transfer via ambulance to the emergency department (Dean and Whyte 2004).

PARTY DRUGS

- 'Party drugs' is a term used to describe substances taken in the context of nightclubs or raves. Three of the main party drugs, amphetamine, cocaine and ecstasy, have been discussed (see above).
- Users are usually experimental, recreational and non-injecting, and are not dependent on psychostimulants.
- It is appropriate to give advice on harm reduction strategies and include advice about the range of possible adverse consequences of regular use such as mood disturbances, paranoid ideation and irritability.

- Brief interventions to reduce the risk of transition to regular use or injecting are also appropriate (see FRAMES model page 487).
* Offer vaccination for hepatitis B and discuss the appropriateness of testing for hepatitis C and HIV serology and the implications of findings.
* Ensure there is awareness of the risk of developing tolerance and dependence with increased frequency of use.
* Give advice on minimizing high risk behaviours including injecting/sex/violence.
* Give advice on the risks arising from poly-drug use.
* Warn patients to pay attention to adequate hydration and cooling in club and dance party settings.

VOLATILE SUBSTANCE ABUSE

- There were 58 deaths associated with volatile substance abuse (VSA) in 2007. Gas fuels are associated with the majority of deaths. There have been 2308 deaths associated with VSA since 1971 (Field-Smith, Butland, Ramsey, et al. 2009).
- Amongst those age 10–14 in the UK, over the period 2000–2007, there were three times as many deaths associated with VSA as with drug misuse (Field-Smith, Butland, Ramsey, et al. 2009).
- Most sniffing is out of curiosity, and stops spontaneously. The sniffing that is most likely to continue is when it is used as an escape from severe family or personal problems (Camoil and Houghton 1998).
- Substances can be stopped abruptly without danger.
- Most programmes adopt strategies that have a overall aim of reducing the harms and risks related to the person's drug use. Some treatment options include counselling, withdrawal and pharmacotherapy. Residential and outpatient programmes are available.
* Explain the dangers: damage to brain, lung, liver and bone marrow; risk of cardiac arrhythmias and sudden death; accidental injury while intoxicated; birth malformations, prematurity and developmental delay.

* Advise about 'safer sniffing', e.g. don't sniff alone, don't put a bag over the head, don't use solvents other than glue as they can be fatal, don't sniff in dangerous places, e.g. rooftops. Stress that sniffing is never safe.
* Mobilize all possible help for the underlying problems.

Re-Solv, the Society for the Prevention of Solvent and Volatile Substance Abuse. National Information Line 01785 810762; www.re-solv.org and the site for children is www.sniffing.org.uk

SMOKING CESSATION

GUIDELINE

West R, McNeill A, Raw M. 2000. Smoking cessation guidelines for health professionals: an update. Thorax 55, 987–999. Online: http://thorax.bmjjournals.com/cgi/content/full/55/12/987

- Smoking remains the largest preventable cause of ill health in the UK, causing over 120,000 deaths per year, around one in five of all deaths (Callum 1998).
- More than one in four deaths between the ages of 35 and 65 are caused by smoking (1:3 for men and 1:5 for women) (Callum 1998).
- Smoking is estimated to be responsible for 90% of lung cancer deaths, the commonest cancer in the UK (21% of all cancer deaths) (Doll, Peto and Wheatley 1994; Department of Health 1998).
- Smoking in pregnancy causes adverse fetal outcomes, such as an increased risk of miscarriage, low birth weight and perinatal death. The risk of sudden infant death syndrome or 'cot-death' is significantly increased by exposure to tobacco smoke (Poswillo 1998).
- Smoking significantly increases the risk of: cancer other than lung cancer (stomach, colon, bladder and kidney), CHD, stroke and vascular dementia, peripheral vascular disease, diabetes, COPD, osteoporotic fractures, gastric ulcer and blindness (Surgeon-General 1989).

- *Passive smoking.* Exposure to 'secondhand smoke' significantly increases the risk of CHD and other diseases.
- In 2007, 22% of adults smoked cigarettes, of whom 73% wanted to give up. There were 60% who had made a serious attempt to give up in the past 5 years (Lader 2008).
- There is no evidence that acupuncture (White, Rampes and Ernst 2001) or hypnosis (Abbot, Stead, White, *et al.* 2001) are effective in assisting patients to stop smoking.
- Brief advice by GPs, drug treatment such as nicotine replacement therapy (NRT), bupropion (Zyban), varenicline (Champix) and behavioural support have all been shown to increase the number of people successfully stopping smoking (West, McNeill and Raw 2000).
- Brief advice (up to 5 minutes) from a GP leads to an increase in the number who have stopped smoking (in addition to those who would have stopped anyway) at 6 months of between 1–3% (Silagy 2001). Approximately 40% of smokers make some form of attempt to quit in response to GP advice (Kreuter 2000; Russell 1979).
- * Discuss with the patient the health risks to themselves and others around them (see above).
- * Explain that smoking cessation greatly reduces the health risks associated with smoking. The risks from smoking decline immediately on cessation. After 10–15 years of abstinence, depending on the number of years as a smoker, the risk of death returns to almost that of a life-long non-smoker (Surgeon-General 1989).

MANAGEMENT PLAN

The following features are essential components of a smoking cessation programme in primary care – *ask, advise, assist, arrange* (West, McNeill and Raw 2000):

- * **ASK** patients about smoking on a regular basis (at least once a year) when they visit the surgery and assess their interest in stopping. Record smoking status and their interest in stopping in the notes.
  - (a) 'Do you smoke?'
  - (b) 'How do you feel about your smoking?'
  - (c) 'Have you ever tried to stop?'
  - (d) 'Are you interested in stopping now?'

- * **ADVISE** all smokers of the value of stopping (at any age) and the risks to health of continuing to smoke. The advice should be clear, firm and personalized, whilst remaining non-judgmental.
  - (a) Do not limit this advice to patients with smoking-related diseases.
  - (b) Try and link the advice to the reasons for the patient consulting and/or relevant to the individual.
  - (c) Reassure patients who have failed on a previous attempt that most do so before finally succeeding (Gourlay 1995).
- * **ASSIST** the smoker if they would like to stop and are *well motivated* by providing further help, advice and referral.
  - (a) Advise them to set a date to stop and stop completely on that date.
  - (b) Offer prescription for NRT, bupropion or varenicline as appropriate for those people planning to quit smoking (see below).
  - (c) Refer for behavioural support at specialist clinic; or
  - (d) Refer to intermediate service (at primary care level) provided by nurses or other health professionals specifically trained and employed to provide smoking cessation support.
- * **ARRANGE** follow-up – although smokers will be followed up by the above support services you may also wish to review the patient yourself 1–2 weeks after their quit date.

DRUG TREATMENT TO AID SMOKING CESSATION

NICOTINE REPLACEMENT THERAPY (NRT)

- NRT increases quit rates by 50–70% regardless of setting and this effect is largely independent of support levels (Stead, Perera and Bullen 2008).
- No form of NRT seems to be more effective than others but smokers given the choice prefer nicotine patches (Cummings, Hyland and Ockene 1997; Shaw, Ferry, Pethica, *et al.* 1998; West, Hajek, Nilsson, *et al.* 2001).
- There *is* evidence of long-term use and dependence with nicotine gum and nasal spray (13–38% using it for 1 year), but there is no evidence of long-term use of patches (Benowitz

1998; Hughes 1989; Blondal, Gudmundsson and Olafsdottir 1999).

- NRT appears to be safe when given to smokers with cardiovascular disease (Benowitz and Gourlay 1997).

BUPROPION

- Bupropion may work by counteracting the effects of nicotine withdrawal by increasing levels of dopamine and noradrenaline in the brain.
- Bupropion has been shown to be at least as effective as NRT when used in smokers of more than 15 cigarettes per day who are well motivated to stop and who also receive regular counselling (Hurt, Sachs and Glover 2001; Jorenby, Leischow, Nides, *et al.* 1999).
- Common side-effects of bupropion include insomnia and dry mouth. Less common side-effects such as seizures have been reported in 1 in 1000 people taking bupropion.
- *CSM warning.* The CSM has issued a reminder that bupropion is contra-indicated in patients with a history of seizures or of eating disorders, a CNS tumour, or who are experiencing acute symptoms of alcohol or benzodiazepine withdrawal. Bupropion should not be prescribed to patients with other risk factors for seizures unless the potential benefit of smoking cessation clearly outweighs the risk. Factors that increase the risk of seizures include concomitant administration of drugs that can lower the seizure threshold (e.g. antidepressants, antimalarials (such as mefloquine and chloroquine), antipsychotics, quinolones, sedating antihistamines, systemic corticosteroids, theophylline, tramadol), alcohol abuse, history of head trauma, diabetes, and use of stimulants and anorectics.
- A provisional list of those drugs that might interact with bupropion was published in 2001 and is available on www.pharmj.com/pdf/zyban.pdf (Cox, Anton and Ferner 2001).

VARENICLINE

- Varenicline is a partial nicotine receptor agonist which patients start 1 week before their quit date and continue for 12 weeks.

- When compared with bupropion the quit rate at 12 weeks was significantly better (1.9-fold) for varenicline (NICE 2007).
- The most commonly reported side-effects have been psychiatric disorders, sleep disturbances and GI upset such as nausea and vomiting.
- The MHRA has reported that depression and suicide-related events have been reported in patients using varenicline who are trying to stop smoking. Patients who are taking varenicline who develop suicidal thoughts or who develop agitation, depressed mood or changes in behaviour should stop their treatment and seek attention. Care should be taken when prescribing varenicline in patients with psychiatric illness.
- The National Institute for Health and Clinical Excellence (NICE) recommends the use of varenicline as an option for smokers who have expressed a desire to quit, and that it should normally be prescribed only as part of a programme of behavioural support (NICE 2008).

BEHAVIOURAL SUPPORT

- Behavioural support further increases the chance of quitting, enabling an additional 1 in 20 smokers to quit for 6 months or more but there is no evidence that individual counselling is more effective than group counselling or vice versa (Lancaster and Stead 2005).
- Evidence from cross-study comparisons suggests that treatment programmes with greater frequency and duration of contact are more effective (West, McNeill and Raw 2000).
- Behavioural support for smokers provided by nurses is effective when they are specifically employed for this purpose but not when it is part of their general duties (Rice and Stead 2001; Steptoe, Doherty, Rink, *et al.* 1999).
- Pro-active telephone counselling enables about 1 in 50 smokers to quit for 6 months or more and may be useful for smokers who are unwilling or unable to attend face-to-face treatment (McAlister, Rabius, Geiger, *et al.* 2004).
- Written self-help materials enable 1 in 100 smokers to abstain for at least 6 months compared with no treatment but have not been shown to improve the success rates of face-to-face treatment (West, McNeill and Raw 2000).

PREGNANT SMOKERS

- For pregnant smokers, referral for support by someone specifically trained and employed for that purpose encourages 1 in 15 to stop smoking for the remainder of the pregnancy (when they would not otherwise have done so) (Lumley, Oliver, Chamberlain, *et al.* 2004; Melvin, Dolan-Mullen, Windsor, *et al.* 2000).
- Support by midwives as part of their normal duties has not been shown to be effective (Hajek, West and Lee 2001; Wisborg, Henriksen and Secher 1998). Support for pregnant women should be on a 1:1 basis, as very few are willing to attend group sessions (West 1994).

- Small studies on the effects of NRT on the foetus have not revealed significant problems (Lambers and Clarke 1996; Linblad, Marsal and Andersson 1988) and it is likely to be considerably safer than smoking.

TELEPHONE SUPPORT AND LEAFLETS

NHS Smoking Helpline 0800 022 4 332; or 0800 169 9 169 (pregnant smokers); or www.smokefree.nhs.uk. Leaflets can be ordered free on this site: choose 'Quit Tools'.
   Quitline tel. 0800 00 22 00 or www.quit.org.uk

References

Abbot, N., Stead, L., White, A., et al., 2001. Hypnotherapy for smoking cessation. Cochrane Database Syst. Rev. (4).

Amato, L., Davioli, M., Ferri, M., et al., 2003. Methadone at tapered doses for the management of opioid withdrawal. Cochrane Database Syst. Rev.

Anderson, P., 1985. Managing alcohol problems in general practice. BMJ 290, 1873–1875.

Anderson, P., 1993. Effectiveness of general practice interventions for patients with harmful alcohol consumption. Br. J. Gen. Pract. 43, 386–389.

Ashworth, M., Gerada, C., 1997. Addiction and dependence II. BMJ 315, 358–360.

Babor, T.F., Higgins-Biddle, J.C., Saunders, J.B., et al., 2001. Audit, the Alcohol Use Disorders Identification Test. World Health Organization (WHO). Available: http://www.who.int (search on 'Alcohol AUDIT').

Baker, A., Kay-Lamkin, F., Lee, N., et al., 2003. A brief cognitive behavioural intervention for regular amphetamine users. Australian Government Department of Health and Ageing, Canberra.

Ball, J., Ross, A., 1991. The effectiveness of methadone maintenance treatment: patients, programs, services and outcome. Springer-Verlag, New York.

Bell, D., 1973. The experimental reproduction of amphetamine psychosis. Arch. Gen. Psychiatry 29, 35–40.

Benowitz, N. (ed.), 1998. Nicotine safety and toxicity. Oxford University Press, New York.

Benowitz, N., Gourlay, S., 1997. Cardiovascular toxicity of nicotine: implications for nicotine replacement therapy. J. Am. Coll. Cardiol. 29, 1422–1431.

Bernadt, M.W., Mumford, J., Taylor, C., et al., 1982. Comparison of questionnaire and laboratory tests in the detection of excessive drinking and alcoholism. Lancet i, 325–328.

Blondal, T., Gudmundsson, L., Olafsdottir, I., 1999. Nicotine nasal spray with nicotine patch for smoking cessation: randomised trial with six year follow up. BMJ 318, 285–289.

Bradley, K., DeBenedetti, A., Volk, R., et al., 2007. AUDIT-C as a brief screen for alcohol misuse in primary care. Alcohol. Clin. Exp. Res. 31 (7), 1208–1217.

Buchan, I., Buckley, E., Deacon, G., et al., 1981. Problem drinkers and their problems. J. R. Coll. Gen. Pract. 31, 151–153.

Callum, C., 1998. The smoking epidemic. Health Education Authority, London.

Camoil, A., Houghton, S., 1998. Volatile solvent use amongst Western Australian adolescents. Adolescence 33, 877–888.

Carmen, B., 2004. Efficacy and safety of naltrexone and acamprosate in the treatment of alcohol dependence: a systematic review. Addiction 99, 811–828.

Chick, J., 1989. Delirium tremens. BMJ 298, 3–4.

Chick, J., Gough, K., Falkowski, W., et al., 1992. Disulfiram treatment of alcoholism. Br. J. Psychiatry 161, 84–89.

Copeland, L., Swift, W., Roffman, R., et al., 2001. A randomised controlled trial of brief interventions for cannabis use disorders. J. Subst. Abuse Treat. 21, 55–64.

Cox, A., Anton, C., Ferner, R., 2001. Take care with Zyban. Pharm. J. 266, 718–722.

Crits-Cristoph, P., Siqueland, L., Blaine, J., et al., 1999. Psychosocial treatments for cocaine dependence: National Institute on Drug Abuse Collaborative Cocaine Treatment Study. Arch. Gen. Psychiatry 56, 493–502.

Cummings, K., Hyland, A., Ockene, J., 1997. Use of the nicotine skin patch by smokers in 20 communities in the US. Tob. Control 6 (Suppl. 2), S63–S70.

Dean, A., Whyte, I., 2004. Emergency management of acute psychostimulant toxicity. In: Baker, A., Lee, N., Jennes, L. (eds), Models of Intervention and Care of Psychostimulant Users, 2nd ed. National Drug Strategy Monograph Series Number 51 Canberra.

Department of Health, 1998. Our healthier nation: a contract for health. The Stationery Office, London.

Department of Health (England) and the devolved administrations, 2007. Drug Misuse and Dependence: UK Guidelines on Clinical Management. Department of Health, the Scottish Government, Welsh Assembly Government and Northern Ireland Executive, London. Available: www.dh.gov.uk (search on 'Drug misuse and dependence').

Department of Health, Home Office, Department for Education and Skills, Department for Culture Media and Sport, 2007. Safe. Sensible. Social. The next steps in the National Alcohol Strategy.

Doll, R., Peto, R., Wheatley, K., 1994. Mortality in relation to smoking: 40 years' observation on male British doctors. BMJ 309, 901–911.

DVLA, 2009. At-a-glance guide to the current medical standards of fitness to drive. DVLA, Swansea.

Faggiano, F., Vigna-Tagliant, F., Versino, E., et al., 2003. Methadone maintenance at different dosages for opioid dependence. Cochrane Database Syst. Rev.

Farrell, M., Ward, J., Mattick, R., 1994. Methadone maintenance

treatment in opiate dependence: a review. BMJ 309, 997–1001.

Feeney, G.F., Connor, J.P., 2008. Wernicke-Korsakoff syndrome (WKS) in Australia: no room for complacency. Drug Alcohol Rev. 27 (4), 388–392.

Fergusson, D., Poulton, R., Smith, P., et al., 2006. Cannabis and psychosis. BMJ 332, 172–175.

Field-Smith, M., Butland, B., Ramsey, J., et al., 2009. Trends in death associated with abuse of volatile substances 1971-2007: St George's Medical School. Available: www.vsareport.org.

Fleming, M., Mundt, M., French, M., et al., 2002. Brief physician advice for problem drinkers: long-term efficacy and benefit-cost analysis. Alcohol Clin. Exp. Res. 26, 36–43.

Ford, C., 2004. Guidance for working with cocaine and crack users in primary care. Royal College of General Practitioners.

Garbutt, J., West, S., Carey, T., 1999. Pharmacological treatment of alcohol dependence. JAMA 281, 1318–1325.

Gossop, M., Marsden, J., Stewart, D., et al., 2003. The National Treatment Outcome Research Study (NTORS): 4-5 year follow-up results. Addiction 98 (3), 291–303.

Gourlay, S., 1995. Double-blind trial of repeated treatment with transdermal nicotine replacement for relapsed smokers. BMJ 311, 363–366.

Gowing, L., Ali, R., White, J., 2003. Buprenorphine for the management of opioid withdrawal. Cochrane Database Syst. Rev.

Gowing, L., Farrell, M., Ali, R., et al., 2003. Alpha 2 adrenergic agonists for the management of opioid withdrawal. Cochrane Database Syst. Rev.

Haigh, R., Hibbert, G., 1990. Where and when to detoxify single homeless drinkers. BMJ 301, 848–849.

Hajek, P., West, R., Lee, A., 2001. Randomised control trial of a midwife-delivered brief smoking cessation intervention in pregnancy. Addiction 96, 485–494.

Hall, W., Degenhardt, L., 2001. Cannabis use and psychosis: a review of clinical and epidemiological evidence. Aust. N. Z. J. Psychiatry 31, 659–668.

Higgins, S., Sigmon, S., Wong, C., et al., 2003. Community reinforcement therapy for cocaine-dependent outpatients. Arch. Gen. Psychiatry 60, 1043–1052.

Hodgson, R., Alwyn, T., John, B., et al., 2002. The FAST Alcohol Screening Test. Alcohol 37, 61–66.

Hughes, J., 1989. Dependence potential and abuse liability of nicotine replacement therapies. Biomed. Pharmacother. 43, 11–17.

Hughes, J., Cook, C., 1997. The efficacy of disulfiram: a review of outcome studies. Addiction 92, 381–395.

Hurt, R., Sachs, D., Glover, E., 2001. A comparison of sustained-release buprorion and placebo for smoking cessation. N. Engl. J. Med. 337, 1195–1202.

Jenner, L., Baker, A., Whyte, I., et al., 2004. Management of patients with psychostimulant use problems: guidelines for general practitioners. Australian Government of Health and Ageing, Canberra.

Jenner, L., Kavanagh, D., Greenaway, L., et al., 1998. The Dual Diagnosis Consortium Report. Alcohol and Drugs Training and Research Unit, Brisbane.

Jorenby, D., Leischow, S., Nides, M., et al., 1999. A controlled trial of sustained-release bupropion, a nicotine patch, or both for smoking cessation. N. Engl. J. Med. 340, 685–691.

Kan, C., Breteler, M., Zitman, F., 1997. High prevalence of benzodiazepine dependence in outpatient users, based on the

DSM-III and ICD-10 criteria. Acta Psychiatr. Scand. 96, 85–93.

Kaner, E., Dickinson, H., Beyer, F., et al., 2007. Effectiveness of brief alcohol interventions in primary care populations. Cochrane Database Syst. Rev. (2).

Kreuter, M., 2000. How does physician advice influence patient behaviour? Arch. Fam. Med. 9, 426–433.

Lader, D., 2008. Smoking-related Behaviour and Attitudes. Office for National Statistics, London.

Lambers, D., Clarke, K., 1996. The maternal and foetal physiologic effects of nicotine. Semin. Perinatol. 20, 115–126.

Lancaster, T., Stead, L., 2005. Individual behavioural counselling for smoking cessation. Cochrane Database Syst. Rev. (4).

Linblad, A., Marsal, K., Andersson, K., 1988. Effect of nicotine of human fetal blood flow. Obstet. Gynecol. 72, 371–382.

Lingford-Hughes, A., Welch, S., Nutt, D., 2004. Evidence-based guidelines for the pharmacological management of substance misuse, addiction and comorbidity: recommendations from the British Association of Psychopharmacology. J. Psychopharm. 18, 292–335.

Lintzeris, N., 2002. Buprenorphine dosing regimes in the management of outpatient heroin withdrawal. Drug Alcohol Rev. 21, 39–45.

Lintzeris, N., Bammer, G., Rushworth, L., 2003. Buprenorphine dosing regime for inpatient heroin withdrawal: a symptom triggered dose titration study. Drug Alcohol Depend. 70, 287–294.

Lintzeris, N., Bell, J., Bammer, G., et al., 2002. A randomised controlled trial of buprenorphine in the ambulatory management of heroin withdrawal. Addiction 97, 1395–1404.

Longabaugh, R., Wirtz, P., Zweben, A., et al., 1998. Network support for drinking, Alcoholics Anonymous and long-term matching effects. Addiction 93, 1313–1333.

Lumley, J., Oliver, S., Chamberlain, C., et al., 2004. Interventions for promoting smoking cessation during pregnancy. Cochrane Database Syst. Rev. (4).

McAlister, A., Rabius, V., Geiger, A., et al., 2004. Telephone assistance for smoking cessation: one year cost effectiveness estimations. Tob. Control 13 (1), 85–86.

McKetin, R., Mattick, R., 1998. Attention and memory in illicit amphetamine users: comparisons with non-drug using controls. Drug Alcohol Depend. 50, 181–184.

Marsch, L., 1998. The efficacy of methadone maintenance interventions in reducing illicit opiate use, HIV risk behaviour and criminality: a meta-analysis. Addiction 93, 515–532.

Mattick, R., Breen, C., Kimber, J., et al., 2003. Methadone maintenance therapy versus no opioid replacement therapy for opioid dependence. Cochrane Database Syst. Rev.

Mattick, R., Kimber, J., Breen, C., et al., 2003. Buprenophine maintenance versus placebo or methadone maintenance for opioid dependence. Cochrane Database Syst. Rev.

Mayo-Smith, M., 1997. Pharmacological management of alcohol withdrawal: a meta-analysis and evidence-based practice guideline. JAMA 278 (2), 144–151.

Melvin, C., Dolan-Mullen, P., Windsor, R., et al., 2000. Recommended cessation counselling for pregnant women who smoke: a review of the evidence. Tob Control 9 (Suppl. 3), III80–III84.

MHRA, 2006. Current Problems in Pharmacovigilance 31, Medicine and Healthcare products Regulatory Agency, London.

Miller, W., Meyers, R., Tonigan, J., 1999. Engaging the unmotivated in treatment for alcohol problems: a comparison of three strategies for intervention through family members. J. Consult. Clin. Psychol. 67, 688–697.

Miller, W., Sanchez, V., 1991. Miller, W., Rollnick, S. (eds.), Motivational Interviewing: Preparing People of Change Addictive Behaviour. Guilford Press, New York.

National Health and Medical Research Council, 2009. Australian Alcohol Guidelines to Reduce Health Risks from Drinking Alcohol. NHMRC, Canberra.

National Health Committee (New Zealand), 1999. Guidelines for recognising, assessing and treating alcohol and cannabis abuse in primary care.

NICE, 2007. Varenicline for smoking cessation. National Institute for Health and Clinical Excellence, London. Available: www.nice.org.uk.

NHS Information Centre Lifestyles Statistics, 2009. Statistics on Alcohol: England 2009. Available: http://www.ic.nhs.uk/pubs/Alcohol09.

NICE., 2008. Smoking cessation services. National Institute for Health and Clinical Excellence, London. Available: www.nice.org.uk.

Ockene, J., Adams, A., Hurley, T., et al., 1999. Brief physician and nurse practitioner- delivered counseling for high-risk drinkers: does it work? Arch. Intern. Med. 159, 2198–2205.

Poswillo, D., 1998. Report on the Scientific Committee on Tobacco and Health. Health Education Authority, London.

Prime Minister's Strategy Unit, 2004. Alcohol Harm Reduction Strategy for England: Cabinet Office.

Raistrick, D., 2000. Management of alcohol detoxification. Advances in Psychiatric Treatment 6, 348–355.

Rice, V., Stead, L., 2001. Nursing interventions for smoking cessation (Cochrane Review). Cochrane Database Syst. Rev. (4).

Russell, M., 1979. Effect of general practitioners advice against smoking. BMJ 2, 231–235.

Scottish Intercollegiate Guidelines Network, 2003. Management of harmful drinking and alcohol dependence in primary care. SIGN, Edinburgh. Available: http://www.sign.ac.uk.

Sees, K., Delucchi, K., Masson, C., et al., 2000. Methadone maintenance vs 180-day psychosocially enriched detoxification for treatment of opioid dependence. JAMA 283, 1303–1310.

Shaw, J., Ferry, D., Pethica, D., et al., 1998. Usage patterns of transdermal nicotine when purchased as a non-prescription medicine from pharmacies. Tob. Control 7, 161–167.

Silagy, C., 2001. Physician advice for smoking cessation (Cochrane Review). Cochrane Database Syst. Rev. (4).

Slattery, J., Chick, J., Cochrane, M., et al., 2003. Prevention of relapse in alcohol dependence. Health Technology Assessment Report 3. Health Technology Assessment Board for Scotland, Glasgow.

Srisurapanont, M., Jarusuraisin, N., 2004. Opioid antagonists for alcohol dependence. Cochrane Database Syst. Rev. (4).

Stead, L., Perera, R., Bullen, C., 2008. Nicotine replacement therapy for smoking cessation. Cochrane Database Syst. Rev. (1).

Stephens, R., Roffman, R., Simpson, E., 1994. Treating adult marijuana dependence: a test of the relapse prevention model. J. Consult. Clin. Psychol. 62, 92–99.

Steptoe, A., Doherty, S., Rink, E., et al., 1999. Behavioural counselling in general practice for the promotion of healthy behaviour among adults at increased risk of coronary heart disease: randomised trial. BMJ 319, 943; discussion 47–48.

Stockwell, T., Murphy, D., Hodgson, R., 1983. The severity of alcohol dependence questionnaire: its use, reliability and validity. Br. J. Addict. 78 (2), 45–156.

Surgeon-General, T., 1989. Reducing the health consequences of smoking: 25 years of progress. Department of Health and Human Services, Public Health Service, Centers for Disease Control Office on Smoking and Health, Bethesda, MD.

Swift, W., Hall, W., Teeson, M., 2001a. Characteristics of DSM-IV and ICD-10 cannabis dependence among Australian adults: results from the National Survey of Mental Health and Wellbeing. Drug Alcohol Depend. 63, 147–153.

Swift, W., Hall, W., Teeson, M., 2001b. Cannabis use and dependence among Australian adults: results from the National Survey of Mental Health and Wellbeing. Addiction 96, 737–748.

Tober, G., Strang, J., 2003. Methadone matters: evolving practice of community methadone treatment of opiate addiction. Taylor and Francis, New York.

Washton, A., Resnick, R.B., Geyer, G., 1983. Opiate withdrawal using lofexidine, a clonidine analogue with fewer side-effects. J. Clin. Psychiatry 44, 335–337.

West, R., 1994. Smoking cessation interventions in pregnancy: guidance to purchasers and providers. Health Education Authority, London.

West, R., Hajek, P., Nilsson, F., et al., 2001. Individual differences in preference for and responses to four nicotine replacement products. Psychopharmacology (Berl.) 153, 225–230.

West, R., McNeill, A., Raw, M., 2000. Smoking cessation guidelines for health professionals: an update. Thorax 55, 987–999.

White, A., Rampes, H., Ernst, E., 2001. Acupuncture for smoking cessation (Cochrane review). Cochrane Database Syst. Rev. (4).

WHO Brief Intervention Study Group, 1996. A cross-national trial of brief interventions with heavy drinkers. Am. J. Public Health 86, 948–955.

Wisborg, K., Henriksen, T., Secher, N., 1998. A prospective intervention study of stopping smoking in pregnancy in a routine antenatal care setting. Br. J. Obstet. Gynaecol. 105, 1171–1176.

Chapter 18

Eating disorders

CHAPTER CONTENTS

OBESITY

- The World Health Organization defines overweight as a body mass index (BMI) of 25 kg/m^2 to 29.9 kg/m^2, obesity as ≥ 30 kg/m^2 and seriously obese as ≥ 40.kg/m^2. This can be subdivided into overweight = BMI 25–29.9; obesity I = BMI 30–34.99; obesity II = BMI 35–39.9; obesity III = BMI ≥ 40.

- *Girth* correlates with visceral fat and indirectly measures central adiposity which is an independent predictor of health risk. A girth of > 94 cm in men and > 80 cm in women is associated with increased health risk (Han, van Leer, Seidell, *et al.* 1995).

- Combining BMI and girth is a more accurate predictor where the BMI is below 35 (see Table 18.1).

- *Prevalence.* Over 50% of the UK population are overweight; 15% are obese. This latter figure doubled between 1980 and1995.

- *Mortality* increases exponentially with increasing body weight (Jung 1997). The Framingham study suggests that a BMI ≥ 30 kg/m^2 reduces life expectancy by about 7 years (Peeters, Barendregt, Willekens, *et al.* 2003).

- The risk of coronary heart disease is double if the BMI is > 25 kg/m^2 and nearly quadrupled if ≥ 29 kg/m^2.

- Asians experience greater adverse metabolic changes from overweight than Europeans and the thresholds should be set correspondingly lower (Choo 2002):

DOI: 10.1016/B978-1-4160-5476-4.00018-3

Table 18.1   The effect of combining BMI and girth

	LOW WAIST CIRCUMFERENCE MEN < 94 CM WOMEN < 80 CM	HIGH WAIST CIRCUMFERENCE MEN 94–102 CM WOMEN 80–88 CM	VERY HIGH WAIST CIRCUMFERENCE MEN > 102 CM WOMEN > 88 CM
Overweight	No increased risk	Increased risk	High risk
Obesity I	Increased risk	High risk	Very high risk

Adapted from NICE. 2006. Obesity. Clinical Guideline 43.

(a) overweight = BMI of ≥ 23 kg/m^2;

(b) obese = ≥ 27.5 kg/m^2;

(c) increased girth in men = ≥ 90 cm.

- Obesity is a risk factor for a number of disorders e.g. type 2 diabetes, polycystic ovary syndrome, slipped femoral epiphysis, hypertension and cardiovascular disease. (see Table 18.2). It is likely that all these risk factors are modulated by the 'metabolic syndrome' (see page 228).

- There is now considerable evidence that lifestyle modifications (exercise and diet) can reduce the progression of impaired glucose tolerance to diabetes and hence reduce these risks (Tuomilheto, Lindstrom, Eriksson, *et al.* 2001; Knowler, Barrett-Connor, Fowler, *et al.* 2002; Pan, Li, Hu, *et al.* 1997). Furthermore, it is estimated (SIGN 1996) that a 10 kg loss in weight would lead to falls of total cholesterol by 10%; LDL-cholesterol by 15%; triglycerides by 30%; and a rise of HDL-cholesterol of 8%.

Table 18.2   Relative risk of different diseases in obese versus non–obese people (National Audit Office (NAO) 2001)

DISEASE	RELATIVE RISK IN WOMEN	RELATIVE RISK IN MEN
Type 2 diabetes	12.7	5.2
Hypertension	4.2	2.6
Heart attack	3.2	1.5
Colon cancer	2.7	3
Angina	1.8	1.8
Gallbladder disease	1.8	1.8
Ovarian cancer	1.7	
Stroke	1.3	1.3

OBESITY IN ADULTS

REVIEW

Noël PH, Pugh JA. 2002. Management of overweight and obese adults. BMJ 325, 757–761

GUIDELINE

National Institute for Health and Clinical Excellence. 2006. *Obesity*; 2006. Available: www.nice.org.uk

- Lifestyle strategies that combine a controlled energy diet, increased physical activity and behaviour therapy are successful for weight reduction and maintenance of that weight loss (Nawaz and Katz 2001; NHLBI 1998).

- *Diet*

  (a) In the UK the Food Standards Agency (www.foodstandards.gov.uk) recommends a healthy balanced diet and cautions against low carbohydrate /high fat diets. Most experts recommend a diet high in complex carbohydrates, restricted total fat and moderate in protein. Decreasing the proportion of energy derived from dietary fat by 10% is associated with a reduction in weight of about 6 kg/year (Bray and Popkin 1998). However, 'low fat' products often contain large quantities of simple carbohydrates. Reductions of 500–1000 kcal a day are required to produce weight loss of 0.45–0.9 kg/week.

  (b) Diets that are low carbohydrate, high protein and high fat are popular (Atkins 2002; Sears and Lawren 1995; Steward, Bethea, Andrews, *et al.* 1998). The health risk of these diets is being evaluated and at present, there is insufficient evidence to make recommendations for or against the use of low carbohydrate diets (Bravata, Sanders, Haung, *et al.* 2003). Weight loss with low carbohydrate diets is associated with calorie restriction and duration of diet, not the reduced carbohydrate content (Bray and Popkin 1998).

(c) A 'glycaemic index' based diet is increasingly popular (Brand-Miller, Foster-Powell and McMillan-Price 2005; Gallop and Renton 2005). The principle is to reduce the postprandial rise in blood glucose and consequent insulin demand. There is evidence that a diet high in rapidly absorbed carbohydrates and low in cereal fibre is associated with an increased risk of diabetes (Schulze, Liu, Rimm, *et al.* 2004). The risk may be confined to those who are insulin resistant or predisposed to diabetes (Brand-Miller 2004).

- *Physical activity*. Physical activity results in modest weight loss and improves cardiovascular fitness (NHLBI, 1998). Excessive weight is a disincentive to physical activity (Swinburn and Egger 2004).

MEDICAL CAUSES OF OBESITY

* Consider:
  (a) thyroid disease (although the link between thyroid disease and obesity is overstated);
  (b) polycystic ovary disease (see page 328);
  (c) Cushing's syndrome;
  (d) drug induced obesity, especially: corticosteroids, psychotropic drugs (especially olanzapine and clozapine), antiretroviral agents, and thiozolidinediones (pioglitazone, rosiglitazone), which may cause a 3–4 kg increase.

MANAGEMENT

- Achieving results in primary care is hard. A training programme for practices in the North of England produced improvements in the practitioners' knowledge and behaviour in obesity management but had no effect on their patients' weight (Moore, Summerhill, Greenwood, *et al.* 2003).

- The evidence in favour of benefit from dietary and exercise advice together with motivational and skills training is only fair to good when the intervention is intensive (US Preventative Services Task Force 2003). 'Intensive' means more than one face to face session per month for at least 3 months.

* Educate all patients about the hazards of obesity and the health benefits of modest weight loss (see above).

* Assess the readiness to change:
  (a) Are you currently involved in any effort to lose weight?
  (b) If not currently involved in any effort to lose weight, are you considering trying to lose weight? Have you made any attempts to lose weight? If so what happened?

Patients who are ready to change

* Help set a realistic goal for modest weight loss (see below) followed by a period in which the new weight is maintained (Scottish Intercollegiate Guidelines Network 2003).

* Encourage patients not to give up if goals are not met. Maximum weekly weight loss of 0.5–1 kg is recommended with a long-term goal of losing 5–10% of the original weight.

* See regularly, e.g. monthly, or arrange follow-up by a nurse or dietician.

* Encourage the adoption of long-term lifestyle change and avoidance of the diet mentality. Stress that all family members will benefit from a change in lifestyle.

* Recommend an increase in physical activity incorporating exercise into daily living and planned activity, e.g. brisk walking 30 minutes on most days, walking rather than driving, using stairs instead of lifts. This has been shown to be as effective as structured exercise and is probably more acceptable (Anderson, Wadden, Barlett, *et al.* 1999). Emphasize the other benefits of exercise (see page 689).

* Recommend a stepwise permanent alteration in the diet to a 'healthy' diet with a lower calorie intake (see below).

* *Short-term weight loss*. Discuss the use of 'meal replacement plans' instead of one or two of the

daily meals. They can be effective in short-term weight loss (Heymsfield, van Mierol, van der Knaap, *et al.* 2004). Meal replacements may be an option for those who have struggled to lose weight with more traditional approaches.

* Review the patient against the eligibility criteria for drug therapy (see below).
* Praise a change in behaviour as well as a reduction in weight (see box).
* Do not discourage a patient from a commercial weight loss diet if it suits them. A comparison of four such diets (Dr Atkins' New Diet Revolution, Slim-Fast Plan, Weight Watchers Pure Points Programme, and Rosemary Conley's Eat Yourself Slim Diet and Fitness Plan) found them all equally effective with an average 5.9 kg weight loss over 6 months compared to controls (Truby, Baic, deLooy, *et al.* 2006).

BEHAVIOURAL AND DIETARY ISSUES

Recommend:

(a) reduced portion size using smaller plates;
(b) eating three meals a day, eating slowly, and stopping eating when no longer hungry;
(c) no snacks but if essential change to fruit (fresh or dried), or breakfast cereals with low fat milks.

Overall alteration in dietary constituents:

(a) reduction in dietary fat with advice on interpretation of food labels (> 3 g fat/100 g food);
(b) increase in unrefined carbohydrate;
(c) a modest increase in lean protein if satiety is an issue;
(d) an increase in fruit and vegetables;
(e) avoidance or reduction of high fat/ high sugar convenience foods.
* Advise a diet along the following lines:
  (a) *Fruit and vegetables:* eat five portions a day;
  (b) *Bread, whole-grain cereals, potatoes, pasta, rice:* eat five portions a day;
  (c) *Lean meat, oily fish:* eat in moderation – two portions a day at the most;
  (d) *Fatty or sugary foods and alcohol:* eat as little as possible.

WEIGHT MAINTENANCE

* Encourage patients who lose weight to maintain the loss. The National Weight Control Registry (www.nwcr.ws) found that those who were successful in losing 14 kg or more and maintaining this have certain characteristics:
  (a) the majority were eating a high carbohydrate, low fat diet. Less than 1% were following a high protein, low fat diet;
  (b) most ate their meals at home;
  (c) the majority monitored their intake and levels of activity with a diary;
  (d) the majority ate regular meals and only 4% skipped breakfast;
  (e) the majority engaged in high levels of physical activity.
* Suggest to patients unwilling or unable to lose weight that they aim for weight constancy (i.e. keeping their weight as it is rather than gaining weight) (Pryke and Docherty 2008).

Drug therapies

Every adult who meets the National Institute for Clinical Excellence (NICE) 2006 criteria should be offered orlistat. It can help both weight loss and maintenance but the benefit is modest. Highly motivated trial subjects on orlistat only manage extra weight loss of the order of 2.9 kg over 1–4 years yet obese patients continue to have unrealistically high expectation of the drugs. A useful way of explaining the likely benefit would be that orlistat is likely to achieve the same weight loss as eating an apple a day instead of an ice cream (Williams 2007).

NICE recommends that orlistat should be available as one part of the management of obesity:

■ if the BMI is ≥ 28 kg/m^2 in the presence of risk factors such as diabetes or dyslipidaemia, or a BMI of ≥ 30 kg/m^2 without comorbidities; *and*

■ it is possible to monitor weight loss and adverse effects (specifically pulse and blood pressure).

Treatment should only continue for more than 3 months if there has been a 5% loss in initial body weight. Continuation after 1 year should be something for doctor and patient to decide together after discussing the benefits and limitations of the drug.

As this book was being prepared for publication the other drug licensed for the treatment of obesity in the UK, sibutramine, was suspended from sale. This followed an interim analysis of the SCOUT study (the Sibutramine Cardiovascular OUTcomes study). High risk patients, who were overweight and who had either cardiovascular disease or type 2 diabetes, were given sibutramine for 5 years. The analysis revealed a 16% increase in cardiovascular adverse events, mainly non-fatal stroke and myocardial infarction, compared to placebo (hazard ratio 1.161; 95%CI 1.029-1.311). The Committee for Medicinal Products for Human Use concluded that the weight loss on sibutramine was modest and may not be sustained after treatment cessation.

Doctors across Europe, including the UK, have been advised not to issue new prescriptions for the drug and to review patients who are already on it. Pharmacists have been advised not to dispense it. There is no danger attached to sudden cessation of the drug.

In the US sibutramine remains available, at the time of writing, but the FDA has requested that cardiovascular disease be made a contraindication to the use of the drug.

The findings of the SCOUT study have come as no surprise to some (Williams 2010). Cardiovascular disease was already noted as a contraindication to use of the drug in the UK, and prescribers were cautioned to monitor blood pressure and pulse rate carefully. Rises of > 20 mm Hg in blood pressure and of > 20 beats per minute in pulse rate were known to occur. Sibutramine acts centrally, inhibiting the re-uptake of noradrenaline and serotonin and thus enhancing the appetite-suppressant action of those transmitters. The adverse effects of the drug presumably come from the resultant increase in sympathetic drive to the cardiovascular system. There is no reason why orlistat, which is a lipase inhibitor and works by reducing the absorption of dietary fat, should have the same adverse effects.

SEVERE OBESITY

Gastric surgery is the most effective and cost effective method reducing weight in severe obesity. NICE suggests that surgery is underutilized and that eligible patients are not being referred for potentially beneficial procedures. Referral to an experienced team for gastroplasty or gastric bypass should be considered in patients aged 18 or over with morbid obesity (BMI ≥ 40 kg/m^2) or between 35 and 40 kg/m^2 with major weight related comorbidities. A 40–60% reduction in weight can occur.

NICE makes the following stipulations:

- all appropriate non-surgical measures have been tried and failed over a period of at least 6 months;
- intensive specialist management will be provided;
- they are fit for the operation; and
- they commit to the need for long-term follow-up.

OBESITY IN CHILDREN

GUIDELINES

National Institute for Health and Clinical Excellence. Obesity; clinical guideline 43; 2006. Available: www.nice.org.uk
  Scottish Intercollegiate Guidelines Network. *Management of Obesity in Children and Young People.* SIGN 2003. Available: www.sign.ac.uk

Comment

Ebbeling CB, Pawlak DB, Ludwig DS. 2002. Childhood obesity: public-health crisis, common sense cure. Lancet 360, 473-482

- The prevalence of obesity varies from 10% at the age of 10 to 17% at the age of 15.
- The BMI changes significantly in childhood, being greatest at the age of 1 and at a nadir by around 6 years of age. In the UK, children are accepted as obese if they are above the 98th centile and overweight if above the 91st centile using age related BMI charts, available on www.health-for-all-children.co.uk.
- Waist circumference has been shown to be linked to dyslipidaemia in children, as it is in adults (Flodmark, Svenger and Nilsson-Ehle 1994). Centiles for British children have now been established (McCarthy, Jarrett and Crawley 2001).

COMPLICATIONS/COMORBIDITY OF CHILDHOOD OBESITY

- Obesity in childhood is associated with a clustering of cardiovascular risk factors which has been identified in children as young as 5. Adolescents who die traumatic deaths show evidence of asymptomatic atherosclerosis and these lesions are more advanced in obese individuals (Strong, Malcom, McMahan, et al. 1999). In a British cohort being overweight in childhood increased the risk of death from ischaemic heart disease in adulthood two-fold over 57 years (Gunnell, Frankel, Nanchahal, et al. 1998).

- Type 2 diabetes now accounts for about 50% of new diagnoses in children in some populations (Fagot-Campagna, Pettit, Engelau, et al. 2000). Precocious puberty in girls and hypogonadism in boys is a recognized association as is polycystic ovary syndrome, although whether obesity is primary or secondary in this situation is not known.

- Pulmonary complications – sleep apnoea, asthma and exercise intolerance are common in obese children.

- Serious hepatic, renal musculoskeletal and neurological consequences have been increasingly recognized.

- Psychosocial consequences of obesity in childhood include negative self-image at the age of 5 and decreasing self-esteem in obese adolescents with associated sadness, loneliness, nervousness and high-risk behaviours (Strauss 2000).

MANAGEMENT

* Plot the child's weight and height and girth on centile charts. If the child's expected final height is close to the mid-parental height (see page 120) and the child is well, no investigations are needed. A pathological cause for the obesity (Cushing's disease, juvenile hypothyroidism, Prader-Willi syndrome) would always be associated with short stature (Ledingham and Warrell 2000).

* Explain to the parents and the children, in ways appropriate to them, the risks associated with obesity. Encourage them to visit the change4life NHS site at www.nhs.uk/Change4Life.

* Consider intervention if the child is obese (above the 98th centile) or overweight (above 91st centile) and the family is willing to accept the necessary lifestyle changes.

* Assess those over the 98th centile for comorbidities.

* When the family is unwilling to accept that a change is necessary, give them the appropriate health information and invite them to return.

* **Set goals.** Aim for a static weight in a growing child, rather than weight reduction. If not possible, work towards a decrease in weight gain, so that the target is a decrease in BMI rather than a decrease in weight. In a pubertal child who has attained adult height aim for a weight reduction of 10% as this has been shown to have benefits on cardiovascular risk factors.

BEHAVIOURAL CHANGE

* Explain that gaining weight is a consequence of an imbalance of energy intake and output and that lifestyle changes including exercise, reduction of energy intake and a reduction of sedentary behaviour are necessary.

* Encourage the family to substitute lower energy foods for high energy foods and not to increase the intake of carbohydrate to compensate for the reduction in fat. Avoid fast foods which tend to be rich in fat and sugary drinks. One sugary drink per day of approximately 120 Cal will increase weight by 5 kg/year (Ebbeling, Pawlak and Ludwig 2002). The family should make small changes to their diet over months rather than dramatic changes which are unlikely to be successful.

* Advise the child to increase physical activity, e.g. brisk walking for 30 minutes a day and up to 60 minutes a day in healthy children. Again small increments in activity should be encouraged and those activities the child enjoys, fostered.

* Advise a reduction in sedentary activity especially television viewing. Explain that children who watch television a lot have much higher levels of obesity and that this occurs not only by displacing physical activity but also by often increasing energy intake by the consumption of energy rich snacks. In addition, there is evidence that younger children will select food they have seen advertised and that there are approximately 10 food commercials

per hour in the UK. Reduction of television viewing has been shown to reduce indices of adiposity (Robinson 1999).

* Encourage the parents to give treats other than food so that the changes do not seem all bad.

Refer:

(a) children who may have serious obesity-related morbidity that requires weight loss, e.g. benign intracranial hypertension, sleep apnoea, obesity hypoventilation syndrome, orthopaedic problems and psychosocial morbidity;

(b) children with a suspected underlying medical cause of obesity;

(c) children with BMI > 99.6th centile;

(d) children with height below the 9th centile, unexpectedly short for the family or with slowed growth velocity;

(e) precocious or late puberty (before age 8; or no signs in girls at 13 or in boys at 15).

Drug treatment may be appropriate, especially in children aged 12 and over, but it should only be initiated in specialist settings. Surgery would only be considered in those who have reached or are reaching physiological maturity, and then only according to the same criteria as for adults (see page 509).

FOLLOW-UP

Review the child and family regularly, possibly as often as every 2 weeks. Agree one change that will be made by the time you see them next.

EATING DISORDERS

For details of the diagnosis of eating disorders see *Evidence-based Diagnosis in Primary Care* by A. F. Polmear (editor), published by Butterworth-Heinemann, 2008.

National Institute for Clinical Excellence. *Eating Disorders.* NICE Clinical Guideline No. 9, 2004. Available: www.nice.org.uk (search on 'eating disorders')
   Eating Disorders Unit. Prevalence. Institute of Psychiatry at the Maudsley. Available: www.iop.kcl.ac.uk (search on 'Eating disorders prevalence')

● 60% of adolescents have undertaken a weight loss diet, and 50% of this population pursue an ideal body image thinner than their own.

● The prevalence of 'pure' anorexia nervosa has not changed in time, with a prevalence of up to 0.8% and that of bulimia nervosa up to 4%.

IDENTIFICATION AND SCREENING OF EATING DISORDERS

● Early assessment and intervention is important in reducing long-term risk. The assessment should include physical, psychological and social components.

● About 10% of recognized sufferers are men. They are more likely to be obsessed by shape and flabbiness than by weight.

* Consider an eating disorder in:

(a) young women with a low BMI compared with age norms;

(b) patients consulting with weight concerns who are not overweight;

(c) women with menstrual disturbances or amenorrhoea;

(d) young people with type 1 diabetes (not because of a causal association but because an eating disorder can complicate management of the diabetes);

(e) patients with gastrointestinal symptoms; patients with physical signs of starvation or repeated vomiting;

(f) children and adolescents with poor growth.

* Ask (National Institute of Clinical Excellence 2004):

(a) do you think you have an eating problem? and

(b) do you worry excessively about your weight?

* Ask the patient if anyone else is worried about their eating habits or exercise routine.

Alternatively use the **SCOFF** questionnaire:

■ Do you make yourself **SICK** because you feel uncomfortably full?

■ Do you worry you have lost **CONTROL** over how much you eat?

■ Have you recently lost more than **ONE** stone (14 lb or 7.7 kg) in a 3-month period?

■ Do you believe yourself to be **FAT** when others say you are thin?

■ Would you say **FOOD** dominates your life?

A score of 2 or more indicates possible anorexia nervosa or bulimia. This questionnaire has been shown to have high sensitivity (100%) and specificity (87.5%) (Morgan, Reid and Lacey 1999).

DIAGNOSIS OF ANOREXIA NERVOSA

* Make the diagnosis of anorexia when the following are present:

  (a) a weight < 85% of expected (DSM-IV definition) or a BMI ≤ 17.5 kg/m^2(ICD-10 definition); and

  (b) a fear of gaining weight or becoming fat that is inconsistent with the patient's weight; and

  (c) a distorted self-image.

* Check for other mental features that are often associated: mood changes, obsessive-compulsive features relating to food or weight or shape, low self-esteem.

* Ask about physical exercise. High levels of physical activity, exercise, overactivity (not sitting still, fidgeting, etc.) are recognized weight control techniques used by people with anorexia.

* Check for physical features that are often associated: amenorrhoea or delayed menarche, hypotension, bradycardia, dry skin with lanugo on the trunk, eroded tooth enamel in a patient who induces vomiting.

* Check that there is no physical disorder which better explains the symptoms: hyperthyroidism, stimulant abuse, or malignancy. However, if the cardinal symptoms of anorexia are present any other disease is likely to be present in addition, rather than mimicking anorexia.

* Check that there is no concurrent psychiatric disorder which would need treating in its own right: major depressive illness is common in anorexia. Obsessive-compulsive disorder is present if obsessions or compulsions exist about things unrelated to food, weight or body shape.

* Check FBC, U&Es, LFTs, TFTs. Be aware of the abnormalities that occur in anorexia per se, rather than being an indication of another disorder: normocytic normochromic anaemia, leucopenia, hypokalaemia from vomiting or purging, raised LFTs, or a low free T$_3$ and T$_4$ without an elevation of TSH.

DIAGNOSIS OF BULIMIA

* Make the diagnosis of bulimia when the following are present:

  (a) binge eating, where a binge is the consumption of a large amount of food in a short period of time; and

  (b) attempts to avoid weight gain: inducing vomiting and/or purging with laxatives.

The DSM IV definition requires that these two features have been present at least twice a week for 3 months. The patient is likely to be at or near normal weight, and to be secretive about the bingeing and purging, which make detection much harder than in anorexia.

* Check for other mental features that are often associated: mood changes, obsessive-compulsive features relating to food or weight or shape, low self-esteem.

* Check for eroded dental enamel, and for abrasions on the knuckles due to forcing the fingers down the throat.

* Check that there is no concurrent psychiatric disorder which would need treating in its own right: depression, anxiety, and substance misuse, especially stimulant misuse.

* Check FBC and U&Es. In severe purging there may be hyponatraemia and hypokalaemia.

MANAGEMENT POINTS COMMON TO ALL TYPES OF EATING DISORDER

Diabetes. Refer patients with diabetes and an eating disorder as they have a greatly increased risk of retinopathy and should be closely monitored.

Pregnancy should be monitored more closely throughout the pregnancy and the postpartum period.

Vomiting. Advise patients who are vomiting to avoid brushing their teeth after vomiting, to rinse with a non-acid mouthwash, to limit acidic foods and drinks and to have regular dental reviews.

Laxative abuse. Advise the patient to reduce the laxative gradually. Explain that laxative use does not significantly reduce calorie absorption.

MANAGEMENT OF ANOREXIA NERVOSA

GUIDANCE AND SYSTEMATIC REVIEWS

National Institute for Clinical Excellence. 2004. *Eating Disorders.* NICE Clinical Guideline No. 9. Available: www.nice.org.uk (search on 'Eating disorders')
   Treasure J, Schmidt U. 2005. Anorexia nervosa. *Clinical Evidence.* Issue 12. BMJ Publishing Group, London

Prognosis. In anorexia nervosa 43% recover, while, of those admitted to hospital, 10% die.
   Work up: pulse, blood pressure, FBC, U+Es, TFTs.

* *Severe anorexia.* Admit if there is evidence of severe anorexia:

   (a) BMI< 15 kg/m^2 especially if there has been rapid weight loss;

   (b) serum potassium < 2.5 mmol/l;

   (c) severe bone marrow dysfunction with loss of platelets;

   (d) proximal myopathy;

   (e) significant gastrointestinal symptoms from repeated vomiting;

   (f) significant risk of suicide;

   (g) other complicating factors, e.g. substance or alcohol abuse.

Note: When a person, felt to be at high risk, refuses treatment consider using the Mental Health Act 1983 or the Children Act 1989. The Mental Health Act Commission, in Guidance Note 3 of August 1997, confirmed that, as a mental disorder, anorexia nervosa does fall within the Act and that detention and even compulsory feeding might be justified.

* *Moderate anorexia.* Refer to an eating disorders unit or local psychiatric department if there is evidence of moderate anorexia (BMI 15–17 kg/m^2 with no evidence of system failure). Monitor frequently while waiting for the appointment.
* *Mild anorexia.* Manage in primary care if anorexia is mild (BMI > 17 kg/m^2, and no additional comorbidity). If there is no response after 8 weeks refer to an eating disorders unit or local psychiatric department.

Management in primary care

* See the patient on her own as well as with the family. Explain early on that you will probably be referring her on to the local child and adolescent unit or specialist eating disorder unit at a later stage (to avoid the patient feeling that her first attempt at treatment has failed).
* Expect denial and ambivalence. Ask about the patient's concerns about:
   (a) the negative effects of anorexia nervosa on aspects of life;
   (b) the benefits that anorexia has for her (e.g. feeling of being in control, feeling safe, being able to get care and attention from the family).
* Explain that:
   (a) purging and severe starvation may cause serious physical harm and that anorexia can be life threatening;
   (b) purging and severe dieting are ineffective ways of achieving lasting weight control.
* Weigh the patient regularly and chart their weight. Set manageable goals in agreement with the patient, e.g. a 0.5 kg increase per week. This requires a calorie intake of about 2500 kcal per day.
* *Multivitamins.* Offer an oral multivitamin supplement if the diet is likely to be poor in vitamins.
* Discuss with the patient and parents that a return to normal eating habits may be a distant goal and encourage the family to be patient and consistent.
* Be aware of the increased risk of self-harm, particularly in those who are bingeing and purging. Review patients regularly, particularly if there is likely to be a hiatus in support services.
* Order a DEXA scan for osteoporosis in a woman with prolonged amenorrhoea (see page 279).

RECOMMEND

Treasure J. 1997. *Breaking Free from Anorexia Nervosa: A Survival Guide for Families, Friends and Sufferers.* Psychology Press
   Lask B, Bryant-Waugh R. 2000. *Anorexia Nervosa and Related Eating Disorders in Childhood and Adolescence.* Psychology Press
   Beat (The Eating Disorders Association). *About Eating Disorders.* www.b-eat.co.uk and choose 'About Eating Disorders'
   The Royal College of Psychiatrists. *Eating Disorders and Eating Disorders in Young People.* Available: www.rcpsych.ac.uk
   An information leaflet for carers of people with anorexia nervosa. Available: www.iop.kcl.ac.uk (search on 'Support for carers')

MANAGEMENT OF BULIMIA NERVOSA

GUIDANCE AND SYSTEMATIC REVIEWS

National Institute for Clinical Excellence. 2004. *Eating Disorders.* NICE Clinical Guideline No. 9. Available: www.nice.org.uk (search on 'Eating disorders')
    Hay PJ, Bacaltchuk J. 2005. Bulimia Nervosa. *Clinical Evidence.* Issue 12. BMJ Publishing Group, London

* *Severe bulimia.* Admit, or refer urgently, those with:
  (a) significant electrolyte imbalance;
  (b) comorbidity, especially diabetes.
* *Moderate bulimia.* Manage initially in general practice. A study has shown that patients managed by self-help measures in general practice do as well as those managed by specialist units and may benefit from the earlier intervention (Durand and King 2003).
* Advise the patient or parents to look up information about the condition on www.b-eat.co.uk or www.rcpsych.ac.uk or to buy:
  (a) Cooper P. 2009. *Overcoming Bulimia Nervosa/Binge Eating.* Revised Edition;
  (b) Treasure J, Schmidt U. 1993. *Getting Better Bit(e) by Bit(e): A Survival Kit for Sufferers of Bulimia or Binge Eating Disorders.* Psychology Press.
* Educate the patient about the need to eat regularly throughout the day (three meals plus two snacks) to reduce urges to binge. Recommend keeping a food dairy.
* Set mutually agreed goals to increase the number of meals, the variety of foods and to reduce vomiting and laxatives.
* Help the patient identify triggers for binge eating and develop strategies to manage these trigger events. Recommend that the patient fills in a binge eating diary.
* Elicit the patient's beliefs about weight, shape and eating and encourage them to question their views about body image.
* Arrange counselling if there are factors in the patient's life that warrant it.
* Discuss with the patient the pros and cons of an SSRI, explaining that these can reduce the frequency of binge eating and purging but that the long-term effects are unknown. Give fluoxetine, increasing slowly to 60 mg/day.

* Review regularly. If there is no improvement by 8 weeks refer to the local Child and Adolescent Mental Health Unit or specialist unit.

ATYPICAL EATING DISORDERS INCLUDING BINGE EATING SYNDROME

About 30% of referrals have eating disorders that are not classifiable as anorexia or bulimia. They may be more suitable for management in primary care than the classic syndromes.
    Binge eating syndrome is characterized by:

(a) eating more rapidly than usual;
(b) eating until uncomfortably full;
(c) eating despite not feeling physically hungry;
(d) eating alone because of embarrassment about the quantities of food consumed;
(e) experiencing a negative effect after eating, e.g. disgust, guilt, depression.

* Encourage the patient to follow an evidence-based self-help programme, e.g. Cooper P. 2009. *Overcoming Bulimia Nervosa/Binge Eating.* Revised Edition.
* Consider prescribing a trial of an SSRI, as an alternative or in addition to the self-help programme.
* Review regularly and refer to the local specialist for cognitive behaviour therapy for binge eating disorder (CBT-BED) if there is no progress.

Sub-threshold anorexia

* Manage as for mild anorexia nervosa.

ATHLETES WITH EATING DISORDERS

Birch K. 2005. Female athlete triad. BMJ 330, 244–246

Eating disorders are common in athletes (www.edauk.com/sport/coach.htm). The American College of Sports Medicine recognizes the Female Athlete Triad (American College of Sports Medicine 1997). The defining features are:

■ *Disordered eating:* spectrum of abnormal patterns of eating, including bingeing, purging, food restriction, prolonged fasting, use of diet pills, diuretics and laxatives and other abnormal eating behaviours.

- *Amenorrhoea:* absence of at least three to six consecutive menstrual cycles in women who have already begun menstruating. Primary and secondary amenorrhoea are both more common in women athletes. The cause appears to be related to low energy intake not low levels of bodily fat.
- *Osteoporosis:* secondary to hypo-oestrogenism.

* Be alert to eating disorders in all patients who have high levels of exercise. Do not dismiss menstrual irregularities as a minor consequence of high levels of exercise. The patient needs further assessment.
* Arrange for a DEXA scan for osteoporosis if there has been prolonged amenorrhea.

References

American College of Sports Medicine, 1997. The female athlete triad: disordered eating, amenorrhoea, osteoporosis: call to action. Sports Med. Bulletin 29, 1–9.

Anderson, R.E., Wadden, T.A., Barlett, S.J., et al., 1999. Effects of lifestyle activity vs structured aerobic exercise in obese women. JAMA 281, 335–340.

Atkins, R.C., 2002. Dr Atkins' new diet revolution. Avon Books, New York.

Brand-Miller, J.C., 2004. Postprandial glycemia, glycemic index, and the prevention of type 2 diabetes. Am. J. Clin. Nutr. 80, 243–244.

Brand-Miller, J., Foster-Powell, K., McMillan-Price, J., 2005. The Low GI Diet Revolution: The Definitive Science-Based Weight Loss Plan (New Glucose Revolution). Marlowe.

Bravata, D.M., Sanders, L., Haung, J., et al., 2003. Efficacy and safety of low–carbohydrate diets: a systematic review. JAMA 289, 1837–1850.

Bray, G.A., Popkin, B.M., 1998. Dietary fat intake does affect obesity. Am. J. Nutr. 68, 1157–1173.

Choo, V., 2002. WHO reassesses appropriate body-mass index for Asian populations. Lancet 360, 235.

Durand, M.A., King, M., 2003. Specialist treatment versus self-help for bulimia nervosa: a randomised controlled trial in general practice. Br. J. Gen. Pract. 53, 371–377.

Ebbeling, C.B., Pawlak, D.B., Ludwig, D.S., 2002. Childhood obesity: public-health crisis, common sense cure. Lancet 360, 473–482.

Fagot-Campagna, A., Pettit, D.J., Engelau, M.M., et al., 2000. Type 2 diabetes among North American children and adolescents with marked obesity: an epidemiologic review and a public health perspective. J. Pediatr. 136, 664–672.

Flodmark, C.E., Svenger, T., Nilsson-Ehle, P., 1994. Waist measurement correlates to a potentially atherogenic lipoprotein profile in obese 12–14 year old children. Acta Paediatr. 83, 941–945.

Gallop, R., Renton, H., 2005. The GI Guide: Understanding the Glycaemic Index, Healthy Eating, Lifestyle and Shopping. Virgin.

Gunnell, D.J., Frankel, S.J., Nanchahal, K., et al., 1998. Childhood obesity and adult cardiovascular mortality: a 57-year follow-up study based on Boyd Orr cohort. Am. J. Clin. Nutr. 67, 1111–1118.

Han, T., van Leer, E., Seidell, J., et al., 1995. Waist circumference action levels in the identification of cardiovascular risk factors: prevalence study in a random sample. BMJ 311, 1401–1405.

Heymsfield, S.B., van Mierol, C.A.J., van der Knaap, H.C.M., et al., 2004. Weight management using meal replacement strategy: meta and pooling analysis from six studies. Int. J. Obes. 27, 537–549.

Jung, R.T., 1997. Obesity as a disease. Br. Med. Bull. 53, 307–321.

Knowler, W.C., Barrett-Connor, E., Fowler, S.E., et al., 2002. Reduction in the incidence of type 2 diabetes with lifestyle intervention or metformin. N. Engl. J. Med. 346, 393–403.

Ledingham, J.G.G., Warrell, D.A. (eds), 2000. The Concise Oxford Textbook of Medicine. OUP, Oxford.

McCarthy, H.D., Jarrett, K.V., Crawley, H.F., 2001. The development of waist circumference percentiles in British children aged 5.0 – 16.9 y. Eur. J. Clin. Nutr. 55, 902–907.

McTigue, K.M., Harris, R., Hemphill, B., et al., 2003. Screening and interventions for obesity in adults: summary of the evidence for the U.S. Preventive Services Task Force. Ann. Intern. Med. 139, 949.

Moore, H., Summerhill, C.D., Greenwood, D.C., et al., 2003. Improving management of obesity in primary care: cluster randomised trial. BMJ 327, 1085–1088.

Morgan, J.F., Reid, F., Lacey, J.H., 1999. The SCOFF questionnaire: assessment of a new screening tool for eating disorders. BMJ 319, 1467–1468.

National Audit Office (NAO), 2001. Tackling obesity in England. The Stationery Office, London. www.nao.gov.uk/publications/nao_reports/00-01/0001220.pdf.

National Institute of Clinical Excellence, 2004. Eating Disorders; Quick Reference Guide. NICE. Available: www.nice.org.

Nawaz, H., Katz, D.L., 2001. American College of Preventative Medicine Practice Policy Statement. Weight management counselling of overweight adults. Am. J. Prev. Med. 21, 73–78.

NHLBI, 1998. Executive summary of the clinical guidelines on the identification, evaluation and treatment of overweight and obesity in adults. Arch. Intern. Med. 158, 1855–1867.

Pan, X.R., Li, G.W., Hu, Y.H., et al., 1997. Effects of diet and exercise in preventing NIDDM in people with impaired glucose tolerance. The Da Qing IGT and Diabetes Study. Diabetes Care 20, 537–544.

Peeters, A., Barendregt, J.J., Willekens, F., et al., 2003. Obesity in adulthood and its consequence for life expectancy: a life table analysis. Ann. Intern. Med. 138, 24–32.

Pryke, R., Docherty, A., 2008. Obesity in primary care: evidence for advising weight constancy rather than weight loss in unsuccessful dieters. Br. J. Gen. Pract. 58, 112–117.

Robinson, T.N., 1999. Reducing children's television viewing to prevent obesity. JAMA 282, 1561–1567.

Schulze, M.B., Liu, S., Rimm, E.B., et al., 2004. Glycemic index, glycemic load, and dietary fiber intake and incidence of type 2 diabetes in younger and middle aged women. Am. J. Clin. Nutr. 80, 348–356.

Scottish Intercollegiate Guidelines Network, 2003. Management of obesity in children and young people. SIGN. Available: www.sign.ac.uk.

Sears, B., Lawren, B., 1995. The zone: a dietary road map to lose weight permanently, reset your genetic code, prevent disease, achieve maximum physical performance. Harper Collins, New York.

SIGN, 1996. Obesity in Scotland. Integrating Prevention with Weight Management. Royal College of Physicians, Edinburgh. Available: http://www.sign.ac.uk.

Steward, H.L., Bethea, M.C., Andrews, S.S., et al., 1998. Sugar busters: cut sugar to trim fat. Ballentine Books, New York.

Strauss, R.S., 2000. Childhood obesity and self-esteem. Pediatrics 105, e15.

Strong, J.P., Malcom, G.T., McMahan, C.A., et al., 1999. Prevalence and extent of atherosclerosis in adolescents and young adults: implications for prevention from pathobiological determinants of atherosclerosis in youth. JAMA 281, 727–735.

Swinburn, B., Egger, G., 2004. The runaway weight gain train: Too many accelerators, not enough breaks. BMJ 329, 736–739.

Truby, H., Baic, S., deLooy, A., et al., 2006. Randomised controlled trial of four commercial weight loss programmes in the UK: initial findings from the BBC 'diet trials'. BMJ 332, 1309–1311.

Tuomilheto, J., Lindstrom, J., Eriksson, J.G., et al., 2001. Prevention of type 2 diabetes mellitus by changes in lifestyle among subjects with impaired glucose tolerance. N. Engl. J. Med. 344, 1343–1349.

US Preventative Services Task Force, 2003. Screening for obesity in adults: recommendations and rationale. Ann. Intern. Med. 139, 930–932.

Williams, G., 2007. Orlistat over the counter. BMJ 335, 1163–1164.

Williams, G., 2010. Withdrawal of sibutramine in Europe. BMJ 340, 377–378.

Chapter 19

The management of chronic fatigue syndrome

CHAPTER CONTENTS

SYSTEMATIC REVIEWS AND REPORTS

NICE. 2007. *Chronic Fatigue Syndrome/Myalgic Encephalomyelitis (or Encephalopathy): Diagnosis and Management of CFS/ME in Adults and Children.* National Institute for Health and Clinical Excellence. London. Available: www.nice.org.uk

Effective Health Care. 2002. Interventions for the management of CFS/ME. NHS Centre for Reviews and Dissemination vol 7, no. 4

Carruthers B, Jain A, De Meirleir K, *et al.* 2003. Myalgic encephalomyelitis/chronic fatigue syndrome: clinical working case definition, diagnostic and treatment protocols. J Chronic Fatigue Syndrome 11, 7–115

Very few patients with chronic fatigue have chronic fatigue syndrome (CFS). The syndrome is found to be present in only 0.2–2.6% of patients complaining in primary care of at least 2 weeks fatigue (Reid, Chalder, Cleare, *et al.* 2000). Conversely, those who do have it need an early diagnosis and intensive management of what is a chronic and disabling condition.

* *Make an early diagnosis.* For details of the diagnosis of chronic fatigue syndrome see *Evidence-based Diagnosis in Primary Care* by A. F. Polmear (editor), published by Butterworth-Heinemann, 2008. By definition, the final diagnosis can only be made after symptoms have been present for 6 months. However, a working diagnosis can be made after between 6 and 12 weeks in a patient who shows the characteristic delayed adverse reaction to mental and/or physical exertion. Other

DOI: 10.1016/B978-1-4160-5476-4.00019-5

disorders should have been excluded by the 6 week stage.

* *Is the diagnosis correct?*
  - Check, from the patient's history, that the patient meets criteria for CFS. The only clinical, as opposed to research, case definition is that of the Canadian Expert Medical Consensus Panel (Carruthers, Jain, De Meirleir, *et al.* 2003) (see below). Check that a competent assessment for mental disorders and for physical disease has been carried out. However, the diagnosis should be a positive one, based on the characteristic symptoms, not merely on the exclusion of other disorders.
  - A routine physical examination is unlikely to be helpful if the history has not provided any clues. The yield in one study of fatigue was 2% (Ebell 2001; Lane, Matthews and Manu 1990). Examination for thyroid disease and neurological disorders might occasionally prove useful.
  - The yield from laboratory investigations is unlikely to be high: 5% (Ebell 2001), 8% (Sugarman and Berg 1984), 9% (Ridsdale, Evans, Jerrett, *et al.* 1993) in different studies. Initially check: FBC, ESR, blood sugar and TFTs. Other tests are hugely more likely to result in false positive than true positive results (Koch, van Bokhoven, ter Riet, *et al.* 2009). If symptoms persist at 4 weeks further tests can be ordered, modified by any pointers in the clinical picture: LFTs, urea and electrolytes, calcium, phosphate, magnesium, creatine kinase, ANA, RF, ferritin, endomysial antibodies and serology for infectious mononucleosis and Lyme disease. Check the urine for blood and protein.
  - Be alert for the appearance of red flags, which might indicate a diagnosis other than CFS, e.g. weight loss, persistent lymphadenopathy, focal neurological signs, or objective evidence of arthritis.
* **Assess** the impact that the condition is making on the patient's life so that management can to tailored for that patient.
* **Explain** what little is known about the condition: that it is real; that the cause is unknown but that abnormalities have been found in a number of systems: immune, endocrine, neurological and musculoskeletal.

Explain that, whatever the cause, inactivity can lead to physical deconditioning which in turn leads to even more adverse effects from exertion. While treatment cannot influence the underlying condition it can reduce the effect of this deconditioning.

* **Explain** that, while you cannot offer a cure, there is a lot you can offer in the way of amelioration. A supportive relationship with an explanation of the 'pacing' approach, see below, may be the most valuable things a doctor can offer.
* **Discuss the prognosis** only at the right time with patients and relatives who want to know. The data come from those referred to specialist clinics and so are likely to be more severely affected than those in primary care. In the medium term, 20–50% of adults show some improvement but only 6% return to their 'normal' level of functioning (Reid, Chalder, Cleare, *et al.* 2000). Recovery in 2 years would be considered fast. Even while improving symptoms are likely to fluctuate.
* **Discuss with the carers** the impact of the illness on their lives.
* **Rest and activity.** There is agreement among patients and clinicians that excessive activity and excessive rest exacerbate the condition. Two approaches are possible:
  1. graded exercise, in which the patient follows a supervised course of aerobic activity which is slowly increased according to what the patient can tolerate. This can lead to significant improvement in wellbeing, in reduction of fatigue and in physical functioning (Reid, Chalder, Cleare, *et al.* 2000). However, drop-outs from the programme are high and one study found that 50% of people with severe CFS reported worsening of the condition with graded exercise (Shepherd 2001); or
  2. 'pacing', in which the patient judges each day what his or her exertion limit is, and then exerts within that, say at 70%, thereby avoiding a 'boom and bust' cycle. This applies to both physical and mental exertion.
* **Relaxation techniques** help some patients to pace themselves. The simplest technique is 'palming'. Place the palms of the hands over the closed eyes and press gently for 1 minute.

Counselling may help patients to 'feel OK' about themselves despite such a debilitating illness.

* **Consider referral for cognitive behavioural therapy (CBT) if available**. A Cochrane review (Price and Couper 2004) found three RCTs which gave an NNT of 2 for CBT; i.e. half of the patients receiving the treatment, compared to placebo, had improved in one physical measure about 6 months after completion of treatment. One study in primary care found that psychodynamic counselling was as effective as CBT (Ridsdale, Godfrey, Chalder, *et al.* 2001). However, one study in which follow-up continued for 5 years found no long-term improvement from CBT in some measures including fatigue and physical functioning (Whiting, Bagnall, Sowden, *et al.* 2001). Furthermore, studies which show benefit use the loosest definition of CFS while those that use a tighter definition fail to show benefit. It may be that patients without true CFS are the ones who benefit.

* **Ask regularly about the patient's mood**. Depression and anxiety may need treatment in their own right.

* **Ask about sleep.** It is disturbed in the majority of patients (Morriss, Sharpe, Sharpley, *et al.* 1993). Explain the principles of sleep management (see page 462). Use short courses of sedatives for crises.

* **Treat pain** with medication if necessary but start at half the usual starting dose and increase slowly. Work through a 'ladder' of paracetamol – NSAID – tricyclic – gabapentin. Use baclofen for muscle spasm.

* **Orthostatic hypotension.** The onset of symptoms is often delayed by at least 10 minutes after standing up. Tell the patient to avoid standing up quickly and staying upright for too long, especially after a large meal. Prescribe support stockings provided there is someone to help put them on.

* **Discuss other possible therapies with the patient**. The points to cover are: that evidence for them is poor (see below); that trying one ineffective treatment after another can be demoralizing and can deflect attention from the therapies of proven benefit, as well as delaying the patient's adjustment to the condition.

THE CANADIAN WORKING CASE DEFINITION (CARRUTHERS, JAIN, DE MEIRLEIR, *ET AL.* 2003)

Essential criteria

■ *Fatigue* which may be physical and/or mental; must be new; and must be bad enough to reduce the patient's activity by at least 50%.

■ *Post-exertional malaise and/or fatigue.* The crucial point is the patient's muscular and/or mental fatigability with delayed recovery, often over more than 24 hours. The deterioration may occur some hours after the exertion.

■ *Two or more neurological/cognitive manifestations:* confusion; impaired concentration and short-term memory; disorientation; difficulty with processing information, categorizing and word retrieval; perceptual and sensory disturbances, e.g. spatial instability and disorientation and inability to focus vision. Other manifestations are ataxia, muscle weakness and fasciculation, and overload phenomena, e.g. photophobia, hypersensitivity to noise, emotional overload.

■ *At least one symptom from two of the following three categories:*

1. *autonomic manifestations:* orthostatic hypotension and/or tachycardia; light-headedness; extreme pallor; nausea and irritable bowel syndrome; irritable bladder syndrome; palpitations; exertional dyspnoea;

2. *neuroendocrine manifestations:* loss of thermostatic stability; intolerance of extremes of heat and cold; loss or increase of appetite and/or weight; worsening of symptoms with stress;

3. *immune manifestations:* tender lymph nodes; recurrent sore throat; recurrent flu-like symptoms; general malaise; new sensitivities to food, medication and/or chemicals.

■ It should have been present for at least 6 months, usually has a discrete onset, and is not due to another active disease.

Almost always present

■ *Sleep dysfunction;* it may be unrefreshing with altered diurnal rhythm and be reduced or increased in amount.

■ Pain in joints or muscles or headaches.

Note: This summary omits some details of the definition for which it is necessary to consult the original article.

INTERVENTIONS FOR WHICH EVIDENCE OF BENEFIT IS POOR

- *Antidepressants.* Evidence that they improve fatigue is poor but they may improve depression if it is present (Reid, Chalder, Cleare, *et al.* 2000).
- *Steroids.* Trials of fludrocortisone and hydrocortisone have failed to show any lasting benefit. The temporary benefit from hydrocortisone 25 to 35 mg daily in one trial was only achieved at the cost of adrenal suppression (Reid, Chalder, Cleare, *et al.* 2000).
- *Dietary supplements.* One small RCT appears to show benefit from magnesium injections. Evidence on evening primrose oil is conflicting (Reid, Chalder, Cleare, *et al.* 2000).
- *Immunotherapy.* Studies of IgG given intravenously do not provide clear evidence of benefit nor does the one study of interferon (Reid, Chalder, Cleare, *et al.* 2000). Adverse effects were common.

Note: The results of trials are hard to relate to the spectrum of patient with the condition seen in primary care – they differed in selection of patients, in definitions of the syndrome, in the expertise of therapists and in how outcomes were measured.

PRACTICAL ISSUES

- **Employment.** Ask whether the patient's work is affected. Provide written support if a change to more flexible working, a different job, or sick leave is needed.

- **Practical aids.** Discuss whether aids, such as kitchen gadgets or a book rest or sunglasses, might help and refer to an occupational therapist if help is needed.
- **Immunizations.** There is a strong impression that immunizations can trigger a relapse. If an immunization is necessary, plan it for a time when the patient has time to recover, possibly over several weeks.
- **Driving.** Drivers whose fatigue could affect their ability to drive are obliged to notify the DVLA and their insurance company.
- **Referral.** Most patients can be diagnosed and managed in primary care with direct referral to physiotherapists, occupational therapists and social services. The paucity of specialists with expertise in CFS makes this inevitable. Referral may be necessary when there is doubt about the diagnosis, or when allied conditions, e.g. fibromyalgia or irritable bladder or bowel disease, warrant specialist assessment.

INFORMATION

A Life Worth Living: A Practical Guide to Living with Myalgic Encephalomyelitis (ME), by Dr Michael Midgley, Overton Studios Trust, 1995

Patients' organization

The ME Association, 7 Apollo Office Court, Radclive Road, Gawcott, Bucks MK18 4DF. Helpline: 0870 444 1836. www.meassociation.org.uk

References

Carruthers, B., Jain, A., De Meirleir, K., et al., 2003. Myalgic encephalomyelitis/chronic fatigue syndrome: clinical working case definition, diagnostic and treatment protocols. J. Chronic Fatigue Syndrome 11, 7–115.

Ebell, M., 2001. What is a reasonable initial approach to the patient with fatigue? J. Fam. Pract. 50, 16; discussion 16–17.

Koch, H., van Bokhoven, M., ter Riet, G., et al., 2009. Ordering blood tests for patients with unexplained fatigue in general practice: what does it yield? Br. J. Gen. Pract. 59, 243–249.

Lane, T.J., Matthews, D.A., Manu, P., 1990. The low yield of physical examinations and laboratory investigations of patients with chronic fatigue. Am. J. Med. Sci. 299 (5), 313–318.

Morriss, R., Sharpe, M., Sharpley, A., et al., 1993. Abnormalities of sleep in patients with chronic fatigue syndrome. BMJ 306, 1161–1164.

Price, J., Couper, J., 2004. Cognitive behaviour therapy for chronic fatigue syndrome in adults (Cochrane review). In: The Cochrane Library, Issue 1. Chichester, UK.

Reid, S., Chalder, T., Cleare, A., et al., 2000. Chronic fatigue syndrome. BMJ 320, 292–296.

Ridsdale, L., Evans, A., Jerrett, W., et al., 1993. Patients with fatigue in general practice: a prospective study. BMJ 307, 103–106.

Ridsdale, L., Godfrey, E., Chalder, T., et al., 2001. Chronic fatigue in general practice: is counselling as good as cognitive behaviour therapy? A UK randomised trial. Br. J. Gen. Pract. 51, 19–24.

Shepherd, C., 2001. Pacing and exercise in chronic fatigue syndrome. Physiotherapy 87, 395–396.

Sugarman, J.R., Berg, A.O., 1984. Evaluation of fatigue in a family practice. J. Fam. Pract. 19 (5), 643–647.

Whiting, P., Bagnall, A.M., Sowden, A., et al., 2001. Interventions for the treatment and management of chronic fatigue syndrome. JAMA 286, 1360–1368.

Chapter 20

Ear, nose and throat problems

CHAPTER CONTENTS

THE EAR

PAIN IN THE EAR

* Examine the external canal and drum. If these are normal then the pain is unlikely to be due to ear disease.
* *Consider:*
  (a) mumps;
  (b) cervical lymphadenopathy;
  (c) dental causes;
  (d) sinus pain;
  (e) temporomandibular (TM) joint pain;
  (f) cervical spine pain;
  (g) pharyngeal tumours.

ACUTE OTITIS MEDIA (AOM)

Scottish Intercollegiate Guidelines Network. 2003. *Diagnosis and Management of Childhood Otitis Media in Primary Care.* Available: www.sign.ac.uk

DOI: 10.1016/B978-0-7020-3053-6.00020-9

- Acute otitis media should be distinguished from myringitis and otitis media with effusion (OME).

Pink suffused drum (myringitis)

* Do not give antibiotics.
* Explain that it is part of a viral infection.

Red bulging drum

This is the only specific sign for AOM (Alberta Medical Association 2008).

* Control pain and fever with:
  (a) paracetamol; by suppository if the patient is vomiting; or
  (b) ibuprofen suspension in children over 1 year old.
* Do not give decongestants or antihistamines (Flynn, Griffin and Schultz 2004); steroid/antibiotic ear drops are similarly unhelpful.

Antibiotics in AOM

- 85% of children with acute otitis media (AOM) and otalgia are free of pain within 24 hours, without antibiotics (van Buchem, Dunk and Van't Hof 1981).
- Antibiotics reduce pain and fever at 3–7 days in infants and children under 2 years old and in those with bilateral AOM (Rovers, Glasziou, Appelman, et al. 2006). They reduce the risk of developing contralateral AOM, but have no effect on pain in the first 2 days, and no effect on the incidence of deafness at 1 month.
- Penicillin reduces the number of children with symptoms and signs of AOM at 1–2 weeks (NNT 7) with a small possibility of adverse reactions. There is no significant advantage from broad-spectrum antibiotics (Glasziou, Del Mar, Sanders, et al. 2003), although their use continues, hallowed by consensus although not by research evidence.
- Writing a prescription for antibiotics but suggesting to the parents that they only use it if the otitis media has not resolved in 3 days can reduce the number taking antibiotics to a quarter with only minor delay in the resolution of symptoms. Parents given a delayed prescription are less likely to believe that they

need to consult a doctor in future episodes (Little, Gould, Williamson, et al. 2001).

* *Infants and children under 2.* Consider prescribing antibiotics in this age group, especially those with high fever or vomiting. They are most likely to benefit (Little, Gould, Moore, et al. 2002; Kaleida, Casselbrant, Rockette, et al. 1991). The SIGN guideline recommends the use of amoxicillin or co-amoxiclav because of the likelihood of infection with Haemophilus or Moraxella, and recommends the use of a 5-day course because of the paucity of studies of shorter courses in this age group.
* In older children discuss with the parents the question of whether to prescribe an antibiotic. Explain that the evidence suggests that it is unlikely to be of benefit unless the AOM is bilateral or there is otorrhoea. Recommend 'watchful waiting' or prescribe phenoxymethylpenicillin, suggesting that they only use it if symptoms persist after 3 days.
* If symptoms persist in the presence of a red bulging drum despite phenoxymethylpenicillin, prescribe a second antibiotic (Bloomington 2001). Use amoxicillin, erythromycin or a cephalosporin.
* If a tympanostomy tube is in place, give antibiotics more readily. They can more than halve the duration of the illness (from 8 to 3 days) with an NNT of 3 for freedom from discharge at 1 week (Ruohola, Heikkinen, Meurman, et al. 2003).
* Review in 4–6 weeks for deafness and/or effusion. Half of all children will have an effusion at 1 month and 10% will have an effusion at 3 months. Persistent fluid is not an indication for further antibiotic treatment (van Buchem, Dunk and Van't Hof 1981).

Referral

Refer to ENT if:

(a) deafness or effusion (which may lead to hearing loss) is still present at 3 months;
(b) the patient has five or more attacks of AOM in one winter, or six or more in 1 year (DTB 1995a);
(c) the ear drum is retracted (DTB 1995a);
(d) a perforation is still present at 1 month.

Refer urgently if there is:

(a) a sudden severe hearing loss; or

(b) a sudden onset of dizziness with nystagmus.

AOM prevention

This remains largely unsubstantiated.

* Encourage breastfeeding.
* Feed upright where possible.
* Avoid cigarette smoke exposure (Strachan and Cook 1998).

AOM prophylaxis

There is some evidence to support antibiotic prophylaxis in children with recurrent otitis media (NNT of 9). The type, duration and criteria for antibiotic use are not clear (O'Neill 2001).

MASTOIDITIS

Admit any patient with:

(a) tenderness, redness or oedema over the mastoid; or

(b) vertigo, vomiting, increasing deafness and nystagmus; or

(c) acute otitis media with continuing fever despite antibiotics.

ACUTE FURUNCULOSIS OF THE EXTERNAL CANAL

* Refer if the tympanic membrane is obscured.
* Early cases respond to antibiotic/corticosteroid drops.
* Surrounding cellulitis needs oral antibiotics as well, e.g. flucloxacillin or erythromycin.
* Exclude diabetes.

BLOODY DISCHARGE (BULLOUS MYRINGITIS)

The patient usually suffers severe pain followed by bleeding. A number of serosanguinous bullae appear on the tympanic membrane or surrounding skin.

* Prescribe adequate analgesia and advise the patient to keep the canal dry.
* Reserve broad-spectrum antibiotics for patients with middle ear effusions (Marais and Dale 1997).
* Refer if the patient suffers persisting pain or hearing loss (Biedlingmaier 1994).

HERPES ZOSTER (RAMSAY HUNT SYNDROME)

As well as a vesicular eruption of the auricle or external auditory meatus, the patient may develop facial palsy or hearing loss and vertigo.

* Treat as for shingles anywhere, with oral aciclovir and adequate analgesia (see page 574).
* Arrange ENT assessment of VIIth and VIIIth nerve function.

DISCHARGE FROM THE EAR

OTITIS EXTERNA

* This may be due to bacterial, viral or fungal infection, and a predisposing factor is any scaling skin disorder (e.g. eczema, psoriasis).
  * Clean the canal with a Jobson Horne wool carrier, or by gently syringing and mopping with cotton wool.

Where there is profuse discharge:

* See daily to clean the canal; teach the patient to do it at home with cotton wool wound on to an orange stick. Commercial cotton buds are too thick and hard; or refer for microsuction.
* Prescribe ear drops containing antibacterial agents and steroid (van Balen, Smit, Zuithoff, et al. 2003). If treatment is still needed after 1 week, change to steroid drops alone.
* Consider, as an alternative, advising the patient to buy aluminium acetate drops. One RCT found them to be as effective as polymyxin-neomycin-hydrocortisone drops (Lambert 1981).
* Tell the patient that reinfection is likely if the ear canal is scratched, cotton buds are used or water is allowed to enter the canal. When contact with water is unavoidable, e.g. showering, the meatus should be plugged with cotton wool impregnated with petroleum jelly.
* Make sure that patients prone to recurrent attacks have ear drops at home to use at the onset of symptoms.

If the canal is severely swollen:

* Refer for the insertion of an antibiotic/ corticosteroid wick or insert half-inch ribbon gauze soaked in steroid cream. Change it daily.
* Give oral antibiotics if there is cellulitis of the surrounding tissues.

Refractory otitis externa

This is more likely if there is a history of eczema or seborrhoeic dermatitis. It is usually due to undiagnosed *Candida* or *Aspergillus* infection and may follow prolonged use of topical antibiotics. The canal is filled with blackish spots or brownish-cream deposits.

* Swab for bacteria and fungi.
* Mop or syringe out the debris gently and dry with cotton wool or a Jobson Horne wool carrier.
* Treat with clotrimazole solution 1% instilled t.d.s. and continued for 14 days after the disappearance of obvious infection.

CHRONIC SUPPURATIVE OTITIS MEDIA (CSOM)

* Refer all patients for initial assessment.
* Take an ear swab if antibiotic drops have been used recently. It may show resistant bacteria or fungi.

Central perforations – 'safe disease'

* Manage an acute exacerbation as in otitis externa, but with even more frequent mopping:
  1. mop the ear;
  2. administer antibiotic drops (Acuin, Smith and Mackenzie 2000);
  3. instruct the patient to pump the drops through the perforation by repeated pressure on the tragus.

Attic or marginal perforations – 'unsafe disease'

This carries the highest likelihood of ototoxicity on topical drug treatment:
  1. ensure that the patient is under ENT supervision;
  2. mop and instil drops as above;
  3. refer urgently if vertigo develops; there may be a fistula into a semicircular canal causing vestibulotoxicity.

Antibiotic ear drops and perforation

* There is agreement that antibiotic drops, except possibly those below, are indicated in the presence of middle ear infection and a perforation; yet many patients are still being denied adequate treatment. Only 34% of GPs would give topical antibiotics in the presence of a perforation, and only 14% in the presence of grommets (Bickerton, Roberts and Little 1988).
* There is less agreement about the use of aminoglycosides and polymyxins in the presence of a perforation. Although used by specialists, the CSM warns doctors against prescribing topical aminoglycosides in the presence of a perforation (Committee for Safety of Medicines 1997). It seems wise, therefore, not to do so in primary care.

DEAFNESS

For details of the diagnosis of deafness see *Evidence-based Diagnosis in Primary Care* by A. F. Polmear (editor), published by Butterworth-Heinemann, 2008.

* At least one third of patients over 70 and half of patients over 80 have deafness severe enough to be helped by a hearing aid (i.e. roughly a 35 dB hearing loss at speech frequencies).
* All deaf people, particularly the elderly, may become isolated, depressed and difficult to live with. When complicated by tinnitus, speech discrimination may deteriorate and auditory hallucinations can occur (Hickish 1989).

Assess whether the hearing loss is:

(a) perceptive (lesion of the inner ear or of the eighth cranial nerve); or

(b) conductive (middle or outer ear).

See page 429 for a description of the tests.

PERCEPTIVE DEAFNESS

* Examine the drum and remove any wax which may be contributing.
* Refer patients with:
  (a) *Unilateral deafness of acute onset*. If the patient is seen within 3 weeks of onset, arrange for outpatient assessment within 24 hours. This is most important in patients with barotrauma, especially if they also experienced vertigo. The round window membrane may have ruptured. Even if the cause is thought to be viral, oral steroids can double the recovery (61% achieving at least partial recovery versus 32% with placebo) (Yueh, Shapiro, MacLean, *et al.* 2003).

(b) *Unilateral deafness with a longer history.*
    Referral is less urgent, but the patient may
    have a treatable cause (e.g. acoustic neuroma).

* Be active in detecting deafness and encouraging
  patients to consider a hearing aid.

* Refer patients for a hearing aid early rather than
  late, and encourage them to persevere with it
  once supplied. Deaf patients lose the ability to
  discriminate between sounds, and have to
  relearn this skill. They may take up to 1 year to
  get the full benefit from an aid. One follow-up in
  the UK at between 8 and 16 years found that
  fewer than half were still using an aid
  (Gianopoulos, Stephens and Davis 2002).

* Ask about the effects of any hearing loss. It is
  more reliable than a hearing test in the surgery.

USEFUL QUESTIONS TO SCREEN FOR HEARING LOSS

Do other people mumble a lot?
Do you find yourself frequently saying 'pardon'?
Does the family say the TV is too loud?
Do you miss hearing the doorbell or phone?
Do you occasionally get the wrong end of the stick
in conversation?

* Refer direct to the audiology department for
  a hearing aid if:
  (a) the deafness is chronic, perceptive and
      bilateral; and
  (b) there is no other ear pathology which needs
      ENT assessment first.

* *Lip reading* will help many patients. If not
  available through the local ENT department,
  contact the Association of Teachers of Lip
  Reading to Adults (ATLA), Westwood Park,
  London Road, Little Horkesley, Colchester, CO6
  4BS. Email: ATLA@lipreading.org.uk; website:
  www.lipreading.org.uk.

* *Cochlear implant devices* are most suitable for
  children over 2 and adults with profound or
  severe deafness. Most benefit is seen in those
  people for whom deafness occurrs after
  language and speech is acquired (NICE 2009).
  Refer to a local ENT specialist for onward
  referral (Douek 1990).

* *Aids:* a number of aids are available for deaf
  people, e.g. special telephones, flashing-light
  alarm clocks, loop amplifiers for radio and TV

sets which allow the patient to hear the sound
through their hearing aid, and *typetalk* – a
system by which deaf people can communicate
via textphones and others can communicate
with them.

* *Communication:* explain to the family how to
  communicate with a deaf person:
  (a) face the person when speaking;
  (b) speak clearly without shouting. Shouting may
      distort the sound and make it harder to hear.

Hearing difficulty with normal auditory testing (King-
Kopetzky syndrome or obscure auditory dysfunction) accounts for up to 20% of referrals to audiology departments. Although there is evidence that
there may be many factors involved, the basic
problem is thought to be in 'central processing'
(see web link below). Refer to the ENT department
for assessment and consideration of listening
devices. The following alterations may help:

(a) less noisy listening conditions (e.g. a carpet in
    a classroom),
(b) facing the speaker,
(c) ensuring that the speaker has the listener's
    attention.

PATIENT ADVICE

For access to a range of information on aids, rights and
other help, contact:
    The Royal National Institute for Deaf People (RNID),
19-23 Featherstone Street, London ECIY 8SL; or Floor 3
Crowngate Business Centre, Brook Street, Glasgow
G40 3AP, tel. 0808 808 0123, www.rnid.org.uk
    SIGN Community (British Deaf Association), 1-3
Worship Street, London EC2A 2AB, Tel. (voice) 0207
588 3520. www.bda.org.uk
    Hearing Concern Link (previously British Association
of the Hard of Hearing), Resource Centre, 356
Holloway Road, London N7 6PA. Tel: 020 7700 8177.
www.hearingconcernlink.org.uk
    Obscure auditory dysfunction, www.nidcd.nih.gov/
health/voice/auditory.asp

CONDUCTIVE DEAFNESS

● Assume that all conductive deafness is treatable.
  This is true whether the drum looks normal, as
  in otosclerosis, or abnormal, as in middle ear
  effusion or CSOM.

﹡ Examine the canal and drum.

If wax is present it may be contributing to the deafness, although removal of wax only raises the hearing threshold by at least 10 dB in one third (Memel, Langley, Watkins, *et al.* 2002):

(a) syringe if the wax is soft; or

(b) disimpact hard wax with a wax hook, then syringe the rest if necessary; or

(c) instil drops (tap water is as effective as anything) and syringe after waiting for at least 15 minutes (Hand and Harvey 2004; Browning 2005); or

(d) suggest that the patient instils ear drops (either a proprietary wax softener or water) into the canal for 2–7 nights and then reattends for syringing. Instillation of either an oil-based or a water-based solvent for 1 week will clear wax in 20% of patients (Keane, Wilson, McGrane, *et al.* 1995) and facilitate syringing in the others.

﹡ Refer all patients with conductive deafness not due to wax, with the exception of a recent perforation not due to CSOM. Even then, refer if the perforation has not healed in 6 weeks.

OTITIS MEDIA WITH EFFUSION (OME)

Fluid in the middle ear without signs or symptoms of inflammation can result in hearing loss but a causal link has not been established between glue ear and significant disability (Bandolier 1994).

Children

- This is also known as secretory otitis media, or glue ear.
- Half of affected children resolve spontaneously within 3 months (American Academy of Pediatrics 1997). However, 2–3% of children under 7 have a more prolonged hearing loss due to OME and need specialist assessment.
- Even those having specialist assessment are unlikely to be helped by surgery, the benefits of which are only temporary. Watchful waiting and immediate presurgery testing may reduce inappropriate surgery (NHS Centre for Reviews and Dissemination 1994). For instance, grommets improve hearing 6 months after insertion but very little after 12 months.

Adenoidectomy improves hearing, but for only up to 2 years. Tonsillectomy and/or myringotomy do not help hearing (Agency for Health Care Policy and Research 1994).

- *Antibiotics.* There may be some benefit from antibiotics in the short term but the effect is small, not maintained and outweighed by side-effects (SIGN 2003).
- *Steroids.* There is evidence that oral or topical intranasal steroids lead to quicker resolution of OME in the short term (Butler and van der Voort 2002). Meta-analysis has not confirmed their long term benefit (Agency for Health Care Policy and Research 1994; Butler and van der Voort 2002).
- OME is more common in children whose parents smoke in the same room.
- Antihistamines and decongestants, orally or topically, are of no value (SIGN 2003).

﹡ **Refer** to the community audiology service, once deafness due to OME is discovered, or even merely suspected by the parents, to determine:

(a) severity;

(b) that the deafness is conductive;

(c) the overall disability.

﹡ **Refer** direct to ENT outpatients if:

(a) deafness is persistent, i.e. more than 3 months; or

(b) deafness is severe (i.e. a hearing loss of more than 25 dB or the child is having difficulties with hearing, speech, learning or social functioning because of it); and

(c) medical treatment has failed (e.g. a 4-week trial of antibiotics, with or without oral steroids); or

(d) deafness is associated with persistent pain.

- If a child has other disabilities, refer if there is any degree of deafness because normal hearing is crucial.

Adults

OME may follow a URTI or barotrauma.

﹡ Advise regular autoinflation with a Valsalva manoeuvre.

﹡ Prescribe ephedrine nose drops or a steroid nasal spray if there is generalized rhinitis.

﹡ Refer if the effusion persists for over 6 weeks. A nasopharyngeal tumour must be excluded, especially in Chinese patients.

Grommets

- The majority of grommets are extruded within 9 months, and only need to be reinserted if deafness recurs.
- Discharge should be treated by aural toilet and antibiotic/corticosteroid drops (see page 525).
- Swimming and bathing pose no danger, but diving should be banned.

HEARING TESTS

Rinne's test

A 512 cps tuning fork is struck and held close to the meatus until the patient signals that it can no longer be heard. The base is then applied to the mastoid process.

If the patient cannot hear it, this is a normal or *positive* Rinne's test, i.e. if deafness is present, it is *perceptive*.

If the patient hears the fork applied to the mastoid process, this is a *negative* Rinne's test, i.e. if deafness is present, it is *conductive*.

False negatives can occur in severe unilateral perceptive deafness. Bone conduction appears better than air conduction, but the sound is in fact being heard by the good ear.

Weber's test

Once the side of the deafness has been discovered, apply the tuning fork to the top of the head.

(a) If the sound is heard on the *deaf side*, then the deafness is *conductive*.

(b) If the sound is heard on the *good side*, the deafness is *perceptive*.

Whereas Rinne's test can only detect a hearing loss of 30 dB, Weber's can detect a 5 dB loss.

The 'whisper test'

This is a good screening test and is easily performed (Eekhof, de Bock, de Laat, *et al.* 1996) with 90–100% sensitivity and 70–87% specificity in adults. In children the sensitivity is slightly less but the specificity is higher (Pirozzo, Papinczak and Glasziou 2003).

1. Cover one of the patient's ears with a finger in the meatus. Move it gently to and fro to mask the whisper in that ear.

2. Stand at arms' length with your head behind the patient's other ear.

3. Whisper, and ask the patient to repeat what he or she has heard: for children under 6 years old e.g. 'bread and butter' or 'Father Christmas'; for children over 6 years old multisyllabic numbers, e.g. '362436'. Correctly hearing three out of six numbers is a 'pass'.

GIDDINESS

For details of the diagnosis of dizziness see *Evidence-based Diagnosis in Primary Care* by A. F. Polmear (editor), published by Butterworth-Heinemann, 2008.

The duration and type of symptom will often indicate the cause. It is important to distinguish between vertigo, unsteadiness and the sensation of light-headedness.

UNSTEADINESS

Episodic

(a) Unsteadiness lasting a few seconds indicates a physiological overload of the vestibular or central systems. It occurs most frequently on rapid movement, associated with a minor inadequacy of the proprioceptive or labyrinthine systems. In young people it occurs in the later stages of recovery after head injury, and in the elderly after standing or turning rapidly.

(b) Unsteadiness lasting hours or days is due to temporary impairment of the central connections or decompensation of the vestibular system. It commonly occurs with alcohol or drug overdose, normal doses of tranquillizers or sedatives, and hyperventilation.

Prolonged

Unsteadiness lasting weeks or months is usually due to central or vestibular inadequacy, and is common in the elderly.

VERTIGO

Episodic

(a) *Vertigo lasting only a few seconds or minutes* indicates a short-lived depression or stimulation of the labyrinth or central connections. It is present on sudden changes in posture, and is commonly due to benign positional vertigo (see below).

(b) *Vertigo lasting a few minutes to a few hours* indicates a physiological or metabolic disturbance of the labyrinth. It occurs in Ménière's disease.

Prolonged

Vertigo lasting more than 24 hours. The clinical picture is of severe incapacitating vertigo associated with nausea and vomiting, and is due to:

(a) a peripheral lesion, usually vestibular neuronitis, in which there is no hearing loss (Cooper 1993). Less common causes are an extension of acute or chronic suppurative otitis media, trauma or, in the elderly, vascular lesions of the inner ear; or

(b) a central lesion which is usually associated with other signs, as in multiple sclerosis, stroke, a posterior fossa tumour or secondary deposits in the brain stem.

EXAMINATION

This should include:

(a) taking the patient's temperature and testing for neck stiffness in the acute attack;

(b) inspection of the ear drums for acute or chronic otitis media;

(c) testing the hearing for the deafness of Ménière's disease or acoustic neuroma;

(d) looking for nystagmus. In peripheral lesions the nystagmus will be horizontal with the fast phase towards the healthy side. Looking towards that side will increase the amplitude of the nystagmus. In central lesions the nystagmus may be horizontal, vertical or rotatory;

(e) looking for other neurological signs, especially cerebellar and cranial nerve signs and papilloedema, as in acoustic neuroma or central lesions.

TREATMENT

Acute vertigo

* Give prochlorperazine 12.5 mg i.m. followed by 25 mg suppositories 8-hourly until the vomiting stops. Continue with prochlorperazine 5–10 mg t.d.s orally until the vertigo ceases.

Recurrent vertigo

Treatment should be directed at encouraging central compensation. Labyrinthine sedatives should be tailed off as soon as possible because they may delay this process.

* *Labyrinthine sedatives.* Give labyrinthine sedatives only if the vertigo is due to labyrinthine dysfunction, e.g. cinnarizine 15–30 mg t.d.s., prochlorperazine 5–10 mg t.d.s., or cyclizine 50 mg t.d.s. Diazepam has potent labyrinthine sedative effects but leads to increased unsteadiness if the dizziness is due to vestibular inadequacy.

* Compensation may occur naturally, especially in young people, but can be accelerated by vestibular rehabilitation exercises. One study in primary care found that two 30-minute sessions tripled the number of patients who improved (Yardley, Beech, Zander, *et al.* 1998).

VESTIBULAR REHABILITATION EXERCISES

(a) *In bed*, performed slowly initially then more rapidly:
  - *eye movements* – up and down, side to side, focusing on a finger as it moves from 1 m away to 30 cm away;
  - *head movements* – moving head forwards then backwards and turning from side to side.

(b) *Sitting:* rotating the head; bending down and standing up with eyes open and closed.

(c) *Standing:* throwing a small ball from hand to hand, turning through 360°.

(d) *Moving about:* walking across the room, up and down a slope, up and down stairs with eyes open and then closed.

PATIENT INFORMATION

Dizziness and Balance Problems available from British Brain & Spine Foundation, 7 Winchester House, Cranmer Road, Kennington Park, London SW9 6EJ, Helpline: 0808 808 1000, www.brainandspine.org.uk
  Keeping Our Balance. Available: http://www.tinnitus.org.uk (choose 'Information for everyone')

MÉNIÈRE'S DISEASE

- This is characterized by vertigo associated with at least one of either hearing loss, tinnitus or a feeling of aural fullness. Symptoms may be unilateral. They vary in severity. In the long term, deafness may remain but the vertigo and tinnitus to a lesser degree. Some people develop a severe bilateral disorder and may need surgery.
- The incidence is variably reported but a practice of 6000 patients may see one new case a year (Bandolier 1995).
- A patient with the condition who drives must inform the DVLA. Driving will be permitted once symptoms are controlled.

REFER TO AN ENT CONSULTANT

(a) To confirm diagnosis before starting treatment.

(b) To exclude an acoustic neuroma in patients with persistent unilateral symptoms.

The diagnosis may be made by electrocochleography in an ENT department.

MEDICAL TREATMENT: ACUTE

No RCTs exist for acute management with betahistine, benzodiazepines or anticholinergics. The most recent analysis of betahistine trial data concludes that there is no evidence that it is effective or ineffective in patients with Ménière's disease or syndrome (James and Burton 2001). Earlier work favoured the use of betahistine in doses of 8–16 mg t.d.s., stating that it may decrease the number and duration of attacks of vertigo as well as reduce tinnitus and the feeling of fullness in the ear (Bandolier 1995). Any benefit may take several months to develop.

* *Acute attacks:* give a labyrinthine sedative, e.g. prochlorperazine 5 mg t.d.s. or cinnarizine 30 mg t.d.s.
* *Recurrent attacks:* give betahistine 16 mg t.d.s.
* *Poor response:* consider referral to ENT. Surgical options are:

   (a) sac decompression; or

   (b) selective division of the 8th nerve; or

   (c) labyrinthectomy.

PROPHYLACTIC

- There is no evidence for prophylactic management of Ménière's disease or syndrome (James and Thorp 2001). One trial shows some control of vertigo with diuretics (Bandolier 2000).

PATIENTS' ORGANIZATION

The Ménière's Society, The Rookery, Surrey Hills Business Park, Wotton, Dorking, Surrey, RH5 6QT, UK. Helpline: 0845 120 2975; www.menieres.org.uk

BENIGN POSITIONAL VERTIGO

GUIDELINE

Strickland C, Russell R. 2003. What is the best way to manage benign paroxysmal positional vertigo? J Fam Pract 52, 971–973

- It is usually possible to diagnose this condition from the history and by performing the Hallpike test. Neurological referral is not necessary.

THE HALLPIKE TEST

- Hold the patient's head in both hands and turn it 45° towards the test ear. Support the neck and, maintaining torsion along with fixed gaze, move head rapidly backwards to a head hanging position, 30–45° (optimally) below the horizontal as rapidly as possible.
- Maintain the head hanging position for 30–60 seconds and observe the patient's eyes. If nystagmus is present note the latent period, magnitude and direction of rotation of the fast phase. Maintain that position for about 1 minute after onset to determine if nystagmus adapts, changes direction or alters.
- Return the patient to the upright position while maintaining 45° neck rotation and observe for reversal of the nystagmus.
- Wait till the patient is settled and then repeat on the same side to assess fatigability. Proceed to the opposite side if no nystagmus is seen on the first side or when the patient has settled from the first test.

Note that the nystagmus may only last a few seconds and will not occur at all in some patients, in whom the diagnosis must be made on the history alone. Note also that the patient will experience vertigo at the same time as the nystagmus.

* Explain that the vertigo may last for a few weeks only or may continue with remissions and relapses for many years.
* Do not give labyrinthine sedatives.
* Teach the patient to minimize the vertigo by sitting up or lying down in stages.
* Discuss with the ENT department whether they offer adaptive physiotherapy or Epley's manoeuvre (Hilton and Pinder 2004). The latter involves repeated rapid positioning of the head, the theory being that this moves otoliths out of the labyrinth. It is a safe and effective treatment for BPPV but does not guarantee long-term resolution of symptoms (Lempert, Gresty and Bronstein 1995).

INSTRUCTIONS FOR PERFORMANCE OF THE MODIFIED EPLEY MANOEUVRE

These instructions are for a patient whose left ear is affected. If it is the right ear that is affected, for left read right and for right read left.

1. Sit up on the bed with your head turned 45° to the left, having placed a pillow on the bed so that it will be under your shoulders, not your head, when you lie down.
2. Lie back quickly, keeping your head turned as before. Wait 30 seconds.
3. Turn your head to the other side. Wait 30 seconds.
4. Roll on to your right side. Wait 30 seconds.
5. Sit up without rolling over on to your back, i.e. still facing right.
6. Repeat this three times a day until the symptoms have ceased.

TINNITUS

For details of the diagnosis of tinnitus see *Evidence-based Diagnosis in Primary Care* by A. F. Polmear (editor), published by Butterworth-Heinemann, 2008.

GUIDELINES

Department of Health, 2009. Provision of Services for Adults with Tinnitus: a Good Practice Guide. Available online: www.dh.gov.uk

1–2% of the population has tinnitus that severely affects the quality of life.

* Reassure the patient that 15% of people experience tinnitus. For most, it improves with time. Worry about it can lead to a vicious circle of increasing distress and more intrusive tinnitus.
* Exclude a drug cause, e.g. aspirin, NSAIDs, quinine, loop diuretics, tricyclics and aminoglycosides.

Refer patients with:

(a) sudden onset;
(b) associated vertigo and hearing loss. They may have Ménière's disease or middle ear disease;
(c) unilateral tinnitus, for exclusion of cerebellopontine angle tumours, especially if there is perceptive deafness on the same side (Luxon 1993);
(d) tinnitus due to occupational disease. If confirmed, patients may be entitled to financial benefits.
(e) neck and skull bruits (carotid artery stenosis or AV fistula).
(f) tinnitus severe enough to need specialist devices, e.g. masking.
(g) tinnitus associated with systemic or neurological disease.

TREATMENT

The Centre for Reviews and Dissemination (Dobie 1999) and Bandolier (Bandolier 2000) record their difficulty in drawing conclusions from available studies. However, some patients may benefit from:

(a) tricyclic antidepressants (nortriptyline (Waddell 2004) and amitriptyline);
(b) alprazolam, although some benzodiazepines make symptoms worse;
(c) electrical stimulation over the mastoid.

* Non-specific support and counselling are probably helpful.
* Consider sedation for those unable to sleep.

* Look for depression associated with tinnitus and treat it in its own right. Suicide is known as a consequence of tinnitus. There is no evidence that psychological treatments help tinnitus in the absence of depression.
* *Masking:* there is no research evidence of a significant effect but considerable clinical experience of benefit. Encourage the patient to mask the noise with:
  (a) background radio static on an empty FM frequency;
  (b) background noise from a fan, or recorded sounds from nature;
  (c) a masking device available through ENT departments.
* *Amplification:* a hearing aid may be used to amplify ordinary background noise.
* *Tinnitus retraining therapy* (TRT): this combines a low level noise generator with psychological retraining to reduce the attention that the patient pays to the tinnitus. There is insufficient evidence to suggest benefit.
* *Cognitive behavioural therapy* (CBT) has a positive effect on the way people cope with tinnitus (Martinez Devesa, Waddell, Perera, and Theodoulou 2007). Refer if this is available locally, with a careful explanation that this does not mean you think the tinnitus is imaginary.

PATIENT ORGANIZATIONS

British Tinnitus Association, Ground Floor, Unit 5, Acorn Business Park, Woodseats Close, Sheffield S8 0TB, tel. 0114 279 6600; Helpline 0800 018 0527; www.tinnitus.org.uk
    The Royal National Institute for Deaf People. www.rnid.org.uk (choose 'Information and resources' then 'Tinnitus')

FACIAL PALSY (LOWER MOTOR NEURONE)

Refer urgently if there is evidence of:
(a) middle ear infection or cholesteatoma;
(b) parotid tumour;
(c) cerebellopontine angle tumour, i.e. deafness, loss of facial sensation, diplopia and cerebellar signs;
(d) trauma; or
(e) Ramsay Hunt syndrome (look for herpetic vesicles on the pinna or in the external auditory canal).

BELL'S PALSY

OVERVIEW

Davenport RJ, McKinstry B, Morrison JM, *et al.* 2009. Bell's palsy: new evidence provides a definitive drug therapy strategy. Brit J Gen Pract 59, 569–570

● Characterized by a unilateral facial weakness with the inability to close the affected eye properly. The weakness may be associated with mild pain behind the ear and some hearing loss. The onset is typically hours or days. It is more common in pregnant women, in those with diabetes, and following a recent upper respiratory infection.
● About half recover in 3 months without treatment (Bandolier accessed January 2010).

PATIENT ORGANIZATION

Bell's Palsy Association: www.bellspalsy.org.uk

REFERRAL

(a) If loss of power is complete – refer to an ophthalmic surgeon be seen that day. Tarsorraphy is likely to be needed.
(b) If the eyelid, when closed, does not cover the cornea. Refer to an ophthalmic surgeon.
(c) If recovery has not started at 6 weeks. Refer to an ENT surgeon to look for an underlying cause.
(d) If recovery at 9 months is incomplete. The patient may benefit from cosmetic surgery.

MANAGEMENT IN PRIMARY CARE

* *Protect the eye* with a patch and/or artificial tears. Warn the patient that the eye is not protected by reflex blinking and must be

safeguarded. This is especially true in windy conditions and during sleep.

* *Give oral prednisolone.* Early treatment with prednisolone significantly improves the chance of complete recovery at 3 and 9 months (Sullivan, Swan, Donnan *et al.* 2007). Give 50 mg/day for 10 days provided it can be started within 72 hours of the onset of the palsy.

● *Antiviral treatment.* Giving antiviral medication such as aciclovir, either alone or with prednisolone, is of no benefit (Salinas 2005).

● *Physiotherapy* has no benefit (Teixeira, Soares, Vieira, *et al.* 2008).

● *Surgical decompression* of the nerve is not indicated. There is insufficient evidence that it is beneficial (Salinas 2005).

THE NOSE

SINUSITIS

GUIDELINES AND REVIEWS

American Academy of Pediatrics. 2001. *Clinical Practice Guideline: Management of Sinusitis.* Online. Available: www.guideline.gov

Ahovuo-Saloranta A, Borisenko Ov, Kovanen N, *et al.* 2008. Antibiotics for acute maxillary sinusitis. Cochrane Database of Systematic Reviews, issue 2. Art No.:CD000243. DOI:10.1002/14651858. CD000243. pub2

Young J, de Sutter A, Merenstein D, *et al.* 2008. Antibiotics for adults with clinically diagnosed acute rhinosinusitis: a meta-analysis of individual patient data. Lancet 371, 908–914

● Diagnosis is usually clinical.

For details of the diagnosis of rhinorrhoea see *Evidence-based Diagnosis in Primary Care* by A. F. Polmear (editor), published by Butterworth-Heinemann, 2008.

● X-rays are unlikely to affect management in general practice because of the poor correlation between clinical symptoms and radiological findings (Evans 1994).

MANAGEMENT OF ACUTE SINUSITIS

● *Decongestants* (topical or oral) are used widely but there are no studies which support their use.

● *Antibiotics.* The Cochrane review above found a slight statistical difference in favour of antibiotics. The clinical significance is equivocal with improvement rates of 80% at 2 weeks in patients treated symptomatically (against 90% for patients treated with antibiotics). The *Drug and Therapeutics Bulletin* recommends a policy of no routine antibiotics or of delayed prescribing (DTB 2009). Immediate antibiotics should be reserved for those who are systemically very unwell or are at risk of complications.

● *Intranasal steroids.* A few studies suggest that intranasal steroids may have some benefit as an adjunct to antibiotics in treatment of acute sinusitis and also as treatment for the underlying rhinitis (Kim 2005).

* Advise the patient to:

(a) take simple analgesics;

(b) use steam inhalations.

* Decide whether to give an antibiotic, e.g. phenoxymethylpenicillin or amoxicillin or a cephalosporin for 10 days. A macrolide can be used in patients who are penicillin sensitive. If not responding after 10 days change to a different antibiotic and add metronidazole 400 mg t.d.s. (Kim 2005). Candidates for an antibiotic are those with:

(a) high fever with prior history suggestive of sinusitis; or

(b) tooth pain; or

(c) severe symptoms; or

(d) a known anatomical blockage.

MANAGEMENT OF CHRONIC SINUSITIS (AH–SEE AND EVANS 2007)

* Start treatment with intranasal steroids. Treat any underlying cause or allergy. For greatest effect, the patient should adopt the following position to insert nose drops: kneel with the top of the head on the floor, drip the drops into the nostril and maintain the position for 2 minutes. Insert 2 drops two to three times a day. Maintain treatment for 1–3 months; more prolonged use can lead to systemic side-effects.

Do not give for more than half the year (Lund 1990).

* Give a 10-day course of a beta-lactamase-resistant antibiotic if symptoms do not resolve with topical steroids. In children with proven sinusitis the benefit is modest (NNT = 8) (Morris and Leach 2002). If the response is partial, antibiotics may need to be continued for up to 6 weeks.
* Use a decongestant spray, e.g. xylometazoline, in patients with severe obstruction, for a maximum of 5 days, as an adjunct to the above. Ephedrine nasal drops are less prone to rebound congestion than xylometazoline but less convenient.
* Where there is no evidence of preceding upper respiratory tract infection, consider an upper molar tooth abscess or possible malignancy.

Refer urgently:

(a) for surgical drainage if there is no response to the above regimen;
(b) patients with orbital or facial cellulitis or who are severely ill. They need admission.

THE COMMON COLD

GUIDANCE

Mossad SB. 1998. Treatment of the common cold. BMJ 317, 33–36
   Simasek M, Blandino DA. 2007. Treatment of the common cold. American Family Physician 75(4), 515–520

A consultation about the common cold is an opportunity for the education of the patient in self-treatment as well as discussion of any underlying issues. Evidence does not support the many OTC remedies available, except paracetamol for those with fever or discomfort. However, in the occasional patient where treatment is needed (singers, examinees) the options are as follows:

- Oral first-generation antihistamines will slightly reduce rhinorrhoea and sneezing but with anticholinergic adverse effects, especially sedation.
- Ipratropium bromide nasal spray will reduce rhinorrhoea with a 26% reduction in symptoms at day 4 (NNT 6) but with a risk of nasal dryness

and headache (Hayden, Diamond, Wood, *et al.* 1996).

- There is limited evidence that a single dose of oral decongestant reduces symptoms (Kollar, Schneider, Waksman and Krusinska 2007). Courses longer than 5 days carry the risk of rebound congestion.
- Steam inhalations give subjective benefit but evidence of objective benefit is conflicting (Singh 2006).
- Oral vitamin C has not been shown to have an effect in reducing the duration or severity of symptoms (Hemilä, Chalker, Treacy, *et al.* 2007).
- Oral zinc has shown benefit in some studies and not in others. If it does work, the dose required is above that found in most vitamin preparations.
- *Echinacea*. There is limited evidence that echinacea may improve symptoms (Linde, Barrett, Bauer, *et al.* 2006).
- There is limited evidence that antibiotics are of benefit for purulent nasal discharge but not enough evidence for their routine use (Arroll and Kenealy 2005).

RHINITIS

GUIDANCE

GPIAG opinion sheet no. 6. Available: www.gpiag-asthma.org
   Scadding GK, Durham SR, Mirakian R, *et al.* 2008. British Society for Allergy and Clinical Immunology guidelines for the management of allergic and non-allergic rhinitis. Clinical and Experimental Allergy 38, 19–42

SEASONAL AND PERENNIAL RHINITIS

- Affects 15–20% of the population; 3% of GP consultations are for allergic rhinitis.
- Treatment is best tailored to the individual's symptoms; where possible identify the underlying cause.
- Allergens should be avoided where possible, e.g. by reducing the dust in the house or driving with windows and air vents closed. However, measures to reduce exposure to the house dust mite have been disappointing (Terreehorst, Hak, Oosting, *et al.* 2003).

INTERMITTENT MILD SYMPTOMS OR ACUTE RESPONSE TO ALLERGEN

- Antihistamines reduce the nasal itching, watery hypersecretion and sneezing, but do little for nasal blockage (Pearlman, Lumry, Winder, *et al.* 1995). Intermittent use may be enough.
- * Use an antihistamine nasal spray for rapid relief (Ratner, van Bavel, Martin, *et al.* 1998).
- * Use an oral, minimally sedating H_1-selective antihistamine with a rapid onset, e.g. loratadine, for nasal and non-nasal symptoms.

REGULAR SYMPTOMS

- Antihistamines may be taken regularly, and for some people are all that is necessary.
- Intranasal steroid sprays are the most effective prophylactic treatment. There is often a delayed onset of action possibly up to a week. Combining them with an antihistamine adds no further benefit (Weiner, Abramson and Puy 1998).
- * Instruct the patient on their proper use:
  - (a) use once or twice a day. The patient should point the spray upwards for one puff and backwards for the other, occluding the other nostril;
  - (b) in seasonal rhinitis, start 2 weeks before the beginning of the season;
  - (c) they should be continued until the rhinitis is likely to have subsided.
- * Consider an ipratropium nasal spray, in addition to steroids, where rhinorrhoea is dominant (Sheikh, Panesar and Dhami 2005).
- * *Use sodium cromoglicate eye drops* regularly in patients with allergic conjunctivitis.
- * Consider referral to an allergy specialist (see page 593).

NASAL BLOCKAGE

- * Use a topical decongestant, e.g. ephedrine nasal drops or xylometazoline spray for 5 days, to open the airway enough for the steroid spray to penetrate. Longer use is likely to lead to rebound congestion on stopping.
- * Use betamethasone nasal drops 0.1%. For greatest effect the patient should use these in the 'head down' position (for more information see leaflet on nasal polyps below). Insert 2 drops

two to three times a day for no more than 1 month. More prolonged use can lead to systemic side-effects. Do not give more than six courses a year. Try to maintain improvement after each course with a steroid spray.

SEVERE SYMPTOMS

- * Oral steroids can be given if symptoms warrant them, e.g. at the time of an examination, but courses should not be repeated frequently. Give oral prednisolone 5–10 mg daily, or 30–40 mg daily for 1 week in dire situations. Intramuscular depot injections of steroids (e.g. Kenalog) last for 3 months, with the inevitable pituitary adrenal suppression, and are not recommended for use in rhinitis.
- * Referral is needed for continuing severe symptoms. Nasal endoscopy may reveal pathology, e.g. a polyp, which was not otherwise visible. In addition, patients with nasal deformity may benefit from surgery.

NASAL POLYPS

GUIDELINE

Scadding GK, Durham SR, Mirakian R *et al.* 2008. British Society for Allergy and Clinical Immunology guidelines for the management of rhinosinusitis and nasal polyposis. Clin Exp Allergy 38, 260–275
- Nasal polyps may be associated with asthma and aspirin sensitivity, but if they occur in the presence of rhinitis it is probably coincidental. Cystic fibrosis should be considered in any child under 16 with nasal polyps.
- The initial treatment should be medical.

- * Stop aspirin and consider stopping other NSAIDs; there is some cross-reaction.
- * Give antibiotics if nasal discharge is purulent. Thick, green–brown secretions may indicate fungal infection. This is more likely to be detected on microscopy than by culture.
- * *Steroids.* Give betamethasone drops 0.1%, 2 drops per nostril t.d.s. using the 'head upside down' position (see patient leaflet), alone or with oral prednisolone (0.5 mg/kg for 5–10 days). Significant improvement may occur within 48

hours. Some patients need indefinite prophylaxis with intranasal mometasone or fluticasone, which have lower bioavailability than betamethasone drops. The evidence for oral steroids comes from a single small trial of poor quality (Patiar and Reece 2009).

* The BSACI guidelines (above) recommend that all new presentations be referred to ENT.

Malignancy

A polyp that does not have the typical smooth, pale or slightly reddened appearance may be malignant, especially if unilateral. Refer urgently.

SNORING AND OBSTRUCTIVE SLEEP APNOEA (OSA)

GUIDELINES

Millman RP. 1999. Do you ever take a sleep history? Ann Intern Med 131, 535–536
   Scottish Intercollegiate Guidelines Network. 2003. *Management of Obstructive Sleep Apnoea/Hypopnoea Syndrome in Adults.* SIGN Guideline 73. Available on www.sign.ac.uk
   NICE. 2008. *Continuous Positive Airway Pressure for the Treatment of Obstructive Sleep Apnoea/Hypopnoea Syndrome.* March. www.nice.org.uk

- 25% of middle-aged men are snorers and 10% of middle-aged women. 4% of middle-aged men and 2% of middle-aged women suffer from OSA, with at least five episodes of apnoea/hypopnoea an hour at night plus daytime sleepiness (Young, Palta, Dempsey, *et al.* 1993). For details of the diagnosis of obstructive sleep apnoea see *Evidence-based Diagnosis in Primary Care* by A. F. Polmear (editor), published by Butterworth-Heinemann, 2008.
- Men under 65 who admit to both snoring and daytime sleepiness are twice as likely to die as men with just one of these symptoms and men

without either symptom. The excess deaths are mainly due to cardiovascular disease (Lindberg, Janson, Svardsudd, *et al.* 1998).

- Those with moderate to severe OSAHS or with mild OSAHS and daytime sleepiness are likely to be offered continuous positive airways pressure (CPAP) as therapy of first choice.

Table 20.1 Symptoms and signs in OSA

SYMPTOMS	SIGNS
Loud snoring	Obesity
Restless sleep with recurrent wakening; nightmares	Sinusitis
	Nasal or
Daytime fatigue or poor	nasopharyngeal
concentration; sleepiness; irritability	obstruction
Family history of OSA	Large tonsils
	Large tongue
	Small chin

* Assess daytime sleepiness with the Epworth Sleepiness Scale, available on http://www.sign.ac.uk/guidelines/fulltext/73/annex1.html. Alternatively, patients can score themselves on the British Snoring and Sleep Apnoea Association website (see below).
* Refer to a sleep study centre (or possibly directly to ENT) patients:
  (a) with excessive daytime sleepiness; or
  (b) where a partner reports apnoeic or choking episodes or restless sleep; or
  (c) where loud snoring is causing relationship problems; or
  (d) where curable pathology in the nose could be contributing, e.g. polyps or a deviated septum.
* Be especially ready to refer urgently patients:
  (a) with obstructive sleep apnoea/hypopnoea and COPD;
  (b) with evidence of ventilatory failure;
  (c) who are symptomatic and drive or operate machinery.

Driving

* When OSA is only suspected, warn the patient not to drive when feeling sleepy and not to embark on a drive if very prone to feeling sleepy.

* If the diagnosis is confirmed, the patient should inform the DVLA and insurance company. Driving will only be permitted once a doctor has confirmed that the condition is controlled.

SNORING WITHOUT APNOEA

* Advise patients to make the following lifestyle changes:
  (a) lose weight if obese, especially if the neck circumference is > 43 cm (17 inches).
  (b) avoid alcohol before bed-time;
  (c) stop smoking;
  (d) discontinue night-time sedation;
  (e) sleep on the side; a golf ball sewn into the back of the pyjamas may help this;
  (f) lift the head of the bed up;
  (g) dilate the nostrils using a Nozovent (available from www.britishsnoring.co.uk).
* Examine for nasal obstruction and consider a trial of intranasal steroids.
* Consider whether the patient could be hypothyroid.
* Recommend ear plugs for the partner.
* Refer to ENT in dire cases.

CONTACTS

The British Snoring and Sleep Apnoea Association (BSSAA), Castle Court, 41 London Road, Reigate, RH2 9RJ. Tel. 01737 245638 or UK Freephone 0800 0851097. www.britishsnoring.co.uk
   The British Sleep Society, PO Box 247, Colne, Huntingdon PE28 3UZ, www.sleeping.org.uk
   SATA (The Sleep Apnoea Trust), 7 Bailey Close, High Wycombe HP13 6QA. Tel. 0845 60 60 685 www.sleep-apnoea-trust.org

THE THROAT AND MOUTH

SORE THROAT

GUIDELINE

SIGN 34. 1999. *Management of Sore Throat and Indications for Tonsillectomy*. RCPE, Edinburgh. Available: www.sign.ac.uk

Systematic review

Del Mar C, Glasziou PP, Spinks A. 2006. Antibiotics for sore throat. Cochrane Database of Systematic Reviews, Issue 4. Art. No.: CD000023. DOI: 10.1002/14651858. CD000023.pub3

The following evidence demonstrates the limited value of throat swabs and of antibiotics in the management of sore throat:

* Approximately 20% of sore throats are bacterial, namely beta-haemolytic streptococci group A (GABHS) and groups C and G.
* The incidence is dependent on age. Only 15% are bacterial under the age of 3, while 50% are bacterial between the ages of 4 and 13 (DTB 1995b) and 10% in adults (Cooper, Hoffman, Bartlett, *et al*. 2001).
* The sensitivity and specificity of the throat swab are low, at most 30% and 80% respectively. Up to 40% of adults are carriers of GABHS. A positive swab is therefore not proof of infection.
* Streptococcal tonsillitis cannot reliably be diagnosed clinically, although it is more likely if the patient is < 11 years old with:
  (a) myalgia;
  (b) tender or swollen cervical lymph glands;
  (c) history of fever;
  (d) tonsillar exudates; and is less likely if there is cough or earache (Dobbs 1996).
* Penicillin speeds up recovery only slightly in patients with streptococcal tonsillitis (7 days after the start of treatment penicillin shows no advantage over placebo in relief of symptoms). It does not get patients back to school or work more quickly (Dagnelie, van der Graaf and De Melker, 1996).
* Antibiotics do not protect against the rare non-suppurative complications in patients with streptococcal tonsillitis, namely rheumatic fever (Howie and Foggo 1985) and acute glomerulonephritis (Taylor and Howie 1983; Glasziou and Del Mar 2000) or, if they do, the incidence of those complications in developed countries is so rare that it should not influence management (Del Mar, Glasziou and Spinks 2000).
* Antibiotics *do* protect against the suppurative complications of sore throat, reducing the incidence of acute otitis media by three quarters and of acute sinusitis by a half. However, these

complications are uncommon. It would be necessary to treat 30 children and 145 adults to prevent one case of acute otitis media (Del Mar, Glasziou and Spinks 2000).

- Antibiotics have no effect on the incidence of URTI, whether bacterial or viral, in the subsequent 6 months. The early use of antibiotics may even increase the chance of recurrence (El-Daher, Hijazi, Rawashdeh *et al.* 1991).
- Patients given penicillin for immediate use are more likely to re-attend than those not given antibiotics or given a prescription only to be used 3 days later if symptoms have not resolved (Little, Williamson, Warner, *et al.* 1997; Little, Gould, Williamson, *et al.* 1997).
- If penicillin is used, a 10-day course is more successful than a 5-day course in eradicating streptococci from the throat. However, this seems to be of no clinical importance, since it does not alter the number of sore throats over the following 6 months (Zwart, Rovers, de Melker, *et al.* 2003).
- Patients who are more satisfied with the consultation get better more quickly (Little, Williamson, Warner, *et al.* 1997).

MANAGEMENT

The aim is to:

(a) avoid unnecessarily widespread use of antibiotics, with its disadvantages: the dependence on the GP that it encourages; the possibility of antibiotic resistance and the adverse effects of the drugs;

(b) give the ill patient the possible benefit of early penicillin.

* Recommend lozenges.
* Recommend analgesics and antipyretics (Snow, Mottur-Pilson, Cooper, *et al.* 2001). Paracetamol is the drug of choice (SIGN 1999). It can decrease throat pain after 3 hours by up to 50%. Ibuprofen 400 mg t.d.s may be even more effective (Thomas, Del Mar and Glasziou 2000).
* Check what it is that concerns the patient. Explain the probable viral nature of the condition, and how they can manage subsequent attacks themselves at home (Little, Williamson, Warner, *et al.* 1997).
* If giving a prescription for antibiotics when the indication is arguable, consider recommending

that it only be used if there has been no improvement after 3 days. This can reduce antibiotic use by two thirds (Arroll, Kenealy, Goodyear-Smith, *et al.* 2003).

* Instruct patients to return in 1 week, if still unwell, for a throat swab, FBC and glandular fever antibodies.
* Be alert to the possibility that the sore throat is really an excuse to consult about some more difficult issue.

SPECIAL CASES

The modest benefit of penicillin, even in proven GABHS, makes a decision not to prescribe reasonable in almost all cases.

* *Ill patients*, e.g. with high fever, dysphagia, marked cervical lymphadenopathy and severe pharyngitis:
  (a) Take a throat swab or a rapid antigen test.
  (b) Give phenoxymethylpenicillin 250 mg q.d.s. or 500 mg b.d. for 5 days; or consider giving a cephalosporin. Give erythromycin if the patient is allergic to penicillin.
  (d) Instruct the patient to telephone for the result.
  (e) If pathogenic streptococci are grown, urge the patient to complete the 10-day course.
* *Sore throat associated with stridor or breathing difficulty*: admit immediately (SIGN 1999).
* *Patients with sore throat who are members of a closed community* where there is an outbreak of streptococcal pharyngitis. Treat as 'ill patients'.
* *Patients in severe pain*: consider giving oral prednisolone 60 mg daily for 2 days. It reduces pain at 12 and 24 hours with 57% painfree at 2 days compared to 33% on placebo. The benefit is more marked in sore throat due to streptococcal infection (Kiderman, Yaphe, Bregman, *et al.* 2005).
* *Patients with prolonged tonsillitis:*
  (a) With negative investigations:
    - repeat glandular fever antibodies weekly for 2 more weeks;
    - take blood for an ASO titre. The throat swab may be a false negative.
  (b) With persistent streptococcal infection:
    - give a cephalosporin or co-amoxiclav. Beta-lactamase-producing organisms may be destroying the penicillin.

* *Patients with a past history of rheumatic fever* should already be taking prophylactic penicillin V 250 mg b.d. If they develop a sore throat they should be given a cephalosporin or co-amoxiclav, in case they have beta-lactamase-producing organisms in the pharynx that are destroying the penicillin.
* *Patients on chemotherapy, immunosuppressive drugs or carbimazole.* Check the WBC.
* *Patients with a past history of quinsy.* Treat as 'ill patients'.

VINCENT'S ANGINA

This is an ulcerative gingivostomatitis, which can spread to the tonsils. It is due to an infection with fusiform bacilli and spirochaetes.

* Give metronidazole 400 mg b.d. for 3 days.

INFECTIOUS MONONUCLEOSIS

* Consider prednisolone 40 mg daily orally for 5 days in patients with severe tonsillitis, to enable them to swallow and avoid airway obstruction.
* Consider a high-dose NSAID to improve the general well-being of patients at an important time of their lives, e.g. when taking examinations.
* Avoid ampicillin-based antibiotics, including co-amoxiclav.

ORAL THRUSH

* Confirm with a mouth swab.
* Treat with an oral antifungal without waiting for the swab result.
* Consider a predisposing cause, e.g. diabetes, the use of broad spectrum antibiotics or inhaled steroids, HIV infection or other causes of immunosuppression.

SORE THROAT DUE TO POSTNASAL DRIP

Treat with intranasal steroids (see page 535).

TONSILLECTOMY

* Not all sore throats are due to tonsillitis.
* In children with recurrent severe tonsillitis, surgery offers the chance of avoiding two moderate or severe throat infections in the next 2 years. Children with a history that is less severe benefit less (Marshall 1998).
* There is no convincing evidence for tonsillectomy in adults.

INDICATIONS FOR REFERRAL

> **GUIDELINE**
>
> National Institute for Clinical Excellence. 2001. *Referral Practice: A Guide to Appropriate Referral from Generalist to Specialist Services.* NICE. Available: www.nice.org.uk

(a) *Recurrent acute tonsillitis*, five or more episodes a year. Attacks should be severe enough to interfere with the child's normal functioning.

(b) *Airway obstruction*, especially if there is sleep apnoea.

(c) *Chronic tonsillitis*, for over 3 months, especially if associated with halitosis.

(d) *Quinsy or peritonsillar cellulitis*, after recovery, in patients under age 25 with a history of recurrent tonsillitis.

(e) *Bacterial carriers who have not responded to antibiotics*, e.g. the diphtheria carrier and the carrier of haemolytic streptococcus group A who has had rheumatic fever.

(f) *Unilateral tonsillar enlargement or ulceration* suggestive of a serious underlying disorder, e.g. malignancy.

(g) *Guttate psoriasis* that is exacerbated by recurrent throat infections.

Less severely affected children are unlikely to benefit. A recent RCT found that in moderately affected children, the modest benefit was outweighed by the 7.9% who had surgery-related complications (Paradise, Bluestone, Colborn, *et al.* 2002).

DYSPHAGIA

∗ Check Hb and refer urgently to an ENT or a general surgeon to exclude a local cause.
∗ If the appointment is not imminent, order a barium swallow. This is the one situation where a barium study should precede endoscopy.

HOARSENESS

∗ Refer urgently anyone suffering from hoarseness for more than 3 weeks. Early tumours confined to the vocal cord treated by radiotherapy have an 80–90% chance of 5-year survival.
∗ Consider re-referring a patient with persistent constant hoarseness, even after a normal laryngoscopy performed in the early stages. A previously undetected nodule or carcinoma may now be visible.
∗ Do not diagnose chronic laryngitis in smokers without laryngoscopy. It is they who are also at risk of laryngeal carcinoma.
∗ If laryngoscopy is normal, refer to a speech therapist or voice teacher. Voice abuse is common in teachers, mothers of young children and anyone who shouts.
∗ Distinguish hoarseness from functional dysphonia, in which the patient adopts a whisper for psychological reasons. These patients need laryngoscopy to exclude a pathological cause before urgent referral to a speech therapist, psychiatrist or psychologist.

VOICE TEACHERS

The Voice Care Network UK (VCN UK), 25 The Square, Kenilworth, Warks, CV8 1EF. Tel./Fax 01926 864000. info@voicecare.org.uk, www.voicecare.org.uk

POST–LARYNGECTOMY

REVIEW

Gleeson M, Jani P. 1994. Long-term care of patients who have had a laryngectomy. BMJ 308, 1452–1453

∗ Treat all respiratory infections vigorously, and admit patients early if they are failing to expectorate their secretions.
∗ Check that the patient:
  (a) is attending speech therapy;
  (b) is eating enough. The sense of smell diminishes because the nose is not being used to sniff. Patients can be taught to sniff by speech therapists;
  (c) has been referred to the National Association of Laryngectomee Clubs, 6 Rickett Street, London SW6 1RU, tel. 020 7381 9993. www.laryngectomy.org.uk. Information for laryngectomees, carers and professionals can be found at the website.

THE FEELING OF A LUMP IN THE THROAT

When diagnostic clues are absent:
(a) Treat as oesophagitis for 2 weeks with antacids and/or a PPI.
(b) Refer non-responders to the ENT department in order to exclude a physical cause.
(c) Counsel those with negative findings to try to uncover the cause for their probable globus hystericus.

SORE MOUTH

RED OR WHITE PATCHES IN THE MOUTH

∗ Refer all as erythroplakia or leukoplakia unless the typical skin lesions show that it is lichen planus. The risk of malignancy over 10 years is 3–6% with leukoplakia, and far higher with erythroplakia.

ULCERATED SORE MOUTH

∗ Be aware that ulcers may be associated with skin, genital or eye lesions as part of a larger syndrome.

Primary herpes stomatitis or labialis

SYSTEMATIC REVIEW

Worrall G. 2001. Herpes labialis. *Clinical Evidence*, Issue 5. BMJ Publishing Group, London. Available: http://clinicalevidence.bmj.com

Review

Chon T, Nguyen L. 2007. What are the best treatments for herpes labialis? J Fam Pract 56, 576–578

* *First attack:* if seen within the first 48 hours give an oral antiviral agent, e.g. aciclovir, unless mild. It can halve the time to healing, at least in children.
* *Recurrent attacks:* use an oral antiviral agent. There is a lack of evidence of benefit for topical agents.
* *Prevention of recurrent attacks:*
  (a) sunblock will dramatically reduce the rate of recurrence in those in whom sun is a factor;
  (b) prophylactic oral antivirals probably do reduce the number of attacks and the size and duration of lesions. Either in the prodromal stage, or before a high risk activity such as skiing, give oral aciclovir for 4 days.

Aphthous ulcers

GUIDANCE

Scully C, Gorsky M, Lozada-Nur F. 2003. The diagnosis and management of recurrent aphthous stomatitis: a consensus approach. J Am Dent Assoc 134, 200–207
     Scully C. 2006. Aphthous ulceration. NEJM 355, 165–172

These may be associated with stress, menstruation, poor overall health or, occasionally, coeliac disease. Large single ulcers can reach 1–2 cm in diameter and take 6 weeks to heal, but at 3 weeks some improvement should already be seen.

* Check FBC, iron, B_{12} and folate levels. 20% of patients with recurrent ulcers have low iron, B_{12} or folate levels. Where ulceration is recurrent, check HIV status and antibodies for coeliac disease.
* In milder cases give:
  (a) triamcinalone in cellulose paste (Adcortyl in Orabase), thinly applied two to four times a day;
  (b) hydrocortisone pellets – dissolve one pellet slowly in contact with the ulcer, three to four times a day;
  (c) topical anaesthetic rinse or gel, or antimicrobial mouthwash;

(d) pressurized steroids (asthma inhalers) sprayed directly onto ulcer (an unlicensed use).
* *In more severe cases* consider oral steroids.
* *In recurrent cases* use chlorhexidine mouthwash to reduce the frequency of relapse (Porter and Scully 2007).
* Refer if there are other symptoms (e.g. uveitis, genital ulceration, arthritis, etc.) suggestive of a systemic disease.
* *Continuous aphthous ulceration or severe ulceration.* Refer to an oral medicine specialist. They may benefit from higher strength steroids or immunosuppressants including thalidomide (an unlicensed use).

Traumatic ulcers

(a) Treat the cause.
(b) Try a local anti-inflammatory agent, such as salicylate cream, applied three to four times a day.
* **Refer for biopsy any ulcer which has not healed within 3 weeks after the removal of any local cause. It may be a squamous cell carcinoma.**

GUM DISEASE

In its most severe form, gum disease is acute necrotizing ulcerative gingivitis.

* Give a chlohexidine mouthwash and metronidazole 400 mg b.d. for 5 days.
* Stop smoking.
* Improve oral hygiene.

SORE MOUTH WITHOUT ULCERATION

Dry mouth may be due to anxiety, drugs, dehydration or Sjögren's syndrome.

* Prescribe an artificial saliva product. Do not encourage the sucking of sweets unless they are sugar-free. Caries is already a hazard for patients with a dry mouth.
* *Oral thrush in a patient wearing dentures.* Sterilize the dentures by soaking them overnight in dilute hypochlorite solution, then apply miconazole oral gel q.d.s. to the part of the denture in contact with the gum.
* *Work-up where diagnosis is not clear:* swab for candida and check FBC, B_{12}, folate, and serum iron.

DENTAL PROBLEMS

TOOTHACHE

* Sensitive to hot, cold and sweet stimuli: this is probably due to exposed dentine. Advise the patient to see a dentist.
* Severe pain, touch sensitivity, gingival swelling with or without local lymphadenopathy, and fever: this is a dental abscess. Refer for drainage. If there is likely to be delay, prescribe:
  (a) penicillin V 500 mg q.d.s., or erythromycin 500 mg b.d., or metronidazole 400 mg b.d.; and
  (b) adequate analgesia. Try an NSAID first.

LOSS OF A TOOTH THROUGH TRAUMA

● Re-implantation of a secondary tooth within 12 hours is likely to succeed, and is worth attempting after an even longer time.
  1. Pick the tooth up by its crown, not by the root.
  2. If dirty, wash it in cold water.
  3. Push it back into its socket or under the patient's tongue, or store it in a cup of milk or in the patient's saliva.
  4. Send the patient immediately to a dentist or accident and emergency department for re-implantation.

COMPLICATIONS AFTER EXTRACTION

Haemorrhage

1. Allow the patient to rinse the mouth out.
2. Place a damp gauze swab over the socket and ask the patient to bite hard for 10–15 minutes.
3. If this fails, either suture across the socket with 3.0 silk or refer to a dentist or oral surgeon.

Painful socket, bad taste, halitosis

This usually occurs 4–5 days after an extraction and is due to the clot not forming or being removed and the socket filling with debris that gets infected.

* Refer to a dentist.
* Give strong analgesics.
* Advise the patient to wash the mouth out with warm saline.

* Start antibiotics: penicillin V 500 mg q.d.s. or erythromycin 500 mg b.d. and metronidazole 400 mg b.d.

HALITOSIS

OVERVIEW
Scully C, Porter S, Greenman J. 1994. What to do about halitosis. BMJ 308, 217–218

90% of halitosis is due to bacterial putrefaction in the mouth (Tessier and Kulkarni 1991).

* Encourage mouth hygiene. Trapped food is a common cause of halitosis, especially in denture wearers.
* Treat any local infection. This may be tonsillitis, gingivitis, sinusitis or even bronchiectasis. A dental check is worthwhile even if there is no obvious pathology.
* Look for a furry tongue, although treatment is difficult. Stopping smoking and scrubbing the tongue with a toothbrush may help.
* Check whether the patient suffers from a dry mouth. This may be due to drugs, DXR or Sjögren's syndrome, or to mouth breathing. Sugar-free mints or gum will aid salivation.
* Ask whether the halitosis only occurs when the patient is hungry. Hunger halitosis is well-recognized, although the cause is not clear.
* Consider certain foods as the cause. Patients usually recognize for themselves the connection with garlic or onions, but may not notice the connection with a diet high in dairy products, especially yoghurt.
* If there is no specific pointer to the cause of the trouble, consider an empirical trial of tooth-brushing and flossing after every meal with an antiseptic mouthwash night and morning for 2 weeks at a time. Longer courses put the patient at risk of fungal overgrowth.
* If the above fails, then consider investigating for rare causes such as:
  (a) metabolic disorders; uraemia, ketosis and liver failure;
  (b) small bowel pathology where bacterial overgrowth may be the cause of the halitosis (e.g. blind loop syndrome). Evidence for this

may be haematological (anaemia; iron deficiency; low serum B_{12} and a raised red cell folate) or radiological (barium meal and follow-through);

(c) nasopharyngeal malignancy.

* If small bowel pathology is not suspected, try a 2-week course of antibiotics (amoxicillin or tetracycline). Chronic bacterial overgrowth of the gut may still be the cause. If the condition improves, consider long-term intermittent use of antibiotics.

* Delusional halitosis may be the only complaint of a patient with a hypochondriacal depression. Refer to a psychiatrist.

References

Acuin, J., Smith, A., Mackenzie, I., 2000. Interventions for chronic suppurative otitis media (Cochrane Review). In: The Cochrane Library, Issue 1. Update Software, Oxford.

Agency for Health Care Policy and Research, 1994. Otitis media with effusion: clinical practice guideline No. 12. Agency for Health Care and Public Research (AHCPR), Rockville MD.

Ah-See, K.W., Evans, A.S., 2007. Sinusitis and its management. BMJ 334, 358–361.

Alberta Medical Association, 2008. Guideline for the diagnosis and treatment of acute otitis media in children. Available: www.amda. ab.ca.

American Academy of Pediatrics, 1997. Managing otitis media with effusion in young children. American Academy of Pediatrics. Available: www.ngc.gov.

Arroll, B., Kenealy, T., Goodyear-Smith, F., et al., 2003. Delayed prescriptions. BMJ 327, 1361–1362.

Arroll, B., Kenealy, T., 2005. Antibiotics for the common cold and acute purulent rhinitis. Cochrane Database Syst. Rev. (3), CD000247. DOI: 10.1002/14651858.CD000247.pub2.

Bandolier, 1994. Glue ear – a sticky problem. Bandolier Feb. Available: www.medicine.ox.ac.uk/Bandolier.

Bandolier, 1995. Ménières disease. Bandolier 13. Available:www.medicine.ox.ac.uk/Bandolier.

Bandolier, 2000. Tinnitus and Ménière's update. Bandolier April. Available:www.medicine.ox.ac.uk/Bandolier.

Bandolier. Bell's palsy systematic reviews, Bandolier. Available: www.medicine.ox.ac.uk/bandolier (search on 'Bell's palsy'). Accessed January 2010.

Bickerton, R.C., Roberts, C., Little, J.T., 1988. Survey of general practitioners' treatment of discharging ear. BMJ 296, 1649–1650.

Biedlingmaier, J.F., 1994. Two ear problems you may not need to refer. Otitis externa and bullous myringitis. Postgrad. Med. 96 (5), 141–145.

Bloomington, M.N., 2001. Institute for Clinical Systems Improvement. Diagnosis and treatment of otitis media in children. Available: www.ngc.gov.

Browning, R., 2005. Ear wax. In: Clinical Evidence. BMJ Publishing Group, London.

Butler, C.C., van der Voort, J.H., 2002. Oral or topical nasal steroids for hearing loss associated with otitis media with effusion in children (Cochrane Review). In: The Cochrane Library, Issue 2. Update Software, Oxford.

Committee for Safety of Medicines, 1997. Reminder: ototoxicity with aminoglycoside eardrops. Curr. Prob. Pharmacovigil. 23. Available: www.mca.gov.uk.

Cooper, C.W., 1993. Vestibular neuronitis: a review of a common cause of vertigo in general practice. Br. J. Gen. Pract. 43, 164–167.

Cooper, R.J., Hoffman, J.R., Bartlett, J.G., et al., 2001. Principles of appropriate antibiotic use for acute pharyngitis in adults: background. Ann. Intern. Med. 134, 509–517.

Dagnelie, C.F., van der Graaf, Y., De Melker, R.A., 1996. Do patients with sore throats benefit from penicillin? Br. J. Gen. Pract. 46, 589–593.

Del Mar, C.B., Glasziou, P.P., Spinks, A.B., 2000. Antibiotics for sore throat (Cochrane Review). In: The Cochrane Library, Issue 4. Update Software, Oxford.

Dobbs, F., 1996. A scoring system for predicting group A streptococcal throat infection. Br. J. Gen. Pract. 46, 461–464.

Dobie, R.A., 1999. A review of randomized clinical trials in tinnitus. Laryngoscope 109, 1202–1211. Reviewed in the Database of Abstracts of Reviews of Effectiveness. In: The Cochrane Library, Issue 4. Update Software, Oxford.

Douek, E., 1990. Sensorineural deafness. BMJ 301, 74–75.

DTB, 1995a. Management of acute otitis media and glue ear. Drug Ther. Bull. 33, 12–15.

DTB, 1995b. Diagnosis and treatment of streptococcal sore throat. Drug Ther. Bull. 33, 9–12.

DTB, 2009. Managing acute sinusitis. Drug Ther. Bull. 47, 3 March.

Eekhof, J.A.H., de Bock, G.H., de Laat, J.A., et al., 1996. The whispered voice: the best test for screening for hearing impairment in general practice. Br. J. Gen. Pract. 46, 473–474.

El-Daher, N.T., Hijazi, S.S., Rawashdeh, N.M., et al., 1991. Immediate versus delayed treatment of group A haemolytic streptococcal pharyngitis with penicillin V. Pediatr. Infect. Dis. J. 10, 126–130.

Evans, K.L., 1994. Diagnosis and management of sinusitis. BMJ 309, 1415–1422.

Flynn, C.A., Griffin, G.H., Schultz, J.K., 2004. Decongestants and antihistamines for acute otitis media in children. Cochrane Database Syst. Rev. (3).

Gianopoulos, I., Stephens, D., Davis, A., 2002. Follow up of people fitted with hearing aids after adult hearing screening: the need for support after fitting. BMJ 325, 471.

Glasziou, P., Del Mar, C., 2000. Upper respiratory tract infection: antibiotics. In: Clinical Evidence, Issue 4. BMJ Publishing Group, London. Available: www.clinicalevidence.org.

Glasziou, P.P., Del Mar, C.B., Sanders, S.L., et al., 2003. Antibiotics for acute otitis media in children. Cochrane Database Syst. Rev. (4).

Hand, C., Harvey, I., 2004. The effectiveness of topical preparations for the treatment of earwax: a systematic review. Br. J. Gen. Pract. 54, 862–867.

Hayden, F.G., Diamond, L., Wood, P.B., et al., 1996. Effectiveness and safety of intranasal ipratropium bromide in common colds. A randomised, double-blind, placebo-controlled trial. Ann. Intern. Med. 125, 89–97.

Hemilä, H., Chalker, E., Treacy, B., et al., 2007. Vitamin C for preventing and treating the common cold. Cochrane Database Syst. Rev. (3), CD000980. DOI: 10.1002/14651858.CD000980.pub3.

Hickish, G., 1989. Hearing problems of elderly people. BMJ 299, 1415–1416.

Hilton, M., Pinder, D., 2004. The Epley (canalith repositioning) manoeuvre for benign paroxysmal positional vertigo. Cochrane Database Syst. Rev. (2), CD003162. DOI: 10.1002/14651858.CD003162.pub2.

Howie, J., Foggo, B., 1985. Antibiotics, sore throat and rheumatic fever. J. R. Coll. Gen. Pract. 35, 223–224.

James, A.L., Burton, M.J., 2001. Betahistine for Ménière's disease or syndrome (Cochrane Review). In: The Cochrane Library, Issue 2. Update Software, Oxford.

James, A., Thorp, M., 2001. Ménière's disease. Clinical Evidence, Issue 5. BMJ Publishing Group, London. Available: www.clinicalevidence.org.

Kaleida, P.H., Casselbrant, M.L., Rockette, H.E., et al., 1991. Amoxicillin or myringotomy or both for acute otitis media: results of a randomized clinical trial. Pediatrics 87, 466–474.

Keane, E.M., Wilson, H., McGrane, D., et al., 1995. Use of solvents to disperse ear wax. Br. J. Clin. Pract. 49 (2), 71–72.

Kiderman, A., Yaphe, J., Bregman, J., et al., 2005. Adjuvant prednisolone therapy in pharyngitis: a randomised controlled trial from general practice. Br. J. Gen. Pract. 55, 218–221.

Kim, A.S., 2005. Sinusitis (acute). In: Clinical Evidence. BMJ Publishing Group, London.

Kollar, C., Schneider, H., Waksman, J., Krusinska, E., 2007. Meta-analysis of the efficacy of a single dose of phenylephrine 10 mg compared with placebo in adults with acute nasal congestion due to the common cold. Clin. Ther. 29 (6), 1057–1070.

Lambert, I.J., 1981. A comparison of the treatment of otitis externa with 'Otosporin' and aluminium acetate: a report from a services practice in Cyprus. J. R. Coll. Gen. Pract. 31, 291–294.

Lempert, T., Gresty, M.A., Bronstein, A.M., 1995. Benign positional vertigo: recognition and treatment. BMJ 311, 489–491.

Lindberg, E., Janson, C., Svardsudd, K., et al., 1998. Increased mortality among sleepy snorers: a prospective population based study. Thorax 53, 631–637.

Linde, K., Barrett, B., Bauer, R., et al., 2006. Echinacea for preventing and treating the common cold. Cochrane Database Syst. Rev. (1), CD000530. DOI: 10.1002/14651858.CD000530.pub2.

Little, P., Gould, C., Moore, M., et al., 2002. I. Predictors of poor outcome and benefits from antibiotics in children with acute otitis media: pragmatic randomised trial. BMJ 325, 22.

Little, P., Gould, C., Williamson, I., et al., 1997. Re-attendance and complications in a randomised trial of prescribing strategies for sore throat: the medicalising effect of prescribing antibiotics. BMJ 315, 350–352.

Little, P., Gould, C., Williamson, I., et al., 2001. Pragmatic randomised controlled trial of two prescribing strategies for childhood acute otitis media. BMJ 322, 336–342.

Little, P., Williamson, I., Warner, G., et al., 1997. Open randomized trial of prescribing strategies in managing sore throat. BMJ 1997; 314, 722–727.

Lund, V.J., 1990. Sinusitis. Prescribers Journal 33, 9–12.

Luxon, L.M., 1993. Tinnitus: its causes, diagnosis, and treatment. BMJ 306, 1490–1491.

Marais, J., Dale, B.A.B., 1997. Bullous myringitis: a review. Clin. Otolaryngol. 22, 497–499.

Marshall, T., 1998. A review of tonsillectomy for recurrent throat infection. Br. J. Gen. Pract. 48, 1331–1335.

Martinez Devesa, P., Waddell, A., Perera, R., Theodoulou, M., 2007. Cognitive behavioural therapy for tinnitus. Cochrane Database Syst Rev. (1).

Memel, D., Langley, C., Watkins, C., et al., 2002. Effectiveness of ear syringing in general practice: a randomised controlled trial and patients' experiences. Br. J. Gen. Pract. 52, 906–911.

Morris, P., Leach, A., 2002. Antibiotics for persistent nasal discharge (rhinosinusitis) in children (Cochrane Review). In: The Cochrane Library, Issue 4.

NHS Centre for Reviews and Dissemination, 1994. The treatment of persistent glue ear in children. Eff. Health Care 1 (4), with update 1996. University of York.

NICE, 2009. Cochlear implants for children and adults with severe to profound deafness. National Institute for Health and Clinical Excellence. Available: www.nice. org.uk.

O'Neill, P., 2001. Long term antibiotic treatment. Clinical Evidence, Issue 5. BMJ Publishing Group, London. Available: www.clinicalevidence. com.

Paradise, J.L., Bluestone, C.D., Colborn, D.K., et al., 2002. Tonsillectomy and adenotonsillectomy for recurrent throat infection in moderately affected children. Pediatrics 110, 7–15.

Patiar, S., Reece, P., 2009. Oral steroids for nasal polyps. Cochrane Database Syst. Rev. (2), CD005232. DOI:10.1002/14651858. CD005232.pub2.

Pearlman, D.S., Lumry, W.R., Winder, J.A., et al., 1995. Once daily cetirizine effective in the treatment of seasonal allergic rhinitis in children aged 6–11 years: a randomized double-blind placebo-controlled study. Clin. Pediatr. 36, 209–215.

Pirozzo, S., Papinczak, T., Glasziou, P., 2003. Whispered voice test for screening for hearing impairment in adults and children: systematic review. BMJ 327, 967–970.

Porter, S., Scully, C., 2007. Aphthous ulcers (recurrent). Clin. Evid. June. Available: http:// clinicalevidence.bmj.com.

Ratner, P.H., van Bavel, J.H., Martin, B.G., et al., 1998. A comparison of the efficacy of fluticasone proprionate aqueous nasal spray and loratadine, alone and in combination, for the treatment of seasonal allergic rhinitis. J. Fam. Pract. 47, 118–125.

Rovers, M.M., Glasziou, P., Appelman, C.I., et al., 2006. Antibiotics for acute otitis media: a meta-analysis with individual patient data. Lancet 368, 1429–1435.

Ruohola, A., Heikkinen, T., Meurman, O., et al., 2003. Antibiotic treatment of acute otorrhea through tympanostomy tube: randomized double-blind placebo-controlled study with daily follow-up. Pediatrics 111, 1061–1067.

Salinas, R., 2005. Bell's Palsy Clinical Evidence. BMJ Publishing Group, London.

Sheikh, A., Panesar, S.S., Dhami, S., 2005. Seasonal allergic rhinitis. Clinical Evidence, Issue 12. BMJ Publishing Group, London.

SIGN 34, 1999. Management of sore throat and indications for tonsillectomy. RCPE, Edinburgh. Online. Available: www.sign.ac. uk/guidelines.

SIGN, 2003. Diagnosis and management of childhood otitis media in primary care. Available on www.sign.ac.uk.

Singh, M., 2006. Heated, humidified air for the common cold. Cochrane Database Syst. Rev. (3), CD001728. DOI: 10.1002/14651858.CD001728. pub3.

Snow, V., Mottur-Pilson, C., Cooper, R.J., et al., 2001. Principles of appropriate antibiotic use for acute pharyngitis in adults. Ann. Intern. Med. 134, 506–508.

Strachan, D.P., Cook, D.G., 1998. Parental smoking, middle ear disease and adenotonsillectomy in children. Thorax 53, 50–56.

Sullivan, F.M., Swan, I.R.C., Donnan, P., et al., 2007. Early treatment with prednisolone or acyclovir in Bell's palsy. NEJM 357, 1598–1607.

Taylor, J.L., Howie, J., 1983. Antibiotics, sore throat and acute nephritis. J. R. Coll. Gen. Pract. 33, 783–786.

Teixeira, L.J., Soares, B.G.D.O., Vieira, V.P., et al., 2008. Physical therapy for Bell's palsy. Cochrane Database Syst. Rev. (3), CD006283. DOI:10.1002/14651858.CD006283. pub2.

Terreehorst, I., Hak, E., Oosting, A.J., et al., 2003. Evaluation of impermeable covers for bedding in patients with allergic rhinitis. N. Eng. J. Med. 349, 237–246.

Tessier, J.F., Kulkarni, G.V., 1991. Bad breath: etiology, diagnosis and treatment. Oral Health 81, 9–24.

Thomas, M., Del Mar, C., Glasziou, P., 2000. How effective are treatments other than antibiotics for acute sore throat? Br. J. Gen. Pract. 50, 817–820.

van Balen, F.A.M., Smit, W.M., Zuithoff, N.P.A., et al., 2003. Clinical efficacy of three common treatments in acute otitis externa in primary care: randomised controlled trial. BMJ 327, 1201–1205.

van Buchem, F.L., Dunk, J.H., Van't Hof, M.A., et al., 1981. Therapy of acute otitis media: myringotomy, antibiotics, or neither? A double-blind study in children. Lancet ii, 883–887.

Waddell, A., 2004. Tinnitus. Clinical Evidence Available: www. clinicalevidence.com.

Weiner, J.M., Abramson, M.J., Puy, R.M., 1998. Intranasal corticosteroids versus oral H1 receptor antagonists in allergic rhinitis: systematic review of randomised controlled trials. BMJ 317, 1624–1629.

Yardley, L., Beech, S., Zander, L., et al., 1998. A randomised controlled trial of exercise therapy for dizziness and vertigo in primary care. Br. J. Gen. Pract. 48, 1136–1140.

Young, T., Palta, M., Dempsey, J., et al., 1993. The occurrence of sleep-disordered breathing among middle-aged adults. N. Engl. J. Med. 328, 1230–1235.

Yueh, B., Shapiro, N., MacLean, C.H., et al., 2003. Screening and management of adult hearing loss in primary care. JAMA 289, 1976–1985.

Zwart, S., Rovers, M.M., de Melker, R.A., et al., 2003. Penicillin for acute sore throat in children: randomised double blind trial. BMJ 327, 1324–1327.

Chapter 21

Eye problems

CHAPTER CONTENTS

Patient information leaflets for a number of eye conditions are available from www.moorfields.nhs.uk/publicationsandresources and www.goodhope.org.uk (follow the link to the eye department)

THE GRITTY IRRITABLE RED EYE

ACUTE INFECTIVE CONJUNCTIVITIS

In an adult or child

- The history and examination traditionally give grounds for distinguishing between bacterial and viral infection but there is no evidence to support this (Rietveld, van Weert, ter Riet, *et al.* 2003). Chlamydial infection should be suspected when only one eye is involved.
- Even in proven bacterial conjunctivitis, antibiotics only modestly improve the rate of resolution. Over half will resolve without treatment in 2–5 days (Sheikh and Hurwitz 2005).
- A large UK study of acute infective conjunctivitis in children and adults found in favour of delayed prescribing of chloramphenicol eye drops, where the prescription could be collected after 3 days if the patient still needed it (Everitt, Little and Smith 2006). This was associated with as good a resolution of symptoms as immediate prescribing but with a lower use of antibiotics (53% vs 99%) and less tendency for the patient to think that they should re-attend in the event

of a future eye infection. Conversely, those who received no antibiotic prescription found that their moderate symptoms lasted a day and a half longer (means of 4.8 vs 3.2 days). Also they returned more frequently during that episode than those given a delayed prescription, though they were still less likely to be given antibiotics (30% vs 53%).

● In the above study an eye swab showed bacterial infection in half of the patients but a positive swab was unrelated to any outcome.

If the visual acuity is normal and the cornea is clear, advise the patient to:

* Wipe away discharge.
* Wash hands after touching the eyes.
* Use separate towels. It seems logical to recommend that children should stay away from school even though this is not the recommendation of the Health Protection Agency (Guidelines on the Management of Communicable Diseases in Schools and Nurseries 2008).
* Advise the patient to return in 3 days to collect a prescription for antibiotic drops if symptoms are not resolving. Prescribe chloramphenicol eye drops 2-hourly for 2 days, then four times a day for a further 5 days. Fears of bone marrow aplasia (Doona and Walsh 1995) from topical chloramphenicol seem to be unfounded (Lancaster, Swart and Jick 1998). Fusidic acid has been shown in one RCT to be more effective than chloramphenicol but overall there appears to be no significant difference in rates of clinical or microbiological cure between different topical antibiotics (Smith 2004). Gentamicin is only indicated if there is gram negative infection.
* If symptoms are still present at 1 week but there are no complications, stop all treatment and review weekly. Adenoviral infection typically takes 2–3 weeks to resolve.
* Refer to eye casualty at any stage if the visual acuity is reduced or the cornea is involved.
* *Orbital cellulitis:* admit immediately.

In a neonate

The likelihood and the dangers of sexually transmissible disease are greater.

* If the eye is mildly sticky: take a swab and review.

* If the discharge is purulent: take swabs for viral, bacterial and chlamydial infection and a smear for gonococci. Then start chloramphenicol eye drops hourly and refer for an ophthalmic opinion the same day.
* Admit for intensive antibiotic therapy if:
  (a) herpes simplex, chlamydia or gonococcus is grown; or
  (b) the clinical situation worsens, with a red eye, cloudy cornea, blepharitis, marked preauricular lymphadenopathy or an unwell child.
* Notify as ophthalmia neonatorum.

INSTILLING INTO THE EYE

Instilling drops: pull the lower lid down with the patient looking up. Squeeze one drop onto the lower fornix.
Instilling ointments or gels: as above but squeeze 1 cm onto the inner surface of the lid. Warn the patient it will blur the vision for a short while.

ALLERGIC CONJUNCTIVITIS

Acute

* Reassure the patient that the eye will not be harmed and that the problem will settle soon.
* Give antihistamine drops, e.g. antazoline with xylometazoline, or olopatadine.

Chronic or recurrent allergic eye disease

* Establish, if possible, what the allergen is and reduce or avoid contact.
* Use an antihistamine plus a vasoconstrictor topically, e.g. antazoline with xylometazoline, but only for short periods. Prolonged use of xylometazoline can lead to rebound hyperaemia when it is stopped. Use a pure antihistamine instead, e.g. olopatadine, epinastine or emedastine.
* *Prophylaxis.* Give sodium cromoglicate, nedocromil sodium or lodoxamide drops q.d.s. Benefit may not be seen for 2 weeks. Where symptoms are seasonal, start treatment before the season starts.
* Consider giving an oral non-sedating antihistamine if symptoms are still not controlled.

* *Severe cases not responding to the above:* Consider using a weak topical steroid (e.g. prednisolone) for up to 5 days, but only if:
  (a) the cornea is monitored for dendritic ulceration;
  (b) the patient is referred after 5 days if treatment is not successful.

More prolonged use carries the risk of raised intra-ocular pressure.

* If a patient worsens dramatically after starting to use drops consider contact sensitivity. The usual cause is the preservative in the drops.

BLEPHARITIS

* Reassure the patient that the condition will not threaten sight. Explain that it is caused by an abnormality of secretion from the meibomian glands, and that treatment has to be long-term.
* *Lid hygiene.* Encourage the patient to clean the eyelid margins of debris first by heating the area with a wet warm flannel and then by gently scrubbing the eyelid margins with a cotton bud dipped in a solution of mild baby shampoo diluted 1:3 with warm water. This should be repeated twice a day until symptoms improve and once a week thereafter.
* Treat patients as if they have dry eyes, as the tears evaporate more rapidly. See below for treatment regimen but do not continue if there is no benefit.
* If there is no improvement, give chloramphenicol ointment to be applied to the lid margins b.d. for a month. The inflammation is secondary to hypersensitivity to the cell wall protein of staphylococcus and may require topical steroid and antibiotic drops for a short period. Encourage the patient to continue lid hygiene.
* Treat those not still responding and those with acne rosacea with long courses of oral antibiotics, e.g. oxytetracycline 250 mg b.d. or doxycycline 50 mg o.d.
* Consider referral to an ophthalmologist of those:
  (a) remaining symptomatic despite treatment for a few months;
  (b) who have associated skin disease;
  (c) where there is suspicion of corneal involvement.

DRY EYE

* Treat any blepharitis (see above).
* Check that the patient is not taking any drugs that might exacerbate the condition, e.g. antihistamines.
* Encourage the patient to try to increase the humidity of their environment, if appropriate.
* Encourage the patient to use artificial tears as often as necessary. Start with hypromellose 0.3%. Drops may be needed every 30 minutes. Higher strengths may give relief for longer.
* Add or substitute products that last longer either:
  (a) by clinging to the surface, e.g. carbomers; or
  (b) by increasing the persistence of the tear film, e.g. polyvinyl alcohol.
* Prescribe paraffin-containing ointments, e.g. Lacri-Lube, for use at night.
* Treat with drops containing acetylcysteine if excess mucus is a problem. Warn the patient that it stings.
* Refer:
  (a) urgently if there is a sudden increase in discomfort, redness or deterioration in vision. These patients are at increased risk of microbial keratitis;
  (b) routinely patients who are having to instil drops very frequently. Insertion of punctum plugs may benefit those who have not responded to treatment.

TRAUMA

* Check the visual acuity. Refer if this is diminished or has decreased when next seen.

Foreign body

* Suspect a foreign body in any unilateral red eye with or without a history of 'something going into the eye'.
* Always fully evert the upper eyelid when looking for a foreign body. If a foreign body is seen, it can usually be removed from the conjunctiva without difficulty.
* **If there is a history of pain while hammering metal or of exposure to glass splinters, refer to exclude an intraocular foreign body.**

Corneal foreign body

1. Insert local anaesthetic. Start with proxymetacaine and when the stinging has stopped, deepen the anaesthesia with amethocaine 1% drops. Continue until the drops feel cold but do not sting;
2. Remove the foreign body with a cotton wool bud or the tip of a sterile needle. Do not dig into the cornea; at its centre it is only 1 mm thick;
3. After removal, prescribe antibiotic eye ointment b.d. for 2 days as prophylaxis;
4. Give a cycloplegic, e.g. cyclopentolate 1% drops q.d.s. if pain continues;
5. Do not apply an eye pad (Easty 1993);
6. Examine after 24 hours:
   (a) with fluorescein to be sure the epithelium has healed;
   (b) to exclude a rust ring if the foreign body was metallic. If present, refer to an ophthalmologist urgently for it to be removed.

Chemical burns

These are acid or alkali burns of which alkali (usually in the form of cement, lime, caustic soda or ammonia) are the more serious.

* Irrigate with tap water or normal saline for 20 minutes.
* Examine the cornea with fluorescein and send to eye casualty if it is not clear.
* *Cement.* Look for cement adhering to the eye, under the lids or in the conjunctival fornices. If found, give local anaesthetic drops (e.g. benoxinate) and remove it, however distressing this is to the patient.
* *Detergent.* If the conjunctiva shows punctate epithelial loss, treat with chloramphenicol and review in 3 days.

Ultraviolet light burns

Arc eye is usually due to exposure to UVC through welding or using a sunbed without eye protection.

* Give local anaesthetic drops, e.g. benoxinate *once*, but do not repeat them; they retard corneal healing.

* Give cyclopentolate 1% drops q.d.s. for as long as the pain lasts. Paralyzing the ciliary muscle will relieve some of the pain.
* Treat with chloramphenicol drops 2-hourly for 24 hours and 4-hourly for the next 24 hours.
* Pad the worst of the two eyes. Few patients would tolerate bilateral padding.
* Give sufficient sedatives and analgesics to ensure a night's sleep. Opioids are likely to be needed. Cessation of blinking during sleep enables the corneal epithelium to heal.
* Advise patients not to drive until they have finished the drops (i.e. at least 48 hours).

Corneal abrasion

* Confirm the abrasion with fluorescein dye.
* Check that there is no deeper damage to the eye, e.g. hyphaema.
* Treat with chloramphenicol ointment 2-hourly for 24 hours and then q.d.s. for a further week.
* Give a cycloplegic, e.g. cyclopentolate 1% drops b.d. if pain continues or consider ophthalmic NSAID drops, e.g. diclofenac sodium (Weaver and Terrell 2003).
* Do not apply an eye pad (Easty 1993).
* Give oral analgesia if the pain is severe.
* Refer if the epithelium has not healed after 24 hours if there is infection or 48 hours if there is no evidence of infection. Note that fluoroscein staining lasts for 3–4 days.
* *Recurrent abrasions.* Recurrences tend to occur in the early morning during opening of that eye, when tear secretion is less. Give long-term artificial tears during the day and ointment at night (see dry eyes). Explain that recurrences can continue for months or years. There is limited evidence that tetracycline 250 mg b.d. for 12 weeks and/or topical prednisolone 0.5% q.d.s for 1 week (with specialist approval) can reduce the tendency to recurrence. Refer to an ophthalmologist if not improving. Laser ablation may be needed.

Blunt injuries

Refer all patients who receive blunt injuries, e.g. from a squash ball as this may give rise to bleeding into the anterior chamber of the eye (hyphaema) and the pressure may rise.

PROBLEMS WITH CONTACT LENSES

Conjunctivitis

* Advise the patient to remove the lens and leave it out until recovered.
* Prescribe antibiotic eye drops.
* Arrange for slit-lamp examination to exclude keratitis, either by the lens provider or the local ophthalmology emergency department.
* Check that the patient is cleaning and disinfecting the lenses every night (or using disposable single use lenses).

Corneal abrasion: see above.

Microbial keratitis: refer to the ophthalmology emergency department immediately. There is a risk of perforation and endophthalmitis.

Other problems need slit-lamp examination to distinguish them. Advise the patient to leave the lenses out and contact the lens prescriber, or refer the patient to an ophthalmologist. NHS facilities are available to lens wearers if pathological problems have arisen.

THE PAINFUL RED EYE THAT IS NOT 'GRITTY'

Most need referral to eye casualty:

(a) keratitis, ocular herpes simplex, corneal ulcer, scleritis and uveitis the same day;

(b) acute glaucoma immediately.

The GP may treat:

(a) *Episcleritis* with a topical NSAID if there is discomfort, e.g. diclofenac or flurbiprofen for 2 weeks. Refer if not improved within a month.

(b) *Recurrent uveitis.* Treatment with topical steroids can be started, provided:

■ their use has been previously sanctioned by a consultant. However, their value in anterior uveitis is uncertain and there is no evidence of a difference between topical steroid or non-steroid anti-inflammatory drops in clinical cure rate (Curi, Matos and Pavesio 2004);

■ the visual acuity is normal;

■ a dendritic ulcer is excluded with fluorescein and magnified examination of the cornea;

but arrange for specialist assessment. Ophthalmic supervision is always necessary because intensive topical steroids may be needed. Treat with topical antivirals if the history is suggestive of herpes, while awaiting assessment.

OPHTHALMIC HERPES ZOSTER

* Give a high dose antiviral drug (see page 574) at the first sign of zoster in the ophthalmic division of the trigeminal nerve (i.e. when the rash appears on the forehead, usually before any involvement of the eye). Untreated, about half would develop eye involvement.

* Refer to an ophthalmologist if there is (Opstelten and Zall 2005):

■ Hutchinson's sign (involvement of the nasociliary nerve which supplies the side of the nose and the skin of the inner corner of the eye);

■ a red eye; or

■ visual complaints.

This referral is for an early, but not immediate appointment. The complications for which ophthalmic expertise is needed, e.g. keratitis or uveitis, tend to occur a week or more after the onset of the rash.

* Be alert to the long-term complications of eye involvement:

■ loss of corneal sensation may make the eye vulnerable to neuropathic ulceration or exposure keratopathy;

■ scarring of the eyelid may lead to incomplete closure, putting the cornea at risk.

Patients with either of these problems will need to use lubricating eye ointments long-term.

LASH, LIDS AND LACRIMAL PROBLEMS

ACUTE DACROCYSTITIS

* Treat aggressively for presumed staphylococcal or streptococcal infection, e.g. with flucloxacillin and amoxicillin, for 1 week.
* Review after 24 hours. If the symptoms are worse, refer for an ophthalmological opinion that day.
* Refer once recovered, for an ophthalmological opinion and possible surgery.

CHALAZION

* Advise the patient to use a warm compress, e.g. a face flannel, over the lump and massage towards the lid margin. Antibiotic ointments or drops are traditionally given (on to the eye, in the hope that they will penetrate the chalazion through the conjunctival surface) despite the lack of evidence of benefit.
* Treat secondary infection with oral antibiotics (see dacrocystitis).
* Review the patient, once recovered, and treat any blepharitis present (see above).
* Refer if a hard lump has failed to resolve after 3 months or is particularly troublesome.
* *Prevention of recurrence.* Encourage lid hygiene (see page 551).

STYES

* Treat the infected eyelash follicle with topical antibiotics.
* If there is marked swelling of the lid consider oral antibiotics.

TWITCHING

* *Mykomia.* Reassure the patient that twitching of a small area of the orbicularis muscle is common and is not sinister. It is often exacerbated by tiredness.
* *Facial twitching.* Refer to a neurologist or paediatrician.
* *Blepharospasm.* Forcible contractions of the entire orbicularis muscle should be referred to an ophthalmologist. Further investigation may be necessary (e.g. MRI scan) and botulinum toxin injections can give short-term relief.

WATERY EYE

This may result from stenosis of the nasolacrimal duct or malposition of the lid.

* Treat any infection with topical antibiotics.
* Consider a trial of artificial tears, e.g. carbomer. The patient's natural tears may be too thin and the over watering a compensation for mild soreness.

* Refer patients who are bothered by it to an ophthalmologist. They may benefit from exploration of the nasolacrimal duct or lid surgery. Massage of the lacrimal sac does not help unless there is a mucocoele.

VISUAL ACUITY TESTING

Tests of visual acuity have a reliability of 98%, but only if the following steps are taken:

(a) The Snellen chart should be the recommended distance from the patient for the size of chart used. The distance should be marked and the patient should stand behind the mark.
(b) The chart should be illuminated with 480 lux (e.g. a spotlight).

One study found that few practices fulfilled these criteria (Pandit 1994).

ACUTE DISTURBANCE OF VISION

* Establish that the loss is acute, and not just sudden awareness of a pre-existing field loss, or cataract.
* Distinguish transient from continuing visual losses and treat as appropriate. For migraine, see page 290; for TIA, see page 309.

ACUTE PAINLESS LOSS OF VISION

CENTRAL RETINAL ARTERY OCCLUSION

If seen within 24 hours

* Arrange for the patient to be seen immediately in eye casualty. If any delay is anticipated:
  (a) *Temporal arteritis.* If the history and examination suggest temporal arteritis give 200–300 mg of hydrocortisone or 500 mg of methylprednisolone by slow intravenous injection.
  (b) Give aspirin 300 mg (unless contraindicated).

If seen after 24 hours

There is no treatment for the eye and the object is to try to prevent retinal artery occlusion of the other eye.

* Refer to an ophthalmologist but less urgently.
* Give aspirin 75 mg daily.
* Take blood for an ESR. If the clinical picture suggests temporal arteritis, give steroids while awaiting the result.
* Look for evidence of more widespread cardiovascular disease especially a carotid bruit. Check blood pressure, fasting blood sugar and lipids.
* Consider the possibility that the occlusion was embolic. If so, refer to a vascular surgeon or cardiologist according to where you suspect the embolus originated.

CENTRAL OR BRANCH RETINAL VEIN OCCLUSION

Work-up:
(a) BP;
(b) FBC for polycythaemia and leukaemia;
(c) Serum lipids;
(d) Blood sugar.
* Refer to eye casualty. The patient may need photocoagulation for chronic macular oedema and ischaemia following a branch vein occlusion. Even if no treatment is available, as in central vein occlusion, complications can develop early. 50% develop neovascular glaucoma within 3 months.

VITREOUS HAEMORRHAGE

* Refer for an ophthalmological opinion within 24 hours to establish the cause of the bleeding. Retinal detachment will require surgical removal of the vitreous. Posterior vitreous detachment is self-limiting.
* Check BP, INR (if on warfarin) and fasting blood sugar.

POSTERIOR VITREOUS DETACHMENT AND RETINAL DETACHMENT

* Refer to be seen that day if a patient reports the sudden appearance of a number of floaters. Assess the visual acuity before referral. A reduced visual acuity may indicate a retinal detachment and increases the urgency.

DECREASED VISION WITH PAIN

ACUTE CLOSED ANGLE GLAUCOMA

* Suspect it when:
  - the patient is unwell, with vomiting and eye or head pain; and
  - the eye is red and tender, the cornea hazy and the pupil semi-dilated.

There may be a past history of episodes of blurred vision, associated with haloes round lights, that have been aborted by exposure to a bright light or by going to sleep. In these situations the pupil constricts, pulling the pupillary iris out of the angle.

* Refer suspected cases urgently to eye casualty or admit. If treatment is delayed adhesions may form between the iris and cornea requiring surgical drainage.
* If it is not possible to get the patient to hospital immediately give acetazolamide 500 mg i.v. and instil pilocarpine 4% into the eye.
* Treat nausea and vomiting with prochlorperazine 12.5 mg i.m.
* Do not attempt to dilate the pupil of anyone with suspected acute angle glaucoma.

OPTIC NEURITIS

● Progressive reduction in vision over a few days with pain on eye movements (classically on upgaze). Colours appear washed out. Symptoms may be worse after a hot shower or bath.
● Improvement occurs within 2 weeks and full recovery is usual within 3 months.
● Between 50 and 70% aged 20–40 with retrobulbar neuritis in the UK will develop multiple sclerosis, almost all of them within 5 years. A second episode increases that risk four-fold (Kanski 1989).
* Refer urgently patients having their first attack. Arrange for the patient to be seen again if symptoms are not improving within 2 weeks.
* Refer patients with a second attack to a neurologist because of the chance that this is multiple sclerosis.
* Treat subsequent attacks with high-dose steroids if they seemed helpful previously; only refer if the attack fails to resolve.

ACUTE DISTORTION OF VISION

* Refer urgently. Older patients may have acute wet age-related macular degeneration, especially if that diagnosis has already been made in the other eye. Typically, they report that straight lines appear crooked. If vision is still better than 6/60 they may benefit from intravenous or intraocular injections of one of the newer drugs approved by NICE, or photodynamic therapy (Wormald, Evans, Smeeth, *et al.* 2004) provided they are seen within 10 days of the onset of symptoms. The Royal College of Ophthalmologists recommends that they should undergo retinal angiography within 14 days of the onset of symptoms (Solebo, Augunawela, Dasgupta, *et al.* 2008).

FLOATERS AND FLASHES

* Refer urgently patients who report:
  (a) multiple floaters, especially if associated with flashing lights. They may have a posterior vitreous detachment, which carries a 5% chance of causing a retinal tear;
  (b) the appearance of a single large blob, which then fragments. They may have a vitreous haemorrhage.
* Be more ready to refer if:
  (a) there is a family history of retinal tear or detachment;
  (b) the other eye has already suffered a detachment. Almost a quarter of patients develop a detachment in the second eye;
  (c) the patient has high myopia;
  (d) there is a history of cataract surgery, which increases the risk of retinal detachment nine-fold.
* Refer immediately if there is a field loss or decrease in acuity. These imply that retinal detachment has occurred. It may be visible ophthalmoscopically. Instruct the patient to lie with the face on the side of the detachment (i.e. the side opposite the field defect) on the pillow, while waiting for the ambulance.

Note: Retinal tears are unlikely to be detected by conventional ophthalmoscopy. A normal fundus is therefore no grounds for inaction.

INFORMATION FOR PATIENTS WITH RETINAL DETACHMENT

Understanding Retinal Detachment. Available online from the Royal College of Ophthalmologists; www.rcophth.ac.uk/about/publications/ (choose 'Patient information')

Information for doctors

Kang HK, Luff AJ. 2008. Management of retinal detachment: a guide for non-ophthalmologists. BMJ 336, 1235–1240

HALOES

See acute angle glaucoma above.

GRADUAL LOSS OF VISION

* See if vision improves when looking through a pinhole. If it does, then a refractive error is at least part of the problem.
* Suggest the following to all patients with visual difficulty:
  (a) use adequate lighting (e.g. an angle-poise lamp), especially for reading and close work;
  (b) rearrange the room to sit with the main window behind the patient and the television away from the window.
* Recommend the '*See for yourself* leaflets' available from the RNIB at www.rnib.org.uk and search for 'Leaflets'.

CATARACTS

SYSTEMATIC REVIEWS

Management of cataract. 1996. Effective Health Care 2(3)
  Snellingen T, Evans JR, Ravilla T, Foster A. 2004. Surgical interventions for age-related cataract (Cochrane review). In: The Cochrane Library, Issue 2. John Wiley & Sons, Ltd, Chichester, UK

* *In a child*, refer as a matter of urgency. Any opacity of the ocular media can have a catastrophic effect on the development of vision and should be diagnosed and treated promptly.
* *In a young adult*. Refer but also investigate for diabetes or any other systemic disease that a clinical history might lead you to suspect.
* *In the elderly:*
  ■ Exclude diabetes.
  ■ *Refer to an optician all patients* who have not had a recent refraction. A myopic shift often accompanies the onset of cataract and a change in spectacle lenses can often postpone the need for cataract surgery.
  ■ *Refer to an ophthalmologist* if no improvement in vision is possible with refraction and:
    (a) the patient is having significant visual problems affecting quality of vision, or activities such as driving or reading; and
    (b) the patient is willing to undergo surgery. There is little point in referring those that are happy with their current level of vision and would not accept an invitation for surgery.
* When referring, include the recent report from the optician. This will reduce duplication and allow the ophthalmic department to gauge the urgency of the referral.

Note: There is no absolute Snellen acuity below which surgery is indicated. It depends on the patient's individual needs and circumstances. However, most patients are content with vision that is 6/18 or better unless they drive or do fine work. Furthermore some patients find their cataract is more disabling than would be predicted from the level of Snellen acuity. This happens for instance in cortical cataract when localized opacities scatter light, causing difficulty with reading and with glare when driving. After surgery 85–90% will achieve vision that is adequate for driving (Allen and Vasavada 2006).

PROBLEMS AFTER CATARACT SURGERY

* *A red eye following surgery* may be due to an allergy to the antibiotic and steroid drops given post-operatively. Rarely, in 0.1–0.5%, it is due to post-operative endophthalmitis. It would therefore be prudent to refer promptly any postoperative patient with a red eye especially if there is reduced vision and pain.
* *More long-term deterioration of vision after surgery:* refer the patient back. 20% develop opacification of the posterior capsule within 2 years of operation. They need laser treatment.

AGE–RELATED MACULAR DEGENERATION (AMD)

This occurs in elderly patients who present with progressive loss of central vision and, frequently, distortion effects. When looking at graph paper the squares may look distorted and the lines wavy. The vision is best in dim light. The eye appears normal except for the choroidoretinal atrophy.

* Refer all patients for specialist assessment:
  (a) to confirm the diagnosis and to assess suitability for photodynamic therapy (PDT). Refer urgently those with sudden deterioration (see page 556).
  (b) to provide low vision aids;
  (c) to consider registration as visually handicapped.
* Reassure patients that, although they have lost some of their central reading vision, they will never be completely blind, and that further deterioration will be slow. The average time it takes for vision to deteriorate to < 3/60 (eligible for blind registration) is 5–10 years.
* Encourage the patient to stop smoking. Smokers carry a three- to four-fold increased risk of age-related macular degeneration. There is evidence that stopping smoking reduces the incidence and progression of the disease (Kelly, Thornton, Lyratzopoulos, *et al.* 2004).
* *Prevention.* There is insufficient evidence to support the role of dietary antioxidants for the primary prevention of AMD (Chong, Wong, Kreis, *et al.* 2007). Furthermore, a Cochrane review urges caution in generalizing these findings to other populations and that there may be risks in taking high dose vitamins especially for smokers (increased risk of lung cancer with beta-carotene) (Evans 2004). A further meta-analysis indicates that high dose vitamin E (> 400 IU/day) is associated with a significant increase in all-cause mortality (Miller, Pastor-Barriuso, Dalal, *et al.* 2005).

CHRONIC SIMPLE GLAUCOMA

- Treatment to lower intraocular pressure has been shown to slow the progression of the disease (Wormald 2003).
- Loss of visual acuity is a late sign of chronic glaucoma. By this stage, disc cupping and field loss are likely to be advanced.
- Fundoscopy for glaucomatous cupping is the most effective single screening manoeuvre, and is easily performed by GPs. Pathological cupping is:
  (a) a pale disc with a sharp rim
  (b) oval vertically
  (c) asymmetrical
  (d) characterised by a cup:disc ratio of 1:3 or more, i.e. the wider the cup the more likely it is to be pathological
  (e) associated with angulation and nasalization of blood vessels. Haemorrhages on the optic disc are a poor prognostic sign.
- The incidence rises with age. In the UK it is 1 in 5000 at age 40–49 years, and only really rises over age 60. Over 85, it is 1 in 10.
- The risk increases:
  (a) with a family history (×10);
  (b) in high myopes (×3);
  (c) in diabetics (×3);
  (d) in African Caribbeans;
  (e) in users of topical steroid drops for over 5 days.

SCREENING AND REFERRAL

* *Family history.* Screen those with a first degree relative with glaucoma as follows, or ensure an optician screens them. They are entitled to free NHS eye tests once they are 40 years old:

(a) age 45–65: every 5 years;
(b) age 66–75: every 2 to 3 years;
(c) age 76 onwards: every 1 to 2 years.

* *Screen others over 45* every 5 years, especially those in the other high-risk groups (see above).

* Refer patients with:
  (a) intraocular pressure (IOP) ≥ 26 mmHg. However, patients with raised IOP without cupping or field loss do not necessarily have glaucoma. The majority have ocular hypertension and only develop glaucoma at the rate of 1% per year;
  (b) a normal IOP with pathological cupping or loss of visual fields. Cupping occurs with normal pressures in one fifth to one third of patients with glaucoma.

* Ensure follow-up of patients with an IOP of 22–25 mmHg but no evidence of glaucoma. They are seven times more likely to develop glaucoma than patients with lower pressures (Crick and Tuck 1995).

* *Driving.* Advise the patient to notify the DVLA, if there is significant bilateral visual field loss (Potamitis, Aggarwal, Tsaloumas, *et al.* 1994).

* Treatment is managed by the hospital eye department. It is helpful to know that the aim is to keep the pressure around 15 mmHg, using:

(a) *Prostaglandin analogues* (latanoprost, travoprost and bimatoprost) which increase aqueous outflow through the uveoscleral pathway and can reduce intraocular pressure by 30–35%. Systemic side-effects are minimal; eyelashes may lengthen and darken and light irises may permanently darken.

(b) *Beta blockers* (timolol, carteolol, betaxolol, levobunolol and metipranolol) which reduce the secretion of aqueous. They can cause systemic symptoms and may unmask latent and previously undiagnosed heart failure and airway obstruction (Kirwan, Nightingale, Bunce, *et al.* 2002). Systemic effects can be reduced by finger pressure on the caruncle or by shutting the eyes for several minutes after instilling the drops. This approach may also increase ocular absorption of the drug.

(c) *Carbonic anhydrase inhibitors* (dorzolamide, brinzolamide or oral acetazolamide) which reduce the secretion of aqueous. Oral acetazolamide is the most effective but has significant side-effects. Topical forms have few side-effects. Neither should be used in patients with sulphonamide allergy.

(d) *Parasympathomimetic drugs* (e.g. pilocarpine) which constrict the pupil and pull on the trabecular meshwork increasing the flow. Pilocarpine eye drops frequently cause headaches, but they tend to disappear after the first few weeks of use. Pilocarpine constricts the pupil and may cause blurred vision if central lens opacities are present.

ALLERGY TO DROPS

This may present with intense itching and irritation of the eyes and eyelids which is exacerbated by instillation of the drops. The allergy may be to the active drug or preservative (usually benzalkonium chloride). Stopping treatment (with monitoring of the pressure) should result in rapid improvement. Some topical agents are available in a preservative-free form.

LASER TREATMENT

(a) *Trabeculoplasty* – argon or diode 'burns' are applied to the trabecular meshwork. It is used only where the drainage angle is open, and is effective for a short term and hence used more for elderly patients.

(b) *Iridotomy* – neodymium: ytrium-aluminium-garnet (Nd:YAG) is used to cut holes in the iris in cases of angle closure glaucoma.

(c) *Iridoplasty* – argon laser burns are applied to the peripheral iris causing contraction of tissue and helps to reduce angle occlusion. Used in cases of angle closure glaucoma.

(d) *Ciliary body ablation* – usually with a diode laser to burn the ciliary body and reduce production of aqueous. The process may need to be repeated to keep the pressure low and patients normally need to continue drug treatment.

SURGICAL TREATMENT

(a) *Iridectomy* is performed for difficult or refractory cases of angle closure glaucoma.

(b) *Trabeculectomy* is the most effective glaucoma filtration procedure when medical or laser treatment has failed. A channel is created to allow flow from the anterior chamber. Once it has been performed, bacterial conjunctivitis can develop more readily into endophthalmitis.

VISUAL HANDICAP

- Over two thirds of people who are eligible are not registered as blind or partially sighted. The majority of these receive no social care services whatsoever.
- Two thirds of all people with visual impairment have an additional disability or serious health problem.
- Over 50% of visually impaired people live alone yet few have been offered any training in daily living skills. Almost half of all visually impaired people cannot cook for themselves because of hazards in the kitchen (Royal National Institute for the Blind 2002).

CERTIFICATION AND REGISTRATION

- Certification is by a consultant ophthalmologist on form CV1.
- *Blind certification* is for those with a VA below 3/60, or with a VA of up to and including 6/60 but with gross visual field restriction.
- *Certification as partially sighted* is not defined by statute. It is appropriate for patients with VA of 6/60 or worse with full visual fields, or those with a VA better than that but with restriction of visual fields. A patient with a homonymous hemianopia, for instance, is likely to be eligible.

● *Registration* is voluntary and would normally be offered at the time of certification. Registration entitles a person to a range of benefits and concessions, and help from some local voluntary groups. The receipt of a CVI by the social services department entitles that person to have his or her name added to the register. This also acts as a trigger for social services to arrange an assessment of the person's social care needs.

● Patients with low vision but not certified as blind or partially sighted should be encouraged to self refer to social services using the Low Vision Leaflet (LVL) available on www.library. nhs.uk/Eyes and search on Low Vision Leaflet.

BENEFITS

Registration means that a social worker will contact the patient and provide:

(a) access to a mobility officer, a teacher of braille, and daily living courses;

(b) free radio and cassette aids;

(c) details of the RNIB talking-book service.

In addition, the registered blind (but not necessarily the partially sighted) are eligible for:

(a) a slightly higher rate of income support;

(b) extra Housing Benefit, Income Support, and Council Tax Benefit;

(c) increased income tax allowance;

(d) reduced fares and a Blue Parking Badge;

(e) free sight tests; and

(f) reduction in the TV licence fee.

The Royal National Institute for the Blind (RNIB) provides information, support and advice for anyone with a serious sight problem, tel. 020 7388 1266; website www.rnib.org.uk; helpline 0845 766 99 99 (interpreters are available); email helpline@rnib.org. uk/Textphone users can call via Typetalk 0800 515152. Contact details for Scotland, Wales, Northern Ireland and the regions of England are given on the website

---

PRESCRIBING FOR PATIENTS WITH CONTACT LENSES (MITCHELL AND EDWARDS 2001)

Topical applications

Avoid:

(a) eye ointments;

(b) eye drops containing preservatives (in soft lenses);

(c) topical steroids;

(d) coloured drops: fluorescein and rose bengal;

(e) sympathomimetics.

Systemic drugs

Avoid:

(a) drugs that reduce or alter tear secretion: oral contraceptives, HRT, drugs with anticholinergic activity (e.g. tricyclic antidepressants, beta-blockers, diuretics, isotretinoin;

(b) drugs that reduce blinking: benzodiazepines;

(c) drugs that stain the lens: nitrofurantoin, rifampicin, sulfasalazine;

(d) drugs that are concentrated in the lens and can irritate the eye: aspirin.

PATIENT INFORMATION

The British Contact Lens Association; www.bcla.org.uk/dosanddonts.asp

---

CORRECTIVE SURGERY FOR MYOPIA

This remains a service provided by the private sector that is not regulated. While legally in the UK any registered medical practitioner may perform refractive surgery, the Royal College of Ophthalmologists recommends that it should only be performed by a fully trained ophthalmologist who has undergone additional specialist training in refractive surgery. He or she may or may not also be an NHS consultant.

∗ Advise patients to download the leaflet 'Excimer Laser Refractive Surgery' Available online from the Royal College of Ophthalmologists; www. rcophth.ac.uk/about/publications/ then go to 'Patient information'.

References

Allen, D., Vasavada, A., 2006. Cataract and surgery for cataract. BMJ 333, 128–132.

Chong, E.W.T., Wong, T.Y., Kreis, A. J., et al., 2007. Dietary antioxidants and primary prevention of age related macular degeneration: systematic review and meta-analysis. BMJ 335, 755–799.

Crick, R.P., Tuck, M.W., 1995. How can we improve the detection of glaucoma? BMJ 310, 546–547.

Curi, A., Matos, K., Pavesio, C., 2004. Acute anterior uveitis. Clin. Evid. Available: www.clinicalevidence.com.

Doona, M., Walsh, J.B., 1995. Use of chloramphenicol as topical eye medication: time to cry halt? BMJ 310, 1217–1218.

Easty, D.L., 1993. Is an eye pad needed in cases of corneal abrasion? BMJ 307, 1022.

Evans, J.R., 2004. Antioxidant vitamin and mineral supplements for age-related macular degeneration (Cochrane Review). In: The Cochrane Library, Issue 2.

Everitt, H.A., Little, P.S., Smith, P.W. F., 2006. A randomised controlled trial of management strategies for acute infective conjunctivitis in general practice. BMJ 333, 321–324.

Guidelines on the Management of Communicable Diseases in Schools and Nurseries, 2008. Health Protection Agency. http://www.hpa.org.uk (search for 'schools').

Kanski, J.J., 1989. Clinical Ophthalmology, 2nd ed. Butterworths, London.

Kelly, S., Thornton, J., Lyratzopoulos, G., et al., 2004. Smoking and blindness. BMJ 328, 537–538.

Kirwan, J.F., Nightingale, J.A., Bunce, C., et al., 2002. β Blockers for glaucoma and excess risk of airways obstruction: population based cohort study. BMJ 325, 1396–1397.

Lancaster, T., Swart, A.M., Jick, H., 1998. Risk of serious haematological toxicity with use of chloramphenicol eye drops in a British general practice database. BMJ 316, 667.

Miller, E.R., Pastor-Barriuso, R., Dalal, D., et al., 2005. Meta-analysis: high-dosage vitamin E supplementation may increase all-cause mortality. Ann. Intern. Med. 42, 37–47.

Mitchell, R., Edwards, R., 2001. Prescribing for patients who wear contact lenses. Prescriber July, 40–44.

Opstelten, W., Zall, M.J.W., 2005. Managing ophthalmic herpes zoster in primary care. BMJ 331, 147–151.

Pandit, J.C., 1994. Testing acuity of vision in general practice: reaching recommended standard. BMJ 309, 1408.

Potamitis, T., Aggarwal, R.K., Tsaloumas, M., et al., 1994. Driving, glaucoma and the law. BMJ 309, 1057–1058.

Rietveld, R.P., van Weert, H.C., ter Riet, G., et al., 2003. Diagnostic impact of signs and symptoms in acute infectious conjunctivitis: systematic literature search. BMJ 327, 789.

Royal National Institute for the Blind, 2002. Progress in sight: national standards of social care for visually impaired adults. Available on www.rnib.org.uk. Search for 'Social services'.

Sheikh, A., Hurwitz, B., 2005. Topical antibiotics for bacterial conjunctivitis: Cochrane systematic review and meta-analysis update. Br. J. Gen. Pract. 55, 962–964.

Smith, J., 2004. Bacterial conjunctivitis. Clinical Evidence Available: www.clinicalevidence.com.

Solebo, A.L., Augunawela, R.I., Dasgupta, S., et al., 2008. Recent advances in the treatment of age-related macular degeneration. Br. J. Gen. Pract. 58, 309–310.

Weaver, C.S., Terrell, K.M., 2003. Do ophthalmic nonsteroidal anti-inflammatory drugs reduce the pain associated with simple corneal abrasion without delaying healing? Ann. Emerg. Med. 41, 134–140.

Wormald, R., 2003. Treatment of raised intraocular pressure and prevention of glaucoma. BMJ 326, 723–724.

Wormald, R., Evans, J., Smeeth, L., et al., 2004. Photodynamic therapy for neovascular age-related macular degeneration (Cochrane review). In: The Cochrane Library, Issue 2.

Chapter 22

Skin problems

CHAPTER CONTENTS

ECZEMA AND DERMATITIS

SYSTEMATIC REVIEWS

Smethurst D, Macfarlane S. 2004. Atopic eczema. *Clinical Evidence*. BMJ Publishing Group, London. Available: www.clinicalevidence.org
   Brown S, Reynolds NJ. 2006. Atopic and non-atopic eczema. BMJ 332, 584–588

Guideline

Primary Care Dermatology Society & British Association of Dermatologists. 2006. Guidelines for the Management of Atopic Eczema. Available: www. library.nhs.uk

- The rash of acute eczema is weepy and excoriated, with indistinct margins. In atopic eczema the distribution is symmetrical and can be widespread. It has a predilection for the flexures of the elbows and knees, plus the face in infants.

- Acute dermatitis from contact with irritants is initially confined to the area in contact with the offending agents, but can spread to adjacent areas.
- Chronic dermatitis presents as thickened, erythematous scaling skin. Both the acute and chronic forms are itchy. Scratch marks can be a prominent feature of the clinical appearance, as can lichen planus (see below).
- Either type of rash can occur in sun exposed skin when certain drugs have been taken (e.g. thiazide diuretics, allopurinol).
- Other body systems may be involved, particularly the respiratory system (hay fever and asthma) and the gut in infants (cow's milk allergy).
- Intrinsic predisposing factors include varicose veins (where stasis in the lower limb may cause accumulation of waste products).
- Persistent environmental provocation – particularly to chemicals at work and home – can cause dermatitis. Organic chemicals such as petroleum products, soaps and detergents are common culprits, as are metals (especially nickel, the metal used in much jewellery).

MANAGEMENT

- Controlled studies support the efficacy of topical steroids as the primary treatment of atopic eczema. Use no more frequently than twice daily (NICE 2004a).
- Evidence for the use of emollients is less strong; they have rarely been subjected to rigorous trials (Hoare, Li Wan Po and Williams 2000).
- There is insufficient evidence to recommend evening primrose oil (Hoare, Li Wan Po and Williams 2000). Evidence for many other interventions is poor.
- Find out how the eczema affects the patient's life. Over 50% of eczema sufferers feel that the eczema interferes with their life.
- Explain the nature of the condition and establish the patient's expectations. A complete cure is not realistic, but treatment should give good control and an acceptable quality of life.

60% of children with atopic eczema have grown out of it by adolescence (Williams and Wuthrich 2000).

- Stress the importance of the correct use of emollients or topical steroids. Explain that the dangers of topical steroids are associated with the potent and very potent preparations and, especially, with their prolonged use.
- Advise the patient to return if control deteriorates.
- Find out if there are trigger factors that can be avoided: wool, heat, cold, exercise, preparations containing lanolin, and emotion.
- For the management of hand dermatitis, see below.

EMOLLIENTS

- Explain that emollients (e.g. white soft paraffin, aqueous cream) work by providing a lipid film on the skin, which slows the water loss from it. The most effective time to apply them is after a bath, when the water content of the skin is greatest. They can also be applied at any time. Urea cream works by helping water bind to the skin, and can also be applied at any time.
- Encourage the patient to apply emollients as freely as possible and as frequently as reasonable. A child with widespread eczema will need at least 250 g/week and an adult 500 g/week. The quantity of emollient used should be > 10 times that of topical steroid.
- Use the oiliest preparation that the patient can tolerate. The patient may need one preparation for the body and a less oily one for the hands and face. Preparations with high oil content are not well tolerated in hot, humid climates.
- *Itch.* Consider using preparations with urea or lauromacrogols.
- The patient should use a bath oil and not soap. Soap further depletes the stratum corneum of the lipids that maintain its integrity.
- Consider the use of twice weekly fluticasone 0.05% cream or 0.005% ointment, in addition to emollients, in those prone to frequent relapses. It has been shown to almost triple the time to the next relapse (Berth-Jones, Damstra, Golsch, *et al.* 2003).

TOPICAL STEROIDS

- *Safety*. Hydrocortisone 1% (cream or, preferably, ointment) is safe for all ages and at all sites bar one: the sole exception is the eyelid, where prolonged use may cause glaucoma. Potent preparations should not be prescribed for children, nor for flexures or the face. Their use should be restricted in sites prone to striae; the breasts, abdomen, upper arms and thighs.
- *Rates of absorption* vary according to site: scrotal skin absorbs 40 times more than the palm, with the forehead, axilla, and back absorbing six times, four times and twice as much, respectively.
- *Steroid strength*. More potent steroids should be used as a course of treatment to cope with an exacerbation, rather than as maintenance (see also Infection, below). Once the exacerbation has settled, either:
  - (a) revert to the weakest available steroid, applied just frequently enough to maintain remission. Once daily is often enough; or
  - (b) use a moderately potent steroid intermittently (e.g. twice a week) (Atherton 2003).
- * *Prescribe enough:* to cover the hands twice daily for a month, an adult needs at least 60 g. To cover the trunk or both legs for the same time, 400 g (BNF 2001).
- * *Prescribe within the following maximums:* moderately potent, 100 g/week; potent, 50 g/week; very potent, 25 g/week.
- * *Base*. Use ointments and not creams, except where the patient cannot tolerate the greasiness of ointments. In that case, use an ambiphylic cream such as Locoid Lipocream.
- * *Pompholyx* is relatively resistant to steroids. Use a potent or very potent steroid. Consider occlusion with plastic gloves or bags.
- * *The face*. Restrict steroids to 1% hydrocortisone. Stronger preparations may cause telangiectasia.

Amounts. Patients need to be told how much cream or ointment to apply. Explain the concept of the fingertip unit (FTU); the amount of cream or ointment that covers the finger from tip to distal crease. 1 FTU (=0.5 g) should cover an area equivalent to the palms of two adult hands.

ACUTE EXACERBATIONS

- *Infection* is often the cause of an exacerbation, whether or not there is clinical evidence of it. S. *aureus* is the most frequent pathogen, colonizing 80% of patients with eczema. S. *aureus* may act as an antigen to exacerbate the allergic reaction Use oral antibiotics, e.g. erythromycin or flucloxacillin. Continue them until the exacerbation is over.
- *Herpes simplex*. Discuss with a dermatologist or arrange for the patient to be seen urgently.
- *Excoriations:*
  - (a) Paste bandages are helpful in excoriated or lichenified eczema. Tar bandages are most effective and messiest; ichthammol, or zinc and calamine, may be more acceptable. Bandages can be put on at night on top of steroid ointment. In children they prevent scratching.
  - (b) Gloves may need to be worn in bed as well.
  - (c) 'Wet wrapping' may be helpful. Soak a tubigrip bandage or tubular gauze dressing in emollient, apply it over the eczema, and cover it with a dry bandage.
- *Steroids*. Use a short course of increased strength, as above. If the skin is moist, use a cream rather than an ointment, to permit evaporation.

SECOND LINE TREATMENTS

Antihistamines

Sedative antihistamines will help children sleep, but they have no specific effect on itch (Hoare, Li Wan Po and Williams 2000). If using an antihistamine for sedation, use the highest recommended doses; lower doses often stimulate them. If going above the recommended doses, increase to that level slowly. Regular use leads to tolerance. Use on alternate nights, or use for 2 weeks and then omit for 2 weeks.

Exclusion diets

These may help a small number of children, although what studies there are have failed to show benefit (Charman 2001). Foods commonly implicated are milk, eggs, citrus fruits, colourings, preservatives, nuts, fish, wheat, tomatoes, lamb, chicken and soya. If undertaken at all, an exclusion diet must be conducted under the supervision of a dietician to avoid malnutrition.

House dust mite

Controlling the house dust mite may improve eczema but the reduction in dust levels must be extreme, with synthetic mattress covers, spraying and high filtration vacuuming (Berth-Jones, Damstra, Golsch, *et al.* 2003).

Oral steroids

Oral corticosteroids can be used as rescue therapy while waiting for an urgent consultant opinion. Patients should not be maintained on steroids or courses of steroids for prolonged periods.

Steroid sparing agents

Tacrolimus, a topical immunomodulator, can be used as a steroid sparing agent in moderate to severe cases, or as alternative treatment where the eczema is resistant to steroids. The treatment effect is similar to moderately potent or potent steroids. There is no evidence for its use in children (NICE 2004b). Long-term side-effects are unknown, and there is a theoretical risk of promotion of malignancy, of which the patient should be warned. NICE recommends that, in the UK, it should only be initiated by a physician (including GPs) with a special interest in dermatology. It should not be used in the presence of herpes simplex and patients prone to herpes should be advised about photoprotection. Pimecrolimus is not considered a cost-effective alternative compared with topical steroids (NICE 2004b). However, it is considered clinically effective for children aged 2–16 as second line treatment of moderate atopic eczema on the face and neck that has not been controlled by topical steroids where there is a serious risk of important adverse effects from further topical steroid use. In the UK pimecrolimus, like tacrolimus, should only be initiated by doctors with a special interest and experience in dermatology.

REFERRAL

Refer patients when:

(a) the diagnosis is uncertain;
(b) there is failure to respond to mildly potent steroids in children;
(c) there is failure to respond to potent steroids in adults, or where regular courses of these steroids are needed;
(d) when specialist assistance would be valuable in counselling patients and the family;
(e) for confirmation of contact allergy where job or lifestyle is at stake;
(f) there is a severe acute exacerbation;
(g) there is bacterial infection that has not responded to a course of oral antibiotics;
(h) there is eczema herpeticum.

HAND ECZEMA/DERMATITIS

- The commonest forms of hand eczema/dermatitis are:
  (a) *Irritant contact dermatitis.* This is common in people where repeated washing or wetting and drying of the hands is essential and those who come into contact with chemicals. There may be dryness and chapping with painful cracks and fissures, particularly over the joints. It may progress to a dry shiny skin that splits easily or to acute inflammation with vesicular eruption and possibly secondary infection.
  (b) *Atopic hand dermatitis.* This is more common in people with a history of atopic dermatitis. There may be chapping and irritation of the backs of the hands with later development of eczematous dermatitis: erythema, oedema, crusting scaling and lichenification of the skin
  (c) *Allergic contact dermatitis.* Important contact allergens may be revealed by patch testing and indicated by profession. There may be obvious areas of inflammation related to contact but commonly is indistinguishable from other features of hand eczema.
- The common contact allergens are:
  (a) Nickel – door knobs, handles, scissors, knitting needles, industrial and hairdressing equipment.
  (b) Potassium dichromate- cement, leather articles, industrial machines, oils.
  (c) Balsam of Peru – (sticky vanilla/cinnamon smelling aromatic bark extract) present in many perfumes, creams and food flavourings.
  (d) Colophony (Rosin) – (sticky coniferous sap) present in a number of household products, medications and adhesives.

* General advice:
  (a) Wash hands as infrequently as possible. Use emulsifying ointment not soap but if soap is used, use sparingly. Thoroughly rinse and dry the hands.
  (b) Apply emollients after hand washing.
  (c) Apply water impermeable barrier creams twice a day.
  (d) Avoid contact if possible with possible triggers (e.g. cleaners, fruits, shampoo).
  (e) Where contact is unavoidable wear gloves to suit the need – cotton, vinyl, rubber with cotton liners.
  (f) Remain vigilant after the episode subsides. The skin remains sensitive for many months.
* Prescribe moderately strong steroid ointments, to be used twice daily. Occlusive dressings are commonly used.
* Consider applying 'wet wraps' (wet cotton gauze) for 30 minutes at a time if the inflammation is marked.
* Treat infection if present.
* Refer all those not responding to a dermatologist for patch testing.
* Refer urgently all patients with severe dermatitis. If there is likely to be a delay consider treating with a course of oral steroids.

PATIENT ORGANIZATIONS

The National Eczema Society, Hill House, Highgate Hill, London N19 5NA, tel. 020 7281 3553; helpline 0800 0891122 (Mon to Fri 8.00 am – 8.00 pm), www.eczema.org
   Eczema Association of Australia Inc., PO Box 1784 DC, Cleveland, Queensland, 4163, tel. 07 3206 3633; www.eczema.org.au

---

SEBORRHOEIC ECZEMA AND DANDRUFF

INFANTS

Reassure the parents that the majority of children are better by the age of 1 year.

* *Cradle cap*. Advise the parent to soften skin scales with arachis or olive oil and gently scrape them off.
* Use emollients freely, and mild steroids if erythema is marked (but not on the face).

ADULTS

* Use emollients.
* Treat with topical hydrocortisone 1% for 4–6 weeks. If there is no improvement, treat with ketoconazole cream twice daily for 4 weeks.
* *Scalp*. Treat with selenium sulphide shampoo or ketoconazole shampoo twice weekly for 2–4 weeks.

If available, use lithium gluconate ointment which is more effective than ketaconazole shampoo (Dreno, Chosidow, Revuz, *et al.* 2003).

ACNE

GUIDELINE

MeReC. 1999. The treatment of acne vulgaris: an update. MeReC Bulletin 10(8), 29–32

Review

Purdy S, de Berker D. 2006. Acne. BMJ 333, 949–953

---

* Explain to the patient what is known about the aetiology of the condition:
  (a) an increase in sebum production;
  (b) keratinization of the follicle, resulting in lesions that are not inflamed (blackheads, whiteheads);
  (c) colonization of the pilosebaceous unit with *Propionibacterium acnes*;
  (d) development of inflammation.
* Explain to the patient that the aims of treatment are to:
  (a) prevent scarring, by reducing non-inflammatory and inflammatory lesions;
  (b) reduce the unsightly appearance of the disease; and so
  (c) reduce the psychological stress and social morbidity.
* Explain that the treatment may take several months to work, and that the patient should re-attend until the condition is satisfactory. Encouragement is important. In one study, 80 out of 120 patients admitted they were non-compliant at 3 months (Adami, Inglott, Azzopardi, *et al.* 1998).

* Explain that treatment is to prevent new spots, not to get rid of the spots that already there. Topical treatment must therefore be applied to the whole area at risk, not just to spots that are present.

* Assess the type of acne and treat accordingly:

    (a) *Comedone-dominated acne* is best managed by keratolytic activities such as frequent washing (but not scrubbing, which can increase the inflammation; Leyden 1997), plus topical retinoid, salicylic acid or azelaic acid. Sunlight is effective, but increases the risk of skin cancer in later life. It is a hazard in combination with a retinoid which causes photosensitivity.

    (b) *Pus-dominated acne* responds to benzoyl peroxide, topical or oral antibiotics, and topical or oral retinoids. Sometimes patients must take them for many months to maintain a remission.

DETAILS OF TREATMENT

* Benzoyl peroxide:
    (a) start at a low strength, i.e. 2.5%, and apply at night;
    (b) warn the patient that mild erythema and transient skin irritation are common, and that it may bleach clothes;
    (c) increase the strength gradually to 10% at 2-weekly intervals, but stop at any stage if irritation occurs.

* *Topical antibiotics* work by reducing *P. acnes*. They are no more effective than benzoyl peroxide or tretinoin, but cause less skin irritation (MeReC 1994). Topical tetracycline is the cheapest, but patients who frequent clubs should know that it will fluoresce under ultraviolet light.

* *Azelaic acid cream* is keratolytic, alters the fatty composition of skin lipids and reduces bacterial concentrations. It avoids the problem of bacterial resistance, but can cause local irritation and photosensitization. Use it daily for 1 week then twice a day for at least 8 weeks, but for no more than 6 months (DTB 1993).

* *Reducing inflammation.* Consider nicotinamide (vitamin B$_3$) gel or adapalene gel (a retinoid-like drug) to reduce inflammation.

* *Topical retinoids:*
    (a) start at a low strength (0.025%) every other night. Warn the patient to expect redness and scaling. When it is clear that it is tolerated, increase to nightly, then b.d., then slowly increase the strength of the preparation until a response is seen.
    (b) use the cream on dry and fair skin, the gel on dark and oily skin, especially in severe acne, and the lotion for large areas such as the back;
    (c) avoid direct sunlight and UV lamps. Do not use in pregnancy.

* *Oral antibiotics* may be added to benzoyl peroxide or retinoids, but to reduce the risk of resistance, should not be combined with a different topical antibiotic. Indeed the increasing antibiotic resistance developed by *Proprionibacterium acnes* has moved opinion away from the routine use of oral antibiotics in maintenance (Garner, Eady and Avery 2002).

    (a) Use oxytetracycline 500 mg b.d. or 1 g daily, for 3 months in the first instance.
    (b) Warn the patient that:
        ■ improvement is unlikely before 6 weeks, and it continues for 6 months;
        ■ strict compliance is essential;
        ■ it must be taken at least half an hour before food and, especially, not taken with milk.
    (c) If effective, decrease to 500 mg daily then 250 mg daily, at 3-monthly intervals.
    (d) Reassess 6-monthly whether to stop for 2 months to see if the problem has resolved. If the condition recurs, restart the original antibiotic.
    (e) If a patient responds initially and then worsens, bacteria may have developed resistance. Change to another antibiotic or to a topical alternative. Alternative oral antibiotics are trimethoprim 100–200 mg b.d or doxycyline 100 mg daily. Because of fears of hepatitis and pneumonitis, minocyline should be reserved for when other antibiotics have failed. Even then there is no evidence that it is better than other antibiotics (Garner, Eady, Popescu, *et al.* 2002).

REFERRAL

✱ Refer patients with:

(a) severe acne and acne still failing to respond;

(b) acne cysts, for consideration of intralesional steroid injections;

(c) psychological distress despite full primary care management.

Treatment options include isotretinoin, UV therapy, and high-dose antibiotics. Isotretinoin, while extremely effective, is very expensive, is teratogenic and often causes cracking of the lips and facial dermatitis. It has been linked with depression and suicide (Wysowski, Pitts and Beitz 2001). Close and expert monitoring is essential.

HORMONAL TREATMENT IN WOMEN

✱ Women with acne not on an combined oral contraceptive may benefit from commencing any preparation (Arowojolu, Gallo, Grimes, *et al.* 2004). Preparations utilizing cyproterone acetate as the progestogen (co-cyprindiol) perform more effectively to reduce acne than other preparations, but carry an increased risk of venous thromboembolism. If using co-cyprindiol, note:

(a) it is not licensed as a contraceptive but is effective as such;

(b) if applicable, write 'for contraceptive use' on the prescription to avoid a prescription charge;

(c) treatment is necessary for several months before benefit is seen.

✱ Consider changing women who are on combined oral contraceptives with progestogens that may aggravate acne (i.e. those containing norethisterone or levonorgestrel) to one containing a less androgenic preparation, e.g. desogestrel, gestodene or norgestimate. They too should be counselled about the risks of thrombosis (see pages 349, 351).

(see pages 349, 351).

SELF-HELP GROUP

Acne Support Group, Howard House, The Runway, South Ruislip, Middlesex HA4 6SE. Tel. 0208 841 4747. www.m2w3.com/acne

ACNE ROSACEA

● This eruption occurs on the face in the middle aged. Some patients report persistence of a flushing tendency that they had in their youth.

● The redness is often inflamed and is accompanied by dilated blood vessels.

● There is often hypertrophy of the skin adnexae. The sebaceous glands may form rhinophyma or 'strawberry' nose.

● Eye involvement occurs in more than half of those with rosacea, ranging from dry gritty eyes to blepharitis, episcleritis and, in 5%, keratitis.

MANAGEMENT

● Use topical azelaic acid (administered in the same way as for acne, see above). Improvement continues for up to 15 weeks (Elewski, Fleischer and Pariser 2003). Topical metronidazole, and tetracyclines orally or topically are also affective (van Zuuren, Graber, Hollis, *et al.* 2003).

● Steroids may produce apparent initial response, but rebound erythema can occur after cessation. Hence, this form of treatment should be avoided.

✱ Explain that it should be possible to get rid of the papules and pustules, but often the erythema and telangiectasia remain.

✱ Encourage the patient to avoid triggers if possible, e.g. caffeine, alcohol, temperature changes, sunlight.

✱ *Burning.* Prescribe emollients to reduce the burning sensation.

✱ *Oral antibiotics.* Long-term oxytetracycline is extremely effective. Start with 500 mg b.d. or 1 g daily for 2 months. Half or a quarter of this dose is often sufficient for maintenance.

✱ *Topical antibiotics.* Topical metronidazole is as effective as oral tetracycline, but much more expensive. Topical clindamycin has been shown to be effective, but is not currently licensed for use in this condition.

PSORIASIS

REVIEW

Naldi L, Rzany B. 2004. Chronic plaque psoriasis. *Clinical Evidence*, Issue 4. London: BMJ Publishing Group. (Search data Jan 2003.) Available: www.clinicalevidence.org

Guideline

Psoriasis – General Management. 2006. British Association of Dermatologists, London. Available: www.bad.org.uk

- The characteristic lesion of psoriasis is a thickened plaque of skin that may include prominent scale. If scale is not present, the lesions are thickened and shiny, and have a well-demarcated edge.
- The lesions present in a wide variety of locations. Most common is the presence of large plaques over the extensor aspects of the elbows and knees, and in large areas of the scalp. Large plaques can occur virtually anywhere in the body, except the face. Smaller lesions can occur over virtually any body surface except the face.
- If lesions occur as multiple lesions, it is called *guttate* (drop-like) *psoriasis*. Plaques of psoriasis can recur in areas of previous skin trauma (the *Koebner phenomenon*). *Pustular psoriasis* is a form with small sterile pustules within the plaques.

ASSESSMENT

* Look for systemic disease, notably inflammatory arthritis. The small joints of the hands are most commonly involved. However, other larger joints (singly or symmetrical), and the spine can be affected. Psoriasis is commonly associated with nail pitting.
* Consider the presence of trigger factors, notably trauma, beta-haemolytic streptococcal sore throat, some drugs (beta-blockers, antimalarials and lithium), and emotional upset.

MANAGEMENT

- Emollients and coal tar preparations reduce psoriatic activity.

- Topical steroids improve psoriasis in the short term. These need to be fluorinated steroids, e.g. 0.05% betamethasone valerate used twice daily. In the longer term, while there is a trade-off between benefit and harm, steroids can reduce or nearly eliminate psoriasis in 60% compared to 20% with placebo.
- Other agents which can be used include calcipotriol (44% improvement), topical retinoids (tazarotene), dithranol, methotrexate, ciclosporin, phototherapy and psoralens with UVA (PUVA). Each has either short-term difficulties or long-term harms that may limit their usefulness (Table 22.1).

Patients with mild to moderate psoriasis can usually be managed in primary care, although the patient may appreciate a single specialist appointment to discuss the condition. Do not delay treatment while waiting for a dermatological opinion.

* *Explain* that psoriasis is common, that it is likely to be chronic with remissions and relapses, that it is not contagious and that the intensity of the treatment will depend on how hard the patient wants to work at it.
* Look out for the psychological impact the psoriasis is having and refer for counselling those not coping well.

Table 22.1	Potential harms in selected treatments for psoriasis known to confer benefits
TREATMENT	**POTENTIAL HARM**
Steroids	Skin atrophy, striae, telangiectasia, adrenocortical suppression
Emollients	Local irritation and contact dermatitis
Coal tar preparations	Local irritation and contact dermatitis
Dithranol	Smell, staining and local burning
Topical calcipotriol	Perilesional irritation
Oral retinoids	Mucocutaneous effects: skin dryness, cheilosis, conjunctivitis
	Low grade hepatotoxicity (1%), spinal ligament thickening, teratogenicity
Phototherapy	Photo-ageing, increased skin cancer risk
PUVA	Increased skin cancer risk
Methotrexate	Dose-related myelosuppression, liver fibrosis and pulmonary toxicity
Ciclosporin (oral)	Renal dysfunction, hypertension
Ciclosporin (topical)	Possibly neither renal dysfunction nor hypertension

* *Prescribe the following general measures* for all patients who want treatment, regardless of what other treatment they are using:

(a) a soap substitute, e.g. aqueous cream; and

(b) a tar-based bath additive, e.g. coal tar solution BP; and

(c) an emollient to be used after bathing. Use the oiliest preparation that can be tolerated. This usually means using an oily preparation, e.g. emulsifying ointment, for the body and a cream, e.g. aqueous cream, for the hands and face.

Prescribe enough. A patient with widespread psoriasis may need 500 g of emollient per week.

LOCALIZED PLAQUE PSORIASIS

* Warn the patient that no benefit will be seen for at least 3 weeks.

* Choose between:

(a) *A vitamin D analogue*, e.g. calcipotriol or tacalcitol. They are easier to use than tar or dithranol but more expensive. They do not stain but, like dithranol, cannot be used on the face or flexures. Observe the maximum total dose of each drug, e.g. calcipotriol 100 g/week, to avoid hypercalcaemia.

(b) *A tar-based cream.* Small plaques may respond to a 1–5% proprietary coal tar preparation once or twice a day but large thick plaques need a strong coal tar dressing, e.g. 7.5% coal tar paste BP, covered with a dressing. Few patients are prepared to tolerate this when there are other more effective and convenient treatments.

(c) *A tar and steroid mixture.* This is a halfway house, which attempts to reap the benefits of tar and steroids while using low strengths of both in order to reduce adverse effects. It may suit some patients with mild psoriasis.

(d) *Short-contact dithranol.* This is more effective than coal tar, but harder work. Start at 0.1% for creams and 0.5% for wax sticks. Apply daily for 30 minutes, then wash off and apply an emollient to stop the skin drying out. Longer contact is no more effective. Increase the strength by doubling it weekly, up to 2%, provided 'burning' does not occur. If there is burning omit the dithranol for a few days, use emollients until the erythema subsides, then restart dithranol.

Warnings:

■ Do not apply to sensitive skin, e.g. the flexures or the face, and avoid putting it on normal skin around the plaques;

■ It stains! Rinse it off the skin, and the bath, afterwards and wear an old dressing gown during the 30 minutes that the dithranol is applied. Wash hands at the end of each day's treatment.

(e) *A topical retinoid*, e.g. tazarotene. Irritation is common but can be reduced if care is taken not to get it on normal skin.

(f) *A topical steroid.* This is the first-line treatment for the face or flexures. Use 1% hydrocortisone on the face but use a moderately potent steroid elsewhere, e.g. 0.025% betamethasone valerate. Other than the face and flexures, steroids are not first line because of the problems of rebound exacerbation and skin thinning (see box below). Restrict use to 100 g/month and impose regular breaks from use (see box).

(g) Tacrolimus ointment, although not licensed. is helpful in flexural psoriasis, although not in the treatment of plaques.

GUIDELINES FOR THE USE OF TOPICAL STEROIDS IN PSORIASIS

From: Greaves 1997.

■ Do not use steroids for more than 4 weeks without review.

■ Do not use potent steroids regularly for ≥ 7 days.

■ Do not give repeat prescriptions without review.

■ Do not give ≥ 100 g per month of a moderately potent steroid.

■ Try to rotate steroids with alternative treatments.

■ Only use potent or very potent steroids under specialist supervision.

WIDESPREAD PLAQUE PSORIASIS

* Refer. Systemic treatment will probably be needed.

SCALP PSORIASIS

* Shampoo daily with a tar shampoo, e.g. Polytar.

* *Exacerbations.* Continue coal tar shampoo and also apply a daily steroid scalp application or calcipotriol scalp solution twice a day (but not prior to shampooing). Diprosalic scalp application has the advantage of combining a steroid with salicylic acid, which helps get rid of scale.

* *Severe crusting.* Use a coconut oil compound (Cocois) every night, washed out with a tar shampoo in the morning. It is messy and smelly, will need to be covered with a shower cap to avoid staining the pillow, and should be reduced to twice weekly applications as soon as a response is achieved.

THE HAIRLINE

* Use a moderately potent, or even a potent steroid cream, with a warning that it must not be used on the face.

SOLES AND PALMS

* Use a potent steroid ointment possibly combined with salicylic acid, e.g. Diprosalic ointment. Response is likely to be poor.
* Consider a course of oral tetracycline.

GUTTATE PSORIASIS

Guttate psoriasis should resolve in a few months without treatment. If treatment is needed:

* Use an emollient for dryness.
* Use a mild tar and steroid cream or calcipotriol to suppress the lesions if the patient prefers a more active approach.
* Refer early for phototherapy if the psoriasis is widespread and troubles the patient.

REFERRAL

Refer when:

(a) the diagnosis is uncertain;
(b) the psoriasis is severe;
(c) the psoriasis fails to respond to the above treatments;
(d) the patient needs increasing amounts or strengths of topical steroids;
(e) the psoriasis affects sites which are difficult to treat e.g. face, palms, soles, genitalia;
(f) the patient needs more intensive education or counselling than is possible in primary care;

(g) there is psoriatic arthropathy;
(h) there is widespread guttate psoriasis;
(i) there is generalized pustular or erythrodermic psoriasis. Referral is urgent: it may be life-threatening. It is especially likely to occur if potent steroids are used and then withdrawn.

PATIENT GROUPS

Australia: Psoriasis Association Inc. 16 Musgrave Street, Kirra, Queensland 4225, tel. 61 7 5599 1166 or email info@psoriasis.org.au. Website: www.psoriasis.org.au

New Zealand: Psoriasis Association of New Zealand Inc. PO Box 44007, Lower Hutt, Wellington 6315. Tel. (04) 568 7139. Email psoriasis@xtra.co.nz Available: www.everybody.co.nz/support/psoriasis.html

UK: Psoriasis Association. Dick Coles House, 2 Queensbridge, Northampton NN4 7BF. Tel. 0845 676 0076. www.psoriasis-association.org.uk

Patient literature

British Association of Dermatologists. *Psoriasis – An Overview and Topical Treatment for Psoriasis.* Available: www.bad.org.uk

SKIN INFECTIONS

VIRAL INFECTIONS

WARTS (OTHER THAN GENITAL WARTS)

SYSTEMATIC REVIEWS

Gibbs S, Harvey I, Sterling JC, Stark R. 2006. Local treatments for cutaneous warts. The Cochrane Database of Systematic Reviews, Issue 3. Art. No.: CD001781. DOI: 10.1002/14651858.CD001781.

DTB. 1998. Tackling warts on the hands and feet. Drug Ther Bull 36, 22–24

● Human papilloma virus (HPV) causes a wide range of different lesions, from cauliflower-like lesions to flat mosaic lesions. Many wart infections are completely asymptomatic, yet shed virus to transmit them.

- Genital warts are of greatest concern because they are associated with malignancy, particularly some subtypes with cervical cancer.
- Warts will probably always remit spontaneously but the time to remission may be very variable.
- First-line topical treatment remains salicylic acid or lactic acid (e.g. 17% lactic acid and 17% salicylic acid in collodion). Between 67% and 84% of warts are cleared by 3 months of daily treatment (DTB 1998a).
- Duct tape occlusion for up to 2 months has been shown to be more effective than cryotherapy (Focht III, Spicer and Fairchok 2002). In that study three quarters of those to which duct tape was applied had resolved in 4 weeks.
- Surgical treatment includes a wide range of destructive methods, including cryotherapy, cautery, laser treatment, and excision. They may be no more effective than chemical methods.
- There is not enough evidence to establish whether any one is superior to another (either in establishing cure or reducing the chance of recurrence, which ranges from 5–35%), or that treatment reduces infectivity (among genital warts).
- * If the patient is not troubled by the wart, suggest that it is left alone. The majority will disappear spontaneously as immunity is gained. However, if the patient elects for treatment, explain that either the patient can occlude the wart with duct tape, or a topical agent can be applied. The wart must be rubbed down with an emery board before the application. Pare down thick warts with a scalpel in the surgery.
- * Choose agents from the following groups. Explain that 3 months treatment may be needed and that the agent should not touch normal skin.
  - (a) salicylic acid for a wart anywhere except on the face;
  - (b) podophyllin, glutaraldehyde or formalin for plantar warts.
  - * Plantar warts. Prescribe a salicylic acid gel for children who wish to use swimming pools, and give them a note to confirm that they do not need a verruca sock.
  - * Filiform warts. Curette them under local anaesthetic.
  - * Plane warts should be left to resolve spontaneously.

- * Surgery. Warts not responding to treatment after 3 months, or those that are a particular nuisance, are candidates for freezing or curettage and cautery. Children under 10 tolerate these procedures badly.

REFERRAL

Refer:

(a) if the diagnosis is uncertain, especially if sites other than hands, feet or face are affected;

(b) if the patient is immunosuppressed;

(c) when there is a sudden widespread eruption of warts. Malignancy or immunodeficiency may be the cause;

(d) warts that have failed to clear after 3 months intensive topical treatment;

(e) facial warts if cryotherapy is not available.

HERPES SIMPLEX LABIALIS

SYSTEMATIC REVIEW

Worrall G. 2006. Herpes labialis. *Clinical Evidence*, October. Available: www.clinicalevidence.com

- Topical aciclovir appears to speed resolution, with agents in a lipophilic base more effective than those of a hydrophilic base. The evidence is better for recurrent than first attacks. Application has to commence immediately symptoms appear to achieve any effect.
- Oral aciclovir (200 mg five times daily for 10 days), valaciclovir (500 mg three times daily for 7 days) and famciclovir (250 mg three times daily for 7 days) similarly reduce the duration of the disease.
- Topical local anaesthetic cream (e.g. Xylocaine gel) may ease the pain.
- There is some evidence that a course of oral aciclovir or famciclovir before exposure to intense UV light reduces the incidence and duration of attacks. Sunscreen prophylaxis similarly reduces the risk of attacks.

HERPES ZOSTER

SYSTEMATIC REVIEWS

Lancaster T, Silagy C, Gray S. 1995. Primary care management of acute herpes zoster: systematic review of evidence from randomized controlled trials. Br J Gen Pract 45, 39–45

Yaphe J, Lancaster T. 2001. Postherpetic neuralgia. *Clinical Evidence*, Issue 5. BMJ Publishing Group, London. Available: www.clinicalevidence.org

- The prevention of post-herpetic neuralgia (PHN) and the prompt treatment of ophthalmic zoster (see page 553) are the most important issues. PHN follows shingles in 50% of patients aged over 60 and 75% of patients over 70, of whom half will still be suffering 1 year later (Bandolier 1995).

- Oral aciclovir (800 mg five times daily for 5 days), famciclovir (250 mg t.d.s. for 7 days), and valaciclovir (1 g t.d.s for 7 days) taken within 72 hours of the appearance of the rash can shorten the duration and severity of the rash, and reduce the risk of persistent post-herpetic pain. The latter two have better bioavailability than aciclovir and may be more effective in reducing the risk of PHN (Kost and Straus 1996; DTB 1998b).

ACUTE HERPES ZOSTER

- * The patient with zoster on exposed skin should remain isolated until the last lesion scabs over. They can transmit the virus to non-immune individuals, who can contract chickenpox.

- * Give adequate analgesia. Opioids may be required. Always co-prescribe a stimulant laxative, e.g. senna.

- * Oral antiviral agents. Prescribe at high dose for 7 days, starting within 72 hours of the start of the rash, for:
  - (a) ophthalmic zoster; or zoster in the first division of the trigeminal nerve before it has begun to involve the eye; or
  - (b) the immunocompromised; or
  - (c) patients in moderate to severe acute pain; or

- (d) older patients, e.g. over age 50.
    Starting the drug after 72 hours may be of value if new vesicles are still appearing.
- * *Corticosteroids/idoxuridine*. The evidence is too weak to recommend their use.

For treatment of PHN, see page 678.

BACTERIAL INFECTIONS

- * Check for diabetes in recurrent or unusually severe skin infections.
- * Topical antibiotics inevitably lead to colonization of the skin with resistant organisms. Do not therefore use antibiotics topically which may be needed systemically.
- * Topical neomycin, if used for less than 10 days, rarely leads to allergy.

CELLULITIS AND ERYSIPELAS

SYSTEMATIC REVIEW

Morris A. 2004. Cellulitis and erysipelas. *Clinical Evidence*. Available: www.clinicalevidence.com

- * Use oral penicillin or erythromycin. Antibiotics effective against streptococcus (penicillin, ceftriaxone, roxithromycin and flucloxacillin) are equally useful, so penicillin is usually the drug of choice. Oral versus intravenous antibiotics have not been tested in a controlled trial.
- * Narrow-spectrum penicillin derivatives (flucloxacillin and dicloxacillin) can cause elevation of hepatic enzymes and should not be used as first line therapies.
- * There is no good evidence that routine microbiological tests improve treatment outcomes (Morris 2001).

Erysipelas is a specific form of cellulitis. It is a superficial skin infection which migrates through lymphatics, and which can cause lymphatic damage. It commonly occurs below the knee, and frequently recurs. *Streptococcus pyogenes* is the usual pathogen. Standard treatment is benzylpenicillin sodium (penicillin G) although newer oral regimens have proved more effective (Bernard, Chosidow and Vaillant 2002). Hospitalization and intravenous antibiotics may be required, particularly for elderly patients, diabetics, patients with leucocytosis or vascular insufficiency (Musette, Benichou, Noblesse, *et al.* 2004). Prolonged courses of antibiotics may be required to eradicate it.

IMPETIGO

SYSTEMATIC REVIEW

Koning S, Verhagen AP, van Suijlekom-Smit LWA *et al.* 2003. Interventions for impetigo. The Cochrane Database of Systematic Reviews, Issue 2. Art. No.: CD003261. DOI: 10.1002

* Treat isolated lesions with topical antibiotic preparations, such as mupirocin, fucidic acid, neomycin or soframycin.
* *Widespread lesions:* give oral antibiotics, e.g. cephalexin or erythromycin. Erythromycin is superior to penicillin.
* It is traditional to reduce the skin bacterial load with regular baths using an antiseptic solution or soap and to reduce the nasal and perianal carry rates of staphylococcus by the use of topical antibacterial agents but without any evidence of benefit.
* Treat all family members simultaneously if cross-infection is a problem. Children should not attend school until the lesions have crusted over and there is no discharge.

OTHER BACTERIAL INFECTIONS

* *Boils* should be drained. Daily washes with chlorhexidine may prevent spread. Oral cephalexin or flucloxacillin are needed for ill patients.
* *Recurrent staphylococcal skin infections.* Patients with recurrent staphylococcal infections often carry staphylococci in sites not cleared by systemic antibiotics, especially the nose and the perineum. Bath daily with triclosan bath concentrate. Prescribe chlorhexidine and neomycin nasal cream or mupirocin nasal ointment.
* *Hidradenitis suppuritiva.* If the axilla is infected, give:
  (a) erythromycin 500 mg b.d. or oxytetracycline 500 mg b.d. for 1 month in the first instance, but 6 months treatment may be needed; or
  (b) topical clindamycin for 3 months.

* *Erythrasma* is due to a corynebacterium, and is often mistaken for axillary tinea. Use a topical imidazole or oral tetracycline or erythromycin for 2 weeks.
* Hair follicles:
  (a) *folliculitis:* use topical antiseptics or topical antibiotics;
  (b) *furunculosis:* use oral antibiotics (e.g. cephalexin or flucloxacillin).
* *Caruncle.* Refer for surgical excision and drainage. The patient will also need antibiotics if unwell, or if there is associated cellulitis. Reduce the risk of recurrence by clearing the skin and nose of pathogenic staphylococci as above.

FUNGAL INFECTIONS

SYSTEMATIC REVIEW

Crawford F, Hollis S. 2007. Topical treatments for fungal infections of the skin and nails of the foot. Cochrane Database of Systematic Reviews, Issue 3. Art No.: CD001434.DOI:10.1002/14651858.CD001434.pub2.

Guidance

Clinical Knowledge Summaries. Fungal infection - skin. Accessed May 2009. Available: www.cks.library.nhs.uk (search on 'Fungal')

* The clinical picture is usually diagnostic, but if confirmation is needed send skin scrapings for fungal microscopy and culture as described below for nail infection. 5 mm^2 of skin flakes are needed.
* Fungal infections usually flourish in moist sites. Explain skin hygiene: keep the skin dry and clean, avoid tight-fitting clothing, wash clothes and bedclothes frequently. Do not share towels.
* There is little to choose between the topical imidazoles: clotrimazole, econazole and miconazole. Ketoconazole is slightly more expensive. Terbinafine is yet more expensive but appears to be slightly more effective (Crawford, Hart, Bell-Syer, *et al.* 2001) and need only be applied for 1 week.
  * Use imidazoles for 2 weeks after clinical healing to avoid recurrence.

- Nystatin is effective against yeasts, but not against other fungi.
- Oral itraconazole and terbinafine should only be used for severe fungal infections.

CANDIDIASIS

- Occurs in napkin dermatitis, intertrigo and angular stomatitis. Use nystatin cream, or an imidazole, with a steroid if there is inflammation.

PITYRIASIS VERSICOLOR

* Explain that:
  (a) it does not need treatment if the patient does not mind the appearance;
  (b) killing the organism, which can be done by means of topical or even systemic antifungals, will not solve the cosmetic issue until old discoloured skin has been desquamated in the usual way; and will not prevent recurrence in susceptible people if treatment is stopped.
* If the patient wishes treatment, use a low toxicity fungal poison such as zinc pyridinethione, selenium sulfide, or a sulpha compound, often made up into a shampoo, which can be used several times a week indefinitely.
* *If there is extensive skin involvement,* consider using ketoconazole 200 mg, itraconazole 200 mg daily for 5 days.

SEBORRHOEIC DERMATITIS AND DANDRUFF

See page 567.

TINEA CAPITIS

* Send scrapings of skin and broken hairs before starting treatment. Use oral itraconazole or terbinafine for 4 weeks. Oral ketoconazole and fluconazole have been used but are limited by their adverse effects (Higgins, Fuller and Smith 2000). Only griseofulvin is licensed in the UK for the treatment of tinea capitis but a longer course is needed than with the other antifungal agents (Fuller, Child, Midgley, *et al.* 2003). Topical antifungals are ineffective.

* If the diagnosis is confirmed, screen close contacts for tinea capitis and corporis. Disinfect combs. Exclude the affected child from school until started on treatment.

TINEA PEDIS, CRURIS AND CORPORIS

(a) Stress the importance of drying any moist areas.
(b) Use an imidazole cream for 3 weeks or terbinafine cream for 1 week.
(c) Consider oral terbinafine in resistant cases.
(d) Avoid relapse by using dusting powders.

FUNGAL INFECTIONS OF NAILS

GUIDANCE

Clinical Knowledge Summaries. Fungal infection – nails. Accessed May 2009. Available: www.cks.library. nhs.uk (search on 'Fungal')

* Most people are not troubled by it. Oral antifungals are not without side-effects.
* Be more ready to treat in someone more vulnerable to secondary bacterial infection, e.g. someone with diabetes, or peripheral vascular disease, or immunodeficiency.
* Explain basic footcare: keep the nails short, avoid long periods when the feet are wet, wear well-fitting shoes, treat any athlete's foot, wear 'shower shoes' in a communal shower. Consult a podiatrist if unable to remove enough distorted nail for comfort.
* If planning drug treatment, confirm the diagnosis by sending scrapings, taken with a blunt scalpel, or nail clippings. These should be transported in a folded square of paper and not refrigerated. Pus from the nail fold is valuable in chronic paronychia. Specify microscopy and culture for fungi. However, a false negative occurs in 30% of cases. Repeat the test if clinical suspicion remains high.
* Dermatophyte infection (infection with *Trichophyton* species). Give terbinafine 250 mg daily for 6 weeks (fingernails) or 3 months (toenails). Patients who prefer not to take oral

drugs, or whose disease is confined to one or two nails, may use amorolfine nail lacquer or tioconazole nail solution.

* Infection with yeasts, non-dermatophyte moulds or mixed infections. Only accept that the non-dermatophyte is the cause of the infection if two samples, taken at different times, are positive. They often colonize nails already infected with a dermatophyte. Give itraconazole 200 mg daily for 3 months or 'pulsed', i.e. 200 mg b.d. for 1 week every month for 2 (fingernails) or 3 (toenails) months.

* Explain that the infection may continue to respond after the end of the course of treatment. Terbinafine and itraconazole persist in nail keratin for up to 9 months after the end of treatment.

LICHEN PLANUS

● This condition may follow contact sensitivity to certain chemicals and drugs, or in response to chronic graft-versus-host disease.

● The rash is a collection of dark shiny, pearly papules about 2–4 mm across. They have a lacy pattern on the surface. The papules are distributed most commonly to flexor surfaces of the body, most commonly the wrist.

● The lesions are self-limiting and usually resolve in a year.

* Examine the mouth and genital mucosa. Asymptomatic white lines across the buccal, anal or genital mucosa confirm the diagnosis.

* If drugs are suspected, they should be withdrawn.

* Topical steroids may assist in reducing the size of the papules.

ALOPECIA

WITH SCARRING

* Take skin scrapings. Treat with antifungals if positive. If negative, refer for skin biopsy for conditions such as discoid lupus erythematosus.

PATCHY WITHOUT SCARRING

* *If there is a rash*, scrape off scales and send for microscopy. If positive, treat with oral itraconazole or terbinafine.

* *Alopecia areata*. Reassure the patient that regrowth is likely to occur within 1 year. Steroid creams are often prescribed, but there is little evidence of value.

* *Trichotillomania*. Consider mechanical damage, especially in children.

DIFFUSE WITHOUT SCARRING

● 80% of men and 35% of women have frontal/temporal pattern balding by the age of 60. Men usually progress to baldness of the crown; women do so less often.

Topical minoxidil 1 ml b.d. or oral finasteride 1 mg daily will slow hair loss, and may restore hair in some patients. Finasteride is an antiandrogenic agent, and may reduce libido and ejaculate volume, and produce gynaecomastia. Most side-effects appear mild (Libecco and Bergfeld 2004).

WORK-UP WHEN HAIR LOSS IS UNEXPECTED

(a) FBC;
(b) ferritin;
(c) TFTs;
(d) calcium and phosphate.

* Exclude drugs as a cause, e.g. cytotoxics, anticoagulants, antithyroid drugs, retinoids.

* *Acute hair loss*. Explain that there is a cycle in the growth of each hair. Stress and illness can bring the majority of hairs to the end of the cycle at the same time so that they all fall out. They will then regrow together.

* *Postpartum acute hair loss*. Explain that the hairs have been held back in their natural cycle during pregnancy, and that now that the pregnancy is over they have caught up and come out at the same time. They will regrow, but it may take many months. Exclude anaemia and thyroid dysfunction.

* Consider referral for counselling, which may be available through the local dermatology department, and for a wig. Advise men with male pattern baldness that minoxidil lotion will

reduce the loss in 70% of cases and promote new hair growth in 30%, with a good cosmetic result in 10%. Results from finasteride are similar or possibly slightly better. They are only available in the UK on a private prescription, and should be used for 3 months before judging benefit. Once stopped the benefit is lost.

- Discuss the option of surgery.

SELF-HELP GROUPS

Hairline International: the Alopecia Patients' Society, Lyons Court, 1668 High Street, Knowle, Solihull, West Midlands B93 0LY, tel. 01564 775281. www. hairlineinternational.com

Alopecia Areata Support Association (Australia), PO Box 89, Camberwell, Victoria 3124, Melbourne, Australia, tel. 03 9513 8580; http://home.vicnet.net. au/~aasa/

SKIN INFESTATIONS

SCABIES

SYSTEMATIC REVIEW

Walker GJA, Johnstone PW. 2007. Interventions for treating scabies. The Cochrane Database of Systematic Reviews, Issue 2. Art. No.: CD000320. DOI: 10.1002/ 14651858.CD000320.pub2.

- Pyrethrin (permethrin) has been found to cure 90% of affected individuals. It is more effective than gamma benzene hexachloride or crotamiton though both these latter agents are effective in their own right.
- Malathion may be effective, but there is no RCT evidence.
- Gamma benzene hexachloride may have rare adverse events: aplastic anaemia and fits in patients treated for extensive disease. In the UK it is not prescribable and in the US its neurotoxicity is considered sufficiently hazardous to advise caution in patients weighing < 110 pounds, which makes it unsuitable for most children. However, in Australia the rarity of the risk means that it is considered an acceptable treatment, particularly

for the rare Norwegian scabies mite, which shows resistance to other treatments.

- * Treat all members of a household and all sexual contacts simultaneously. Where transmission is sexual, screen for other STDs (see page 70).
- * *Instructions:*
  1. Apply the selected treatment to all areas below the neck before retiring, and wash off in the morning. Children and those with compromised immunity need to have the cream applied to the neck, face, ears and scalp as well. Wash all bedclothes, bed linen and underclothes in hot water that day.
  2. Repeat the treatment in 1 week to eradicate the hatched mites.
- * Give appropriate antibiotics (cephalexin or erythromycin) if pustules are present.

Note: The itch may persist longer than the mites. Repeated use of antiscabetic lotions does *not* accelerate resolution. Specific antipruritic measures are more appropriate.

LICE

HEAD LICE

- Overuse of insecticides has led to resistance. Current guidelines stress that treatment should only be given if a living, i.e. moving, louse is found. Nits are egg cases stuck to hairs and do not necessarily mean there is active infestation.
- *Bug-busting* (wet-combing of the hair to remove lice) is ineffective as treatment (Roberts, Casey, Morgan, *et al.* 2000). The place of wet-combing is in detection (see box below).
  - * Make sure the whole household is checked and ask the parents to notify the school nurse so that the rest of the class can be examined. UK guidelines stress that the affected child should not be excluded from school. Any transmission will already have taken place.
  - * Prescribe the recommended parasiticidal preparation: malathion, permethrin or carbaryl. Health districts will rotate from one preparation to the other every 3 years to avoid resistance. It is important to cooperate with this policy. Local chemists or the local pharmaceutical advisers will know the current recommendations.

* *Practicalities*: two applications are needed 7 days apart; lotions, liquids or creme rinses should be used, not shampoos.

Note: Asthmatics or young children should use aqueous malathion.

Note: Carbaryl has been found to cause cancer in laboratory animals after prolonged exposure to high doses. There is therefore a theoretical risk that it may be carcinogenic in humans, although the CMO advises that any risk is exceedingly small (Chief Medical Officer 1995).

DETECTION COMBING

1. Buy a fine-tooth detector comb.
2. Wash the hair and leave it wet. Comb first with an ordinary comb then with the detector comb, beginning at the top of the head. The comb must be touching the scalp and be drawn right to the ends of the hairs.
3. Look for lice on the comb.
4. Continue to comb until the whole scalp and all the hair has been covered – it should take 10–15 minutes.
5. If you find something that could be a louse, stick it to a piece of paper with clear sticky tape and take it to a nurse, doctor or pharmacist for confirmation.

PATIENT INFORMATION

The National Pediculosis Association: www.headlice.org

GENITAL LICE (CRAB LICE)

● Treat all intimate contacts. It is usually spread by sexual contact in adults, but finding it in a child does not necessarily raise suspicion of sexual abuse. It can survive for 24 hours in clothes or bedding.
● Use aqueous preparations of malathion, permethrin, phenothrin or malathion to the whole body, not just the pubic hair, for 12 hours and repeated after 7 days.

BODY LICE

● Wash clothes in hot water. No other treatment is necessary.

PAPULAR URTICARIA

FLEAS

● Deflea the cat, dog or rabbit.
● Treat the house. Spray insecticide on carpets and soft furnishings, and around where the pet sleeps.

BED BUGS

● Wash bed linen.
● Call in the environmental health-department to treat the house. The bugs live behind wallpaper and skirting boards, not in the beds themselves.

ANIMAL MITES

● Treat the pet, who is likely to have signs of the disease (e.g. mange).

BIRD MITES

● Clear birds' nests from outside the bedroom window if bird mites are suspected.

MALIGNANCY

There are three main groups of primary skin cancer:

1. basal cell carcinoma (BCC), arising from the basal cells of the germinal layer;
2. squamous cell carcinoma (SCC) arising from squamous cells; and
3. melanoma, arising from pigmented cells (melanocytes).

Although all are common in white-skinned people living in sunny climates, the prognosis of each is very different.

BASAL CELL CARCINOMAS (BCCS)

SYSTEMATIC REVIEW

Bath-Hextall F, Bong J, Perkins W, *et al.* 2004. Interventions for basal cell carcinoma of the skin: systematic review. BMJ 329, 705–708

- These are the most common skin cancers. They are most common on head and upper trunk.
- Although they do not metastasize without undergoing squamous transformation, delay in diagnosis can lead to disaster from loss of wide areas of tissue, or underlying organs such as the eye.
- A trial of sun-screen failed to show benefit for preventive BCCs.

MANAGEMENT

* If there is any doubt about diagnosis, biopsy is indicated.
* Treatment is by excision. Radiotherapy is used less than in the past because it appears to be less effective than surgery with a worse cosmetic effect.
* Superficial ones can be treated with local destruction, such as liquid nitrogen cryotherapy or imiquimod cream. Facial lesions should be excised due to the small risk of local spread along neurovascular bundles to deep tissues including the brain.
* Warn patients that they are at increased risk of other skin cancers and that they should be especially diligent about preventative measures (Wong, Strange and Lear 2003).

SQUAMOUS CELL CARCINOMAS (SCCS)

SYSTEMATIC REVIEW

Green A, Marks R. 2004. Squamous cell carcinoma of the skin (non-metastatic). *Clinical Evidence.* BMJ Publishing Group. Available: www.clinicalevidence.com

These are also common skin cancers. They are most common on sun-exposed areas including extremities.

- There is good evidence that daily use of sunscreens reduces SCC (and solar keratosis) formation compared to just patient discretionary use.
* *Referral.* In the UK, urgent referral, to be seen within 2 weeks, is indicated for any patient with:

(a) an indurated lesion in which there has been documented expansion over the last 1–2 months; or
(b) a positive biopsy; or
(c) any new or growing skin lesion in a patient who is immunosuppressed.

* If there is any doubt about diagnosis, biopsy is indicated.
* Treatment is by excision (SCCs are much less radiosensitive to superficial X-ray therapy than BCCs).
* Stress the importance of further prevention. Use of a sun-screen has been shown to decrease the later formation of SCCs in a randomized trial. Use of a hat and clothing is even more effective in avoiding solar damage.

MELANOMA

For details of the diagnosis of pigmented skin lesions see *Evidence-based Diagnosis in Primary Care* by A. F. Polmear (editor), published by Butterworth-Heinemann, 2008.

- Melanomas are the most dangerous form of skin cancer, and are also related to past sun exposure.
- Of several forms, the most common is the superficial spreading melanoma (SSM) for which early diagnosis of thin lesions is critical because it conveys a much better prognosis compared to those left to grow thicker. Nodular, and acral forms (on palms and feet) carry a worse prognosis, although this is very variable.
- They are pigmented (except in the case of the rare amelanotic form). SSMs especially can be hard to distinguish from benign skin naevi ('moles'), and also flat seborrhoeic keratoses.
- Special distinguishing characteristics of melanomas include asymmetry, size greater than 6 mm, irregular edges or surface, or non-uniform pigmentation. Unfortunately, early SSMs are often difficult to diagnose.

MANAGEMENT

* If there is any doubt about diagnosis, biopsy.
* In the UK, patients qualify for referral urgently, to be seen within 2 weeks, if they have a pigmented lesion which shows one or more of

the following: growing in size, changing shape, irregular outline, changing colour, mixed colour, ulceration, or inflammation.

* Definitive treatment is by excision of the lesion plus, a margin of between 1 and 2 cm of healthy tissue (Haigh, DiFronzo and McCready 2003).

Lesions with a histology report indicating less than 0.75 mm thickness have a very good prognosis.

There is no evidence that any immunotherapy, chemotherapy or radiotherapy provides any significant improvement in mortality or morbidity.

SOLAR KERATOSES (ACTINIC KERATOSES)

GUIDELINE

Stockfleth E, Kerl H. 2006. Guidelines for the management of actinic keratoses. Eur J Dermatol 16, 599–606

Solar keratoses (SKs) are keratotic lesions on sun-exposed skin caused by solar damage.

- Sunscreen applied daily reduces the risk of solar keratoses developing (Green and Marks 2004).
- They may be precursors of SCCs. However, most SKs spontaneously remit without progress into SCCs. Fewer than 1 in 1000 SKs transform into SCCs (Marks, Rennie and Selwood 1988). Moreover, many SCCs arise from previously normal skin rather than SKs.
- Some patients worry about skin cancer (for which SKs are indeed a risk factor), and the hardness of the lesions can be irritating on clothing.
- Treating SKs as a preventive to developing SCCs is unjustified.
- * If there is any doubt about the diagnosis of cancer, biopsy.
- * Consider destructive treatment of SKs (by cryotherapy, or excision biopsy if there is diagnostic doubt) for local symptomatic treatment.
- * Symptomatic treatment of SKs can also be achieved by use of topical applications such as salicylic ointment (5%) or urea cream (10%) or colchicine cream (1%) (Grimaitre, Etienne, Fathi, *et al*. 2000) or by topical diclofenac.

* *5-fluorouracil cream (5-FU):* people with damaged skin can benefit from applying 5-FU daily to affected areas, such as the forehead or forearms. Stop the cream after 2–3 weeks, when the patient experiences an inflammatory reaction. The skin will then regenerate, leaving a cosmetically improved surface. Only prescribe it if reasonably experienced in its use. Before treatment:

(a) warn the patient that the treatment is unpleasant; the inflammatory reaction will cause erythema and possibly ulceration;

(b) check carefully for malignancy in the area; 5-FU can mask an SCC or a BCC.

HYPERHIDROSIS

GENERALIZED HYPERHIDROSIS

A cause is not usually found, but, especially in those with an onset in adult life, consider:

(a) autonomic nervous system imbalance, as in the menopause;

(b) autonomic neuropathy, with areas of hypohidrosis and compensatory hyperhidrosis elsewhere;

(c) hyperthyroidism;

(d) hyperpituitarism.

HYPERHIDROSIS OF THE PALMS, SOLES AND AXILLAE

* Use daily aluminium chloride hexahydrate applied at night to dry skin and washed off in the morning, until benefit is achieved. Do not apply within 12 hours of shaving or using depilatories. Use hydrocortisone cream if the preparation causes irritation. Reduce to weekly applications once control is achieved.

* For treatment failures, discuss the availability of iontophoresis or injections of botulinum toxin with the local physiotherapy department or dermatologist (Simpson 1988).

* Otherwise consider referral for sympathectomy for palmar sweating and axillary skin excision for axillary sweating. Both have their problems; infection following skin excision, and surgical disasters following sympathectomy.

* If odour is a problem apply an antibacterial b.d., e.g. chlorhexidine cream or dusting powder.
* Recommend the Hyperhidrosis Support Group UK at www.hyperhidrosisuk.org

GRAVITATIONAL ULCERS

SYSTEMATIC REVIEWS

Nelson EA, Cullum N, Jones J. 2001. Venous leg ulcers. *Clinical Evidence*, Issue 5. BMJ Publishing Group, London. Available: www.clinicalevidence.org
   O'Meara S, Cullum N, Nelson EA. 2009. Compression for venous ulcers. The Cochrane Database of Systematic Reviews, Issue 1. DOI: 10.1002/14651858. CD00265
   Compression therapy for venous leg ulcers. Effective Health Care 1997; 3 (4)

* Firm, but not excessive compression dressings of the legs have been shown to reduce healing time. Compression devices (e.g. TED stockings) also reduce recurrence of venous ulcers.
* The type of dressing used does not appear to influence healing time but multicomponent systems are more effective than single component systems, especially if an elastic layer is included.
* Pentoxifylline and flavinoids improve healing rates but they are not recommended by current guidelines (RCN Institute, Centre for Evidence Based Nursing, University of York and School of Nursing, Midwifery and Health Visiting, University of Manchester 1998; British Association of Dermatologists and the Royal College of Physicians of London 1995).

MANAGEMENT

* *Check the arterial supply* before compression bandages are applied. The ratio of ankle to brachial systolic blood pressure (ABI) (see page 437) should be measured by Doppler. Compression should not be applied if the ratio is less than 0.8. Palpation of foot pulses may miss significant arterial insufficiency.

* Check the Hb and fasting sugar in all patients, and possibly the serum iron in patients with chronic ulcers that fail to heal.
* Agree, with the responsible nursing staff, a practice policy for the treatment of gravitational ulcers using multilayer compression bandaging capable of being left on for a week at a time.
* *General measures.* Encourage mobility. Elevate the leg when sitting; footstools are not sufficient elevation. Raise the foot of the bed.
* *Infection.* Take a swab and clean the ulcer as above. If the ulcer is foul-smelling, start metronidazole 400 mg b.d. for 7 days. If there is evidence of cellulitis, use appropriate oral antibiotics (e.g. erythromycin). A positive swab does not necessarily mean infection (Thompson and Smith 1994). Do not use topical antibiotics: they are ineffective and give rise to sensitization.
* *Prevention.* Once the ulcer is healed, the patient must be obsessional about wearing a support stocking of at least medium strength (18–24 mmHg at the ankle). Even then, one-third of ulcers relapse in the first year after healing.

REFERRAL

* Refer all patients with a poor arterial supply (ABI < 0.8) for further investigation by a vascular surgeon.
* *Consider varicose vein surgery* in any patient with prominent incompetent perforators or varicosities:
  (a) *before* the skin ulcerates; or
  (b) *after* the skin has healed; or
  (c) *while the ulcer is present*. Venous surgery has increased healing from 57% to 89% (Wilson 1989).
* *Consider referral for grafting* for any ulcer that is failing to improve after 3 months, or which has not healed after 1 year.
* Consider biopsy of the edge of a non-healing ulcer if no progress is made with other treatment modes. Non-healing ulcers are rarely the presenting symptom of large skin cancers, usually basal cell carcinomas.

PRESCRIBING A COMPRESSION STOCKING (EFFECTIVE HEALTH CARE 1997)

Is there a medical contraindication?

* Check that the ABI is not below 0.8.
* Check that there is not marked oedema. The pressure of a stocking may cause tissue damage. Control the oedema by medical means or compression bandages first.
* Check that the patient does not have a condition which is associated with small vessel disease: diabetes or rheumatoid arthritis. Compression may close off these already compromised small arteries.
* Check that the patient does not have an allergy to nylon or rubber. If the patient does have an allergy, prescribe a stocking with a high percentage of cotton or prescribe a cotton tubular bandage to be worn under the stocking.

Is there a practical problem?

* Can the patient pull the stockings on and off? If not, can a carer? A metal frame can make it easier, as can the use of talcum powder or a silky socklet to reduce friction between the stocking and the foot or leg.
* Is the shape of the leg suitable for an off-the-peg stocking? Patients with very thin legs, or with oddly shaped legs (e.g. the champagne-bottle leg of chronic venous insufficiency) need stockings that are made to measure by a hospital appliance department.

What stocking should be prescribed in those who are suitable?

* Class 3 (25–30 mmHg at the ankle) is most likely to be effective if the patient can tolerate it.
* 'Below knee' is more easily tolerated and is usually adequate, especially if the problem is limited to the foot and calf. 'Above knee' stockings are harder to put on but may give some comfort to patients with arthritic knees.
* Check the patient's preference for open-toe or closed-toe stockings.
* Record the following measurements and include them on the prescription: ankle circumference at its narrowest point; calf circumference at its widest point; length of the leg from the base of the heel to just below the knee.
* Once it is clear that the patient can tolerate the stockings, prescribe a spare, so that one can be washed while the other is being worn. Prescribe a new pair every 4–6 months: they lose their compression.

URTICARIA

GUIDELINES

Grattan CEH, Humphreys F. 2007. *Guidelines for Evaluation and Management of Urticaria in Adults and Children.* British Association of Dermatologists. Available: www.bad.org.uk
  Powell RJ, Du Toit GL, Siddique N, *et al.* 2007. BSACI guidelines for the management of chronic urticaria and angio-oedema. Clin Exp All 37, 631–650.

* Distinguish 'ordinary' urticaria from physical urticaria and contact urticaria. The management of the last two is to avoid the stimulus.

MANAGEMENT OF ORDINARY URTICARIA

* Attempt to identify an allergen from the history. Skin prick tests and radioallergosorbent testing (RAST) may be able to confirm a clinical suspicion. Biological allergens are the most common triggers. These include drugs (antibiotics, salicylates), insect stings, ingestion of certain foods (including nuts, fish and shellfish, fruits), and preservatives (e.g. tartrazine).
* Avoid drugs which can worsen urticaria, e.g. aspirin and codeine.
* Avoid aggravating physical factors, e.g. cold, heat or stress.
* Offer soothing lotions, e.g. calamine.
* Give a non-sedating antihistamine. Try at least two before abandoning them; individual responses vary. Consider moving to a higher dose if the standard dose is insufficiently effective but there are no adverse effects. A sedating antihistamine may be more helpful at night. In chronic urticaria, give the drug for 3–6 months before weaning off over several weeks. In acute intermittent urticaria the antihistamine can be taken as needed, or prophylactically if an attack can be predicted.
* Consider adding an H_2-receptor antagonist if the antihistamine alone is insufficient.

* Oral corticosteroids can shorten an episode of acute urticaria. Give prednisolone 50 mg/day for 3 days but not long term.
* Refer patients whose chronic urticaria is sufficiently troublesome. Even their prognosis is not bad; referred patients have a 50% chance of being symptom-free without treatment in 6 months (Champion, Roberts, Carpenter, *et al.* 1969).

SELF–HELP GROUP

Allergy UK. 3 White Oak Square, London Road, Swanley, Kent BR8 7AG. Tel. 01322 619898. Helpline 01322 619864. www.allergyuk.org

Professional organization with patient information: The Australasian Society of Clinical Immunology and Allergy (ASCIA). PO Box 450, Balgowlah, NSW 2093, Australia, tel. 02 9907 9773; www.allergy.org.au

---

References

Adami, M., Inglott, A., Azzopardi, L., et al., 1998. Acne management in community practice. Pharm. J. 261, R20.

Arowojolu, A.O., Gallo, M.F., Grimes, D.A., et al., 2004. Combined oral contraceptive pills for treatment of acne. Cochrane Database Syst. Rev. (3), CD004425. DOI: 10.1002/14651858.CD004425. pub2. Available: www.nelh.nhs. uk/cochrane.asp.

Atherton, D., 2003. Topical corticosteroids in atopic dermatitis. BMJ 327, 942–943.

Bandolier, 1995. Does treating acute herpes zoster in primary care stop post-herpetic neuralgia? Bandolier 17, 133.

Bernard, P., Chosidow, O., Vaillant, L.; French Erysipelas Study Group, 2002. Oral pristinamycin versus standard penicillin regimen to treat erysipelas in adults: randomised, non-inferiority, open trial. BMJ 325, 864–868.

Berth-Jones, J., Damstra, R.J., Golsch, S., et al., 2003. Twice weekly fluticasone proprionate added to emollient maintenance treatment to reduce risk of relapse in atopic dermatitis: randomised double blind, parallel group study. BMJ 326, 1367–1370.

BNF, 2001. Topical steroids. Section 13.4. British National Formulary; No. 42. Available: www.bnf.org.

British Association of Dermatologists and the Royal College of

Physicians of London, 1995. Guidelines for the management of chronic venous leg ulceration. Br. J. Dermatol. 132, 446–452.

Champion, R.H., Roberts, S.O.B., Carpenter, R.G., et al., 1969. Urticaria and angio-oedema: a review of 554 patients. Br. J. Dermatol. 81, 588–597.

Charman, C., 2001. Atopic eczema. *Clinical Evidence* Issue 5. BMJ Publishing Group, London. Online. Available: www. clinicalevidence.com.

Chief Medical Officer, 1995. CMO's letter PL/CMO (95)4 Available: www.dh.gov.uk (choose 'CMO letters' then 'Index to CMO letters' then '1995' then 'PL CMO (1995)4: Carbaryl').

Crawford, F., Hart, R., Bell-Syer, S., et al., 2001. Topical treatments for fungal infections of the skin and nails of the foot (Cochrane Review). In: The Cochrane Library. Update Software, Oxford Issue 4. Available: www.nelh.nhs. uk/cochrane.asp.

Dreno, B., Chosidow, O., Revuz, J., et al., 2003. Lithium gluconate 8% vs ketoconazole 2% in the treatment of seborrhoeic dermatitis: a multicentre, randomized study. Br. J. Dermatol. 148, 1230–1236.

DTB, 1993. Azelaic acid – a new topical treatment for acne. Drug Ther. Bull. 31, 50–52.

DTB, 1998a. Tackling warts on the hands and feet. Drug Ther. Bull. 36, 22–24.

DTB, 1998b. Update on drugs for herpes zoster and genital herpes. Drug Ther. Bull. 36.

Effective Health Care, 1997. Compression therapy for venous leg ulcers. Eff. Health Care 3 (4).

Elewski, B.E., Fleischer, A.B., Pariser, D.M., 2003. A comparison of 15% azelaic acid gel and 0.75% metronidazole gel in the topical treatment of papulopustular rosacea. Arch. Dermatol. 139, 1444–1450.

Focht III, D.R., Spicer, C., Fairchok, M.P., 2002. The efficacy of duct tape vs cryotherapy in the treatment of verruca vulgaris (the common wart). Arch. Pediatr. Adolesc. Med. 156, 971–974.

Fuller, L.C., Child, F.J., Midgley, G., et al., 2003. Diagnosis and management of scalp ringworm. BMJ 326, 539–541.

Garner, S., Eady, A., Avery, T., 2002. Robust evidence is needed in treating acne (letter). BMJ 325, 1422.

Garner, S.E., Eady, E.A., Popescu, C., et al., 2002. Minocycline for acne vulgaris: efficacy and safety (Cochrane Review). In: The Cochrane Library, Issue 4. Update Software, Oxford, Available: www.nelh.nhs.uk/cochrane.asp.

Greaves, M.W., 1997. Current management of psoriasis. J. Dermatolog. Treat. 8, 35–36.

Green, A., Marks, R., 2004. Squamous cell carcinoma of the skin (non-metastatic). *Clinical Evidence*, No 12. BMJ Books, Oxford, Online.

Available: www.clinicalevidence. com.

Grimaitre, M., Etienne, A., Fathi, M., et al., 2000. Topical colchicine therapy for actinic keratoses. Dermatology 200 (4), 346–348.

Haigh, P.I., DiFronzo, L.A., McCready, D.R., 2003. Optimal excision margins for primary cutaneous melanoma: a systematic review and meta-analysis. Can. J. Surg. 46, 419–426.

Higgins, E.M., Fuller, L.C., Smith, C. H., 2000. Guidelines for the management of tinea capitis. Br. J. Dermatol. 143, 53–58.

Hoare, C., Li Wan Po, A., Williams, H., 2000. Systematic review of treatments for atopic eczema. Health Technol. Assess. 4, 37. Available: www.ncchta.org.

Kost, R.G., Straus, S.E., 1996. Postherpetic neuralgia – pathogenesis, treatment and prevention. N. Engl. J. Med. 335, 32–42.

Leyden, J.J., 1997. Therapy for acne vulgaris. N. Engl. J. Med. 336, 1156–1162.

Libecco, J.F., Bergfeld, W.F., 2004. Finasteride in the treatment of alopecia. Expert Opin. Pharmacother. 5 (4), 933–940.

Marks, R., Rennie, G., Selwood, T., 1988. Malignant transformation of solar keratoses. Lancet i, 795–797.

MeReC, 1994. Acne vulgaris. MeReC Bulletin 5, 41–44.

Morris, A., 2001. Cellulitis and erysipelas. *Clinical Evidence*, Issue 5. BMJ Publishing Group, London, Available: www.clinicalevidence. org.

Musette, P., Benichou, J., Noblesse, I., et al., 2004. Determinants of severity for superficial cellulitis (erysipelas) of the leg: a retrospective study. Eur. J. Intern. Med. 15, 446–450.

NICE, 2004a. Frequency of applications of topical steroids for atopic eczema. National Institute For Clinical Excellence, London. Online. Available: www.nice. org.uk.

NICE, 2004b. Tacrolimus and pimecrolimus for atopic eczema. National Institute for Clinical Excellence, London. Online. Available: www.nice.org.uk.

RCN Institute, Centre for Evidence Based Nursing, University of York and School of Nursing, Midwifery and Health Visiting, University of Manchester, 1998. The management of patients with venous leg ulcers. Available: www.rcn.org.uk.

Roberts, R.J., Casey, D., Morgan, D. A., et al., 2000. Comparison of wet combing with malathion for treatment of head lice in the UK:

a pragmatic randomised controlled trial. Lancet 356, 540–544.

Simpson, N., 1988. Treating hyperhidrosis. BMJ 296, 1345.

Thompson, P.D., Smith, D.J., 1994. What is infection? Am. J. Surg. 167 (Suppl. 1a), 75–115.

van Zuuren, E.J., Graber, M.A., Hollis, S., et al., 2003. Interventions for rosacea. Cochrane Database Syst. Rev. (4), CD003262. DOI: 10.1002/ 14651858.CD003262.pub2. Available: www.nelh.nhs.uk/ cochrane.asp.

Williams, H.C., Wuthrich, B., 2000. The natural history of atopic dermatitis. In: Williams, H.C. (ed.), Atopic dermatitis. Cambridge University Press, Cambridge.

Wilson, E., 1989. Prevention and treatment of venous leg ulcers. Health Trends 21, 97.

Wong, C.S.M., Strange, R.C., Lear, J. T., 2003. Basal cell carcinoma. BMJ 327, 794–798.

Wysowski, D.K., Pitts, M., Beitz, J., 2001. An analysis of reports of depression and suicide in patients treated with isotretinoin. J. Am. Acad. Dermatol. 45, 515–519.

Chapter 23

Allergic problems

CHAPTER CONTENTS

FOOD ALLERGIES

GUIDELINES/REPORTS

Chapman JA, Bernstein IL, Lee RE, *et al.* 2006. Food allergy: a practice parameter. Ann Allergy Asthma Immunol 96 (3) S2, 1–68
  Royal College of Physicians. 2003. *Allergy: The Unmet Need. A Blueprint for Better Patient Care.* Royal College of Physicians, London

- The UK incidence of severe food allergy is believed to be increasing (Gupta, Sheikh, Strachan and Anderson 2007).
- Adverse reactions to food may result from allergy (hypersensitivity) or intolerance (reactions that are not clearly immunologically mediated) (Sampson 2004).
- The severity of allergic reactions is highly variable, with symptoms ranging from mild urticaria to life-threatening anaphylaxis.
- Patients will often use the term 'allergy' to refer to any of a number of food-related adverse reactions; double-blind, placebo-controlled studies, however, show that only a minority of these reactions have an allergic basis (Sampson 2005; Rona, Keil, Summers, *et al.* 2007).
- In addition to the immediate effects of allergic reactions, food allergies can have a significant impact on patients' everyday lives (Primeau, Kagan, Joseph, *et al.* 2000). Activities such as food shopping, eating outside the home and travelling abroad can become challenging.

DOI: 10.1016/B978-0-7020-3053-6.00023-4

Accurate diagnosis and good long-term management are therefore crucial in maintaining quality of life and minimizing anxiety (Munoz-Furlong 2003).

● Evidence-based guidelines for the diagnosis and management of allergies are available (Chapman, Bernstein, Lee, *et al.* 2006). Note that data from randomized controlled trials are limited in the area of food allergies; these guidelines are based on a systematic review of the best available evidence.

DIAGNOSIS

For details of the diagnosis of food allergy see *Evidence-based Diagnosis in Primary Care* by A. F. Polmear (editor), published by Butterworth-Heinemann, 2008.

● Differentiating food allergy from intolerance is important because the former will typically require meticulous avoidance of the food(s) in question; continued exposure to the triggering food(s) in those with IgE-mediated food allergy increases the risks of major systemic allergic reactions such as anaphylaxis (Wood 1999; Sheikh and Walker 2002).

∗ Attempt to differentiate food allergy from intolerance by the following features of the history and examination:

(a) *Family history:* food allergy usually occurs in those with a personal and/or family history of allergic disorders.

(b) *Type of food:* although almost any food may provoke allergic symptoms in sensitized individuals, most reactions occur in relation to exposure to a small group of foods (Table 23.1) (Teuber, Beyer, Comstock and Wallowitz 2006).

(c) *Speed of onset:* symptoms soon after food intake (usually < 1 hour and often within minutes) are suggestive of allergy.

Table 23.1	Foods commonly responsible for triggering allergic reactions
CHILDREN	**ADULTS**
Milk	Fish and seafood
Egg white	Tree nuts
Peanuts	Peanuts
Wheat	Additives
Soya beans	Fruits

(d) *Effect of re-exposure:* re-exposure to the same food(s) will tend to produce very similar reactions in those with food allergy; the picture is often much more variable in those with intolerance.

(e) *Pollen-food allergy syndrome* (known until recently as oral allergy syndrome) is an IgE-mediated hypersensitivity to raw fruits, root vegetables and some nuts. It is most likely to occur in patients with tree pollen allergy (spring hay fever). Contact urticaria and/or angioedema of the lips and oropharynx occur through a cross-reactivity between specific epitopes in pollens and fresh fruit/vegetables, manifesting as an itchy oropharynx and swelling of the lips and tongue. More severe reactions may occur, but are unusual (Perry, Scurlock and Jones 2006).

(f) *The clinical picture:* food allergy will typically precipitate symptoms suggestive of inflammation of one or more organs including features of angioedema (particularly of lips and tongue), urticaria, conjunctivitis, rhinitis, bronchospasm, gastrointestinal oedema (cramps, vomiting and diarrhoea) and anaphylaxis (Perry, Scurlock and Jones 2006). Food-related symptoms of tiredness, joint and muscle pains, sleep disturbance and emotional upset are all suggestive of a diagnosis of food intolerance.

MANAGEMENT

Symptomatic treatment

∗ Treat symptomatically; if life-threatening features are present (respiratory difficulty or symptoms suggestive of hypotension) then treat as for anaphylaxis (see page 591).

Further management

∗ Attempt to identify unequivocally the food(s) responsible for triggering symptoms. Take a detailed history of reactions from the patient and, if necessary, refer to the list of the most common trigger foods to deduce likely culprits (Table 23.1). Confirm clinical suspicion with objective allergy test (skin-prick test and/or serum-specific IgE).

* Refer to an allergist if provision for suitable testing is unavailable, in the event of diagnostic uncertainty, and/or if the patient has experienced a life-threatening reaction (Durham and Church 2006).
* Recommend the avoidance of food(s) found to trigger symptoms. Advise careful checking of food ingredients (e.g. by reading food labels, asking waiting staff and caterers when eating outside the home).
* Encourage patients to be pro-active in seeking relevant information. For example, organizations such as Allergy UK and the Anaphylaxis Campaign, as well as many larger food manufacturers and catering chains, now publish allergen information online (see, for example, the INFORMALL database: http://foodallergens. ifr.ac.uk/).
* Recommend that patients with pollen-food allergy syndrome avoid the offending fruits and/or vegetables in their raw form; in most cases, the allergen is removed by peeling or destroyed by heating and the peeled/cooked fruits and/or vegetables can then be safely consumed.
* Enlist the help of a dietician to ensure that patients fully understand about the foods that they need to avoid, to help them manage avoidance when eating in and outside the home and to ensure their diet is nutritionally adequate (National Asthma and Respiratory Training Centre 2001).
* Issue self-injectable adrenaline to those with a history of anaphylaxis and recommend a medical identity bracelet/necklace.
* Refer patients with severe food intolerance(s) to a gastroenterologist. Any exclusion diet should be dietician-supervised (Grimshaw 2006).
* Review patient periodically to ensure long-term management is effective.

Reintroducing foods after a period of avoidance

Children with allergy to milk and eggs will commonly develop tolerance to these foods as they grow older. In those with a history of reactions that are not considered to be life threatening, the careful reintroduction of these foods at a later date may be appropriate.

* Consider reintroducing:
   (a) *milk* at the age of 3 years (by which time 85% of children with a history of milk allergy will be tolerant); and
   (b) *eggs* at the age of 6 years (by which time 55–80% of children with a history of egg allergy will be tolerant) (Teuber, Beyer, Comstock and Wallowitz 2006).
* *Persistent symptoms*. Refer to specialist services.

Note: Peanut and fish/seafood allergy is, in the majority of individuals, life-long (Teuber, Beyer, Comstock and Wallowitz 2006), and attempts at reintroduction are not normally recommended.

Prevention

* Strict food and house dust mite allergen avoidance should be considered for prevention of allergy in high-risk infants, as this may reduce allergic diseases in childhood (Arshad, Bateman, Sadeghnejad, *et al.* 2007; Arshad, Matthews, Gant and Hide 1992).
* Encourage lactating mothers of infants with a parent or sibling with an atopic disease to exclusively breastfeed for 4–6 months (Friedman and Zieger 2005).
* Encourage mothers of infants with a parent or sibling with an atopic allergic disease who are unable to exclusively breastfeed to use a hydrolysed cow's milk formula (Friedman and Zieger 2005).

Although those with a family history of allergic disorders have been advised to avoid peanuts during pregnancy, lactation, weaning and until the age of at least 3 years (Friedman and Zieger 2005; Fiocchi, Assa'ad and Bahna 2006), there is concern that this may actually be increasing the risk of peanut allergy through preventing the development of immunological tolerance (Du Toit, Katz, Sasieni, *et al.* 2008).

USEFUL CONTACTS

For patients

The Anaphylaxis Campaign, PO Box 275, Farnborough, Hampshire GU14 6SX Tel. 01252 546100; Helpline: 01252 542029; fax 01252 377140; email: info@anaphylaxis.org.uk; website: www. anaphylaxis.org.uk

Allergy UK. 3 White Oak Square, London Road, Swanley, Kent, BR8 7AG. Helpline: 01322 619898; fax 01322 470330; email: info@allergyuk.org; website: www.allergyuk.org

The Informall Database A searchable database with information on allergenic foods for professionals and lay people; website:

foodallergens.ifr.ac.uk/

MedicAlert Foundation. 1 Bridge Wharf, 156 Caledonian Road, London N1 9UU. Freephone 0800 581420; fax 020 7278 0647; email: info@medicalert.org.uk; website: www.medicalert.org.uk

Supermarkets can provide information on products that are 'free from' certain ingredients.

For professionals

British Society for Allergy and Clinical Immunology. Elliott House, 10–12 Allington Street, London, SW1E 5EH. Tel. 0207 808 7135; fax 0207 808 7139; website: www.bsaci.org

Education for Health. The Athenaeum, 10 Church Street, Warwick CV34 4AB. Tel. 01926 493313; email: info@educationforhealth.org; website: www.educationforhealth.org

NHS Clinical Knowledge Summaries provide evidence-based information and practical 'know how' about the common conditions managed in primary care; website: http://cks.library.nhs.uk/clinical_topics/by_clinical_specialty/allergies

Skills for Health has developed competences to describe what health professionals need to do, what they need to know and which skills they need to carry out activities related to the diagnosis and management of allergy. These are available on their website: http://tools.skillsforhealth.org.uk/suite/show/id/69

ANAPHYLAXIS

GUIDELINES

Joint Task Force on Practice Parameters; American Academy of Allergy, Asthma and Immunology; American College of Allergy, Asthma and Immunology; and Joint Council of Allergy, Asthma, and Immunology. 2005. The diagnosis and management of anaphylaxis: an updated practice parameter. J Allergy Clin Immunol 115(3 suppl), S483–S523

Muraro A., Roberts G, Clark A, *et al.* 2007. The management of anaphylaxis in childhood: position paper of the European Academy of Allergology and Clinical Immunology. Allergy 62, 857–871

Working Group of the Resuscitation Council (UK). 2008. *Emergency Treatment of Anaphylactic Reactions. Guidelines for Healthcare Providers.* London: Resuscitation Council (UK). Available: www.resus.org.uk/pages/reaction.pdf

- Anaphylaxis is a severe, life-threatening generalized or systemic hypersensitivity reaction (Johannson, Bieber, Dahl, *et al.* 2004). It is rapid in onset and may cause death (Sampson, Munoz-Furlong, Campbell, *et al.* 2006).

- Anaphylaxis is commonly triggered by foods, drugs, insect venom and latex. It may also be induced by exercise. Some cases are idiopathic.

- The UK incidence of anaphylaxis is believed to be increasing rapidly (Gupta, Sheikh, Strachan and Anderson 2007; Department of Health 2006).

- It is estimated that there are between 10 and 30 deaths from anaphylaxis in the UK each year, many of which are potentially preventable (Pumphrey and Gowland 2007; Newton 2006).

- The classification of reactions into anaphylactic (IgE-mediated hypersensitivity reactions) and anaphylactoid (non-IgE-mediated mast cell degranulation) is of little practical relevance to the management of anaphylaxis and is now largely avoided.

- Evidence-based guidelines for the management of anaphylaxis are available (Joint Task Force on Practice Parameters; American Academy of Allergy, Asthma and Immunology; American College of Allergy, Asthma and Immunology; and Joint Council of Allergy, Asthma, and Immunology 2005; Working Group of the Resuscitation Council (UK) 2008; Muraro, Roberts, Clark, *et al.* 2007; Sheikh and Walker 2005; Choo and Sheikh 2007; Nurmatov, Worth and Sheikh 2008), though note that randomized controlled trials of commonly recommended treatments have not been conducted (Sheikh, Shehata, Brown and Simons 2008; Sheikh, ten Broek, Brown and Simons 2007; Sheikh,

Simons and Choo 2009). Guidelines are based on the best available evidence.

- Anaphylaxis can have a significant long-term impact on a patient's everyday life beyond the immediate ill-effects of a reaction. Managing an unfamiliar set of risks may be challenging for patients, particularly immediately after diagnosis. The possibility of further reactions can lead to increased anxiety. Allergen avoidance requires careful vigilance, and may adversely affect the patient's family and social life. Good long-term management is therefore essential in maintaining quality of life (Panesar, Walker and Sheikh 2003; Akeson, Worth and Sheikh 2007; Avery, King, Knight and Hourihane 2003; Mandell, Curtis, Gold and Hardie 2002).

DIAGNOSIS

- Anaphylaxis presents a range of signs and symptoms, causing difficulties in diagnosis. A diagnosis is likely when all three of the following criteria are met:
  - sudden onset and rapid progression of symptoms;
  - life-threatening airway and/or breathing and/or circulation problems;
  - skin and/or mucosal changes (flushing, urticaria, angioedema).
- There may also be gastrointestinal symptoms such as vomiting. Exposure to a known allergen for the patient supports the diagnosis (Working Group of the Resuscitation Council (UK) 2008).
- Skin or mucosal changes alone are not a sign of an anaphylactic reaction. Furthermore, these changes can be subtle or absent in some anaphylactic reactions.
- Anaphylaxis is a variety of allergic reaction, not a type of disease. Diagnosis of an anaphylactic reaction should always be followed up by investigation into the underlying cause.

MANAGEMENT

- Management is best considered in two stages: treatment of the acute attack and follow-up care (Muraro, Roberts, Clark, et al. 2007; Simons 2006).

Acute management (see Table 23.2)

The key steps for the treatment of an anaphylactic reaction are shown in the algorithm (Appendix 27).

1. Commence life support (basic and advanced) if indicated.
2. Give oxygen.
3. Give adrenaline (epinephrine) 1:1000 solution (i.m.) if not already administered (many patients with a history of anaphylaxis will have been issued with adrenaline for self-injection). The Resuscitation Council cautions against the use of the i.v. route except by experienced practitioners treating profound shock (Working Group of the Resuscitation Council (UK) 2008).
4. Give inhaled beta$_2$-agonist if there is severe bronchospasm.
5. Repeat adrenaline 5 minutes after first dose if there is no clinical improvement.
6. Give chlorphenamine i.m. (or by slow i.v. injection).
7. Give i.v. crystalloid fluid infusion if symptoms of hypotension persist (a repeat dose may be necessary) (Working Group of the Resuscitation Council (UK) 2008).
8. Give hydrocortisone i.m. (or by slow i.v. injection).

Table 23.2	Route of administration and drug dosage for agents used in the emergency treatment of anaphylaxis
DRUG (ROUTE OF ADMINISTRATION)	**AGE-RELATED DOSAGE**
Adrenaline 1:1000 (i.m.)	< 6 months: 150 mcg (0.15 ml) > 6 months–6 years: 150 mcg (0.15 ml) 6–12 years: 300 mcg (0.3 ml) > 12 years (small or prepubertal child): 300 mcg (0.3 ml) > 12 years: 500 mcg (0.5 ml)
Chlorfeniramine (i.m. or slow i.v.)	< 6 months: 250 mcg/kg 6 months–6 years: 2.5 mcg 6–12 years: 5 mcg > 12 years 10 mcg
Hydrocortisone (i.m. or slow i.v.)	< 6 months: 25 mcg 6 months–6 years: 50 mcg 6–12 years: 100 mcg > 12 years: 200 mcg
Crystalloid fluid (i.v.)	Children: 20 ml/kg of body weight Adults: 500–1000 ml

9. Following treatment, the patient should be observed for a minimum of 6 hours in a clinical area suitable for resuscitation if necessary (Working Group of the Resuscitation Council (UK) 2008).

* *Trigger*. Refer to an allergist in order to identify the trigger objectively and for consideration of desensitization therapy (Working Group of the Resuscitation Council (UK) 2008; Muraro, Roberts, Clark, *et al.* 2007). This will involve a detailed history and subsequent investigations, which may include skin-prick testing, serum-specific IgE tests and allergen challenge.

* *Allergen avoidance*. Reinforce any allergen advice issued to patients and families, tailored to individual age and circumstances; dietetic referral may be indicated in cases of food allergy. Encourage patient/parent to be pro-active in seeking relevant information, e.g. checking product labels on foods, pharmaceuticals and cosmetic products. Advise avoidance, where possible, of products carrying 'may contain' allergen labels.

* *Adrenaline*. Issue adrenaline for self-administration (for example, EpiPen, Anapen or Ana-Guard) and educate the patient on when and how to use it. Delayed use of adrenaline can lead to fatality (Pumphrey and Gowland 2007), so advise patients not to hesitate in self-administering. In addition to verbal explanation, use a trainer autoinjector and ask the patient to demonstrate its correct use. Ensure autoinjector dosage is correct (both EpiPen and Anapen are available in 'junior' versions for patients weighing 15–30 kg). Advise patients to take note of their autoinjector expiry date, and make arrangements for repeat prescription. Note that adrenaline auto-injector users can subscribe to an expiry alert service by letter, email or sms text message (see useful contacts below). Multiple autoinjectors may need to be prescribed to cover different sites, such as one for home and one for school or the workplace.

* *Alert bracelet*. Recommend purchase of a medical identity bracelet/necklace or smart card documenting history of anaphylaxis and that adrenaline is carried.

* *Asthma control*. Optimize asthma management in those with a history of asthma, as the risk of

fatality is increased in this group (Pumphrey and Gowland 2007).

* Liaise with nursery/school/school nurse/work as appropriate (Vickers, Maynard and Ewan 1997).

* Review the patient 6 months after diagnosis, and thereafter every year, and following any subsequent reactions. Reviews should be used to support patients' self-management as appropriate: for example, reinforcing allergen avoidance advice, encouraging carrying adrenaline auto-injector, re-training in auto-injector use, or referring to specialist for re-testing. A management plan incorporating training in adrenaline use, support and follow-up may prove useful (Muraro, Roberts, Clark, *et al.* 2007; Choo and Sheikh 2007; Nurmatov, Worth and Sheikh 2008; Hourihane 2001).

USEFUL CONTACTS

For patients

The Anaphylaxis Campaign, PO Box 275, Farnborough, Hampshire GU14 6SX. Tel. 01252 546100; Helpline: 01252 542029; fax 01252 377140; email: info@anaphylaxis.org.uk; website: www.anaphylaxis.org.uk

Allergy UK. 3 White Oak Square, London Road, Swanley, Kent, BR8 7AG. Helpline: 01322 619898; fax 01322 470330; email: info@allergyuk.org; website: www.allergyuk.org

MedicAlert Foundation. 1 Bridge Wharf, 156 Caledonian Road, London N1 9UU. Freephone 0800 581420; fax 020 7278 0647; email: info@medicalert.org.uk; website: www.medicalert.org.uk

Supermarkets can provide information on products that are 'free from' certain ingredients (see Table 23.2).

For professionals

British Society for Allergy and Clinical Immunology. Elliott House, 10–12 Allington Street, London, SW1E 5EH. Tel. 0207 808 7135; fax 0207 808 7139; website: www.bsaci.org

Education for Health. The Athenaeum, 10 Church Street, Warwick CV34 4AB. Tel. 01926

493313; email: info@educationforhealth.org; website: www.educationforhealth.org

Adrenaline prescribing information. Includes auto-injector demonstration and details of expiry

alert system; websites: http://www.alk-lifeline.co.uk/pages/home.aspx; www.anapen.co.uk

References

Akeson, N., Worth, A., Sheikh, A., 2007. The psychological impact of anaphylaxis on young people and their parents. Clin. Exp. Allergy 37, 1213–1220.

Arshad, S.H., Bateman, B., Sadeghnejad, A., et al., 2007. Prevention of allergic disease during childhood by allergen avoidance: the Isle of Wight prevention study. J. Allergy Clin. Immunol. 119, 307–313.

Arshad, S.H., Matthews, S.M., Gant, C., Hide, D.W., 1992. Effect of allergen avoidance on development of allergic disorders in infancy. Lancet 339, 1493–1497.

Avery, N.J., King, R.M., Knight, S., Hourihane, J.O.B., 2003. Assessment of quality of life in children with peanut allergy. Pediatr. Allergy Immunol. 14, 378–382.

Chapman, J.A., Bernstein, I.L., Lee, R.E., et al., 2006. Food allergy: a practice parameter. Ann. Allergy Asthma Immunol. 96 (3) S2, 1–68.

Choo, K., Sheikh, A., 2007. Action plans for the long-term management of anaphylaxis: a systematic review of effectiveness. Clin. Exp. Allergy 37, 1090–1094.

Department of Health, 2006. A review of services for allergy. Department of Health, London.

Du Toit, G., Katz, Y., Sasieni, P., et al., 2008. Early consumption of peanuts in infancy is associated with a low prevalence of peanut allergy. J. Allergy Clin. Immunol. 122, 984–991.

Durham, S.R., Church, M.K., 2006. Principles of allergy diagnosis. In: Holgate, S.T., Church, M.K., Lichtenstein, L.M. (eds), Allergy.

3rd ed. Mosby Elsevier, Philadelphia, pp. 3–16.

Fiocchi, A., Assa'ad, A., Bahna, S., 2006. Food allergy and the introduction of solid foods to infants: a consensus document. Ann. Allergy Asthma Immunol. 97, 10–21.

Friedman, N.J., Zieger, R.S., 2005. The role of breast-feeding in the development of allergies and asthma. J. Allergy Clin. Immunol. 115, 1238–1248.

Grimshaw, K.E.C., 2006. Dietary management of food allergy in children. Proc. Nutr. Soc. 65, 412–417.

Gupta, R., Sheikh, A., Strachan, D.P., Anderson, H.R., 2007. Time trends in allergic disorders in the UK. Thorax 62, 91–96.

Hourihane, J., 2001. Community management of severe allergies must be integrated and comprehensive, and must consist of more than just epinephrine. Allergy 56, 1023–1025.

Johannson, S.G.O., Bieber, T., Dahl, R., et al., 2004. Revised nomenclature for allergy for global use: report of the Nomenclature Review Committee of the World Allergy Organization, October 2003. J. Allergy Clin. Immunol. 113, 832–836.

Joint Task Force on Practice Parameters; American Academy of Allergy, Asthma and Immunology; American College of Allergy, Asthma and Immunology; and Joint Council of Allergy, Asthma, and Immunology, 2005. The diagnosis and management of anaphylaxis: an updated practice parameter.

J. Allergy Clin. Immunol. 115 (Suppl. 3), S483–S523.

Mandell, D., Curtis, R., Gold, M., Hardie, S., 2002. Families coping with a diagnosis of anaphylaxis in a child. Allergy Clin. Immunol. Int. 14, 96–101.

Munoz-Furlong, A., 2003. Daily coping strategies for patients and their families. Pediatrics 111, 1654–1661.

Muraro, A., Roberts, G., Clark, A., et al., 2007. The management of anaphylaxis in childhood: position paper of the European academy of Allergology and clinical immunology. Allergy 62, 857–871.

National Asthma and Respiratory Training Centre, 2001. Management of allergy in primary care. NARTC, Warwick: Unit 8.

Newton, J., 2006. An epidemiological report for the Department of Health's review of services for allergy. Department of Health, London.

Nurmatov, U., Worth, A., Sheikh, A., 2008. Anaphylaxis management plans for the acute and long term management of anaphylaxis: a systematic review. J. Allergy Clin. Immunol. 122, 353–361.

Panesar, S., Walker, S., Sheikh, A., 2003. Primary care management of anaphylaxis. Prim. Care Resp. J. 12, 124–126.

Perry, T.T., Scurlock, A.M., Jones, S.M., 2006. Clinical manifestations of food allergic disease. In: Malecki, S.J., Burks, A.W., Helm, R.M. (eds), Food Allergy. ASM Press, Washington DC, pp. 3–17.

Primeau, M.N., Kagan, R., Joseph, L., et al., 2000. The psychological burden of peanut allergy as perceived by adults with peanut allergy and the parents of peanut-allergic children. Clin. Exp. Allergy 30, 1135–1143.

Pumphrey, R.S.H., Gowland, M.H., 2007. Further fatal allergic reactions to food in the United Kingdom, 1999–2006. J. Allergy Clin. Immunol. 119, 1018–1019.

Rona, R.J., Keil, T., Summers, C., et al., 2007. The prevalence of food allergy: a meta-analysis. J. Allergy Clin. Immunol. 120, 638–646.

Sampson, H.A., 2004. Update of food allergy. J. Allergy Clin. Immunol. 113, 805–819.

Sampson, H.A., 2005. Food allergy: accurately identifying clinical reactivity. Allergy 60 (Suppl. 79), 19–24.

Sampson, H.A., Munoz-Furlong, A., Campbell, R.L., et al., 2006. Second symposium on the definition and management of anaphylaxis: summary report. J. Allergy Clin. Immunol. 117, 391–397.

Sheikh, A., Shehata, Y.A., Brown, S.G.A., Simons, F.E.R., 2008. Adrenaline (epinephrine) for the treatment of anaphylaxis with and without shock. Cochrane Database Syst. Rev. (4), CD006312. DOI: 10.1002/14651858.CD006312.pub2.

Sheikh, A., Simons, F.E.R., Choo, K.J.L., 2009. Glucocorticoids for the treatment of anaphylaxis (Protocol). Cochrane Database Syst. Rev. (1), CD007596. DOI: 10.1002/14651858.CD007596.

Sheikh, A., ten Broek, V.M., Brown, S. G.A., Simons, F.E.R., 2007. H1-antihistamines for the treatment of anaphylaxis with and without shock. Cochrane Database Syst. Rev. (1), CD006160. DOI: 10.1002/14651858.CD006160.pub2.

Sheikh, A., Walker, S., 2002. Ten-minute consultation: food allergy. BMJ 325, 1337.

Sheikh, A., Walker, S., 2005. Ten minute consultation: anaphylaxis. BMJ 331, 30.

Simons, F.E.R., 2006. Anaphylaxis, killer allergy: long-term management in the community. J. Allergy Clin. Immunol. 117, 367–377.

Teuber, S.S., Beyer, K., Comstock, S., Wallowitz, M., 2006. The big eight foods: clinical and epidemiological overview. In: Malecki, S.J., Burks, A.W., Helm, R.M. (Eds.), Food Allergy. ASM Press, Washington DC, pp. 49–79.

Vickers, D.W., Maynard, L., Ewan, P.W., 1997. Management of children with potential anaphylactic reactions in the community: a training package and proposal for good practice. Clin. Exp. Allergy 27, 898–903.

Wood, S.F., 1999. GP Guide to the Diagnosis and Management of Allergic Disorders in Children. Mosby, London.

Working Group of the Resuscitation Council (UK), 2008. Emergency treatment of anaphylactic reactions. Guidelines for healthcare providers. London: Resuscitation Council (UK). Available: www.resus.org.uk/pages/reaction.pdf.

Chapter 24

Older people

CHAPTER CONTENTS

DOI: 10.1016/B978-0-7020-3053-6.00024-6

KEEPING OLDER PEOPLE HEALTHY

SCREENING AND PREVENTION

* Continue screening programmes for mammography and cervical screening until older age. There is little evidence that screening is no longer worthwhile and most programmes recommend continuing to age 75 years, although in the UK *routine* screening ends at 65.
* Screening for, and management of, hypertension in particular and cardiovascular disease in general is more important for older people (Curb, Pressel, Cutler, *et al*. 1996) as they are at higher absolute risk. Treating 10 older people with hypertension and diabetes, or 20 older people with hypertension alone, for 5 years will prevent one cardiovascular event.
* Influenza and pneumococcal vaccination are recommended in the UK and elsewhere for all persons aged 65 years and over.

SMOKING

* Advise smoking cessation for all older people. Stopping reduces mortality by 50% (Curb, Pressel, Cutler, *et al*. 1996). Simple advice from primary care doctors is effective in smoking cessation (Vetter and Ford 1990).

ALCOHOL

● Although alcohol consumption decreases with age, 17% of men and 7% of older women exceed safe limits. 1–5% of older people who drink more than occasionally report that they are 'problem drinkers' and males more so than females (DHSS 1994).

- Alcohol misuse amongst older people contributes to falls, stroke, depression and osteoporosis.
- Simple advice from the GP is effective in reducing alcohol consumption (Anderson 1993).

EXERCISE

- 30–60 minutes of sustained low level activity, such as walking, on at least 3 days per week (Manley 1996) will result in moderate health benefits such as reduced fatigue, weight loss, increased socialization, improved control of type 2 diabetes, and less shortness of breath on exertion (Rooney 1993).
- Those who exercise develop disability at a quarter of the rate of those who do not exercise, even though the exercisers have a higher rate of fractures and short-term disability related to their exercise behaviour. This improvement is still present after 9 years. A study of medical care costs found that they were a quarter less in the exercising group. Even the very old benefit, with improvements in muscle strength, gait velocity and stair climbing ability (Elon 1996).
- * Advise regular, safe, physical activity as part of daily activities. Simple advice delivered in primary care is effective in increasing activity for older patients (Kerse, Jolley, Arroll, et al. 1999; Elley, Kerse, Arroll, et al. 2003).
- * Recommend exercise which mimics the activities of daily living (ADL) such as repetitive sit to stand and walking. This is more acceptable and beneficial for older people.
- * Referral to physiotherapy for specific strength and balance training will reduce falls by 40% in women over age 80 years (Campbell, Robertson, Gardner, et al. 1997).
- * Participation in group based tai chi chuan for older people is associated with fitness outcomes, including improvements in maximal oxygen uptake (VO_2 max), muscular strength and flexibility as well as reducing the risk of falls (Wolf, Barnhart, Kutner, et al. 1996; Jin 1992; Li, Harmer, McAuley, et al. 2001; Lan, Lai, Wong, et al. 1996).

NUTRITION

DoH. 2004. Food and Health Action Plan. Department of Health. Available http://www.dh.gov.uk/PolicyAndGuidance/HealthAndSocialCareTopics/HealthyLiving/FoodAndHealthActionPlan/fs/en

- The National Diet and Nutrition Survey (1989) in the UK indicated that, in those over the age of 65:
  - (a) average intake of vitamins and minerals was above recommended levels except for some in residential and nursing homes;
  - (b) vitamin D status was poor in some, particularly those in residential and nursing homes;
  - (c) poor oral health, especially a lack of natural teeth, was associated with poor diet and nutritional status;
  - (d) average intake of sugars and saturated fatty acids exceeded recommended levels;
  - (e) average fibre intake was lower than recommended.
- Among independent older people 3% of men and 6% of women are underweight, and in nursing and residential care, these figures rise to 16% and 15% respectively (Finch, Doyle, Lowe, et al. 1998).
- Poorer households consume:
  - (a) less of the following: fruit and vegetables, salads, wholemeal bread, whole grain and high fibre cereals, and oily fish;
  - (b) more of the following: white bread, full fat milk, table sugar and processed meat products often high in fat.
- A national survey of older people in private households (Department of Health 1992) found the following:
  - (a) over half reported long-standing illness or disability;
  - (b) one in five had difficulty seeing, even with glasses;
  - (c) one in 10 were unable to walk down the road or manage stairs;
  - (d) one in five had been seen by a hospital doctor in the preceding 3 months;

(e) half of the women and a quarter of the men aged 85 years and over were not able to cook a main meal alone;

(f) only one in 10 received 'meals on wheels'.

* Assess the risk of dietary deficiencies in older patients especially those with chronic diseases, poor dentition, poor mobility, on low incomes, and housebound.

* Have a low threshold for checking the vitamin B_{12} status of older people especially if they develop neuropsychiatric symptoms (see page 635).

* Consider checking a patient's vitamin D status. Vitamin D deficiency is common in older people as the skin decreases in capacity to synthesize the provitamin calcidol, exacerbated by their low exposure to sunlight. Serious deficiencies are common in the elderly house-bound. Poor muscle strength and weakness is associated with vitamin D deficiency and this weakness may contribute to the risk of falls. Supplementation with 800 IU significantly reduces the incidence of falls (Venning 2005).

* Advise patients, no matter what age, to maintain a healthy diet including at least five portions of fruit and vegetables a day (see page 690). There is evidence that the modified Mediterranean diet is associated with increased survival among older people (Trichopoulou 2005). Refer to a dietician if there is concern about dietary intake. Ask the patient to do a food diary for a week prior to being seen.

* Advise isolated patients to contact social services and local NGOs (e.g. Age Concern). Eating with others may not only offer more interaction and reduce loneliness but there is evidence that family style meals may improve nutrition in older people (Nijs, de Graaf, Kok, et al. 2006).

MANAGING FRAILTY

● Frailty is best regarded as 'a condition or syndrome which results from a multi-system reduction in reserve capacity to the extent that a number of physiological systems are close to, or passed the threshold of symptomatic clinical failure. As a consequence, the frail person is at increased risk of disability and death from minor external stresses' (Campbell and Buchner 1997).

● General practice, as part of the primary healthcare network, is well placed to detect and treat emerging frailty and prevent further deterioration.

● The Nottingham Extended Activities of Daily Living (EADL; see Appendix 30) scale may be useful in detecting unsuspected functional decline (see page 621).

● Comprehensive geriatric assessment is associated with improved outcomes for older people, such as reducing hospital admission, re-admission, survival rates as well as improved physical and cognitive functioning (Stuck, Sui, Weiland, et al. 1993; Robinson and Turnock 1998; Nikolaus, Specht-Leible, Bach et al. 1999).

● One specific form of frailty is the decline in renal function with age; a decline which has implications for the prescribing of drugs that are renally excreted and for the management of conditions which, in themselves, impair renal function. A rise in serum creatinine is a late sign of renal impairment; estimation of the GRF is more useful (see page 425).

EARLY INTERVENTION

● Preventive home visits by health professionals or lay people trained in case-finding reduce mortality and admission to residential care and may promote independence and improve quality of life for frail older people (Elkan, Kendrick, Dewey, et al. 2001).

● Effective management of minor ailments, such as painful foot problems, may halt declining mobility and improve long-term outcomes.

● Physical therapy aimed at reducing functional impairment in older people with moderate frailty will delay functional decline, i.e. in ADL score (Gill, Baker, Gottschalk, et al. 2002).

● Maximizing the management of chronic problems and minimizing polypharmacy may halt functional decline. The UK National Service Framework recommends an annual review of medication for people aged 75 and over, with a 6-monthly review for those taking four or more medicines.

SUPPORTING OLDER PEOPLE AT HOME

- There is considerable variation in the availability of services for older people internationally and within countries, both in formal and informal provision. Generally, there is a multitude of services available aimed at either maintaining function or providing rehabilitation.
- Services can be accessed either by direct referral or through specialist geriatric services.
- A comprehensive assessment is recommended before referring to services.
- In general, services are accessed in the UK through a social worker; in Australia by direct referral or through geriatric assessment services; and in New Zealand through the needs assessment service coordinator.

DIFFICULTY MAINTAINING LIVING ARRANGEMENTS

- * Refer to an occupational therapist for assessment of activities of daily living (ADL) function at home and provision of equipment.
- * Refer to a social worker to arrange a home carer for housework.
- * Refer to a social worker for Meals-on-Wheels (daily hot food or weekly frozen meal deliveries).
- * Refer to a podiatrist/chiropodist for foot care.

ISOLATION

- * Refer to Age Concern for provision of a volunteer/befriending service.
- * Refer to a social worker for day centre placement.
- * Refer to Dial-a-Driver or social worker to access a subsidized taxi service.

CARER STRESS (see page 626)

- * Ask any carer specifically how they are coping.
- * Ascertain the source of any stress.
- * Refer for access to respite services, including day and night respite, and residential home placement for short periods.
- * Refer for home care for personal assistance.
- * Refer to an occupational therapist, for assessment of ADL function and equipment.

FUNCTIONAL DETERIORATION AT HOME

Refer to:

(a) a geriatrician for comprehensive assessment;

(b) a day hospital, for multidisciplinary assessment and treatment;

(c) physiotherapy for musculoskeletal assessment and exercises (Gill, Baker, Gottschalk, *et al.* 2002);

(d) occupational therapy for ADL functional assessment, provision of equipment and treatment;

(e) a social worker for personal home care;

(f) the district nurses for a bathing service;

(g) a speech language therapist if the condition affects communication or swallowing;

(h) a dietician.

POOR RECOVERY AFTER AN ACUTE EPISODE

- * Consider referral to:

(a) the appropriate hospital service;

(b) the district nursing service;

(c) the occupational therapist, physiotherapist for functional assessment and provision of equipment;

(d) the social worker for temporary provision of personal care and housework.

SUICIDE (O'CONNELL, CHIN, CUNNINGHAM, *ET AL.* 2004)

- Elderly people have a higher risk of completed suicide than any other age group (56 per 100,000) with a male to female ration of 4:1.
- The ratio of parasuicide to completed suicide is much lower suggesting that suicidal behaviour in older people has a much greater degree of intent.
- The main psychological factor associated with suicide in older people is recurrent major depression.
- Poor physical health and disability seem to be associated with the 'wish to die'.
- * Consider identifying all those with a known history of depressive disorder and question directly as to whether they have considered suicide (see page 459). Treat and/or refer as appropriate.
- * Screen those patients with significant comorbidities.

ACUTE CONFUSION, AGITATION, LOSS OF MOBILITY

- A change in mental or physical status of usually well independent older people should be taken seriously and treated urgently. Symptoms of serious illness are often masked and fever is seldom higher than 37.5°C even in overwhelming infection.
- Acute change can be due to serious disease without overt symptomatology related to that disease. Confusion can be as simple as 'the patient has suddenly changed, something is wrong, the level of function has deteriorated'.
- Agitation may occur and can be defined as 'inappropriate verbal, vocal, or motor activity that is not explained by needs' and may be due to undiagnosed pain, acute illness, or simply the inability to communicate needs.
- A loss of mobility or 'taken to bed' may be due to serious illness.
- Establishing the onset of deterioration and prior function is essential to identify delirium characterized by a fluctuating level of consciousness, disorientation, and global cognitive deficit. This is almost always due to an organic cause, usually infection.
- The classic triad of confusion, incontinence and falls should alert the clinician to the presence of serious illness (Mold 1996).

CONFIRMATION OF THE PRESENCE OF AN ACUTE CONFUSIONAL STATE

For details of the diagnosis of delirium see *Evidence-based Diagnosis in Primary Care* by A. F. Polmear (editor), published by Butterworth-Heinemann, 2008.

The simplest formal assessment is the Confusion Assessment Method (CAM) which states that the patient has delirium if:

- there was an acute onset with a fluctuating course;
- there is inattention; and
- there is either disorganized thinking or an altered level of consciousness. Consciousness may be depressed or the patient may be hyperalert.

The CAM has a sensitivity of at least 94% and a specificity of at least 90% (LR+ 9.4; LR− 0.07) for the diagnosis of delirium, when used by non-psychiatrists and compared to psychiatrists as the gold standard (Inouye, van Dyck, Alessi, *et al.* 1990).

DIAGNOSIS OF THE CAUSE OF THE CONFUSION

A diagnosis of acute serious illness or medication toxicity should be assumed until proven otherwise. There are many causes for acute confusion including (O'Keefe and Sanson 1998):

(a) infection, most commonly, pneumonia and urinary tract infection;

(b) cardiovascular disorder, especially myocardial infarction and congestive heart failure;

(c) neurological disorder, most commonly stroke;

(d) medication interaction or toxicity, particularly psychotropic or cardiovascular medications;

(e) acute alcohol withdrawal;

(f) acute psychiatric disorder, including psychosis;

(g) electrolyte disturbance, dehydration, hyponatraemia;

(h) endocrine disorder, thyroid disease, diabetes;

(i) acute change in hearing or vision;

(j) faecal impaction or retention of urine;

(k) neoplasia;

(l) acute surgical emergency, such as peritonitis from appendicitis or gallbladder disease;

(m) undiagnosed fracture;

(n) hypothermia.

SPECIFIC EVALUATION

A thorough history and physical examination are necessary including:

(a) history of prior functional level, social support, medications and medical problems. Involving caregivers or family member to get a history may be necessary;

(b) examination of cardiovascular and neurological systems;

(c) musculo-skeletal examination, especially for those with reduced mobility. Suspect undiagnosed fracture after apparent minor injury with excessive disability;

(d) abdominal examination to exclude an acute abdomen;

(e) rectal examination;

(f) examination of the fundi;

(g) rectal temperature;

(h) investigations will be guided by the history and physical examination (see box below).

POSSIBLE INVESTIGATIONS

FBC and ESR

Creatinine, eGFR, and electrolytes

LFTs

TFTs

B_{12}

MSU

Blood glucose

Calcium

Blood cultures

ECG

CXR and other X-rays as suggested by the examination

MANAGEMENT

Delirium, acute confusion

* Refer for admission to an acute medical ward or geriatric assessment ward if the diagnosis cannot be clearly identified and the patient cannot be managed at home, or if a diagnosis is made e.g. pneumonia or stroke, which requires admission.

If treating the patient at home:

* Treat any infection with an appropriate antibiotic.

* Stop medications with potential toxicity, especially sedative/hypnotics if they are suspected of causing acute confusion.

* Treat dehydration with fluids with attention to cardiovascular function.

* Deal with faecal impaction in the usual way, with attention to follow-up bowel function. Fluids, exercise and fibre are all needed for adequate bowel function in older people.

Agitation

* Treat the cause as above, especially undiagnosed pain.

* Refer for admission to geriatric or psychogeriatric assessment ward if the patient cannot be managed at home.

* Refer to a psychiatrist for evaluation if psychosis is suspected.

* If no cause is found and the patient has underlying dementia, see below (page 602).

* Behavioural management is useful for any agitated patient including:

    (a) allowing wandering in a safe environment;

    (b) relocation to alternative living arrangements if agitation becomes a constant problem and cannot be managed in the current living arrangement;

    (c) encouraging participation in usual activities;

    (d) avoiding confrontation if aggression is a feature;

    (e) avoiding physical restraint; it worsens agitation and can cause injury.

* See page 604 for services available.

* *Medication.* Reserve antipsychotics, typical or atypical, for patients who are so agitated that they pose a risk to themselves or to others. They are associated with increased mortality, especially from stroke and sudden cardiac death. Haloperidol may be associated with less risk than the atypicals.

* Avoid benzodiazepines. Even short-acting benzodiazepines accumulate in the older person and worsen the confusion. They increase the risk of injury from falling, with patients on higher doses of certain drugs, (oxazepam, flurazepam and chlordiazepoxide) having the highest risk (Tamblyn, Abrahamowicz, du Berger, *et al.* 2005).

Loss of mobility

* Treat acute illness as for acute confusion above.

* If minor injury is the cause, and significant disability has resulted and there is no fracture:

    (a) give adequate pain relief;

    (b) mobilize as soon as possible;

    (c) refer to community physiotherapy or outpatient department or day hospital services for rehabilitation (Forster, Young and Langhorne 2002).

* Consider giving vitamin D 800 units daily with calcium co-supplementation. This may reduce the risk of hip fracture in frail older people (Gillespie, Avenell, Henry, *et al.* 2002) (see page 280).

* Refer the patient to a day hospital, which can improve overall functional outcome and reduce service utilization when compared with no comprehensive care (Forster, Young and Langhorne 2002).
* Refer for comprehensive inpatient geriatric assessment and management if overall function has deteriorated without apparent cause (Stuck, Sui, Wieland, *et al.* 1993).

SUBACUTE DETERIORATION WITHOUT ACUTE ILLNESS: DEPRESSION OR DEMENTIA

* Deterioration in mental or physical status can be slow and progressive and not apparently due to acute illness (i.e. not delirium).
* If the onset is slow and workup has not shown a treatable acute cause then the differential diagnoses of dementia and depression must be considered.

DIAGNOSIS

* The diagnosis of depression is often missed in older people as the prominence of physical symptoms compounds the diagnosis.
* Dementia is of more insidious onset than depression.
* In depression cognitive and physical deterioration is worse in the mornings.
* In depression insight is present; in dementia it is rare.
* Orientation is poor in dementia and preserved in depression.
* Memory loss is characteristically worse for recent events in dementia, but can be similar for recent and remote events in depression.

SPECIFIC EVALUATION

* Ask about a family and personal history of depression.
* Ask about recent significant events. Bereavement and relocation predispose to social isolation and depression.
* Check functional status and independence in living activities.
* Check the patient's social and financial supports.

* Ask about driving. Specific driving assessment may be necessary later.
* The geriatric depression scale is useful in diagnosing depression in those without severe dementia (Montorio and Izal 1996).
* Assess the patient's cognitive state formally using one or both of the following tests or use the TYM test (see page 602):
  * *Clock drawing* is a useful, non-threatening test of mental function. Simply draw a circle and ask the patient to 'make it into a clock with the time at 10 to two'. If numbers are not spread throughout all four quadrants then the test is positive for dementia.
  * A standardized mental test score, such as the Abbreviated Mental Test Score, see box. It is only reliable if used precisely (Holmes and Gilbody 1996). A more well-validated but time-consuming score is the MMSE (see below).

ABBREVIATED MENTAL TEST SCORE

Each question scores 1. A score of 6 or less suggests dementia.

1. Age (*exact number of years*);
2. Time (*to the nearest hour*);
3. A simple address, e.g. 42 West Street, to be repeated by the patient at the end of the test;
4. Year (*the current year*);
5. The place (*exact address or the name of the surgery or hospital*);
6. Recognition of two persons present (*by name or role*);
7. Date of birth (*correct day and month*);
8. Year of the First World War (*1914 or 1918 is enough*);
9. Name of the monarch (*must be current monarch*);
10. Count backwards from 20 to 1 (with no mistakes, or with mistakes which the patient corrects without prompting).

MANAGEMENT

* Treatment of dementia is outlined in the next section.
* Refer for geriatric medical or geriatric psychiatric assessment if the diagnosis is not clear.

* Treat depression, if present, with:
  (a) an antidepressant (see page 454) (Wilson, Mottram, Sivanranthan, *et al*. 2002); and/or
  (b) psychological therapy including cognitive behaviour therapy. Poor access to publicly funded counselling services may limit its availability.
* Follow-up is essential to ensure recovery of function.

DEMENTIA

For details of the diagnosis of dementia see *Evidence-based Diagnosis in Primary Care* by A. F. Polmear (editor), published by Butterworth-Heinemann, 2008.

GUIDELINES

Practice parameter: diagnosis of dementia (an evidence-based review). Report of the Quality Standards Subcommittee of the American Academy of Neurology. Neurology 2001, 56, 1143–1153, and 1154–1166.

NICE. 2006. *Dementia: Supporting People with Dementia and their Carers in Health and Social Care*. Clinical Guideline 42. Available on www.nice.org.uk

Burns A, Illiffe S. 2009. Dementia. BMJ 338, 405–409

* Dementia affects 10% of those over age 65 years and 20% of those over age 80 years.
* Absolute numbers of those with dementia will increase exponentially in the next two decades as the world population ages.
* New therapies recently available and currently under investigation mean that identification of early dementia may become important in the future.
* A UK parliamentary committee report (House of Commons 2008) has criticized the whole range of dementia care:
  (a) poor diagnosis – only a third receive a formal diagnosis;
  (b) fragmented home support;
  (c) untrained staff in care homes; and
  (d) a failure to recognize and manage dementia in hospitals.

DIAGNOSIS

* Suspect dementia when the patient has:
  (a) impairment in short and long-term memory, abstract thinking, judgment, other higher cortical function or personality change; and
  (b) the disturbance is severe enough to interfere significantly with work, social activities or relationships; and
  (c) delirium is absent (American Psychiatric Association 1987).
* Confirm it with a formal assessment. NICE mentions:
  (a) 6-item cognitive impairment test;
  (b) the General Practitioner Assessment of Cognition (GPCOG);
  (c) the 7-minute screen;
  (d) Mini Mental State Examination (MMSE).

A good combination is the Abbreviated Mental Test Score plus the clock drawing test (see above). The former tests orientation and memory while the latter tests praxis and spatial perception.

A promising new test is the TYM ('test your memory') test (Brown, Pengas, Dawson, *et al*. 2009). It has three advantages over the tests currently in use: it tests many different cognitive domains; it is performed by the patient alone, taking less than a minute of the doctor's or nurse's time to score it; and it is sensitive for the detection of early Alzheimer's disease. Using a score of ≤ 42 out of 50 as positive it is 93% sensitive and 86% specific for Alzheimer's disease. The original article and the test itself are available on www.bmj.com and on www.tymtest.com

* Determine, from the history and examination, whether it is possible to decide on the cause of the dementia (see below). This entails examination of the patient's mental state and cognition, a neurological and cardiovascular examination and a screen for depression. However, many patients have atypical or non-specific presentations.
* Exclude the few cases of reversible cognitive impairment as detailed below. The box lists the clinical features of the types of dementia.

TYPES OF DEMENTIA LISTED IN ORDER OF PREVALENCE

Dementia – Alzheimer's type
  ◼ Accounts for the majority of dementia cases.
  ◼ Insidious onset over several years.
  ◼ Global deficits.

Vascular dementia

■ Accounts for 10% of dementia cases, although 29–41% of dementia cases autopsied have some vascular pathology.

■ Stepwise progression.

■ Bilateral neurological signs.

■ A history of cardiovascular disease suggests vascular dementia.

■ Risk factors, or a history of risk factors for cardiovascular make vascular dementia more likely.

Dementia with Lewy bodies

Dementia plus the following:

■ Balance and gait disorder.

■ Prominent hallucinations and delusions.

■ Sensitivity to antipsychotics.

■ Fluctuations in alertness.

Frontotemporal dementia

■ Early loss of personal awareness.

■ Early loss of social awareness.

■ Hyperorality.

■ Stereotyped, perseverative behaviours.

Prion disease (Creutzfeld–Jakob disease; CJD)

■ Rapidly progressive symptoms.

■ Characteristic EEG pattern of periodic sharp wave complexes.

■ Pathological brain tissue diagnosis.

■ CSF 14-3-3 protein (high sensitivity and specificity for diagnosis of CJD).

Specific evaluation

* Take a history from a caregiver or a source other than the patient. Objective assessment of change (e.g. from the carer) may help support the diagnosis. Use the Informant Questionnaire on Cognitive Decline in the Elderly (IQCODE): http://cmhr.anu.edu.au/ageing/Iqcode/download/pdf/shortEnglish.pdf.

* Screen for depression.

* Examine the patient's mental state, cognition, neurological system.

* Examine the cardiovascular system.

* Investigations:

  (a) vitamin B_{12} level;

  (b) thyroid function;

  (c) FBC, creatinine, eGFR, electrolytes, LFTs, calcium, glucose, ESR;

  (d) CXR, MSU;

  (e) syphilis screening may no longer be needed unless there is a specific risk factor or they are from certain parts of the USA.

* Imaging with CT or MRI scan. Availability will limit access in some regions.

Other options are not recommended or not appropriate for primary care. Imaging with single photon emission computerized tomography (SPECT) or positron emission tomography (PET) is not recommended for routine use. Genetic testing and genotyping is not currently recommended. The CSF 14-3-3 protein may become available and is useful for confirming or rejecting the diagnosis of CJD in clinically appropriate circumstances.

MANAGEMENT

General

* It is widely accepted that patients with dementia should be assessed by a psychogeriatrician or geriatrician.

* Cognition, function, mood and behaviour as well as general health should be re-evaluated in patients with dementia every 6 months.

* Prognosis. If the family wishes to know, explain that a diagnosis of AD reduces life expectancy in a way that depends on the person's age. At age 65 median survival with AD is 8 years; at 90 at is 3 years (Brookmeyer, Corrada, Curriero, et al. 2002).

* Driving. Advise the patient to inform the DVLA and their insurance company. If there is reasonable concern about public safety the GPs should inform the DVLA themselves. Download and give to the patient, the leaflet Driving and Dementia available from http://alzheimers.org.uk/downloads/Driving_dementia_lwd.pdf. Indicate that the maximum time driving might be allowed is 3 years (Breen, Breen, Moore, et al. 2007).

Training the carers (see also page 626)

* Refer for intensive long-term education and support for caregivers (if available) to delay time to residential care placement. A meta-analysis has shown that interventions designed to support carers can improve their mental health as well resulting in the patient with AD staying

at home longer (Brodaty, Green and Koschera 2003).

* Explain the principles of reality orientation and how to cope with a dementing person(see below).
* If the patient is not already too impaired, explain how he or she can reduce the impact of the condition on their lives (see page 606).
* If sleep is a problem, train the carers in sleep hygiene practices: (advice about exercise, sleep at regular times, avoiding naps (see page 463). This has been shown to improve sleep patterns with daytime benefits as well. To achieve these benefits the carers will need considerable support (McCurry, Gibbons, Logsdon, *et al.* 2003).
* Refer for home support (see supporting older people at home page 598).
* Consider referral for placement in dementia-specific long-term care. This reduces behavioural problems and use of chemical and physical restraints.
* Consider whether the patient might be in pain. Many older patients suffer from painful conditions. A patient with dementia may be unable to communicate that pain is a problem. Look out for signs of distress (frowning, looking frightened, aggression, agitation or withdrawal) and give an analgesic if pain could be the cause (Scherder, Oosterman, Swaab, *et al.* 2005).

For patients in residential care

* Offer residential care staff education about the behavioural management patients with AD.
* Explain that a safe wandering space is essential for the older person with dementia to avoid agitation and unnecessary restraint, although there is no direct evidence of benefit (Price, Hermans and Grimley Evans 2002). This is especially useful for 'sundowning' (increased agitation in the late afternoon).
* Scheduled toileting and prompted voiding reduces urinary incontinence.
* Music therapy, simulated natural sounds and intensive multimodality group training may improve overall function.

Psychosocial interventions

The main cognitive approaches that can play a role are as follows:

(a) Reality orientation; this is based on the belief that continual, repetitive reminders will keep the patient stimulated and better orientated. There is some evidence of improved cognition and behaviour in dementia sufferers (Spector, Orrell, Davies, *et al.* 2000).
(b) Memory enhancement strategies; these include setting shorter term goals, maintaining a social circle and family role.
(c) Presenting dementia as a disability that can be accommodated and emphasizing continuing abilities.

General principles for carers:

(a) treat the patient with respect and dignity and address the patient as though you expect them to understand;
(b) recognize the patient's level of capability but do not talk down or treat them as a child;
(c) encourage all attempts at personal care and activities of daily living;
(d) when talking, look directly at the person and maintain eye contact;
(e) use short sentences expressing one thing at a time;
(f) do not use implied messages; say exactly what is meant;
(g) if not understood, repeat the message a different way. Do not shout and do not rush them;
(h) mention names of familiar people, the date, week and time in all conversations;
(i) reward the patient's attempts with a smile or compliment.

Reality orientation in the patient's home could include:

(a) a large clock and a calendar visible at all times;
(b) wearing a watch with a date display;
(c) having stimulating materials available, e.g. newspapers and magazines;
(d) a reality orientation board with a schedule of daily activities and reminders, e.g. appointments, at what time to expect a carer that day, as well a reminder of the day and date.

Medications for cognitive symptoms

Alzheimer's disease (Doody, Stevens, Beck, *et al.* 2001)

Cholinesterase inhibitors have been shown to improve cognition and global functioning in patients with Alzheimer's disease. The improvements are small and come at the cost of an increase in adverse effects. The benefits are greatest for those in whom the disease is moderate or moderately severe.

NICE has issued the following guidance on their use by the NHS in the UK (September 2007) (NICE 2007):

- Donepezil, galantamine and rivastigmine may be used in moderately severe Alzheimer's disease.
- Memantine may be used in moderately severe to severe Alzheimer's disease but only as part of a clinical trial.
- The severity of the condition may be assessed using the MMSE, where 'moderate' to 'moderately severe' are represented by scores of 10–20 points (see Table 24.1). However, the MMSE should not be used if another condition makes it unreliable (e.g. learning difficulties, sensory impairment or linguistic problems).
- The drug should be initiated by a specialist in the care of patients with dementia.
- A patient given the drug should be reviewed 6 monthly with an MMSE score and global, functional and behavioural assessment. Carers' views should be sought. The drug may be continued only if the MMSE score remains at or above 10 and the patient's condition is such that it is felt that the drug is having a worthwhile effect.
- A patient already started on one of the above drugs may continue it for as long as seems appropriate, even if the criteria above are not met.

Families may ask their GP's opinion of various drugs that can be bought over the counter; for instance:

- *Vitamin E* may slow the progression of AD, although evidence is limited (Tabet, Birks, Grimley Evans, *et al.* 2002).
- *Gingko biloba*. There is limited evidence of benefit in cognitive function from taking gingko biloba and no evidence of increased harm. 'Over the counter' preparations vary considerably in potency compared to the pure product used in RCTs (Warner, Butler and Arya 2005). Relatives can be warned that the chance of benefit is small.

Ischaemic vascular dementia and mixed dementia

Evidence-based data supporting pharmacological efficacy of agents to treat non-AD dementia are less strong than for AD. However, some research shows that patients with vascular dementia benefit from galantamine (Erkinjuntti, Kurz, Gauthier, *et al.* 2002) and from donepezil (Malouf and Birks 2004) although they are not licensed for this condition.

✳ Offer all the measures appropriate for the secondary prevention of cardiovascular disease (see page 168), if the patient's condition and life expectancy warrant it. Blood pressure control with perindopril and indapamide has been shown to slow cognitive decline and reduce disability (Fransen, Anderson, Chalmers, *et al.* 2003). However, other interventions, e.g. aspirin, may not halt cognitive decline although they are likely to reduce the risk of CVD (Rands, Orrel, Spector, *et al.* 2005).

Medication for behavioural symptoms

The treatment of *delirium*, an acute change in mental status characterized by fluctuation in level of consciousness, is empirical. It is more complex in those with dementia (Britton and Russell 2002).

✳ Look for an organic cause, most commonly undiagnosed pain, infection and cardiovascular disorder, as with well older people.
✳ Use behavioural and environmental modification. 'Reality orientation' (presenting orientation information based on time, place and person related) has been shown in one systematic review of small RCTs to improve behaviour (Spector, Orrell, Davies, *et al.* 2000).
✳ Treat *agitation and psychosis as follows:*
  (a) *Mild* – trazodone, carbamazepine, sodium valproate, SSRIs.
  (b) *Severe agitation or if psychosis* is present – the choice is between haloperidol and

Table 24.1	Grading of severity in Alzheimer's disease according to the Mini Mental State Examination (MMSE)
SEVERITY	**MMSE SCORE**
Mild	21–26
Moderate	15–20
Moderately severe	10–14
Severe	< 10

risperidone. Their use is associated with a small increase in the risk of cerebrovascular disease and death. This risk may be greater with risperidone than with haloperidol but the latter is more likely to cause sedation and parkinsonian symptoms (Schneider, Dagerman and Insel 2005).

(c) *Severe behavioural disturbance which poses a risk to the patient or to others* – haloperidol in low dose and for the shortest possible time.

* Withdraw an antipsychotic from a patient with dementia, unless the need for it is overwhelming. A UK RCT in patients with dementia on antipsychotic treatment found that those whose antipsychotic medication was switched to placebo had a better chance of surviving over 12 months than those in whom the medication was continued (Ballard, Hanney, Theodoulou, *et al.* 2009).

* *Treat depression* with SSRIs or mirtazapine although the evidence is sparse (Bains, Birks and Dening 2002).

Teaching the patient to cope with cognitive impairment

● In the early stages of cognitive impairment the patient can be taught how to minimise the functional disability. A simple analogy, such as 'if you had a limp you'd use a stick – but since it's your memory that's not so good you need to learn ways to help it' may help the patient to accept the concept. Another phrase that is readily understood is 'use it or lose it'.

● Family and carers should be involved in this process from the beginning. It will help to overcome their frustration at living with a cognitively impaired relative and, as the patient becomes more impaired, they can take over some of the tasks.

● Cognitive impairment is embarrassing and frustrating. The natural tendency is to try to cover it up. The approach outlined below depends on the opposite: accepting it and adopting techniques to minimize its effect.

* Advise the patient to:
  (a) do things when you are most alert;
  (b) take rest;
  (c) use relaxation techniques to reduce stress;
  (d) take regular exercise; exercise three or more times a week is associated with significantly

less decline in cognitive loss (Larson, Wang, Bowen, *et al.* 2006);

  (e) keep active, e.g. household jobs, visiting, reading, etc;
  (f) be involved in sports, music and other activities that involve co-ordination;
  (g) keep a regular routine;
  (h) learn to live with pain and not expect all pain to be relieved but use analgesics when necessary, particularly for night pain;
  (i) express feelings;
  (j) eat well balanced meals;
  (k) reduce alcohol intake;
  (l) consider counselling.

Memory difficulties

Memory involves learning, storage and recall. There is little that can be done to improve the storage of memory but there are techniques to improve learning and recall.

* Advise the patient to:
  (a) avoid undermining their confidence. Remember 'no-one's memory is perfect'! If you forget something don't get too upset about it;
  (b) reduce alcohol and avoid sedatives;
  (c) try to concentrate in a place free of distractions;
  (d) try to motivate yourself to learn. Make sure you understand and remember all the information;
  (e) improve retention by rehearsing/repeating information and by making associations to improve retention;
  (f) learn one new thing at a time and try to avoid the confusion that comes with information overload;
  (g) when learning something study for short periods and frequently rather than long periods;
  (h) use memory aids, e.g. dry wipe boards, 'Post-it' note pads, diaries, a calendar and alarms.

Anxiety, moodiness and irritability

* Advise the patient to:
  (a) identify the sources of aggravation and try to come up with a simple solution;

(b) practice talking to oneself, e.g. stay calm, relax etc.;

(c) leave the situation explaining that you will need to calm down and go back to it later;

(d) use relaxation techniques (e.g. tapes, therapy, counting to 10);

(e) take regular exercise;

(f) get things 'off your chest' by talking or writing.

Difficulty in initiating activities

∗ Advise the patient to:

(a) improve your organizational skills (daily routines, use of a diary, avoid putting things off, priority lists, break the task into smaller tasks, use simple methods to achieve things, ask for help or delegate, take time and not to rush, if necessary involve others in decision making);

(b) involve others so they can help motivate you;

(c) reward yourself when steps are completed. Do this frequently and make the goals reasonable;

(d) if orientation is a problem use maps, landmarks, plan routes and written directions.

Reading

Having to re-read something several times is common. This may be a result of concentration or memory problems but may also result from a change in the brain's ability to handle a lot of information.

∗ Advise the patient to try:

(a) moving their finger under each word at a comfortable pace;

(b) blocking off the words underneath the sentence with a sheet of paper;

(c) creating a window, in card, that only allows one line to read at a time;

(d) taking notes to help focus and concentrate on the important parts;

(e) reading larger print;

(f) testing themselves about what they have read.

Problems in social situations

They may have difficulties in understanding certain social situations and jump to conclusions that are inappropriate.

∗ Advise the patient to:

(a) clarify what was meant;

(b) explain what they believe was said;

(c) get feedback from others;

(d) recognize problem situations or people and plan how to respond beforehand;

(e) communicate openly and honestly; above all respect the others' position;

(f) give the 'benefit of the doubt' to others and assume they mean no harm.

Different patterns of cognitive impairment require different specific approaches. See entries under Alzheimer's disease, Parkinson's disease and Huntington's disease.

Financial and legal aspects (UK)

∗ Assess whether the patient is eligible for exemption from the Council tax (see pgno 6).

∗ Assess whether it is appropriate for someone else to be given power of attorney (see pages 18 and 614).

SUPPORT GROUPS

Alzheimer's New Zealand, PO Box 2808, Christchurch, New Zealand, tel. 64 3 365 1590; www.alzheimers.org.nz

Alzheimer's Association Australia, PO Box 108, Higgins 2615, tel. 61 2 6254 4233; www.alzheimers.org.au

Alzheimer's Society, Gordon House, 10 Greencoat Place, London SW1P 1PH, Helpline 0845 300 0336; www.alzheimers.org.uk

Details of Alzheimer's Associations in other countries can be found on the website of the Alzheimer's Disease International. www.alz.co.uk

Age Concern New Zealand, PO Box 10-688, Wellington, New Zealand, tel. 64 4 471 2709; www.ageconcern.org.nz

Age Concern England, Astral House, 1268 London Road, London SW16 4ER, tel. 020 8765 7200; www.ageconcern.org.uk

Details of other UK branches of Age Concern can be found on the UK website above

FALLS

GUIDELINES

American Geriatrics Society, British Geriatrics Society, American Academy of Orthopaedic Surgeons Panel on Falls Prevention. 2001. Guideline for the prevention of falls in older persons. J Am Geriatric Soc 49, 664–672

National Institute for Clinical Excellence. 2004. *Falls: The Assessment and Prevention of Falls in Older People.* NICE Clinical Guideline 21

Falls are serious and common for those over age 75 years. Risk factors have been identified and specific interventions proven to reduce falls.

RISK FACTORS

(a) age over 80 years;
(b) cognitive impairment;
(c) history of fall and fall-related injury;
(d) arthritis;
(e) depression;
(f) use of mobility aid;
(g) gait and balance impairment;
(h) lower limb muscle weakness;
(i) visual deficit;
(j) impaired daily functioning, or a low score on the Nottingham EADL scale (see page 621);
(k) use of psychotropic medications.

Those with multiple risk factors are at a higher risk of falls.

DIAGNOSIS

* Ask older people (aged 75 and older) routinely, once a year, 'have you had a fall in the last year?'
* Perform a simple gait assessment (see below).
* Distinguish between 'hot' and 'cold' falls.
  (a) 'Hot' falls result from major medical conditions such as stroke, myocardial infarction or seizure. Treatment of the acute illness usually entails admission to hospital.
  (b) 'Cold' falls occur in the absence of serious acute illness. This part of the chapter deals

with management of cold falls and those with high risk of falls.
* Refer anyone with a recent 'cold' fall, or with recurrent falls in the last year, or with an abnormality of gait or balance, for falls risk assessment. The UK *National Service Framework for Older People* (Department of Health 2001) recommends that this should take place in a specialist falls centre.

Specific evaluation

A falls risk assessment includes:
(a) history of fall circumstances;
(b) medication review;
(c) review of chronic medical problems including alcohol misuse;
(d) examination of:
  ■ vision;
  ■ gait and balance (see below);
  ■ lower leg strength;
  ■ neurological system, especially proprioceptive and coordination function and including mental status;
  ■ cardiovascular system, especially heart rate and rhythm, lying and standing blood pressure and the murmurs of valvular disease;
(e) the environment in which the falls occurred, with attention to:
  ■ hazards such as loose mats, cords and unstable furniture;
  ■ lighting levels;
(f) assessment of the person's fear of falling and the effect it is having on functional ability;
(g) investigations including FBC and ECG.

SIMPLE GAIT ASSESSMENT

Ask the patient to stand from a chair, without using the arms, walk 3 m, turn around and return (the 'Get Up and Go' test) (Mathias, Nayak and Isaacs 1986). Unsteadiness or difficulty completing this in less than 30 seconds shows a gait and balance deficit and further evaluation is needed.

MANAGEMENT

● Results of the evaluation will guide specific management. Most patients needing intervention will have multiple risk factors.

- Multifactorial intervention is more effective than single intervention in preventing future falls, with a RR of 0.73 (95%CI 0.63 to 0.85) for unselected older people and 0.60 (95%CI 0.50 to 0.73) for those in residential care (Gillespie, Gillespie, Robertson, *et al.* 2003).
- Refer all with a history of loss of consciousness to a physician. Investigations, such as a 24-hour ECG, may reveal a cause. Carotid sinus hypersensitivity can be detected by carotid sinus massage in controlled conditions including cardiac monitoring.
- Ensure that trained professionals conduct the falls prevention programme. A common sense approach, without such training, can be counterproductive. For instance, recommending brisk walking to older people at risk of falling can increase the fracture rate.
- Treat those at high risk of recurrent falls as follows:

Community–dwelling older people at high risk of recurrent falls (Gillespie, Gillespie, Robertson, *et al.* 2003)

- Refer for a programme of muscle strengthening and balance retraining (Robertson, Gardner, Devlin, *et al.* 2001) and advice on use of assistive devices. This depends on the local availability of a falls clinic or falls-related exercise groups.
- Encourage increased exercise such as walking or refer to an exercise programme with a balance component (Lord, Castell, Corcoran, *et al.* 2003).
- Recommend vestibular rehabilitation exercises for those who have a problem with their balance (see box).
- Refer for Tai Chi Chuan exercise. A 15-week course reduces falls by 50% (Wolf, Barnhart, Kutner, *et al.* 1996). The availability of classes may be limited.
- Assess vision and refer if necessary.
- Review medications and reduce psychotropics. Drugs that are especially likely to cause falls are benzodiazepines, tricyclic antidepressants, phenothiazines and butyrophenones, antihypertensives, anticholinergics and hypoglycaemic agents.
- *Home environment.* Assess whether loose carpets, poor lighting or general cluttering of furniture are

increasing the risk. Refer for modification of other environmental hazards according to the availability of occupational therapy (see page 625).
- Review all medical conditions. Treat cardiovascular disorders, including postural hypotension and any cardiac arrhythmia.
- *Osteoporosis.* Consider giving vitamin D_3 800 IU daily with calcium co-supplementation to reduce the risk of vertebral fracture (Gillespie, Avenell, Henry, *et al.* 2002). The vitamin D may, in addition, increase muscle strength and neuro-muscular co-ordination.

Older people in residential care and assisted living settings at high risk of recurrent falls

- Intensive multicomponent interventions including individualized activity programmes, staff education, medical review, hip protective garments and environmental hazard reduction have been successful in reducing falls in residential care (Jensen, Lundin-Olsson, Nyberg, *et al.* 2002; Becker, Kron, Lindemann, *et al.* 2003).
- Refer to physiotherapy for gait and balance training and advice on use of assistive devices. This depends on the availability of physiotherapy services in long-term care.
- Consider giving vitamin D_3 800 IU daily with calcium co-supplementation to reduce the risk of hip fracture (Gillespie, Avenell, Henry, *et al.* 2002).
- Offer hip protective devices and garments to reduce hip fracture (Parker, Gillespie and Gillespie 2002). Follow-up is needed; they are only effective if actually worn.

VESTIBULAR REHABILITATION EXERCISES

(a) *In bed*, performed slowly initially then more rapidly:
   - *eye movements* – up and down, side to side, focusing on a finger as it moves from 1 m away to 30 cm away;
   - *head movements* – moving head forwards then backwards and turning from side to side.
(b) *Sitting:* rotating the head; bending down and standing up with eyes open and closed.
(c) *Standing:* throwing a small ball from hand to hand, turning through 360°.
(d) *Moving about:* walking across the room, up and down a slope, up and down stairs with eyes open and then closed.

LOWER LIMB PROBLEMS

NIGHT CRAMPS (BUTLER, MULKERRIN AND O'KEEFFE 2002)

Nocturnal leg cramps are common occurrences among older, generally healthy adults, 70% of whom experience them at some time.

DIAGNOSIS

Most are idiopathic but they are more common in certain conditions:

- Peripheral vascular disease.
- Renal failure.
- Diabetes.
- Thyroid disease.
- Hypomagnesaemia.
- Hypocalcaemia.
- Hypokalaemia.

POSSIBLE INVESTIGATIONS

FBC and ESR.
Creatinine, eGFR, and electrolytes.
LFTs.
Blood glucose.
Calcium and magnesium.
TFTs.

MANAGEMENT

* Treat the underlying cause whenever possible.
* Look for a drug cause: diuretics, nifedipine, beta-agonists, steroids, morphine, cimetidine, penacillamine, statins and lithium have all been implicated.
* Explain the technique to abort a cramp as it is starting: forcibly stretch the muscle that is in spasm. Thus, for cramp in the calf, the patient should stand up with the leg straight and forcibly dorsiflex the foot by pressing the ball of the foot on the floor.
* Recommend a trial of calf stretching exercises; they have been found helpful in a single uncontrolled trial. The technique is to stand 3 feet from a wall, rest against it with the arms outstretched, then tilt towards it, keeping the heels on the floor, until the stretch is felt in the calves, holding the position for 10 seconds. Do this three times a day, with three stretches each time. If after three days there is improvement, continue it long term.
* *Drug treatment.*
  - Quinine sulphate 200–300 mg at night can modestly reduce the number of cramps, though, if they occur there is no reduction in their duration or severity (Butler, Mulkerrin and O'Keeffe 2002). However, quinine carries the risk of a severe sensitivity reaction in 1 in 1000 to 3500, of which the main manifestation is severe thrombocytopenia. Hepatitis and haemolytic uraemic syndrome have also been described. Finally, it is very dangerous in overdosage. Because of these risks the US Food and Drug Administration has banned its marketing for cramp, but it remains licensed for cramp in the UK. The patient should understand the risks and should realize that it will be necessary to take the drug for 4 weeks before deciding whether it has helped.
  - Other drugs: there is slender evidence that orphenadrine, naftidrofuryl and verapamil may reduce the frequency of cramps. Vitamin E does not appear to help.

RESTLESS LEGS SYNDROME

For details of the diagnosis of restless legs syndrome see *Evidence-based Diagnosis in Primary Care* by A. F. Polmear (editor), published by Butterworth-Heinemann, 2008.

REVIEWS

Chaudhuri KR, Appiah-Kubi LS, Trenkwalder C. 2001. Restless legs syndrome. J Neurol Neurosurg Psychiatry 71, 143–146
    Medcalf P, Bhatia KP. 2006. Restless legs syndrome. BMJ 333, 457–458

● The syndrome is characterized by 'creepy crawly' sensations in the lower limbs. These occur at rest in the evenings or at night and are temporarily relieved by moving the limbs. The minimum diagnostic criteria proposed by the

International Restless Legs Syndrome Study Group (Walters 1995) are:

(a) a desire to move limbs, usually associated with para/dysaesthesia;

(b) motor restlessness;

(c) symptoms worse or exclusively present at rest: partial/temporary relief with activity;

(d) symptoms worse in the evening or at night.

● Iron deficiency with or without anaemia is found in a third of older people with restless legs.

● A positive family history is present in 63–92% of patients with the idiopathic syndrome.

WORK-UP

(a) FBC.

(b) Serum ferritin.

(c) Folic acid.

(d) B_{12}.

(e) Creatinine, eGFR, and electrolytes.

---

* Examine to exclude peripheral neuropathy.
* Review the patient's drugs. Possible causes are neuroleptics, lithium, beta-blockers, calcium-channel blockers, TCAs, phenytoin, and H_2-blockers.
* Explain what to do during an attack: walk about, stretch the legs, have a bath, do something interesting as a distraction, or massage the legs.
* Consider drug treatment for patients with symptoms that are sufficiently severe. Dopaminergic drugs are effective but prone to cause adverse effects. They are unlicensed for this use in the UK. Levodopa itself appears to cause augmentation in up to 85% of users, that is, symptoms appear to start earlier in the day and may spread to the upper limbs. It can also lead to rebound the following morning and is not recommended (DTB 2003). Start each drug with a low dose at first, administered at least 2 hours before the patient goes to bed. If one drug fails, try one from another group. Consider giving domperidone for the first few weeks to reduce nausea. Options are:

(a) a dopamine agonist, e.g. pramipexole, ropinirole, pergolide, bromocriptine, or

cabergoline. Patients on the last three must be monitored for pulmonary, retroperitoneal or pericardial fibrosis. The largest trials have given the following NNTs for complete or almost complete relief: ropinirole 8 (95%CI 4.2 to 99); pergolide 1.9 (95%CI 1.4 to 2.7) (Bandolier 2004). Pramipexole and ropinirole are licensed in the UK;

(b) an antiepileptic, e.g. carbamazepine, or gabapentin, although the DTB review (above) does not find the evidence sufficient to justify their use.

If insomnia is severe add clonazepam 0.5–2 mg nocte but long-term use carries the risk of dependence.

PATIENT SUPPORT AND INFORMATION

The Restless Legs Syndrome Foundation, 819 Second Street SW, Rochester, MN 55902-2985 USA. www.rls.org

The Bandolier Restless Legs website: http://www.medicine.ox.ac.uk/bandolier/ (search on 'Restless legs')

POSTURAL ANKLE OEDEMA

Many patients are given diuretics inappropriately for postural oedema.

* Assess carefully to exclude a cardiac, renal or hepatic cause.
* Treat postural oedema by advising the patient to:

(a) keep active;

(b) elevate legs when sitting; and

(c) use support hosiery.

* Give a diuretic only where the oedema is too severe to permit the patient to pull on a support stocking, and even then only give it for a maximum of 3 weeks.
* Consider a trial without diuretics for those already started on them. In one study, 85% of those suitable were successfully withdrawn from diuretics (de Jonge, Knotternerus, van Zutphen, et al. 1994). Be aware that even patients who do not need their diuretics are likely to suffer an initial increase in oedema as a rebound phenomenon, which may take 6 weeks to settle.

ELDER ABUSE

House of Commons Health Committee. *Elder Abuse, 2003–4.* Available: http://www.publications.parliament. uk/pa/cm200304/cmselect/cmhealth/111/111.pdf

- A UK study has shown the prevalence of abuse in the patient's own home to be significant, with physical abuse in 2%, verbal in 5% and financial in 2% (Ogg and Bennett 1992). 45% of carers of older people in respite care admitted to some form of abuse (Homer and Gilliard 1990).
- There are no statutory guidelines or legislation; however, abuse is a crime. Intervention should always be interdisciplinary.
- Abuse may take the form of:
  - (a) *physical:* hitting, slapping, pushing, kicking, misuse of medication, restraint; or inappropriate sanctions;
  - (b) *psychological:* including emotional abuse, threats or harm or abandonment, deprivation of contact, humiliation, blaming, controlling, intimidation, coercion, harassment, verbal abuse, isolation or withdrawal from services or supportive networks;
  - (c) *sexual:* including rape and sexual assault or sexual acts to which the vulnerable adult has not consented, could not consent to, or was pressurized into consenting to;
  - (d) *financial or material abuse:* theft, fraud, exploitation, pressure in connection with wills, property or inheritance or financial transactions, or the misuse or misappropriation of property, possession or benefits;
  - (e) *neglect and acts of omission:* ignoring medical or physical care needs, failure to provide access to appropriate health, social care or educational services, the withholding of the necessities of life, such as medication, adequate nutrition; and
  - (f) *discriminatory abuse:* racist, sexist, based on a person's disability and other forms of harassment.
- Abuse can occur anywhere:
  - (a) in someone's own home;
  - (b) in a carer's home;
  - (d) in day care;
  - (e) in a residential or nursing home;
  - (f) in hospital.
- Abuse may occur for many reasons.
  - (a) In the home the causes include: poor quality long-term relationships; a carer's inability to provide the level of care needed; a carer with mental or physical health problems.
  - (b) In other setting it may a symptom of a poorly run establishment, especially when staff are inadequately trained and poorly supervised.
- *Suspect abuse when:
  - (a) there is delay in seeking medical help;
  - (b) there are differing histories from patient and carer, especially if explanations are implausible;
  - (c) there are inconsistencies on examination;
  - (d) there are frequent calls for visits by the GP or A&E attendances;
  - (e) the carer does not accompany the patient when that would be expected;
  - (f) there is abnormal behaviour in the presence of the carer, e.g. fear or withdrawal.
- *Discuss the situation with the patient, carer and involved care agencies. Further action will depend on the wishes and competence of the patient and the nature and severity of the abuse.
- *Discuss the case with Action on Elder Abuse (see box below).
- *Download for the patient the leaflets available from Action on Elder Abuse; (available on www. elderabuse.org.uk (choose 'Useful downloads'). For patients who may be being abused in residential or nursing homes download the Commission for Social Care Inspection leaflet 'Abuse of older people – what you can do to stop it' (http://www.csci.org.uk/publications/ general/factsheet_elderabuse.pdf). For a guide to the whole area of elder abuse recommend *Hidden Voices: Older People's Experience of Abuse.*

PROFESSIONAL AND PATIENT INFORMATION

Action on Elder Abuse, Astral House, 1268 London Road, London SW16 4ER, tel. 020 8765 7000; helpline 080 8808 8141; www.elderabuse.org.uk

SEX AND THE ELDERLY (see also page 371)

- Sexual activity is common in the elderly with studies indicating at least 50% of 60–90-year-olds remain sexually active. Although coitus declines in frequency, interest is maintained in different ways (e.g. masturbation, oral sex). There is a shift from genital sex to intimacy.

- In a study looking at the secular trends in health the sexual activity of Swedish 70-year-olds in 1971 was compared with 70-year-olds in 2001. Men and women from the latter group reported higher satisfaction with sexuality, fewer sexual dysfunctions and more positive attitudes to sexuality in later life (Beckman, Waern, Gustafson, *et al.* 2008).

∗ *Men.* Explain the 'normal' changes associated with aging (Masters and Johnson 1970):

  (a) the urgency of sexual interest declines from the late 40s;
  (b) erection is less frequent;
  (c) erection needs more stimulation especially tactile;
  (d) the erection is more difficult to sustain;
  (e) the turgidity of the erection diminishes;
  (f) ejaculation is less forceful;
  (g) the refractory period is longer;
  (h) there may be periods of difficulty establishing an erection and the frequency of these episodes increases over time. However, the pleasure derived from sex may not be significantly altered.

∗ *Women.* Explain the 'normal' changes associated with aging (Masters and Johnson 1966):

  (a) arousal requires more stimulation;
  (b) the lining of the vaginal wall thins and vaginal lubrication decreases;
  (c) there is less vaginal vasocongestion and tensing;
  (d) uterine contractions are fewer;
  (e) clitoral detumescence is rapid;
  (f) the capacity to achieve orgasm remains into old age but the length of time taken to achieve it increases.

∗ Consider the risk of sexually transmitted infection in older people embarking on new relationships and counsel them on the importance of safe sex.

∗ Be willing to discuss sexual issues with all but particularly with:

  (a) women undergoing gynaecological operations;
  (b) men undergoing prostate treatment;
  (c) patients who have severe arthritis (changing position and timing of analgesia may be needed);
  (d) patients who have had a stroke or myocardial infarction.

RESIDENTIAL AND NURSING HOMES

Kamel HK. 2001. Sexuality in aging: focus on the institutionalised elderly. Ann Long-term Care 9, 64–72

- Patients in nursing or residential homes continue to have an interest in sexual activity. Sexual behaviour is often seen as a problem rather than an expression of a need for love and intimacy. Men with dementia are more likely to exhibit inappropriate sexual behaviour.

∗ *'Inappropriate behaviour'.* Advise staff about sexuality in the elderly and advise them against unintentionally giving cues that may be misinterpreted (e.g. when washing them). In addition consider:

  (a) *behavioural approaches:* e.g. tell the patient that the behaviour is inappropriate, isolate them from residents of the sex they are subjecting, use clothing that opens at the back for males who expose their genitals;
  (b) *drug therapy:* there is little evidence but consider in very difficult cases: SSRIs, antiandrogens (cyproterone acetate), progestogens (medoxyprogesterone acetate) or oestrogens. Cyproterone is the only drug that has a licence for 'hypersexuality and sexual deviation'.

PATIENT LITERATURE

Available: www.relate.org.uk (choose 'Useful books' then 'Sex problems'):
Zilbergeld B. *Better Than Ever: Time for Love and Sex*
Williamson ML. *Great Sex After 40: Strategies for Lifelong Fulfilment*

LEGAL ASPECTS

POWER OF ATTORNEY

At an early stage of declining mental function, suggest to the family that they consult a solicitor about a lasting power of attorney (LPA) *before* the patient is incapable of signing the form. In order to sign, the patient must be capable of understanding the implications of so doing, and may be capable of this even if incapable of managing his or her affairs. If it is left too late, it is then necessary to apply to the Court of Protection to appoint a receiver, and this is much more cumbersome. The LPA must be registered before it can be used. Note that this is different from the registration of the older power, the enduring power of attorney (EPA) which only becomes necessary when the person who signed it is, or is becoming, incapable of managing his or her own affairs (see page 18).

> For more information about enduring power of attorney, lasting power of attorney, court of Protection and other relevant legal aspects in the UK go to the Public Guardianship Office website www.guardianship.gov.uk (choose 'Forms' then 'Publications').

DETENTION OF AN OLDER PERSON

> **GUIDELINE**
>
> UK: Section 47 of the National Assistance Act and Article 10, The Human Rights Act 1999

The National Assistance Act allows for the 'detention and maintenance in suitable premises of persons in need of care and attention'. It enables a local authority to seek an order from a magistrates court for the removal of a person from his or her home on the grounds that:

(a) he is suffering from a grave chronic disease or, being aged, infirm or physically incapacitated, is living in insanitary conditions;

(b) he is unable to look after himself and is not receiving proper care and attention from anyone else; and

(c) his removal is necessary in his own interests or for preventing injury to the health or, serious nuisance to, other persons.

Following the court hearing, an order can be made to remove a person by a specified officer of the appropriate authority. The order authorizes the person's detention and maintenance, but does not provide for medical treatment to be given without the person's consent. The initial order can last up to 3 months although it can be extended. If after 6 weeks an appeal is successful, the order can be revoked.

There is now some discussion that the Human Rights Act 1999, which came into force on 2 October 2000, will prove contrary to the National Assistance Act, as Section 6 (1) of the former makes it unlawful for a public authority to act in a way which goes against the European Convention on Human Rights, such as everyone has the right to 'liberty and security of person' and 'respect for his private and family life, his home and his correspondence.' However, if the person is removed under Section 47, this can be undertaken under 'protection for health,' although it remains a possibility that removals may be appealed at some stage in the future.

* Refer for comprehensive assessment by social worker, geriatrician, or psychogeriatrician, as part of application to the magistrate. This is not technically required under the Act.

Note: The Act should not be used for patients with mental disorder, who are covered by the Mental Health Act (see page 472).

* In Australia and New Zealand, refer to the local geriatric assessment team if there is a need for legal intervention to ensure patient safety and well-being.

MENTAL CAPACITY

See page 17.

References

American Psychiatric Association, 1987. Diagnostic and Statistical Manual of Mental Disorder, 3rd ed., revised. American Psychiatric Association, Washington DC.

Anderson, P., 1993. Effectiveness of general practice interventions for patients with harmful alcohol consumption. Br. J. Gen. Pract. 43, 386–389.

Bains, J., Birks, J.S., Dening, T.R., 2002. The efficacy of antidepressants in the treatment of depression in dementia (Cochrane Review). In: The Cochrane Library, Issue 4. Update Software, Oxford.

Ballard, C., Hanney, M.L., Theodoulou, M., et al., 2009. The dementia antipsychotic withdrawal trial (DART-AD): long-term follow-up of a randomised placebo-controlled trial. Lancet Neurol. 8, 151–157.

Bandolier, 2004. Restless legs: impact and treatment update. July. Available: http://www.medicine.ox.ac.uk/bandolier (search on 'restless legs').

Becker, C., Kron, M., Lindemann, U., et al., 2003. Effectiveness of a multifaceted intervention on falls in nursing home residents. J. Am. Geriatr. Soc. 51, 306–313.

Beckman, N., Waern, M., Gustafson, D., et al., 2008. Secular trends in self reported sexual activity and satisfaction in Swedish 70 year olds; cross sectional survey of four populations, 1971–2001. BMJ 337, 151–154.

Breen, D.A., Breen, D.P., Moore, J.W., et al., 2007. Driving and dementia. BMJ 334, 1365–1369.

Britton, A., Russell, R., 2002. Multidisciplinary team interventions for delirium in patients with chronic cognitive impairment (Cochrane Review). In: The Cochrane Library, Issue 1. Update Software, Oxford.

Brodaty, H., Green, A., Koschera, A., 2003. Meta-analysis of psychosocial interventions for caregivers of people with dementia. J. Am. Geriatr. Soc. 51, 657–664.

Brookmeyer, R., Corrada, M.M., Curriero, F.C., et al., 2002. Survival following a diagnosis of Alzheimer disease. Arch. Neurol. 59, 1764–1767.

Brown, J., Pengas, G., Dawson, K., et al., 2009. Self administered cognitive screening test (TYM) for detection of Alzheimer's disease: cross sectional study. BMJ 338, b2030.

Butler, J.V., Mulkerrin, E.C., O'Keeffe, S.T., 2002. Nocturnal leg cramps in older people. Postgrad. Med. J. 78, 596–598.

Campbell, A., Buchner, D., 1997. Unstable disability and the fluctuation of frailty. Age Ageing 26, 315–318.

Campbell, A., Robertson, M., Gardner, M., et al., 1997. Randomised controlled trial of a general practice programme of home based exercise to prevent falls in elderly women. BMJ 315, 1065–1069.

Curb, J., Pressel, S., Cutler, J., et al., 1996. Effect of diuretic-based antihypertensive treatment on cardiovascular disease risk in older diabetic patients with isolated systolic hypertension. Systolic Hypertension in the Elderly Program Cooperative Research Group. J. Am. Med. Assoc. 276, 1886–1892.

de Jonge, J., Knotternerus, J.A., van Zutphen, W.M., et al., 1994. Short term effect of withdrawal of diuretic drugs prescribed for ankle oedema. BMJ 308, 511–513.

Department of Health, 1992. Report on Health and Social Subjects 31– The Nutrition of Elderly People. Committee on Medical Aspects of Food Policy, HMSO.

Department of Health, 2001. National Service Framework for Older People. Department of Health, London. www.doh.gov.uk/nsf/olderpeople.htm.

DHSS, 1994. Living in Britain: Results from the 1994 General Household Survey. HMSO, Norwich.

Doody, R., Stevens, J., Beck, C., et al., 2001. Practice parameter: management of dementia (an evidence-based review). Report of the Quality Standards Subcommittee of the American Academy of Neurology. Neurology 56, 1154–1166.

DTB, 2003. Managing patients with restless legs. Drug Ther. Bull. 41, 81–88.

Elkan, R., Kendrick, D., Dewey, M., et al., 2001. Effectiveness of home based support for older people: systematic review and meta-analysis. Commentary: When, where, and why do preventive home visits. BMJ 323, 719.

Elley, C.R., Kerse, N., Arroll, B., et al., 2003. Effectiveness of counselling patients on physical activity in general practice: cluster randomised controlled trial. BMJ 326, 793.

Elon, R.D., 1996. Geriatric medicine. BMJ 312, 561–563.

Erkinjuntti, T., Kurz, A., Gauthier, S., et al., 2002. Efficacy of galantamine in probable vascular dementia and Alzheimer's disease combined with cerebrovascular disease: a randomised trial. Lancet 359, 1283–1290.

Finch, S., Doyle, W., Lowe, C., et al., 1998. National Diet and Nutrition Survey: People aged 65 Years and Over: Volume 1: Report of the Diet and Nutrition Survey. The Stationery Office, London.

Forster, A., Young, J., Langhorne, P., 2002. Medical day hospital care for the elderly versus alternative forms of care (Cochrane Review).

In: The Cochrane Library, Issue 1. Update Software, Oxford.

Fransen, M., Anderson, C., Chalmers, J., et al., 2003. Effects of a perindopril-based blood pressure-lowering regimen on disability and dependency in 6105 patients with cerebrovascular disease: a randomized controlled trial. Stroke 34, 2333–2338.

Gill, T., Baker, D., Gottschalk, M., et al., 2002. A program to prevent functional decline in physically frail, elderly persons who live at home. N. Engl. J. Med. 347, 1068–1074.

Gillespie, W., Avenell, A., Henry, D., et al., 2002. Vitamin D and vitamin D analogues for preventing fractures associated with involutional and post-menopausal osteoporosis (Cochrane Review). In: The Cochrane Library, Issue 1. Update Software, Oxford.

Gillespie, L., Gillespie, W., Robertson, M., et al., 2003. Interventions for preventing falls in elderly people (Cochrane Review). In: The Cochrane Library, Issue 4. Update Software, Oxford.

Holmes, J., Gilbody, S., 1996. Differences in use of the abbreviated mental test score by geriatricians and psychiatrists. BMJ 313, 465.

Homer, A., Gilliard, C., 1990. Abuse of elderly people by their carers. BMJ 301, 1359–1362.

House of Commons, 2008. Public Select Committee. Improving services and support for people with dementia. Sixth report. www.publications.parliament.uk/pa/cm200708/cmselect/cmpubacc/228/228.pdf

Inouye, S., van Dyck, C., Alessi, C., et al., 1990. Clarifying confusion: the confusion assessment method. A new method for detection of delirium. Ann. Intern. Med. 113, 941–948.

Jensen, J., Lundin-Olsson, L., Nyberg, L., et al., 2002. Fall and injury prevention in older people living in residential care facilities. Ann. Intern. Med. 136, 733–741.

Jin, P.T., 1992. Efficacy of tai chi, brisk walking, meditation, and reading in reducing mental and emotional stress. J. Psychosom. Res. 36, 361–370.

Kerse, N., Jolley, D., Arroll, B., et al., 1999. Improving health behaviours of the elderly: a randomised controlled trial of a general practice educational intervention. Br. Med. J. 319, 683–687.

Lan, C., Lai, J., Wong, M., et al., 1996. Cardiorespiratory function, flexibility, and body composition among geriatric tai chi chuan practitioners. Arch. Phys. Med. Rehabil. 77, 612–616.

Larson, E., Wang, L., Bowen, J., et al., 2006. Exercise is associated with reduced risk for incident dementia among persons 65 years of age and older. Ann. Intern. Med. 144, 73–81.

Li, F., Harmer, P., McAuley, E., et al., 2001. Tai chi, self efficacy and physical function in the elderly. Prev. Sci. 2, 229–239.

Lord, S.R., Castell, S., Corcoran, J., et al., 2003. The effect of group exercise on physical functioning and falls in frail older people living in retirement villages: a randomized, controlled trial. J. Am. Geriatr. Soc. 51, 1685–1692.

Malouf, R., Birks, J., 2004. Donepezil for vascular cognitive impairment (Cochrane Review). In: The Cochrane Library, Issue 1. John Wiley, Chichester, UK.

Manley, A., 1996. Physical Activity and Health. A Report of the Surgeon General. Department of Health and Human Services, Pittsburgh, US.

Masters, W.H., Johnson, V.E., 1966. Human Sexual Response. Several different publishers since 1966.

Masters, W.H., Johnson, V.E., 1970. Human Sexual Inadequacy. Several different publishers since 1970.

Mathias, S., Nayak, U., Isaacs, B., 1986. Balance in elderly patients: the 'Get up and Go' test. Arch. Phys. Med. Rehabil. 67, 387–389.

McCurry, S.M., Gibbons, L.E., Logsdon, R.G., et al., 2003. Training caregivers to change the sleep hygiene practices of patients with dementia: the NITE-AD project. J. Am. Geriatr. Soc. 51, 1455–1460.

Mold, J., 1996. Principles of geriatric care. American Health Consultants. Primary Care Reports 2, 2-9.

Montorio, I., Izal, M., 1996. The Geriatric Depression Scale: a review of its development and utility. Int. Psychogeriatr. 8, 103–112.

NICE, 2007. Donepezil, galantamine, rivastigmine (review) and memantine for the treatment of Alzheimer's disease (amended). Technology appraisal guidance 111 (amended). September.

Nijs, K.A., de Graaf, C., Kok, F.J., et al., 2006. Effect of family style mealtimes on quality of life, physical performance, and body weight of nursing home residents: cluster randomised controlled trial. BMJ 332, 1180–1183.

Nikolaus, T., Specht-Leible, N., Bach, M., et al., 1999. A randomized trial of comprehensive geriatric assessment and home intervention in the care of hospitalized patients. Age Ageing 28, 543–550.

O'Connell, H., Chin, A.V., Cunningham, C., et al., 2004. Suicide in older people. BMJ 329, 895–899.

O'Keefe, K., Sanson, T., 1998. Elderly patients with altered mental status. Emerg. Med. Clin. North Am. 16, 701–715.

Ogg, J., Bennett, G., 1992. Elder abuse in Britain. BMJ 305, 998–999.

Parker, M., Gillespie, L., Gillespie, W., 2002. Hip protectors for preventing hip fractures in the elderly (Cochrane Review). In: The Cochrane Library, Issue 1. Update Software, Oxford.

Price, J., Hermans, D., Grimley Evans, J., 2002. Subjective barriers to prevent wandering of cognitively impaired people (Cochrane Review). In: The Cochrane Library, Issue 1. Update Software, Oxford.

Rands, G., Orrel, M., Spector, A., et al., 2005. Aspirin for vascular dementia. Cochrane Database Syst. Rev. (1) The Cochrane Collaboration. John Wiley.

Robertson, M.C., Gardner, M.M., Devlin, N., et al., 2001. Effectiveness and economic evaluation of a nurse delivered home exercise programme to prevent falls. 2: Controlled trial in multiple centres. BMJ 322, 701–704.

Robinson, J., Turnock, T., 1998. Investing in Rehabilitation; Review Findings. King's Fund, London.

Rooney, E., 1993. Exercise for older patients: why it's worth the effort. Geriatrics 48, 68–72.

Scherder, E., Oosterman, J., Swaab, D., et al., 2005. Recent developments in pain in dementia. BMJ 330, 461–464.

Schneider, L.S., Dagerman, K.S., Insel, P., 2005. Risk of death with atypical antipsychotic drug treatment for dementia. JAMA 294, 1934–1943.

Spector, A., Orrell, M., Davies, S., et al., 2000. Reality orientation for dementia. Cochrane Database Syst. Rev. (3). John Wiley.

Stuck, A.E., Sui, A., Wieland, G.D., et al., 1993. Comprehensive geriatric assessment: a meta-analysis of controlled trials. Lancet 342, 1032–1036.

Tabet, N., Birks, J., Grimley Evans, J., et al., 2002. Vitamin E for Alzheimer's disease (Cochrane Review). In: The Cochrane Library, Issue 1. Update Software, Oxford.

Tamblyn, R., Abrahamowicz, M., du Berger, R., et al., 2005. A 5-year prospective assessment of the risk associated with individual benzodiazepines and doses in new elderly users. JAGS 53, 233–241.

Trichopoulou, A., for members of the EPIC – Elderly Prospective Study Group, 2005. Modified Mediterranean diet and survival: EPIC-elderly prospective cohort study. BMJ 330, 991–995.

Venning, G., 2005. Recent developments in vitamin D deficiency and muscle weakness among elderly people. BMJ 330, 524–526.

Vetter, N., Ford, D., 1990. Smoking prevention among people aged 60 and over: a randomized controlled trial. Age Ageing 19, 164–168.

Walters, A., 1995. Towards a better definition of restless legs syndrome. The International Restless Legs Syndrome Study Group. Mov. Disord. 10, 634–642.

Warner, J., Butler, R., Arya, P., 2005. Dementia. Clinical Evidence, Issue 12. BMJ Publishing Group, London.

Wilson, K., Mottram, P., Sivanranthan, A., et al., 2002. Antidepressants versus placebo for the depressed elderly (Cochrane review). In: The Cochrane Library, Issue 1. Update Software, Oxford.

Wolf, S., Barnhart, H., Kutner, N., et al., 1996. Reducing frailty and falls in older persons: an investigation of Tai Chi and computerized balance training. Atlanta FICSIT Group. Frailty and Injuries: Cooperative Studies of Intervention Techniques. J. Am. Geriatric. Soc. 44, 489–497.

Chapter 25

Disability

CHAPTER CONTENTS

PHYSICAL DISABILITY AND REHABILITATION

- A person is defined as disabled if blind, deaf, dumb, or suffering from mental disorder, or substantially and permanently handicapped by illness, injury or congenital deformity or other such disabilities (Chronically Sick and Disabled Persons Act 1970).
- Clear evidence exists for the benefit of rehabilitation in patients with stroke (Outpatient Service Trialists 2003), heart disease (Joliffe, Rees, Taylor, *et al.* 2001), COPD (Lacasse, Goldstein, Lasserton and Martin 2006), multiple sclerosis (Khan, Turner-Stokes, Ng and Kilpatrick 2007) and falls (Gillespie, Gillespie, Robertson, *et al.* 2003; Howe, Rochester, Jackson, *et al.* 2007).
- Physiotherapy and occupational therapy are effective in the management of rheumatoid arthritis (Steultjens, Dekker, Bouler, *et al.* 2004), ankylosing spondylitis (Dagfinrud, Hagen and Kvein 2004) and osteoarthritis (Fransen, McConnell and Bell 2001).
- The provision of equipment and alterations to the home can improve independence and quality of life and are cost-effective interventions (Heywood and Turner 2007).

Every person with a significant physical disability needs:

(a) an assessment of overall abilities in all aspects of daily life
(b) an understanding of their life goals and aspirations

© 2011 Elsevier Ltd.
DOI: 10.1016/B978-0-7020-3053-6.00025-8

The GP needs to become familiar with the medical condition that has caused the disability. Where the condition is a rarity, the GP will not gain the confidence of the family without this knowledge and will not be able to take a proactive role.

When making an assessment, check the following:

(a) Can the person's physical state be improved?

(b) Can the person's mental state, including self-esteem, be improved?

(c) Can the person's ability to live independently be improved?

(d) Can the person's mobility inside and outside be improved?

(e) Is there any work that the person may be able to undertake?

(f) Can the person be helped to enjoy leisure and social activities?

(g) What roles can the person fulfil in their family and local community?

(h) Would the carer benefit from more support?

(i) Can the person's or carer's financial state be improved (see Chapter 1)?

INFORMATION AND ORGANIZATIONS ON DISABILITY

If only I had known that a year ago. . . A guide for newly disabled people and their family and friends. RADAR Feb 2007

Royal Association for Disability and Rehabilitation (RADAR), 12 City Forum, 250 City Road, London EC1V 8AF, tel. 020 7250 3222; email: radar@radar.org.uk website: www.radar.org.uk

Disablement Information and Advice Line (DIAL), A network of 140 local disability information and advice services. St Catherine's, Tickhill Road, Doncaster, South Yorkshire DN4 8QN, tel. 01302 310123; e-mail: enquiries@DIALuk.org.uk; website: www.dialuk.info

Disability Rights Commission. An independent body established in 2000 by Act of Parliament to stop discrimination and to promote equal opportunity for disabled people. Website: www.drc-gb.org

---

REFERRAL

Consider referral to the appropriate agency if:

(a) the cause of the disability is unknown; or

(b) there is new impairment, disability or handicap; or

(c) there is deterioration in existing impairment, disability and handicap; or

(d) the disabled person and/or their carer are barely coping.

POOR PROGRESS

Consider:

(a) unidentified medical problems, e.g. anaemia, heart failure, hypothyroidism, Parkinson's disease;

(b) occult depression;

(c) occult dementia that may be masked by intact social skills;

(d) communication problems, e.g. poor vision or hearing.

ELIGIBILITY FOR SERVICES

Section 2 of the Chronically Sick and Disabled Persons Act 1970 lists the arrangements that the Local Authority has a **duty** to make:

(a) the provision of practical assistance for that person in his or her home;

(b) the provision for that person of, or assistance to that person in obtaining wireless, television, library or similar recreational facilities;

(c) the provision for that person of lectures, games, outings and taking advantage of educational facilities that are available;

(d) the provision of facilities or assistance in travelling to and from his or her home for the purposes of participating in any services provided;

(e) the provision of assistance for that person in arranging for the carrying out of any works of adaptation in the home or the provision of additional facilities designed to secure his or her greater safety, comfort or convenience;

(f) facilitating the taking of holidays;

(g) the provision of meals for that person in his or her home or elsewhere;

(h) the provision for that person in obtaining a telephone and any special equipment necessary to enable him or her to use a telephone (Dimond 1997).

WHERE REHABILITATION SERVICES CAN BE LOCATED

With the overall reduction of hospital bed numbers there has been expansion of rehabilitation services accessible to the GP and provided in community settings. GPs need to be familiar with the provision in their local area. Awareness of the eligibility criteria of the different services are essential in managing patients' expectations.

(a) *Social Services* for the physical disability, occupational therapy or sensory impairment services.

(b) *Intermediate care:* often integrated health and social services multidisciplinary teams for time limited periods of rehabilitation or reablement. They may provide home-based services or alternative beds outside the acute hospital setting.

(c) *Community rehabilitation teams:* for specific clinical conditions such as stroke, physical disability, learning disability, etc.

(d) *Secondary care and tertiary services:* a range of outpatient or specialist services for wheelchair assessment, specialist seating and tissue viability, orthotics and prosthetics, environmental control systems and communication aids, management of spasticity.

ASSESSMENT OF LEVEL OF DISABILITY AND DEPENDENCY

In addition to the assessment of the underlying condition a broader picture of how the person is coping with managing daily tasks can assist in deciding where referrals need to be made. Activities of daily living can be categorized into:

(a) *personal care:* feeding, dressing, toileting, grooming and indoor mobility;

(b) *extended care:* managing domestic tasks and the wider environment in cooking, shopping, working and socializing.

1. *The Community Dependency Index (CDI)* (see Appendix 29) is a standardized assessment of personal care and is recommended when:

    (a) there is high level dependency, the patient is predominantly housebound and reliant on informal carers;

    (b) when a package of care from statutory services appears to be indicated. The CDI will help decide on the frequency and extent of support needed.

A score of less than 75 usually represents a moderate disability and a score of less than 50 represents a severe disability (Eakin and Baird 1995; Ward, Macaulay, Jagger and Harper 1998).

2. *The Nottingham Extended Activities of Daily Living Questionnaire* (see Appendix 30) is more appropriate when there are low or moderate levels of dependency and the person is able to access the wider environment (Gladman 1992).

ASSESSMENT OF THE HOME ENVIRONMENT

Refer for an OT assessment if the home environment is presenting a barrier to the person managing daily tasks independently. The following are the most common areas that the GP can observe, or ask questions about, to identify difficulties:

- Access
    - Are the steps and stairs at the entrance way and within the house negotiable by the person?
    - Is there level access or do thresholds or door widths present a barrier?
    - Is there adequate space to manoeuvre in corridors and in rooms with mobility equipment?
    - Do the floor coverings present a hazard?
- Controls
    - Can the person reach sockets and light switches?
    - Is the home adequately heated?
    - Is the lighting, door and window security adequate?
    - Can the person get to the door to respond to callers?
- Kitchen
    - Can the person reach the oven and hob to handle hot items safely?
    - Can the person reach into both high and low cupboards?
    - Is the sink and work surface a suitable height?
    - Can the person open jars and tins, and prepare vegetables?
- Toilet and bathroom
    - Is the person able to get in and out of the bath/ shower?
    - Can the person get on and off the toilet?
    - Can the person manage taps?
- Bedroom and living rooms
    - Can the person get in and out of his or her bed and chair?

- Can the person easily reach the telephone from his or her bed or chair?
- Has the person had any accidents in the home?

> **SELF ASSESSMENT FOR PATIENTS ON REDUCING HOME HAZARDS**
>
> Clemson L. *Westmead Home Safety Assessment* (Clemson, Fitzgerald and Heard 1999). Forms can be purchased through www.worldretailstore.com

ROLE OF GP IN REHABILITATION ASSESSMENT

Detailed information on the person's disability, diagnosis and prognosis is required to enable the therapist or rehabilitation team to plan appropriate short- and long-term interventions. The relationship between a GP or therapist and a person with physical disability is more of a partnership with the person being the expert in managing their daily routines. The person has more choice and control of the range of interventions with direct payments and individual budgets for care, respite, equipment and potentially adaptations in the home. In complex cases it is useful to discuss the options to reach realistic solutions and to ensure resources are appropriately allocated. The success of any rehabilitation programme relies on the aspirations of the person and their motivation to reach their goals. Recognition of what stage the individual is at in the 'cycle of change' is essential to bring about changes in health-related behaviours (Diclemente, Prochaska and Norcross 1994). GPs and therapists should use consultative and motivational approaches to promote self-care and self-management (Tomkins and Collins 2005).

Promoting self-care and self-management is dependent on the strategies used for informing and educating and involving people and their families in this approach.

To improve health literacy

- Provision of printed leaflets and health information packages.
- Access to computer based and internet health information.
- Patient decision aids.
- Targeted approaches to tackle low levels of health literacy in disadvantaged groups.

To improve self-care

- Self-management education.
- Self-monitoring and self-administered treatment.
- Self-help groups and peer support.
- Patient access to personal health information.
- Patient centred telecare and telehealth (Coulter and Ellins 2007).

COMMUNITY INTERVENTIONS

Following assessment the therapist or rehabilitation team may:

(a) plan interventions to reduce the impairment and prevent complications through goal-focused, person-centred activity programmes that are graded, reviewed and progressed;

(b) reduce the disability through advice on, and in some cases supply of, specialist equipment and teaching alternative coping strategies;

(c) reduce environmental barriers by recommending adaptations to the home or workplace or if necessary provide rehousing reports;

(d) support the fulfilment of roles in the family and local community.

These broad areas of intervention relate to the World Health Organization's definition of health including impairment, activity (formerly disability) and participation (formerly handicap) as well as wellbeing. A holistic rehabilitation programme is likely to address all these areas and is covered in more detail in the rest of this section.

Throughout, advice, support and training can be given to formal and informal carers alongside liaison with other involved parties.

COMMUNITY REHABILITATION

The following areas of rehabilitation may be included in a person's programme. Referrals for specific services may be made either by the GP or the therapist, or for some services the therapist may need to approach the GP for authorization.

(a) *Physical rehabilitation:* programmes to improve balance, co-ordination, circulation, muscle power and joint range of movement, reduce pain, maintain positioning, seating, the management of tone and spasms, referral for orthotics. Passive movements need to be completed regularly by a carer trained by the therapist to prevent contractures. GPs and therapists will need to work closely together to achieve optimum dosage of medication for spasticity in order to reduce spasm without reducing tone to such an extent that function is adversely effected. Exercise referral schemes and community education classes can be an alternative or follow-up to a rehabilitation programme as well as secondary prevention for many long-term conditions.

(b) *Cognitive rehabilitation:* programmes to develop skills in problem solving, addressing perceptual difficulties such as hemianopia, agnosia and dyspraxia, memory strategies, compensation techniques, improving attention, body image and spatial awareness. Cognitive behavioural therapy can be appropriate for anxiety and depression, difficulties adjusting to disability, problems related to work or in relationships and in managing chronic problems such as pain.

(c) *Vocational rehabilitation:* assessment of vocational aptitudes, referral to the Job Centre Plus either by the GP or by a potential employer for assessment and advice from the disability employment advisor. The advisor can make recommendations to an employer on what equipment, adaptation of the work environment and practical support of an assistant is needed and this may be financially supported through an access to work or a job introduction scheme (see page 4).

(d) *Community access:* refer for shop mobility schemes, taxi-card schemes, dial-a-ride, driving assessment centres for people who want to return to driving or to learn to drive with a disability, or to the motability scheme for adaptation of a vehicle for a disabled person as a driver or as a passenger (see page 13).

(e) *Leisure:* the importance of leisure activities for self-esteem and motivation should not be overlooked; accessing clubs and community education classes, socializing, volunteering and a balance of active and sedentary pastimes.

COMMUNITY EQUIPMENT SERVICES

A wide range of large-scale equipment can be loaned to patients for use both in the long term and short term. Increasingly, health and social services are required to integrate their provision into a single service (Department of Health 2001/008). Small-scale equipment such as dressing, feeding and kitchen equipment may not be available for loan. GPs can encourage patients to return equipment that they no longer use. Commonly available equipment includes:

(a) *nursing equipment:* hoists, beds, pressure-relieving equipment, commodes, urinals, palliative care equipment;

(b) *mobility and positioning equipment:* sticks, crutches, frames, wheelchairs, cushions, wedges, transfer belts and boards, multiglide sheets;

(c) *daily living equipment:* toilet seats and frames, bath boards, seats and hoists, trolleys, perching stools, bed and chair raisers, modified cutlery, tap turners;

(d) *minor works:* integrated community equipment services are also required to provide minor works up to the value of £1000. This could include grab rails, bannisters, half steps, ramps, door widening, door entry systems, keysafes, repositioning electric sockets and switches, and lever taps.

ALTERNATIVE SOURCES OF EQUIPMENT

Online self-assessment:

Online self-assessment tool and directory of equipment suppliers provided by the Disabled Living Foundation. Website: www.asksara.org.uk/welcome.php

Retail outlets

Look up Yellow Pages index under 'Disabled equipment and vehicles'

Mail order catalogues for equipment

Nottingham Rehab Supplies, Findel House, Excelsior Road, Ashby Park, Ashby de la Zouch, Leicestershire LE65 1NG, tel. 0845 120 4522. Website: www.nrs-uk.co.uk

Chester Care Catalogue by Homecraft Roylan, Nunn Brook Road, Huthwaite, Sutton-in-Ashield, Notts, NG17 2HU, tel. 08702 423305. Website: www.homecraft-roylan.com

Mail order catalogues for special shoes

Hotter Comfort Concept, tel. 0800 525 893. www.hottershoes.com

Cosyfeet, 5 The Tanyard, Leigh Road, Street, Somerset BA16 0HR, tel. 01458 447275. Email: comfort@cosyfeet.co.uk. Website: www.cosyfeet.com

Mail order catalogues for adapted clothes:

www.makoa.org/clothing.htm is a website listing approx 20 suppliers of adapted clothing

Assistive technologies for profound disability

GPs and therapists will need to consider the need for, and know where to refer for, the following:

(a) communication aids;

(b) environmental control systems;

(c) telecare and telehealth systems;

(d) wheelchairs.

Communication aids

Electronic communication aids use computer technology to produce synthetic speech and/or digital script for aphasic patients.

Environmental control systems

An environmental control system should be considered for people with a high level of disability such that they are unable to manage using a standard telephone, TV remote controls, light switches and door or window handles. The electronic equipment is operated through a single switch to provide control of an individually selected range of functions that could include TV and music centres, door entry systems, door, window and curtain opening/closing, telephones, pagers, and alarms, profiling beds and reclining chairs, and turning any electrical appliance on and off. The equipment is remote controlled, both infrared and/or radio wave. The person will need to have the cognitive ability to learn to use the equipment, be motivated to use it and derive some functional independence and safety.

Telecare and telehealth

The most simple and widely available telecare systems are the personal alarms. These require activation by the user to send the signal through the telephone system to a call centre who then mobilizes a response, generally from family or friends that are key holders. However, the range

of assistive technology has now expanded and can provide passive monitoring such as through falls detectors, movement detectors, pressure pad monitors, wander guards and medication reminder devices. The response mechanisms can also be escalated from family to include wardens, care agencies and intermediate care services. Telecare needs to be considered to help support the person to remain at home as long as possible and can be an alternative to moving to sheltered accommodation or a residential home. Telecare equipment is increasingly being made available through integrated community equipment services (Audit Commission 2004; Department of Health 2004).

Telehealth supports the monitoring of symptoms and uses web technology for the transmission of results or even remote consultations. Monitoring can include peak flow, spirometer, blood pressure, pulse oximeter, glucometer, PT/INR, fluid status, weight and activity levels.

Wheelchairs

GPs and therapists can requisition the issuing of a manual wheelchair from a standard limited range. Assessment needs to include the frequency and location of use, height and weight of the person, whether the person will self propel, fitness of the main carer for attendant-propelled wheelchairs, whether the wheelchair will be transported in a car and, if being used in the home, whether any adaptations to the house are required.

If the person has a very clear idea of a non-standard type of wheelchair he or she requires, the person should be advised about *the voucher scheme*. There are two options:

(a) *The independent option* to contribute to the cost of a more expensive wheelchair of the person's choice. The person will own the wheelchair and be responsible for its maintenance and repair.

(b) *The partnership option* to contribute to the cost of a more expensive wheelchair of the person's choice from a range selected by the local wheelchair service. The NHS will own the wheelchair and be responsible for its maintenance and repair (Department of Health accessed 2010).

Powered wheelchairs

● Referral should be made to the local wheelchair service for electrically powered indoor chairs

(EPIC), electrically powered indoor/outdoor chairs (EPIOC) and special seating clinics for wheelchair postural supports.

- OTs can advise on suitable outdoor electric scooters. Patients who receive mobility allowance can use this to hire or hire/purchase a scooter through the Motability scheme (www.motability.co.uk).
- All people who use powered vehicles in public spaces should be advised to take out at least third party liability insurance.

For people who depend on these assistive technologies, a 24-hour call-out service for breakdown maintenance and servicing arrangement is essential (Audit Commission 2000). Also a person who uses a combination of an electric wheelchair, communication aid and an environmental control system is likely to need the services of a rehabilitation engineer to integrate the switching mechanisms for all equipment.

HOME ADAPTATION

Assistance towards housing adaptations for people with permanent and substantial physical disability is available via the Disabled Facilities Grant or for some council home tenants they may be funded directly by the council. The OT's role is to assess and make specific recommendations on what is necessary and appropriate (Thorpe 2006). It is then the decision of the Home Improvement Agency on what adaptations are reasonable and practical. The grant process is lengthy and works cannot be started prior to grant approval. The disabled person is means tested and may be required to make a contribution to the costs. The grant limit is £25,000 in England and £30,000 in Wales, although the government has announced it will increase this. For any works more than the grant limit the local council may use its discretionary powers under the Regulatory Reform (Housing Assistance) Order 2002.

INDICATIONS FOR MANDATORY GRANTS

(a) Access in, out and around the property to the principal rooms: kitchen, bathroom, toilet, living room, bedroom.
(b) To ensure the safety of the disabled person and his or her carer.

(c) Access to essential facilities: bathing, cooking, lighting, heating.
(d) To enable the disabled person to care for dependants or vice versa.

Some of the adaptations completed most frequently include ramps and level thresholds, stairlifts, overhead tracking hoists, level access showers, special toilets and wheelchair accessible kitchens.

Discretionary grants and loans

These options can include assistance to move to a new property, preferential rate loans to top-up the mandatory grant for meeting the costs of a home owner's contribution, and equity release loans. Councils are required to publish their local housing strategy.

Repairs grants

These grants or loans can be available for properties in serious disrepair. The disabled person should be advised to apply direct to the council. In all cases the council will need to check that the proposed works are necessary, appropriate, reasonable and practical.

For information on the grants and loan schemes in operation, apply to the local council's housing or environmental health services or the Home Improvement Agency.

OTHER SOURCES OF INFORMATION FOR ADAPTATIONS AND EQUIPMENT

People who have above the financial savings threshold for grants or who are in receipt of compensation may wish to seek assistance privately to avoid waiting for assessment and advice. Alternatives could include the following:

(a) *Private and independent OTs:* lists obtainable through College of Occupational Therapists (UK), 106–114 Borough High Street, Southwark, London, SE1 1LB, tel. 020 7357 6480; www.cot.co.uk.
(b) *Independent Living Centres* and *Disability Resource Centres.* These are listed by the Disabled Living Centres Council, 1st Floor, Winchester House, 11 Cranmer Road, London, SW9 6EJ,

tel: 0207 820 0567. Website: www.lboro.ac.uk/info/usabilitynet/dlcc.html.

(c) *National exhibitions:* Naidex, Independent Living, Care and Rehabilitation.

(d) *Centre for Accessible Environments* for architectural advice, consultancy, training and publications for new build homes, public buildings and spaces. Nutmeg House, 60 Gainsford Street, London SE1 2NY, tel. 020 7357 8182; email cae@ globalnet.co.uk.

(e) *Disabled Living Foundation* – a registered charity that provides information on equipment that promotes independence. It runs an equipment centre, telephone helpline, training events and publishes the Hamilton Index, a comprehensive database of equipment and suppliers (available on subscription), tel. 020 7289 6111; email info@dlf.org.uk; www.dlf.org.uk.

(f) *Foundations* is the national co-ordinating body for home improvement agencies. Home Improvement Agencies are dedicated to offering home repair and adaptation for older and disabled people to live independently in their own homes for as long as they wish. Foundations, Bleaklow House, Howard Town Mill, Glossop, Derbyshire SK13 8HT. Tel. 01457 891909. email: foundations@cel.co.uk; www.cel.co.uk/foundations/.

(g) *Joseph Rowntree Foundation* for research on housing and social issues. Details of Part M building standards, lifetime home standards and smart homes are on their website. The Homestead, 40 Water End, York, North Yorkshire YO30 6WP, tel. 01904 629241; email: info@ jrf.org.uk; www.jrf.org.uk.

(h) Mandelstram M. *How to get Equipment for Disability*, 3rd edition. London: Jessica Kingsley and Kogan Page for the Disabled Living Foundation, 1993.

SUPPORTS FOR HOME LIVING

Refer to social services for:

(a) home care assessment, identification of needs, commissioning care through independent care agencies for personal care tasks, 24-hour live-in carer schemes, direct payments, individual budgets;

(b) meals;

(c) respite care including sitting service, day care and short or long stays in residential/nursing homes;

(d) assessment of carer's needs.

CARERS

GUIDELINE

The National Strategy for Carers. 2001. Department of Health, London. Available: www.carers.gov.uk

- 6 million people in the UK are carers, of these 1.5 million care for more than 20 hours per week. Family and friends provide 70% of the care. The Australian Bureau of Statistics (Australian Bureau of Statistics 1998) estimates that there are 2.3 million carers in Australia, or one in every five households. Of these carers, about 500,000 are providing substantial or full-time care.

- Caring imposes a strain on the health of the carer. 20% have never had a break from caring, and 65% admit that their own health has suffered (Department of Health 2001).

- Carers need good information on the needs and treatment of the person they are caring for. One study found that only a third of carers had received any information, training or guidance in relation to the patient's medication, dressings or other healthcare needs (Department of Health 2001).

SERVICES

In the UK, the Carers and Disabled Children Act 2000, (available: www.carers.gov.uk):

(a) gives carers the right to an assessment in their own right, even if the person they care for has refused an assessment themselves. This is a mandatory duty on local authorities;

(b) allows councils to be innovative and creative in providing carers services focused on the outcomes carers want to see;

(c) gives local authorities a power (not a duty) to provide direct payments to carers (for services to them); to carers with parental responsibilities for services to disabled children; and to

16–17-year-old disabled young people for their own services;

(d) gives local authorities a power (not a duty) to offer vouchers for short-term breaks.

COMMON PROBLEMS FOR CARERS

(a) Poor health and exhaustion.

(b) A restricted social life.

(c) Damage to their relationships with the person with care needs or with their partner.

(d) Emotional problems:
- anger with the situation, with the person they are caring for, and with those who provide services;
- feeling undervalued, especially by health professionals.

(e) Financial limitations:
- loss of earnings;
- increased wear and tear on clothing, upholstery, etc.;
- the need to purchase special items;
- increased heating and laundry bills.

* Consider whether keeping an index of carers would help to foster an awareness of their needs in the practice.

* During every consultation with a patient or carer consider:
  (a) whether the carer and patient know everything they need to know about the illness. Information can, however, only be passed to the carer with the patient's consent;
  (b) whether more is expected of the carer than he or she has been educated for, e.g. simple nursing procedures;
  (c) the impact of caring under the categories above.

* *Referral.* Discuss with every carer the need for extra support, with a view to referral to Social Services for assessment. Recommend *How to get help in looking after someone: a carer's guide to carer's assessment.* Available: www.carers.gov. uk/carersleaflet.htm.

* Direct the carer to appropriate local or national voluntary organizations to provide emotional support as well as practical advice (e.g. eligibility for financial benefits or the provision of breaks).

SUPPORT AND ADVICE FOR CARERS

Australia:

Carers Australia: www.carersaustralia.com.au
   Carer Resource Centres: freecall 1800 242 636 (10 a.m.–4 p.m. Monday to Friday). Provide support and information for carers
   Carer Respite Centres: freecall 1800 059 059. Provide emergency assistance 24 hours per day
   Telephone Interpreter Service: 13 1450

UK:

CarersUK, 20 Great Dover Street, London SE1 4LX, Tel. 020 7378 4999 Carers' Line 0808 808 7777, Email: info@carersuk.org. www.carersuk.org.uk
   Princess Royal Trust for Carers: 0844 800 4361; www.carers.org
   Crossroads – Caring for Carers: tel. 0845 450 0350; www.crossroads.org.uk
   Contact a Family, 209-211 City Road, London EC1V 1JN; tel. 020 7608 8700; Helpline 0808 808 3555; email: info@cafamily.org.uk; www.cafamily.org.uk for families with disabled children, especially those with rare diseases

PEOPLE WITH LEARNING DISABILITY (UK) OR INTELLECTUAL DISABILITY (AUSTRALIA AND NEW ZEALAND)

- Poor communication is a major barrier to care. It can be minimized by people with an intellectual disability, where able, or their carers, providing high quality health information. Clinicians can only make informed assessments and management recommendations if symptoms or signs, such as records of seizures, behaviour, bowel chart or menstruation, and past history, are clearly documented. It is the responsibility of paid carers and their organizations to provide such information (Lennox, Diggens and Ugoni 1997).

- The GP is the professional most in contact with people with an intellectual disability and the one responsible for the provision of medical care. Proactive care is especially important as, at times, such patients will not seek care or be able to describe subjective experience crucial to assessment and diagnosis. 'Over-investigations' may be indicated where a clear history is lacking.

● The possibility that the aetiology of an individual's disability can be identified becomes more likely as genetic knowledge increases. Accurate diagnosis may have major ramifications for the family and for the person with the disability.

● There are high levels of undiagnosed and undermanaged conditions (Beange, McElduff and Baker 1995). The RCGP has recommended regular medical review (Royal College of General Practitioners 1990) and some evidence exists to support yearly health review by GPs (Lennox, Green, Diggens and Ugoni 2001; Webb and Rogers 1999).

* Refer when the suspicion of learning disability arises. Re-refer if there is weight change, change in behaviour or if the patient's carer or a close relative dies (WHO 2004).

* Check the aetiology of the patient's condition, if it is unknown:

(a) Send blood for karyotyping and screening for fragile X.

(b) Send urine for screening for inborn errors of metabolism.

(c) Consider review by a genetics service.

AREAS OF CONCERN (BEANGE, LENNOX AND PARMENTER 1999)

(a) Gastrointestinal disorders
  ■ *Constipation* is present in up to 70%, with the attendant risk of faecal impaction, atonic bowel and obstruction.
  ■ *Reflux oesophagitis* is present in 30% of people with an intellectual disability with an IQ less than 50. The use of anticonvulsants and cerebral palsy appear to predispose patients to develop reflux oesophagitis (Bohmer, Klinkenberg-Knol, Niezen-de Boer and Meuwissen 1997). The prevalence of *H. pylori* is high, with up to 90% in institutional populations affected.
  ■ Dysphagia – is common especially where neuromotor disturbance is a feature.

(b) *Dental care:* is often poor. Dental disease is found in up to 86%.

(c) *Visual impairment:* is present in 19–44% of adults. Eye pathology is common (Webb and Rogers 1999).

(d) *Hearing impairment:* is present in 12–36% of adults, yet regular screening is not commonly performed. Wax impaction is common.

(e) *Epilepsy:*
  * The risk of death is increased 3.6 times, when compared to non-disabled people with epilepsy. Under- and overdiagnosis occurs.
  * Assessment should include past history of treatment, investigation, identification of seizure type and assessment of the standard of support that is needed. In particular, the service must ensure that:
    ■ the prescribed medication is given;
    ■ carers are adequately trained to provide rescue medication;
    ■ an experienced staff or family member attends the consultation and provides an adequate history and can describe the impact of the epilepsy on the person's quality of life;
    ■ the risk of bathing or showering has been assessed;
    ■ a management plan for acute seizures has been agreed;
    ■ the impact of the epilepsy in the patient's social setting has been assessed.

(f) *Nutrition, inactivity and obesity:* obesity in this population has been found to be between 10 and 40% (Webb and Rogers 1999; Beange, Lennox and Parmenter 1999; Bohmer, Klinkenberg-Knol, Niezen-de Boer and Meuwissen 1997; Rimmer and Yamaki 2006; Carmeli, Merrick 2007).
  * Ensure that adequate exercise is made available.
  * Check for nutritional deficiencies associated with difficulties with feeding and swallowing.

(g) *Psychiatric disorders:* the lifetime prevalence is probably 30–40%. Unrecognized grief reaction, post-traumatic stress, depression and anxiety disorders are common.

(h) *Medication:* inadequate review, polypharmacy and side-effects are all common.

(i) *Behaviour change:* may indicate an unrecognized physical or mental health problem *per se* and/or be secondary to changes in the environment.

(j) *Unrecognized pain:* with musculoskeletal and other sources of pain unreported.

(k) *Women's health:* menstrual management can often be taught and medications avoided. Cervical smears are indicated where women fulfil the criteria for screening, in particular that they have at some time in their life been sexually active.

(l) *Men's health:* check for undescended testes.

(m) *Osteoporosis and osteomalacia:* is more common (Centre, McElduff and Beange 1994) in people with an intellectual disability, and especially those with Down syndrome. Some risk factors for osteoporosis such as immobility, use of anticonvulsants, hypogonadism and poor diet, are more common in this population.

(n) *Hypothyroidism:* is present in 15% of people with Down syndrome and may also be increased in the non-Down syndrome population with intellectual disability.

(o) *Health screening/promotion* activities: may have been omitted.
  * Check that the patient's immunizations meet national standards. Ensure, especially, that hepatitis A and B, influenza and pneumococcus are covered where indicated. The Australian National Health and Medical Research Council (NH&MRC 2000) and the UK Department of Health recommend hepatitis A and B immunization where people with learning disability live in residential care facilities, especially in large institutions.
  * Cervical smears and mammography are all indicated as per national guidelines.

DOWN SYNDROME

GUIDELINES

Cohen WI, for the Down Syndrome Medical Interest Group. Health care guidelines for individuals with Down syndrome: 1999 Revision. Down Syndrome Quarterly, 4(3). Available: http://www.denison.edu (search on 'Down syndrome'). General health information - www.ds-health.com/
  DSMIG Surveillance Essentials Development Group. Basic medical surveillance essentials for people with Down's syndrome, 1999–2000. Available: www.dsmig.org.uk

Patients with Down syndrome need regular surveillance. This may not occur even if they see a paediatrician. Topics that need attention are:

(a) *Cardiac problems* are present in 50%, mostly endocardial cushion defects, some of them life-threatening and treatable.
  * All babies need a cardiological assessment, as the cardiac abnormality may not be clinically easy to detect.
  * Refer again at the age of 18; the patient may have developed mitral valve prolapse or aortic regurgitation despite normal findings at an earlier assessment.
  * Give antibiotics, along the lines set out on page 163, to all adults with Down syndrome who:
    ■ are known to have a cardiac defect prone to SBE; or
    ■ who have not had an echocardiogram since early childhood.

(b) *Eye problems* are very common and include stenotic nasolacrimal ducts, blepharitis, conjunctivitis, cataracts (from birth and increasing throughout life), keratoconus and refractory errors.

 * Routine evaluations should begin at 6 months of age (USA) or in the second year of life (UK), and be performed annually (USA) or every 2 years (UK) thereafter.

(c) *Hearing and ENT problems:* over 50% of people with Down syndrome have a significant hearing impairment. If undetected it is likely to be a significant cause of preventable secondary handicap.

 * Ensure the patient has a hearing assessment before 6 months of age then yearly until age 3 and 2–5 yearly thereafter (USA) or between 6 and 10 months, yearly until age 5, then every 2 years for life (UK).

(d) *Thyroid diseases:* up to 40% have thyroid dysfunction at some time in their lives. About 7% have current hypothyroidism, while in others it is subclinical. The clinical diagnosis can be difficult (Dinani and Carpenter 1990).

 * Check TFTs every 1–2 years. If the TSH is only mildly raised but the thyroxine (T_4) is normal and the patient is clinically euthyroid, check antithyroid antibodies and give T_4 only if they are raised.

(e) *Sleep apnoea:* is common and may result from excessive lymphoid tissue in the nasopharynx. The usual symptoms of sleep apnoea may be present or just behaviour change.

 * Refer for sleep and ENT assessment if concerned.

(f) *Growth:* the average height at any age is around the 2nd centile for the general population.

 Deviations from this expected height may indicate congenital heart disease, upper airways obstruction, coeliac disease, hypothyroidism or poor nutrition because of feeding problems.

 * Chart height and weight on charts specific for Down syndrome.

 * Refer those who fall significantly below their expected centile.

 * Manage obesity with advice about exercise and diet.

(g) *Alzheimer's-type dementia:* is increasingly present from middle age.

 * Exclude depression and other reversible causes of functional deterioration, especially hypothyroidism.

(h) *Osteoporosis:* appears to be more common.

 * Review dietary calcium and check levels of oestradiol, progesterone, FSH, LH, TSH, vitamin D and testosterone. Consider assessing the bone mineral density.

(i) *Infections and immunodeficiency:* are both common. Frequent respiratory infections may be due to low IgG levels.

 * Check IgG levels if there are recurrent or chronic infections. Levels of IgG subclasses must be measured. In Down syndrome, subclasses 2 and 4 may be low yet the total IgG normal.

 * Give influenza and pneumococcus immunizations.

(j) *Atlantoaxial instability:* ligamentous laxity occurs in 14% and about 1% suffer from acute or chronic neurological problems due to instability of the cervical spine. Cervical spine X-rays in children are not helpful in predicting subsequent acute dislocation or subluxation at the atlantoaxial joint.

 * Do not ban sport: there is no evidence that it increases the risk of cervical spine injury in this group any more than in the general population.

 * Refer urgently anyone with Down syndrome who develops:

  ■ pain behind the ear or elsewhere in the neck;

  ■ an abnormal head posture;

  ■ torticollis;

  ■ a deterioration in gait, manipulative skills or bowel or bladder control.

(k) *Gastrointestinal disorders:* congenital abnormalities, such as duodenal atresia and imperforate anus, partial upper GI obstruction, tracheo-esophageal fistula and pyloric stenosis are all more common as are chronic constipation and Hirschsprung disease. Between 7% and 16% have coeliac disease.

(l) *Skin:* alopecia areata, vitiligo and fungal infections are common.

(m) *Depression:* appears to be more common. Exclude hypothyroidism.

(n) *Bereavement:* many patients with Down syndrome live with elderly parents, and are strongly attached to, and dependent on them. In addition, when a parent dies they may be unable to understand death or their own grief. They may find things even harder if they are sent away in a mistaken attempt to spare their feelings. This problem can be reduced by getting the patient used to other people, and to staying away for short periods.

References

Audit Commission, 2000. Fully Equipped. Audit Commission Publications, London.

Audit Commission, 2004. Assistive Technology, Older People - Independence and Wellbeing. Audit Commission Publications.

Australian Bureau of Statistics, 1998. Disability, Ageing and Carers, Australia. Summary of findings. Australian Bureau of Statistics, Canberra, p. 25.

Beange, H., Lennox, N., Parmenter, T., 1999. Health targets for people with intellectual disability. J. Intellect. Dev. Disabil. 24, 283–297.

Beange, H., McElduff, A., Baker, W., 1995. Medical disorders of adults with mental retardation: A population study. Am. J. Ment. Retard. 99, 595–604.

Bohmer, C.J., Klinkenberg-Knol, E.C., Niezen-de Boer, R.C., Meuwissen, S.G., 1997. The prevalence of gastro-oesophageal reflux disease based on non-specific symptoms in institutionalized, intellectually disabled individuals. Eur. J. Gastroenterol. Hepatol. 9, 187–190.

Carmeli, E., Merrick, J., 2007. Aging, exercise and persons with intellectual disability. International J. Disability Human Dev. 6, 11–14.

Centre, J., McElduff, A., Beange, H., 1994. Osteoporosis in groups with intellectual disability. Aust. N. Z. J. Dev. Disabil. 19, 251–258.

Clemson, L., Fitzgerald, M., Heard, R., 1999. Content validity of an assessment tool to identify home fall hazards: the Westmead Home Safety Assessment. Br. J. Occ. Ther. 62, 171–179.

Coulter, A., Ellins, J., 2007. Effectiveness of strategies for informing, educating and involving patients. BMJ 335, 24–27.

Dagfinrud, H., Hagen, K.B., Kvein, T.K., 2004. Physiotherapy interventions for ankylosing spondylitis. Cochrane Database Syst. Rev. (4), CD002822.

Department of Health, 2001. National Strategy for Carers. Department of Health, London. Available: www.carers.gov.uk.

Department of Health, 2001/008. Community equipment services, HSC 2001/008. DoH, London.

Department of Health, 2004. Telecare – Getting started. DoH, London.

Department of Health, Wheelchair voucher scheme. Available: www.direct.gov.uk (choose 'Disabled people' then search on 'Wheelchair voucher scheme'). Accessed 2010.

Diclemente, C.C., Prochaska, J.O., Norcross, J., 1994. Changing for Good. Harper Collins, New York.

Dimond, B.C., 1997. Legal aspects of occupational therapy. Blackwell Science, Oxford.

Dinani, S., Carpenter, S., 1990. Down's syndrome and thyroid disorder. J. Ment. Defic. Res. 34, 187–193.

Eakin, P., Baird, H., 1995. The Community Dependency Index: a standardised assessment of need and measure of outcome for community occupational therapy. Br. J. Occ. Ther. 58, 17–22.

Fransen, M., McConnell, S., Bell, M., 2001. Exercise for osteoarthritis of the hip or knee. Cochrane Database Syst. Rev. (2), CD004376.

Gillespie, L.D., Gillespie, W.J., Robertson, M.C., et al., 2003. Interventions for preventing falls in elderly people. Cochrane Database Syst. Rev. (4), CD000340.

Gladman, J.R., 1992. The Extended Activities of Daily Living Scale: a further validation. Disabil. Rehabil. 14, 41–43.

Heywood, F., Turner, L., 2007. Better Outcomes, Lower Costs: Implications for Health and Social Care Budgets of Investment in Housing, Adaptations, Improvements and Equipment: A review of the evidence. Office for Disability Issues.

Howe, T.E., Rochester, L., Jackson, A., et al., 2007. Exercise for improving balance in older people. Cochrane Database Syst. Rev. (4), CD004963.

Joliffe, J.A., Rees, K., Taylor, R.S., et al., 2001. Exercised based rehabilitation for coronary heart disease. Cochrane Database Syst. Rev. (1), CD001800.

Khan, F., Turner-Stokes, L., Ng, L., Kilpatrick, T., 2007. Multidisciplinary rehabilitation for adults with multiple sclerosis. Cochrane Database Syst. Rev. (2), CD006036.

Lacasse, Y., Goldstein, R., Lasserton, T.J., Martin, S., 2006. Pulmonary rehabilitation for chronic obstructive airways disease. Cochrane Database Syst. Rev. (4), CD003793.

Lennox, N., Diggens, J., Ugoni, A., 1997. The general practice care of people with intellectual disability: barriers and solutions. J. Intellect. Disabil. Res. 41, 380–390.

Lennox, N., Green, M., Diggens, J., Ugoni, A., 2001. Audit and comprehensive health assessment programme in the primary healthcare of adults with intellectual disability: a pilot study. J. Intellect. Disabil. Res. 45, 226–232.

NH&MRC, 2000. The Australian Immunisation Handbook, seventh ed. National Health and Medical Research Council, Australian Government Publishing Service, Canberra.

Outpatient Service Trialists, 2003. Therapy based rehabilitation services for stroke patients at home. Cochrane Database Syst. Rev. (1), CD002925.

Royal College of General Practitioners, 1990. Primary care for people with a mental handicap. Occasional Paper 47. Royal College of General Practitioners, London.

Rimmer, J., Yamaki, K., 2006. Obesity and intellectual disability. Ment. Retard. Dev. Disabil. Res. Rev. 12, 22–27.

Steultjens, E.M.J., Dekker, J., Bouler, L.M., et al., 2004. Occupational therapy for rheumatoid arthritis. Cochrane Database Syst. Rev. (1), CD003114.

Thorpe, S., Habinteg Housing Association, 2006. Wheelchair Housing Design. BRE Press.

Tomkins, S., Collins, A., 2005. Promoting Optimal Self Care. Dorset and Somerset Strategic Health Authority.

Ward, G., Macaulay, F., Jagger, C., Harper, W., 1998. Standardised assessment: a comparison of the Community Dependency Index and the Barthel Index with an elderly hip fracture population. Br. J. Occ. Ther. 61, 121–126.

Webb, O., Rogers, L., 1999. Health screening for people with intellectual disability: the New Zealand experience. J. Intellect. Disabil. Res. 43, 497–503.

WHO, 2004. Guide to Mental and Neurological Health in Primary Care – Learning Disability. Available: http://www.whoguidemhpcuk.org.

Chapter 26

Haematology

CHAPTER CONTENTS

ANAEMIAS

For details of the diagnosis of anaemia see *Evidence-based Diagnosis in Primary Care* by A. F. Polmear (editor), published by Butterworth-Heinemann, 2008.

HYPOCHROMIC MICROCYTIC ANAEMIA

Goddard A F, James MW, McIntyre A S, Scott BB. 2005. *Guidelines for the Management of Iron Deficiency Anaemia.* British Society of Gastroenterology. www.bsg.org.uk/clinical_prac/guidelines.htm

DIAGNOSIS OF IRON DEFICIENCY

(a) Anaemia (WHO) Hb < 13 Hb g/dl (male); < 12 g/dl (female).
(b) MCV < 77 fl, MCHC < 32 g/dl.
(c) Serum ferritin < 15 mcg/l.
(d) Serum iron < 14 μmol/l (male), < 11 μmol/l (female), and TIBC > 75 μmol/l; (for iron assays check local laboratory's normal range).

DOI: 10.1016/B978-0-7020-3053-6.00026-X

WORK-UP OF ESTABLISHED IRON DEFICIENCY ANAEMIA

(a) History and examination including evidence of GI blood loss, menstrual blood loss, malabsorption, dietary deficiency and drug history (especially NSAIDS).

(b) Rectal examination.

(c) Urine dipstick for blood.

(d) *H. pylori* serology.

(e) Coeliac serology.

(f) Hb electrophoresis if thalassaemia is possible.

● Around 1 mcg/l of serum ferritin corresponds to 8 mg of stored iron. A ferritin value of 20 mcg/l is within the normal range (15–300 mcg/l). If, however, the haemoglobin level was reduced to 9.5 g/l, for instance, stores would not contain enough iron to support a rise in haemoglobin to 12.5 g/l.

● A serum ferritin < 15 mcg/l indicates that iron deficiency is present and a level of 25 mcg/l is highly suggestive.

● *In patients with chronic disease* a serum ferritin cut-off value of < 50 mcg/l is still consistent with iron deficiency. In this situation the serum transferrin is also low. A therapeutic trial of iron for 3 months may be helpful. Increased reticulocytes after a week and a rise in haemoglobin after 3 weeks indicates iron deficiency.

MANAGEMENT

* Refer to a gastroenterologist (under the 2 week rule) patients of any age with:

  (a) significant iron deficiency anaemia without obvious cause (Hb < 11 g/dl in men, or < 10 g/dl in postmenopausal women). In one study, 84% of patients with no obvious cause from the history had a GI cause (28% upper, 24% lower and 29% upper and lower) (Hardwick and Armstrong 1997). Referral is recommended even if the patient admits to a poor diet (Goddard, McIntyre and Scott 2000);

  (b) dyspepsia with a proven anaemia.

* *Women under the age of 45.* Treat women with menorrhagia with iron but refer to a gynaecologist if they do not respond to treatment. Iron deficiency anaemia occurs in 5–10% of menstruating women (World Health Organization 1992).

* *Menstruating women over the age of 45* should be treated as above but beware of assuming that menorrhagia is the cause of the anaemia. If in doubt, refer to a gastroenterologist, as well, for further investigation.

IRON SUPPLEMENTATION

* Give a ferrous compound, e.g. ferrous sulphate 200 mg b.d. or t.d.s., taken after food to reduce the GI side-effects and improve adherence. Avoid modified-release preparations; they may release their iron beyond the duodenum and upper jejunum, where absorption is best.

* Warn patients that their stools will turn black.

* Advise patients to avoid foods that might reduce absorption, e.g. rich in tannates (tea) or phytates (bran or cereal) and medications that might reduce acidity in the stomach (antacids, PPIs and H_2 blockers).

* Check the haemoglobin after 3 weeks. It should rise by 0.1 g/dl per day, starting 10 days after the start of treatment (approx 2 g/dl in the first 4 weeks).

* Continue treatment for 3 months after the haemoglobin has returned to normal.

FAILURE TO RESPOND

* Check that the patient is taking the tablets.

* Review the diagnosis. A serum ferritin < 15 mcg/l is only 59% sensitive and 99% specific for iron deficiency anaemia. This means that it will only detect just over half of those who have it, with one false positive diagnosis in every 100 positives. A cut-off of 100 mcg/l will detect 94% of cases but at the expense of false positives in 29% (Griner 1999). Transferrin index, if available, is more reliable.

* Are there other deficiencies as well as iron, e.g. folic acid?

* Look for underlying chronic disease, which is inhibiting a response to the iron.

* Look for continuing blood loss or malabsorption.

* Check *H. pylori* serology if not already done. *H. pylori* colonization may impair iron absorption and increase iron loss.

* Refer if no reason is found.

TRANSFUSION

* Admit for transfusion only if the patient is decompensating, or if blood loss is continuing at a rate that is too fast for supplementation to keep up. There is no absolute level at which patients require transfusion. Every patient will have a different requirement according to the time over which the anaemia has developed and the ability of the heart and lungs to cope.

NORMOCHROMIC NORMOCYTIC ANAEMIA

CHARACTERISTICS

(a) Normochromic, normocytic or mildly hypochromic (MCV rarely < 75 fL).
(b) Mild and non-progressive anaemia rarely < 9.0 g/dl.
(c) Reduced serum iron and TIBC.
(d) Serum ferritin normal or raised.

CAUSES

(a) Chronic infection;
(b) chronic inflammation, e.g. rheumatoid arthritis or polymyalgia rheumatica (PMR);
(c) malignancy;
(d) hypothyroidism, hyperthyroidism, adrenal or pituitary insufficiency, hypogonadism;
(e) chronic renal failure;
(f) mild iron deficiency; particularly likely if the serum ferritin is low normal.

WORK–UP

(a) FBC, ESR and CRP, blood film, reticulocyte count.
(b) Serum ferritin.
(c) U&Es; electrolytes, eGFR.
(d) TFTs.
(e) CXR.

Note: In elderly patients the classic red blood cell features of microcytosis in iron deficiency and macrocytosis in vitamin B_{12} or folate deficiency occur less commonly. The mean cell volume (MCV) is probably less helpful in elderly people (Elis, Ravid, Manor, *et al.* 1996; Seward, Safran, Marton, *et al.* 1990).

MACROCYTIC ANAEMIA

REVIEWS

Hopffbrand V, Prowan D. 1997. Macrocytic anaemias. BMJ 314, 430–433
   Oh RC, Brown DL. 2003. Vitamin B_{12} deficiency. Am Fam Physician 67, 979–986, 993–994

DIAGNOSIS

MCV > 100 fL.

CAUSES

Modest elevation (101–110 fL) is usually due to:

(a) alcohol misuse;
(b) HIV infection;
(c) liver disease;
(d) hypothyroidism;
(e) cytotoxic drugs; or
(f) haemopoietic stem cell disorders, although B_{12} or folate deficiency are possible.

Severe elevation (> 130 fL) is likely to be due to B_{12} or folate deficiency.
   From the history and examination, check:

(a) *Diet.* Only a diet free of all animal produce, i.e. a vegan diet, can lead to vitamin B_{12} deficiency, but folic acid deficiency can occur in those who eat few green vegetables and cereals and little liver, especially if there is increased cell turnover or during pregnancy.
(b) *Alcohol intake.*
(c) *Evidence of hypothyroidism or liver disease.*
(d) *Bowel symptoms.* Malabsorption may cause folic acid deficiency and, rarely, B_{12} deficiency.
(e) *Previous surgery.* Gastrectomy or ileal resection will lead to B_{12} deficiency.
(f) *A personal or family history* of conditions related to pernicious anaemia: Hashimoto's thyroiditis, Addison's disease or diabetes.
(g) *Prolonged use of H_2 antagonists or PPIs* (Bradford and Taylor 1999).

Note: Macrocytosis without anaemia is most likely to be due to excess alcohol intake.

(a) Serum vitamin B_{12} and red cell folate.

(b) LFTs, including GGT.

(c) TFTs.

(d) Reticulocyte count.

(e) Serum ferritin (to exclude coexistent iron deficiency).

(f) If the vitamin B_{12} is low check:
- parietal cell and intrinsic factor autoantibodies;
- homocysteine and methylmalonic acid levels (if available). They are raised in almost all cases of B_{12} deficiency. When both are measured the sensitivity for detecting true B_{12} deficiency in a patient with a low or low-normal serum B_{12} level is 99.8% (individual sensitivities are methylmalonic acid 98.4% and homocysteine 95.9%). Methylmalonic acid is highly specific but homocysteine much less so.

However, if the serum folate is also low, treat with folic acid and repeat the B_{12} level. It may have been depressed by the folate deficiency.

Serum B_{12} is an insensitive and fairly nonspecific guide to whether the tissues are B_{12} deficient. Oh and Brown (see 'Reviews' above) suggest the following approach:
- Serum B_{12} below 100 pg/ml: accept that the patient is B_{12} deficient.
- Serum B_{12} 100–400 pg/ml and either the serum homocysteine or methylmalonic acid is raised: give oral B_{12}. If the levels of homocysteine and methylmalonic acid fall to normal, the patient is B_{12} deficient.

MANAGEMENT

Vitamin B_{12} deficiency

* Refer urgently all patients with dyspepsia and pernicious anaemia to a gastroenterologist or directly for endoscopy (DOH 2000).

* Refer young patients to a haematologist, whether or not intrinsic factor antibodies are positive.

* Refer older patients if the intrinsic factor antibodies are negative and they are fit enough for further investigations.

* Give B_{12} without referral to older patients with positive intrinsic factor antibodies or in whom a Schilling test would be inappropriate.

* Treat with at least six injections of hydroxycobalamin 1 mg over 2 weeks. There is no value in more frequent injections. Continue life-long prophylaxis with hydroxycobalamin 1mg i.m. every 3 months. Improvement in appetite and well-being occur within days, the reticulocyte count peaks at about 7 days and the haemoglobin should rise by 2–3 g a fortnight. Check the Hb fortnightly until normal.

* People anaemic because of dietary deficiency should be encouraged to eat bread fortified with B_{12}, or to take oral B_{12} supplements. Large doses of oral vitamin B_{12} 1000–2000 mcg daily for 2 weeks then 1000 mcg daily for life are effective (Oh and Brown 2003; Lederle 1998) but are not licensed in the UK.

* Treat any co-existing hypothyroidism which otherwise will limit the response.

Folic acid deficiency

* Refer to a gastroenterologist unless a dietary cause is obvious or there is increased cell turnover, e.g. haemolysis or pregnancy.

* Give 5 mg daily for 4 months and continue for life unless the cause has been corrected. One tablet (5 mg) per week is enough in the prophylaxis of haemolytic anaemia.

* Check that a serum B_{12} has been organized. It is customary to caution against giving folic acid to a patient with macrocytic anaemia until B_{12} deficiency has been excluded lest the folic acid precipitate the neurological effects of B_{12} deficiency. A full diagnosis of the cause of the macrocytosis is clearly essential, but the fear of precipitating neurological damage is probably unfounded (Dickinson 1995).

* Give iron supplements to all patients with a haemoglobin of 8 g/dl or below or in those in whom the serum ferritin is also low.

ABSENT SPLEEN

Davies JM, Barnes R, Milligan D. 2002. Update of guideline for the prevention and treatment of infection in patients with an absent or dysfunctional spleen. Clinical Medicine (Journal of the Royal College of Physicians of London) 2, 440–443. Available: www.bcshguidelines.com

* Give all patients with functional hyposplenism:
  (a) pneumococcal immunization, repeated every 5 years;
  (b) a single dose of *Haemophilus influenza* B vaccine, or three doses in infants;
  (c) a single dose of meningococcal group C conjugate vaccine, or three doses in infants < 5 months old, or two doses in infants aged 5–12 months;
  (d) influenza vaccine annually;
  (e) life-long prophylactic antibiotics (phenoxymethylpenicillin 500 mg b.d. or erythromycin 250 mg b.d.).
* *Infection*. Be more ready than usual to admit hyposplenic patients if they develop systemic infection.
* Advise patients to carry written information to alert health professionals and possibly carry an alert bracelet.
* Advise the patient about the risk of overseas travel especially malaria, unusual infections and animal bites.
* Document the functional hyposplenism and risk of infection as well as the vaccination status.

HAEMOCHROMATOSIS

● In the UK about 250,000 people have a genetic predisposition to haemochromatosis but only about 5000 are currently diagnosed. There is evidence that many times this number have tissue damage and disease caused by iron overload.

Candidates for screening

■ Patients with unexplained manifestations of liver disease, or a known cause of liver disease, with abnormalities of serum ferritin or transferrin index.

■ Patients with type 2 diabetes if they have hepatomegaly, elevated enzymes, atypical cardiac disease or early onset sexual dysfunction.

■ Patients with the triad of early onset atypical arthropathy, cardiac disease and male sexual dysfunction.

■ First degree relatives of known cases of haemochromatosis.

* Check the transferrin saturation after an overnight fast. If > 50%, refer to a haematologist or hepatologist. A raised serum ferritin confirms increased iron stores but may be elevated in other conditions.

PATIENT SUPPORT

The Haemochromatosis Society, Hollybush House, Hadley Green Road, Barnet, Herts EN5 5PR. Tel. 020 8449 1363. www.haemochromatosis.org.uk

THROMBOCYTOPENIA

GUIDELINE

British Committee for Standards in Haematology. General Haematology Task Force. 2003. Guidelines for the investigation and management of idiopathic thrombocytopenic purpura in adults, children and in pregnancy. Br J Haematol 120, 574–596. Available: www.bcshguidelines.com

* Admit patients with thrombocytopenia and mucocutaneous bleeding.
* Contact the haematologist if a patient has:
  (a) a platelet count below $60 \times 10^9/l$; or
  (b) evidence of bone marrow failure.

In a well patient with thrombocytopenia on one sample, repeat the sample and ask for a film.

* If there is still thrombocytopenia:
  (a) Check U&Es, LFTs, B_{12}, folic acid, and, after counselling, HIV status.
  (b) Ask about alcohol consumption and drugs especially aspirin, HRT, oestrogens, clopidogrel.
  (c) Ask if there is a family history of bleeding disorder or known thrombocytopenia.
  (d) Ask if there is a personal history of bleeding especially after dental extraction.
  (e) Check for evidence of malignancy and evidence of autoimmune disease, e.g. SLE.
  (f) Refer all patients with a confirmed platelet count $< 100 \times 10^9/l$ to a haematologist.

RECOMMENDATIONS FOR 'SAFE' PLATELET COUNTS IN ADULTS

■ Dentistry $\geq 10 \times 10^9/l$
■ Extractions $\geq 30 \times 10^9/l$
■ Minor surgery $\geq 50 \times 10^9/l$

- Major surgery $\geq 80 \times 10^9/l$
- Pregnancy:
  - (a) $> 50 \times 10^9/l$ is safe for normal delivery
  - (b) $> 80 \times 10^9/l$ is safe for Caesarean section, spinal or epidural anaesthesia where coagulation is otherwise normal.

PREGNANCY

Gestational thrombocytopaenia. Platelet counts tend to fall during pregnancy and levels of $120–150 \times 10^9/l$ are not uncommon especially in the third trimester.

* Refer all women with a confirmed platelet count $< 100 \times 10^9/l$ to a haematologist.

HAEMATOLOGICAL PROBLEMS IN ETHNIC MINORITIES

The following conditions may be found in people whose family originates from an area where malaria is or was once common (see Table 26.1).

HAEMOGLOBINOPATHIES

* The basic screen is: FBC, haemoglobin electrophoresis and sickle test.

THALASSAEMIA

UK Thalassaemia Society. 2008. *Standards for the Clinical Care of Children and Adults with Thalassaemia in the UK.* Available: www.ukts.org (choose 'Publications')

- The management of a patient with thalassaemia disease is a matter for secondary care. The aim of treatment is to maintain the haemoglobin above 9.5–10 g/dl by transfusion; to maintain folic acid levels; and to reduce the damage done by iron overload using chelation therapy. Bone marrow transplant and splenectomy are further options.

- A patient with thalassaemia disease who arrives from abroad to stay in the UK should be referred urgently to the nearest specialist thalassaemia centre.

- The GP needs to be aware of the acute and chronic complications that may occur, e.g. cardiac failure; endocrine deficiency (diabetes, hypothyroidism, hypoparathyroidism and hypogonadism); viral hepatitis; fracture from osteoporosis; leg ulcers; bacterial infections.

- There are 200,000 people in the UK with thalassaemia trait (thalassaemia minor). They may well be detected by the GP because of mild hypochromic microcytic anaemia with a normal or raised red cell count and a normal ferritin in a patient from an ethnic group at increased risk of the condition (see Table 26.2).

MANAGEMENT OF THALASSAEMIA TRAIT IN PRIMARY CARE

* Confirm the diagnosis by serum electrophoresis.
* Explain the nature of the condition. The website of the UK Thalassaemia Society is excellent but is inevitably dominated by information about thalassaemia major and intermedia.

Table 26.1 Haemoglobinopathies common in the UK

CONDITION	ORIGINS OF THOSE AT RISK	MANAGEMENT	SELF–HELP GROUPS
Thalassaemia disease	Mediterranean, Middle East, Indian subcontinent, South East Asia	Transfusion and desferrioxamine	UK Thalassaemia Society, tel. 0208 882 0011; www.ukts.org
Thalassaemia trait		Genetic counselling and prenatal diagnosis	
Sickle-cell disease	Central and West Africa, Caribbean and, occasionally, Mediterranean, Middle East and Indian subcontinent	Penicillin and folic acid lifelong prophylaxis	Sickle Cell Society, tel. 020 8961 7795; www.sicklecellsociety.org
		Pneumococcal, meningococcal C and Hib vaccine	
		Avoid factors which precipitate crises	
		Strong analgesia for crises	
Sickle-cell trait		Genetic counselling and prenatal diagnosis	

Table 26.2	Frequency of β-thalassaemia trait
AREA OF ORIGIN	FREQUENCY OF β-THALASSAEMIA TRAIT
Greece	1 in 7
Italy	1 in 10
Turkey	1 in 12
South Asia	1 in 20
Africa (including Afro-Caribbeans)	1 in 20–50
English of north European origin	1 in 1000

* Give oral folic acid during times of stress: infection, other illnesses, pregnancy, poor nutrition.
* Avoid giving iron and warn the patient not to let any other doctor give iron because of the mild anaemia.
* Discuss the implications for having children, if appropriate. Briefly, there is only a problem if the partner is also a carrier of the trait. If so, there is a 1 in 4 chance of a child with thalassaemia disease, a 1 in 2 chance of a child with the trait, and a 1 in 4 chance of a normal child. Refer for genetic counselling if both partners are known to have the trait.

SICKLE-CELL DISEASE

It is estimated that there are about 12,000 people with sickle-cell disease in the UK (Yardumian and Crawley 2001).

* Screen potential carriers antenatally, see page 380. In the UK all babies are screened at birth.
* Refer to hospital urgently any patient with sickle-cell disease who presents with:
  (a) severe pain;
  (b) systemic illness (fever, generally unwell, dehydration, unable to drink because of vomiting). The patient may be immunocompromised because of multiple splenic infarcts. Children under the age of 3 are at most risk of overwhelming infection;
  (c) abdominal pain, especially if associated with rapid enlargement of the spleen;
  (d) worsening anaemia;
  (e) acute chest symptoms (breathlessness, cough, chest pain);
  (f) a neurological or ocular event;
  (g) priapism.

* Manage less severe attacks at home with:
  (a) analgesia, ranging from paracetamol to parenteral morphine plus an antiemetic; and
  (b) an NSAID; and
  (c) oral hydration.
* Be on the look-out for chronic complications: pulmonary fibrosis, renal impairment, proliferative retinopathy, avascular necrosis, especially of the hip, and leg ulcers.
* Advise all parents of children with sickle-cell disease to take steps to avoid crises by making sure that they guard against cold and dehydration, and seek early treatment for infection.
* Ensure that the child:
  (a) is taking prophylactic penicillin from the age of 3 months. This is usually given in a b.d. dosage, e.g. a 6–12-year-old would receive 250 mg b.d. The prophylaxis is maintained until at least the age of 5 (Meremikwu 2005) and probably for life;
  (b) has received the pneumococcal vaccination appropriate for his or her age, i.e. conjugated vaccine up to the age of 2 and unconjugated vaccine thereafter. Repeat it 3-yearly until the child reaches the age of 10, and then 5–10 yearly;
  (c) receives all other childhood vaccines;
  (d) is immunized every autumn against influenza.
* Consider giving folic acid supplements, according to the local policy.

VENOUS THROMBOEMBOLISM (VTE)

GUIDELINE

Walker ID, Greaves M, Preston FE. 2001. Investigation and management of heritable thrombophilia. Br J Haematol 114, 512–518. Available: www.bcshguidelines.com

* 5% of the UK population is heterozygous for the commonest hereditary form of thrombophilia: factor V Leiden. It carries a four-fold increased risk of VTE and accounts for 20–40% of VTE in the UK (Greaves 2001).
* Acquired causes of VTE are common, e.g. cancer, myeloproliferative diseases, SLE.

- In both hereditary and acquired forms, a trigger is usually also present, e.g. immobility, pregnancy, combined oral contraception, the post-operative state. For details of the diagnosis of thrombophilia see *Evidence-based Diagnosis in Primary Care* by A. F. Polmear (editor), published by Butterworth-Heinemann, 2008.

PATIENTS AT RISK OF VTE

* Give all patients at high risk of VTE, lifestyle advice to reduce that risk.
* Consider referring the following for investigation for thrombophilia (DTB 1995):
  (a) DVT aged under 40;
  (b) recurrent DVT or superficial thrombophlebitis;
  (c) unusual DVT, e.g. mesenteric vein thrombosis;
  (d) skin necrosis in association with venous thrombosis;
  (e) those with a VTE and a first degree relative who has had a VTE;
  (f) recurrent fetal loss ($\times 3$);
  (g) unexplained neonatal thrombosis.
* In borderline cases the GP may choose to screen the patient with a FBC, prothrombin time, APTT and a fibrinogen concentration.

Patients diagnosed with thrombophilia

* Recommend: *Thrombophilia: information for patients and their relatives*. Available: www.bcshguidelines.com (choose 'Current guidelines').
* Recommend that the patient with a past history of VTE or proven thrombophilia carry a card giving details of the condition.
* *Preconception*. Refer all women with a known history of thrombophilia, who are contemplating pregnancy, for preconceptual advice, preferably to a unit specializing in thrombophilia. Those on long-term anticoagulants should be informed of the risk of fetal complications associated with maternal coumarin ingestion. A pregnancy test should be organized if they are 3 or more days late with a period, and immediate referral made if positive.

* *Pregnancy*. All women at risk should wear graduated compression stockings throughout their pregnancy and for 6–12 weeks afterwards. All pregnant women at risk should be referred urgently for consideration of low molecular weight heparin injections or warfarin.

Implications of a diagnosis of thrombophilia

(a) Patients can benefit from prophylactic measures at times when they are at high risk of VTE: in pregnancy; following trauma or surgery; on long-haul flights. Women can avoid the oral contraceptive pill.
(b) Should a thrombosis occur, anticoagulants are needed for the same duration and intensity as in patients without the condition.
(c) Prophylactic anticoagulants are not indicated; the risk of serious haemorrhage considerably outweighs the risk of fatal VTE.
(d) Identification of an inherited disorder may prejudice life insurance.

Population screening is therefore not justified and screening of family members may not be, unless a female relative is considering starting the combined oral contraceptive.

MANAGEMENT OF VTE

- Initial management of confirmed VTE at home with low molecular weight heparin appears to be cost effective (Othieno, Affan and Okpo 2007). Routine monitoring is not needed.
* Refer patients with suspected VTE for specialist assessment. Clinical diagnosis is unreliable. For details of the diagnosis of VTE see *Evidence-based Diagnosis in Primary Care* by A. F. Polmear (editor), published by Butterworth-Heinemann, 2008.
* Continue the specialist's treatment if VTE is confirmed; either low molecular weight heparin or warfarin.
* Prescribe a calf-length elastic compression stocking if the DVT is in the leg. If the patient is prepared to wear it for 2 years it will reduce the risk of post-thrombotic syndrome, at least in patients with proximal DVTs (Brandjes, Buller, Heijboer, *et al.* 1997).

Warfarin (DTB 1992; Baglin, Keeling and Watson 2006; Baglin, Cousins, Keeling, *et al.* 2006)

Practicalities

Timing and frequency of prothrombin times

Patients should take their warfarin in the evening and have blood taken in the morning. Prothrombin time should be checked weekly for 3–4 weeks, then every 6–8 weeks if control is good. Warfarin needs often change with the change of lifestyle following discharge from hospital. Revert to weekly checks for 4 weeks, even in patients previously well controlled.

Starting and discontinuation of anticoagulation

- For patients who do not require rapid anticoagulation a slow-loading regimen (3 mg a day for a week and then titrated to INR or 2 mg/day for 2 weeks then titrated to INR) is safe and achieves therapeutic anticoagulation within 3–4 weeks in the majority of patients (Baglin, Keeling and Watson 2006).
- Simple regimens are probably safer especially in the elderly, e.g. where the patient takes 4 mg/day four 1 mg tablets is less confusing than one 3 mg and one 1 mg tablet.
- Oral anticoagulant therapy can be discontinued abruptly when the period of therapy is completed.

TARGET INR FOR DIFFERENT CLINICAL INDICATIONS (see also Tables 26.3 and 26.4)

The annual incidence of major bleeding in patients who take warfarin for more than 6 months is 2–3% with an estimated case fatality rate of 9% (Linkins, Choi and Douketis 2003).

Major bleeding occurs in more patients taking warfarin for 6 months than 3 months (Campbell, Bentley, Prescott, *et al.* 2007).

The frequency of recurrence of VTE at 2–3 years is similar in patients taking 3 months or 12 months anticoagulation (Agnelli, Prandoni, Santamaria, *et al.* 2001; Agnelli, Prandoni, Becattini, *et al.* 2003).

The management of poor control (Baglin, Keeling and Watson 2006)

Recommendations for avoiding haemorrhage

(a) Major bleeding

   ✳ Stop warfarin; ADMIT.

Table 26.3 Target INR for different clinical indications

INDICATION	TARGET INR	DURATION OF ANTICOAGULATION
Pulmonary embolus	2.5	6 months
Proximal deep vein thrombosis	2.5	6 months*
Calf vein thrombus	2.5	3 months
Recurrence of venous thromboembolism when no longer on warfarin	2.5	Consider long term
Recurrence of venous thromboembolism while on warfarin	3.5	Consider long term
Antiphospholipid syndrome	2.5	Consider long term
Atrial fibrillation	2.5	Long term
Cardioversion	2.5 or 3.0	3 weeks before and 4 weeks after procedure
Mural thrombus	2.5	3 months
Cardiomyopathy	2.5	Long term
Mechanical prosthetic heart valve	3.0 or 2.5	Long term

*Shortening treatment to 3 months is recommended if circumstances indicate that the risk:benefit ratio favours this, for example if a reversible precipitating factor was present and there are risk factors for bleeding (e.g. age > 65 years).

Table 26.4 Warfarin: maximum recall periods during maintenance therapy

One high INR	Recall in 7–14 days (stop treatment for 1–3 days) (maximum 1 week in prosthetic valve patients)
One low INR	Recall in 7–14 days
One therapeutic INR	Recall in 4 weeks
Two therapeutic INRs	Recall in 6 weeks
Three therapeutic INRs	Recall in 8 weeks, except patients with a prosthetic valve
Four therapeutic INRs	Recall in 10 weeks, except patients with a prosthetic valve
Five therapeutic INRs	Recall in 12 weeks, except patients with a prosthetic valve

Patients with a prosthetic heart valve, after discharge from hospital may need more frequent INR monitoring in the first few weeks.

* If there is likely to be a delay give phytomenadione (vitamin K_1) 5–10 mg by slow intravenous injection.

(b) INR > 8.0, no bleeding or minor bleeding

  * Stop warfarin, measure the INR every 2–3 days, restart when INR < 5.0.

  * If there are other risk factors for bleeding give phytomenadione (vitamin K_1) 500 mcg by slow intravenous injection or 5 mg by mouth (for partial reversal of anticoagulation give smaller oral doses of phytomenadione for example 0.5–2.5 mg using the intravenous preparation orally); repeat dose of phytomenadione if INR still too high after 24 hours.

(c) INR 6.0-8.0, no bleeding or minor bleeding

  * Stop warfarin, measure the INR every 2–3 days, restart when INR < 5.0.

(d) INR < 6.0 but more than 0.5 units above target value

  * Reduce dose or stop warfarin, measure the INR every 2–3 days, restart when INR < 5.0.

(e) Unexpected bleeding at therapeutic levels

  * Consider the possibility of an underlying cause, for example unsuspected gastrointestinal tract pathology.

Other points:

* Reversal of warfarin with vitamin K can cause prolonged warfarin resistance. In patients at high risk of thromboembolism (e.g. with mechanical heart valves) assess the need for vitamin K on an individual basis.

* *Apparent need for a high dose.* If the dose goes above 9 mg/day, suspect poor compliance, drug interaction or abnormal warfarin handling. Check the warfarin level. Advise about diet. Some vegetables contain high quantities of natural vitamin K. The patient need not avoid these foods but needs to remain consistent in their intake.

* *Drug interactions.* Check the INR 3–5 days after starting a new drug unless it is known not to affect the INR.

Dental procedures (Perry, Nokes and Heliwell 2006)
Oral anticoagulants should not be discontinued in the majority of patients requiring out-patient dental surgery including dental extraction.

* Check INR 72 hours prior to dental surgery or scaling. There is no need to check the INR prior to non-invasive procedures.

* *Single dose of antibiotics:* where the patient is stably anticoagulated (INR 2.5) there is no need to alter the anticoagulant regimen.

* *Course of antibiotics:* check the INR 2–3 days after starting treatment.

* *NSAIDs.* Patients taking warfarin should not be prescribed non-selective NSAIDs or COX-2 inhibitors as analgesia following dental surgery.

References

Agnelli, G., Prandoni, P., Becattini, C., et al., 2003. Extended oral anticoagulant therapy after a first episode of pulmonary embolism. Ann. Intern. Med. 139, 19–25.

Agnelli, G., Prandoni, P., Santamaria, M., et al., 2001. Three months versus one year of oral anticoagulant therapy for idiopathic deep venous thrombosis. Warfarin Optimal Duration Italian Trial Investigators. N. Engl. J. Med. 345, 165–169.

Baglin, T., Cousins, D., Keeling, D., et al., 2006. Recommendations from the British Committee for Standards in Haematology and National Patient Safety Agency. Br. J. Haematol. 136, 26–29. Available: www.bcshguidelines.com.

Baglin, T., Keeling, D., Watson, H., 2006. British Committee for Standards in Haematology. Guidelines on oral anticoagulation (warfarin): third edition - 2005 update. Br. J. Haematol. 132, 277–285. Available: http://www.bcshguidelines.com.

Bradford, G., Taylor, C., 1999. Omeprazole and vitamin B12 deficiency. Ann. Pharmacother. 33, 641.

Brandjes, D., Buller, H., Heijboer, H., et al., 1997. Randomised trial of effect of compression stockings in patients with symptomatic proximal-vein thrombosis. Lancet 349, 759–762.

Campbell, I., Bentley, D., Prescott, R., et al., 2007. Anticoagulation for three versus six months in patients with deep vein thrombosis or pulmonary embolism, or both: randomised trial. BMJ 334, 674.

Dickinson, C., 1995. Does folic acid harm people with vitamin B12 deficiency? QJM 88, 357–364.

DOH, 2000. Guidelines for the urgent referral of patients with suspected cancer. Department of Health,

London. Available on www.dh.
gov.uk/cancer/referral.htm.

DTB, 1995. Management of patients
with thrombophilia. Drug Ther.
Bull. 33, 6–8.

DTB, 1992. How to anticoagulate.
Drug Ther. Bull. 30, 77–80.

Elis, A., Ravid, M., Manor, Y., et al.,
1996. Clinical approach to
"idiopathic" normocytic-
normochromic anemia. J. Am.
Geriatr. Soc. 44, 832–834.

Goddard, A., McIntyre, A., Scott, B.,
2000. Guidelines for the
management of iron deficiency
anaemia. British Society of
Gastroenterology. www.bsg.org.
uk/clinical_prac/guidelines.htm.

Greaves, M., 2001. Thrombophilia.
Clin. Med. 1, 432–435.

Griner, P.F., 1999. Microcytosis. In:
Black, E.R., Bordley, D.R., Tape, T.G.,
Panzer, R.J. (eds), Diagnostic
Strategies for Common Medical
Problems. 2nd ed. American
College of Physicians,
Philadelphia.

Hardwick, R., Armstrong, C., 1997.
Synchronous upper and lower
gastrointestinal endoscopy is an
effective method of investigating
iron deficiency anaemia. Br. J.
Surg. 84, 1725–1728.

Lederle, F., 1998. Oral cobalamin for
pernicious anaemia: back from the
verge of extinction. J. Am. Geriatr.
Soc. 46, 1125–1127.

Linkins, L., Choi, P., Douketis, J.,
2003. Clinical impact of bleeding
in patients taking oral
anticoagulant therapy for venous
thromboembolism: a meta-
analysis. Ann. Intern. Med. 139,
893–900.

Meremikwu, M., 2005. Sickle cell
disease. *Clinical Evidence*. BMJ
Publishing Group, London.

Oh, R., Brown, D., 2003. Vitamin B12
deficiency. Am. Fam. Physician
67, 979–986.

Othieno, R., Affan, M., Okpo, E.,
2007. Home versus in-patient
treatment for deep vein

thrombosis (Cochrane Review).
Cochrane Database Syst. Rev. (3).

Perry, D., Nokes, T., Heliwell, P.,
2006. Guidelines for the
management of patients on oral
anticoagulants requiring dental
surgery. British Committee for
Standards in Haematology.
Available: www.bcshguidelines.
com.

Seward, S., Safran, C., Marton, K.,
et al., 1990. Does the mean
corpuscular volume help
physicians evaluate hospitalized
patients with anemia? J. Gen.
Intern. Med. 5, 187–191.

World Health Organization, 1992.
The prevalence of anaemia in
women: a tabulation of available
information, 2nd ed. WHO,
Geneva.

Yardumian, A., Crawley, C., 2001.
Sickle cell disease. Clin. Med. 1,
441–446.

Chapter 27

Cancer and palliative care in patients with cancer

CHAPTER CONTENTS

CANCER

THE ROLE OF THE GP IN A FOLLOW-UP REVIEW OF A PATIENT WITH CANCER

* Check that the patient has as much information about the cancer as he or she wishes to have. Sensitivity and respect for individual wishes are fundamental in the communication process. Prognostic information needs to relate to that individual patient and alters for each patient with the stage of the illness. Patients and relatives prefer the doctor to (Kirk, Kirk and Kristjanson 2004):

   (a) play it straight;
   (b) stay the course;
   (c) give time;
   (d) show they care;
   (e) make it clear;
   (f) pace information.

* Check that the avenues of communication are clear to both GP and patient; specifically that a key worker has been identified. For those cancers where such a post exists this is likely to be a specialist nurse.
* Enquire about the patient's emotional state. Distress which is more than an expected reaction to the diagnosis may need specific treatment.
* Check the impact the diagnosis, and the patient's condition, is having on the family. When the patient is unwell or the prognosis is poor, try to see the carer alone.
* Encourage the patient to understand and manage their own care and recommend local

© 2011 Elsevier Ltd.
DOI: 10.1016/B978-0-7020-3053-6.00027-1

and national support organizations (see below). Patients value contact with survivors of similar cancers.

* *Finances.* Explain that they are eligible for free prescriptions (form FP92A) and may be eligible for other benefits (see page 6).
* Move to the inauguration of palliative care early, when it becomes apparent that treatment will not be curative.

SOURCES OF INFORMATION FOR PROFESSIONALS

National Cancer Institute (US) www.cancer.gov
   National Electronic Library for Health. http://library.nhs.uk/cancer
   The sources of information for patients below all include information for professionals

PATIENT INFORMATION AND SUPPORT

CancerBACUP (British Association for Cancer United Patients), 3 Bath Place, Rivington Street, London EC2A 3RJ, tel. 0808 800 1234; www.cancerbacup.org.uk
   Cancerhelp (produced by Cancer Research UK) for patients and families. www.cancerhelp.org.uk
   American Cancer Society. www.cancer.org
   Mywavelength. This is a free, web-based support network where patients can get in touch with other people who have the same cancer type. Choose 'C' for cancer and choose the cancer type. www.mywavelength.com
   Riprap is for children and teenagers: www.riprap.org.uk

The sections on individual cancers that follow concentrate on information that will be useful to the GP in the management of patients, most of whom will also be under specialist care, but who may come to the GP to discuss their prognosis or with the first presentation of a recurrence.

BREAST CANCER

* Women with breast cancer should have a family history taken, in order to judge whether their cancer puts other women in the family at increased risk (see page 435).

* Women with breast cancer may die from the disease even after a remission of over 5 years. This excess mortality over their contemporaries is present even 20–40 years after diagnosis and initial treatment (Sainsbury, Haward, Rider, *et al.* 1995). Survival is best if the tumour is:
  (a) small (less than 2 cm): 5-year survival 95%. With larger tumours (more than 2 cm) the 5-year survival is 80%;
  (b) tubular or mucinous;
  (c) low grade (well differentiated). High grade (poorly differentiated) tumours carry poorer prognosis;
  (d) oestrogen receptor positive; they are more likely to respond to hormone therapy.
* Young women (under the age of 35) tend to develop aggressive tumours with a 5-year survival of less than 50%.

Table 27.1	Staging and prognosis in breast cancer	
STAGE	TNM	5-YEAR SURVIVAL (AMERICAN JOINT COMMISSION ON CANCER AND INTERNATIONAL UNION AGAINST CANCER 2010)
0	Tis (tumour in situ)	100%
1	T1, N0, M0	98%
2A	T0-2, N0-1, M0	88%
2B	T2-3, N0-1, M0	76%
3A	T0-T3, N2, M0	56%
3B	T4, any N, M0; any T, N3, M0	49%
4	Any T, any N, M1	16%

For a description of the TNM scoring see next page.

LIKELY PRESENTATIONS OF RECURRENT DISEASE

(a) Nodules in the skin or in the scar.
(b) Nodes in the axilla or neck.
(c) Contralateral breast cancer.
(d) Bone pain, especially spinal.
(e) Cough or breathlessness from pulmonary metastases.

(f) Constitutional symptoms secondary to hypercalcaemia (lassitude, anorexia, constipation, nausea).

(g) Neurological or behavioural problems secondary to brain metastases.

(h) Anaemia from marrow infiltration.

Table 27.2	Common sites of metastases in breast cancer	
COMMON SITES	COMMON PRESENTATIONS	MEDIAN SURVIVAL TIME (MONTHS) (LEONARD, RODGER AND DIXON 1994)
Soft tissue	Lumps	19
Bone	Pathological fracture, spinal cord compression Symptoms of hypercalcaemia	15
Lung	Breathlessness, cough	10
Liver	Abdominal pain	8
Brain	Headache, confusion, behavioural change, focal signs	3

TNM scoring in carcinoma of the breast (T = tumour, N = nodes, M = metastases.)

SCORE	DESCRIPTION
Tis (Tumour in situ)	Ductal carcinoma in situ, LCIS, Paget's disease of the nipple
T0	No evidence of primary tumour
T1	The tumour is 2 cm or less in diameter, with no skin involvement – except in the case of Paget's disease where it is confined to the nipple with no nipple retraction or fixation
T2	Tumour greater than 2 cm but less than 5 cm
T3	Tumour greater than 5 cm in greatest diameter, less than 10 cm
T4	Greater than 10 cm, or skin or chest wall involvement or peau d'orange
N0	No palpable ipsilateral axillary nodes
N1	Palpable, ipsilateral axillary nodes
N2	Ipsilateral axillary nodal metastases fixed to one another or to other structures
N3	Metastases to ipsilateral internal mammary nodes
M0	No evidence of metastases
M1	Distant metastases (includes ipsilateral supraclavicular nodes)

SUPPORT ORGANIZATIONS

Breast Cancer Care, Kiln House, 210 New Kings Road, London SW6 4NZ, Helpline: 0808 800 6000, tel: 020 7384 2984, Fax: 020 7384 3387, email: info@breastcancercare.org.uk; website: www. breastcancercare.org.uk

Breast Cancer Care (Scotland), 4th Floor, 40 St Enoch Square, Glasgow, G1 4DH, tel: 0845 0771 892, Fax: 0141 221 9499, email: sco@breastcancercare.org.uk Website: www. breastcancercare.org.uk

Lymphoedema Support Network, St Luke's Crypt, Sydney Street, London SW3 6NH, tel: 0207 351 4480, website: www.lymphoedema.org

OVARIAN CANCER

- The overall survival rate is around 30%. Despite high response rates to chemotherapy (55–75%), relapse is common within 2 years.
- *Histological grading*: grade 1 (low-grade or well differentiated) tumours usually grow slowly and are less likely to spread. Grade 2 (moderate grade) and grade 3 (high grade or poorly differentiated) are likely to grow more quickly and are more likely to spread.
- *Increasing age* worsens the prognosis. Patients under 50 in all stages have considerably better 5-year survival than older patients (40% compared to 15%). Women over 65 have 5-year relative survival rates of almost half those of women under 65.
- Patients who respond to platinum-based therapy initially and then experience relapse after a significant platinum-free interval have a good chance of responding again to platinum-based treatment (response rates of up to 60% are reported).
- Patients who are considered platinum-resistant (disease progression on platinum therapy or recurrence shortly after completion of initial therapy) are treated, at relapse or progression, with drugs that have been shown to be active in resistant disease. If paclitaxel was not used first line, then it is the second line drug of choice. NICE guidelines recommend liposomal doxorubicin or topotecan, in the second line

treatment. Response rates are around 20% with a progression free survival of around 4–5 months.

- Patients who relapse after 6 months may be treated with the same regimen (response rate around 20%).

Table 27.3	Prognosis in ovarian cancer according to stage and histological grade	
STAGE	**DESCRIPTION**	**PROGNOSIS (5-YEAR SURVIVAL) AND LIKELY TREATMENT**
Stage 1	Limited to the ovaries	
1a	Limited within the capsule of one ovary. No malignant ascites	Grade 1 – 90–100% Grade 3 – as 1c surgery
1b	Limited within the capsule of both ovaries. No malignant ascites	Grade 1 – 90–100% Grade 3 – as 1c surgery
1c	1a or 1b and either there is some cancer on the surface of at least one ovary or malignant ascites or positive peritoneal washings or the ovary ruptures before or during surgery	Poorer prognosis Surgery usually with adjuvant chemotherapy
Stage 2	Extended outside the ovary or ovaries but within the pelvis	50% Surgery then chemotherapy
Stage 3	Spread outside the pelvis into the abdominal cavity (including superficial liver metastases) or positive retroperitoneal or inguinal nodes	15–20% Debulking surgery followed by chemotherapy
Stage 4	Distant metastases	5–10%

LIKELY PRESENTATIONS OF RECURRENT DISEASE

(a) Cough, breathlessness and pleuritic pain from pulmonary and pleural metastases.

(b) Pelvic and inguinal nodes.

(c) Small and large bowel obstruction and ascites (one third of patients with ascites also have pleural effusion).

* Check CA 125 levels if a recurrence is suspected. They are not specific for ovarian metastases but a raised level increases the probability that symptoms are due to a recurrence.

SUPPORT ORGANIZATIONS

Gynae C. 1, Bolingbroke Road, Swindon, Wiltshire, SN2 2LB; tel: 01793 322005. Email: gynaec@wilts. communigate.co.uk or Gynae_C@yahoo.com. Website: http://www.communigate.co.uk/wilts/gynaec/

Ovacome, Elizabeth Garrett Anderson Hospital, London, WC1E 6DH Tel. 0207 380 9589, E-mail: ovacome@ovacome.org.uk. Website: www.ovacome. org.uk

OESOPHAGEAL CANCER

The overall 5-year survival is between 5 and 10%.

TNM scoring in carcinoma of the oesophagus (T = tumour, N = nodes, M = metastases)	
T1	Tumour invading lamina propria or submucosa
T2	Tumour invading muscularis propria
T3	Tumour invading adventitia
T4	Tumour invading adjacent structures
N0	No nodes
N1	Regional nodes
M0	No distant metastases
Lower third oesophagus	Coeliac nodes
M1a	Other distant metastases
M1b	
Upper third oesophagus	Cervical nodes
M1a	Other distant metastases
M1b	
Middle third oesophagus	Distant metastases including non-regional nodes
M1b	

Table 27.4	Staging and prognosis of oesophageal cancer	
STAGE	**DEFINITION**	**5-YEAR SURVIVAL**
1	T1, N0, M0	50%
2a	T2-3, N0, M0	10–30%
2b	T1-2, N1, M0	Subsequent stages have increasingly worse prognosis
3	T3, N1, M0 or T4, any N, M0	
4	Any T, any N, M1	

BARRETT'S OESOPHAGUS

- The annual risk of carcinoma is 0.5%. Surveillance may be performed every 1–2 years but has a low yield of carcinoma. In one study 143 patients with Barrett's oesophagus had annual endoscopy for 10 years (Macdonald, Wicks and Playford 2000). Only one case of carcinoma was detected. The chance of dying from an unrelated illness was far greater.
- High grade dysplasia carries a 40–50% risk of progression to invasive cancer in 5 years. Resection may be offered.

LIKELY PROBLEMS AFTER TREATMENT OF OESOPHAGEAL CANCER

(a) Dysphagia either from obstruction by the tumour or nodes.
(b) Pain – directly from the tumour or oesophageal reflux.
(c) Malnutrition.
(d) Aspiration if there is a fistula or regurgitation is a problem.

GASTRIC CANCER

Only 20% of patients have operable tumours at diagnosis and in this group the 5-year survival is 10–20%.

TNM scoring in carcinoma of the stomach (T = tumour, N = nodes, M = metastases)

Tis	In situ
T1	Limited to lamina propria or submucosa
T2	Invading muscularis propria (2a), or subserosa (2b)
T3	Invasion through the serosa but not of adjacent structures
T4	Invasion of adjacent structures
N1	1–6 nodes involved
N2	7–15 nodes involved
N3	> 15 nodes involved
M0	No distant metastases
M1	Distant metastases

Table 27.5   Staging and prognosis in gastric cancer

STAGE	DEFINITION	5-YEAR SURVIVAL
0	Tis, N0, M0	90%
1a	T1, N0, M0	70%
1b	T1, N1, M0; T2, N0, M0	
2	T1, N2, M0; T2, N1, M0; T3, N0, M0	40%
3a	T2, N2, M0; T3, N1, M0; T4, N0, M0	15%
3b	T3, N2, M0	
4	T4, N1–3, M0; T1–3, N3, M0; any T, any N, M1	< 5%

LIKELY PRESENTATIONS OF RECURRENCE

(a) Jaundice, hepatomegaly, or right hypochondrial pain from liver metastases. The pain responds poorly to opioids but may respond to NSAIDs or steroids.
(b) Ascites from peritoneal spread.
(c) Breathlessness from lung metastases.
(d) Nonspecific back pain and abdominal pain from involvement of the coeliac plexus.

LIKELY PROBLEMS OF ADVANCED GASTRIC CANCER

(a) Severe epigastric pain.
(b) Obstruction.
(c) Ascites.
(d) Steatorrhoea from invasion of the pancreas.
(e) Anorexia, dysphagia, nausea and vomiting.

COLORECTAL CANCER

The overall 5-year survival is around 40%.

TNM scoring in colorectal carcinoma (T = tumour, N = nodes, M = metastases)	
T1	Invading submucosa
T2	Invading muscularis propria
T3	Invading subserosa or non-peritonealized pericolic/perirectal tissues
T4a	Invading visceral peritoneum
T4b	Invading other organs
N0	No lymph nodes involved
N1	1–3 regional nodes
N2	4 or more regional nodes
M0	No metastases
M1	Distant metastases

Survival rates may be improved with adjuvant chemotherapy (5-fluorouracil (5FU) and folinic acid (FA)) as follows:

- Stage 2 – uncertain effect – trials in progress.
- Stage 3 – improves absolute 5-year survival by 10%.
- Stage 4 - response in 20–30%, with improvement in median survival of 6 months and symptom-free period improved from 2 months to 10 months.

Oxalplatin and irinotecan, added to 5FU/FA, improve response rates further.

FOLLOW–UP OF COLORECTAL CANCER

GUIDELINES

Schofield JH, Steele RJ. 2002. Guideline for follow up after resection of colorectal cancer. Gut 51(suppl V), v3–v5.

NICE. Improving outcomes in colorectal cancers – manual update. Available: www.nice.org.uk

- 80% of recurrences occur within the first 2 years after surgery and it is traditional to undertake more intensive follow-up during this period. However, the majority of local and distant recurrences are symptomatic at the time of discovery and patients may wait for their follow-up appointments to disclose symptoms.
- Only about 30% of patients with recurrent disease are suitable for surgery and the survival results are poor.
- Although the responsibility for follow-up is usually with specialists the results of one RCT indicate no greater mortality or morbidity in those followed-up in general practice.
- Patients with colorectal cancer have a predisposition to further adenomas and a second primary cancer in the remaining large bowel. Colonoscopy is recommended:
  (a) after resection to establish if polyps or further primary cancer are present;
  (b) at 5-yearly intervals if they are 'polyp free' until the age of 70;
  (c) more frequently if five or more adenomas are found.
- * Refer if there are any symptoms of primary bowel cancer, i.e. a mass, rectal bleeding, a change in bowel habit to looser stools or increased frequency, or iron deficiency anaemia without obvious cause.
- * Consider checking carcinoembryonic antigen (CEA) levels in those patients who had a raised CEA at diagnosis, unless it is being checked by the specialist clinic. Refer if the level is rising.

Table 27.6 Staging and prognosis of colorectal cancer with possible treatments

Stage 0	Confined to the mucosa		
Stage 1 (Dukes' A)	Into the submucosa or muscularis propria	T1-2, N0, M0	> 90% surgery
Stage 2 (Dukes' B)			
Stage 2a (Dukes' B)	Though the outer layer	T3, N0, M0	60–80% surgery
Stage 2b (Dukes' B)	Though the outer layer onto adjoining structures but no lymph nodes affected	T4, N0, M0	60–80% surgery
Stage 3 (Dukes' C)	Local lymph node involvement	T1or 2, N1 or 2, M0	Up to 40% Surgery and adjuvant chemotherapy
Stage 4	Distant spread	Any T, any N, M1	< 5%

However, there is no evidence that the lead time provided by monitoring confers any survival benefit.

✳ Examine the liver for metastases.

SUPPORT ORGANIZATIONS

British Colostomy Association, 15 Station Road, Reading, Berkshire RG1 1LG. Tel. 0800 3284257 (24 hour helpline). Fax: 01189 569095. Website: www. bcass.org.uk. Email: sue@bcass.org.uk

LUNG CANCER

● 80% die within a year of diagnosis and overall 5-year survival is around 5%.

TNM scoring in lung cancer (T = tumour, N = nodes, M = metastases)

TMN SCORE	DESCRIPTION
TX	Positive cytology, primary tumour not apparent on imaging or bronchoscopy
T0	No evidence of primary tumour
TIS	Carcinoma in situ
T1	Tumour < 3 cm surrounded by, but not invading, lung or visceral pleura
T2	Tumour > 2 cm from the carina with any of the following: > 3 cm, involving bronchus, or invading the visceral pleura
T3	Tumour of any size invading the chest wall, diaphragm, pericardium, mediastinal pleura, or bronchus, or is < 2 cm from carina (without involvement)
T4	Tumour of any size involving mediastinum, heart, great vessels, carina, trachea, oesophagus, vertebral body, or tumour with malignant pleural or pericardial effusion or satellite nodules within the ipsilateral lobe
NX	Regional nodes cannot be assessed
N0	No regional node metastases
N1	Metastases to ipsilateral peribronchial and/or ipsilateral hilar lymph nodes and intrapulmonary nodes
N2	Metastases to ipsilateral mediastinal and /or sub-carinal lymph nodes
N3	Metastases to contralateral mediastinal or hilar, scalene or supraclavicular nodes
MX	Presence of distant metastases cannot be assessed
M0	No distant metastases
M1	Distant metastases present, including nodules in different lobes

Table 27.7 Staging and prognosis for non-small cell lung cancer

STAGE	TNM	5-YEAR SURVIVAL (%)
Stage IA	T1, N0, M0	60
Stage IB	T2, N0, M0	35–40
Stage IIA	T1, N1, M0	30–35
Stage IIB	T2, N1, M0	25
	T3, N0, M0	20
Stage IIIA	T1-3, N2, M0	10–15
	T3, N1, M0	10
Stage IIIB	T1-3, N3, M0	0–7
	T4, N0-3, M0	0–7
Stage IV	Any T, any N, M1	0–1

Table 27.8 Staging for small cell lung cancer

Limited disease (LD)	Confined to one hemithorax, involving ipsilateral and/or contralateral hilar, mediastinal or supraclavicular nodes, and patients with ipsilateral pleural effusion	With chemotherapy, median survival is 12–15 months
Extensive disease (ED)	All patients with metastases in the contralateral lung and distant metastases	With chemotherapy, median survival is 8–10 months

POSSIBLE PARANEOPLASTIC COMPLICATIONS

(a) Proximal muscle group myopathy (Eaton-Lambert syndrome).
(b) SIADH, ectopic ACTH production.
(c) Clubbing, hypertrophic pulmonary osteoarthropathy, polymyositis.
(d) Anaemia, thrombocytopaenia, thrombocytosis, migratory thrombophlebitis.
(e) Peripheral neuropathy, cortical or cerebellar degeneration.
(f) Dermatomyositis, acanthosis nigricans.

POSSIBLE CHEST PROBLEMS

(a) Pleural effusion and pleuritic pain.
(b) Distal atelectasis and recurrent or persistent pneumonias.

(c) Recurrent laryngeal nerve palsy causing hoarseness.

(d) Horner's syndrome (constricted pupil, anhidrosis, ptosis).

(e) Horner's syndrome plus shoulder pain (in Pancoast's tumour).

(f) Superior vena cava obstruction.

LIKELY PRESENTATIONS OF RECURRENT DISEASE:

(a) Brain.

(b) Bone.

(c) Liver.

(d) Adrenal glands.

(e) Bone marrow.

(f) Bowel obstruction.

(g) Fistulae between bowel and skin or bladder.

SUPPORT ORGANIZATIONS
British Lung Foundation, 73–75 Goswell Road, London, EC1V 7ER, Tel: 0207 688 5555. Fax: 0208 688 5556. Enquiries: enquiries@blf-uk.org. Website: www.lunguk.org   Roy Castle Lung Cancer Foundation, 200 London Road, Liverpool L3 9TA. Helpline: 0800 358 7200 (office hours). Website: www.roycastle.org

PROSTATE CANCER

See also page 420.

TNM scoring in carcinoma of the prostate (T = tumour, N = nodes, M = metastases)	
TNM SCORE	**DESCRIPTION**
T1	Not palpable or visible on imaging
T1a	Incidental finding involving < 5% of resected tissue
T1b	Incidental finding involving > 5% of resected tissue
T1c	Needle biopsy positive
T2	Confined to the prostate
T2a	Half of one lobe involved
T2b	More than one half of one lobe involved
T2c	Both lobes involved
T3	Invading through the prostate capsule
T3a	Extracapsular spread
T3b	Invasion of the seminal vesicle(s)
T4	Tumour fixed or invades adjacent structures (bladder neck, external sphincter, rectum, levator muscles or pelvic wall)
N1	Regional nodes (below the bifurcation of common iliac arteries)
M1a	Non-regional nodes
M1b	Bone
M1c	Other site

HISTOLOGICAL GRADING (GLEASON SCORES)

Values range from 2–10, where 2 corresponds to a well differentiated tumour and 10 corresponds to a very poorly differentiated tumour. Patients with low grade lesions (2–4) have 15-year survival of about 94% whereas those with higher grade lesions (7–10) have a 15-year survival of 15–50%.

Most men diagnosed with prostate cancer die from other causes. The predicted 15-year cancer mortality with a Gleason score of 6 is around 10% whereas mortality from other causes is around 60%. Radical treatment is likely to have a small impact on survival with considerable long-term morbidity.

Watchful waiting is often chosen in those who:

(a) are over 70 years of age;

(b) have low Gleason scores (7 or below);

(c) have comorbidity and a life expectancy of less than 15 years.

Hormonal therapy and palliative radiotherapy may be offered if the patient develops symptomatic disease.

Active surveillance is performed to tailor treatment to the individual:

(a) in younger patients who are fit for radical surgery;

(b) with early stage disease (T1-2, Low Gleason scores ≤ 7, PSA< 15).

Patients are frequently monitored with PSA testing, DRE and repeat biopsies. Patients with rapid doubling of PSA with an increased Gleason score may be offered radical treatment.

Radical prostatectomy has a disease free survival rate at 10 years of about 75%. However, incontinence occurs in around 15% and impotence in 30% with modern techniques. Urethral stricture occurs in around 5%.

Table 27.9   Examples of staging and prognosis for carcinoma of the prostate

STAGE	DESCRIPTION OF THE T SCORE	5-YEAR RECURRENCE RATE FOLLOWING LOCAL THERAPY
PSA < 10, Gleason ≤ 6, T1, T2a	Not clinical enlarged or tumour found in < 5% of resected tissue	6–20%
PSA 10–20, Gleason 7, T2b, T3a	More than half of one lobe involved or extracapsular spread	35–60%
PSA > 20, Gleason 8–10, T3b	Invasion of the seminal vesicle(s)	50–100%

Radiotherapy may be performed on its own but increasingly is combined with 3–6 months of hormonal therapy followed by 3 years hormonal therapy. Acute side-effects of radiotherapy especially fatigue, proctitis and increased frequency of bowel movements. Long-term side-effects are impotence in around 30% and incontinence < 1%.

Brachytherapy (insertion of radioactive seeds or temporary implants) is most likely to be offered to patients with: Gleason score ≤ 6, PSA < 10, a TNM score of T1–2, minimal obstructive symptoms and a small prostate volume. 80% are free of PSA relapse at 5 years and 70% at 10 years. Side-effects include impotence in 30%, incontinence in 1%, transient retention of urine and transient proctitis.

LIKELY PRESENTATIONS OF RECURRENT DISEASE

(a) Bone pain, pathological fracture and cord compression.
(b) Anaemia and thrombocytopaenia from marrow infiltration.
(c) Haematuria and perineal pain.
(d) Lymphoedema from nodal disease.
(e) Obstructive uropathy.

SIDE-EFFECTS OF TREATMENT

(a) Bladder outflow problems.
(b) Impotence.
(c) Hot flushes from androgen withdrawal. Venlafaxine and gabapentin may ease symptoms but their use is outside licence (see page 336).
(d) Gynaecomastia.

PATIENT ORGANIZATIONS

The Prostate Cancer Charity, 3 Angel Walk, London, W6 9HX. Tel. 020 8222 7622, helpline: 0845 300 8383. Email: info@prostate-cancer.org.uk; website: http://www.prostate-cancer.org.uk
   Prostate Cancer Support Association (PSA) BM Box 9434, London WC1N 3XX. Tel. 0845 601 0766, 9am–7pm M-F. Email: psagensec@blotholm.org.uk. Website: http://www.prostatecancersupport.info

BLADDER CANCER

TNM scoring in carcinoma of the bladder (T = tumour, N = nodes, M = metastases)	
TNM SCORE	**DESCRIPTION**
Tx	Primary tumour impossible to assess
Ta	Non-invasive papillary tumour
Tis	Flat tumour 'in situ'
T1	Invading subepithelial tissue only
T2	Invading muscularis
2a	Superficial muscle
2b	Deep muscle
T3	Extends beyond the muscularis
T3a	Micoscopically
T3b	Extravesical mass
T4a	Invading prostate, uterus or vagina
T4b	Invading pelvic wall, abdominal wall
N1	Single node ≤ 2 cm
N2	Single node > 2–5 cm, multiple nodes ≤ 5 cm
N3	Any node > 5 cm
M1	Distant metastases

Histological grading: grade 1 (low-grade or well differentiated) usually grow slowly and are less likely to spread; grade 2 (moderate grade) and grade 3 (high grade or poorly differentiated) are likely to grow more quickly and are more likely to spread.

Table 27.10	Staging and prognosis of bladder cancer	
STAGE	**TNM SCORE**	**5-YEAR SURVIVAL**
Carcinoma in situ	Tis	See below
1	T1, N0, M0	See below
2	T2a/b, N0, M0	60–75%
3	T3a/b, T4a, N0, M0	20–40%
4	T4b, N0, M0; any T, N1-3; any T, any N, M1	5–10%

Early bladder cancer (Tis, Ta, T1)

- All cured by surgery, immunotherapy or chemotherapy.
- Grade 1 more likely to be cured whereas grades 2 or 3 more likely to recur.
- Overall all superficial tumours 65% will recur, of these 45% will be more serious disease.
- Most Ta tumours are grade 1 and most recurrences are superficial that can be removed.
- Most T1 are grade 2–3 and more likely to become invasive if not treated (50%).

Invasive bladder cancer (T2, T3)

- Overall 5-year survival rate for surgery is 45%, improved to 50% with neoadjuvant chemotherapy.
- Radical radiotherapy has a lower overall 5-year survival rate of 35–40% but has the benefit of retention of bladder function in 70%. Acute side-effects include diarrhoea and cystitis. Later effects include radiation proctitis, bladder neck obstruction and haematuria.

Likely symptoms after treatment

(a) Frequency, dysuria and incontinence.
(b) Bladder spasms with severe suprapubic pain.

Likely presentations of recurrent disease

(a) Pelvic or intra-abdominal nodes.
(b) Liver.
(c) Lung.
(d) Bone.

(e) Adrenal glands.
(f) Intestine.

REACTIONS AND SIDE-EFFECTS OF TREATMENT

RADIOTHERAPY

* Explain to the patient that they may become very emotional during and after treatment and that this is normal.
* Recognize that once treatment is completed they may feel they have lost their support network.

Tiredness

- This is usually worse towards the end of the course of treatment. With brain tumours the tiredness is more pronounced and is maximal 1–2 weeks after treatment.
- Tiredness continues for some months after treatment finishes.
* Advise patients to:
  (a) plan to take a 1–2 hour sleep after a radiotherapy session;
  (b) adjust their lives to minimize the energy expended;
  (c) take short regular walks or some other form of exercise.

Eating and drinking

* Advise the patient to:
  (a) maintain their fluid intake;
  (b) eat small amounts often;
  (c) ignore worries about high fat foods;
  (d) alter the diet to suit swallowing ability;
  (e) consider giving food supplements.

Skin

* Advise the patient to:
  (a) seek advice from the radiology team about washing. If this is not forthcoming, advise them to gently wash the treatment area with warm water and simple soap. Dry by dabbing with a towel or air drying;

(b) avoid talc which may irritate and increase the skin reaction to radiotherapy;

(c) wear loose clothing made with natural fibre;

(d) avoid sun exposure of the treatment area and protect with sunscreen cream.

CHEMOTHERAPY

* *Common side-effects of chemotherapy drugs.* Go to www.cancerhelp.org.uk (choose 'Cancer treatments' then 'Chemotherapy' then 'Side-effects of specific cancer drugs').

Fatigue

* Advise the patient that:

(a) most people regain their normal energy levels 6–12 months after treatment ends, but it may take longer;

(b) fatigue may significantly affect the patient's life mentally, physically, emotionally and spiritually;

(c) fatigue is worse in those who have a combination of treatments, advanced cancer, or are elderly;

(d) fatigue is worse about 10 days after each dose of chemotherapy, i.e. at the same time as the white count is lowest.

Lowered resistance to infection

* Prescribe antibiotics for patients on chemotherapy at a much lower threshold. Resistance is lowered during the treatment and for many months afterwards.

* Check the FBC in patients with infection.

* Refer urgently:

(a) a patient with a temperature reading of 38°C;

(b) unexplained hypotension or tachycardia;

(c) rigors;

(d) a patient who feels generally unwell.

Nausea and vomiting

* Admit patients with nausea 7–14 days after chemotherapy especially if they have an i.v. line in place. It can be a presenting sign of sepsis.

* Treat most patients with antiemetics but admit if they do not come under control or they are dehydrated.

Diarrhoea

This is particularly common with 5FU and capecitabine.

* Assess for dehydration. Patients passing stool five to six times a day may need admission.

* Check for neutropenia. If present, admit.

Constipation

This can be caused by vinca-alkaloids and 5HT-3 antiemetics, e.g. granisetron. See page 208 for management.

* Check FBC. If there is neutropenia do not order enemas.

Stomatitis (sore ulcerated mouth)

Symptoms may occur 4–7 days after chemotherapy and can last a further 7–10 days. Difflam or sucralfate mouthwash or treatments used for aphthous ulcers may help (see page 542).

Depression

* Explain that 25% of patients become depressed and that they should return if this occurs.

Cognitive functions

* Explain that concentration and memory may vary during treatment and that for some this continues after treatment.

PALLIATIVE CARE IN PATIENTS WITH CANCER

REVIEW

O'Neill B, Fallon M. 1997. ABC of palliative care. BMJ 315, 801–804

Guidelines

Scottish Intercollegiate Guidelines Network and the Scottish Cancer Therapy Network. 2008. *Control of Pain in Adults with Cancer.* SIGN, June. Online. Available: www.sign.ac.uk

National Council for Palliative Care. 2003. *Guidelines for Managing Cancer Pain in Adults*, 3rd edition. Can be ordered from www.ncpc.org.uk (choose 'publications' then 'clinical guidelines and research')

National Institute for Health and Clinical Excellence. 2004. *Improving Supportive and Palliative Care for Adults with Cancer*. March. Online. Available: www.nice.org.uk

Watson M, Lucas C, Hoy A, Back I. 2005. *Oxford Handbook of Palliative Care*. Oxford University Press

The World Health Organization defines palliative care as the 'active total care of patients whose disease is not responsive to curative treatment' (WHO 1990). Control of pain, of other symptoms and of psychological, social and spiritual problems is paramount. The goal of palliative care is the achievement of the best quality of life for patients and their families. Palliative care should not be reserved for the terminal stages; it may be appropriate as soon as an incurable disease is diagnosed. Palliative care is necessarily multidisciplinary and requires effective communication with patients, their families and others involved in their care.

The NICE guideline (above) recommends that palliative care be systematically organized, e.g. along the lines of the Macmillan Cancer Relief Gold Standards Framework (www.macmillan.org.uk choose 'Health professionals' then 'Primary care' then 'Gold standards framework') or The Liverpool Care Pathway (www.lcp-mariecurie.org.uk, choose 'Example pathways' then 'Community').

TALKING TO THE PATIENT

Sensitivity and respect are fundamental to the communication process (Kirk, Kirk and Kristjanson 2004). It is important to find out what the individual wishes are before embarking on any discussion.

* *Breaking bad news.* Patients will dictate the pace at which they want to receive details of the diagnosis. A stepwise approach beginning with a 'warning shot' may be helpful. They may not wish to hear the whole diagnosis straight away. At any stage they may be more concerned with practical aspects of their care.
* Give patients every opportunity to ask about their illness. Useful questions to ask are: 'is there anything you want to ask me about your illness?' and 'have you any particular worries about your illness?'
* *Denial* may be a valid coping mechanism for those who are unable or not yet ready to adapt to the reality of a terminal illness. Denial is rarely complete or fixed. Empathetic listening and responding to a patient's concerns may allow the patient to feel safe enough to let the painful reality into their conscious thinking.
* *'Please don't tell him he has cancer.'* Collusion is a means of protecting another from pain. It is most often seen between patients and relatives but may also occur between professionals. Honest discussion allows patients to be reassured and to readjust hopes and aims for the future.
* *Anger, guilt and blame.* Acknowledging the emotion and exploring the issue with a patient and his or her family will help them to move on.
* *Fears.* Explore patients' fears about their illness. It will be possible to reassure them about the degree to which many of their symptoms can be relieved.
* *False reassurance* can undermine the relationship in the future. Do not guarantee to control their pain all the time. 5% of patients have uncontrollable pain.
* Encourage the patient and relative to contact support agencies for more information and be prepared to discuss the disease and prognosis at any stage.
* *Express hope.* There is a need for hopeful but realistic messages. If patient and family recognize that there is no possibility of cure, focus on what can be done to improve the quality of life.
* *Dying.* Ask whether there are specific aspects that the professional team should be aware of. This is especially important in ethnic minorities (Gatrad, Brown, Notta, *et al.* 2003). Ethnic minority groups are much less likely to use palliative care services than white patients (Hill and Penso 1995).
* *Place of death.* At an appropriate time ask the patient where they would like to die and if the response is 'at home', ask what their feelings are about hospice admission, if home management becomes difficult.

THE HOME

* Try to keep the patient from adopting an invalid role before it is essential. Encourage the family to eat, watch television, etc. with the patient.
* Some rearrangement of the home may be necessary, especially sleeping near the toilet or providing a commode. District nursing services or social services may be able to help.

NUTRITION

● Food and nourishment are an important part of health and well-being. Feeding relatives who are ill is a part of the caring and nurturing process and provides a tangible and practical role for the family. Appetite in patients with advanced cancer is often limited and unpredictable. This is frequently the cause of carer anxiety and sometime family conflict.
● Some patients and families adopt strict diets, e.g. vegetarian, vegan or complementary therapy diets. In individual cases physical and psychological benefits have been reported but often the rigorous regimes become burdensome for weak patients and their exhausted carers.
● *Oesophageal stents.* Patients treated palliatively with stents for oesophageal cancer require a liquid/pureed diet with the provision of fizzy drinks after eating to avoid stent blockage.

● *Food supplements.* A large range of food supplements/meal replacements are available but their value is not proven. There is a large wastage and it is important to establish the patient's preferences and prescribe small quantities.
● Food and fluids are seldom needed at the very end of life. The family is likely to need reassurance about this.
* Advise the patient to increase their intake of vitamin C. Vitamin C intake is often low and patients with low plasma levels have a shorter survival (Maryland, Bennett and Keith 2005).

FINANCIAL ASPECTS

* *Free prescriptions* are available for patients (Form FP92A for patients under retirement age).
* *Disability Living Allowance and Attendance Allowance under the Special Rules (DS1500)* are available for patients unlikely to live more than 6 months (see page 6).
* *Macmillan Cancer Relief Grants* are available for people with cancer who have a low income and little capital. Application must be by a professional on a form available from: 89 Albert Embankment, London SE1 7UK; www.macmillan.org; email: cancerline@macmillan.org.uk.

SUPPORT

* *Psychological support* has been shown to improve emotional and physical symptoms although not to affect the medical outcome (Fallowfield 1995). This may be available as part of the hospital oncology service. Alternatively, the national cancer self-help groups have details of local branches.
* *The palliative care/community hospice team* should be involved early in the illness if this facility exists locally. An early meeting of all the professionals involved in the patient's care is necessary in order to establish one person as the key worker, with responsibility for ensuring that all the different aspects of the patient's care are being covered.
* *Hospice admission* may be needed at some stage, for symptom control, as a respite for the carer or

for the terminal stage. Encourage patients and relatives to visit the hospice early in the illness. Remember, however, that most patients in the UK wish to die at home, although only a quarter do so (Thorpe 1993).

THE DYING PATIENT

The terminal phase may be recognized first by the patient themselves. Indicators are:

(a) progressive weight loss;

(b) profound weakness;

(c) drowsiness and reduced cognition;

(d) diminished intake of food and fluids.

* Discuss with the patient and relatives, the situation and the question of resuscitation.

* Ask again about preferred place of death.

* *Out of hours*. Inform the out of hours team about the situation and current drug regimen.

* *Assess medication*. Many medications for comorbid conditions can be reduced or stopped. Discuss with the relatives and patient the need to re-evaluate the drug regimen and that in most cases stopping medication will not hasten death. However, the psychological consequences of stopping medication need to be borne in mind (Stevenson, Abernethy, Miller, *et al.* 2004).

PROVISION OF PALLIATIVE CARE DRUGS OUT OF HOURS

● In the terminal stages, deterioration in the clinical condition may be rapid. The GP needs to think proactively about medication. Sufficient supplies of drugs to cover the out of hours period (possibly allowing for an increased dose) should be available. Drugs not previously used (e.g. hyoscine and midazolam) may be required, and it may be appropriate to leave these in the patient's home for administration by a visiting doctor.

● Despite difficulties with controlled drugs, there is a place for assembling palliative care bags which might include drugs, palliative care equipment (e.g. syringe driver, catheter, needles and gloves) and useful information on crisis management, palliative support telephone numbers, etc.

THE PALLIATIVE CARE BAG (THOMAS 2001)

Drugs to consider include:

Non-controlled drugs

Midazolam

Haloperidol

Cyclizine

Hyoscine hydrobromide or butylbromide

Glycopyrronium bromide

Levomepromazine

Rectal diazepam

Water for injection

Controlled drugs

Diamorphine

Local conditions will determine where these bags are kept

SYMPTOM CONTROL

Twycross R, Wilcock A, Charlesworth S, Dickman A. 2002. *Palliative Care Formulary*. Radcliffe Medical Press
Watson M, Lucas C, Hoy A, Back I. 2005. *Oxford Handbook of Palliative Care*. Oxford University Press

● Patients with cancer experience psychological as well as physical symptoms. Most patients will have more than one symptom (see Table 27.11). For details of the diagnosis of symptoms in palliative care see *Evidence-based Diagnosis in Primary Care* by A. F. Polmear (editor), published by Butterworth-Heinemann, 2008.

Prescribing outside a drug licence (Twycross, Wilcock, Charlesworth, *et al.* 2002). The prescriber may wish

Table 27.11	Common symptoms in cancer patients		
PHYSICAL	**%**	**PSYCHOLOGICAL**	**%**
Lack of energy	73	Worrying	72
Pain	63	Feeling sad	67
Drowsiness	60	Feeling nervous	62
Dry mouth	55	Difficulty sleeping	53
Nausea	45	Feeling irritable	47
Anorexia	45	Difficulty concentrating	40

to discuss use of a drug outside its licence with a specialist. When using a drug outside its licence, a doctor should:

(a) record in the patient's notes the reason for the decision to prescribe outside the licensed indications;

(b) where possible explain, in sufficient detail, the position to the patient (and family where appropriate), to allow them to give informed consent;

(c) inform other professionals (e.g. pharmacists) involved to avoid misunderstandings.

PAIN

GUIDELINE

National Council for Hospice and Specialist Palliative Care Services. 2003. *Guidelines for Managing Cancer Pain in Adults*. NCHSPCS, London

Aims of pain management

- Achieve a level of pain control that is acceptable to the patient.
- Assess pain and evaluate the effectiveness of management promptly.
- Be aware of the components of total pain.
- Relieve pain at night, at rest, and on movement.
- Provide patients and their carers with up-to-date information on using pain relieving drugs.
- Support and encourage carers.

- Most patients with cancer pain have more than one pain. The pains may be from different sources, and the pains from any one source may be of several different types, e.g. neuropathic or due to tissue damage (nociceptive). The treatment of each of these is different.

- Depression, anxiety, fear and anger all contribute to the perception of pain. The failure to deal with the patient's emotional state can lead to inappropriately high but ineffective doses of morphine.

- With effective assessment and a systematic approach to the choice of analgesics, over 80% of cancer pain can be controlled with the use of inexpensive drugs administered by mouth. For most of the 80%, the relief will be good, for a

minority it will only be moderate. Consideration must always be given to treating the underlying cause of the pain by means of surgery, radiotherapy, chemotherapy or other appropriate measures.

- Involving the patient in the assessment of pain, and in decisions about the treatment of pain, seems to lead to more satisfactory pain control.

* Fully assess the cause and type of each pain experienced by the patient. However, analgesia should not wait for investigations to be completed.

* Assess the severity of the pain, or rather, accept the patient's assessment of it. Repeat the assessment daily until the situation is stable. Professionals tend to underestimate pain, especially severe pain (Scottish Intercollegiate Guidelines Network and the Scottish Cancer Therapy Network 2000). Studies suggest that formal assessment of pain leads to improved management. Outcome measures are usually based on a verbal rating scale, a numerical rating scale or a visual analogue scale. Patients with advanced disease may have difficulty in completing scales, the most common reason for this being cognitive impairment. Some measures such as the Palliative Care Outcome Scale are designed to take this difficulty into account (Hearn and Higginson 1999). This is a verbal rating scale which considers not only the symptom but more importantly the impact the symptom is having upon the individual. It has been validated in inpatient, outpatient and community settings. There is a good correlation between patient, carer and staff ratings, which is important when considering a frail population who may not be able to complete the scale themselves.

VERBAL RATING SCALE

Ask: Over the past 3 days have you been affected by pain?

Score	Answer
0	Not at all;
1	Slightly – but not bothered by it;
2	Moderately – pain limits some activity;
3	Severely – activities or concentration markedly affected;
4	Overwhelmingly – unable to think of anything else.

* Assess the way that the patient's emotional and spiritual state is contributing to their perception of pain. Patients will often try to hide their feelings from their family, and even from their doctors. Ask specific questions, rather than relying on an unspoken assessment. For instance, asking 'do you feel low most of the time?' and 'do you feel tense, or restless or frightened most of the time?' will allow the patient to admit to depression and anxiety if they are present. A question like 'how has this illness affected the way you feel about yourself?' may allow the patient to talk about more spiritual issues.
* Explain the cause(s) of the pain and your treatment plan to the patient and family. Leave a written pain management plan with the patient, even if it just gives the patient instructions about how to use the medication for breakthrough pain (National Council for Palliative Care 2003).
* Enlist the help of anyone available to combat loneliness, boredom and despair.

PRINCIPLES OF ANALGESIC USE

* Use an effective drug in adequate doses and at regular intervals.
* Start at the step of the WHO ladder appropriate for the patient's pain. Do not hesitate to consult a palliative care consultant in cases of severe pain.
* Add a co-analgesic to the ladder at any step if necessary.

Route of administration

(a) Give drugs orally by choice; if this is not possible then;
(b) Give drugs rectally or transdermally; or
(c) Give drugs intramuscularly in the very short-term, but a subcutaneous syringe driver is preferable for anything longer than a few hours.

Choice of drug

* Use the WHO analgesic ladder:

Step 1: non-opioid analgesia, e.g. paracetamol ± a NSAID;

Step 2: Opioid for mild to moderate pain, e.g. codeine 30–60 mg or dihydrocodeine 30–60 mg ± paracetamol and an NSAID;

Step 3: Opioid for moderate to severe pain, e.g. morphine ± paracetamol and an NSAID.

* If a patient's pain is not controlled on a step move up the ladder. Do not change to another drug on the same step of the ladder.
* If the patient needs an NSAID but is at high risk of gastrointestinal ulceration, co-prescribe a proton pump inhibitor.

STRONG OPIOIDS

GUIDELINES

Expert Working Group of the European Association for Palliative Care. 1996. Morphine in cancer pain: modes of administration. BMJ 312, 823–826
    Working Group of the Ethical Issues in Medicine Committee of the Royal College of Physicians. 2000. *Principles of Pain Control in Palliative Care for Adults.* London: Royal College of Physicians. Available: www.rcplondon.ac.uk

Tolerance and addiction

* Both patients and professionals may have fears about the use of strong opioids. These should be discussed.
* Tolerance to opioids is rarely seen in managing cancer pain. A need for increasing doses is usually due to progression of the disease.
* Psychological dependence or addiction is not a problem except in patients with pre-existing addiction.
* *Titration of dose.* Titrate the dose required using a formulation with rapid onset and short duration. The dose may need to be changed daily until control is achieved (see oral morphine below).
* *Maintenance.* Once stabilized, change to a controlled-release drug.
* *Reduction of dose.* If a patient on large doses of morphine is given radiotherapy or a nerve block, watch for evidence that the pain is subsiding. If it does, reduce the dose by one third in the first instance, once it is clear that the intervention has succeeded. Deprived of pain the patient will become more sensitive to morphine, and may suffer symptoms of morphine toxicity, e.g. confusion,

hallucinations, myoclonus, nausea, sedation, and rarely respiratory depression.

Side-effects of opioids

✳ Warn patients of the side-effects of opioids and treat as necessary:

(a) *sedation:* this usually resolves within a few days;

(b) *nausea and vomiting:* an antiemetic, e.g. metoclopramide or haloperidol, should be prescribed routinely, to be taken as needed, when opioids are started or when their dose is increased. It can usually be stopped 5–10 days later;

(c) *constipation:* prescribe a laxative prophylactically. Use a stimulant and/or a softening agent;

(d) *dry mouth:* this is often the most troublesome symptom. Recommend simple measures, e.g. cool drinks, sucking sweets, etc.;

(e) *cerebral toxicity* (see below).

Oral morphine

● Morphine is the most commonly used strong opioid analgesic.

● Immediate-release preparations are better when more intensive titration of the dose is needed. They can be given as tablets or solution.

✳ Start at 5–10 mg 4-hourly, or higher if the pain was uncontrolled on high doses of weak opioids (for guidance on doses in the elderly or renal impaired patient see below). Note that:

(a) the dose needed may be 5–150 mg or more, 4-hourly;

(b) if pain returns before the next dose, increase the strength and *not* the frequency of doses. Make increases of 30–50% of the previous dose each time;

(c) *breakthrough pain:* authorize, for every patient on morphine, extra doses for breakthrough pain, with each extra dose equal to the patient's 4-hourly dose. The patient should wait 30 minutes and take a further dose if the response is insufficient. If breakthrough pain is frequent, increase the 24-hour dosage;

(d) *painful procedures:* if cover is needed for a painful procedure, use a drug that is rapid in onset and short acting, e.g. a fentanyl lozenge. This works in 15 minutes. Alternatively, if there is sufficient time, give an extra dose of morphine 30–60 minutes before, as for breakthrough pain;

(e) *other opioid analgesics:* buprenorphine can act as antagonist to morphine and is probably best avoided in a patient on morphine. Pethidine leads to the accumulation of the toxic metabolite norpethidine and should not be used.

Modified-release (MR) morphine is best for the patient with stable requirements; it gives steady blood levels and good compliance. Tablets should not be crushed. Where there is a difficulty in swallowing, liquid controlled-release formulations can be used.

(a) The dose needed may be from 20–400 mg daily.

(b) Preparations designed for 12-hourly and 24-hourly use are available. Calculate the total daily requirement and give as two doses 12 hours apart or one dose daily depending on the preparation.

(c) Continue to use normal release morphine for breakthrough pain.

Morphine in the elderly and those with renal impairment

✳ Contact the palliative care team for advice.

✳ Start at 2.5–5 mg 4-hourly.

✳ Morphine may be cleared more slowly than in the younger patient. Dosage intervals may be lengthened to 6 hours, and changes of dose should only be made after 3 days, since the drug may accumulate over that time before reaching a steady state.

✳ Do not use sustained release preparations unless renal function and doses are stable.

Patients unable to take oral drugs

Consider:

(a) *suppositories:* either morphine 15 mg 4-hourly or oxycodone 8-hourly (see below for equivalence);

(b) *diamorphine injection:* which is over 10 times more soluble than morphine. Give subcutaneous injections 4-hourly in the very short term; i.m. injections are more painful. In the longer term, use a syringe driver (see page 664);

(c) *transdermal drugs:* see page 666.

Opioid equivalents

Warning: Use Table 27.12 as a rough guide only. Equivalents vary from one individual to another as absorption varies.

If there is poor response to morphine

* Is the cause of the pain one which means that morphine is less likely to help (e.g. nerve pain)?
* Is the blood level of morphine correct? For instance: is the dose appropriate? is the drug being absorbed or is it being lost through vomiting, gastric stasis or diarrhoea?
* Are there psychological and spiritual factors that need attention?
* Consider:
  (a) hypercalcaemia;
  (b) bone/joint pain especially if the pain is movement related;
  (c) neuropathic pain;
  (d) skin pain;
  (e) gut pain.

If increasing the dose of morphine is effective but side-effects are intolerable

Intolerable side-effects include:

(a) agitation;
(b) seeing shadows in the periphery of the visual field;
(c) vivid dreams;

Table 27.12 Morphine equivalents

The following are approximately equivalent to oral morphine 15 mg:
Rectal morphine 15 mg
Oral diamorphine 10 mg
Parenteral diamorphine 5 mg
Parenteral oxycodone 5 mg
Oral oxycodone 10 mg
Rectal oxycodone 30 mg
Oral hydromorphone 2 mg
Oral codeine 200 mg
Oral dihydrocodeine 150 mg
Oral tramadol 75 mg

(d) visual and auditory hallucinations;
(e) confusion;
(f) myoclonic jerks.

Note: Agitated confusion may be interpreted as being due to pain and higher doses of opioids given.

* Consider:
  (a) reduction of the dose of opioids;
  (b) *opioid rotation.* Change to an alternative opioid with equivalent pain relief;
  (c) whether the patient is well hydrated;
  (d) using haloperidol for agitation.

It may be possible to increase the dose of opioid once symptoms have resolved.

Alternatives to morphine

If the patient has adverse effects with morphine consider:

■ Hydromorphone, which is about seven times stronger than morphine. Titrate with hydromorphone normal release capsules and then convert to controlled release capsules.
■ Oxycodone, which is up to one and a half times stronger than hydromorphone. Titrate as with hydromorphone.

If the patient is unable to take oral morphine and a syringe driver is not appropriate:

■ Fentanyl and buprenorphine transdermally see below. Buprenorphine may have advantages if renal function is impaired.

The patient seems to be in total pain

* Exclude and treat, if possible:
  (a) other physical symptoms, e.g. nausea or a sore mouth;
  (b) depression or extreme anxiety;
  (c) spiritual anxieties or family relationship difficulties.

Co-analgesics (or adjuvant drugs)

● Co-analgesics are most often used for neuropathic pain but they may help in pain of any type.

Tricyclic antidepressants, e.g. amitriptyline

1. Start at 25 mg at night (10 mg in the elderly).

2. Warn the patient that it will be several days before any benefit is felt; 50–90% of patients achieve at least 50% reduction in the severity of the pain (McQuay and Moore 1997). The NNT for antidepressants in neuropathic pain is 3 (Collins, Moore, McQuay, *et al.* 2000).

3. Warn the patient that side-effects may occur, especially dry mouth and drowsiness.

4. Increase the dose fortnightly until a good response is achieved. This is likely to be at 75 mg or below, although occasionally it is worth continuing up to 150 mg daily. The effective dose is likely to be lower than that required for depression.

5. Continue treatment for 2 months after the pain has stopped, then tail it off over a month.

Anticonvulsants

Gabapentin and pregabalin are the only anticonvulsants licensed for the treatment of all types of neuropathic pain. Pregabalin may have fewer side-effects than gabapentin. However, sodium valproate, carbamazepine and clonazepam have been in widespread use for many years.

1. Start with low doses, and increase until relief of symptoms is achieved or until blood levels are in the therapeutic range for epilepsy (see Appendix 16).

2. Continue this dose for 6 weeks before abandoning as ineffective.

3. If one drug fails it is not helpful to try another (McQuay, Carroll, Jadad, *et al.* 1995).

Non-pharmacological approaches

* Consider psychological techniques of which the best evidence lies with CBT. This may be available through the local pain clinic or via the palliative care team.

* Be prepared to support a patient who wishes to use alternative therapies: for instance acupuncture, transcutaneous electrical nerve stimulation (TENS), herbal medicine, homeopathy, relaxation therapy, music therapy, massage or hypnotherapy. There is no evidence of benefit for any of these over placebo in cancer pain; yet patients seem to benefit from them and, given the situation, even a placebo response is better than no response at all.

SPECIAL TYPES OF PAIN

BONE PAIN

* *Radiotherapy* is the most effective treatment for localized bony secondaries. It will take 2–3 weeks to work with about a third obtaining at least 50% pain relief with a median duration of pain relief of 12 weeks (McQuay, Carroll and Moore 1997). As the pain starts to ease, remember to reduce the dose of morphine as above.

* *NSAIDs* should be used in high doses, e.g. naproxen 500 mg t.d.s. orally or rectally.

* *Opioids* are often less effective than NSAIDs. Do not persevere if side-effects occur without benefit.

* *Nerve blocks* are helpful in the medium term if a nerve is accessible, e.g. intercostal block for rib pain or epidural block for vertebral pain.

* *Bisphosphonates.* Give orally or consider admission for the intravenous infusion of a bisphosphonate. There is no evidence as to which route is more effective and the maximum pain relief is likely by 4 weeks. The NNT is 6 (Wong and Wiffen 2005). See also page 280. In some situations a specialist will recommend prophylactic bisphosphonates (Ross, Saunders, Edmonds, *et al.* 2003). They can significantly decrease pathological fractures (vertebral and non-vertebral), hypercalcaemia and the need for radiotherapy. There is no effect on the incidence of spinal cord compression. They need to be given for 6 months for this effect to be demonstrated. The use of bisphosphonates has been shown to increase significantly the time to the first skeletal event but not to increase survival.

* *Drugs for neuropathic pain* (see adjuvant drugs page 662). There is evidence that this is a unique pain relating to destruction of nerve endings in the bone and hyperexcitability in the spinal cord (Urch 2004).

* *Radioactive strontium* should be considered in patients with widespread bony metastases.

* *Pathological fractures.* The pain may be greatly reduced by internal fixation followed by radiotherapy.

INCIDENT PAIN (PAIN ON MOVEMENT BUT ABSENT AT REST)

* Do not increase the 24-hour opioid dose. The increase in side-effects may outweigh the benefit. Consider giving breakthrough analgesia as above before the patient is moved.
* Fentanyl lozenges. Start at 200 mcg regardless of the opioid dose. Analgesia starts after 5–15 minutes and lasts up to 2 hours.
* Consider co-analgesics.
* *Physiotherapy*. Refer to improve muscle tone and rehabilitation.
* *Orthopaedic surgeon*. Refer for surgical stabilization of the affected area. Internal stabilization of long bones may produce considerable benefit, even in advanced disease.

NEUROPATHIC PAIN (PAIN DUE TO NERVE DAMAGE)

Examples are nerve injury, and compression or infiltration of nerve by tumour. Neuropathic pain may be improved but is often not completely relieved by non-opioid or opioid analgesics. Co-analgesics are often required.

* Co-analgesics. Start a tricyclic antidepressants as soon as the diagnosis of neuropathic pain is made. Add, or change to, an anticonvulsant if necessary (see co-analgesics, page 662).
* *Use conventional analgesics* in addition. A consensus is emerging that they can be of benefit in neuropathic pain (DTB 2000).
* *Pain clinic*. Consider referral to a pain clinic.
* *Consider steroids*, e.g. dexamethasone 8 mg daily, if inflammation is contributing to the nerve damage.
* Consider using non-drug methods, e.g. TENS, acupuncture, physiotherapy and occupational therapy. Some patients find them helpful despite the lack of good evidence to support their use, whether for pain, dyspnoea, nausea or vomiting at the end of life (Pan, Morrison, Ness, *et al.* 2000).

VISCERAL PAIN

Although initially managed by analgesics, invasive techniques should be considered at an early stage:

(a) *Epidural and intrathecal catheters* can deliver opioids and local anaesthetics direct to the spinal cord to give effective analgesia in lower limb and abdominal pain with few adverse effects.
(b) *Pancreatic carcinoma or other upper abdominal tumours*. Coeliac axis block may have a place early in the disease.
(c) *Pelvic tumours*. These may give rise to bladder and rectal tenesmus and severe perineal pain. Response to opioids is poor, although muscle relaxants and anticholinergics may have some value. Sacral nerve root block may prove effective.

SYRINGE DRIVERS (see Table 27.13)

* Indications include:
  (a) persistent nausea or vomiting;
  (b) difficulty swallowing;
  (c) intestinal obstruction;
  (d) comatose patient.
* *Timescale*. No individual infusion solution should be used for more than 24 hours (to minimize the risk of infection).
* Skin reactions:
  (a) Do not use chlorpromazine, prochlorperazine or diazepam;
  (b) Be cautious with cyclizine and levomepromazine; both can cause local irritation;
  (c) Add a small dose of dexamethasone (0.5 mg daily) to the solution if irritation is a problem and increase the dilution by using a larger volume syringe.
* *Combinations*. The following can be mixed with diamorphine: cyclizine, dexamethasone, haloperidol, hyoscine, levopromazine, midazolam and metoclopramide, but see Appendix 31 for details.

CONVERTING FROM A FENTANYL PATCH TO DIAMORPHINE VIA A SYRINGE DRIVER

(a) Remove the patch and give half the hourly dose of the patch in mg of diamorphine over the first 24 hours. Then double the dose. For example, if changing from fentanyl patch 200 mcg/hour, give diamorphine 100 mg/24 hours for the first 24 hours then 200 mg/24 hours thereafter. Warn

Table 27.13   Drugs commonly used in a syringe driver indications and doses.

SYMPTOM	24-HOUR DOSE
	Nausea and vomiting
Haloperidol	2.5–10 mg
Levopromazine	5–25 mg (less sedating and may be effective)
	25–200 mg (sedation in 50% of patients)
Cyclizine	150 mg (see Appendix 27 re: mixing ability with diamorphine)
Metoclopramide	30–100 mg (may cause skin reactions)
Octreotide	300–600 mg
	Excessive respiratory secretions/colic (bowel)
Hyoscine hydrobromide	0.6–2.4 mg (occasionally causes agitation)
Hyoscine butylbromide	20–60 mg
Glycopyrronium	0.6–1.2 mg
	Restlessness/Confusion
Haloperidol	5–15 mg
Levopromazine	50–200 mg
Midazolam	20–100 mg (sedative and anticonvulsant)
	Convulsions
	Continue with antiepiletic if already being taken and can be taken orally
Midazolam	20–40 mg
	Pain
Diamorphine	For dose, see text. The strength may go up to 250 mg/ml. In doses of up to 40 mg/ml, either water or physiological saline can be used as a diluent. Above 40 mg/ml, only water can be used. If the dose needs to be increased, increase it by 30–50% in a fresh syringe for a new 24-hour period
Oxycodone	Half the total daily dose of oral oxycodone or numerically same total dose as parenteral diamorphine
	Raised intracranial pressure
Dexamethasone	4–16 mg in a separate syringe driver over 6–8 hours. If given over 24 hours restlessness is increased

the patient that they may feel drowsy for 24 hours. Alternatively:

(b) Keep the patch on and give twice the breakthrough pain dose over 24 hours. This is most suitable if the patient is moribund but in pain. (e.g. fentanyl 100 mcg/hour ≡ breakthrough dose of 20 mg diamorphine, therefore give 40 mg diamorphine over 24 hours).

Breakthrough pain

● *Patients on diamorphine.* Give a subcutaneous bolus injection roughly one sixth of the total daily dose of diamorphine (e.g. if giving 300 mg diamorphine/24 hours, give 50 mg diamorphine s.c. or 150 mg orally).

● *Patients on oral morphine.* Give a dose roughly one sixth of the total daily dose (e.g. total daily dose 180 mg give 30 mg oral morphine or 10 mg diamorphine s.c.).

● *Patients on fentanyl patches.*

(a) *Diamorphine.* Divide the patch strength by five and give as mg of diamorphine (fentanyl patch 100 mcg/hour: give 20 mg diamorphine).

(b) *Oral morphine.* Divide the patch strength by two and give as mg of morphine (e.g. fentanyl 100 mcg/hour give 50 mg morphine orally).

(c) *Other opioids.* Calculate the oral morphine breakthrough dose and then convert (e.g. fentanyl 200 mcg/hour ≡ 100 mg oral morphine ≡ 50 mg oral oxycodone).

TRANSDERMAL ANALGESIA

Moving from oral drugs to a patch or to a syringe driver is never simple. Inexperienced GPs would do well to take specialist advice.

FENTANYL

Fentanyl patches should only be used for patients whose pain is stable, because of the time taken to titrate the dose. When the patch is first applied it will take 12–18 hours before maximal analgesia is seen. The dose of the patch should not be increased until it is due to be changed, but an immediate release opioid should always be prescribed for breakthrough pain. Also once a patch is removed there will continue to be some absorption of fentanyl from the skin for a further 12–18 hours.

(a) If on 4 hourly morphine apply the patch and continue the 4 hourly morphine for 12 hours.

(b) If on 12 hourly morphine apply the patch at the same time as the last dose of morphine.

(c) If on 24 hourly morphine apply the patch 12 hours after the last dose.

Note that fentanyl is less constipating than morphine and the laxative dose should be halved.

BUPRENORPHINE

■ Buprenorphine patch 35 mcg/hour ≡ dihydrocodeine 120–240 mg, or morphine 30–60 mg per 24 hours.

■ Buprenorphine patch 52.5 mcg/hour ≡ dihydrocodeine 360 mg, morphine 90 mg per 24 hours.

■ Buprenorphine patch 70 mcg/hour ≡ dihydrocodeine 400 mg, morphine 120 mg per 24 hours.

The dose should not be adjusted for 24 hours. If necessary give 200–400 mcg sublingually for breakthrough pain. It takes about 30 hours for the plasma level to be reduced by half on removing the patch.

NAUSEA AND VOMITING

> **GUIDELINE**
>
> Clinical Knowledge Summaries. 2009. *Palliative Care: Nausea and Vomiting*. Available: http://cks.library.nhs.uk/palliative_cancer_care_nausea_vomiting

Nausea has a prevalence of 20–30% in all patients with advanced cancer, rising to 70% in the last week of life. Differentiation of the likely cause is vital so that reversible factors may be addressed and the right type of antiemetic chosen, see Table 27.14.

1. *Evaluation of the patient*

   ✳ Consider particularly:

   (a) the timing of symptoms (with smell of food or after large meal). If worse in the early morning consider raised intracranial pressure;

   (b) the type of vomiting (regurgitation, or vomiting);

   (c) the content of the vomit (faeculent, bile stained, undigested food, etc.);

   (d) the drug regimen. Several drugs may be implicated by a variety of mechanisms including:

   ■ GI irritation (e.g. NSAIDs, antibiotics);

   ■ gastric stasis (e.g. opioids, tricyclics, phenothiazines);

   ■ chemoreceptor trigger zone stimulation (e.g. opioids, digoxin, antibiotics, cytotoxics);

   ■ 5-HT$_3$ receptor stimulation (e.g. cytotoxics, SSRIs).

Table 27.14 First line antiemetics			
CLINICAL PROBLEM	**DRUG**	**ORAL DOSE**	**DOSES BY OTHER ROUTES**
Gastritis, or gastric stasis. Chemotherapy	Metoclopramide	10–20 mg q.d.s.	s.c.: 40–100 mg/24 hours
Functional bowel obstruction	Domperidone	20 mg b.d. to 30 mg t.d.s.	rectally: 60 mg b.d.
'Toxic' causes, e.g. radiotherapy, hypercalcaemia, morphine	Haloperidol	1–2 mg nocte or b.d.	s.c.: 5 mg/24 hours
Mechanical bowel obstruction, raised intracranial pressure, motion sickness	Cyclizine	50 mg t.d.s.	rectally: 100 mg t.d.s. s.c.: 150 mg/24 hours

* *Cerebral metastases.* Check the fundi for papilloedema and refer if there is any suspicion of raised intracranial pressure. Radiotherapy can improve symptoms in 80% but itself can induce nausea.
* Examine the mouth, pharynx and abdomen and the degree of hydration.
* Check U&Es, and serum calcium.

2. *Correct any reversible causes:*
   (a) *hypercalcaemia:* rehydrate and give a bisphosphate. Bisphosphonates normalize calcium in about 70% of patients with minimal side-effects (Saunders, Ross, Broadley, *et al.* 2004);
   (b) *infection:* consider antibiotics;
   (c) *raised intracranial pressure:* give dexamethasone;
   (d) *gastric irritation/ulceration:* stop NSAIDs, give a proton pump inhibitor;
   (e) *constipation:* treat with laxatives;
   (f) *anxiety:* empathize and give explanation and reassurance.

3. *Non-drug measures* might include:
   (a) control of malodorous discharge from fungating tumour;
   (b) calm environment away from food;
   (c) avoidance of exposure to foods causing nausea;
   (d) small meals;
   (e) acupuncture/acupressure over the P6 point at the wrist.

4. *Drug treatment*

There is no universal antiemetic. Instead the choice of drug depends upon the postulated cause of the problem. In practice, the initial decision is a choice between three first line antiemetics depending upon the clinical problem (Table 27.14).

Remember that:

(a) The final common pathway for the action of prokinetic drugs is cholinergic. Anticholinergic drugs (including cyclizine) block their action.
(b) If more than one antiemetic is required, choose a combination with complementary actions and effects (e.g. cyclizine and haloperidol). Drugs such as levomepromazine have an action at multiple receptors and may replace drug combinations.

(c) Vomiting may prevent adequate treatment of other symptoms, e.g. pain. If the patient is vomiting or nauseated for most of the time then the drug should be given by a non-oral route (e.g. continuous s.c. infusion or sometimes rectally).

If there is still inadequate symptom control, other drugs may need to be considered:

(a) *Dexamethasone* is most often used in combination with other antiemetics. Dose: 4–8 mg daily (orally or s.c.).
(b) *Levomepromazine* is the most broad-spectrum antiemetic available. It may be sedating, particularly in higher doses and causes postural hypotension in the elderly. Dose: 6.25–12.5 mg stat (orally or s.c.) then 12.5–50 mg over 24 hours. If preferred, the dose may be given once daily at bedtime.
(c) *5-HT$_3$ antagonists* (ondansetron, granisetron and tropisetron). They have similar efficacy and tolerability and few side-effects apart from severe constipation. They are rarely indicated in the palliative care setting.
(d) *Benzodiazepines* may be particularly useful in anticipatory vomiting. Lorazepam is useful as it is available in a 1 mg sublingual tablet obviating the need for swallowing.
(e) *Other phenothiazines.* Prochlorperazine may be given buccally but not subcutaneously. There is a risk of dystonic reactions particularly in adolescents and those with AIDS. Chlorpromazine has a wide spectrum of receptor affinity but does not share the potent 5-HT$_2$ antagonistic properties of levomepromazine.
(f) *Domperidone* does not cross the blood–brain barrier so has fewer central effects than metoclopramide. Give 10–20 mg t.d.s. orally (maximum 80 mg daily), or 30 mg b.d. rectally.

Whichever drug regimen is chosen, if a subcutaneous infusion is used, consider changing to an oral regime once good control has been achieved and maintained for 72 hours. Continue antiemetics indefinitely unless the cause resolves.

IN MALIGNANT BOWEL OBSTRUCTION

* *Surgery.* Never exclude referral for palliative surgery as an option in patients with advanced cancer who develop obstruction.

∗ *Nasogastric suction* should only be used in those being considered for surgery and those with high obstruction who respond poorly to drug treatment. The latter may benefit from a venting gastrostomy.

∗ Stop osmotic and stimulant laxatives.

∗ *Prokinetic anti-emetics* should be used with care if bowel obstruction is suspected as they may increase gut colic. However, if the patient does not have colic and is passing flatus, start a prokinetic emetic (e.g. metoclopramide 30–60 mg/24 hours via syringe driver) and discuss with the specialist the use of dexamethasone 8–16 mg via a syringe driver over 6–8 hours (Feuer and Broadley 1999).

∗ *For patients with colic*: hyoscine butylbromide 60–120 mg or glycopyrronium 0.4–2.4 mg as an antisecretory agent and antispasmodic, levomepromazine 6.25–50 mg/24 hours as an antiemetic, both given via a syringe driver.

OTHER SYMPTOMS

ANOREXIA AND WEAKNESS

∗ Exclude reversible causes, e.g. a drug effect or depression. Ensure that pain is controlled.

∗ Good mouth care is essential. Ill fitting dentures, secondary to weight loss, can often be relined and improved.

∗ Consider metoclopramide if the patient feels full after eating only a small amount.

∗ Consider appetite stimulants, e.g. dexamethasone 2–4 mg daily (if the prognosis is felt to be short) or a progestogen such as megestrol 320–480 mg daily or medroxyprogesterone acetate 40–800 mg daily if the prognosis is longer.

CONSTIPATION

Clinical Knowledge Summaries. 2009. *Palliative Care: Constipation*. Available: http://cks.library.nhs.uk/palliative_cancer_care_constipation

Constipation can lead to abdominal pain and increased use of constipating analgesics. Overflow diarrhoea, urinary retention or 'overflow' incontinence may occur.

∗ *Prevention*. Use stimulant and softening laxatives in combination especially when prescribing includes opioids. Possible combinations are:
  (a) three senna tabs plus 15 ml of lactulose;
  (b) three senna tabs plus 300 mg docusate;
  (c) co-danthramer capsules or 30 ml of syrup;
  (d) four co-danthramer strong capsules or 10 ml of strong syrup;
  (e) three co-danthrusate capsules.

∗ Avoid bulking agents, which are especially ineffective in constipation due to opioids.

∗ Be prepared to give high doses of laxatives to patients on high doses of opioids, e.g. senna 10 tablets at night or bisacodyl four tablets at night, or co-danthrusate three capsules q.d.s. but be aware of the tablet burden and consider adding macrogol before increasing the dose. Effective doses may be outside the licence.

∗ High faecal impaction may be treated with an oral regime of macrogol 3350, eight sachets in 1 litre of water drunk over 6 hours daily for up to 3 days.

∗ Low faecal impaction (stool in the rectum). Consider:
  (a) suppositories: bisacodyl for soft stools, glycerol or glycerol plus bisacodyl for hard stools;
  (b) micro-enema's e.g. docusate or sodium citrate.

∗ 'Poor response'. Consider sodium phosphate enema or an arachis oil retention enema placed high in the rectum if the rectum is empty. The latter can be left overnight and a sodium phosphate or sodium citrate enema given the next day.

DIARRHOEA

∗ Exclude impaction with faecal overflow. These patients require rectal laxatives with a stool softener. Stimulant laxatives may cause colic.

∗ Check that the patient is not taking a high dose of laxative intermittently.

∗ Use loperamide 2–16 mg/day, or codeine 10–60 mg every 4 hours.

* *Malabsorption due to pancreatic carcinoma* – use pancreatic enzyme supplements with an H_2-receptor antagonist or proton pump inhibitor.
* *Radiotherapy-induced or chologenic diarrhoea* – use colestyramine 12–24 g/day.

PSYCHIATRIC REACTIONS

At around the time of diagnosis and with advanced disease 50% of patients with cancer experience levels of anxiety and depression severe enough to adversely affect the quality of life.

Depression

Patients with malignant disease suffering from major depression respond as well to antidepressants as those with no physical illness.

* Check that poorly treated symptoms are not contributing to the depression. Look for specific problems, e.g. low sodium, which may be causing depression.
* Check that the issues covered on page 656 have been addressed.
* Treat with an antidepressant.

Anxiety

* *Physical causes.* Look for a physical cause, e.g. pain, pulmonary embolism, internal haemorrhage, drug or alcohol withdrawal.
* Treat with:
  (a) a benzodiazepine; or
  (b) haloperidol, which may be of particular value if the patient is confused; or
  (c) a tricyclic antidepressant for chronic low-grade anxiety.
* *Severe acute anxiety* is more likely to be secondary to a physical cause, and may need lorazepam 1–3 mg orally or midazolam 5–10 mg s.c.

Agitated confusion

Centeno C, Sanz A, Bruera E. 2004. Delirium in advanced cancer patients. Palliative Medicine 18, 184–194

Delirium, with the exception of terminal delirium, is reversible in 50% of cases. It is profoundly upsetting for family and friends to observe and they require full support and explanation.

* Consider causes that need treatment in their own right: infection, constipation, retention of urine, poorly treated physical symptoms, oversedation, hypercalcaemia, hypoglycaemia, hyponatraemia, hypernatraemia or cerebral oedema.
* Review all drugs that could be contributing to the delirium especially opioids. Consider changing to another opioid with equivalent pain relief.
* Use:
  (a) *haloperidol* 1.5–10 mg orally once a day. This is non-sedating and remains the gold standard. The extrapyramidal side-effects may be lower if administered parenterally (Vella-Brincat and Macleod 2004);
  (b) *levomepromazine* 25–50 mg orally or 12.5–25 mg i.m., 4-hourly, in very agitated patients;
  (c) *midazolam*. It has a short half life and rapid onset of action and can be given to achieve control while investigations are proceeding; dose 20–50 mg per 24 hours via syringe driver or 2.5–5 mg s.c. every 6–8 hours; or
  (d) *diazepam*, orally or rectally. Beware that benzodiazepines may aggravate rather than alleviate delirium.
     If the above are not effective involve the specialist, unless this has already been done. Other options are:
  (e) *risperidone* in low doses (0.5–1 mg every 12 hours) especially in brain tumour-induced behavioural disorders, in other organic brain syndromes and in the elderly.
  (f) *olanzapine*. It is more sedative than risperidone, has few pharmacological interactions and can be given at night-time; dose 5–12 mg/day.
* If the confusion is primarily nocturnal, use a single night-time dose.
* Consider withdrawing the sedative after a few days if the cause was treatable, e.g. dehydration or infection.
* *Long-term heavy sedation.* Give haloperidol 10–30 mg with midazolam 30–60 mg over 24 hours, by syringe driver.

* *Complicated delirium in the terminal days* may need the addition of phenobarbital (200–600 mg daily) via a separate syringe driver.

RESPIRATORY SYMPTOMS

Clinical Knowledge Summaries. 2009. *Palliative Care: Cough and Dyspnoea.* Accessed online. http://cks. library.nhs.uk/palliative_cancer_care_cough
http://cks.library.nhs.uk/palliative_cancer_care-dyspnoea

Cough

Cough has a prevalence of 33% in all types of cancer. It may have malignant or non-malignant causes. It is a exhausting symptoms which, if controlled, will benefit the patient and carers.

* *Infection.* Treat infection if present.
* *Simple measures* such as nebulized saline are often comforting.
* *Cough suppressants.* Give pholcodine linctus 10 ml 4-hourly. If the patient is already on a strong opioid, increase the dose of that instead. Severe cough may justify the use of diamorphine for that indication alone. Methadone is traditional, but has an excessively long half-life. It can be of value at night, but there is a risk of accumulation.
* *Antimuscarinics.* These can be used to reduce salivary secretions. Give hyoscine hydrobromide 0.2–0.4 mg s.c. stat. or 1.2–2.4 mg sc over 24 hours.

Breathlessness

Dyspnoea has a prevalence of 50% in people with any type of cancer and the prevalence increases as the point of death approaches.

* Consider investigation if appropriate, e.g. as a minimum a full blood count and chest X-ray.
* Treat an underlying cause where appropriate (e.g. pleural effusion, SVC obstruction).
* *Simple non-pharmacological measures* such as sitting the patient upright and arranging cool airflow across the patient's face (e.g. with a fan

or opening a window). Oxygen may be appropriate.
* Refer to a breathlessness clinic or for relaxation therapy, if available. Breathless clinics have been shown to produce highly significant improvements in patient's breathlessness, functional capacity, activity levels and stress levels (Corner, Plant, A'Hern, *et al.* 1996; Bredin, Corner, Krishnasamy, *et al.* 1999).
* Give a *benzodiazepine* as an anxiolytic, e.g. lorazepam 0.5–2 mg sublingually (outside license) to achieve rapid control, followed by oral diazepam 5–10 mg daily or midazolam; or
* Give an opioid (e.g. morphine 2.5 mg 4-hourly). If the patient is already taking an opioid, increase the dose by 30% every 2–3 days until symptoms are controlled.
* Corticosteroids may be considered although no studies support their use. They should be discontinued if there is no benefit.

Other respiratory symptoms

* *Hiccup:*
  (a) reduce gastric distension with metoclopramide or domperidone;
  (b) relax smooth muscle with nifedipine sublingually stat and then 5 mg t.d.s.;
  (c) suppress the central hiccup reflex with baclofen;
  (d) as a last resort use chlorpromazine 25–50 mg orally or i.m. q.d.s.
* *Death rattle.* Reposition the patient on one side. Give hyoscine hydrobromide 200–600 mcg 4–6-hourly s.c., or hyoscine butylbromide 20–80 mg per 24 hours via a syringe driver or glycopyrronium bromide 200 mcg s.c. stat. Start treatment early, i.e. at the first signs of moist breathing.
* *Haemoptysis:*
  (a) Consider referral for radiotherapy for bronchial tumours;
  (b) Consider tranexamic acid (1 g t.d.s.) to reduce bleeding;
  (c) Plan a course of action in case massive haemoptysis occurs. Emergency admission might be appropriate for the patient who is not otherwise terminal. Otherwise, lie the patient on the side of the tumour and give intravenous diamorphine and benzodiazepine (for dyspnoea and anxiety).

* *Stridor* from obstruction of the larynx or airway. Give high-dose dexamethasone (16 mg daily).
* *Pleural or chest wall pain.* Consider the need for radiotherapy or intercostal nerve block. Prescribe an NSAID unless already taken.
* *Severe breathlessness and a sensation of drowning* may be due to superior vena caval obstruction.
  (a) Give high-dose oral steroids (stop after 5 days if not effective).
  (b) Admit for radiotherapy if appropriate.
  (c) Use low-dose morphine to relieve dyspnoea.
  (d) Consider benzodiazepines.

SPINAL CORD COMPRESSION

● Spinal cord compression may present as severe unremitting back pain, nerve root irritation, weakness of the legs, urinary hesitancy and constipation.
● Maintain a high level of clinical suspicion in patients with known vertebral metastases or patients with cancer of the prostate or breast.
● Loss of sphincter control is a poor prognostic indicator for recovery of function.
* Commence dexamethasone 16 mg/day.
* Refer urgently for MRI, with a view to radiotherapy or laminectomy, if the patient's condition warrants it. If treatment is commenced within 24–48 hours of the onset of symptoms, neurological damage may be reversible.

ITCH

* *Dry skin.* Use any moisturising agent, e.g. emulsifying ointment. Apply it copiously and often. A sedative antihistamine may help, e.g. hydroxyzine.
* Check ferritin levels and a full blood count. Iron deficiency even without anaemia should be treated.
* Check serum creatinine and eGFR. Renal failure may contribute. Odansetron and mirtazepine may be of value.
* *Paroxetine.* Consider prescribing paroxetine in patients with advanced cancer (Zylicz, Smits and Krajnik 1998) although it is unlicensed for this use.

* *Obstructive jaundice.* Use stanozolol 5 mg daily. Colestyramine is less helpful and harder to take.

INSOMNIA

* Use:
  (a) a short- to medium-acting benzodiazepine or similar (e.g. zolpidem, zopiclone or zaleplon); or
  (b) amitriptyline 25–50 mg at night, which may help pain as well; or
  (c) a neuroleptic, e.g. levomepromazine. It will help concurrent agitation or nausea.

MOUTH AND THROAT PROBLEMS

Clinical Knowledge Summaries. 2009. *Palliative Cancer Care: Oral.* Available: http://cks.library.nhs.uk/palliative_cancer_care_oral

Dry mouth was reported in 90% of patients with advanced cancer. Oral problems are common and often predictable following chemotherapy and head and neck radiotherapy. Routine mouth care reduces the risk of problems developing. Drugs are a common cause of dry mouth.

* *Dysphagia.* If there is also oral candida, assume that dysphagia is due to oesophageal candida and use fluconazole 50 mg daily for 7 days. Also consider obstructive tumour or neuromuscular causes.
* *Aphthous ulcers.* See page 542.
* *Dryness.* Assess whether the patient is dehydrated and correct if possible. Use crushed ice, semifrozen juices or tonic water, pineapple chunks or artificial saliva, e.g. Glandosane spray. Use petroleum jelly for cracked lips, but avoid lemon glycerine combinations that increase the dryness overall.
* *Pain/soreness.* Use:
  (a) local anaesthetic, e.g. benzydamine oral rinse or local anaesthetic lozenges or spray;
  (b) coating agents, e.g. sucralfate suspension as a mouthwash, carmellose paste or carbenoxolone mouthwash.
* *Dirty mouth.* Encourage:
  (a) regular brushing with a soft toothbrush;
  (b) mouthwashes to remove debris;

(c) chewing unsweetened pineapple chunks (fresh or tinned) if the tongue is coated. The proteolytic enzyme annanase will clear the tongue in days.

* *Foul smell.* Use oral metronidazole 400 mg b.d. or rectal 500 mg b.d.

CACHEXIA/ANOREXIA/ASTHENIA

The combination of anorexia, muscle wasting and weakness and severe physical and mental fatigue is common in palliative care.

* Exclude possibly treatable contributing causes, e.g. dyspepsia, oral thrush, anxiety/depression, constipation and pain.
* Check serum electrolytes and calcium levels.
* Reassure the patient that it is common to feel full with smaller quantities of food. Suggest to the relatives that any small amounts of food the patient enjoys are offered more frequently.
* Discuss with the patient and relatives the role of enteral food supplements.
* Consider enlisting the help of a dietician.
* *Drug treatment.* Discuss with the palliative care team and consider:
  (a) corticosteroids, e.g. dexamethasone 2–4 mg/ day. This may stimulate appetite and reduce nausea as well as having a general euphoric effect. However, the effects wear off after a few weeks and side-effects are common.
  (b) progestogens, e.g. megestrol acetate 80–160 mg/day. This is expensive but improves appetite and nutritional status after a few weeks. The effect is maintained for months.
  (c) prokinetic drugs, e.g. metoclopramide 10 mg q.d.s., particularly if there is gastric stasis.

RAISED INTRACRANIAL PRESSURE

* Dexamethasone 16 mg/day for 5 days, reducing to 4 mg/day over 2 weeks. Avoid an evening dose, which can cause insomnia. Monitor closely as symptoms may recur on reduction of dose, especially if the underlying tumour has not been treated or has responded to treatment.
* *Nausea.* Cyclizine is the antiemetic of choice.

MUSCLE SPASM

* Use:
  (a) dantrolene 25 mg/day increasing to a maximum of 400 mg/day;
  (b) baclofen 5 mg t.d.s. increasing to a maximum of 100 mg/day; or
  (c) diazepam 2–10 mg t.d.s.

BLADDER SPASM

* Treat any infection.
* Give:
  (a) oxybutynin 5 mg b.d./t.d.s.; or
  (b) amitriptyline 25 mg at night increasing to 75 mg;
  (c) *catheter in situ.* The specialist service may have access to bupivacaine bladder washouts.

MALIGNANT ULCER

* *If smelly:*
  (a) give metronidazole topically or orally. Topical gel is much more expensive than tablets, and is only indicated in those who cannot tolerate the latter (DTB 1992);
  (b) refer to the community nursing team.
* *If bleeding:*
  (a) *acute.* Pack with gauze soaked in adrenaline 1 in 1000;
  (b) *long term.* Consider referral for radiotherapy. Apply topically:
    ■ sucralfate suspension (tightly applied on a non-adherent dressing); or
    ■ tranexamic acid (use the injection solution on a non-adherent dressing).
* *If dirty:* consider debridement with a polysaccharide, hydrocolloid or hydrogel dressing.
* *Excessive discharge.* Use dressings with high absorbency, e.g. calcium alginate. A watery discharge may respond to high-dose topical steroids once daily for a week.

LYMPHOEDEMA

* *Active or passive movements of the limb* should be performed regularly, i.e. 2-hourly in the daytime.

* *Skin dryness.* Maintain skin hydration with a moisturizer.
* *Breaks in the skin.* Protect them from infection with antiseptic cream.
* *Cellulitis.* Treat with elevation and antibiotics. Use penicillin; infection is usually due to streptococcus. A patient with repeated infections should have a supply of penicillin at home. Antibiotics may need to be continued for several months.

Reducing lymphoedema

* Consider:
  (a) *Massage.* This can be done by the patient or carer, or by an electrical massager, for about 20 minutes twice a day. It is contraindicated if the skin is damaged, for instance by tumour or infection. Massage is done from areas of congestion to areas of normal drainage; or from the area of normal drainage to the areas of obstruction. The latter approach is attempting to open up the lymphatic channels.
  (b) *Support* should be from high-compression, low-stretch materials. A single layer is usually adequate. Do not apply compression to the lower limb if the ankle brachial pressure index is < 0.8 (see page 437).
  (c) Gentle exercises performed regularly.
  (d) Compression pumps and low compression bandaging may be required for long-standing lymphoedema.
* Contact the palliative care team or lymphoedema nurse.

SELF-HELP GROUP

Lymphoedema Support Network, St Luke's Crypt, Sydney Street, London SW3 6NH, tel. 0207 351 4480; www.lymphoedema.org

LIVING WILL (ADVANCE DIRECTIVE) (see page 22)

Patients may wish to state their wishes about medical treatment should they develop:

(a) a life-threatening condition; or
(b) permanent mental impairment; or
(c) permanent unconsciousness.

DO NOT ATTEMPT RESUSCITATION POLICY (DNAR)

Every area has its own DNAR policy based on *'Decisions Relating to Cardiopulmonary Resuscitation. A Joint Statement from the British Medical Association, Resuscitation Council (UK) and the Royal College of Nursing. 2007'.*

* Discuss with the patient and relatives their feelings about cardiopulmonary resuscitation (CPR) before they reach an advanced stage.
* Advise the patient or relative to view the section on the cancer bacup site on CPR. www.cancerbacup.org.uk/Resourcessupport/Advancedcancer/CPRforpeoplewithcancer
* Contact the 'out of hours 'service, ambulance service and district nurses and fax a copy to all parties.

WITHHOLDING AND WITHDRAWING LIFE-PROLONGING TREATMENTS

The General Medical Council of the UK has issued guidance on this issue, available on www.gmc-uk.org. The guidance states the principle that, while doctors must show respect for human life, they should avoid treatments where prolonging life would provide no net benefit to the patient. The guidance discusses the issues of who is competent to make the decision to withhold or stop treatment. It strongly makes the point that, in a situation of doubt, treatment may reasonably be started and then, when it has become clear that it is of no net benefit to the patient, stopped. Despite the fact that some professionals, and patients and their families, find stopping treatment more difficult than not starting it, the moral issue is the same in both situations.

References

American Joint Commission on Cancer and International Union Against Cancer: http://imaginis.com/breasthealth/staging.asp. Accessed January 2010.

Bredin, M., Corner, J., Krishnasamy, M., et al., 1999. Multicentre randomised controlled trial of nursing intervention for breathlessness in patients with lung cancer. BMJ 318, 888–889.

Collins, S.L., Moore, R.A., McQuay, H.J., et al., 2000. Antidepressants and anticonvulsants for diabetic neuropathy and post herpetic neuralgia: a quantitative systematic review. J. Pain Symptom Manage. 20, 449–458.

Corner, J., Plant, H., A'Hern, R., et al., 1996. Non-pharmacological intervention for breathlessness in lung cancer. Palliat. Med. 299, 305–308.

DTB, 1992. Metronidazole gel for smelly tumours. Drug Ther. Bull. 30, 18–19.

DTB, 2000. Drug treatment of neuropathic pain. Drug Ther. Bull. 38 (Dec), 89–93.

Fallowfield, L., 1995. Psychosocial interventions in cancer. BMJ 311, 1316–1317.

Feuer, D.J., Broadley, K.E., 1999. Corticosteroids for the resolution of malignant bowel obstruction in advanced gynaecological and gastrointestinal cancer. Cochrane Database Syst. Rev. (3).

Gatrad, A.R., Brown, E., Notta, H., et al., 2003. Palliative care needs of minorities. BMJ 327, 176–177.

Hearn, J., Higginson, I.J., 1999. Development and validation of a core outcome measure for palliative care: the palliative care outcome scale. Qual. Health Care 8, 219–227.

Hill, D., Penso, D., 1995. Opening Doors: Improving Access to Specialist and Palliative Care Services by Members of the Black and Minority Ethnic Communities. National Council for Hospice and Specialist Care Services, London.

Kirk, P., Kirk, I., Kristjanson, L.J., 2004. What do patients receiving palliative care for cancer and their families want to be told? A Canadian and Australian qualitative study. BMJ 328, 1343–1350.

Leonard, R.C., Rodger, A., Dixon, J.M., 1994. ABC of breast diseases. Metastatic breast cancer. BMJ 309, 1501–1504.

Macdonald, C.E., Wicks, A.C., Playford, R.J., 2000. Final results from 10 year cohort of patients undergoing surveillance for Barrett's oesophagus: observational study. BMJ 321, 1252–1255.

Maryland, M.C., Bennett, M.I., Keith, A., 2005. Vitamin C deficiency in cancer patients. Palliat. Med. 19, 17–20.

McQuay, H., Carroll, D., Jadad, A.R., et al., 1995. Anticonvulsant drugs for the management of pain: a systematic review. BMJ 311, 1047–1052.

McQuay, H.J., Carroll, D., Moore, R.A., 1997. Radiotherapy for painful bone metastases: a systematic review. Clin. Oncol. 9, 150–154.

McQuay, H.J., Moore, R.A., 1997. Antidepressants and chronic pain. BMJ 314, 763–764.

National Council for Palliative Care, 2003. Guidelines for managing cancer pain in adults, 3rd ed. Available: www.ncpc.org.uk (choose 'Publications' then 'Clinical guidelines and research').

Pan, C.X., Morrison, R.S., Ness, J., et al., 2000. Complementary and alternative medicine in the management of pain, dyspnoea, and nausea and vomiting near the end of life: a systematic review. J. Pain Symptom Manage. 20, 374–387.

Ross, J.R., Saunders, Y., Edmonds, P.M., et al., 2003. Systematic review of role of bisphosphonates on skeletal morbidity in metastatic cancer. BMJ 327, 469–484.

Sainsbury, R., Haward, B., Rider, L., et al., 1995. Influence of clinician workload and patterns of treatment on survival from breast cancer. Lancet 345, 1265–1270.

Saunders, Y., Ross, J.R., Broadley, K.E., et al., 2004. Systematic review of bisphosphonates for hypercalcaemia of malignancy. Palliat. Care 18, 418–430.

Scottish Intercollegiate Guidelines Network and the Scottish Cancer Therapy Network, 2000. Control of pain in patients with cancer: SIGN. Available: www.sign.ac.uk.

Stevenson, J., Abernethy, A.P., Miller, C., et al., 2004. Managing comorbidities in patients at the end of life. BMJ 329, 909–912.

Thomas, K., 2001. Macmillan Cancer Relief Report: Out of Hours Palliative Care in the Community. March.

Thorpe, G., 1993. Enabling more dying people to remain at home. BMJ 307, 915–918.

Twycross, R., Wilcock, A., Charlesworth, S., et al., 2002. Palliative Care Formulary. Radcliffe Medical Press.

Urch, C., 2004. The pathophysiology of cancer-induced bone pain: current understanding. Palliat. Care 18, 267–274.

Vella-Brincat, J., Macleod, A.D., 2004. Haloperidol in palliative care. Palliat. Med. 18, 195–201.

WHO, 1990. Cancer pain relief and palliative care. World Health Organization, Geneva.

Wong, R., Wiffen, P.J., 2005. Bisphosphonates for relief of pain secondary to bone metastases. Cochrane Database Syst. Rev. www.thecochranelibrary.com.

Zylicz, Z., Smits, C., Krajnik, M., 1998. Paroxetine for pruritis in advanced cancer. J. Pain Symptom Manage. 16, 121–124.

Chapter 28

Management of pain

CHAPTER CONTENTS

© 2011 Elsevier Ltd.

DOI: 10.1016/B978-0-7020-3053-6.00028-3

ACUTE PAIN

ADULTS

Use the WHO 'analgesic ladder' starting at the most appropriate level for the pain:

- Step 1: *paracetamol*, or an *NSAID*, or both.
- Step 2: *codeine* or *dihydrocodeine*. Use doses that are significantly more effective than paracetamol alone, e.g. 30–60 mg codeine or dihydrocodeine 30 mg.
- Step 3: *a strong opioid* (though strong opioids are controversial in non-malignant pain). Once the decision to use an opioid has been made, morphine or diamorphine in adequate doses are usually most appropriate. Adequate doses are likely to be well above 10 mg. The Oxford analgesic League Table shows that morphine 10 mg IM is no more effective than ibuprofen 400 mg orally (Oxford Pain Site accessed 2010).
- Some patients with swallowing difficulties or severe constipation may be better managed using a transdermal preparation (buprenorphine or fentanyl). Patients who experience significant side-effects from morphine may be treated successfully with oxycodone.
- *A co-analgesic*, sometimes called an adjuvant analgesic, (a tricyclic antidepressant or an anticonvulsant) may be added to any of the three steps in pain of any type, although they are most helpful in neuropathic pain (see page 677). There is increasing evidence of the value of combining opioids with adjuvants for synergistic activity. They work in a number of

ways to dampen down peripheral sensitization of nerve endings but also spinal synaptic transmission.

NSAIDs

NSAIDs are widely used effective analgesics in acute pain of any cause. At doses of ibuprofen 600–800 mg t.d.s. they are more powerful than paracetamol (Oxford Pain Site accessed 2010). Given parenterally or rectally, they are first line treatment for renal and biliary colic and are very helpful in acute severe musculoskeletal pain, e.g. diclofenac 75 mg i.m. or 100 mg rectally. Diclofenac injection may be repeated after half an hour. Even diclofenac suppositories have been shown to be superior to i.m. pethidine in renal colic (Thompson, Pike, Chumas, et al. 1989). Suppositories have the advantage over injections of not causing sterile abscesses.

NSAIDs and adverse effects (see page 266)

Cyclo-oxygenase-2 selective inhibitors (coxibs) and some non-selective NSAIDs (e.g. high-dose diclofenac and high-dose ibuprofen) increase the risk of thrombotic events. Non-selective NSAIDs increase the risk of GI ulceration more than do coxibs, but coxibs also carry some risk.

* Tailor the choice of NSAID to the patient. A good choice for a patient with cardiovascular disease is ibuprofen 400 mg t.d.s. or naproxen 500 mg b.d. A good choice for a patient with a past history of peptic ulceration is ibuprofen 400 mg t.d.s. plus a proton pump inhibitor, or a coxib plus a proton pump inhibitor.

INFANTS AND YOUNG CHILDREN

REVIEWS

Treating moderate and severe pain in infants. Drug Ther Bull March 1994, 32, 21–4
   The British National Formulary for Children. 2008. BMJ Publishing Group, RPS Publishing, RCPCH Publishing Ltd., London. Available: www.bnfc.org

● Infants, even neonates, feel pain and need analgesia in the same way as older children (Anon. 1989).

● Paracetamol is licensed for children from 3 months old and for children 2 months old, for use with immunization. The rectal route is effective and safe.

● Ibuprofen is effective as an antipyretic and analgesic in children (Marriott, Stephenson, Hull, *et al.* 1991) although only licensed for children aged 1 and over. Paracetamol can be co-prescribed.

* Explain to the child the cause of the pain and likely duration. Pain and fear are closely related, especially in children. It is important to be honest and not pretend that all pain will be removed.

CHRONIC NON–MALIGNANT PAIN

Three concepts are crucial to successful management:

● *Relating the drug treatment to the type of pain.* The treatment of neuropathic pain is different from the treatment of tissue-damage (nociceptive) pain. Even within nociceptive pain, some types respond better to NSAIDs than to analgesics, e.g. dysmenorrhoea and arthritic pain. This is independent of their anti-inflammatory effect (MeReC 1993).

● *Total pain.* There are always physical, psychological, social, emotional and spiritual elements in pain (Clark 1999). The psychological component may be the understandable anger, fear and misery likely to be found in anyone with chronic pain, or the significant psychiatric illness, especially depression, present in up to 50%. This will intensify the pain that is felt. In addition, pain can lead to changes in behaviour, which in turn alter the family dynamics. All these components of the 'chronic pain syndrome' must be addressed. Psychological treatment, especially cognitive behavioural therapy, has been shown to be helpful (McQuay, Moore, Ecclestone, et al 1997).

● *Measurement of pain intensity.* Formal measurement of perceived pain intensity can guide the physician in the tailoring of medication as well as demonstrating improvement to the patient and carer, if there has been any. The simplest way to assess and document the severity of pain is to ask the patient to score it on a scale of 1 to 10, either verbally or by drawing a 10 cm line, marked from 1 to 10 and asking the patient to mark the position of the pain on the line, where 0 is no pain and 10 the worse possible pain imaginable. Patients tend to score mild pain as < 3, moderate pain between 3 and 5.5 and severe pain above 5.5 (Collins, Moore, McQuay 1997). Pain scores above 5 usually interfere with the patient's functioning (Serlin, Mendoza, Nakamura, *et al.* 1995). Professionals tend to underestimate pain, especially severe pain, while carers tend to overestimate it (Grossman, Sheidler, Sweeden, *et al.* 1991).

GENERAL PRINCIPLES OF MANAGEMENT

* Explain the reason for the pain. Pain clinics sometimes find that patients are more concerned about this than about pain relief.
* Explain that treatment is unlikely to abolish pain completely, but that the aim is to stop it from affecting the quality of the patient's life.
* Explore the psychological component with the patient and the family. If the patient seems to think you are implying that it's all 'in the mind', make it clear that you know the pain is real.

NOCICEPTIVE PAIN (PAIN DUE TO TISSUE DAMAGE)

* *Use the analgesic ladder* as above, but not usually beyond dihydrocodeine 120 mg/day. Most pain specialists will not use strong opioids for this condition because of tolerance, addiction and side-effects. Others feel there is a place for opioids in patients with intractable pain which is interfering with life, where the diagnosis is proven, the pain is opioid-sensitive, and where there are no psychological contraindications. A recent meta-analysis showed that strong, but not weak, opioids were superior to naproxen

and to nortriptyline (Furlan, Sandoval, Mailis-Gagnon, *et al.* 2006). Another meta-analysis has shown that opioids improve the quality of life as well as relieving pain, but longer term studies are needed (Devulder, Richaz and Nataraja 2005). For the practicalities of opioid use, see page 660.

* *NSAIDs.* Consider adding an NSAID to the chosen analgesic (see page 676).
* *Adjuvant analgesics.* Consider adding a tricyclic antidepressant (see below). Co-analgesics are sometimes helpful (see below), although not as helpful as in neuropathic pain.
* *Pain clinic.* Consider referral to a pain clinic for further physical, as well as psychological, interventions. Transcutaneous electrical neural stimulation (TENS) is widely used in pain clinics, although evidence for benefit is not strong. Nerve blocks may be extremely helpful in certain situations, e.g. epidural injection for low back pain, caudal injection for coccidynia, intercostal block for rib pain and brachial plexus block for arm pain. Nerve destruction is little used because of the problem of deafferentation pain that it can cause.

NEUROPATHIC PAIN (PAIN DUE TO NERVE DAMAGE)

Examples of neuropathic pain are nerve injury, compression or infiltration of nerve by tumour, shingles, and diabetic neuropathy. It is characterized by one or more of the following:

(a) a burning or aching quality;

(b) an element of 'shooting' pain;

(c) autonomic instability; vasoconstriction or vasodilation;

(d) allodynia (severe pain from mild stimuli) – this is diagnostic;

(e) sensory loss, especially pain in an area of numbness.

Conventional wisdom is that neuropathic pain responds poorly to analgesics, including opioids. A meta-analysis, however, suggests that this is a misconception, possibly due to the fact that, while single doses and short courses of opioids are ineffective, longer courses (at least 8 days) show significant benefit. Adverse effects, however, are common and none of the studies has extended over 56 days nor addressed the issue of dependency (Eisenberg, McNicol and Carr 2005).

A recent review of guidelines reported that first-line treatments are antidepressants and certain anticonvulsants but that opioids and tramadol are second line and in certain clinical situations could become first-line (O'Connor and Dworkin 2009).

PRINCIPLES OF MANAGEMENT

* *Simple analgesic.* Give paracetamol and/or an NSAID.
* *Adjuvant analgesic.* Add a tricyclic antidepressant and/or an anticonvulsant. The evidence of benefit from other antidepressants is poor.
* *Opioid.* If still in pain, institute a trial of a weak opioid.
* *Pain clinic.* Refer to a pain clinic.

Tricylic antidepressants, e.g. amitriptyline

* Start at 25 mg o.n. (10 mg in the elderly) as soon as the diagnosis of neuropathic pain is made.
* Warn the patient that it will be 1–7 days before there is benefit. The NNT is 3; i.e. one in three patients will have at least 50% relief which they would not have had with placebo (DTB 2000).
* Warn the patient that side-effects may occur, especially dry mouth and drowsiness.
* Increase the dose fortnightly until a good response is achieved. If there is a response it is likely to be at 75 mg or below, although occasionally it is worth continuing up to 150 mg daily. The effective dose is likely to be lower than that required for depression.
* Continue treatment for 2 months after the pain has stopped, then tail it off over a month. Do not change to another tricyclic if amitriptyline fails; most are likely to be less successful (DTB 2000).

Anticonvulsants

* Use gabapentin, pregabalin, carbamazepine or valproate. Carbamazepine and gabapentin have overall NNTs of approximately 3 (Wiffen, Collins, McQuay, *et al.* 2000). The evidence for phenytoin is less clear (DTB 2000). Gabapentin has the advantage of fewer drug interactions which is important in patients with comorbidity, especially HIV neuropathy.
* Start with low doses, and increase until relief of symptoms is achieved or until blood levels are in the therapeutic range for epilepsy (see Appendix 16).
* Continue this dose for 6 weeks before abandoning as ineffective. If one drug fails it is not helpful to try another (McQuay, Carroll, Jadad, *et al.* 1995). Only gabapentin and pregabalin are licensed for all neuropathic pain while carbamazepine and phenytoin are licensed for trigeminal neuralgia.

POST-HERPETIC NEURALGIA (PHN)

See also page 574.

* Give conventional analgesics, e.g. paracetamol. Most will not respond, in which case stop the drug. Do not proceed up the analgesic ladder beyond a trial of a weak opioid.
* Give tricyclic antidepressants (see above) to all patients with severe pain and to others who are at high risk of PHN. Starting amitriptyline early appears to reduce the severity of PHN should it develop later (Bowsher 1994).
* If tricyclic antidepressants do not give adequate relief, consider:
  (a) *an anticonvulsant* e.g. gabapentin (see above);
  (b) *a local anaesthetic cream* (e.g. Emla) to be applied thickly at night and covered with clingfilm. It may be removed in the morning, and benefit will last for some of the day (Rowbotham, Davies, Verkempinck, *et al.* 1989);
  (c) *capsaicin cream* q.d.s. for up to 8 weeks. In one trial 39% reported at least moderate relief after 6 weeks against 6% on placebo (DTB 2000). An unpleasant burning sensation is likely for the first 1–2 weeks, and can be reduced by applying Emla cream before the capsaicin.
* Refer patients still in pain after 8 weeks. Stellate ganglion block may reduce pain. In one uncontrolled study it was associated with freedom from pain in 40% of those referred before 1 year although in only 22% of those referred after 1 year (Milligan and Nash 1985).

TRIGEMINAL NEURALGIA

Patients often describe this as 'the worst pain in the world' (Bennetto, Patel and Fuller 2007).

* Refer patients with atypical symptoms; or who are relatively young; or who do not respond to first line medical treatment. They need imaging to discover the 5–10% in whom the neuralgia is secondary to tumour, multiple sclerosis, bony abnormalities, or A-V malformations. Almost all other patients are found to have an aberrant arterial, or occasionally venous, loop which is pressing on the trigeminal nerve.

* Explain that the course of the disease is variable with remissions and relapses. A third of patients only ever have one attack. After a first episode 65% have a second within 5 years, with similar delays for subsequent attacks.

* Use carbamazepine first line, starting with 100 mg nocte or b.d., and increasing until relief is achieved or the maximum dose of 1.6 g daily is reached.

* Change to oxcarbazepine if benefit is obtained but adverse effects are troublesome.

* If there is no response to carbamazepine change to gabapentin. Alternatives are lamotrigine or baclofen. If there is a partial response to carbamazepine, combine it with an anticonvulsant.

* Refer, if medical treatment is unsatisfactory, for consideration of surgery. The choice lies between some kind of nerve ablation, which is safe but may lead to numbness and eventual relapse; and microvascular decompression, which has a lower relapse rate, less risk of numbness, but a slightly higher risk of serious adverse effects.

* Recommend the Trigeminal Neuralgia Association UK on www.tna.org.uk which provides information about the condition and about patient support groups.

REFLEX SYMPATHETIC DYSTROPHY

● This is a pain syndrome, usually affecting an extremity, following trauma (even minimal trauma). It is characterized by swelling, discoloration, temperature changes, abnormal sensitivity, sweating and loss of function. X-rays may show osteopenia. Early recognition, pain control and mobilization are thought to be associated with a better prognosis (Paice 1989).

* Refer to a pain clinic as soon as the diagnosis is made. A trial of mild analgesics is worthwhile but usually unhelpful. A pain clinic is likely to try intravenous regional sympathetic blockade but evidence of benefit is poor (Jadad, Carroll, Glynn, *et al.* 1995).

DIABETIC POLYNEUROPATHY (JUDE AND SCHAPER 2007)

* Explore the patient's perception of the pain and the impact it is having. Address and treat anxiety, depression and disturbed sleep.

* Encourage the patient to work to optimize their blood glucose control. Large variations in blood glucose appear to exacerbate pain.

* Treat with a tricyclic antidepressant (as above) if there are no contraindications.

* Consider adding an anticonvulsant (gabapentin, or pregabalin) or the antidepressant duloxetine.

* Consider an opioid.

CENTRAL PAIN

This may be of brain or spinal cord origin. Stroke is the commonest cause. The onset of pain may be delayed for up to 3 years after the event. It is particularly difficult to treat, and early referral to a pain clinic would be wise.

* Use:
  (a) amitriptyline (see above);
  (b) anticonvulsants (see above);
  (c) a neuroleptic, e.g. perphenazine. In a patient already on low-dose amitriptyline, the compound preparation Triptafen is convenient.

* Consider discussing with a pain specialist, the use of methadone or ketamine. They are antagonists at the NMDA receptors, which appear to be sensitized in chronic pain.

References

Anon. 1989. Pain relief in babies – a not so simple problem. Matern. Child Health J. April 121–122.

Bennetto, L., Patel, N.K., Fuller, G., 2007. Trigeminal neuralgia and its management. BMJ 334, 201–215.

Bowsher, D., 1994. Post-herpetic neuralgia in older patients. Incidence and optimal treatment. Drugs Aging 5, 411–418.

Clark, D., 1999. "Total pain", disciplinary power and the body in the work of Cicely Saunders, 1958–1967. Soc. Sci. Med. 49, 727–736.

Collins, S.L., Moore, R.A., McQuay, H.J., 1997. The visual analogue pain intensity scale: what is moderate pain in millimetres? Pain 72, 95–97.

Devulder, J., Richaz, U., Nataraja, S.H., 2005. Impact of long-term use of opioids on quality of life in patients with chronic, nonmalignant pain. Curr. Med. Res. Opin. 21, 1555–1568.

DTB, 2000. Drug treatment of neuropathic pain. Drug Ther. Bull. 38, 89–93.

Eisenberg, E., McNicol, E.D., Carr, D.B., 2005. Efficacy and safety of opioid agonists in the treatment of neuropathic pain of nonmalignant origin. JAMA 293, 3043–3052.

Furlan, A.D., Sandoval, J.A., Mailis-Gagnon, A., et al., 2006. Opioids for chronic noncancer pain: a meta-analysis of effectiveness and side effects. CMAJ 174, 1589–1594.

Grossman, S.A., Sheidler, V.R., Sweeden, K., et al., 1991. Correlation of patient and caregiver ratings of cancer pain. J. Pain Symptom Manage. 6, 53–57.

Jadad, A.R., Carroll, D., Glynn, C.J., et al., 1995. Intravenous regional sympathetic blockade for pain relief in reflex sympathetic dystrophy: a systematic review and a randomised, double-blind crossover study. J. Pain Symptom Manage. 10, 13–20.

Jude, E.B., Schaper, N., 2007. Treating painful diabetic polyneuropathy. BMJ 335, 57–58.

McQuay, H.J., Moore, R.A., Eccleston, C., et al., 1997. Systematic review of outpatient services for chronic pain control. Health Technol. Assess. 1 (6), i–iv, 1–135.

McQuay, H.J., Carroll, D., Jadad, A.R., et al., 1995. Anticonvulsant drugs for the management of pain: a systematic review. BMJ 311, 1047–1052.

Marriott, S.C., Stephenson, T.J., Hull, D., et al., 1991. A dose-ranging study of ibuprofen syrup as an antipyretic. Arch. Dis. Child. 66 (Suppl.), 1037–1042.

MeReC, 1993. Combination Analgesics. MeReC Bulletin 4, 45–47.

Milligan, N.S., Nash, T.P., 1985. Treatment of post-herpetic neuralgia: a review of 77 consecutive cases. Pain 23, 381–386.

O'Connor, A.B., Dworkin, R.H., 2009. Treatment of neuropathic pain: an overview of recent guidelines. Am J Med 122 (Suppl 10), S22–32.

Oxford Pain Site accessed 2010. www.medicine.ox.ac.uk/bandolier (choose Oxford pain site, then acute pain, then analgesic league table).

Paice, E., 1989. Reflex sympathetic dystrophy. BMJ 310, 1645–1648.

Rowbotham, M.C., Davies, P.S., Verkempinck, C., et al., 1989. Topical lidocaine reduces pain in post-herpetic neuralgia. Pain 38, 297–301.

Serlin, R.C., Mendoza, T.R., Nakamura, Y., et al., 1995. When is cancer pain mild, moderate or severe? Grading pain severity by its interference with function. Pain 61, 277–284.

Thompson, J.F., Pike, J.M., Chumas, P.O., et al., 1989. Rectal diclofenac compared with pethidine injection in acute renal colic. BMJ 299, 1140–1141.

Wiffen, P., Collins, S., McQuay, H., et al., 2000. Anticonvulsant drugs for acute and chronic pain. Cochrane Database Syst. Rev. (3).

Chapter 29

Death and bereavement

CHAPTER CONTENTS

BEREAVEMENT

SYSTEMATIC REVIEW

Woof WR, Carter YH. 1997. The grieving adult and the general practitioner: a literature review in two parts. Br J Gen Pract 47, 443–8, 509–14

The GP is in a unique position to:

(a) help the bereaved to express their feelings and come to terms with their loss at a pace that is appropriate for that person. At times, even the avoidance of emotion may be part of that adaptation;

(b) encourage the bereaved to begin life again after an appropriate time;

(c) detect and treat pathological grief.

PATHOLOGICAL GRIEF

Expect it when:

(a) death was sudden or stigmatized (e.g. suicide or AIDS);

(b) death was, or was seen by the survivor to have been, avoidable;

(c) death is unexplained, as in cot death, miscarriage or stillbirth;

(d) the bereaved is socially isolated or has economic difficulties;

(e) the relationship was of either a dependent or ambivalent nature. Excessive pining may follow the former, and excessive guilt the latter;

© 2011 Elsevier Ltd.

DOI: 10.1016/B978-0-7020-3053-6.00029-5

(f) the person is vulnerable by reason of personality, previous mental illness or bereavement, or poor physical health.

Consider it when:

(a) the bereaved appears to be stuck in a state of denial, anger or depression, rather than moving towards acceptance. Most people will have overcome denial by 2 months, anger by 6 months and depression by 12 months, although these timings are a crude guide only;

(b) guilt is anything more than transitory;

(c) the depth of grief makes the patient unable to discuss his or her feelings;

(d) the bereaved is suicidal, rather than just 'looking forward to joining' the deceased;

(e) the bereaved is using alcohol or drugs to cope with the loss.

MANAGEMENT

Before the death

If the family is willing and time permits, it is helpful for them to discuss openly their feelings with the dying, especially sharing any resentments they have about the past which, if not expressed now, might lead to prolonged guilt or anger later. Love, too, can be expressed at this stage, and the bereaved will not feel when it is too late that the dead person 'never knew how much I loved him/her'.

At the time of death

* Encourage the family to see the dead person and express any unfinished business.
* Inform the family about the registration of the death, and how to contact a funeral director (see page 685).

After the death

After a bereavement, the minimum should be one visit with an invitation to talk further at a later stage.

* Show concern and talk through the last illness. Encourage the patient to express any anger or guilt about what happened. Acknowledge anything you think could have been done better, without waiting for the relatives to bring it up. Where possible, reassure the bereaved that they did everything possible to help.
* Explain that many different emotions may follow bereavement, and that none is abnormal. Specifically, explain that it is common to continue to hear and look for the deceased, and that this is not a sign of madness.
* *Pathological grief.* If pathological grief is present, the GP should arrange for support (from a counsellor, psychologist or psychiatrist as appropriate).
* *Drugs.* Avoid using regular tranquillizers and discourage alcohol (a number of people given benzodiazepines at bereavement continue long-term use). Antidepressants will be needed where bereavement has triggered a depressive illness.
* Tell the bereaved about people or organizations who can help, e.g. counsellor, health visitor, Cruse, the clergy (addresses of the main organizations are given below).
* Recommend reading, e.g. *A Death in the Family* by Jean Richardson (1979), published by Lion Publishing, or *the leaflet Bereavement*, by the Royal College of Psychiatrists.
* Give an invitation for review some 6 weeks later.
* Note the event in the notes of the whole family. Record the actual date in the summary of the spouse or consort, in order to spot the significance of symptoms presenting at that time in future years.

PATIENT ORGANIZATIONS

Cruse Bereavement Care, 0844 477 9400; email: helpline@cruse.org.uk website: www.crusebereavementcare.org.uk

Sudden Death Support Association, Yew Tree Farm, Part Lane, Swallowfield, Reading, Berkshire, RG7 1TB. Tel: 01189 888099

For parents who have lost a child

The Child Death Helpline, tel. 0800 282986; www.childdeathhelpline.org.uk

Compassionate Friends, tel. 0845 123 2304; www.tcf.org.uk for the parents of children who have died (at any age)

LITERATURE

Royal College of Psychiatry. *Bereavement.* Available: www.rcpsych.ac.uk (search on 'Bereavement')

The National Association of Bereavement Services, 2 Plough Yard, London EC2A, tel. 020 7709 9090

For professionals: *The WHO Guide to Mental Health in Primary Care: Bereavement and Loss.* Online. Available: www.mentalneurologicalprimarycare.org (search on 'bereavement')

COT DEATH

Early contact and follow-up will help reduce feelings of isolation and misdirected anger. Close liaison with the health visitor is essential.

* Explain that many reactions may occur, including hearing the baby cry, having aching arms and waking at night as though to attend to the baby.
* *Post-mortem.* Explain that a post-mortem examination will be necessary, and that the parents will have to make a statement to the police. Explain the role of the coroner, and that there may have to be an inquest. Explain that the police will have to visit, ask questions and may take away bedding. Reassure them that this is routine and that they are not under suspicion.
* Download a copy of 'When a baby dies suddenly and unexpectedly' available from www.fsid.org.uk (search on 'When a baby dies suddenly and unexpectedly')
* *Breastfeeding.* Give advice about stopping lactation (see page 402).
* *Hypnotics.* Offer a small number of benzodiazepines to help sleep if the patient is becoming exhausted.
* *Identical twins.* The survivor is at higher risk, and short-term admission should be considered.
* *Other siblings* will need support. Give guidance on the emotional needs of brothers and sisters.
* *Paediatrician.* Inform the paediatrician designated for cot death or the community paediatrician. Inform the child health department so no further appointment for immunizations are sent.
* *Follow-up.* Ensure that the parents have been given an appointment to discuss the death with a paediatrician, and arrange to see them yourself afterwards.

PROFESSIONAL AND PATIENT INFORMATION

The Foundation for the Study of Infant Deaths, 35 Belgrave Square, London SW1X 8QB, tel. 0207 233 2090; Helpline: 0808 802 6868, email: support@fsid.org.uk; website: www.fsid.org.uk

Parent 24-hour Cot Death helpline, tel. 0207 235 1721.

SANDS (Stillbirth and Neonatal Death Society), 28 Portland Place, London W1N 4DE, helpline: 0207 436 5881; www.uk-sands.org

BEREAVED CHILDREN

* Children are 'concrete' thinkers, and do not develop the adult concept of death until the age of 9 or 10. This means that they do not realize that it happens to everyone, and that the dead person will never come back. Between the ages of 3 and 6 they are egocentric and go through a phase of antagonism to the parent of the same sex, and if that parent dies they may feel they caused the death.
* Bereaved children have a high morbidity; 40–50% have behavioural symptoms at 1 year, and up to 10% develop quite severe mental illness later in life.
* Try to match the explanation to the child's level of understanding. Explain that, although doctors are able to help with most illnesses, some are too severe to cure.
* Encourage the whole family to talk about the dead person in front of the child, thereby giving the child permission to express his or her feelings.
* Explain to the parents that children are more likely to express their feelings through play and art than verbally. They should make sure that play leaders and teachers are alert to what has happened.

＊ Viewing the body and attending the funeral can help the child to realize that the person is really dead.

BOOKS FOR AND ABOUT BEREAVED CHILDREN

Winston's Wish is a charity dedicated to childhood bereavement. Address: The Clara Burgess Centre, Gloucestershire Royal Hospital, Gloucester. Tel 01242 515157 or 0845 203040. Email: info@winstonswish.org.uk Website: www. winstonswish.org.uk. The website has details of books and pamphlets for bereaved children and for families who have lost a child. On the website search on 'useful reading'.

Varley S. 1992. *Badger's Parting Gifts.* HarperTrophy. This illustrated book is suitable for children from pre-school age onwards. It is available from www.amazon.co.uk where reviews of the book by parents can be read.

The Royal College of Psychiatrists lists books and leaflets about bereavement. Go to www.rcpsych.ac.uk and search on 'bereavement'.

SUICIDE

● Because the death is sudden, perhaps unexpected and possibly violent, particularly intense feelings of shock and distress may occur in survivors.
● Suicide carries a stigma, which may make those bereaved reluctant to seek support.
● Guilt is a common reaction to suicide. A GP may feel that he or she has failed their patient. A relative may feel guilt that they were unable to prevent the death, or guilt at their relief after years of caring for a mentally ill relative. Anger against 'helping' professions is a common response to bereavement.

SUPPORT ORGANIZATIONS

The Samaritans, tel. 08457 909090. www.samaritans. org.uk

Survivors of bereavement by suicide. helpline 0844 561 6855; www.uk-sobs.org.uk

Literature

The website of Survivors of Bereavement by Suicide lists and reviews books on suicide. Go to www.uk-sobs. org.uk and choose 'Book Reviews'.

Royal College of Psychiatrists. *Factsheet 25. Suicide and Attempted Suicide: For Parents and Teachers.* Available: www.rcpsych.ac.uk (search on 'suicide').

Wertheimer A. 2001. *A Special Scar: The Experiences of People Bereaved by Suicide.* Routledge, London

MURDER

SUPPORT FOR RELATIVES

Support after murder or manslaughter (SAMM). Helpline 9am – 9pm 0845 872 3440. Email support@samm.org.uk. Website www.samm.org.uk

DEATH RITUALS OF DIFFERENT CULTURES

● *Buddhism:* cremation is arranged at a time determined by monks; no fundamental objections to post-mortem examination.
● *Christianity:* cremation or burial; no fundamental objections to post-mortem examination.
● *Hinduism:* body is cremated; post-mortem examination is felt to be disrespectful.
● *Islam:* the body should be touched only by Muslims; non-Muslims should wear disposable gloves when touching the body. Burial should be carried out within 24 hours.
● *Judaism:* burial within 24 hours; post-mortem only in exceptional cases.
● *Sikhism:* cremation within 24 hours.

It is important to establish from the family:

(a) What are the preferred rituals for management of the dying, the dead body, the disposal of the body and rituals to commemorate loss?
(b) What are their beliefs about what happens after death?
(c) What do they believe is the appropriate emotional expression of a loss?

(d) Are there any gender rules for handling the death?

(e) Are certain deaths particularly traumatic or stigmatized?

ASPECTS OF DEATH

Home Office: The General Register Office. 2008. *Guidance for Doctors Completing Medical Certificates of Cause of Death in England and Wales.* Available: www.gro.gov.uk/medcert/

CERTIFICATION

Refer to the coroner cases where:

(a) The cause of the death is unknown.

(b) The deceased was not seen by the certifying doctor either after death or in the 14 days before death (28 days in Northern Ireland).

(c) The death was violent, unnatural or suspicious.

(d) The death may be due to an accident (whenever it occurred).

(e) The death may be due to self-neglect or neglect by others.

(f) The death may be due to an industrial disease, or related to the deceased's employment.

(g) The death may be due to an abortion.

(h) The death may have occurred during an operation or before recovery from the effects of an anaesthetic, or was related to a medical treatment or procedure.

(i) The death may be a suicide or was otherwise self-induced.

(j) The death occurred during or shortly after detention in police or prison custody or while detained under the Mental Health Act.

Referral is not obligatory but is helpful when:

(a) The relatives are considering a complaint.

(b) The deceased was in receipt of a service or industrial disability pension and where the cause of death is related to that disability, or where the pensioner was in receipt of a constant attendance allowance. It will assist a claim for a funeral grant and widow's pension.

If the death is to be a coroner's case or if the GP is uncertain:

(a) Do not allow the body to be moved from the place of death. The police will do this.

(b) Contact the coroner's office (out of normal hours, ring the police station). Uniformed officers will attend the scene of death. Warn the relatives of this, and explain that this does not (necessarily) mean that something has gone wrong.

The coroner may organize a post-mortem and/or issue a death certificate; or advise the GP to issue a certificate (the GP should initial the back of the certificate).

If the death is not a coroner's case:

* Discuss the death with the relatives, and explain that they can now telephone the funeral directors.

* Issue the death certificate or, if another doctor will be signing it, tell the relatives to contact that doctor.

* Recommend the leaflet What to do After a Death (available from *the Citizens Advice Bureau* on www.adviceguide.org.uk (search on 'death').

In Scotland, for 'coroner' read 'procurator fiscal'.

PRACTICAL ASPECTS OF THE COMPLETION OF MEDICAL CERTIFICATES OF CAUSE OF DEATH IN ENGLAND AND WALES (MCCD)

The structure of the MCCD (Examples are taken from the Guidance for doctors completing Medical Certificates of Cause of Death in England and Wales. 2008. Available: www.gro.gov.uk/ medcert)

The disease or condition thought to be the underlying cause should appear in the lowest completed line of part I see Table 29.1.

More than three conditions in a sequence can be included by adding more than one condition on a line, e.g.

Ia. Post-transplant lymphoma.

Ib. Immunosuppression following renal transplant 15 years ago.

Ic. Glomerulonephrosis due to insulin dependent diabetes mellitus.

II. Recurrent urinary tract infections.

Insulin dependent diabetes with renal complications is the underlying cause.

Table 29.1	Example of a completed medical certificate
I (a) Disease or condition leading directly to death	Intraperitoneal haemorrhage
(b) Other disease or condition, if any, leading to I(a)	Ruptured metastatic deposit in liver
(c) Other disease or condition, if any, leading to I(b)	Primary adenocarcinoma of ascending colon
II Other significant conditions **Contributing to death** but not related to the disease or condition causing it	Non–insulin dependent diabetes mellitus

The colon cancer on line 1(c) led directly to the liver metastases on line 1(b), which ruptured, causing the fatal haemorrhage on 1(a). Adenocarcinoma of the colon is the underlying cause of death.

Acceptable and unacceptable causes of death

* **Old age** should only be given as the **sole** cause of death in very limited circumstances. These are that:
  (a) You have personally cared for the deceased over a long period (years, or many months).
  (b) You have observed a gradual decline in your patient's general health and functioning.
  (c) You are not aware of any identifiable disease or injury that contributed to the death.
  (d) You are certain that there is no reason that the death should be reported to the coroner.
  Refer all patients dying under the age of 80 if you consider 'old age' or 'senility' is justifiable on the certificate. 'Frailty of old age' should be treated in the same way.

* Avoid 'natural causes' and organ failure alone, instead give the underlying cause, e.g.
  Ia. Liver failure.
  Ib. Hepatocellular carcinoma.
  Ic. Chronic hepatitis B infection.

* Avoid terminal events, modes of dying and other vague terms.

* Avoid the term 'cerebrovascular accident'. Consider using terms such as 'stroke' or 'cerebral infarction' if no more specific description can be given. Include antecedent conditions or treatments, e.g. atrial fibrillation, artificial heart valves.

* *Neoplasms.* Specify the histological type and anatomical site of the cancer, e.g.
  Ia. Carcinomatosis.
  Ib. Small cell carcinoma of left main bronchus.
  Ic. Heavy smoker for 40 years.
  II. Hypertension, cerebral arteriosclerosis, ischaemic heart disease.

* Avoid ambiguity about the primary site if both primary and secondary cancer sites are mentioned. If using the term 'metastatic' or 'metastases' indicate whether this is to or from the named site, e.g.
  Ia. Intraperitoneal haemorrhage.
  Ib. Metastases in liver.
  Ic. From primary adenocarcinoma of ascending colon.

* *Diabetes.* Specify whether type I or type II, e.g.
  Ia. End-stage renal failure.
  Ib. Diabetic nephropathy.
  Ic. Insulin dependent diabetes mellitus.

* *Deaths involving infections and communicable diseases.*
  ■ If the cause of death was from a notifiable disease or there is uncertainty if the disease is notifiable contact the local Health Protection Unit (HPU).
  ■ In deaths from infectious diseases state:
    (a) The manifestation or body site, e.g. pneumonia, pyelonephritis, hepatitis, meningitis, septicaemia, or wound infection.
    (b) The infecting organism, e.g. pneumococcus, influenza A virus, meningococcus.
    (c) Antibiotic resistance, if relevant, e.g. methicillin resistant *Staphylococcus aureus* (MRSA), or multiple drug resistant *Mycobacterium tuberculosis.*
    (d) The source and/or route of infection, if known, e.g. food poisoning, needle sharing, contaminated blood products, post-operative, community or hospital acquired, or healthcare associated infection.

* Health care associated infections(HCAI)
  ■ If a healthcare associated infection was a part of the sequence leading to death it should be included in part I: e.g.
    Ia. Clostridium difficile pseudomembranous colitis.
    Ib. Multiple antibiotic therapy.

Ic. Community acquired pneumonia with severe sepsis.

II. Immobility, polymyalgia rheumatica, osteoporosis.

■ If a HCAI contributed but was not part of the direct sequence it should be included in part II, e.g.

Ia. Carcinomatosis and renal failure.

Ib. Adenocarcinoma of the prostate.

II. Chronic obstructive airways disease and catheter associated Escherichia coli urinary tract infection.

✱ *Pneumonia.* Specify, where possible, whether it was lobar or bronchopneumonia and whether primarily hypostatic, or related to aspiration and the organism involved, e.g.

Ia. Pneumococcal pneumonia.

Ib. Influenza A.

Ic.

II. Ischaemic heart disease.

✱ *Bronchopneumonia.* If using the term bronchopneumonia include in the sequence in part I any predisposing conditions, especially those that may have led to paralysis, immobility, depressed immunity or wasting, as well as chronic respiratory conditions such as chronic bronchitis, e.g.

Ia. Bronchopneumonia.

Ib. Immobility and wasting.

Ic. Alzheimer's disease.

✱ *Injury.* If the coroner instructs you, as the patient's clinician, to certify, include details as to how the injury occurred and where it happened, such as at home, in the street, or at work, e.g.

Ia. Pulmonary embolism.

Ib. Fractured neck of femur.

Ic. Tripped on loose floor rug at home.

II. Left sided weakness and difficulty with balance since haemorrhagic stroke 5 years ago; hemiarthroplasty 2 days after fracture.

✱ *Substance misuse.* Refer deaths due to acute or chronic **poisoning**, by **any** substance, and deaths involving drug dependence or misuse of substances other than alcohol and tobacco must be referred. Deaths from diseases related to chronic alcohol or tobacco use need not be referred to the coroner, provided the disease is clearly stated on the MCCD, e.g.

Ia. Carcinomatosis.

Ib. Bronchogenic carcinoma upper lobe left lung.

Ic. Smoked 30 cigarettes a day.

II. Chronic bronchitis and ischaemic heart disease.

DONATION OF EYES, BODIES AND ORGANS

DONATION OF EYES

Telephone the local ophthalmology unit. The eyes should be removed within 24 hours of death. Most people who die could become corneal donors. The only medical conditions restricting donation are viral diseases, motor neurone disease, active leukaemias or lymphomas, previous intraocular surgery, ocular infection or malignancy.

DONATION OF BODIES FOR DISSECTION OR RESEARCH

Advise the patient to download the leaflet *How to donate a body* from the Human Tissue Authority's website www.hta.gov.uk/donations/ howtodonateyourbodytomedicalscience.cfm

An alternative is to donate the brain alone. Brains from those with and without neurological disorders are needed. There are specific brain banks for specific diseases or the donation can be made to the MRC London Brain Bank for Neurodegenerative Diseases. An information pack is available from Brainbank@iop.kcl.ac.uk.

DONATION OF ORGANS

A person can indicate their agreement to donation by joining the NHS Organ Donor Register and by carrying a donor card. Go to www.uktransplant. org.uk and choose how to become a donor and carrying a donor card. If no record of consent exists, the HT Act permits consent to be obtained from the person nominated by the deceased person to act on his or her behalf; or if one does not exist, from a person in a 'qualifying relationship' – such as a partner or other relative or friend.

Chapter **30**

Health promotion

CHAPTER CONTENTS

This section brings together information about how the risk of disease can be reduced by a healthy lifestyle. Some of the information is also to be found elsewhere in the book under the relevant disease. The purpose of this section is to answer the questions: 'why should I change my lifestyle?' or, for a practice, 'why should we give lifestyle advice?'

EXERCISE

OVERVIEW

Department of Health. 2001. *Exercise Referral Systems: A National Quality Assurance Framework*. DoH, London. Available: www.dh.gov.uk (search on 'Exercise referrals')

- There is considerable evidence that moving from a sedentary to a more active lifestyle improves health.
- Exercise advice is more likely to be effective if appropriate to the individual; for example, although some will join a gym, many more will be able to adapt to walking to work or walking the children to school, walking up moving escalators, walking up stairs instead of using the lift, doing the housework at 'double time'.
- Once an individual has started to change it is important for them to stay motivated. The following may help:
  (a) keeping a diary;
  (b) setting short- and long-term goals;

DOI: 10.1016/B978-0-7020-3053-6.00030-1

(c) reminding oneself of why the change was initiated, e.g. to lose weight, to feel healthy;

(d) visualization – picturing oneself achieving the goal;

(e) getting pleasure out of the exercise and reminding oneself of how one feels after exercise.

* Advise patients that exercise reduces the risk *of the following*.

(a) *CHD*. Physically inactive people have about double the risk of CHD (Department of Health 2001). Exercise must be vigorous (for 20 minutes, three times a week) or moderate, e.g. brisk walking (for 30 minutes five times a week) (Powell and Pratt 1996). The exercise may be broken into separate bouts as long as they are for at least 10 minutes each. In the short term, the risk of myocardial infarction is halved (British Heart Foundation 1991) with less risk of death if it does occur, but this benefit is lost if exercise is stopped. Exercise continued for over 1 year improves the coronary collateral circulation enough to be demonstrable on a thallium scan. Regular physical activity prevents or delays the development of high blood pressure and reduces blood pressure in people with hypertension (Manson, Hu, Rich-Edwards, *et al.* 1999).

(b) *Diabetes*. Time spent in a sedentary manner (e.g. watching television) significantly increases the risk of developing type 2 diabetes (Hu, Letzmann, Stampfer, *et al.* 2001). Conversely, the risk of developing diabetes may be reduced by more than 50% in those who undertake regular moderate exercise (Perry, Wannamethe, Walker, *et al.* 1995; Hu, Stampfer, Solomon, *et al.* 1999).

(c) *Cancer*. It is postulated that adoption of an active lifestyle could reduce all-cause cancer by 45% (Shephard and Futcher 1997). There is strong evidence that physically active men and women have about half the risk of colonic cancer, and women possibly 30% of the risk of breast cancer, compared to sedentary counterparts (CMO 2004; Davey Smith, Shipley, Batty, *et al.* 2000; Batty 2000).

(d) *Osteoporosis*. Exercise will increase bone density, even in women over 70. It should be weight bearing, for at least 30 minutes per day. If practised at least three times a week, fracture rates are halved. Conversely, immobilization produces irreversible bone loss.

(e) *Depression*. There is evidence that exercise reduces the intensity of depression (Martinsen, Medhus and Sandvik 1985), and that depression is more common in those who are physically inactive (Farmer, Locke, Moscicki, *et al.* 1985). Both short- and long-term exercise reduce the intensity of depression (North, McCullagh and Zung vu Tran 1990).

(f) *Disability in older people*. Those who exercise develop disability at a quarter of the rate of those who do not exercise, even though the exercisers have a higher rate of fractures and short-term disability related to their exercise behaviour. This difference is still present after 9 years. Medical care costs are reduced by a quarter in those who exercise. Even the very old benefit, with improvements in muscle strength, gait velocity and stair-climbing ability (Elon 1996).

(g) *Falls in older people* are reduced by a multifactorial intervention approach that includes exercise and balance training (Tinetti, Baker, McAvay, *et al.* 1994).

Exercise of moderate intensity equates to 60–85% of the maximum age-adjusted heart rate. Maximum age-adjusted heart rate = 220 – age in years. The patient will feel slightly breathless and warmer than usual.

Excessive exercise may:

(a) increase the risk of upper respiratory infection (Shephard and Shek 1999);

(b) be associated with poor nutrition and osteoporosis (see 'The female athlete triad', page 514).

DIET

A modified Mediterranean diet has been shown to be associated with a reduction in mortality of 7% in a population aged over 60 (Trichopoulou 2005). This incorporates: a high intake of vegetables, legumes, fruits, relatively unrefined cereals; a moderate or high intake of fish; a low intake of saturated lipids but a high intake of unsaturated lipids, especially olive oil; a low to moderate intake of dairy products; a low intake of meat; and a modest intake of alcohol.

The COMA report recommends major changes in the national pattern of food consumption (Report of the Cardiovascular Review Group of the Committee on Medical Aspects of Food Policy (COMA) 1994).

- *A higher fruit and vegetable intake* (five or more servings daily) helps provide protection against:
  (a) cardiovascular disease; increasing fruit and vegetables by two servings per day may decrease cardiovascular risk by 30%;
  (b) macular degeneration and cataract;
  (c) cancers, including breast, colorectal and stomach;
  (d) diverticular disease;
  (e) diabetes;
  (f) blood pressure (Appel, Moore, Obarzanek, *et al.* 1997; John, Ziebland, Yudkin, *et al.* 2002).

The UK policy is to advise five portions (5 × 80 g) of a variety of fruit and vegetables a day. The benefits stem not only from individual components but also the interaction between these components. Dietary supplements containing isolated minerals and vitamins do not appear to have the same benefits and some studies indicate they may cause harm (Department of Health 1998). For more information about five-a-day and what constitutes a 'portion', go to www.nhs.uk and search on 'five a day'.

- *A higher intake of starch carbohydrates and non-starch polysaccharides* (e.g. potatoes, bread, pulses and pasta) helps provide protection against:
  (a) cardiovascular disease;
  (b) cancers, including breast and colorectal.

- *Reduced intake of saturated fat* (by an average of 11 g per day) and total fat (by 15 g per day). The COMA report recommends simple measures, e.g. reduction in fatty meat and meat products, high-fat dairy products and full-fat spreads, with increased use of skimmed milks and low-fat spreads. High fat intake increases the risk of:
  (a) CHD: modest reductions in saturated fat and salt intake may reduce cardiovascular disease;
  (b) cancers: including colorectal, prostate and breast;
  (c) large bowel disease;
  (d) osteoarthritis.

- *Altered fat intake.* Eating fatty fish may reduce CHD deaths by up to 30%. The COMA report recommends eating at least two portions of fish per week, at least one of which should be fatty, and replacing fats rich in saturated fatty acids with fats and oils low in saturates and rich in monounsaturates.

- *Reduced sodium.* The COMA report recommends an average reduction of salt intake of about 3 g/day. They recommend not adding salt to food and consuming low-salt foods where possible. Common sources of salt are nuts, crisps, canned foods and bread. High sodium intake increases the risk of:
  (a) stroke;
  (b) hypertension;
  (c) stomach cancer;
  (d) osteoporosis.

OBESITY

- The World Health Organization defines overweight as a body mass index (BMI) of 25 kg/m^2 to 29.9 kg/m^2, obesity as $\geq$ 30 kg/m^2 and seriously obese as $\geq$ 40 kg/m^2. See also page 505.

- *Girth* correlates with visceral fat and indirectly measures central adiposity, which is an independent predictor of health risk. A girth of > 94 cm in men and > 80 cm in women is associated with increased health risk (Han, van Leer, Seidell, *et al.* 1995).

- *Prevalence.* Over 50% of the UK population are overweight; 15% are obese. This latter figure doubled between 1980 and 1995.

- *Mortality* increases exponentially with increasing body weight (Jung 1997). The Framingham study suggests that a BMI $\geq$ 30 kg/m^2 reduces life expectancy by about 7 years (Peeters, Barendregt, Willekens, *et al.* 2003).

- The risk of CHD is double if the BMI is > 25 kg/m^2 and nearly quadrupled if = 29 kg/m^2. Asians with a BMI of 22–23 kg/m^2 have an increased risk and > 27.5 kg/m^2 a high risk (Choo 2002).

- Obesity is a risk factor for a number of disorders, e.g. type 2 diabetes, polycystic ovary syndrome, slipped femoral epiphysis, hypertension and cardiovascular disease (see Table 30.1). It is likely that all these risk factors are modulated by the 'metabolic syndrome' (see page 228).

Table 30.1	Relative risk of different diseases in obese versus non–obese people	
DISEASE	**RELATIVE RISK IN WOMEN**	**RELATIVE RISK IN MEN**
Type 2 diabetes	12.7	5.2
Hypertension	4.2	2.6
Heart attack	3.2	1.5
Colon cancer	2.7	3
Angina	1.8	1.8
Gall bladder disease	1.8	1.8
Ovarian cancer	1.7	
Stroke	1.3	1.3

Based on The National Audit Office (NAO). 2001. *Tackling Obesity in England*. The Stationery Office, London. Available: www.google.co.uk (search on 'tackling obesity in England').

● There is now considerable evidence that lifestyle modifications (exercise and diet) can reduce the progression of impaired glucose tolerance to diabetes and hence reduce these risks (Tuomilheto, Lindstrom, Eriksson, *et al.* 2001; Knowler, Barrett–Connor, Fowler, *et al.* 2002; Pan, Li, Hu, *et al.* 1997). Furthermore, it is estimated (SIGN 1996) that a 10 kg loss in weight would lead to falls of total cholesterol by 10%; LDL-cholesterol by 15%; triglycerides by 30%; and a rise of HDL-cholesterol of 8%.

ALCOHOL

Modest alcohol intake (1–3 units a day) protects against CHD (Meister, Whelan and Kava 2000), heart failure (Abramson, Williams, Krumholz, *et al.* 2001) and ischaemic stroke (Sacco, Elkind, Boden-Albala, *et al.* 1999; Berger, Arjani, Kase, *et al.* 1999), but promoting alcohol for this purpose could be hazardous and needs to be balanced against the adverse effects of alcohol.

(a) *CHD*. Keep alcohol intake within safe limits – up to 4 units per day for men and 3 for women, with a daily tally rather than a weekly one (Gaziano and Hennekens 1995) (see also 'Binge drinking', below, and page 486). A higher intake raises LDL cholesterol, triglyceride, blood pressure and calorie intake.

(b) *Cancer*. Several cancers show evidence of a dose–response relation with alcohol intake, e.g. mouth, pharynx, larynx, oesophagus and liver.

In others, there is a possible relationship, e.g. breast and rectum (the latter beer only). Studies indicate that the cancer risk of alcohol multiplies, instead of merely adding to, the risk from smoking (Austoker 1994a). It is estimated that a woman drinking two units of alcohol a day has a lifetime risk of developing breast cancer that is 8% higher than a woman who drinks 1 unit a day (Committee on Carcinogenicity 2004).

(c) *Binge drinking* has been shown to be associated with a seven times higher risk of 'external death' (violence, suicides, injuries, poisonings), and a five times higher risk of fatal myocardial infarction (Kauhanen, Kaplan, Goldberg, *et al.* 1997). Approximately 6% of UK breast cancers could be prevented by reducing intake to a very low level (less than 1 unit a week) (Gaziano and Hennekens 1995). The increase in risk for head and neck cancers can be identified at intakes at and above 40 g/day (≡5 units) (HDA 2002). It has been estimated that 80–90% of cancers of the oral cavity, pharynx and larynx can be avoided by abstaining from smoking or alcohol (Seitz and Homann 2001).

SMOKING

Smoking increases the risk of *the following*.

(a) *Cancers*, including lung (90% are smokers; people smoking 25 cigarettes per day have 25 times the risk), stomach, colon, bladder and renal pelvis (increased five times).

(b) *CHD*. Men under the age of 65 who smoke > 25 cigarettes a day have three times the risk of dying from CHD compared to non-smokers. There is evidence that women who smoke have a 50% higher risk of dying from CHD than men (Prescott, Hippe, Schnohr, *et al.* 1998). The increase in risk is reversible. Someone who smokes 20 a day or less and stops has a risk of CHD 10 years later almost the same as one who has never smoked.

(c) *Stroke and vascular dementia*. Stroke risk is increased almost four times in women smoking > 25 cigarettes a day.

(d) *Peripheral vascular disease*, which is up to twice as common as in non-smokers.

(e) *Diabetes*. Current smoking roughly doubles the risk of developing diabetes (Perry,

Wannamethe, Walker, *et al.* 1995; Rimm, Chan, Stampfer, *et al.* 1995).

(f) *COPD.* Almost all patients with COPD are (or have been) smokers. The rate of fall of FEV_1 is reduced if a patient stops smoking.

(g) *Osteoporotic fractures.* Postmenopausal bone loss is greater in smokers than non-smokers. The risk of hip fracture is estimated to be 17% greater at age 60, 41% greater at age 70 and 71% greater at age 80 in female smokers. The data on men are limited, but the effect appears to be similar (Law and Hackshaw 1997).

(h) *Gastric ulcers,* which are up to twice as common in smokers.

(i) *A poorer outcome of pregnancy.* There is a 60–70% increased risk of ectopic pregnancy, placental abruption, placenta praevia and premature rupture of membranes (Castles, Adams, Melvin, *et al.* 1999). There is a significantly increased risk of miscarriage, low birthweight, admission to a neonatal intensive care unit, perinatal death and sudden infant death syndrome (DiFranza and Lew 1995). Cancers may also be more prevalent in infants of mothers who smoke through their pregnancy (Boffetta, Tredaniel and Greco 2000).

(j) *Blindness.* Smokers carry a three- to four-fold increased risk of age-related macular degeneration, giving 54,000 extra cases of visual impairment in those aged > 69 in the UK. There is evidence that stopping smoking reduces the incidence and progression of the disease (Kelly, Thornton, Lyratzopoulos, *et al.* 2004).

PASSIVE SMOKING (DAVIS 1994; SCIENTIFIC COMMITTEE ON TOBACCO AND HEALTH 1998)

Passive smoking increases the risk of:

(a) *CHD:* the risk is increased by about 25% (He, Vupputuri, Allen, *et al.* 1999);

(b) *lung cancer:* the risk is increased by about 15–25% (Copas and Shi 2000; Taylor, Cumming, Woodward, *et al.* 2001);

(c) respiratory illness and decreased lung function (Spitzer, Lawrence, Dales, *et al.* 1990);

(d) *low-birthweight infants:* infants born to non-smoking women exposed to environmental tobacco smoke are two to four times more likely to be of low birthweight (Misra and Nguyen 1999).

In children

(a) *Respiratory illness.* Children who grow up in households where one or both parents smoke have a significantly higher risk of (Cook and Strachan 1999):

- aged 0–2: wheeze, lower respiratory tract infection and hospital admission for lower respiratory tract infection;
- aged 5–16: asthma, other respiratory symptoms (cough, phlegm, breathlessness), decreased FEV_1;
- recurrent otitis media and middle ear effusion.

(b) *Sudden infant death* (Cook and Strachan 1999).

(c) *Cancer.* The results of exposure to paternal smoke suggest an increased risk of brain tumours and lymphomas (Boffetta, Tredaniel and Greco 2000).

SUN EXPOSURE (AUSTOKER 1994b; ARMSTRONG AND KRICKER 2001)

- Basal cell carcinoma (BCC), squamous cell carcinoma (SCC) and melanoma are all caused by sun exposure.
- The incidence is higher in fair-skinned, sun-sensitive, rather than darker-skinned, less sun-sensitive people.
- The risk increases with increasing solar radiation.
- The highest incidences are on the most sun-exposed parts of the body and lowest densities on the least sun-exposed parts.
- Occupational exposure is associated mainly with SCC, and recreational sun exposure is associated mainly with melanoma and BCC.
- Risk is increased if there is a history of sunburn or the presence of benign skin damage.
- There is evidence that sunscreens reduce the incidence of squamous cell carcinoma and solar keratosis. It is more effective if applied to exposed areas every morning and reapplied after heavy sweating, bathing or prolonged sun exposure (Green 2001).
- The sunscreen should protect against ultraviolet A and B. In patients at high risk, suggest a sun protection factor (SPF) of at least 15 (DTB 1990). Sunscreens should be liberally applied, and reapplied every 2 hours if exposure to the sun continues.

- Fine-woven cotton clothing and hats also screen the skin.
- Exposure to sunlight should be rationed and strong midday sun avoided.
- Children should be protected against strong sunlight at all times. Use a sunscreen with a high sun protection factor (×15), and additional protection against ultraviolet A radiation.
- Do not use sunbeds and sunlamps.

LIFESTYLE CHANGES APPROPRIATE IN SPECIFIC DISEASES

Information about the lifestyle changes that are appropriate in specific diseases are as follows.

(a) Interventions to reduce cardiovascular disease (see page 166).

(b) Intervention to reduce diabetes (see page 228).

(c) **Interventions to reduce the risk of cancer.**
Up to 75% of cancer deaths may be preventable either by lifestyle interventions or early detection. The following lifestyle interventions are known to reduce the risk of cancer although their effect is not accurately quantified:

- *Stopping smoking* (thought to contribute to about a third of all cancers) (Cancer Research UK 2004). Stopping smoking for 10 years halves the risk and the longer the cessation the lower the risk.
- *Dietary changes.* It has been estimated that dietary changes could help prevent up to a third of all cancers (Maynard, Gunnell, Emmett, *et al.* 2003). The strongest evidence is for at least a 50% increase in fruit and vegetable intake (see above).
- *Obesity* is linked to physical activity and diet and has been estimated to contribute to 10% of cancers.
- *Exercise* has a protective effect on colon cancer (CMO 2004; Davey Smith, Shipley, Batty, *et al.* 2000; Batty 2000). The risk in the most active individuals is about 40–50% lower than the least active.
- *Alcohol* is thought to be a major cause in about 3% of all cancers, and 6% of breast cancers, in the UK (HDA 2002).
- *Exposure to sun.* Melanoma accounts for about 2% of cancer cases in the UK (approximately 6,000 cases); non-melanoma skin cancer for about 40,000 cases.

References

Abramson, J.L., Williams, S.A., Krumholz, H.M., et al., 2001. Moderate alcohol consumption and risk of heart failure among older persons. JAMA 285, 1971–1977.

Appel, L., Moore, T., Obarzanek, E., et al., 1997. A clinical trial of the effects of dietary patterns on blood pressure. N. Engl. J. Med. 336, 1117–1123.

Armstrong, B.K., Kricker, A., 2001. The epidemiology of UV induced skin cancer. J. Photochem. Photobiol. B 63, 8–18.

Austoker, J., 1994a. Cancer prevention in primary care: reducing alcohol intake. BMJ 308, 1549–1552.

Austoker, J., 1994b. Melanoma: prevention and early diagnosis. BMJ 308, 1682–1686.

Batty, D., 2000. Does physical activity prevent cancer? BMJ 321, 1424–1425.

Berger, K., Arjani, U.A., Kase, C.S., et al., 1999. Light to moderate alcohol consumption and the risk of stroke among U.S. male physicians. N. Engl. J. Med. 341, 1557–1564.

Boffetta, P., Tredaniel, J., Greco, A., 2000. Risk of childhood cancer and adult lung cancer after childhood exposure to passive smoke: a meta-analysis. Environ. Health Perspect. 108, 73–82.

British Heart Foundation, 1991. Working Group Report. British Heart Foundation, London.

Cancer Research UK, 2002. Smoking and Cancer. CRUK, London.

Cancer Research UK, 2004. Cancer stats, incidence UK. CRUK, London.

Castles, A., Adams, E.K., Melvin, C., et al., 1999. Effects of smoking during pregnancy. Five meta-analyses. Am. J. Prev. Med. 3, 208–215.

Choo, V., 2002. WHO reassesses appropriate body-mass index for Asian populations. Lancet 360, 235.

CMO, 2004. At Least Five a Week: Evidence of the Impact of Physical Activity and its Relationship to Health. Department of Health, London.

Committee on Carcinogenicity, 2004. Consumption of Alcoholic Beverages and Risk of Breast Cancer in Women. Department of

Health, London. Available: www. advisorybodies.doh.gov.uk (search for 'COC/04/S5').

Cook, D.G., Strachan, D.P., 1999. Summary of effects of parental smoking on the respiratory health of children and implications for research. Thorax 54, 357–366.

Copas, J.B., Shi, J.Q., 2000. Reanalysis of epidemiological evidence on lung cancer and passive smoking. BMJ 320, 417–418.

Davey Smith, G., Shipley, M.J., Batty, G.D., et al., 2000. Physical activity and cause specific mortality in the Whitehall study. Public Health 114, 308–315.

Davis, R.M., 1994. Passive smoking: history repeats itself. BMJ 315, 961–962.

Department of Health, 1998. Nutritional Aspects of the Development of Cancer. HMSO, London.

Department of Health, 2001. Exercise Referral Systems: A National Quality Assurance Framework. DoH, London. Available: www. dh.gov.uk (search on 'exercise referrals').

DiFranza, J.R., Lew, R.A., 1995. Effect of maternal cigarette smoking on pregnancy complications and sudden infant death syndrome. J. Fam. Pract. 40, 385–394.

DTB, 1990. Topical sunscreens. Drug Ther. Bull. 28, 61–62.

Elon, R.D., 1996. Geriatric medicine. BMJ 312, 561–563.

Farmer, M.E., Locke, B.Z., Moscicki, C.K., et al., 1985. Physical activity and depressive symptoms: the NHANES 1 epidemiologic follow-up study. Am. J. Epidemiol. 128, 1340–1351.

Gaziano, J.M., Hennekens, C., 1995. Royal Colleges' advice on alcohol consumption. BMJ 311, 3–4.

Green, A., 2001. Squamous cell carcinoma of the skin: non-metastatic. Does the use of sunscreen help to prevent cutaneous squamous cell carcinoma? Clinical Evidence, Issue 5. Update Software, Oxford.

Han, T., van Leer, E., Seidell, J., et al., 1995. Waist circumference action levels in the identification of cardiovascular risk factors: prevalence study in a random sample. BMJ 311, 1401–1405.

HDA, 2002. Cancer Prevention: a Resource to Support Local Action in Delivering the NHS Cancer Plan. Health Development Agency, London. Available: www. publichealth.nice.org.uk (search on 'Cancer prevention').

He, J., Vupputuri, S., Allen, K., et al., 1999. Passive smoking and the risk of coronary heart disease—a meta-analysis of epidemiologic studies. N. Engl. J. Med. 340, 920–926.

Hu, F.B., Letzmann, M.F., Stampfer, M.J., et al., 2001. Physical activity and television watching in relation to risk for type 2 diabetes mellitus in men. Arch. Intern. Med. 161, 1542–1548.

Hu, F.B., Stampfer, M.J., Solomon, C., et al., 1999. Walking compared to vigorous physical activity and risk of type 2 diabetes in women. JAMA 282, 1433–1439.

John, J., Ziebland, S., Yudkin, P., et al., 2002. Effects of fruit and vegetable consumption on plasma antioxidant concentrations and blood pressure: a randomised controlled trial. Lancet 359, 1969–1974.

Jung, R.T., 1997. Obesity as a disease. Br. Med. Bull. 53, 307–321.

Kauhanen, J., Kaplan, G.A., Goldberg, D.E., et al., 1997. Beer binging and mortality: results from the Kuopio ischaemic heart disease risk factor study, a prospective population based study. BMJ 315, 846–851.

Kelly, S., Thornton, J., Lyratzopoulos, G., et al., 2004. Smoking and blindness. BMJ 328, 537–538.

Knowler, W.C., Barrett–Connor, E., Fowler, S.E., et al., 2002. Reduction in the incidence of type 2 diabetes with lifestyle intervention or metformin. N. Engl. J. Med. 346, 393–403.

Law, M.R., Hackshaw, A.K., 1997. A meta-analysis of cigarette smoking, bone mineral density and risk of hip fracture: recognition of a major effect. BMJ 315, 841–846.

Manson, J.E., Hu, F.B., Rich–Edwards, J.W., et al., 1999. A prospective study of walking as compared with vigorous exercise in the prevention of coronary heart disease in women. N. Engl. J. Med. 341, 650–658.

Martinsen, E.W., Medhus, A., Sandvik, L., 1985. Effects of aerobic exercise on depression: a controlled study. BMJ 291, 109.

Maynard, M., Gunnell, D., Emmett, P., et al., 2003. Fruit, vegetables and antioxidants in childhood and risk of adult cancer: the Boyd Orr cohort. J. Epidemiol. Community Health 57, 218–225.

Meister, K.A., Whelan, E.M., Kava, R., 2000. The health effects of moderate alcohol intake in humans: an epidemiologic review. CRC Crit. Rev. Clin. Lab. Sci. 37, 261–296.

Misra, D.P., Nguyen, R.H., 1999. Environmental tobacco smoke and low birth weight: a hazard in the workplace? Environ. Health Perspect. 107 (Suppl. 6), 897–904.

North, T.C., McCullagh, P., Zung vu Tran, A., 1990. The effect of exercise on depression. Exerc. Sport Sci. Rev. 80, 379–416.

Pan, X.R., Li, G.W., Hu, Y.H., et al., 1997. Effects of diet and exercise in preventing NIDDM in people with impaired glucose tolerance. The Da Qing IGT and Diabetes Study. Diabetes Care 20, 537–544.

Peeters, A., Barendregt, J.J., Willekens, F., et al., 2003. Obesity in adulthood and its consequence for life expectancy: a life table analysis. Ann. Intern. Med. 138, 24–32.

Perry, I.J., Wannamethe, S.G., Walker, M.K., et al., 1995. Prospective study of risk factors for development of non-insulin dependent diabetes in middle-aged British men. BMJ 310, 560–564.

Powell, K.E., Pratt, M., 1996. Physical activity and health. BMJ 313, 126–127.

Prescott, E., Hippe, M., Schnohr, P., et al., 1998. Smoking and the risk of myocardial infarction in women and men: longitudinal population study. BMJ 316, 1043–1047.

Report of the Cardiovascular Review Group of the Committee on Medical Aspects of Food Policy (COMA), 1994. Nutritional Aspects of Cardiovascular Disease. Report of Health and Social Subjects, 46. DoH, London.

Rimm, E.B., Chan, J., Stampfer, M.J., et al., 1995. Prospective study of cigarette smoking, alcohol use, and the risk of diabetes in men. BMJ 310, 555–559.

Sacco, R., Elkind, M., Boden–Albala, B., et al., 1999. The protective effect of moderate alcohol consumption on ischemic stroke. JAMA 281, 53–60.

Scientific Committee on Tobacco and Health, 1998. Report of the Scientific Committee on Tobacco and Health. Stationery Office, London.

Seitz, H.-K., Homann, N., 2001. Effect of alcohol on the orogastro-intestinal tract, the pancreas and the liver. In: Heather, N., Peters, T.J., Stockwell, T. (eds), International Handbook of Alcohol Dependence and Problems. Wiley, Chichester.

Shephard, R.J., Futcher, R., 1997. Physical activity and cancer: how may protection be maximized? Crit. Rev. Oncog. 8, 219–272.

Shephard, R.J., Shek, P.N., 1999. Exercise, immunity, and susceptibility to infection: a J-shaped relationship? The Physician and Sports Medicine. Available: www.physsportsmed. com.

SIGN, 1996. Obesity in Scotland. Integrating Prevention with Weight Management. Scottish Intercollegiate Guidelines Network, Edinburgh.

Spitzer, W.O., Lawrence, V., Dales, R., et al., 1990. Links between passive smoking and disease: a best-evidence synthesis. A report of the Working Group on Passive Smoking. Clin. Invest. Med. 1, 17–42.

Taylor, R., Cumming, R., Woodward, A., et al., 2001. Passive smoking and lung cancer: a cumulative meta-analysis. Aust. N. Z. J. Public Health 3, 203–211.

Tinetti, M.E., Baker, D.I., McAvay, G., et al., 1994. A multifactorial intervention to reduce the risk of falling among elderly people living in the community. N. Engl. J. Med. 330, 1769–1773.

Trichopoulou, A., 2005. Modified Mediterranean diet and survival: EPIC-elderly prospective cohort study. BMJ 330, 991–995.

Tuomilheto, J., Lindstrom, J., Eriksson, J.G., et al., 2001. Prevention of type 2 diabetes mellitus by changes in lifestyle among subjects with impaired glucose tolerance. N. Engl. J. Med. 344, 1343–1349.

Appendices

Appendix 1 ROUTINE SCHEDULE OF IMMUNISATIONS

AGE	IMMUNIZATION
2 months	DTaP/ IPV/ Hib and PCV
3 months	DTaP/ IPV/ Hib and Men C
4 months	DTaP/ IPV/ Hib and Men C and PCV
12 months	Hib/MenC
13–15 months	MMR and PCV
3 years 4 months–5 years (preschool)	DTaP/ IPV, or dTaP/ IPV, and MMR
13–18 years	Td/ IPV plus MMR (two doses) and Men C (one dose) if not already given
18–24 years	Men C (one dose) if not already given
65 onwards	Flu annually and PCV once
Girls aged 12–13	Cervarix

aP = acellular pertussis; D = diphtheria; d = low dose diphtheria; flu = influenza; Hib = *H. influenzae* b; IPV = inactivated polio vaccine; Men C = meningococcal C; MMR = mumps, measles and rubella; PCV = pneumococcal vaccine; T = tetanus.

Appendix 2 INCUBATION PERIOD AND INFECTIVITY OF COMMON DISEASES

DISEASE	INCUBATION PERIOD	PERIOD OF INFECTIVITY	EXCLUSION FROM SCHOOL OR NURSERY
Bacillary dysentery	1–7 days	Mean 7 days	Children under 5: 1 negative stool. Others, until 24 hours after last diarrhoea
Campylobacter	1–10 days	1–3 weeks	For 24 hours after last diarrhoea
Cryptosporidiosis	1–14 days	2–4 weeks	For 24 hours after last diarrhoea
Enteroviral infection	2–3 days	1–2 weeks	None
E. coli enteritis	2–48 hours or longer	12 days or longer	24 hours after last diarrhoea 48 hours if aged < 5 or with poor hygiene. However, with *E. coli* 0157 exclude until 2 negative stools.
Gastroenteritis (rotaviral)	2–4 days	6–10 days	24 hours from last diarrhoea or vomiting
Gastroenteritis (adenoviral)	8–10 days	7–14 days	24 hours from last diarrhoea or vomiting

Continued

Appendix 2   INCUBATION PERIOD AND INFECTIVITY OF COMMON DISEASES—Cont'd

DISEASE	INCUBATION PERIOD	PERIOD OF INFECTIVITY	EXCLUSION FROM SCHOOL OR NURSERY
Gastroenteritis (Norwalk virus)	4–77 hours	0–3 days	3 days after onset
Gastroenteritis (unidentified)	N/A	N/A	For duration of the illness
Giardiasis	5–20 days	2 weeks	24 hours from last diarrhoea
Salmonellosis	4 hours to 5 days	Adults 4 weeks (median). Children under 5 up to 1 year	Children under 5: 1 negative stool. Others, until 24 hours after last diarrhoea
Typhoid and paratyphoid	3–56 days	2 weeks to indefinite	Until 24 hours after last diarrhoea
Other diseases			
Chickenpox	11–20 days	–4 to +5 days	5 days from start of rash
Conjunctivitis	3–29 days	2 weeks	None
Haemophilus influenzae	4–5 days	Indefinite (untreated)	24 hours from start of antibiotics
Head lice	N/A	Indefinite (untreated)	None
Hand, foot and mouth disease	3–5 days	7 days	None
Hepatitis A	2–6 weeks	–17 days to +2 weeks	Only exclude children < 5 years old, for 5 days from start of illness.
Hepatitis B	6 weeks to 6 months or longer		From onset to appearance of anti-HBe
Herpes simplex	1–6 days	1–8 weeks (primary infection) 1–3 days (recurrence)	None
Impetigo	N/A	N/A	Until lesions crusted
Infectious mononucleosis	33–49 days	At least 2 months	None
Influenza	1–3 days	? 1–3 weeks	None
Measles	9–18 days	–2 to +3 days	From prodromal symptoms to 5 days after the onset of the rash
Meningococcal disease	N/A	Indefinite (untreated) < 2 days (treated)	For the duration of the illness
Meningococcal infection	2–10 days		Until 48 hours after starting treatment
Mumps	15–24 days	Days –6 to +4	3 days before to 5 days after the start of the swelling
Pertussis	5–21 days	6 weeks or more, or 1 week if given a macrolide	7 days after exposure to 3 weeks after the onset of typical cough (shortened to 7 days with a macrolide)
Rabies	9 days to 9 weeks (possibly up to 2 years)	Until death	N/A
Rubella	15–20 days	Day 1 to 6	1 week before the rash appears to 5 days after
Scabies	7–27 days	Indefinite until treated	Until effectively treated
Scarlet fever	½–5 days	3 days if treated	10–21 days after the onset of the rash; 5 days after penicillin started
Rabies	9 days to 9 weeks (possibly up to 2 years)	Until death	N/A
Rubella	15–20 days	Day 1 to 6	1 week before the rash appears to 5 days after
Scabies	7–27 days	Indefinite until treated	Until effectively treated
Scarlet fever	½–5 days	3 days if treated	10–21 days after the onset of the rash; 5 days after penicillin started
Slapped cheek disease	13–18 days	–6 to –3 i.e. prodrome only	None
Streptococcal pharyngitis	½–5 days	Indefinite (untreated)	None
Tetanus	4–21 days	Not contagious	None
Threadworms	2–4 weeks	Indefinite	None
Tinea	2–4 weeks	Indefinite	None
Tuberculosis	4 weeks to years	Smear positive: until 2 weeks after starting treatment	Until 2 weeks after starting treatment (but none if smear negative)
Warts	1–24 months	While present	None

Appendix 3 A SUGGESTED TABLE OF IMMUNISATIONS FOR TRAVEL

This schedule is for an adult who has been fully immunised as a child according to the UK recommendations. Few travellers will need all the immunisations below; they should only be given if appropriate to the travel planned.

Day 0	Rabies, Japanese encephalitis, tick-borne encephalitis, hepatitis B
Day 7	Rabies, Japanese encephalitis
Day 14	Tick-borne encephalitis
Day 28	Rabies, Japanese encephalitis, hepatitis B
At some point in the above schedule (either together or spread out over the month). Immunisation early in the month (at least 1 week before departure) will allow time for immunity to develop	BCG, cholera, hepatitis A, meningococcal ACWY, polio, tetanus and diphtheria (as Td), typhoid, yellow fever

If exposure to risk continues, further immunisations against hepatitis B will be needed at 2 months and at 1 year from the first dose, and against tick-borne encephalitis at 9 months to 1 year after the last dose.

Appendix 4 NOTIFICATION OF INFECTIOUS DISEASES

The notification of the following diseases is required by law in the UK, and the doctor is not excused from notification by considerations of confidentiality. The following list applies to England and Wales, with variations for Scotland and Northern Ireland indicated.

Acute encephalitis*	Plague
Acute poliomyelitis	Relapsing fever
Anthrax	Rubella
Cholera	Scarlet fever
Diphtheria	Smallpox
Dysentery (amoebic or bacillary)	Tetanus[†]
Food poisoning	Tuberculosis
Suspected food poisoning	Typhoid fever
Leprosy*[†]	Typhus
Leptospirosis[†]	Viral haemorrhagic fever
Malaria[†]	Viral hepatitis
Measles	Whooping cough
Meningitis	Yellow fever*
Meningococcal septicaemia	
Mumps	
Ophthalmia neonatorum*[†]	
Paratyphoid fever	

*Not notifiable in Scotland, where chickenpox, erysipelas, Legionella infection, Lyme disease, membranous croup, puerperal fever and toxoplasmosis are notifiable.
[†]Not notifiable in Northern Ireland, where chickenpox, gastroenteritis in children under 2 years old, and Legionella infection are notifiable.

Appendix 5 CHILD HEALTH PROMOTION

HISTORY AND EXAMINATION	HEALTH EDUCATION
Neonatal examination	
(a) Elicit and consider concerns expressed by the parents	(a) Feeding and nutrition
(b) Review family history, pregnancy and birth	(b) Sleeping position
(c) Assess risk of hearing defect and refer accordingly	(c) Baby care
(d) Full physical examination, including weight and head circumference	(d) Sibling management

Continued

Appendix 5   CHILD HEALTH PROMOTION—Cont'd

HISTORY AND EXAMINATION	HEALTH EDUCATION
(e) Check for CDH and testicular descent (f) Inspect eyes, check red reflex (g) Check PKU and thyroid tests have been done (h) Screen for haemoglobinopathy, if relevant	(e) Crying and sleep problems (f) Transport in a car
First 2 weeks	
In addition to the neonatal examination: (a) Assess the level of support and assistance that each new parent is likely to require	(a) Nutrition (b) The effects of passive smoking (c) Accident prevention – bathing, scalding by feeds, fires (d) Immunisation
6–8 weeks	
(a) Check history, review growth and development and ask about parental concerns. (b) Physical examination, weight, head circumference (and length, if indicated). (c) Check for CDH (d) Enquire about concerns regarding vision, squint and hearing (e) Check whether the baby is in the high-risk category for hearing loss and refer if necessary (f) Discuss and perform immunisations	(a) Immunisation (b) Nutrition (c) Dangers of fires, falls, overheating and scalds (d) Recognition of illness and what to do
2, 3 and 4 months	
(a) Primary immunisations	
6–9 months	
(a) Enquire about parental concerns regarding health and development, vision and hearing (b) Look for evidence of CDH (c) Check for testicular descent (d) Observe visual behaviour and look for squint (e) Distraction test for hearing (HV)	(a) Accident prevention –choking, scalds and burns (including sunburn), falls (b) Anticipate increased mobility (e.g. safety gates, guards, etc.) (c) Nutrition (d) Dental prophylaxis (e) Reinforce advice about safety in cars and passive smoking (f) Developmental needs
18–24 months	
(a) Enquire about parental concerns particularly regarding behaviour, vision and hearing (b) Confirm that the child is walking with a normal gait, and that speech and comprehension are appropriate for age (c) Arrange detailed vision, hearing or language assessment if indicated (d) Remember the prevalence of iron deficiency anaemia (e) Measure height Note: Inform the community paediatric services if there is any anxiety about a child's educational potential	(a) Accident prevention – falls from heights, drowning, poisoning, road safety (b) Nutrition (c) Developmental needs – language and play (d) Need to mix with other children – playgroup, etc. (e) Avoidance and management of behaviour problems
36–54 months	
(a) Enquiry and discussion about vision, squint, hearing and behaviour, language acquisition and development (b) Discuss, if appropriate, whether the child is likely to have special educational problems and refer as appropriate (c) Measure the height and chart it (d) Refer for hearing test if concerned	(a) Accidents – fires, roads, drowning (b) Road safety (c) Preparation for school (d) Nutrition and dental care

Adapted from annex to DOH letter PL/CMO(92)3, PL/CNO(92)3, with permission.

Appendix 6 STAGES OF CHILD DEVELOPMENT

Summary of development: birth to 16 weeks

	0–4 WEEKS	6–8 WEEKS	12–16 WEEKS
Social	Watches mother and may smile	Responsive smile by 6 weeks and vocalises	Recognises family, shows pleasure
Motor			
Ventral suspension	Head hangs down until 3–4 weeks then up momentarily	Head held in horizontal plane, and briefly up by 8 weeks	Head maintained well above plane of body by 12 weeks
Prone	Head to side, pelvis high, knees drawn up under abdomen	Chin up intermittently at 6 weeks, well up at 8 weeks Pelvis flat	Head and shoulders up, and chest by 16 weeks Weight on forearms
Supine	Head to side, limbs flexed or ATNR* posture	ATNR posture common but head to midline by 8 weeks	ATNR declining Head and hands now to midline
Pull-to-sit	Complete head lag	Less head lag	Slight head lag
Held sitting	Very round back Head drops forward	Back rounded Head briefly up	Back straighter and head up
Held standing	Walking and placing reflexes present until 6 weeks	Sags at hips and knees, getting head up by 8 weeks	Increasingly bears weight on legs
Hands	Strong grasp reflex Hands often closed	Grasp reflex present but slight by 8 weeks. Fingers extend more often	Grasp reflex fades between 12 and 16 weeks Can hold rattle briefly
Vision	Blink and pupil reflexes Eye righting reflex Random movements but can fixate	Smoother conjugate eye movements Fixates on face/objects and follows through 45°–90°	Follows through 130° Hand regard common (12–20 weeks)
Vocalisation/ hearing	Cries, stills or startles to sounds	Eyes turn to sounds Starts vocalising	Varied coos, squeals and laughs Turns to sounds

*ATNR: asymmetric tonic neck reflex

Summary of development: 4–10 months

	4–6 MONTHS	6–8 MONTHS	8–10 MONTHS
Personal and social behaviour	Responsive to all comers Smiles at self in mirror Excited at approach of food	Discriminates between family and strangers Attracts attention Hand feeds biscuit	Wary of strangers Waves bye-bye Attempts to use spoon
Gross motor	No head lag in traction Rolls prone to supine Back straight in supported sitting	Lifts head up in supine Rolls supine to prone/creeps Sits without lateral support Bears weight on feet (5–8 months)	Sits steadily, pivots and leans Can get from prone to sitting Pulls self to stand and crawls
Fine motor and vision	Reaches and grasps toys (4–6 months) Plays with toes Very alert visually	Transfers cube hand to hand (5–7 months) Can hold two cubes Any squint reported after 6 months is abnormal	Pincer grasp of pellet (8–12 months) Releases object and looks for it (7–11 months) Points at 1 mm sweet
Language and hearing	Varied sounds and squeals Consonants such as ba or da	Starts to babble da-da Turns to sounds (4–8 months)	Varied babble ma-ma, ba-ba, da-da Indicates and understands 'No' Locates sounds well

Appendix 6 STAGES OF CHILD DEVELOPMENT—Cont'd

Summary of development: 12–24 months

	12–15 MONTHS	18–24 MONTHS
Personal and social behaviour	Shows affection and may be shy Indicates wants, points, claps hands (10–18 months) Mouthing stops (12–15 months) Enjoys casting (12–15 months) May manage cup and spoon with spills (10–17 months)	Becoming egocentric, clinging and resistant Loves domestic mimicry Definitely stopped mouthing and casting (by 18 months) Helps undress Independent with cup and spoon (15–24 months)
Gross motor	Walks holding on (8–12 months) Walks alone (11–15 months)	Walks well (12–18 months) Climbs stairs, kneels (14–22 months)
Fine motor and vision	Fine pincer grasp Bangs bricks together (8–14 months) Holds two cubes Scribbles (12–18 months)	May show hand preference (after 15 months) Builds 2 to 3 cubes Turns pages (15–24 months)
Language and hearing	Mama, Dada, with meaning (9–15 months) Three to four clear words (12–18 months)	Can point to 3 parts of body, has 6 to 20 words and jargon (15–24 months)

Summary of development: 2–5 years

	2–3 YEARS	3–4 YEARS	5 YEARS OLD
Personal and social skills	Enjoys solitary play, alongside peers, not sharing Possessive: tantrums if thwarted Feeds quite neatly, using spoon and fork or fingers May be clean and dry by day, with supervision, or may refuse to cooperate	Plays with peers, sharing toys Enjoys make-believe play Shows concern and sympathy for others, and able to take turns by 4 years Easily manages spoon and fork and then knife Mostly dry day and night Can wash hands, dress and undress by 4 years, except fastenings	Plays complicated cooperative games Makes friends Comforts playmates and siblings in distress Almost completely independent in self-help skills now Can carry out simple domestic tasks and run errands
Gross motor	Now very mobile Runs, kicks ball, tries to throw Walks up and down stairs two feet to a step Propels tricycle by pushing with feet on floor	Up stairs one foot per step at 3, and down by 4 years Can walk, then run on tip-toe, and hop, by 4 years Enjoys climbing, pedals a tricycle skilfully	Enjoys running, jumping, climbing, swings and slides, and starting to play ball games Can stand on one leg, hop 10 times and heel-toe walk a narrow line
Fine motor and vision	Neat prehension, and controlled release Tower of 6–8 bricks Holds pencil in fist Circular scribble (24 months) copies vertical line, imitates circle (30 months) Simple puzzles and can thread large beads Difficult age to test vision Recognises two-dimensional symbols and may match letters at 30 months	Tower of 9–10 and imitates 3 cube bridge at 3 years, steps or gate by 4 years Awkward tripod grasp of pencil at 3 years – copies circle and imitates cross Dynamic tripod after 4 years; draws man with head, trunk and legs Can do letter-matching vision tests, using linear charts, each eye separately, by 3½ to 4 years	Can write name, copy a square and a triangle Draws man with detailed features and limbs Can fold paper and use scissors to cut out shapes Performs Snellen chart type of vision test
Language and hearing	Listens to simple stories and understands two-part instructions Can say 50–100 single words and join two to three: (Daddy gone car) Many questions – what? and who? Long monologues, still some jargon, enjoys nursery rhymes and jingles Toy tests of hearing or may point to named pictures	Intelligible but immature speech, 3–5 word sentences, knows name and sex, at 3 years Long stories, constant more abstract questions, grammar mostly correct, and speech clear, by 4 years Knows age and address, 6+ colours and can count to 4+ Can do cooperative (conditioned) hearing tests	Enjoys riddles and jokes Understands negatives and complex questions and instructions Gives long descriptions and explanations Speech easily intelligible with few errors Manages full audiometry and speech discrimination now

Appendix 7 STAGES OF PUBERTY

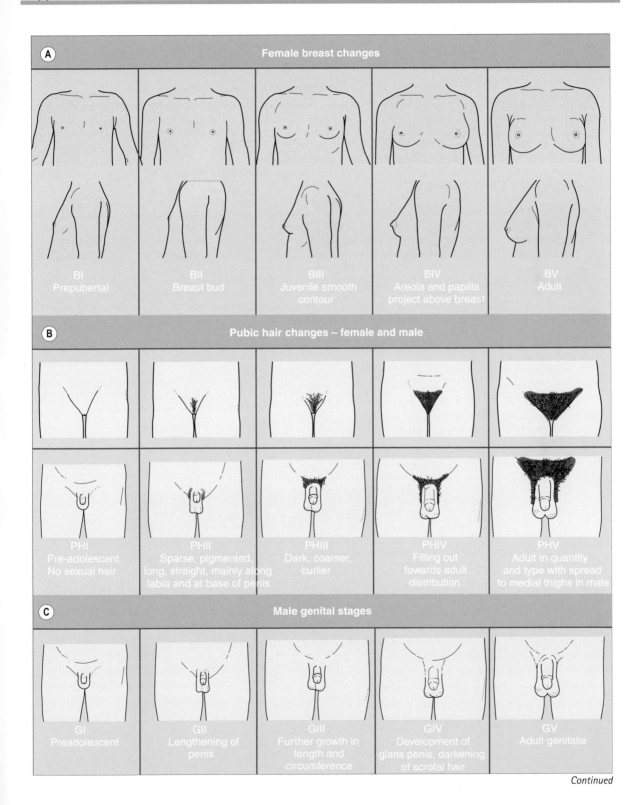

A   Female breast changes

BI
Prepubertal

BII
Breast bud

BIII
Juvenile smooth
contour

BIV
Areola and papilla
project above breast

BV
Adult

B   Pubic hair changes – female and male

PHI
Pre-adolescent
No sexual hair

PHII
Sparse, pigmented,
long, straight, mainly along
labia and at base of penis

PHIII
Dark, coarser,
curlier

PHIV
Filling out
towards adult
distribution

PHV
Adult in quantity
and type with spread
to medial thighs in male

C   Male genital stages

GI
Preadolescent

GII
Lengthening of
penis

GIII
Further growth in
length and
circumference

GIV
Development of
glans penis, darkening
of scrotal hair

GV
Adult genitalia

Continued

Appendix 7 STAGES OF PUBERTY—Cont'd

(a) The stages of breast development in a female. Stage 1 (BI): Preadolescent: elevation in papilla only. Stage 2 (BII): Breast bud stage: elevation of breast and papilla as a small mound. Enlargement of areolar diameter. Stage 3 (BIII): Further enlargement and elevation of breast and areola, with no separation of their contours. Stage 4 (BIV): Projection of areola and papilla to form a secondary mound above the level of the breast. Stage 5 (BV): Mature stage; projection of papilla only, due to recession of the areola to the general contour of the breast. (This last stage may not be reached in women until after their first pregnancy.)

(b) Pubic hair development: male and female. Stage 1 (PHI): Preadolescent. The vellus over the pubes is not further developed than that over the abdominal wall, i.e. no pubic hair. Stage 2 (PHII): Sparse growth of long, slightly pigmented downy hair, straight or slightly curled, chiefly at the base of the penis or along the labia. Stage 3 (PHIII): Considerably darker, coarser and more curled. The hair spreads sparsely over the junction of the pubes. Stage 4 (PHIV): Hair now adult in type, but area covered is still considerably smaller than in the adult. No spread to the medial surface of the thighs. Stage 5 (PHV): Adult in quantity and type with distribution of the horizontal (or classically feminine) pattern. Spread to medial surface of thighs but not up linea alba or elsewhere above the base of the inverse triangle (spread up linea alba occurs later and is rated Stage 6).

(c) Male genital development. Stage 1 (GI): Preadolescent: testes, scrotum and penis are of about the same size and proportion as in early childhood. Stage 2 (GII): Enlargement of scrotum and testes. Skin of scrotum reddens and changes in texture. Little or no enlargement of penis at this stage. Stage 3 (GIII): Enlargement of penis, which occurs at first mainly in length. Further growth of testes and scrotum. Stage 4 (GIV): Increased size of penis with growth in breadth and development of glans. Testes and scrotum larger; scrotal skin darkened. Stage 5 (GV): Genitalia adult in size and shape. (The volume of the adult testis varies in size from 12 to 25 mL.)
Both sexes: axillary hair. Stage 1: Preadolescent. No axillary hair. Stage 2: Scanty growth of slightly pigmented hair. Stage 3: Hair adult in quality and quantity.

With permission from Lissauer T, Clayden G. Illustrated Textbook of Paediatrics. 3rd edition. London: Mosby; 2005

Appendix 8 PREDICTED NORMAL PEAK FLOW VALUES IN CHILDREN (UNDER 15 YEARS OF AGE)

HEIGHT		PEAK FLOWS (L/MIN)
(CM)	(FT IN)	
91	3–0	100
99	3–3	120
107	3–6	140
114	3–9	170
122	4–0	210
130	4–3	250
137	4–6	285
145	4–9	325
152	5–0	360
160	5–3	400
168	5–6	440
175	5–9	480

Appendix 9 PEAK EXPIRATORY FLOW IN NORMAL SUBJECTS

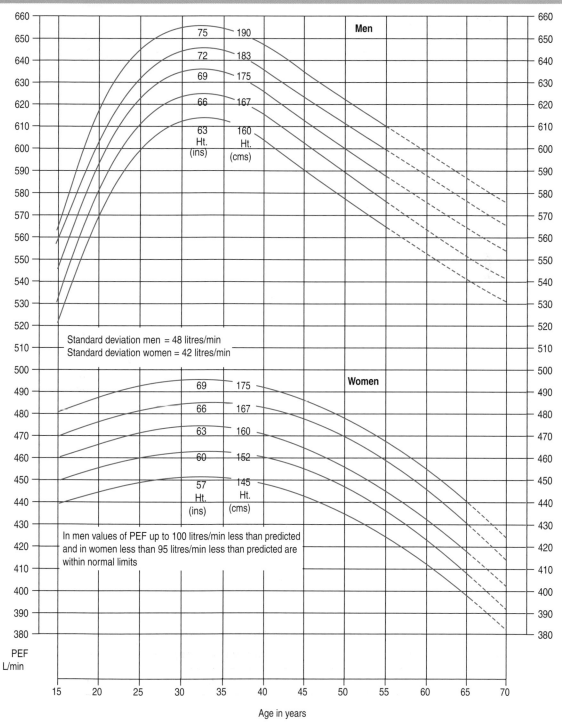

Appendix 10 FEV$_1$/FVC CHARTS

Females

AGE (YEARS)		HEIGHT (M)							
		1.45	1.50	1.55	1.60	1.65	1.70	1.75	1.80
25	FEV$_1$	2.5	2.7	2.9	3.1	3.4	3.6	3.8	4.0
	FVC	2.9	3.1	3.3	3.6	3.8	4.0	4.2	4.4
30	FEV$_1$	2.4	2.6	2.8	3.0	3.2	3.4	3.7	3.9
	FVC	2.8	3.0	3.2	3.4	3.6	3.9	4.1	4.3
35	FEV$_1$	2.3	2.5	2.7	2.9	3.1	3.3	3.5	3.7
	FVC	2.6	2.9	3.1	3.3	3.5	3.7	4.0	4.2
40	FEV$_1$	2.1	2.3	2.6	2.8	3.0	3.2	3.4	3.6
	FVC	2.5	2.7	2.9	3.2	3.4	3.6	3.8	4.0
45	FEV$_1$	2.0	2.2	2.4	2.6	2.9	3.1	3.3	3.5
	FVC	2.4	2.6	2.8	3.0	3.3	3.5	3.7	3.9
50	FEV$_1$	1.9	2.1	2.3	2.5	2.7	2.9	3.2	3.4
	FVC	2.2	2.5	2.7	2.9	3.1	3.3	3.6	3.8
55	FEV$_1$	1.8	2.0	2.2	2.4	2.6	2.8	3.0	3.2
	FVC	2.1	2.3	2.6	2.8	3.0	3.2	3.4	3.7
60	FEV$_1$	1.6	1.8	2.1	2.3	2.5	2.7	2.9	3.1
	FVC	2.0	2.2	2.4	2.6	2.9	3.1	3.3	3.5
65	FEV$_1$	1.5	1.7	1.9	2.1	2.4	2.6	2.8	3.0
	FVC	1.8	2.1	2.3	2.5	2.7	3.0	3.2	3.4
70	FEV$_1$	1.4	1.6	1.8	2.0	2.2	2.4	2.7	2.9
	FVC	1.7	1.9	2.2	2.4	2.6	2.8	3.0	3.3

Males

AGE (YEARS)		HEIGHT (M)							
		1.55	1.60	1.65	1.70	1.75	1.80	1.85	1.90
25	FEV$_1$	3.4	3.6	3.8	4.1	4.3	4.5	4.7	5.0
	FVC	3.9	4.2	4.5	4.8	5.1	5.4	5.7	6.0
30	FEV$_1$	3.3	3.5	3.7	3.9	4.2	4.4	4.6	4.8
	FVC	3.8	4.1	4.4	4.7	5.0	5.3	5.5	5.8
35	FEV$_1$	3.1	3.3	3.6	3.8	4.0	4.2	4.5	4.7
	FVC	3.7	4.0	4.3	4.5	4.8	5.1	5.4	5.7
40	FEV$_1$	3.0	3.2	3.4	3.6	3.9	4.1	4.3	4.5
	FVC	3.6	3.8	4.1	4.4	4.7	5.0	5.3	5.6
45	FEV$_1$	2.8	3.0	3.3	3.5	3.7	3.9	4.2	4.4
	FVC	3.4	3.7	4.0	4.3	4.6	4.9	5.2	5.4
50	FEV$_1$	2.7	2.9	3.1	3.3	3.6	3.8	4.0	4.2
	FVC	3.3	3.6	3.9	4.2	4.4	4.7	5.0	5.3
55	FEV$_1$	2.5	2.8	3.0	3.2	3.4	3.7	3.9	4.1
	FVC	3.2	3.5	3.7	4.0	4.3	4.6	4.9	5.2
60	FEV$_1$	2.4	2.6	2.8	3.1	3.3	3.5	3.7	4.0
	FVC	3.0	3.3	3.6	3.9	4.2	4.5	4.8	5.0
65	FEV$_1$	2.2	2.5	2.7	2.9	3.1	3.4	3.6	3.8
	FVC	2.9	3.2	3.5	3.8	4.1	4.3	4.6	4.9
70	FEV$_1$	2.1	2.3	2.5	2.8	3.0	3.2	3.4	3.7
	FVC	2.8	3.1	3.3	3.6	3.9	4.2	4.4	4.8

Appendix 10 FEV$_1$/FVC CHARTS—Cont'd

Girls

HEIGHT		FEV$_1$	FVC
METRES	INCHES		
0.80	32	0.41	0.46
0.90	35	0.56	0.64
1.00	39	0.75	0.86
1.10	43	0.98	1.11
1.20	47	1.24	1.43
1.30	51	1.55	1.79
1.40	55	1.90	2.20
1.50	59	2.29	2.68
1.60	63	2.73	3.22
1.70	67	3.23	3.82
1.80	71	3.77	4.48

Boys

HEIGHT		FEV$_1$	FVC
METRES	INCHES		
0.80	32	0.40	0.46
0.90	35	0.56	0.65
1.00	39	0.76	0.89
1.10	43	1.00	1.17
1.20	47	1.28	1.52
1.30	51	1.61	1.92
1.40	55	2.00	2.38
1.50	59	2.43	2.92
1.60	63	2.93	3.53
1.70	67	3.49	4.22
1.80	71	4.11	4.99

Appendix 11A SUMMARY OF STEPWISE MANAGEMENT OF ASTHMA IN ADULTS

Patients should start treatment at the step most appropriate to the initial severity of their asthma. Check concordance and reconsider diagnosis if response to treatment is unexpectedly poor.

MOVE UP TO IMPROVE CONTROL AS NEEDED

MOVE DOWN TO FIND AND MAINTAIN LOWEST CONTROLLING STEP

STEP 1
Mild intermittent asthma

Inhaled short-acting β_2 agonist as required

STEP 2
Regular preventer therapy

Add inhaled steroid 200-800 mcg/day*

400 mcg is an appropriate starting dose for many patients

Start at dose of inhaled steroid appropriate to severity of disease.

STEP 3
Initial add-on therapy

1. Add inhaled long-acting β_2 agonist (LABA)
2. Assess control of asthma:
   - **good response to LABA** - continue LABA
   - **benefit from LABA but control still inadequate** - continue LABA and increase inhaled steroid dose to 800 mcg/day* (if not already on this dose)
   - **no response to LABA** - stop LABA and increase inhaled steroid to 800 mcg/day.*If control still inadequate, institute trial of other therapies, leukotriene receptor antagonist or SR theophylline

STEP 4
Persistent poor control

Consider trials of:
- increasing inhaled steroid up to 2000 mcg/day*
- addition of a fourth drug e.g. leukotriene receptor antagonist, SR theophylline, β_2 agonist tablet

STEP 5
Continuous or frequent use of oral steroids

Use daily steroid tablet in lowest dose providing adequate control

Maintain high dose inhaled steroid at 2000 mcg/day*

Consider other treatments to minimise the use of steroid tablets

Refer patient for specialist care

* **BDP or equivalent**

SYMPTOMS   vs   TREATMENT

Appendix 11B SUMMARY OF STEPWISE MANAGEMENT OF ASTHMA IN CHILDREN AGED 5–12

Patients should start treatment at the step most appropriate to the initial severity of their asthma. Check concordance and reconsider diagnosis if response to treatment is unexpectedly poor.

MOVE UP TO IMPROVE CONTROL AS NEEDED

MOVE DOWN TO FIND AND MAINTAIN LOWEST CONTROLLING STEP

STEP 1
Mild intermittent asthma

Inhaled short-acting β_2 agonist as required

STEP 2
Regular preventer therapy

Add inhaled steroid 200–400 mcg/day* (other preventer drug if inhaled steroid cannot be used) 200 mcg is an appropriate starting dose for many patients

Start at dose of inhaled steroid appropriate to severity of disease.

STEP 3
Initial add-on therapy

1. Add inhaled long-acting β_2 agonist (LABA)
2. Assess control of asthma:
   - good response to LABA
     - continue LABA
   - benefit from LABA but control still inadequate
     - continue LABA and increase inhaled steroid dose to 400 mcg/day* (if not already on this dose)
   - no response to LABA
     - stop LABA and increase inhaled steroid to 400 mcg/day.* If control still inadequate, institute trial of other therapies, leukotriene receptor antagonist or SR theophylline

STEP 4
Persistent poor control

Increase inhaled steroid up to 800 mcg/day*

STEP 5
Continuous or frequent use of oral steroids

Use daily steroid tablet in lowest dose providing adequate control

Maintain high dose inhaled steroid at 800 mcg/day*

Refer to respiratory paediatrician

SYMPTOMS   vs   TREATMENT

* BDP or equivalent

Reproduced with permission from Scottish Intercollegiate Guidelines Network and the British Thoracic Society. British Guideline on the Management of Asthma. SIGN Guideline No. 101. Edinburgh: SIGN; 2008, revised 2009. Available online: www.sign.ac.uk/

Appendix 11C SUMMARY OF STEPWISE MANAGEMENT OF ASTHMA IN CHILDREN UNDER 5

MOVE UP TO IMPROVE CONTROL AS NEEDED

Patients should start treatment at the step most appropriate to the initial severity of their asthma. Check concordance and reconsider diagnosis if response to treatment is unexpectedly poor.

MOVE DOWN TO FIND AND MAINTAIN LOWEST CONTROLLING STEP

Inhaled short-acting β₂ agonist as required

STEP 1
Mild intermittent asthma

Add inhaled steroid 200–400 mcg/day*†
or leukotriene receptor antagonist if inhaled steroid cannot be used.

Start at dose of inhaled steroid appropriate to severity of disease.

STEP 2
Regular preventer therapy

In those children taking inhaled steroids 200–400 mcg/day consider addition of leukotriene receptor antagonist.

In those children taking a leukotriene receptor antagonist alone reconsider addition of an inhaled steroid 200–400 mcg/day.

In children under 2 years consider proceeding to step 4.

STEP 3
Initial add-on therapy

Refer to respiratory paediatrician.

STEP 4
Persistent poor control

SYMPTOMS vs **TREATMENT**

* BDP or equivalent
† Higher nominal doses may be required if drug delivery is difficult

Management of acute severe asthma in adults in general practice

Many deaths from asthma are preventable. Delay can be fatal. Factors leading to poor outcome include:

- Clinical staff. Failing to assess severity by objective measurement
- Patients or relatives failing to appreciate severity
- Under-use of corticosteriods

Regard each emergency asthma consultation as for acute severe asthma until shown otherwise.

Assess and record:

- Peak expiratory flow (PEF)
- Symptoms and response to self treatment
- Heart and respiratory rates
- Oxygen saturation (by pulse oximetry)

Caution: Patients with severe or life threatening attacks may not be distressed and may not have all the abnormalities listed below. The presence of any should alert the doctor.

Moderate asthma	Acute severe asthma	Life threatening asthma

INITIAL ASSESSMENT

PEF > 50-75% best or predicted	PEF 33-50% best or predicted	PEF < 33% best or predicted

FURTHER ASSESSMENT

■ $SpO_2 \geq 92\%$	■ $SpO_2 \geq 92\%$	■ $SpO_2 < 92\%$
■ Speech normal	■ Can't complete sentences	■ Silent chest, cyanosis or poor respiratory effort
■ Respiration < 25 breaths/min	■ Respiration ≥ 25 breaths/min	■ Arrhythmia or hypotension
■ Pulse < 110 beats/min	■ Pulse ≥ 110 beats/min	■ Exhaustion, altered consciousness

MANAGEMENT

Treat at home or in surgery and ASSESS RESPONSE TO TREATMENT	Consider admission	Arrange immediate ADMISSION

TREATMENT

■ β_2 bronchodilator:- - Via spacer (give 4 puffs initially and give a further 2 puffs every 2 minutes according to response up to maximum of 10 puffs) If PEF > 50-75% predicted/best: ■ nebuliser (preferably oxygen driven) (salbutamol 5 mg or terbutaline 10 mg) ■ Give prednisolone 40-50 mg ■ Continue or step up usual treatment If good response to first treatment *(symptoms improved, respiration and pulse settling and PEF > 50%) continue or step up usual treatment and continue prednisolone*	■ Oxygen to maintain SpO_2 94-98% if available ■ β_2 bronchodilator: - nebuliser (preferably oxygen driven) (salbutamol 5 mg or terbutaline 10 mg) - Or via spacer (give 4 puffs initially and give a further 2 puffs every 2 minutes according to response up to maximum of 10 puffs) ■ Prednisolone 40-50 mg or IV hydrocortisone 100 mg ■ **If no response in acute severe asthma: ADMIT**	■ Oxygen to maintain SpO_2 94-98% ■ β_2 bronchodilator and ipratropium: - nebuliser (preferably oxygen driven) (salbutamol 5 mg or terbutaline 10 mg) and (ipratropium 0.5 mg) - Or via spacer (give 4 puffs initially and give a further 2 puffs every 2 minutes according to response up to maximum of 10 puffs) ■ Prednisolone 40-50 mg or IV hydrocortisone 100 mg immediately

Admit to hospital if any: ■ life threatening features ■ features of acute severe asthma present after initial treatment ■ previous near-fatal asthma Lower threshold for admission if **afternoon or evening attack, recent nocturnal symptoms or hospital admission, previous severe attacks, patient unable to assess own condition, or concern over social circumstances.**	**If admitting the patient to hospital:** ■ Stay with patient until ambulance arrives ■ Send written assessment and referral details to hospital ■ β_2 bronchodilator via oxygen-driven nebuliser in ambulance	**Follow up after treatment or discharge from hospital:** ■ **GP review within 48 hours** ■ Monitor symptoms and PEF ■ Check inhaler technique ■ Written asthma action plan ■ Modify treatment according to guidelines for chronic persistent asthma ■ Address potentially preventable contributors to admission

Appendix 11E   MANAGEMENT OF ACUTE ASTHMA IN CHILDREN IN GENERAL PRACTICE

Management of acute asthma in children in general practice

Age 2–5 years

ASSESS ASTHMA SEVERITY

Moderate asthma
- $SpO_2 \geq 92\%$
- Able to talk
- Heart rate ≤ 140/min
- Respiratory rate ≤ 40/min

Severe asthma
- $SpO_2 < 92\%$
- Too breathless to talk
- Heart rate > 140/min
- Respiratory rate > 40/min
- Use of accessory neck muscles

Life threatening asthma
$SpO_2 < 92\%$ plus any of:
- Silent chest
- Poor respiratory effort
- Agitation
- Altered consciousness
- Cyanosis

- β_2 agonist 2–10 puffs via spacer ± facemask
- Consider soluble prednisolone 20 mg

- Oxygen via face mask
- 2–10 puffs of β_2 agonist [give 2 puffs, every 2 minutes according to response up to maximum of 10 puffs] or nebulised salbutamol 2.5 mg or terbutaline 5 mg
- Soluble prednisolone 20 mg

- Oxygen via face mask
- Nebulise:
  - salbutamol 2.5 mg or terbutaline 5 mg
  +
  - ipratropium 0.25 mg
- Soluble prednisolone 20 mg or IV hydrocortisone 50 mg

Increase β_2 agonist dose by 2 puffs every 2 minutes according to response up to 10 puffs

Assess response to treatment 15 mins after β_2 agonist

IF POOR RESPONSE ARRANGE ADMISSION

IF POOR RESPONSE REPEAT β_2 AGONIST AND ARRANGE ADMISSION

REPEAT β_2 AGONIST VIA OXYGEN-DRIVEN NEBULISER WHILST ARRANGING IMMEDIATE HOSPITAL ADMISSION

GOOD RESPONSE
- Continue β_2 agonist via spacer or nebuliser, as needed but not exceeding 4-hourly
- **If symptoms are not controlled repeat β_2 agonist and refer to hospital**
- Continue prednisolone for up to 3 days
- Arrange follow-up clinic visit

POOR RESPONSE
- Stay with patient until ambulance arrives
- Send written assessment and referral details
- Repeat β_2 agonist via oxygen-driven nebuliser in ambulance

NB: If a patient has signs and symptoms across categories, always treat according to their most severe features

LOWER THRESHOLD FOR ADMISSION IF:
- Attack in late afternoon or at night
- Recent hospital admission or previous severe attack
- Concern over social circumstances or ability to cope at home

---

Age > 5 years

ASSESS ASTHMA SEVERITY

Moderate asthma
- $SpO_2 \geq 92\%$
- PEF ≥ 50% best or predicted
- Able to talk
- Heart rate ≤ 125/min
- Respiratory rate ≤ 30/min

Severe asthma
- $SpO_2 < 92\%$
- PEF 33–50% best or predicted
- Too breathless to talk
- Heart rate > 125/min
- Respiratory rate > 30/min
- Use of accessory neck muscles

Life threatening asthma
$SpO_2 < 92\%$ plus any of:
- PEF < 33% best or predicted
- Silent chest
- Poor respiratory effort
- Agitation
- Altered consciousness
- Cyanosis

- β_2 agonist 2–10 puffs via spacer
- Consider soluble prednisolone 30–40 mg

- Oxygen via face mask
- 2–10 puffs of β_2 agonist [give 2 puffs, every 2 minutes according to response up to maximum of 10 puffs] or nebulised salbutamol 2.5–5 mg or terbutaline 5–10 mg
- Soluble prednisolone 30–40 mg

- Oxygen via face mask
- Nebulise:
  - salbutamol 5 mg or terbutaline 10 mg
  +
  - ipratropium 0.25 mg
- Soluble prednisolone 30–40 mg or IV hydrocortisone 100 mg

Increase β_2 agonist dose by 2 puffs every 2 minutes according to response up to 10 puffs

Assess response to treatment 15 mins after β_2 agonist

IF POOR RESPONSE ARRANGE ADMISSION

IF POOR RESPONSE REPEAT β_2 AGONIST AND ARRANGE ADMISSION

REPEAT β_2 AGONIST VIA OXYGEN-DRIVEN NEBULISER WHILST ARRANGING IMMEDIATE HOSPITAL ADMISSION

GOOD RESPONSE
- Continue β_2 agonist via spacer or nebuliser, as needed but not exceeding 4-hourly
- **If symptoms are not controlled repeat β_2 agonist and refer to hospital**
- Continue prednisolone for up to 3 days
- Arrange follow-up clinic visit

POOR RESPONSE
- Stay with patient until ambulance arrives
- Send written assessment and referral details
- Repeat β_2 agonist via oxygen-driven nebuliser in ambulance

NB: If a patient has signs and symptoms across categories, always treat according to their most severe features

LOWER THRESHOLD FOR ADMISSION IF:
- Attack in late afternoon or at night
- Recent hospital admission or previous severe attack
- Concern over social circumstances or ability to cope at home

---

Reproduced with permission from Scottish Intercollegiate Guidelines Network and the British Thoracic Society. British Guideline on the Management of Asthma. SIGN Guideline No. 101.

Appendix 12 CARE PATHWAY FOR RESPIRATORY TRACT INFECTIONS

Care pathway for respiratory tract infections (RTI's)

At the first face-to-face contact in primary care, including walk-in centres and emergency departments, offer a clinical assessment, including:
• history (presenting symptoms, use of over-the-counter or self medication, previous medical history, relevant risk factors, relevant comorbidities
• examination as needed to establish diagnosis

Address patients' or parents'/carers' concerns and expectations when agreeing the use of the three antibiotic strategies (no prescribing, delayed prescribing and immediate prescribing)

Agree a no antibiotic or delayed antibiotic prescribing strategy for patients with acute otitis media, acute sore throat/acute pharyngitis/acute tonsillitis, common cold, acute rhinosinusitis or acute cough/acute bronchitis

However, also consider an immediate prescribing strategy for the following subgroups,depending on the severity of the RTI

The patient is at risk of developing complications

No antibiotic prescribing
Offer patients:
• reassurance that antibiotics are not needed immediately because they will make little difference to symptoms and may have side effects, for example, diarrhoea, vomiting and rash
• a clinical review if the RTI worsens or becomes prolonged

Delayed antibiotic prescribing
Offer patients:
• reassurance that antibiotics are not needed immediately because they will make little difference to symptoms and may have side effects, for example, diarrhoea, vomiting and rash
• advice about using the delayed prescription if symptoms do not settle or get significantly worse
• advice about re-consulting if symptoms get significantly worse despite using the delayed prescription
The delayed prescription with instructions can either be given to the patient or collected at a later date

No antibiotic, delayed antibiotic or immediate antibiotic prescribing
Depending on clinical assessment of severity, also consider an immediate prescribing strategy for:
• children younger than 2 years with bilateral acute otitis media
• children with otorrhoea who have acute otitis media
• patients with acute sore throat/acute pharyngitis/acute tonsillitis when 3 or more Centor criteria* are present

Immediate antibiotic prescribing or further investigation and/or management
Offer immediate antibiotics or further investigation/management for patients who:
• are systemically very unwell
• have symptoms and signs suggestive of serious illness and/or complications (particularly pneumonia, mastoiditis, peritonsillar abscess, peritonsillar cellulitis, intraorbital or intracranial complications
• are at high risk of serious complications because of pre-existing comorbidity. This includes patients with significant heart, lung, renal, liver or neuromuscular disease, immunosuppression, cystic fibrosis, and young children who were born prematurely
• are older than 65 years with acute cough and 2 or more of the following, or older than 80 years with acute cough and 1 or more of the following:
  – hospitalisation in previous year
  – type 1 or type 2 diabetes
  – history of congestive heart failure
  – current use of oral glucocorticoids

Offer all patients:
• advice about the usual natural history of the illness and average total illness length
  – acute otitis media: 4 days
  – acute sore throat/acute pharyngitis/acute tonsilitis: 1 week
  – common cold: 1½ weeks
  – acute rhinosinusitis: 2½ weeks
  – acute cough/acute bronchitis: 3 weeks

• advice about managing symptoms including fever (particularly analgesics and antipyretics). For information about fever in children younger than 5 years, refer to 'Feverish illness in children' (NICE clinical guideline 47).

*Centor criteria are: presence of tonsillar exudate, tender anterior lymphadenopathy or lymphadenitis, history of fever and an absence of cough

Reproduced with permission from NICE Clinical Guideline No. 69: Respiratory Tract Infections - antibiotic prescribing. July 2008.

Appendix 13 MONITORING PATIENTS TAKING DISEASE MODIFYING ANTIRHEUMATIC DRUGS (DMARDS)

> **Guideline:** Chakravarty K, McDonald H, Pullar T, et al. BSR/BHPR guideline for disease-modifying anti-rheumatic drug (DMARD) therapy in consultation with the British Association of Dermatologists. *Rheumatology* (Oxford). 2008;47:924-925. http://rheumatology.oxfordjournals.org/cgi/data/kel216a/DC1/1. The tables below are reproduced from this guideline with the permission of Oxford University Press.

Note that in addition to absolute values for haematological indices a rapid fall or a consistent downward trend in any value should prompt caution and extra vigilance.

Methotrexate

* **Pre-treatment assessment:** FBC, U&E, LFT and CXR (unless CXR done within the last 6 months). Consider pulmonary function tests in selected patients.
* **Monitor** FBC, U&E, LFT every 2 weeks until dose of methotrexate and monitoring stable for 6 weeks; thereafter monthly until the dose and disease is stable for 1 yr.
* Thereafter **reduce the monitoring frequency,** based on clinical judgement with due consideration for risk factors including age, comorbidity, renal impairment, etc when monthly monitoring is to continue.

Threshold for action	Action to be taken
WBC $< 3.5\ 10^9/l$	Withhold until discussed with specialist team.
Neutrophils $< 2.0\ 10^9/l$	Withhold until discussed with specialist team.
Platelets $< 150\ 10^9/l$	Withhold until discussed with specialist team.
AST, ALT > twice upper limit of reference range	Withhold until discussed with specialist team.
Albumin - unexplained fall (in absence of active disease)	Withhold until discussed with specialist team.
Rash or oral ulceration, nausea and vomiting, or diarrhoea	Withhold until discussed with specialist team.
New or increasing dyspnoea or dry cough	Withhold and discuss urgently with specialist team.
MCV> 105 fl	Withhold and check serum B_{12}, Folate and TFTs and discuss with specialist team if necessary.
Mild to moderate renal impairment	Withhold until discussed with specialist team
Severe sore throat, abnormal bruising	Immediate FBC and withhold until the result of FBC is available.

Sulfasalazine

* **Pre-treatment assessment:** FBC, U&E's creatinine, LFTs.
* **Monitoring:** FBC and LFTs monthly for the first 3 months and 3 monthly thereafter. If, following the first year, dose and blood results have been stable, frequency of blood tests can be reduced to every 6 months for the second year of treatment. Thereafter, monitoring of blood for toxicity may be stopped.
* Patient should be asked about the presence of rash or oral ulceration at each visit.
* **Following dose changes:** Repeat FBC, LFT one month after dose increases

Threshold for action	Action to be taken
WBC < 3.5 10^9/l	Withhold until discussed with specialist team.
Neutrophils < 2.0 10^9/l	Withhold until discussed with specialist team.
Platelets < 150 10^9/l	Withhold until discussed with specialist team.
AST, ALT > twice upper limit of reference range	Withhold until discussed with specialist team.
MCV > 105 fl	Check B_{12}, folate and TSH. If abnormal, treat any underlying abnormality. If normal, discuss with the specialist team.
Nausea/dizziness/headache	If possible continue, may have to reduce dose or stop if symptoms severe. Discuss with specialist team.
Abnormal bruising or severe sore throat	Check FBC immediately and withhold until results available. Discuss with the specialist team, if necessary.
Unexplained acute widespread rash	Withhold. Seek urgent specialist (preferably dermatological) advice.
Oral ulceration	Withhold until discussed with specialist team.

Gold

Pretreatment assessment: FBC, urinalysis, U&E's, LFT's.
Monitoring: Monthly FBC and urinalysis. Patient should be asked about the presence of rash or oral ulceration at each visit.

Threshold for action	Action to be taken
WBC < 3.5x10^9 /l	withhold until discussed with rheumatologist
Neutrophils < 2.0x10^9 /l	withhold until discussed with rheumatologist
Platelets < 150x10^9 /l	withhold until discussed with rheumatologist
Eosinophilia > 0.5x10^9/l	Caution: increase vigilance
Proteinuria 2+ or more	Check MSU: If evidence of infection, treat appropriately. If sterile and 2+ proteinuria or more persists, withhold until discussed with rheumatologist
Rash or oral ulceration	withhold until discussed with rheumatologist
Abnormal bruising or sore throat	withhold until FBC result available

Leflunomide

(a) Pre-treatment assessment FBC, U&E's creatinine and LFTs. Blood pressure and weight.

(b) Monitoring FBC, LFTs every month for 6 months and, if stable, 2 monthly thereafter. Blood checks should be continued at least once a month, if co-prescribed with another immunosuppressant or potentially hepatotoxic agent. Blood pressure and weight should be checked at each monitoring visit.

Threshold for action	Action to be taken
WBC< 3.5 10^9/1	Withhold until discussed with specialist team.
Neutrophils< 2.0 10^9/l	Withhold until discussed with specialist team.
Platelets< 150 10^9/l	Withhold until discussed with specialist team.
AST, ALT between two and three times the upper limit of reference range.	If the current dose is more than 10mg daily reduce the dose to 10mg daily and recheck weekly until normalized. If the AST & ALT is returning to normal, leave on 10mg a day. If LFTs remain elevated withdraw the drug and discuss with the specialist team.
AST, ALT more than three times the upper limit of reference range	Recheck LFTs within 72 h, if still more than three times the reference range, stop drug and consider referral for washout.
Rash or itch	Consider dosage reduction with or without antihistamines; if severe, stop and consider referral for washout
Hair loss	Consider dosage reduction; if severe, stop and consider washout
Abnormal bruising or severe sore throat	Check FBC immediately and withhold until results are available.
Hypertension If BP$> 140/90$	treat in line with NICE guidance. If BP remains uncontrolled, stop leflunomide and consider washout
Headache	If severe, consider dosage reduction. If headaches persist, stop and consider washout
GI upset (nausea, diarrhoea)	If loading dose has been used, give symptomatic treatment. If steady state has been reached, give symptomatic treatment and consider dosage reduction. If symptoms are severe or persistent, stop and consider washout
Weight loss	Monitor carefully. If $> 10\%$ weight loss with no other cause identified, reduce dosage or stop and consider washout
Breathlessness	If increasing shortness of breath occurs, stop leflunomide and consider washout

Appendix 14 Dermatomes and Myotomes

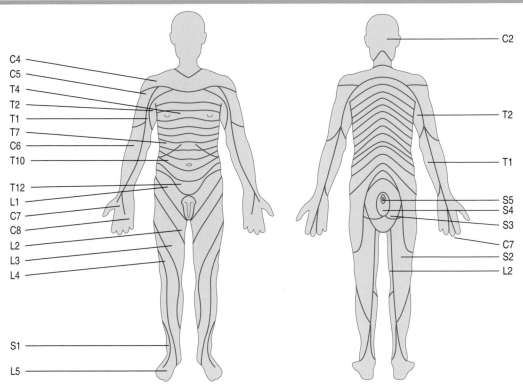

Muscle group	Nerve supply	Reflexes
Diaphragm	C(3), 4, (5)	
Shoulder abductors	C5	
Elbow flexors	C5, 6	Biceps jerk C5, 6
Supinators/pronators	C6	Supinator jerk C6
Wrist extensors	C6	
Wrist flexors	C7	
Elbow extensors	C7	Triceps jerk C7
Finger extensors	C7	
Finger flexors	C8	
Intrinsic hand muscles	T1	Abdominal reflex T8–12
Hip flexors	L1, 2	
Hip adductors	L2, 3	
Knee extensors	L3, 4	Knee jerk L3, 4
Ankle dorsiflexors	L4, 5	
Toe extensors	L5	
Knee flexors	L4, 5 S1	
Ankle plantar flexors	S1, 2	Ankle jerk S1, 2
Toe flexors	S1, 2	
Anal sphincter	S2, 3, 4	Bulbocavernosus reflex S3, 4
		Anal reflex S5
		Plantar reflex

Appendix 15 TESTING PERIPHERAL NERVES

NERVE ROOT	MUSCLE	TEST — BY ASKING THE PATIENT TO
C3, 4	Trapezius	Shrug shoulder, adduct scapula
C4, 5	Rhomboids	Brace shoulder back
C5, 6, 7	Serratus anterior	Push forward against resistance
C5, 6, 7, 8	Pectoralis major (clavicular head)	Adduct arm from above horizontal and forward
C6, 7, 8 T1	Pectoralis major (sternocostal head)	Adduct arm below horizontal
C5	Supraspinatus	Abduct arm the first 15°
C5, 6	Infraspinatus	Externally rotate arm, elbow at side
C6, 7, 8	Latissimus dorsi	Adduct horizontal and lateral arm
C5, 6	Biceps	Flex supinated forearm
C5, 6	Deltoid	Abduct arm between 15° and 90°
Radial nerve		
C7, 8	Triceps	Extend elbow against resistance
C5, 6	Brachioradialis	Flex elbow with forearm half way between pronation and supination
C6, 7	Extensor carpi radialis longus	Extend wrist to radial side with fingers extended
C5, 6	Supinator	Arm by side, resist hand pronation
C7, 8	Extensor digitorum	Keep fingers extended at MCP joint
C7, 8	Extensor carpi ulnaris	Extend wrist to ulnar side
C7, 8	Abductor pollicis longus	Abduct thumb at 90° to palm
C7, 8	Extensor pollicis brevis	Extend thumb at MCP joint
C7, 8	Extensor pollicis longus	Resist thumb flexion at IP joint
Median nerve		
C6, 7	Pronator teres	Keep arm pronated against resistance
C6, 7, 8	Flexor carpi radialis	Flex wrist towards radial side
C7, 8, T1	Flexor digitorum sublimis	Resist extension at PIP joint (while you fix the proximal phalanx)
C8, T1	Flexor digitorum profundus I and II	Resist extension at the DIP joint
C8, T1	Flexor pollicis longus	Resist thumb extension at interphalangeal joint (fix proximal phalanx)
C8, T1	Abductor pollicis brevis	Abduct thumb (nail at 90° to palm)
C8, T1	Opponens pollicis	Thumb touches 5th finger-tip (nail parallel to palm)
C8, T1	1st and 2nd lumbricals	Extend PIP joint against resistance with MCP joint held hyperextended
Ulnar nerve		
C7, 8	Flexor carpi ulnaris	Abducting little finger, see tendon when all fingers extended
C8, T1	Flexor digitorum profundus III and IV	Fix middle phalanx of little finger, resisting extension of distal phalanx
C8, T1	Dorsal interossei	Abduct fingers (use index finger)
C8, T1	Palmar interossei	Adduct fingers (use index finger)
C8, T1	Adductor pollicis	Adduct thumb (nail at 90° to palm)
C8, T1	Abductor digiti minimi	Abduct little finger
C8, T1	Opponens digiti minimi	With fingers extended, carry little finger in front of other fingers
Nerve Root		
L4,5, S1	Gluteus medius and minimus (superior gluteal nerve)	Internal rotation at hip, hip abduction
L5, S1, 2	Gluteus maximus (inferior gluteal nerve)	Extension at hip (lie prone)
L2, 3, 4	Adductors (obturator nerve)	Adduct leg against resistance

Femoral nerve		
L1, 2, 3	Iliopsoas	Flex hip with knee flexed and lower leg supported (patient lies on back)
L2, 3	Sartorius	Flex knee with hip externally rotated
L2, 3, 4	Quadriceps femoris	Extend knee against resistance
Sciatic nerve		
L4, 5, S1, 2	Hamstrings	Flex knee against resistance
L4, 5	Tibialis posterior	Invert plantar-flexed foot
L4, 5	Tibialis anterior	Dorsiflex ankle
L5, S1	Extensor digitorum longus	Dorsiflex toes against resistance
L5, S1	Extensor hallucis longus	Dorsiflex hallux against resistance
L5, S1	Peroneus longus and brevis	Exert foot against resistance
S1	Extensor digitorum brevis	Dorsiflex hallux (muscle of foot)
S1, 2	Gastrocnemius	Plantar flex ankle joint
S1, 2	Flexor digitorum longus	Flex terminal joints of toes
S1, 2	Small muscles of foot	Make sole of foot into a cup

Source: Medical Research Council. *Aids to the Examination of the Peripheral Nervous System* (1976) London: HMSO; 1976. Crown copyright material is reproduced with the permission of the Controller of HMSO and the Queen's Printer for Scotland.

Appendix 16 DRUG LEVELS

DRUG	THERAPEUTIC RANGE
For the following drugs, blood should be taken pre-dose:	
Carbamazepine	4–12 mg/L
Ethosuximide	40–100 mg/L
Phenobarbital	20–40 mg/L
Phenytoin	10–20 mg/L (child: 6–14 mg/L)
Primidone	As for phenobarbital
Theophylline	10–20 mg/L
For the following drugs, blood should be taken at the times indicated:	
Digoxin (8–12 hours after last dose)	0.6–2.0 µl/L toxicity 1.8–3.0 µg/L
Lithium (12 hours after last dose)	0.4–1.0 mmol/L
Valproate (2 hours after last dose)	50–100 mg/L

Appendix 17 CHECKLIST TO GUIDE THE REVIEW OF A PATIENT WITH MULTIPLE SCLEROSIS

This is not a list of questions to be asked of every person with MS on every occasion. It is a list to remind clinicians of the wide range of potential problems that people with MS may face, and which should be actively considered as appropriate. A positive answer should lead to more detailed assessment and management.

INITIAL QUESTION

It is best to start by asking an open-ended question such as:

'Since you were last seen or assessed has any activity you used to undertake been limited, stopped or affected?'

Activity domains

Then, especially if nothing has been identified, it is worth asking questions directly, choosing from the list below those appropriate to the situation based on your knowledge of the person with MS:

'Are you still able to undertake, as far as you wish:

- vocational activities (work, education, other occupation)?
- leisure activities?
- family roles?
- shopping and other community activities?
- household and domestic activities?
- washing, dressing, using toilet?
- getting about (either by walking or in other ways) and getting in and out of your house?
- controlling your environment (opening doors, switching things on and off, using the phone)?'

If restrictions are identified, then the reasons for these should be identified as far as possible considering impairments (see below), and social and physical factors (contexts).

Common impairments

It is worth asking about specific impairments from the list below, again adapting to the situation and what you already know:

'Since you were last seen have you developed any new problems with:

- fatigue, endurance, being overtired?
- speech and communication?
- balance and falling?
- chewing and swallowing food and drink?
- unintended change in weight?
- pain or painful abnormal sensations?
- control over your bladder or bowels?
- control over your movement?
- vision and your eyes?
- thinking, remembering?
- your mood?
- your sexual function or partnership relations?
- how you get on in social situations?'

Final question

Finally, it is always worth finishing with a further open-ended question:

'Are there any other new problems that you think might be due to MS that concern you?'.

Reproduced with permission from NICE Clinical Guidelines No. 3. *Management of multiples sclerosis in primary and secondary care.*

Appendix 18 OBSTETRICAL TABLE

	1	2	3	4	5	6	7	8	9	10	11	12	13	14	15	16	17	18	19	20	21	22	23	24	25	26	27	28	29	30	31	
January	1	2	3	4	5	6	7	8	9	10	11	12	13	14	15	16	17	18	19	20	21	22	23	24	25	26	27	28	29	30	31	January
October	8	9	10	11	12	13	14	15	16	17	18	19	20	21	22	23	24	25	26	27	28	29	30	31	1	2	3	4	5	6	7	November
February	1	2	3	4	5	6	7	8	9	10	11	12	13	14	15	16	17	18	19	20	21	22	23	24	25	26	27	28	–	–	–	February
November	8	9	10	11	12	13	14	15	16	17	18	19	20	21	22	23	24	25	26	27	28	29	30	1	2	3	4	5	–	–	–	December
March	1	2	3	4	5	6	7	8	9	10	11	12	13	14	15	16	17	18	19	20	21	22	23	24	25	26	27	28	29	30	31	March
December	6	7	8	9	10	11	12	13	14	15	16	17	18	19	20	21	22	23	24	25	26	27	28	29	30	31	1	2	3	4	5	January
April	1	2	3	4	5	6	7	8	9	10	11	12	13	14	15	16	17	18	19	20	21	22	23	24	25	26	27	28	29	30	–	April
January	6	7	8	9	10	11	12	13	14	15	16	17	18	19	20	21	22	23	24	25	26	27	28	29	30	31	1	2	3	4	–	February
May	1	2	3	4	5	6	7	8	9	10	11	12	13	14	15	16	17	18	19	20	21	22	23	24	25	26	27	28	29	30	31	May
February	5	6	7	8	9	10	11	12	13	14	15	16	17	18	19	20	21	22	23	24	25	26	27	28	1	2	3	4	5	6	7	March
June	1	2	3	4	5	6	7	8	9	10	11	12	13	14	15	16	17	18	19	20	21	22	23	24	25	26	27	28	29	30	–	June
March	8	9	10	11	12	13	14	15	16	17	18	19	20	21	22	23	24	25	26	27	28	29	30	31	1	2	3	4	5	6	–	April
July	1	2	3	4	5	6	7	8	9	10	11	12	13	14	15	16	17	18	19	20	21	22	23	24	25	26	27	28	29	30	31	July
April	7	8	9	10	11	12	13	14	15	16	17	18	19	20	21	22	23	24	25	26	27	28	29	30	1	2	3	4	5	6	7	May
August	1	2	3	4	5	6	7	8	9	10	11	12	13	14	15	16	17	18	19	20	21	22	23	24	25	26	27	28	29	30	31	August
May	8	9	10	11	12	13	14	15	16	17	18	19	20	21	22	23	24	25	26	27	28	29	30	31	1	2	3	4	5	6	7	June
September	1	2	3	4	5	6	7	8	9	10	11	12	13	14	15	16	17	18	19	20	21	22	23	24	25	26	27	28	29	30	–	September
June	8	9	10	11	12	13	14	15	16	17	18	19	20	21	22	23	24	25	26	27	28	29	30	1	2	3	4	5	6	7	–	July
October	1	2	3	4	5	6	7	8	9	10	11	12	13	14	15	16	17	18	19	20	21	22	23	24	25	26	27	28	29	30	31	October
July	8	9	10	11	12	13	14	15	16	17	18	19	20	21	22	23	24	25	26	27	28	29	30	31	1	2	3	4	5	6	7	August
November	1	2	3	4	5	6	7	8	9	10	11	12	13	14	15	16	17	18	19	20	21	22	23	24	25	26	27	28	29	30	–	November
August	8	9	10	11	12	13	14	15	16	17	18	19	20	21	22	23	24	25	26	27	28	29	30	31	1	2	3	4	5	6	–	September
December	1	2	3	4	5	6	7	8	9	10	11	12	13	14	15	16	17	18	19	20	21	22	23	24	25	26	27	28	29	30	31	December
September	7	8	9	10	11	12	13	14	15	16	17	18	19	20	21	22	23	24	25	26	27	28	29	30	1	2	3	4	5	6	7	October

The rows in the table are in pairs. Find the date of the first day of the patient's last menstrual period in the top row of a pair. The date immediately below it is the expected date of delivery.

Appendix 19 IMMUNISATIONS IN PREGNANCY

Immunisations Contraindicated in Pregnancy	
Vaccine	Comments
BCG	Live mycobacterium
Cholera (oral)	No evidence of safety; benefit unlikely to outweigh theoretical risk
Measles	Live virus. Avoid pregnancy for 3 months after vaccination
Mumps	Live virus. Avoid pregnancy for 3 months after vaccination
Rubella	Live virus. Avoid pregnancy for 3 months after vaccination
Typhoid Ty21a	Live bacterium
Varicella	Live virus. Consider giving VZIG if exposed to chickenpox in pregnancy
Yellow fever	Live virus. Give patient a written waiver if travelling to a country requiring a certificate. If risk of contracting the disease is high the patient may choose to have the immunisation.

Immunisations which may be given in pregnancy if patient and physician judge that the potential benefit outweighs the risk
That risk is theoretical. In almost all of these immunisations there is no evidence either way. If deciding to give the immunisation, it may be thought prudent to waiting until the second or third trimester in case a reaction to the vaccine were to trigger a first trimester miscarriage.

Vaccine	Comments
Diphtheria/tetanus	
Hepatitis A	The patient may choose immunoglobulin as a safer alternative
Hepatitis B	
Immunoglobulin	
Influenza	The vaccine is positively indicated in pregnant women at risk. They are more prone to pulmonary complications than non-pregnant women.
Japanese encephalitis	Inactivated virus but there is no consensus on its safety
Meningococcus	
Pneumococcus	
Polio (oral)	Paralysis seems more likely in pregnancy than in the non-pregnant woman. Neonatal infection carries a high mortality rate.
Rabies	
Typhoid (Vi capsular polysaccharide)	

Adapted from: Centers for Disease Control and Prevention. CDC Health Information for International Travel 2008. Mosby; Atlanta, Georgia; NICE. *Antenatal care: routine care for the healthy pregnant woman.* National Collaborating Centre for Women's and Children's Health. Commissioned by the National Institute for Health and Clinical Excellence. Clinical Guideline 62; 2008. http://www.nice.org.uk and Martinez L (ed). International Travel and Health. World Health Organization, Geneva; 2002.

Appendix 20 EDINBURGH POSTNATAL DEPRESSION SCALE

Instructions for users

1. The mother is asked to underline the response which comes closest to how she has been feeling in the previous 7 days.
2. All 10 items must be completed.
3. Care should be taken to avoid the possibility of the mother discussing her answers with others.
4. The mother should complete the scale herself, unless she has limited English or has difficulty with reading.
5. The EPDS may be used at 6–8 weeks to screen postnatal women. The child health clinic, postnatal check-up or a home visit may provide suitable opportunities for its completion.

Scoring the EPDS

- Response categories are scored 0, 1, 2 and 3 according to increased severity of the symptom.
- Items marked with an asterisk are reverse scored (i.e. 3, 2, 1 and 0). The total score is calculated by adding together the scores for each of the 10 items.
- Mothers who score above a threshold 12/13 are likely to be suffering from a depressive illness of varying severity. Nevertheless, the EPDS score should not override clinical judgement. A careful clinical assessment should be carried out to confirm the diagnosis. The scale indicates how the mother has felt during the previous week, and in doubtful cases it may be usefully repeated after 2 weeks. The scale will not detect mothers with anxiety neuroses, phobias or personality disorders.

As you have recently had a baby, we would like to know how you are feeling. Please UNDERLINE the answer which comes closest to how you have felt IN THE PAST 7 DAYS, not just how you feel today. Here is an example, already completed.
I have felt happy:
Yes, all the time
<u>Yes, most of the time</u>
No, not very often
No, not at all
This would mean: 'I have felt happy most of the time' during the past week. Please complete the other questions in the same way.

In the past 7 days:

1. I have been able to laugh and see the funny side of things:
   As much as I always could
   Not quite so much now
   Definitely not so much now
   Not at all
2. I have looked forward with enjoyment to things:
   As much as I ever did
   Rather less than I used to
   Definitely less than I used to
   Hardly at all
3. *I have blamed myself unnecessarily when things went wrong:
   Yes, most of the time
   Yes, some of the time
   Not very often
   No, never
4. *I have been anxious or worried for no good reason:
   No, not at all
   Hardly ever
   Yes, sometimes
   Yes, very often

Continued

Appendix 20   EDINBURGH POSTNATAL DEPRESSION SCALE—Cont'd

5. *I have felt scared or panicky for no very good reason:
   Yes, quite a lot
   Yes, sometimes
   No, not much
   No, not at all
6. *Things have been getting on top of me:
   Yes, most of the time I haven't been able to cope at all
   Yes, sometimes I haven't been coping as well as usual
   No, most of the time I have coped quite well
   No, I have been coping as well as ever
7. *I have been so unhappy that I have had difficulty sleeping:
   Yes, most of the time
   Yes, sometimes
   Not very often
   No, not at all
8. *I have felt sad or miserable:
   Yes, most of the time
   Yes, quite often
   Not very often
   No, not at all
9. *I have been so unhappy that I have been crying:
   Yes, most of the time
   Yes, quite often
   Only occasionally
   No, never
10. *The thought of harming myself has occurred to me:
   Yes, quite often
   Sometimes
   Hardly ever Never

Appendix 21 ADMISSION PROCEDURES FOR PATIENTS WITH MENTAL HEALTH PROBLEMS

Compulsory admission

The team needed to complete a Section 2 or Section 3 consists of:

(a) the GP;
(b) an approved social worker (ASW);
(c) an approved psychiatrist (duty consultant or specialist registrar).
The procedure to follow between 9 a.m. to 5 p.m. for assessment of a patient who may need to be sectioned from home might be as follows:

✳ Obtain relevant information from a partner who may know the patient better.
✳ Review the records to assess:
   (a) risk of violence;
   (b) past history of outcomes of previous sections;
   (c) previous responses to treatment.
✳ Phone the family or carer to obtain their assessment of the:
   (a) current situation and urgency;
   (b) need for police support;
   (c) risk of violence, access to weapons.

✳ Ensure the patient is at home and someone is in to allow access.
✳ Explain the procedure and arrange a time to visit.
✳ Contact the duty ASW and duty psychiatrist:
  (a) provide basic information: name, date of birth, address, past history, current problem, reason for assessment, phone number of patient, name of carer or relative at home, how to contact you in the next few hours, name of key worker, any known risk of violence or self harm;
  (b) decide on the need for police support;
  (c) arrange a time to meet together at the home.
✳ If a joint visit is not possible decide:
  (a) when each will visit;
  (b) how to discuss assessments and decide on need for sectioning;
  (c) where to leave the section form for GP to sign, e.g. will it be left with relative or brought to surgery?
✳ If the GP visits first, take the section forms and complete, if appropriate.
✳ Avoid sedating patient as this makes subsequent assessment difficult.
✳ Avoid asking the relative to sign Section 2 or 4, as this increases guilt and may disrupt future relationships.
✳ If the two doctors cannot do a joint assessment, they must examine the patient within 5 days of each other.
✳ Organise a hospital bed (the ASW is responsible for arranging transport).
✳ If the GP and ASW disagree on the need for sectioning:
  (a) record the basis of each decision in writing;
  (b) identify a home care plan;
  (c) decide who will reassess and when;
  (d) instruct the carer in what to do if the situation changes.
✳ Ask family or carer to make a GP follow-up appointment to find out how they are coping and what has happened to the patient, and future plans.
✳ Complete item of service claim form.

Voluntary admission

✳ If patient is known to hospital staff and a bed is available and the patient accepts admission: arrange admission, write a letter, organise transport.
✳ If patient is known to hospital staff but there are no beds available: contact the bed manager or psychiatric nurse manager.
  1. If a bed is found, arrange admission as above.
  2. If a bed is not immediately available and a 2-hour delay is acceptable, if supported by CPN or crisis team:
    (a) arrange for the hospital to phone you and family when bed available;
    (b) write letter and give to patient or relative;
    (c) ask the family to phone the GP if they have not heard from hospital in 2 hours.
  3. If a bed is not immediately available and a delay is not acceptable:
    (a) phone the A & E psychiatric registrar or A & E mental health nurse;
    (b) consider referral to A & E;
    (c) other local options (to be entered here).
✳ If the patient not known to hospital staff: if Monday to Friday, 9 a.m. to 5 p.m. then:
  (a) check catchment area and relevant consultant (in London phone Emergency Bed Service: 020 7407 7181 to obtain this information);
  (b) phone the consultant on pager or mobile or contact his or her secretary to ask the psychiatrist to phone you ASAP:
    –if the consultant is available arrange for domiciliary visit or admission;
    –if consultant not available, phone the SHO or registrar and proceed as above;
    –if out of hours, follow the local protocol for voluntary admission if available.

Note: The out of hours service should ensure that the protocol is in the doctor's bag.

Appendix 22 THE EARLY WARNING FORM FOR USE IN PSYCHOTIC ILLNESS

EARLY WARNING SIGNS

Name: ....

I am at risk of developing episodes of: ....

....

My early warning signs are (e.g. changes in sleep, eating/drinking or mood, becoming quiet or loud or more withdrawn):

1. ....

2. ....

3. ....

Whenever I have any of these signs I will respond by:

....

....

My health worker is: ....   Phone ....

My home contact is: ....   Phone ....

My advocacy contact is: ....   Phone ....

If I have any concerns about my illness I will contact:

.... immediately.

Reproduced with permission from Falloon IRH et al. Managing Stress in Families: Cognitive and Behavioural Strategies for Enhancing Coping Skills. London: Routledge; 1993.

Appendix 23 AUDIT

The Alcohol Use Disorders Identification Test: Interview Version

Initially give an explanation of the content and purpose of the questions and the need for accurate answers. Read questions as written. Record answers carefully. Begin the AUDIT by saying "Now I am going to ask you some questions about your use of alcoholic beverages during this past year." Explain what is meant by "alcoholic beverages" by using local examples of beer, wine, vodka, etc. Code answers in terms of "standard drinks". Place the correct answer number in the box at the right.

1. How often do you have a drink containing alcohol?
   (0) Never [Skip to Qs 9-10]
   (1) Monthly or less
   (2) 2 to 4 times a month
   (3) 2 to 3 times a week
   (4) 4 or more times a week

2. How many drinks containing alcohol do you have on a typical day when you are drinking?
   (0) 1 or 2
   (1) 3 or 4
   (2) 5 or 6
   (3) 7, 8, or 9
   (4) 10 or more

3. How often do you have six or more drinks on one occasion?
   (0) Never
   (1) Less than monthly
   (2) Monthly
   (3) Weekly
   (4) Daily or almost daily

Skip to Questions 9 and 10 if Total Score for Questions 2 and 3 = 0

4. How often during the last year have you found that you were not able to stop drinking once you had started?
   (0) Never
   (1) Less than monthly
   (2) Monthly
   (3) Weekly
   (4) Daily or almost daily

5. How often during the last year have you failed to do what was normally expected from you because of drinking?
   (0) Never
   (1) Less than monthly
   (2) Monthly
   (3) Weekly
   (4) Daily or almost daily

6. How often during the last year have you needed a first drink in the morning to get yourself going after a heavy drinking session?
   (0) Never
   (1) Less than monthly
   (2) Monthly
   (3) Weekly
   (4) Daily or almost daily

7. How often during the last year have you had a feeling of guilt or remorse after drinking?
   (0) Never
   (1) Less than monthly
   (2) Monthly
   (3) Weekly
   (4) Daily or almost daily

8. How often during the last year have you been unable to remember what happened the night before because you had been drinking?
   (0) Never
   (1) Less than monthly
   (2) Monthly
   (3) Weekly
   (4) Daily or almost daily

9. Have you or someone else been injured as a result of your drinking?
   (0) No
   (2) Yes, but not in the last year
   (4) Yes, during the last year

10. Has a relative or friend or a doctor or another health worker been concerned about your drinking or suggested you cut down?
    (0) No
    (2) Yes, but not in the last year
    (4) Yes, during the last year

Record total of specific items here:

An AUDIT score in the range of 8-15 represent a medium level of alcohol problems where brief interventions would be appropriate. Scores of 16 and above represent a high level of alcohol problems with higher levels of intervention and monitoring recommended. Scores of 20 or more suggest dependent drinking and merits further assessment.[1]
AUDIT-C uses the first three questions only. If the score is 3 or more then complete the full questionnaire.

---

[1]Babor TF, Higgins-Biddle JC, Saunders JB, et al. *Audit, the Alcohol Use Disorders Identification Test*: World Health Organization (WHO), 2001. Online: www.who.int and search on "Alcohol AUDIT".

Appendix 24 INTERNATIONAL PROSTATE SYMPTOM SCORE (IPSS)

	NOT AT ALL	LESS THAN ONE TIME IN FIVE	LESS THAN HALF THE TIME	ABOUT HALF THE TIME	MORE THAN HALF THE TIME	ALMOST ALWAYS	
1. Incomplete emptying Over the past month, how often have you had a sensation of not emptying your bladder completely after you have finished urinating?	0	1	2	3	4	5	
2. Frequency Over the past month, how often have you had to urinate again less than 2 hours after you finished urinating?	0	1	2	3	4	5	
3. Intermittency Over the past month, how often have you found you stopped and started again several times when you urinated?	0	1	2	3	4	5	
4. Urgency Over the past month, how often have you found it difficult to postpone urination or felt sudden urges to urinate?	0	1	2	3	4	5	
5. Weak stream Over the past month, how often have you had a weak urinary stream?	0	1	2	3	4	5	
6. Straining Over the past month, how often have you had to push or strain to begin urination?	0	1	2	3	4	5	
	None	Once	Twice	Three times	Four times	Five times or more	
7. Nocturia Over the past month, how many times did you typically get up to urinate from the time you went to bed at night to the time you got up in the morning?	0	1	2	3	4	5	

(scoring items 1–7: 0–7 = mild; 8–19 = moderate; 20–35 = severe)

Quality of life	Delighted	Pleased	Mostly satisfied	No strong feelings either way	Mostly dissatisfied	Unhappy	Terrible
If you were to spend the rest of your life with urinary conditions just the way they are now, how would you feel about it?	0	1	2	3	4	5	6

Appendix 25 BODY MASS INDEX

Box mass index $= W/H^2$

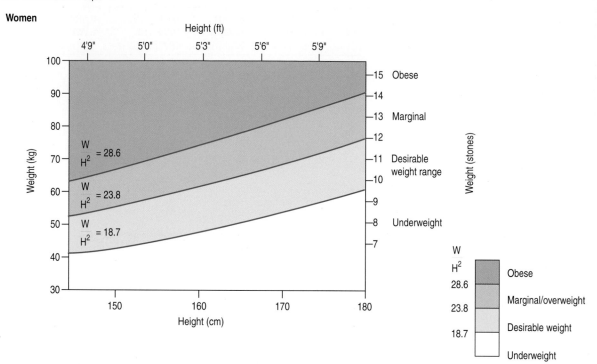

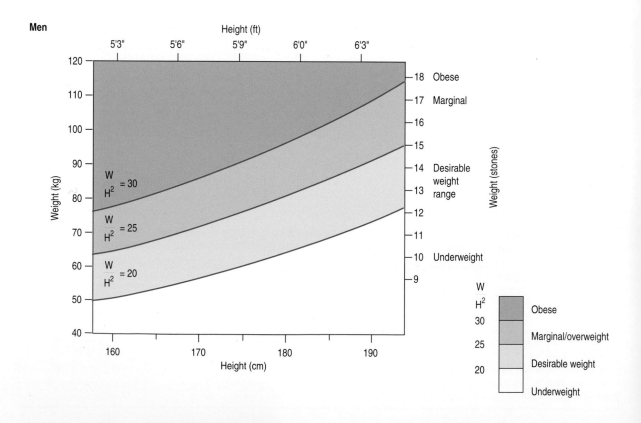

Appendix 26 REFERENCE RANGES FOR YOUNG ADULTS

Reference ranges vary according to laboratory and test method. The following are given as typical ranges but if the laboratory performing the test gives a range that differs from these it should be used instead. The range will also vary according to age and gender.

Blood

BIOCHEMISTRY AND IMMUNOLOGY			
Serum or plasma		Immunoglobulins:	
Acid phosphatase:		IgG	6–13g/L
total	1–5 iu/L	IgM	0.5–2.0 g/L
prostatic	0–1 iu/L	IgA	1.0–4.0 g/L
ACTH	10–80ng/L	Lactate dehydrogenase	70–250 iu/L
Alkaline phosphatase	30–300 iu/L	Magnesium	0.7–1.0 mmol/L
Alanine aminotransferase	5–35 iu/L	Osmolality	280–295 mosmol/kg
Amylase	< 120 u/L	Phosphate (inorganic)	0.8–1.4 mmol/L
Asparate aminotransferase	5–35 iu/L	Potassium	3.4–5.2 mmol/L
Bicarbonate	21–26 mmol/L	Prolactin	Male: 80–400 mu/L
Bilirubin	< 17 mmol/L		Female: 90–520 mu/L
Calcium	2.26–2.60 mmol/L		Postmenopausal female:
Chloride	95–105 mmol/L	Protein:	80–280 mu/L
Cholesterol	< 5.5 mmol/L	total	60–80 g/L
Complement:		albumin	35–50 g/L
C3	0.69–1.5 mg/L	PSA	0–4 ng/mL
C4	0.12–0.27 mg/L	Sodium	133–145 mmol/L
		Total thyroxine	70–140 nmol/L
Cortisol:		free T4	10–26 pmol/L
9.00 a.m.	130–690 nmol/L	Free T3	3–9 pmol/L
midnight	half the a.m. value	Tri-iodothyronine	1.2–3.0 nmol/L
Creatinine	70–130 mol/L	TSH	0.3–3.8 mu/L
Creatine kinase	< 200 iu/L	Triglycerides**	< 0.55–1.90 mmol/L
α-fetoprotein	< 10 ku/L	Urea	2.5–6.7 mmol/L
γ-glutamyl transferase:		Uric acid:	
men	11–51 iu/L	men	0.15–0.42 mmol/L
women	7–33 iu/L	women	0.10–0.36 mmol/L
Glucose (fasting)	3.4–5.5 mmol/L		
Growth hormone	< 5.5 mu/L	*Arterial blood gases*	
		pH	7.35–7.45
		PaO_2	12–14 kPa
		$PaCO_2$	4.6–6.0 kPa

*to convert cholesterol from mmol/L into mg/dL multiply by 39.
**to convert triglycerides from mmol/L into mg/dL multiply by 89.

Continued

Appendix 26 REFERENCE RANGES FOR YOUNG ADULTS—Cont'd

Haematology	
Haemoglobin	13.5–18.0 g/dL (men)
	11.5–16.0 g/dL (women)
MCV	82–98 fL
MCH	26.7–33.0 pg
MCHC	31.4–35.0 g/dL
WBC	$3.2–11.0 \times 10^9$/L
Neutrophils	$1.9–7.7 \times 10^9$/L
Monocytes	$0.1–0.9 \times 10^9$/L
Eosinophils	$0.0–0.4 \times 10^9$/L
Basophils	$0.2–0.8 \times 10^9$/L
Platelets	$120–400 \times 10^9$/L
Reticulocytes	$25–100 \times 10^9$/L (or $< 2\%$)
Ferritin	30–230 µg/L (male)
	6–80 µg/L (female)
	14–180 µg/L (post-menopausal female)

Urine	
Sodium	100–250 mmol/24 hours
Potassium	14–120 mmol/24 hours
Albumin:	
– microalbuminuria	20–200 mg/L
– proteinuria	> 200 mg/L
Albumin/creatinine ratio:	
– microalbuminuria	2.5 mg/mmol (men) or 3.5 mg/mmol (women) to 30 mg/mmol
– proteinuria	> 30 mg/mmol
Creatinine clearance	85–125 mL/min (men); 75–115 mL/min (women)
Osmolality	350–1000 mosmol/kg

Reproduced from Working Group of the Resuscitation Council (UK). Emergency treatment of anaphylactic reactions. Guidelines for healthcare providers. London: Resuscitation Council (UK), 2008, by permission of the Resuscitation Council.

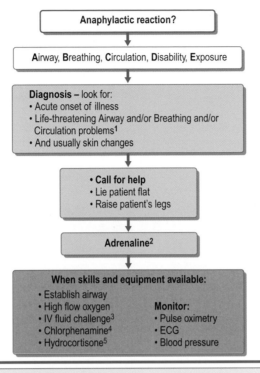

Anaphylactic reaction?

Airway, Breathing, Circulation, Disability, Exposure

Diagnosis – look for:
• Acute onset of illness
• Life-threatening Airway and/or Breathing and/or Circulation problems[1]
• And usually skin changes

• **Call for help**
• Lie patient flat
• Raise patient's legs

Adrenaline[2]

When skills and equipment available:
• Establish airway
• High flow oxygen
• IV fluid challenge[3]   **Monitor:**
• Chlorphenamine[4]   • Pulse oximetry
• Hydrocortisone[5]   • ECG
                                  • Blood pressure

[1] **Life-threatening problems:**
Airway: swelling, hoarseness, stridor
Breathing: rapid breathing, wheeze, fatigue, cyanosis, $SpO_2 < 92\%$, confusion
Circulation: pale, clammy, low blood pressure, faintness, drowsy/coma

[2] Adrenaline *(give IM unless experienced with IV adrenaline)*
IM doses of 1:1000 adrenaline (repeat after 5 mins if no better)
• Adult   500 micrograms IM (0.5mL)
• Child more than 12 years   500 micrograms IM (0.5mL)
• Child 6–12 years   300 micrograms IM (0.3mL)
• Child less than 6 years   150 micrograms IM (0.15mL)
Adrenaline IV to be given **only by experienced specialists**
Titrate: Adults 50 micrograms; children 1 microgram/kg

[3] IV fluid challenge:
Adult - 500–1000mL
Child - crystalloid 20 mL/kg

Stop IV colloid if this might be the cause of anaphylaxis

	[4] Chlorphenamine (IM or slow IV)	[5] Hydrocortisone (IM or slow IV)
Adult or child more than 12 years	10 mg	200 mg
Child 6–12 years	5 mg	100 mg
Child 6 months–6 years	2.5 mg	50 mg
Child less than 6 months	250 micrograms/kg	25 mg

Appendix 28 PROBLEMS ASSOCIATED WITH SPECIFIC CAUSES OF DISABILITY

	AUDIOVISUAL	ENDOCRINE	PSYCHIATRIC/ PSYCHOLOGICAL	CNS	CARDIOVASCULAR	MUSCULAR/ SKELETAL AND SKIN	OTHER	INHERITANCE
Cerebral palsy 1:500	Visual impairment Hearing impairment		Depression Variable intellectual capacity	Epilepsy		Orthopaedic problems Neuromuscular problems	Genitourinary problems Incontinence Constipation Dental problems Recurrent aspiration Oesophagitis, gastroesophageal reflux ± bleeding/ anaemia Swallowing/eating difficulties	
Down syndrome 1:700	Visual impairment (multifactorial), cataracts Hearing impairment (multifactorial) Annual assessments recommended	Hypothyroidism Annual TFT recommended	Depression Alzheimer's type dementia (clinical onset uncommon before 40 years)	Epilepsy Usually clonic/ tonic	Congenital heart defects (present in 40 to 50%)	Atlantoaxial instability Skin disorders, alopecia, eczema	Blood dyscrasias Childhood leukaemia Sleep apnoea Increased susceptibility to infections Coeliac disease	Most cases are sporadic; 4% due to translocation involving chromosome 21 or rarely parental mosaicism
Prader–Willi 1:10,000–25,000	Strabismus Myopia	NIDDM (secondary to obesity) Hypogonadism Delayed puberty	Hyperphagia Impulse control difficulties Self-injury			Scoliosis, kyphosis Hypotonia Skin picking	Infantile failure to thrive, then hyperphagia and severe obesity High tolerance to pain Decreased ability to vomit Sleep apnoea Osteoporosis Undescended testes Dental abnormalities	Atypical. Most cases are sporadic

Syndrome (incidence)	Sensory	Behaviour/Intellectual	Neurological	Cardiac	Musculoskeletal	Other	Inheritance
Fragile X 1:6000	Visual impairment (multifactorial) Hearing impairment Recurrent ear infections	Attention deficit/hyperactivity Variable intellectual capacity Disabled in social functioning	Epilepsy Usually clonic/tonic, complex partial	Aortic dilatation, mitral valve prolapse (related to connective tissue dysplasia)	Connective tissue dysplasia Scoliosis Congenital hip dislocation	Hernias (CT related) Abnormalities of speech and language	X-linked
Phenylketonuria 1:10,000–20,000		Variable intellectual capacity Phobic anxiety Disabled in social functioning	Epilepsy Hyperactivity Tremor and pyramidal tract signs Extrapyramidal syndromes			Eczema	Autosomal recessive
Angelman syndrome 1:10,000	Glaucoma	Easily excitable Hyperactive	Severe developmental delay Epilepsy		Joint contractures and scoliosis (in adults)	Speech impairment Movement and balance disorder Characteristic EEG changes	Variety of genetic mechanisms on chromosome 15
Williams ? < 1:20,000	Hyperacusis Strabismus	Variable intellectual capacity Attention deficit problems in childhood	Perceptual and motor function reduced	Cardiac abnormalities Hypertension CVAs Chronic hemiparesis	Joint contractures Scoliosis Hypotonia	Renal abnormalities	Microdeletion on chromosome 7
Rett 1:14,000 Females	Refractory errors	Severe intellectual disability	Epilepsy Vasomotor instability	Prolonged QT interval	Osteopenia Fractures Scoliosis	Hyperventilation Apnoea Reflux Feeding difficulties Growth failure	Usually sporadic X-linked
Noonan < 1:10,000	Strabismus Refractive errors Vision/hearing impairments	Mild intellectual disability	Epilepsy	Pulmonary valvular stenosis ASD, VSD, PDA	Scoliosis Talipes equinovarus Pectus carinatum/excavatum	Abnormal clotting factors, platelet dysfunction Undescended tests, deficient spermatogenesis Lymphangiectasia Hepatosplenomegaly Cubitus valgus, hand abnormalities	Autosomal dominant, may be sporadic

Continued

Appendix 28   PROBLEMS ASSOCIATED WITH SPECIFIC CAUSES OF DISABILITY—Cont'd

	AUDIOVISUAL	ENDOCRINE	PSYCHIATRIC/ PSYCHOLOGICAL	CNS	CARDIOVASCULAR	MUSCULAR/ SKELETAL AND SKIN	OTHER	INHERITANCE
Tuberous sclerosis 1:6000–17,000	Retinal tumours Eye rhabdomyomatas		Variable intellectual capacity Behavioural difficulties Sleep problems	Cerebral astrocytomas Epilepsy	Rhabdomyomatas Hypertension	Bone Rhabdomyomata	Kidney and lung hamartomata Polycystic kidneys Liver rhabdomyomata Liver rhabdomyomata Dental abnormalities Skin lesions	Autosomal dominant
Neurofibromatosis 1:300	Hearing impairment (glioma affecting auditory nerve)	Various endocrine abnormalities	Variable intellectual capacity	Variable clinical phenomena depeneding on site of the tumours Epilepsy		Skeletal abnormalities especially kyphoscoliosis	Variable clinical phenomena depending on the location of the neurofibroma Tumours are susceptible to malignant change Other varieties of tumours may be associated	Autosomal dominant

Adapted from an original unpublished version by Michael Kew and Glyn Jones and reproduced with the kind permission of the University of Queensland

Appendix 29 THE COMMUNITY DEPENDENCY INDEX

© Professor Pamela Eakin, reproduced with permission.
Score the patient under the following nine headings. A score < 75 suggests moderate disability; < 50 suggests severe disability.

Personal toilet

5 = Client can wash hands and face, comb hair, clean teeth and shave. Must be able to get to water, brushes, without help and operate them independently.
0 = Any help or supervision needed or difficulty with personal toilet.

Feeding

10 = Independent. The client can feed himself a meal from a tray or table when someone puts the food within reach. He must put on his own assistive device if this is needed, cut up food, spread butter and so on. He must accomplish this in a reasonable time (that is acceptable to the client).
5 = Food must be cut for the client or some help is necessary with the items above. Unreasonable time or effort required if feeds independently.
0 = Client unable to feed himself.

Moving from (wheel)chair to bed and return

15 = Independent in all phases of this activity.
Chair: client can safely stand up from sitting in his chair (high chair allowed) without help from another person, and sit down again. Client must be able to get in/out bed without help, and, once in bed be able to turn and move up and down in the bed as necessary. Client
Or wheelchair: client can safely approach the bed in his wheelchair, lock brakes, lift footrests, transfer safely to the bed and lie down. Once in bed he must be able to turn and move up and down the bed as necessary. Client must be able to transfer back into the wheelchair safely including changing the position of the wheelchair for the return transfer.
10 = Client can independently sit down and stand up from chair, or transfer in and out of a wheelchair, but still has difficulty or needs help in bed.
5 = Help or supervision needed to ensure client's safety in all parts of this activity; or client performs all or parts of this activity with difficulty.
0 = Client unable to perform this activity.

Getting on and off the toilet or commode (during day and night)

10 = Client is able to reach the toilet/commode area unassisted. He is able to transfer on and off the commode, fasten and unfasten clothes, prevent spoiling of clothes, use toilet paper without help. He may use equipment or stable fittings for support if needed (e.g. rail, raised toilet seat or side of bath). If he uses a commode he must be able to position it for use, empty it and clean it out.
5 = Client has difficulty with part of this activity or client needs help because of imbalance or in handling clothes or in using toilet paper or in flushing the toilet.
0 = Client needs help to empty the commode or is not able to transfer.
Note: If the client can use the toilet independently during the day but has the commode at night, which someone else empties, then score = 5.

Walking 50 yards outside the house or using a wheelchair

Walking
15 = Client gets in/out of the house unassisted. He can walk at least 50 yards without help or supervision outside his home. He may wear braces and prostheses and use walking aids. He must be able to reach and operate aids without help.
10 = Client has difficulty or needs minimal help or supervision in any of the above but can walk at least 50 yards.
Wheelchair
5 = Client cannot walk but can propel a wheelchair independently. He must be able to go round corners and turn around. He must be able to get in and out of the house independently (access). He must be able to push the wheelchair at least 50 yards. If the wheelchair is used indoors he must be able to manoeuvre himself to a table, bed or toilet. Do not score for wheelchair use if the client gets a score for walking.
0 = Client unable to walk or propel a wheelchair for 50 yards.

Continued

Appendix 29   THE COMMUNITY DEPENDENCY INDEX—Cont'd

Dressing and undressing

10 = Client is able to put on and remove and fasten all clothing and tie shoelaces (adaptations/aids allowed). This activity includes putting on and removing prostheses, braces and corsets where these are prescribed. Special clothing, such as slip-on shoes or dresses that open down the front may be used where necessary.

5 = Client has difficulty or needs help in putting on and removing or fastening any clothing. Where helped he must do at least half the work himself. He must accomplish this in a reasonable time.

0 = Client needs help with all or most of dressing.

Bathing self

5 = Client can use a bath or shower. He must be able to do all the steps involved in whichever method is employed without another person helping him. Verbal supervision is allowed.

0 = Client has difficulty or needs help.

Note: Where the client's home does not have bathing/shower facilities, score 5 for using a bath/shower in another facility or having an all-over wash if independent. Where client has an all over wash because he is unable to use the bath/shower then score = 0.

Ascending and descending stairs

10 = Client is able to get up and down stairs safely, without help or supervision. He may and should use the handrails and walking aids when needed. He must be able to carry walking aids up and down the stairs if needed. If a stair lift or vertical lift is used, the client must be able to use it without help or supervision (including transfers).

5 = Client has difficulty, needs help or supervision in any one of the above items.

0 = Client unable to climb the stairs.

Note: If the client does not have stairs in the house, count as 10 because they are not an obstacle to independence in the home, even if they are obstacles in the community.

Continence of bowels

10 = Client is able to control bowels and has no accidents. He can use a suppository or take an enema when necessary (e.g. spinal cord injury). He can manage external devices (e.g. colostomy).

5 = Client needs help with any of the above.

0 = Client does not have bowel control.

Continence of bladder

10 = Client able to control his bladder day and night. Clients who wear external device and leg bag must put them on independently, clean and empty the bag and stay dry day and night.

5 = Client has control of bladder, but cannot get to the toilet or commode in time (e.g. due to poor mobility) or needs help with an external device.

0 = Client does not have bladder control.

Appendix 30 NOTTINGHAM EXTENDED ACTIVITIES OF DAILY LIVING QUESTIONNAIRE (EADL)

Score the patient on each item on a scale of 0 to 3 where '3' represents independent function, '2' represents alone with difficulty, '1' represents alone with help, and '0' represents unable.

SUBSCALE	ITEM
Mobility	1. Do you walk around outside?
	2. Do you climb stairs?
	3. Do you get in and out of the car?
	4. Do you walk over uneven ground?
	5. Do you cross roads?
	6. Do you travel on public transport?
Kitchen	7. Do you manage to feed yourself?
	8. Do you manage to make yourself a hot snack?
	9. Do you take hot drinks from one room to another?
	10. Do you do the washing up?
	11. Do you make yourself a hot drink?
Domestic	12. Do you manage your own money when you are out?
	13. Do you wash small items of clothing?
	14. Do you do your own housework?
	15. Do you do your own shopping?
	16. Do you do a full clothes wash?
Leisure	17. Do you read newspapers or books?
	18. Do you use the telephone?
	19. Do you write letters?
	20. Do you go out socially?
	21. Do you manage your own garden?
	22. Do you drive a car?
	Total (0–66)

Appendix 31 DRUG STABILITIES IN SYRINGE DRIVERS

Notes on using tables of drug mixture stabilities

- The following tables are separated into mixtures containing two or three drugs, ordered by diamorphine first, then the other drugs in alphabetical order.
- The maximum dose for each drug in each syringe size is given. Provided the doses for every drug in the combination is less than or equal to these maximum values, then the mixture is stable for 24 hours. Above the maximum doses stated the solution is either unstable or has not been tested and it is not possible to say whether it is stable or not.
- The following combinations are not stable:

  (a) diamorphine, dexamethasone and levomepromazine;
  (b) diamorphine, dexamethasone and midazolam;
  (c) diamorphine, cyclizine and metoclopramide;
  (d) octreotide and levomepromazine;
  (e) octreotide and cyclizine;
  (f) octreotide and dexamethasone;
  (g) diamorphine, metoclopramide and ondansetron.

Two drug combinations for subcutaneous infusion which are stable for 24 hours
Diluent: Water for injections BP

DRUG COMBINATION	MAXIMUM DOSE (MG) KNOWN TO BE STABLE IN:			COMMENTS
	8 ML IN A 10 ML SYRINGE	14 ML IN A 20 ML SYRINGE	17 ML IN A 30 ML SYRINGE	
Diamorphine and cyclizine	160 160* If diamorphine dose > 160, cyclizine dose must be no more than 80	280 280* If diamorphine dose > 280, cyclizine dose must be no more than 140	340 340* If diamorphine dose > 340, cyclizine dose must be no more than 170	If exceed these doses then likely to get precipitate *Maximum recommended daily dose 150
Diamorphine and dexamethasone	400 3.2	700 5.6	850 6.8	Can precipitate if undiluted drugs are mixed during preparation
Diamorphine and haloperidol	400 32	– 	–	If exceed these doses then likely to get precipitate
Diamorphine and hyoscine HBr	1200 3.2	–	–	–
Diamorphine and hyoscine butylbromide (Buscopan)	1200 160	–	–	–
Diamorphine and ketorolac	47 40	82 74	90 90	–
Diamorphine and levomepromazine (Nozinan)	400 80	700 140	850 170	Mixture can be irritant, dilute to largest possible volume

				Comments
Diamorphine and metoclopramide	1200 40	2100 70	2550 85	Mixture can be irritant dilute to largest possible volume
Diamorphine and midazolam	400 16	700 28	850 34	–
Diamorphine and octreotide	200 0.9	350 1.6	425 1.9	–
Diamorphine and ondansetron	40 5	70 9	85 11	

Three drug combinations for subcutaneous infusion which are stable for 24 hours
Diluent: Water for injections BP

				Comments
Diamorphine and cyclizine and haloperidol	160 160 16	280 280 28	340 340 34	Above these doses the mixture is likely to precipitate
Diamorphine and dexamethasone and dexamethasone and haloperidol	400 3.2 8	700 5.6 14	850 6.8 17	Only stable if diamorphine and haloperidol are well diluted before dexamethasone is added Use only if no other options
Diamorphine and dexamethasone and metoclopramide	400 3.2 24	700 5.6 42	850 6.8 51	–
Diamorphine and haloperidol and midazolam	560 4 32	980 7 56	1190 8.5 68	–
Diamorphine and hyoscine butylbromide (Buscopan) and midazolam	560 4 22	980 7 39	1190 8.5 48	Hyoscine butylbromide is usually used at doses of 60–120 mg. Stability data at these concentrations is not known in three drug combinations
Diamorphine and levomepromazine and metoclopramide	400 80 24	700 140 42	850 170 51	–

Appendix 32 GUIDELINES FOR THE URGENT REFERRAL OF PATIENTS WITH SUSPECTED CANCER

CANCER TYPE	REFERRAL GUIDELINES

Lung cancer	*Urgent referral for chest X-ray*
	
	● Haemoptysis
	● *Unexplained* or persistent (more than 3 weeks):
	  – cough
	  – chest/shoulder pain
	  – dyspnoea
	  – weight loss
	  – chest signs
	  – hoarseness
	  – finger clubbing
	  – features suggestive of metastasis from a lung cancer (e.g. brain, bone, liver or skin)
	  – cervical/supraclavicular lymphadenopathy
	  – unexplained change in symptoms in someone with underlying chronic respiratory disease
	
	Urgent referral to a chest physician
	Any of the following:
	
	● Chest X-ray suggestive/suspicious of lung cancer (including pleural effusion and slowly resolving consolidation)
	● Persistent haemoptysis in smokers/ex-smokers over 40 years of age
	● High suspicion of lung cancer despite normal chest X-ray
	● History of asbestos exposure and recent onset of chest pain, shortness of breath or unexplained systemic symptoms where a chest X-ray indicates pleural effusion, pleural mass or any suspicious lung pathology
	● Signs of superior vena caval obstruction (swelling of face/neck with fixed elevation of jugular venous pressure) (consider immediate referral)
	● Stridor (consider immediate referral)

Upper GI cancer	*Urgent referral*
	
	● Dysphagia – food sticking on swallowing (any age)
	● Dyspepsia at any age combined with one or more of the following:
	  – chronic GI bleeding
	  – progressive unintentional weight loss
	  – iron deficiency anaemia
	  – persistent vomiting
	  – suspicious barium meal result
	● Unexplained upper abdominal pain and weight loss, with or without back pain
	● Upper abdominal mass
	● Obstructive jaundice (depending on clinical state)
	● Consider urgent referral for those with unexplained worsening of dyspepsia combined with at least one of the following:
	  – Barrett's oesophagus
	  – peptic ulcer surgery over 20 years ago
	  – known dysplasia, atrophic gastritis, intestinal metaplasia

Continued

Lower GI cancer

- Consider urgent referral for those without dyspepsia who have:
  - persistent vomiting and weight loss
  - unexplained weight loss and iron deficiency anaemia
- Refer urgently for endoscopy patients age 55 years or above with unexplained and persistent recent-onset dyspepsia alone.

Urgent referral

All ages

- A definite palpable right-sided abdominal mass consistent with involvement of the large bowel
- A definite palpable rectal (not pelvic) mass
- Men with unexplained iron deficiency anaemia and an Hb of 11 g/100 mL or below
- Women who are not menstruating with unexplained iron deficiency anaemia and an Hb of 10 g/100 mL or below

40 years old and over

- Rectal bleeding *with* a change in bowel habit to looser stools and/or increased frequency of defecation persistent for 6 weeks

60 years old and over

- Rectal bleeding for at least 6 weeks *without* a change in bowel habit and *without* anal symptoms'
- Change of bowel habit to looser stools and/or increased frequency of defecation, *without* rectal bleeding and persistent for 6 weeks

Breast cancer

Urgent referral

- Patients with a discrete hard lump with fixation
- Women aged 30 or older with a discrete lump that persists after their next period, or presents after the menopause
- Women aged < 30 with a lump that enlarges, or is fixed and hard, or in whom there are other reasons for concern e.g. family history
- Those with a lump or with suspicious symptoms and a past history of breast cancer.
- Those with unilateral eczematous skin or nipple change that does not respond to topical treatment
- Those with nipple distortion of recent onset
- Those with spontaneous unilateral bloody nipple discharge
- Men aged 50 and older with a unilateral, firm subareolar mass.

Conditions that require referral – but not necessarily urgently

- Discrete lump in a younger women (age < 30 years)
- breast pain not responding to initial treatment and/or with unexplained persistent symptoms

Gynaecological cancer

Urgent referral

- Clinical features suggestive of cervical cancer on examination
- Unexplained vulval lump
- Vulval bleeding due to ulceration
- Postmenopausal bleeding (PMB) in a women who is not on HRT
- On tamoxifen with PMB
- On HRT: persistent or unexplained bleeding for more than 6 weeks after stopping HRT

Appendix 32 GUIDELINES FOR THE URGENT REFERRAL OF PATIENTS WITH SUSPECTED CANCER—Cont'd

CANCER TYPE	REFERRAL GUIDELINES
	Consider urgent referral:
	● Persistent intermenstrual bleeding and negative pelvic examination
	Urgent ultrasound scan (USS):
	● Palpable abdominal or pelvic mass that is not obviously uterine fibroids or gastrointestinal or urological. If the scan suggests cancer, or if urgent USS is not available, urgent referral should be made
Urological cancers	*Urgent referral* **Prostate:**
	– hard irregular prostate typical of carcinoma
	– normal prostate but rising or raised age-specific PSA, with or without lower urinary tract symptoms
	Bladder and kidney:
	– painless macroscopic haematuria
	– age 40 and over with recurrent or persistent urinary tract infection associated with haematuria
	– unexplained microscopic haematuria in adults aged 50 years and over
	– abdominal mass identified clinically or on imaging thought to arise from the urinary tract
	Testis:
	– swelling or mass in the body of the testis
	Penis:
	– any suspected penile cancer
	Non-urgent referral of microscopic haematuria in a patient aged < 50
	– to a renal physician if there is proteinuria or a raised serum creatinine
	– to a urologist if there is no proteinuria and serum creatinine is normal
Haematological cancers	*Urgent referral*
	● Blood count/film reported as suggestive of acute leukaemia (immediate referral)
	● Spinal cord compression or renal failure suspected of being due to myeloma (immediate referral)
	● Persistent unexplained splenomegaly
Skin cancers	*Urgent referral:*
	● A lesion suspected to be melanoma
	● Suspicion of squamous cell carcinoma:
	– non-healing keratinising or crusted tumours > 1 cm with significant induration on palpation
	– patients in whom squamous cell carcinoma has been diagnosed from a biopsy undertaken in general practice
	– after an organ transplant with new or growing cutaneous lesions

Continued

Head and neck cancer

Urgent referral:

- Unexplained lump in the neck that is of recent onset or a previously undiagnosed lump that has changed over 3 to 6 weeks
- Unexplained persistent swelling in the parotid or submandibular gland
- Unexplained persistent sore or painful throat
- Unexplained persistent pain in the head or neck for > 4 weeks associated with otalgia (ear ache) but a normal otoscopy
- Unexplained ulceration of oral mucosa or mass persisting for > 3 weeks
- Unexplained red and white patches of the oral mucosa (including suspected lichen planus) that are painful or swollen or bleeding
- Any other patients with persistent symptoms or signs (> 6 weeks) related to the oral cavity in whom a definitive diagnosis of a benign lesion cannot be made
- Unexplained tooth mobility lasting > 3 weeks (to a dentist)
- Hoarseness for > 3 weeks. Order urgent chest X-ray. If positive, refer to a team specialising in the management of lung cancer. If negative, refer urgently to a team specialising in head and neck cancer

Thyroid cancer

- Tracheal compression due to thyroid swelling (immediate referral)
- Solitary nodule increasing in size
- Thyroid swelling associated with:
  – history of neck irradiation
  – family history of an endocrine tumour
  – unexplained hoarseness or voice changes
  – cervical lymphadenopathy
  – pre-pubertal patient or patient aged 65 or older

Brain tumours

Urgent referral: when a brain tumour is suspected in a patient with:

  – progressive neurological deficit
  – new onset seizures
  – headaches
  – mental changes
  – cranial nerve palsy
  – unilateral sensorineural deafness

- Headaches of recent onset with features suggestive of raised intracranial pressure e.g. vomiting, drowsiness, posture-related headache, pulse-synchronous tinnitus or other focal or non-focal neurological symptoms
- A new, qualitatively different, unexplained headache that becomes progressively severe
- Suspected recent-onset seizures (refer to neurologist)

Consider urgent referral when there is rapid progression of:

- Subacute focal neurological deficit
- Unexplained cognitive impairment, and/or behavioural disturbance
- Personality change

Sarcoma

Urgent referral

Suspected spontaneous fracture needs immediate X-ray. Refer if it suggests possible cancer A palpable lump with one or more of the following characteristics:

  – size > 5cm

Appendix 32 GUIDELINES FOR THE URGENT REFERRAL OF PATIENTS WITH SUSPECTED CANCER—Cont'd

CANCER TYPE	REFERRAL GUIDELINES
	– painful
	– increasing in size
	– deep to fascia, fixed or immobile
	– recurrence after previous excision
	● Suspected Kaposi's sarcoma in a patient who has HIV
	● Increasing, unexplained or persistent bone pain or tenderness, particularly pain at rest, (especially if not in the joint) or an unexplained limp. Investigate urgently first
Children's cancers	
General	*Urgent referral*
	● When a child presents 3 or more times with the same problem and investigation reveals no clear diagnosis
	● Persistent back pain after investigation and taking parental anxiety into account
Leukaemia	● Unexplained petechiae (refer immediately)
	● Hepatosplenomegaly (refer immediately)
	● Take blood for FBC and film (and refer urgently if positive) if any of the following is present:
	– fatigue
	– pallor
	– unexplained irritability
	– unexplained fever
	– persistent or recurrent upper respiratory tract infections
	– generalised lymphadenopathy
	– persistent or unexplained bone pain
	– unexplained bruising
Lymphoma	● Hepatosplenomegaly (immediate referral)
	● Mediastinal or hilar mass on chest X-ray (immediate referral)
	● Lymphadenopathy (particularly if there is no evidence of previous local infection) with at least one of the following:
	– nodes > 2 cm in size
	– non-tender, firm/hard nodes
	– progressively enlarging
	– associated with other signs of general ill health, fever and/or weight loss
	– involves axillary nodes (in the absence of any local infection or dermatitis) or supraclavicular nodes
	● Shortness of breath and unexplained petechiae or hepatosplenomegaly
Brain and CNS tumours	*Urgent referral*
	● Altered level of consciousness (immediate referral)
	● Headache and vomiting that cause early morning waking or occur on waking (immediate referral)
	● Children aged < 2 with any of the following (immediate referral):
	– bulging fontanelle
	– extensor attacks
	– persistent vomiting
	– new-onset seizures

Children of any age with any of the following (immediate or urgent referral):

- new-onset seizures
- cranial nerve abnormalities
- visual disturbance
- gait abnormality
- motor or sensory signs
- unexplained deteriorating school performance or developmental milestones
- unexplained behavioural and/or mood changes
- Children age 2 and older, and young people, with persistent headache where you cannot carry out an adequate neurological examination
- Children < 2 years old with any of the following:
  - abnormal increase in head size
  - arrest or regression of motor development
  - altered behaviour
  - abnormal eye movements
  - lack of visual following
  - poor feeding or failure to thrive
  - squint (where the urgency will depend on other factors)

Neuroblastoma   *Refer urgently children with:*

- proptosis
- unexplained back pain
- leg weakness
- unexplained urinary retention

Wilms' tumour   *Refer urgently* children with haematuria

Soft tissue sarcoma   *Refer urgently* children with an unexplained mass if associated with one or more of the following characteristics:

- non-tender
- progressively enlarging
- size > 2 cm in maximum diameter
- or deep to fascia
- associated with enlarging regional lymph node

Bone sarcoma   *Refer* children or young people with rest pain, back pain or unexplained limp (discuss with paeditrician). Refer urgently if there is persistent localised bone pain and/or swelling and X-ray suggests cancer

Retinoblastoma   *Refer urgently* children with a white pupillary reflex, a new squint or change in visual acuity suggestive of cancer, or any visual problems and a family history of retinoblastoma

Index

Notes: Page numbers followed by *t* refers to tables and *b* refers boxes.